Burket's

ORAL MEDICINE

12th edition

Burket's

ORAL MEDICINE

12th edition

Michael Glick, DMD, FDS RCSEd
William M. Feagans Chair
Dean and Professor of Oral Medicine
School of Dental Medicine
State University of New York
University at Buffalo
Buffalo, New York

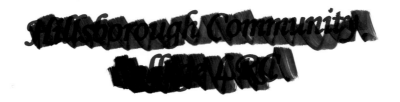

2015
People's Medical Publishing House—USA
Shelton, Connecticut

People's Medical Publishing House-USA
2 Enterprise Drive, Suite 509
Shelton, CT 06484
Tel: 203-402-0646
Fax: 203-402-0854
E-mail: info@pmph-usa.com

PMPH-USA

14 15 16 17/**JPBros**/9 8 7 6 5 4 3 2 1

ISBN-13	978-1-60795-188-9
ISBN-10	1-60795-188-6
eISBN-13	978-1-60795-280-0

Printed in India by Replika Press Pvt. Ltd.
Editor: Linda H. Mehta; Copyeditor/Typesetter: diacriTech; Cover designer: Mary McKeon

Library of Congress Cataloging-in-Publication Data
Burket's oral medicine / [edited by] Michael Glick. -- 12th edition.
      p. ; cm.
   Oral medicine
   Includes bibliographical references and index.
   ISBN 978-1-60795-188-9—ISBN 1-60795-188-6—ISBN 978-1-60795-280-0 (eISBN)
   I. Glick, Michael, editor. II. Title: Oral medicine.
   [DNLM: 1. Mouth Diseases. 2. Diagnosis, Oral—methods. WU 140]
   RK308

   617.5'22—dc23
                                                                                2014032898

Sales and Distribution

Canada
Login Canada
300 Saulteaux Cr., Winnipeg, MB
R3J 3T2
Phone: 1.800.665.1148
Fax: 1.800.665.0103
www.lb.ca

Foreign Rights
John Scott & Company
International Publisher's Agency
P.O. Box 878
Kimberton, PA 19442, USA
Tel: 610-827-1640
Fax: 610-827-1671
rights@johnscottco.us

United Kingdom, Europe, Middle East, Africa
Eurospan Limited
3, Henrietta Street, Covent Garden,
London WC2E 8LU, UK
Within the UK: 0800 526830
Outside the UK: +44 (0)20 7845 0868
http://www.eurospanbookstore.com

Singapore, Thailand, Philippines,
Indonesia, Vietnam, Pacific Rim, Korea
McGraw-Hill Education
60 Tuas Basin Link
Singapore 638775
Tel: 65-6863-1580
Fax: 65-6862-3354
www.mheducation.com.sg

Australia, New Zealand, Papua
New Guinea, Fiji, Tonga, Solomon
Islands, Cook Islands
Woodslane Pty Limited
10 Apollo Street
Warriewood NSW 2102
Australia
Tel: 612-8445-2300
Fax: 612-9997-5850
www.woodsland.com.au

India, Bangladesh, Pakistan, Sri Lanka, Malaysia
Jaypee Brothers Medical Publishers (P) Ltd.
4838, 24 Ansari Road, Darya Ganj
New Delhi- 110002, India
Phone: +91 11 23272143
Fax: +91 11 23276490
www.jaypeebrothers.com

People's Republic of China
People's Medical Publishing House
International Trade Department
No. 19, Pan Jia Yuan Nan Li
Chaoyang District
Beijing 100021, P.R. China
Tel: 8610-67653342
Fax: 8610-67691034
www.pmph.com/en/

Notice: The authors and publisher have made every effort to ensure that the patient care recommended herein, including choice of drugs and drug dosages, is in accord with the accepted standard and practice at the time of publication. However, since research and regulation constantly change clinical standards, the reader is urged to check the product information sheet included in the package of each drug, which includes recommended doses, warnings, and contraindications. This is particularly important with new or infrequently used drugs. Any treatment regimen, particularly one involving medication, involves inherent risk that must be weighed on a case-by-case basis against the benefits anticipated. The reader is cautioned that the purpose of this book is to inform and enlighten; the information contained herein is not intended as, and should not be employed as, a substitute for individual diagnosis and treatment.

DEDICATION

In memory of my mother, Siv Glück, who encouraged me to be the best person I could be; and my friend and colleague Jonathan Ship, whose life sadly ended much too early.
For my father, Dan Glück, with love and appreciation.

CONTENTS

Alfredo Aguirre, DDS, MS [6]
School of Dental Medicine
State University of New York
University at Buffalo
Buffalo, New York

Sunday O. Akintoye, BDS, DDS, MS [23]
Associate Professor
Department of Oral Medicine
Director, Oral Medicine Research Program
University of Pennsylvania School of Dental Medicine
Philadelphia, Pennsylvania

Faizan Alawi, DDS [6]
Associate Professor of Pathology
Director, Penn Oral Pathology Services
University of Pennsylvania School of
    Dental Medicine
Philadelphia, Pennsylvania

Sowmya Ananthan, BDS, DMD, MSD [12]
Clinical Assistant Professor
Divisions of Temporomandibular Disorders and Orofacial
    Pain & Oral Medicine
Rutgers School of Dental Medicine
Newark, New Jersey

Robert Anolik, MD [14]
President and Director of Clinical Research
Allergy and Asthma Specialists
Blue Bell, Pennsylvania

Jane C. Atkinson, DDS [2, 20]
Center for Clinical Research
Division of Extramural Research
National Institute of Dental and Craniofacial Research
National Institutes of Health
Bethesda, Maryland

Rafael Benoliel, BDS, LDS RCSEng [12]
Professor and Associate Dean for Research
Department of Diagnostic Sciences
Rutgers School of Dental School
Rutgers State University of New Jersey
Newark, New Jersey

Bruce Blasberg, DMD, FRCD(C) [11]
Professor Emeritus, Dentistry
Faculty of Dentistry
University of British Columbia
Vancouver, British Columbia, Canada

Leah M. Bowers, DMD [10]
Resident, Department of Oral Medicine
Carolinas Medical Center
Charlotte, North Carolina

Michael T. Brennan, DDS, MHS, FDS RCSEd [10]
Professor and Director, Carolinas Medical Center
Charlotte, North Carolina

Stephen Challacombe, BDS, PhD, FDS RCSEd, FRCPath [20]
Professor of Mucosal Immunology, Oral Microbiology and
    Oral Medicine
Kings College London
London, England

K. C. Chan, DMD, MS, FRCD(C) [7]
Clinical Assistant Professor of Oral and Maxillofacial
    Pathology, Radiology and Medicine
New York University College of Dentistry
New York, New York

Katharine Ciarrocca, DMD, MSEd [26]
Assistant Professor of Oral Medicine
Georgia Regents University
Augusta, Georgia

Mary A. Cutting, MS, RAC [2]
Center for Clinical Research
Division of Extramural Research
National Institute of Dental and Craniofacial Research
National Institutes of Health
Bethesda, Maryland

Scott S. De Rossi, DMD [13, 17]
Chairman, Diagnostic Sciences
Department of Oral Health and Diagnostic Sciences
Georgia Regents University
Augusta, Georgia

Sandhya Desai, MD [14]
Family Medicine Specialist
Scripps Coastal Medical Center
Carlsbad, California

Matthew J. Diamond, DO, MS, FACP [17]
Assistant Professor of Nephrology, Hypertension, and
    Transplant Medicine
Georgia Health Sciences University
Augusta, Georgia

**Mark Donaldson, BSc (Pharm), RPh, PharmD,
FASHP, FACHE [3]**
Director of Pharmacy Services
    Northwest Healthcare
Kalispell, Montana
Clinical Professor
Skaggs School of Pharmacy
University of Montana
Missoula, Montana
Clinical Assistant Professor
Oregon Health and Sciences University
School of Dentistry
Portland, Oregon

Sharon Elad, DMD, MSc [8]
Professor and Chair, Division of Oral Medicine
Eastman Institute for Oral Health
Professor of Oncology
Wilmot Cancer Center
University of Rochester Medical Center
Rochester, New York

Eli Eliav, DMD, MSc, PhD [12]
Director, Eastman Institute for Oral Health
University of Rochester Medical Center
Vice Dean for Oral Health
School of Dentistry and Medicine
Rochester, New York

**Joel Epstein, DMD, MSD, FRCD(C),
FDS RCSEd [8]**
Diplomat, American Board of Oral Medicine
Consulting Staff, Division of Otolaryngology and
    Head and Neck Surgery
City of Hope
Duarte, California

Dena Fischer, DDS, MSD, MS [2]
Center for Clinical Research
Division of Extramural Research
National Institute of Dental and Craniofacial Research
National Institutes of Health
Bethesda, Maryland

Philip C. Fox, DDS, FDS RCSEd [10]
President, PC Fox Consulting LLC
Cabin John, Maryland

Michael Glick, DMD, FDS RCSEd [Ed, 1, 14]
William M. Feagans Chair
Dean and Professor of Oral Medicine
School of Dental Medicine
State University of New York
University at Buffalo
Buffalo, New York

Jason Goodchild, DMD [3]
Clinical Associate Professor, Department of Oral Medicine
University of Pennsylvania School of Dental Medicine
Philadelphia, Pennsylvania
Clinical Assistant Professor, Division of Oral Diagnosis
Department of Diagnostic Sciences
New Jersey Dental School
Newark, New Jersey

Martin S. Greenberg, DDS, FDS RCSEd [1, 4, 11]
Professor Emeritus Department of Oral Medicine
University of Pennsylvania School of Dental Medicine
Philadelphia, Pennsylvania

Nidhi Gulati, MD [26]
Medical Director, Georgia War Veterans Nursing Home
Assistant Professor, Department of Family Medicine
Medical College of Georgia
Assistant Professor, Department of Biobehavioral Nursing
Georgia Regents University College of Nursing
Augusta, Georgia

Holli A. Hamilton, MD, MPH [2]
Senior Medical Officer
Division of Extramural Research
National Institute of Dental and Craniofacial Research
National Institutes of Health
Bethesda, Maryland

Palle Holmstrup, DDS, PhD, DrOdont [5]
Professor and Chairman, Section of Periodontology,
    Microbiology and Community Dentistry
Department of Odontology
School of Dentistry, Faculty of Health Sciences
University of Copenhagen
Copenhagen, Denmark

Michaell A. Huber, DDS [18, 22]
Associate Professor, Department of Comprehensive
    Dentistry
University of Texas Health Science Center
    Dental School
San Antonio, Texas

Matin M. Imanguli, MD, DDS [20]
Center for Clinical Research
Division of Extramural Research
National Institute of Dental and Craniofacial Research
National Institutes of Health
Bethesda, Maryland

Siri Beier Jensen, DDS, PhD [9]
Associate Professor
Section of Oral Medicine, Clinical Oral Physiology,
    Oral Pathology & Anatomy
School of Dentistry, Faculty of Health Sciences
University of Copenhagen
Copenhagen, Denmark

Mats Jontell, DDS, PhD, FDS RCSEd [1, 5]
Professor of Oral Medicine and Pathology
Chairman of the Department of Continuing Education
Institute of Odontology at Sahlgrenska Academy
University of Gothenburg
Gothenburg, Sweden

Junad Khan BDS, MPH, PhD [12]
Assistant Professor, Department of Diagnostic Sciences
Rutgers School of Dental Medicine
Newark, New Jersey

A. Ross Kerr, DDS, MSD [7]
Department of Surgical Sciences (Oral and Maxillofacial
    Surgery)
NYU Langone Medical Center
New York, New York

Ernest W.N. Lam, DMD, MSc, PhD, FRCD(C) [28]
Professor and the Dr. Lloyd & Mrs. Kay Chapman Chair
    in Clinical Sciences
Graduate Program Director and Head
Discipline of Oral and Maxillofacial Radiology
Faculty of Dentistry
The University of Toronto
Toronto, Ontario, Canada

Mark Lepore, MD [14]
Vice President, Clinical Development, Inhalation
Lupin Pharmaceuticals
Philadelphia, Pennsylvania

Laszlo Littmann, MD, PhD [15]
Department of Internal Medicine
Carolinas Medical Center
Charlotte, North Carolina

Peter B. Lockhart, DDS, FDS RCPS, RCSEd [15]
Professor and Chair Emeritus of Oral Medicine
Carolinas Medical Center
Charlotte, North Carolina

Lina M. Mejia, DDS [16]
Associate Professor, Oral Medicine and Diagnostic
    Sciences
College of Dental Medicine
Nova Southeastern University
Fort Lauderdale, Florida

Mark McLean, BMed, PhD, FRACP [23]
Professor and Chair, Department of Medicine
University of Western Sydney
Penrith, New South Wales, Australia

Niki Moutsopoulos, DDS, PhD [20]
Assistant Clinical Investigator
Oral Immunity and Infection Unit
National Institute of Dental and Craniofacial Research
National Institutes of Health
Bethesda, Maryland

Ali Naji, MD, PhD [21]
J. William White Professor of Surgery
Director, Kidney/Pancreas Transplant Programs
Associate Director, Institute for Diabetes, Obesity, and
    Metabolism
University of Pennsylvania School of Medicine
Philidelphia, Pennsylvania

Joel J. Napeñas, DDS, FDS RCSEd [19]
Assistant Professor, Division of Oral Medicine and
    Radiology
Schulich School of Medicine and Dentistry
Western University
London, Ontario, Canada
Department of Oral Medicine
Carolinas Medical Center
Charlotte, North Carolina

Mahvash Navazesh, DMD [25]
Associate Dean, Academic Affairs and
    Student Life
Herman Ostrow School of Dentistry
University of Southern California
Los Angeles, California

Richard Ohrbach, DDS, PhD [11]
Associate Professor, Department of Oral Diagnostic
 Sciences
School of Dental Medicine
State University of New York
University at Buffalo
Buffalo, New York

Pragna Patel, PhD [25]
Professor of Biochemistry & Molecular Biology and
 Dentistry
Institute of Genetic Medicine
Keck School of Medicine
University of Southern California
Los Angeles, California

Lauren L. Patton, DDS FDS RCSEd [19]
Professor and Chair, Department of
 Dental Ecology
UNC School of Dentistry
The University of North Carolina
Chapel Hill, North Carolina

Douglas E. Peterson, DMD, PhD, FDS RCSEd [9]
Professor of Oral Medicine
School of Dental Medicine
Co-Chair, Head & Neck Cancer and Oral Oncology
 Program
Neag Comprehensive Cancer Center
University of Connecticut
Farmington, Connecticut

Joan A. Phelan, DDS [7]
Professor, Oral and Maxillofacial Pathology,
 Radiology and Medicine
New York University College of Dentistry
New York, New York

Stanley R. Pillemer, MD [20]
Senior Consultant
American Biopharma Corporation
Gaithersburg, Maryland

Andres Pinto, DMD, MPH [21]
Associate Professor and Chair, Oral and
 Maxillofacial Medicine and
 Diagnostic Sciences
Case Western Reserve University School of Dental
 Medicine
Cleveland, Ohio

David L. Porter, MD [21]
Director, Blood and Marrow Transplantation
Hospital of the University of Pennsylvania
Philadelphia, Pennsylvania

J. Ned Pruitt II, MD [13]
Director, MCG Neurology Residency Program
Associate Professor, Department of Neurology
Georgia Regents Medical Center
Augusta, Georgia

Spencer W. Redding, DDS, MEd [22]
Department of Comprehensive Dentistry
University of Texas Health Science Center
San Antonio Dental School
San Antonio, Texas

Vidya Sankar, DMD, MHS, FDS RCSEd [18, 22]
Department of Comprehensive Dentistry
University of Texas Health Science Center
San Antonio Dental School
San Antonio, Texas

Frank A. Scannapieco, PhD, DMD [14]
Professor and Chair, Department of Oral Biology
School of Dental Medicine
State University of New York
University at Buffalo
Buffalo, New York

**Mark Schifter, BDS, MDSc (Oral Med), M SND,
RCSEd, FFD RCSI (Oral Med), FRACDS
(Oral Med) [23]**
Staff Specialist and Head, Department of Oral Medicine,
 Oral Pathology, and Special Needs Dentistry
Westmead Centre for Oral Health
Westmead Hospital
Westmead, NSW, Australia

Jonathan A. Ship, DMD, FDS RCSEd [1]*
Director, Bluestone Center for Clinical Research
Professor of Oral and Maxillofacial Pathology, Radiology
 and Medicine
New York University College of Dentistry
New York, New York
*Deceased

Michael A. Siegel, DDS, MS, FDS RCSEd [16]
Professor and Chair, Department of Diagnostic Sciences
College of Dental Medicine
Professor, Internal Medicine (Dermatology)
College of Osteopathic Medicine
Nova Southeastern University
Fort Lauderdale, Florida

David A. Sirois, DMD, PhD [24]
Associate Professor, Oral & Maxillofacial Pathology,
 Radiology and Medicine
New York University College of Dentistry
Associate Professor of Neurology
New York University School of Medicine
New York, New York

Harold C. Slavkin, DDS [25]
Founding Director, USC Center for Craniofacial Molecular Biology
Professor, Ostrow School of Dentistry
University of Southern California
Los Angeles, California

Thomas P. Sollecito, DMD [21]
Professor and Chairman, Department of Oral Medicine
University of Pennsylvania School of Dental Medicine
Philadelphia, Pennsylvania

Lynn W. Solomon, DDS, MS [16]
Associate Professor, Department of Oral Medicine and Diagnostic Sciences
College of Dental Medicine
Nova Southeastern University
Fort Lauderdale, Florida

Eric T. Stoopler, DMD, FDS RCSEd, FDS RCSEng [24]
Associate Professor of Oral Medicine
Director, Postdoctoral Oral Medicine Program
University of Pennsylvania School of Dental Medicine
Attending Physician, Department of Oral & Maxillofacial Surgery
University of Pennsylvania Health System
Philadelphia, Pennsylvania

Jose Luis Tapia, DDS, MS [6]
Assistant Professor, Oral Diagnostic Sciences
School of Dental Medicine
State University of New York
University at Buffalo
Buffalo, New York

Patrick Vannelli, MD [14]
Physician, Private Practice
Allergy & Asthma Specialists
Blue Bell, Pennsylvania

Sook Bin Woo, DMD, MMSc, FDS RCSEd [4, 22]
Associate Professor, Oral Medicine, Infection, and Immunity
Director, Advanced Graduate Education Program in Oral and Maxillofacial Pathology
Division of Oral Medicine and Dentistry
Brigham and Women's Hospital
Boston, Massachusetts

Mark J. Wrobel, PharmD [3]
Clinical Assistant Professor
Director, PharmD Advisement
SUNY at Buffalo School of Pharmacy and Pharmaceutical Sciences
SUNY at Buffalo School of Dental Medicine
Buffalo, New York

Juan F. Yepes, DDS, MD, MPH, MS, DrPH, FDS RCSEd [27]
Associate Professor of Pediatric Dentistry
Department of Pediatric Dentistry
Riley Hospital for Children
Indiana University School of Dentistry
Indianapolis, Indiana

Julyana Gomes Zagury, DMD, MSD [12]
Clinical Assistant Professor
Division of Temporomandibular Disorders and Orofacial Pain Department of Diagnostic Sciences
Rutgers School of Dental Medicine
Newark, New Jersey

In the introduction to the first edition of *Burket's Oral Medicine* published in 1946, Dr. Appleton, Dean of the School of Dentistry at the University of Pennsylvania, wrote "The practitioner of medicine, physician and internist, would do well to read at least the Table of Contents. If he does that, I believe he'll delve deeper. It should convince him that the mouth contains much more than the doubly unruly tongue. There are many situations and ways in which he can help the neighboring dentist, and the dentist can in turn help him. Both physician and dentist will benefit, but the patient would benefit most." Although our knowledge of oral medicine has dramatically increased in the past 70 years, this new 12th edition could have been introduced in a similar fashion. Oral medicine is at the forefront of interprofessional education and practice, and the 12th edition of *Burket's Oral Medicine* will be a resource to all health professionals.

In order to reflect changes in the reach of the discipline of oral medicine, the 12th edition of this seminal text includes five new chapters: Research Design and Evaluation, Oral Complications of Cancer Therapy, Geriatric Oral Medicine,

Pediatric Oral Medicine, and Radiologic Interpretations, and 28 new contributors. Together, the more than 70 contributors of the chapters included in the 12th edition represent seven countries and present a text truly international in scope.

Due to the complexity of the "art and science" of the field of oral medicine, there will be inconsistencies among the chapters in cases in which lack of evidence for specific protocols results in reliance on clinical judgment. Such discrepancies add rather than detract from our knowledge base and, when found, were left as is.

The 12th edition of this definitive text on oral medicine delivers indispensable content to students, residents, and clinicians from many different health disciplines seeking to advance their knowledge in this exciting field of healthcare delivery. The text offers support with necessary diagnostic skills, basic research, and clinical advice needed to treat medically complex dental patients, as well as a myriad of oral complications.

—Michael Glick, DMD
Buffalo, New York

Introduction to Oral Medicine and Oral Diagnosis: Evaluation of the Dental Patient

Michael Glick, DMD, FDS RCSEd

Martin S. Greenberg, DDS, FDS RCSEd

Mats Jontell, DDS, PhD, FDS RCSEd

Jonathan A. Ship, DMD, FDS RCSEd*

❐ INFORMATION GATHERING
  Medical History
  Patient Examination
  Consultations
❐ ESTABLISHING A DIFFERENTIAL AND FINAL DIAGNOSIS
❐ FORMULATING A PLAN OF ACTION
  Medical Risk Assessment
  Modification of Dental Care for Medically Complex Patients
  Monitoring and Evaluating Underlying Medical Conditions

❐ ORAL MEDICINE CONSULTATIONS
❐ THE DENTAL AND MEDICAL RECORD: ORGANIZATION, CONFIDENTIALITY, AND INFORMED CONSENT
  Organization
  Problem-Oriented Record
  Condition Diagram
  The SOAP Note
  Confidentiality
  Informed Consent
❐ ELECTRONIC HEALTH RECORDS

Oral medicine is a specialized discipline within dentistry that focuses on provision of dental care for medically complex patients, and the diagnosis and management of medical disorders involving the mouth, jaws, and salivary glands. Offering care to a patient seeking diagnosis and treatment is a responsibility that entails both broad and detailed knowledge and should only be provided by a health-care professional with appropriate training and experience.

Clinicians are presently caring for an aging population who are living longer with complications of chronic illnesses and multiple comorbidities, and having endured complex surgical procedures while taking multiple medications. This population of patients requires oral health professionals with an increased knowledge of medical diseases and their effect on oral diseases and provision of oral health care. What previously was considered the purview of hospital-based dentists has become a common occurrence in general and specialty dental practice. Oral health is an integral part of total health, and oral health professionals must adapt to

---

* Deceased

these demographic changes by increasing their knowledge of medicine related to oral and dental health care.[1]

Technological advances are influencing all aspects of patient interactions, from our initial contact with a patient, through medical history taking, diagnosis, and treatment options. Electronic health records (EHRs) afford a means for sharing health information among multiple clinicians caring for the same patient and can provide point-of-care algorithms for eliciting and using health information.[2] Modern imaging techniques such as computed tomography and magnetic resonance imaging provide more detailed information but require increased interpretation skills. Technology is a means to acquire more sophisticated data but requires increased training for accurate interpretation; and yet, the most important skills for accurate diagnosis remain an experienced clinician who has developed the skills to listen and examine.

The initial encounter with a patient will influence all subsequent care. The skilled, experienced practitioner has learned to elicit the clinical, laboratory, and other necessary information required for an accurate diagnosis. Performing a diagnostic evaluation, including a patient interview and a physical examination, is an art as well as a skill. Although mastering a patient evaluation can be assisted by specific clinical protocols, the experienced practitioner will add his or her own skills to the diagnostic methodology.

A variety of accessible sources of health-care information are now readily available to patients, and many will use this information to self-diagnose, as well as demand specific treatments.[3] Although, a patient-centered approach is encouraged, in which a patient's preferences and values will influence care, the practitioner has the responsibility for treatment decisions and needs to educate the patient to make informed, scientific- and evidence-based choices.

Obtaining, evaluating, and assessing a patient's oral and overall health status is the obligation of the treating oral health-care professional. This process can arbitrarily be divided into four major overlapping parts:

1. Information gathering
2. Establishing a differential and final diagnosis
3. Formulating a plan of action
4. Initiating treatment and follow-up

INFORMATION GATHERING

An appropriate interpretation of the information collected through a medical history and patient examination achieves several important objectives; it affords an opportunity for

1. gathering the information necessary for establishing the diagnosis of the patient's chief complaint (CC)
2. assessing the influence of the patient's systemic health on patient's oral health
3. detecting underlying systemic conditions that the patient may or may not be aware of
4. providing a basis for determining whether dental treatment might affect the systemic health of the patient
5. providing a basis for determining necessary modifications to routine dental care
6. monitoring known medical conditions

Medical History

Obtaining an appropriate and accurate medical history is the *sine qua non* of all patient care. A patient's medical history is elicited through a systematic review of the patient's chief or primary complaint, a detailed history related to this complaint, information about past and present medical conditions, pertinent social and family histories, and a review of symptoms by organ system. A medical history also includes biographic and demographic data used to identify the patient.

There is no universally agreed upon method for obtaining a medical history, but a systematic approach will help the practitioner to gather all necessary information without overlooking important facts. The nature of the patient's oral health visit (i.e., initial dental visit, complex diagnostic problem, emergency, elective continuous care, or recall) often dictates how the history is obtained. The two most common means of obtaining initial patient information are a patient-self- administered preprinted health questionnaire or by recording information during a systematic health interview without the benefit of having the patient fill out a questionnaire. The use of self-administered screening questionnaires is the most commonly used method in dental settings (Figure 1-1). This technique can be useful in gathering background medical information, but the accurate diagnosis of a specific oral complaint requires a history of the present illness and other information that is necessary to obtain verbally. The challenge in any health-care setting is to use a questionnaire that has enough items to obtain the essential medical information but is not too long to deter a patient's willingness and ability to fill it out. These questionnaires should be constructed in a manner that allows the clinician to query the patient about the most essential and relevant required information yet provides a starting point for a dialogue with the patient about other pertinent information not included on the health form. Preprinted self-administered health questionnaires are readily available, standardized, and easy to administer and do not require significant "chair time." They give the clinician a starting point for a dialogue to conduct more in-depth medical queries but are restricted to the questions chosen on the form and are therefore limited in scope. The questions on the form can be misunderstood by the patient, resulting in inaccurate information, and they require a specific level of reading comprehension. Preprinted forms cover broad areas without necessarily focusing on particular problems pertinent to an individual patient's specific medical condition. Therefore, the use of these forms requires that the provider has sufficient background knowledge to understand reason for the questions on the forms. Furthermore, the provider needs to realize that a given standard history form necessitates timely and appropriate follow-up questions, especially when positive responses have been elicited. An established routine for performing and recording the history and examination should be followed conscientiously.

The oral health-care professional has a responsibility to obtain relevant medical and dental health information, yet the patient cannot always be relied upon to know this information or provide an accurate and comprehensive assessment of his or her medical or dental status.

All medical information obtained and recorded in an oral health-care setting is considered confidential and constitutes a legal document. Although it is appropriate for the patient to fill out a history form in the waiting room, any discussion of the patient's responses must take place in a private setting. Furthermore, access to the written or electronic (if applicable) record must be limited to office personnel who are directly responsible for the patient's care. Any other release of private information should be approved, in writing, by the patient and retained by the dentist as part of the patient's medical record.

Changes in a patient's health status or medication regimen should be reviewed at each office visit prior to initiating dental care. This is important as medical status and medication regimens often change. The monitoring of patients' compliance with suggested medical treatment guidelines and prescribed medications is part of the oral health-care professional's responsibilities.[4] The following strategies are common to all methods of history taking

- review available patient information prior to meeting the patient;
- make the patient feel comfortable and pay attention to the patient's concerns; do not rush the interview process;
- pay attention to the patient; greet the patient; use the patient's name; ensure privacy; sit rather than stand; maintain eye contact as often as possible; do not concentrate chiefly on entering the information into an EHR as this may distract the clinician from listening to pertinent information;
- use the patient's own words to describe her primary reason(s) ("CC") to seek care/consultation;
- use open-ended questions that allow the patient to express herself;
- although all information should be collected in a systematic fashion, the order is not as important as is initiating a dialogue with the patient about her health;
- create a timeline of the reported patient-related events; an accurate chronology is an extremely important element to establish a causative relationship.

The medical history traditionally consists of the following subcategories:

1. *Identification*: Name, date and time of the visit, date of birth, gender, ethnicity, occupation, contact information of a primary care physician, and referral source.
2. *CC*: The main reason for the patient seeking care or consultation—recorded in the patient's own words.
3. *History of present illness*: A chronologic account of events; state of health before the presentation of the present problem; description of the first signs and symptoms and how they may have changed; description of occurrences of amelioration or exacerbation; previous clinicians consulted and prior treatment. For those who favor mnemonics, nine dimensions of a medical problem can be easily recalled using OLD CHARTS (Onset, Location/radiation, Duration, Character, Habits, Aggravating factors, Reliving factors, Timing, and Severity). (Modification of Reference 5).
4. *Medical history*: General health; childhood illnesses; major adult illnesses; immunizations; surgeries (date, reason, and outcome); pregnancies (gravid); births (para); medications (prescribed medications, over-the-counter medications, supplements, and home remedies); and allergies.
5. *Family history*: Blood relatives with illnesses similar to the patient's concern; specific genetic disorders, cardiovascular diseases, diabetes mellitus, different types of cancers.
6. *Personal and social history*: Birthplace; marital status; children; habits (tobacco use, alcohol use, recreational drug use); sexual history; occupation; religious preferences that may have an impact on types of care.
7. *Review of systems (ROS)*: Identifies symptoms in different body systems (Table 1-1).

The ROS is a comprehensive and systematic review of subjective symptoms affecting different bodily systems. It is an essential component for identifying patients with an undiagnosed disease that will affect dental treatment or associated symptoms that will help determine the primary diagnosis; for example, identifying a patient with skin, genital, or conjunctival lesions who also has oral mucosal disease or a patient with anesthesia, parasthesia, or weakness who also complaints of orofacial pain. The clinician records both negative and positive responses. Direct questioning of the patient should be aimed at collecting additional data to assess the severity of a patient's medical conditions, monitor changes in medical conditions, and assist in confirming or ruling out those disease processes that may be associated with a patient's symptoms.

Patient Examination

The examination of the patient represents the second stage of the evaluation and assessment process. An established routine for examination decreases the possibility of overlooking undiscovered pathologic conditions. The examination is most conveniently carried out with the patient seated in a dental chair, with the head supported. When dental charting is involved,

FIGURE 1-1 Health history questionnaire.

Health History Form

ADA American Dental Association®
America's leading advocate for oral health

Email: _____ Today's Date: _____

As required by law, our office adheres to written policies and procedures to protect the privacy of information about you that we create, receive or maintain. Your answers are for our records only and will be kept confidential subject to applicable laws. Please note that you will be asked some questions about your responses to this questionnaire and there may be additional questions concerning your health. This information is vital to allow us to provide appropriate care for you. This office does not use this information to discriminate.

Name:			Home Phone: *Include area code*	Business/Cell Phone: *Include area code*
Last	*First*	*Middle*	( )	( )

Address:	City:	State:	Zip:
Mailing address			

Occupation:	Height:	Weight:	Date of Birth:	Sex: M F

SS# or Patient ID:	Emergency Contact:	Relationship:	Home Phone: *Include area code* ( )	Cell Phone: *Include area code* ( )

If you are completing this form for another person, what is your relationship to that person?

Your Name _____ *Relationship* _____

Do you have any of the following diseases or problems: *(Check DK if you Don't Know the answer to the the question)*

	Yes	No	DK
Active Tuberculosis	☐	☐	☐
Persistent cough greater than a 3 week duration	☐	☐	☐
Cough that produces blood	☐	☐	☐
Been exposed to anyone with tuberculosis	☐	☐	☐

If you answer yes to any of the 4 items above, please stop and return this form to the receptionist.

Dental Information *For the following questions, please mark (X) your responses to the following questions.*

	Yes	No	DK		Yes	No	DK
Do your gums bleed when you brush or floss?	☐	☐	☐	Do you have earaches or neck pains?	☐	☐	☐
Are your teeth sensitive to cold, hot, sweets or pressure?	☐	☐	☐	Do you have any clicking, popping or discomfort in the jaw?	☐	☐	☐
Is your mouth dry?	☐	☐	☐	Do you brux or grind your teeth?	☐	☐	☐
Have you had any periodontal (gum) treatments?	☐	☐	☐	Do you have sores or ulcers in your mouth?	☐	☐	☐
Have you ever had orthodontic (braces) treatment?	☐	☐	☐	Do you wear dentures or partials?	☐	☐	☐
Have you had any problems associated with previous dental treatment?	☐	☐	☐	Do you participate in active recreational activities?	☐	☐	☐
Is your home water supply fluoridated?	☐	☐	☐	Have you ever had a serious injury to your head or mouth?	☐	☐	☐
Do you drink bottled or filtered water?	☐	☐	☐	Date of your last dental exam:			
If yes, how often? *Circle one:* DAILY / WEEKLY / OCCASIONALLY				What was done at that time?			
Are you currently experiencing dental pain or discomfort?	☐	☐	☐	Date of last dental x-rays:			

What is the reason for your dental visit today?

How do you feel about your smile?

Medical Information *Please mark (X) your response to indicate if you have or have not had any of the following diseases or problems.*

	Yes	No	DK		Yes	No	DK
Are you now under the care of a physician?	☐	☐	☐	Have you had a serious illness, operation or been hospitalized in the past 5 years?	☐	☐	☐
Physician Name:	Phone: *Include area code* ( )			If yes, what was the illness or problem?			
Address/City/State/Zip:							
				Are you taking or have you recently taken any prescription or over the counter medicine(s)?	☐	☐	☐
Are you in good health?	☐	☐	☐	If so, please list all, including vitamins, natural or herbal preparations and/or dietary supplements:			
Has there been any change in your general health within the past year?	☐	☐	☐				
If yes, what condition is being treated?				_____			
				_____			
Date of last physical exam:				_____			

© 2012 American Dental Association
Form S500

Medical Information
Please mark (X) your response to indicate if you have or have not had any of the following diseases or problems.

(Check DK if you Don't Know the answer to the question)

	Yes	No	DK		Yes	No	DK
Do you wear contact lenses?	□	□	□	Do you use controlled substances (drugs)?	□	□	□

Joint Replacement. Have you had an orthopedic total joint (hip, knee, elbow, finger) replacement? ☐ ☐ ☐
Date: _____ If yes, have you had any complications? _____

Are you taking or scheduled to begin taking an antiresorptive agent (like Fosamax®, Actonel®, Atelvia, Boniva®, Reclast, Prolia) for osteoporosis or Paget's disease? ☐ ☐ ☐

Since 2001, were you treated or are you presently scheduled to begin treatment with an antiresorptive agent (like Aredia®, Zometa®, XGEVA) for bone pain, hypercalcemia or skeletal complications resulting from Paget's disease, multiple myeloma or metastatic cancer? ☐ ☐ ☐
Date Treatment began: _____

Do you use tobacco (smoking, snuff, chew, bidis)? ☐ ☐ ☐
If so, how interested are you in stopping?
Circle one: VERY / SOMEWHAT / NOT INTERESTED

Do you drink alcoholic beverages? ☐ ☐ ☐
If yes, how much alcohol did you drink in the last 24 hours? _____
If yes, how much do you typically drink i n a week? _____

WOMEN ONLY Are you:
Pregnant? ☐ ☐ ☐
Number of weeks: _____
Taking birth control pills or hormonal replacement? ☐ ☐ ☐
Nursing? ☐ ☐ ☐

Allergies. Are you allergic to or have you had a reaction to:
To all **yes** responses, specify type of reaction.

	Yes	No	DK		Yes	No	DK
Local anesthetics _____	□	□	□	Metals _____	□	□	□
Aspirin _____	□	□	□	Latex (rubber) _____	□	□	□
Penicillin or other antibiotics _____	□	□	□	Iodine _____	□	□	□
Barbiturates, sedatives, or sleeping pills _____	□	□	□	Hay fever/seasonal _____	□	□	□
Sulfa drugs _____	□	□	□	Animals _____	□	□	□
Codeine or other narcotics _____	□	□	□	Food _____	□	□	□
				Other _____	□	□	□

Please mark (X) your response to indicate if you have or have not had any of the following diseases or problems.

	Yes	No	DK		Yes	No	DK		Yes	No	DK
Artificial (prosthetic) heart valve	□	□	□	Autoimmune disease	□	□	□	Glaucoma	□	□	□
Previous infective endocarditis	□	□	□	Rheumatoid arthritis	□	□	□	Hepatitis, jaundice or liver disease	□	□	□
Damaged valves in transplanted heart	□	□	□	Systemic lupus erythematosus	□	□	□	Epilepsy	□	□	□
Congenital heart disease (CHD)				Asthma	□	□	□	Fainting spells or seizures	□	□	□
Unrepaired, cyanotic CHD	□	□	□	Bronchitis	□	□	□	Neurological disorders	□	□	□
Repaired (completely) in last 6 months	□	□	□	Emphysema	□	□	□	If yes, specify:_____			
Repaired CHD with residual defects	□	□	□	Sinus trouble	□	□	□	Sleep disorder	□	□	□
				Tuberculosis	□	□	□	Do you snore?	□	□	□

Except for the conditions listed above, antibiotic prophylaxis is no longer recommended for any other form of CHD.

	Yes	No	DK		Yes	No	DK		Yes	No	DK
Cardiovascular disease	□	□	□	Mitral valve prolapse	□	□	□	Cancer/Chemotherapy/ Radiation Treatment	□	□	□
Angina	□	□	□	Pacemaker	□	□	□	Chest pain upon exertion	□	□	□
Arteriosclerosis	□	□	□	Rheumatic fever	□	□	□	Chronic pain	□	□	□
Congestive heart failure	□	□	□	Rheumatic heart disease	□	□	□	Diabetes Type I or II	□	□	□
Damaged heart valves	□	□	□	Abnormal bleeding	□	□	□	Eating disorder	□	□	□
Heart attack	□	□	□	Anemia	□	□	□	Malnutrition	□	□	□
Heart murmur	□	□	□	Blood transfusion	□	□	□	Gastrointestinal disease	□	□	□
Low blood pressure	□	□	□	If yes, date:_____				G.E. Reflux/persistent heartburn	□	□	□
High blood pressure	□	□	□	Hemophilia	□	□	□	Ulcers	□	□	□
Other congenital heart defects	□	□	□	AIDS or HIV infection	□	□	□	Thyroid problems	□	□	□
				Arthritis	□	□	□	Stroke	□	□	□

Additional right column:
Mental health disorders Specify: _____ □ □ □
Recurrent Infections □ □ □
Type of infection: _____
Kidney problems □ □ □
Night sweats □ □ □
Osteoporosis □ □ □
Persistent swollen glands in neck □ □ □
Severe headaches/ migraines □ □ □
Severe or rapid weight loss □ □ □
Sexually transmitted disease □ □ □
Excessive urination □ □ □

Has a physician or previous dentist recommended that you take antibiotics prior to your dental treatment? ☐ ☐ ☐
Name of physician or dentist making recommendation: _____
Phone: *Include area code* ( )

Do you have any disease, condition, or problem not listed above that you think I should know about? ☐ ☐ ☐
Please explain:

NOTE: Both doctor and patient are encouraged to discuss any and all relevant patient health issues prior to treatment.
I certify that I have read and understand the above and that the information given on this form is accurate. I understand the importance of a truthful health history and that my dentist and his/her staff will rely on this information for treating me. I acknowledge that my questions, if any, about inquiries set forth above have been answered to my satisfaction. I will not hold my dentist, or any other member of his/her staff, responsible for any action they take or do not take because of errors or omissions that I may have made in the completion of this form.

Signature of Patient/Legal Guardian: _____ Date: _____

Signature of Dentist: _____ Date: _____

FOR COMPLETION BY DENTIST
Comments: _____

TABLE 1-1	Review of Systems Is a Systematic Approach to Ascertain Mostly Subjective Symptoms Associated With the Different Body Systems

General: Weight changes, malaise fatigue, night sweats
Head: Headaches, tenderness, sinus problems
Eyes: Changes in vision, photophobia, blurring, diplopia, spots, discharge
Ears: Hearing changes, tinnitus, pain, discharge, vertigo
Nose: Epistaxis, obstructions
Throat: Hoarseness, soreness
Respiratory: Chest pain, wheezing, dyspnea, cough, hemoptysis
Cardiovascular: Chest pain, dyspnea, orthopnea (number of pillows needed to sleep comfortably), edema, claudication
Dermatologic: Rashes, pruritus, lesions, skin cancer (epidermoid carcinoma, melanoma)
Gastrointestinal: Changes in appetite, dysphagia, nausea, vomiting, hematemesis, indigestion, pain, diarrhea, constipation, melena, hematochezia, bloating, hemorrhoids, jaundice
Genitourinary: Changes in urinary frequency or urgency, dysuria, hematuria, nocturia, incontinence, discharge, impotence
Gynecologic: Menstrual changes (frequency, duration, flow, last menstrual period), dysmenorrhea, menopause
Endocrine: Polyuria, polydipsia, polyphagia, temperature intolerance, pigmentations
Musculoskeletal: Muscle and joint pain, deformities, joint swellings, spasms, changes in range of motion
Hematologic: Easy bruising, epistaxis, spontaneous gingival bleeding, increased bleeding after trauma
Lymphatic: Swollen or enlarged lymph nodes
Neuropsychiatric: Syncope, seizures, weakness (unilateral and bilateral), changes in coordination, sensations, memory, mood, or sleep pattern, emotional disturbances, history of psychiatric therapy

having an assistant record the findings saves time and limits cross-contamination. Before seating the patient, the clinician should observe the patient's general appearance and gait and should note any physical deformities or impediments.

The routine oral examination should be carried out at least once annually or at each recall visit. This includes a thorough inspection and, when appropriate, palpation, auscultation, and percussion of the exposed surface structures of the head, neck, and face and a detailed examination of the oral cavity, dentition, oropharynx, and adnexal structures. Laboratory studies and additional special examination of other organ systems may be required for the evaluation of patients with orofacial pain, oral mucosal disease, or signs and symptoms suggestive of otorhinologic or salivary gland disorders or pathologies suggestive of a systemic etiology. A less comprehensive but equally thorough inspection of the face and oral and oropharyngeal mucosae should be carried out at each dental visit. The tendency for the oral health professional to focus on only the tooth or jaw quadrant in question should be strongly resisted.

Each visit should be initiated by a deliberate inspection of the entire face and oral cavity prior to the scheduled or emergency procedure. The importance of this approach in the early detection of head and neck cancer and in promoting the image of the dentist as the responsible clinician of the oral cavity cannot be overstated (see Chapter 8, "Oral and Oropharyngeal Cancer").

Examination carried out in the dental office is traditionally restricted to that of the superficial tissues of the oral cavity, head, and neck and the exposed parts of the extremities. On occasion, evaluation of an oral lesion logically leads to an inquiry about similar lesions on other skin or mucosal surfaces or about the enlargement of other regional groups of lymph nodes. Although these inquiries can usually be satisfied directly by questioning the patient, the oral health professional may also quite appropriately request permission from the patient to examine axillary nodes or other

skin surfaces provided that the examination is carried out competently and there is adequate privacy for the patient. A male oral health professional should have a female assistant present in the case of a female patient; a female oral health professional should have a male assistant present in the case of a male patient. Similar precautions should be followed when it is necessary for a patient to remove tight clothing for accurate measurement of blood pressure. A complete physical examination should not be attempted when facilities are lacking or when religious or other customs prohibit it.

The degree of responsibility accorded to the oral health professional in carrying out a complete physical examination varies from institution to institution, hospital to hospital, state to state, and country to country.

The examination procedure in a dental office setting includes five areas:

1. Registration of vital signs (respiratory rate, temperature, pain level, pulse, and blood pressure)
2. Examination of the head, neck, and oral cavity, including salivary glands, temporomandibular joints, and head and neck lymph nodes
3. Examination of cranial nerve function
4. Special examination of other organ systems
5. Requisition of appropriate laboratory studies

Consultations

Consultations with other health-care professionals are initiated when additional information is necessary to assess a patient's health status. Consent from the patient is needed before a consultation is initiated.[6] All verbal and written consultation should be documented in the patient's record. A consultation letter should identify the patient and contain a brief overview of the patient's pertinent medical history and a request for specific medical information (Figure 1-2). A physician cannot "clear" a patient for treatment.[7]

A physician's advice and recommendation may be helpful in managing a dental patient, but the responsibility to provide safe and appropriate care lies ultimately with the oral health-care provider.

Patients for whom a dentist may need to obtain medical consultation include (1) the patient with known medical problems who is scheduled for either inpatient or outpatient dental treatment and cannot adequately describe all of his or her medical problems; (2) the patient in whom abnormalities are detected during history taking, on physical examination, or through a laboratory study of which the patient is not aware; (3) the patient who has a high risk for the development of particular medical problems; and (4) the patient for whom additional medical information is required that may impact the provision of dental care or assist in the diagnosis of an orofacial problem.

When there is a need for a specific consultation, the consultant should be selected for appropriateness to the particular problem, and the problem and the specific questions to be answered should be clearly transmitted to the consultant in writing. Adequate details of the planned dental procedure, including, when appropriate, expected amount of bleeding; an assessment of time and stress to the patient; expected period of posttreatment disability; and details of the particular symptom, sign, or laboratory abnormality that gave rise to the consultation should be provided to the consultant. The written request should be brief and should specify the particular concern and items of information needed from the consultant. Importantly, requests for "medical clearance" should be avoided.[7]

ESTABLISHING A DIFFERENTIAL AND FINAL DIAGNOSIS

Before establishing a final diagnosis in the orofacial region, the oral health-care professional often needs to formulate a differential diagnosis based on the history and physical examination findings. The disorders included in the differential diagnosis will determine which laboratory tests, such as biopsies, blood tests, or imaging studies, are required to reach a final diagnosis.

The rapidity and accuracy with which a diagnosis or set of diagnoses can be achieved depends on the history and examination data that have been collected and on the clinician's knowledge and ability to match these clinical data with

---

Consultation

Date: February 26, 2007

To: John Doc, MD

From: Martin Dent, DMD

Patient name and DOB: Oscar Jones; DOB – February 1, 1945

Summary and request:

A 62-year-old African American man presents to our dental office for multiple extractions. This is a very stressful procedure with anticipated bleeding from multiple intraoral sites. Local anesthesia will be used and will include 3.6–7.2 mL of 2% lidocaine with 1:100,000 concentration of epinephrine.

Examination revealed a slightly overweight male in no apparent distress. His BP was 172/100 mm Hg, with a pulse of 65 beats/min with regular rate and rhythm.

His medical history is remarkable for multiple medical problems, including hypertension ×20 years; multiple angina attacks, the last one in 1998; reported history of renal disease; and multiple medications.

Review of systems is remarkable for polyurea, polydipsia, and occasional shortness of breath at rest.

Please advise as to the patient's hypertensive control, stable versus unstable angina, any other type of cardiovascular diseases or target organ damage, type and severity of renal disease, possible diabetes mellitus, and types and regimen of medications.

Patient signature and date:

_____

Oral health-care professional signature and date:

_____

Please return this consultation to:

_____

FIGURE 1-2   Consultation.

suspected disease processes. Experienced clinicians who have an extensive knowledge of human physiology, disease etiology, and a broad knowledge of the relevant literature can usually rapidly establish a correct diagnosis. Such "mental models" of disease syndromes also increase the efficiency with which experienced clinicians gather and evaluate clinical data and focus supplemental questioning and testing at all stages of the diagnostic process.

For effective treatment, as well as for health insurance and medicolegal reasons, it is important that a diagnosis (or diagnostic summary) is entered into the patient's record after the detailed history and physical, radiographic, and laboratory examination data. When more than one health problem is identified, the diagnosis for the primary complaint (i.e., the stated problem for which the patient sought medical or dental advice) is usually listed first, followed by subsidiary diagnoses of concurrent problems. Previously diagnosed conditions that remain as actual or potential problems are also included, with the qualification "by history," "previously diagnosed," or "treated" to indicate their status. Problems that were identified but not clearly diagnosed during the current evaluation can also be listed with the comment "to be ruled out." Because oral medicine is concerned with regional problems that may or may not be modified by concurrent systemic disease, it is common for the list of diagnoses to include both oral lesions and systemic problems of actual or potential significance in the etiology or management of oral lesions. Items in the medical history that do not relate to the current problem and that are not of major health significance usually are not included in the diagnostic summary. For example, a diagnosis might read as follows:

1. Alveolar abscess, mandibular left first molar
2. Rampant generalized dental caries secondary to radiation-induced salivary hypofunction
3. Carcinoma of the tonsillar fossa, by history, excised and treated with 65 Gy two years ago
4. Cirrhosis and prolonged prothrombin time, by history
5. Hyperglycemia; R/O (rule out) diabetes

A definite diagnosis cannot always be made, despite a careful review of all history, clinical, and laboratory data. In such cases, a descriptive term (rather than a formal diagnosis) may be used for the patient's symptoms or lesion, with the added word "idiopathic," "unexplained," or (in the case of symptoms without apparent physical abnormality) "functional" or "symptomatic." The clinician must decide what terminology to use in conversing with the patient and whether to clearly identify this diagnosis as "undetermined." Irrespective of that decision, it is important to recognize the equivocal nature of the patient's problem and to schedule additional evaluation, by referral to another consultant, additional testing, or placement of the patient on recall for follow-up studies.

Unfortunately, there is no generally accepted system for identifying and classifying diseases, and diagnoses are often written with concerns related to third-party reimbursement and medicolegal and local peer review, as well as for the purpose of accurately describing and communicating the patient's disease status. Within different specialties, attempts have been made to achieve conformity of professional expressions and language.

Some standardization of diagnoses has been achieved in the United States as a result of the introduction in 1983 of the diagnosis-related group (DRG) system as an obligatory cost-containment measure for the reimbursement of hospitals for inpatient care. In August 2006, the Centers for Medicare and Medicaid Services (CMS) issued a final ruling that initiated a transition plan for replacing, at the time, existing CMS DRGs with a classification methodology that more accurately reflects a patient's severity of disease. Beyond cost containment, patient grouping classifications also are used for epidemiologic monitoring, clinical management, and comparison of hospital activity and as a prospective payment system. Yet, groupings are mostly based on medical diagnoses, such as the *International Classification of Diseases, Tenth Revision* (ICD-10).[8] ICD-11 is expected to be available in 2017.

Although scientifically derived, the DRG system is designed for fiscal use rather than as a system for the accurate classification of disease. It also emphasizes procedures rather than diseases and has a number of serious flaws in its classification and coding system. The ICD system, by contrast, was developed from attempts at establishing an internationally accepted list of causes of death and has undergone numerous revisions in the past 160 years, related to the various emphases placed on clinical, anatomic, biochemical, and perceived etiologic classification of disease at different times and different locations. There is still no official set of operational criteria for assigning the various diagnoses included in the ICD. In addition, the categories for symptoms, lesions, and procedures applicable to oral cavity conditions are limited and often outdated. Medicare and other third-party reimbursers are usually concerned only with diagnoses of those conditions that were actively diagnosed or treated at a given visit; concurrent problems not specifically addressed at that visit are omitted from the reimbursement diagnosis, even if they are of major health significance. The clinician, therefore, must address a number of concerns in formulating a diagnosis, selecting appropriate language for recording diagnoses on the chart, and documenting requests for third-party reimbursement.

The patient (or, when appropriate, a responsible family member or guardian) should also be informed of the diagnosis, as well as the results of the examinations and tests carried out. Because patients' anxieties frequently emphasize the possibility of a potentially serious diagnosis, it is important to point out (when the facts allow) that the biopsy specimen revealed no evidence of a malignant growth, the blood test revealed no abnormality, and no evidence of diseases, such as diabetes, anemia, leukemia, or other cancer, was found. Equally important is the necessity to explain to the patient the nature, significance, and treatment of any lesion or disease that has been diagnosed.

Medical risk assessment of patients before dental treatment offers the opportunity for greatly improving dental services for patients with compromised health. It does require considerably more clinical training and understanding of the natural history and clinical features of systemic disease processes than have been customarily taught in predoctoral dental education programs[9]; however, a partial solution to this problem has been achieved through undergraduate assignments in hospital dentistry and (most important) through hospital-based dental general practice dentistry, oral medicine, and oral and maxillofacial surgery residency programs. It is hoped that revisions in dental predoctoral curricula will recognize this need and provide greater emphasis on both the pathophysiology of systemic disease and the practical clinical evaluation and management of medically complex patients in the dental student's program.

FORMULATING A PLAN OF ACTION

Medical Risk Assessment

The information gathering described above is also designed to help the oral health professional (1) recognize a general health status that may affect dental treatment; (2) make informed judgments on the risk of dental procedures; and (3) identify the need for medical consultation to provide assistance in diagnosing or treating systemic disease that may be an etiologic factor in oral disease or that is likely to be worsened by the proposed dental treatment. The end point of the diagnostic process and the formulation of a plan of action is usually not a simple process. To minimize any adverse events, an assessment of any special risks associated with a patient's compromised medical status that could be triggered by the planned anesthetic, diagnostic, or medical or surgical treatment procedure must be entered in the patient record—usually as an addendum to the plan of treatment. This process of medical risk assessment is the responsibility of all clinicians prior to initiating any treatment or intervention and applies to outpatient and inpatient situations.

A routine of initial history taking and physical examination is essential for all dental patients as even the apparently healthy patient may on evaluation be found to have a history or examination findings of sufficient significance to cause the oral health professional to modify the plan of treatment, change a medication, or even defer a particular intervention until additional diagnostic data are available. To respect the familiar medical axiom *primum non nocere* (first, do no harm), all procedures carried out and all prescriptions given to a patient should be preceded by the oral health professional's conscious consideration of the risk of the particular procedure. Establishing a formal medical risk assessment ensures a continuous evaluation process by the clinician. A summary of the medical risk assessment, delineating potential risks to the patient due to the proposed plan of action, should be entered in the patient record.

The oral health professional traditionally arrives at a decision for or against dental treatment for a medically complex patient by requesting the patient's physician to "clear the patient for dental care." Unfortunately, in many cases, the physician is provided with little information about the nature of the proposed dental treatment (type of treatment, amount of local anesthetics, anticipated bleeding, etc.) and may have insufficient data (other than personal experience with dental care) on which to judge the stress (physical or psychological) likely to be associated with the proposed dental treatment. The response of a given patient to specific dental interventions may also be unpredictable, particularly when the patient has a number of comorbidities and is taking multiple medications. In addition, the practitioner identified by the patient as her physician may not have adequate or complete data from all previous medical evaluations—a requisite to make an informed judgment on the patient's likely response to dental care. All too frequently, the oral health professional receives the brief comment "OK for dental care," which suggests that a recommendation for safe dental care is often given casually and subjectively rather than being based on objective physiologic data. As mentioned earlier, another health professional cannot from a legal standpoint "clear" a patient for any dental procedure.[7]

More importantly, the practice of having the patient "cleared" for dental care confuses the issue of responsibility for untoward events occurring during dental treatment. Although the dentist often must rely on the physician or a consultant for expert diagnostic information and for an opinion about the advisability of dental treatment or the need for special precautions, the oral health professional retains the primary responsibility for the procedures actually carried out and for the immediate management of any unexpected or unfavorable complication, that is, the safety of the patient. The oral health professional is most familiar with the procedures she is carrying out, as well as with their likely complications, but the oral health professional must also be able to assess a patient for medical or other problems that are likely to set the stage for the development of complications. Therefore, physicians can only advise on what types of modifications are necessary to treat a patient; it is ultimately the responsibility of the treating oral health-care professional to ensure a patient's safety.

Numerous protocols have been proposed to facilitate efficient and accurate preoperative assessment of medical risk.[10–12] Many of the earlier guides were developed for the assessment of risks associated with general anesthesia or major surgery and focus on mortality as the dependent variable; guides for the assessment of hazards associated with dental or oral surgical procedures performed under local or regional anesthesia usually take the same approach. Of these, the most commonly used is the American Society of Anesthesiologists (ASA) Physical Scoring System (Table 1-2).[13] Although scores such as the ASA classification are commonly included in the preoperative evaluation of patients admitted to hospitals for

TABLE 1-2	American Society of Anesthesiologists' Physical Status Classification
P1	A normal healthy person
P2	A patient with a mild disease
P3	A patient with a severe systemic disease that limits activity but is not incapacitating
P4	A patient with an incapacitating systemic disease that is a constant threat to life
P5	A moribund patient who is not expected to survive without the operation
P6	A declared brain-dead patient whose organs are being removed for donor purposes

In the event of an emergency, precede the number with an "e."
Adapted from American Society of Anesthesiologists.[22]

dental surgery, they use relatively broad risk categories, and their applicability to both inpatient and outpatient dental procedures is limited. Furthermore, in medicine, the ASA score is used to assess a patient's ability to tolerate general anesthesia and should not be used to predict complications associated with the actual surgery. Thus, using an ASA score for medical risk assessment in a dental setting is not appropriate. The validity of preanesthetic risk assessment has also been questioned by several authors in light of data, suggesting that the "demonstrable competence" of the anesthetist can also be a significant factor in anesthetic outcome.[14]

A more appropriate medical assessment for dental care, the Medical Complexity Status (MCS), was specifically developed for dental patients and has been used successfully for patients with medical problems ranging from nonsignificant to very complex diseases and conditions.[11] The MCS protocol is based on the premise that very few complications will arise during provision of routine dental care in an outpatient setting to patients with stable or controlled medical conditions. However, modification of dental care may be still necessary and should be based on the level of the anticipated complication. The MCS classification and protocol, with examples, are described in more detail in Table 1-3.

Modification of Dental Care for Medically Complex Patients

In this book, many different medical conditions are discussed, and protocols for the modification of dental care are suggested. Yet the assessment of risk to any medically complex patient follows similar guidelines. It is helpful to focus on the following three questions, which will change according to the severity of the underlying disease or condition:

1. What is the likelihood that the patient will experience an adverse event due to dental treatment?
2. What is the nature and severity of the potential adverse event?
3. What is the most appropriate setting in which to treat the patient?

Each of these questions can be subdivided into smaller entities, which will facilitate the assessment of the patient.

The four major concerns that must be addressed when assessing the likelihood of the patient experiencing an adverse event are as follows:

1. Possible impaired hemostasis
2. Possible susceptibility to infections
3. Drug actions and drug interactions
4. The patient's ability to withstand the stress and trauma of the dental procedure

Patients are designated to a MCS category at their initial dental visit, which may be modified during subsequent visits according to patients' changing medical status. Based on several critical items—MCS category, experience of the oral health-care professional, the patient's ability to tolerate dental care, adequacy of the dental facility—a determination of where the patient is best treated should be made: (1) a non-hospital-based outpatient setting; (2) a hospital-based outpatient setting; (3) an inpatient short-procedure unit setting; or (4) an inpatient operating room setting. Most medically complex patients can be safely treated when the aforementioned factors have been addressed.

The diagnostic procedures (obtaining and recording the patient's medical history, examining the patient, establishing a differential diagnosis, acquiring the additional information required to make a final diagnosis, such as relevant laboratory and imaging studies and consultations from other clinicians) outlined in the preceding pages are designed to assist the oral health-care professional in establishing a plan of treatment directed at those disease processes that have been identified as responsible for the patient's symptoms. A plan of treatment of this type, which is directed at the causes of the patient's symptoms rather than at the symptoms themselves, is often referred to as rational, scientific, or definitive (in contrast to symptomatic, which denotes a treatment plan directed at the relief of symptoms, irrespective of their causes).

The plan of treatment (similar to the diagnostic summary) should be entered in the patient's record and explained to the patient in detail. This encompasses the procedure, chances for cure (prognosis), complications and side effects, and required time and expense. As initially formulated, the plan of treatment usually lists recommended procedures for the control of current disease as well as preventive measures designed to limit the recurrence or progression of the disease process over time. For medicolegal reasons, the treatment that is most likely to eradicate the disease and preserve as much function as possible (i.e., the ideal treatment) is usually entered in the chart, even if the clinician realizes that compromises may be necessary to obtain the patient's consent to treatment. It is also unreasonable for the clinician to prejudge a patient's decision as to how much time, energy, and expense should be expended on treating the patient's disease or how much discomfort and pain the patient is willing to tolerate in achieving a cure. Patient involvement in deciding the final treatment plan is highly suggested to achieve a satisfactory outcome. Such an approach has been promulgated by the Institute of Medicine as "patient-centered care" and is defined as

TABLE 1-3 Medical Complexity Status Classification and Protocol

Major categories

MCS 0 Patients with no medical problems

MCS 1 Patients with controlled or stable medical conditions

MCS 2 Patients with uncontrolled or unstable medical conditions

MCS 3 Patients with medical conditions associated with acute exacerbation, resulting in high risk of mortality

Subcategories

A. No anticipated complications

B. Minor complications are anticipated. "Minor complications" are defined as complications that can be successfully addressed in the dental chair.

C. Major complications are anticipated. "Major complications" are defined as complications that should be addressed by a medical provider and may sometimes require a hospital setting.

Examples of different MCS categories

MCS–0

A healthy patient

MCS–1A

A patient with controlled hypertension
(No modifications to routine dental care are necessary.)

MCS–1B

A patient with epilepsy (petite mal) that is controlled with medications
(The patient's epilepsy status is controlled, but if the patient has a seizure, it will pass without any interventions from the oral health-care practitioner. It would be pertinent to avoid any dental treatment that may bring about a seizure.)

MCS–1C

A patient with a penicillin allergy
(The allergy will not change a stable condition, but if penicillin is given, a major complication may ensue.)

MCS–2A

A patient with hypertension and a blood pressure of 150/95 mm Hg but without any target organ disease (see Chapter 15, "Diseases of the Cardiovascular System")
(The patient's hypertension is by definition not controlled, i.e., above 140/90 mm Hg. Yet this level of blood pressure, in an otherwise healthy patient, does not justify instituting any dental treatment modifications.)

MCS–2B (see Chapter 23, "Diabetes Mellitus and Endocrine Diseases")

A patient with diabetes mellitus and a glycosylated hemoglobin of 11%
(Because of the patient's poor long-term glycemic control, the patient may be more susceptible to infections and poor wound healing. Dental modifications, such as possible antibiotics before a surgical procedure, may be indicated.)

MCS–2C

A patient with uncompensated congestive heart failure
(Because of the patient's compromised medical condition, it is important to avoid placing the patient in a supine position in the dental chair as this may induce severe respiratory problems for the patient.)

MCS–3

A patient with unstable angina

"Providing care that is respectful of and responsive to individual patient preferences, needs, and values, and ensuring that patient values guide all clinical decisions."[15]

The plan of treatment may be itemized according to the components of the diagnostic summary and is usually written prominently in the patient record to serve as a guide for the scheduling of further treatment visits. If the plan is complex or if there are reasonable treatment alternatives, a copy should also be given to the patient to allow consideration of the various implications of the plan of treatment he or she has been asked to agree to. Modifications of the ideal plan of treatment, agreed on by patient and clinician, should also be entered in the chart, together with a signed disclaimer from the patient if the modified plan of treatment is likely to be significantly less effective or unlikely to eradicate a major health problem.

Monitoring and Evaluating Underlying Medical Conditions

Several major medical conditions can be monitored by oral health-care personnel.[16,17] Signs and symptoms of systemic conditions, the types of medications taken, and the patient's compliance with medications can reveal how well a patient's underlying medical condition is being controlled. Signs of medical conditions are elicited by physical examination, which includes measurements of blood pressure and pulse and laboratory or other diagnostic evaluations. Symptoms are elicited through a ROS, whereby subjective symptoms that may indicate changes in a patient's medical status are ascertained. A list of the patient's present medications, changes in medications and daily doses, and a record of the patient's compliance with medications usually provide a good indicator of how a medical condition is being managed. The combined information on signs, symptoms, and medications is ultimately used to determine the level of control and status of the patient's medical condition.

ORAL MEDICINE CONSULTATIONS

Both custom and health insurance reimbursement systems recognize the need of individual practitioners to request the assistance of a colleague who may have more experience with the treatment of a particular clinical problem or who has received advanced training in a medical or dental specialty pertinent to the patient's problem. However, this practice of specialist consultation is usually limited to defined problems, with the expectation that the patient will return to the referring primary care clinician once the nature of the problem has been identified (diagnostic consultation) and appropriate treatment has been prescribed or performed (consultation for diagnosis and treatment).

There are three categories of oral medicine consultations:

1. Diagnosis and nonsurgical treatment of orofacial problems. This includes oral mucosal disease, temporomandibular and myofascial dysfunction, chronic jaw and facial pain, dental anomalies and jaw bone lesions, salivary hypofunction and other salivary gland disorders, and disorders of oral sensation, such as dysgeusia, dysesthesia, and glossodynia.
2. Dental treatment of patients with medical problems that affect the oral cavity or for whom modification of standard dental treatment is required to avoid adverse events.
3. Seeking an opinion on the management of dental disease that does not respond to standard treatment, such as rampant dental caries or periodontal disease in which there is a likelihood that systemic disease is an etiologic cofactor.

In response to a consultation request, the diagnostic procedures outlined in this chapter are followed, with the referral problem listed as the CC and with supplementary questioning (i.e., history of the present illness) directed to the exact nature, mode of development, prior diagnostic evaluation/treatment, and associated symptoms of the primary complaint. A thorough examination of the head, neck, and oral cavity is essential and should be fully documented, and the ROS should include a thorough exploration of any associated symptoms. When pertinent, existing laboratory, radiographic, and medical records should be reviewed and documented in the consultation record, and any additional testing or specialized examinations should be ordered.

A comprehensive consultation always includes a written report of the consultant's examination, usually preceded by a history of the problem under investigation and any items from the medical or dental history that may be pertinent to the problem. A formal diagnostic summary follows, together with the consultant's opinion on appropriate treatment and management of the issue. Any other previously unrecognized abnormalities or significant health disorder should also be xcommunicated to the referring clinician. When a biopsy or initial treatment is required before a definitive diagnosis is possible, and when the terms of the consultation request are not clear, a discussion of the initial findings with the referring clinician is often appropriate before proceeding. Likewise, the consultant usually discusses the details of his or her report with the patient unless the referring dentist specifies otherwise. In community practice, patients are sometimes referred for consultation by telephone or are simply directed to arrange an appointment with a consultant and acquaint him or her with the details of the problem at that time; a written report is still necessary to clearly identify the consultant's recommendations, which otherwise may not be transmitted accurately by the patient.

In hospital practice, the consultant is always advisory to the patient's attending oral health professional or physician, and the recommendations listed at the end of the consultation report are not implemented unless specifically authorized by the attending physician, even though the consultation report becomes a part of the patient's official hospital record. For some oral lesions and mucosal abnormalities, a brief history and examination of the lesion will readily identify the problem, and only a short written report is required; this accelerated procedure is referred to as a limited consultation.

THE DENTAL AND MEDICAL RECORD: ORGANIZATION, CONFIDENTIALITY, AND INFORMED CONSENT

The patient's record is customarily organized according to the components of the history, physical examination, diagnostic summary, plan of treatment, and medical risk assessment described in the preceding pages. Test results (diagnostic laboratory tests, radiographic examinations, and consultation and biopsy reports) are filed after this, followed by dated progress notes recorded in sequence. Separate sheets are incorporated into the record for the following: (1) a summary of medications prescribed for or dispensed to the patient, (2) a description of surgical procedures, (3) the anesthetic record, (4) a list of types of radiographic exposures, and (5) a list of the patient's problems and the proposed and actual treatment. This pattern of organization of the patient's record may be modified according to local custom and varying approaches to patient evaluation and diagnostic methodology taught in different institutions.

Organization

In recent years, educators have explored a number of methods for organizing and categorizing clinical data, with the aim of maximizing the matching of the clinical data with the "mental models" of disease syndromes referred to earlier in this chapter. The problem-oriented record (POR) and the condition diagram are two such approaches; both use unique methods for establishing a diagnosis and also involve a reorganization of the clinical record.

Problem-Oriented Record

The POR focuses on problems requiring treatment rather than on traditional diagnoses. It stresses the importance of complete and accurate collecting of clinical data, with the emphasis on recording abnormal findings rather than on compiling the extensive lists of normal and abnormal data that are characteristic of more traditional methods (consisting of narration, checklists, questionnaires, and analysis summaries). Problems can be subjective (symptoms), objective (abnormal clinical signs), or otherwise clinically significant (e.g., psychosocial) and need not be described in prescribed diagnostic categories. Once the patient's problems have been identified, priorities are established for further diagnostic evaluation or treatment of each problem. These decisions (or assessments) are based on likely causes for each problem, risk analysis of the problem's severity, cost and benefit to the patient as a result of correcting the problem, and the patient's stated desires. The plan of treatment is formulated as a list of possible solutions for each problem. As more information is obtained, the problem list can be updated, and problems can be combined and even reformulated into recognized disease categories. The POR is helpful in organizing a set of complex clinical data about an individual patient, maintaining an up-to-date record of both acute and chronic problems, ensuring that all of the patient's problems are addressed, and ensuring that preventive and active therapy is provided. It is also adaptable to computerized patient-tracking programs. However, without any scientifically based or accepted nomenclature and operational criteria for the formulation of the problem list, data cannot be compared across patients or clinicians. An additional concern that has been put forth is the reliance of a POR to "automatically" generate a diagnosis.[18] Although the POR will allow for a systematic approach to delineate specific problems, clinicians need to be able to synthesize findings into an appropriate diagnosis.[19]

Despite these shortcomings, two features of the POR have received wide acceptance and are often incorporated into more traditionally organized records: the collection of data and the generation of a problem list. The value of a problem list for individual patient care is generally acknowledged and is considered a necessary component of the hospital record in institutions accredited by the Joint Commission on Accreditation of Healthcare Organizations.

Condition Diagram

The condition diagram uses a standardized approach to categorizing and diagramming the clinical data, formulating a differential diagnosis, prevention factors, and interventions (treatment or further diagnostic procedures). It relies heavily on graphic or nonnarrative categorization of clinical data and provides students with a concise strategy for summarizing the "universe of the patient's problems" at a given time. Although currently used in only a limited number of institutions, the graphic method of conceptualizing a patient's problems is supported by both educational theory and its proven success with medical students.

The SOAP Note

The four components of a problem—subjective, objective, assessment, and plan (SOAP)—are referred to as the SOAP mnemonic for organizing progress notes or summarizing an outpatient encounter (see Figure 1-3). The components of the SOAP mnemonic are as follows:

- S or subjective: The patient's complaint, symptoms, and medical history (a brief review)
- O or objective: The clinical examination, including a brief generalized examination, and then a focused evaluation of the CC or the area of the procedure to be undertaken
- A or assessment: The diagnosis (or differential diagnosis) for the specific problem being addressed
- P or plan: The treatment either recommended or performed

The SOAP note is a useful tool for organizing progress notes in the patient record for routine office procedures and follow-up appointments. It is also quite useful in a hospital record when a limited oral medicine consultation must be documented.

S—"I have had severe pain in a lower right tooth since last night."
O—Examination reveals tooth #30 with large caries lesion; #30 not responding to cold or heat stimulation; #30 sensitive to percussion (9, on a 1–10 scale). Afebrile, pulse 68, respiration 18, blood pressure 125/85. No enlarged lymph nodes. Radiograph shows large radiolucent area surrounding the apex of the mesial root of tooth #30.
A—Irreversible pulpitis in tooth #30.
P—Root canal therapy, with subsequent post/core build-up and a fixed prosthesis.
Confidentiality of patient records

FIGURE 1-3 Example of a SOAP note.

Confidentiality

Patients provide dentists and physicians with confidential dental, medical, and psychosocial information with the understanding that the information (1) may be necessary for effective diagnosis and treatment, (2) will remain confidential, and (3) will not be released to other individuals without the patient's specific permission. This information may also be entered into the patient's record and shared with other clinical personnel involved in the patient's treatment unless the patient specifically requests otherwise. Patients are willing to share such information with their dentists and physicians only to the extent that they believe that this contract is being honored.

There are also specific circumstances in which the confidentiality of clinical information is protected by law and may be released to authorized individuals only after compliance with legally defined requirements for informed consent (e.g., psychiatric records and confidential HIV-related information). Conversely, some medical information that is considered to be of public health significance is a matter of public record when reported to the local health authorities (e.g., clinical or laboratory confirmation of reportable infectious diseases such as syphilis, hepatitis, or AIDS). Courts may also have the power to subpoena medical and dental records under defined circumstances, and records of patients participating in clinical research trials may be subject to inspection by a pharmaceutical sponsor or an appropriate drug regulatory authority. Dentists are generally authorized to obtain and record information about a patient to the extent that the information may be pertinent to the diagnosis of oral disease and its effective treatment. The copying of a patient's record for use in clinical seminars, case presentations, and scientific presentations is a common and acceptable practice provided that the patient is not identified in any way.

Conversations about patients, discussion with a colleague about a patient's personal problems, and correspondence about a patient should be limited to those occasions when information essential to the patient's treatment has to be transmitted. Lecturers and writers who use clinical cases to illustrate a topic should avoid mention of any item by which a patient might be identified and should omit confidential information. Conversations about patients, however casual, should never be held where they could possibly be overheard by unauthorized individuals, and discussion of patients with nonclinical colleagues, friends, family, and others should always be kept to a minimum and should never include confidential patient information.

Informed Consent

Prior consent of the patient is needed for all diagnostic and treatment procedures, with the exception of those considered necessary for treatment of a life-threatening emergency in a comatose patient.[20] In dentistry, such consent is more often implied than formally obtained, although written consent is generally considered necessary for all surgical procedures (however minor), the administration of general anesthetics, and clinical research.

Consent of the patient is often required before clinical records are transmitted to another dental office or institution. In the United States, security control over electronic transmission of patient records has since 1996 been governed by the Health Insurance Portability and Accountability Act. The creation and transmission of electronic records are an evolving process that is mainly dependent on technological advances and fast movement of the integration of electronic patient information.[21]

There may also be specific laws that discourage discrimination against individuals infected with HIV by requiring specific written consent from the patient before any HIV-related testing can be carried out and before any HIV-related information can be released to insurance companies, other practitioners, family members, and fellow workers.[22,23]

Oral health-care professionals treating patients whom they believe may be infected with HIV must therefore be cognizant of local law and custom when they request HIV-related information from a patient's physician, and they must establish procedures in their own offices to protect this information from unauthorized release. In response to requests for the release of psychiatric records or HIV-related information, hospital medical record departments commonly supply the practitioner with the necessary additional forms for the patient to sign before the records are released. Psychiatric information that is released is usually restricted to the patient's diagnoses and medications.

ELECTRONIC HEALTH RECORDS

The oral health-care sector has in recent decades undergone extensive computerization with focus on the EHR. However, EHR specifically developed for oral medicine are virtually nonexistent, due to low commercial incentives, and instead, oral medicine clinicians often have to rely on the use of electronic records that are developed for general dentistry or medicine. It is desirable that these records have the capability to incorporate modules created to allow structured recording of information related to oral medicine. This is of great importance for the discipline of oral medicine to take advantage of benefits provided by EHR. EHR systems can incorporate many capabilities, but the following specific functionalities hold great promise in improving oral medicine healthcare.

1. To facilitate registration of structured recording of patient data:

   Registration of clinical data using a digital form ensures consistent information collection from patient to patient, and at the same time minimizes loss of important information. It is essential that the clinical information recorded have high reliability and validity. *Reliability* is the extent to which, for example, a repeated question yields the same answer. If independent practitioners are not able to replicate questions to yield consistent answers, it is not possible to draw conclusions or make claims about the generalizability of their clinical data. *Validity* refers to how collected data reflect precise answers, that is, the degree of closeness of a measurement to its true value. Unfortunately, most data in EHR are not tested for reliability and validity, which weakens the potential for evaluation and research. Any EHR designed for oral medicine should have the capability to allow for continuous modification and needs and should be evaluated for reliability and validity before introduction in a clinical setting. Assessment of validity and reliability should be a continuous process.

Many EHRs allow registration of free text, which makes extraction of information more difficult and therefore becomes less useful for clinical evaluation and research. However, free text may have its place in EHRs as it allows the record to become more readable and understandable. Some clinical information is too specific to be captured by predetermined items. Thus, when developing an oral medicine EHR, a distinction need to be made between information necessary for health analysis and information essential to understand the clinical findings of a particular patient.

2. To facilitate the visualization of the data as needed:

Oral medicine is a discipline that is image oriented with clinical images, radiologic images, and histopathologic images. EHRs developed for general dental care may not offer access to these types of images.

A limitation of the conventional paper record is the lack of an easy method of compiling clinical information. Poor penmanship may further lessen the ability to compile and evaluate data. Unfortunately, most EHR has an interface that is not always designed to fully utilize the benefits that an electronic tool can provide. This is usually not due to lack of technical solutions but due to the difficulty of defining a successful treatment outcome.

3. To facilitate clinical follow-up of both individual patients and larger patient groups to provide the basis for clinical development and research

The capability to convert collected clinical datasets into new evidence-based knowledge is the prime rational to justify the substantial financial investments made to implement EHR. However, most available EHRs do not prioritize this feature and therefore do not effectively support the compilation and analysis of the recorded information. This deficiency is probably due to attempts to reproduce traditional paper records as the framework and conventional analogous interfaces. The information recorded in most current EHRs cannot, even with considerable effort, facilitate clinical decisions. Furthermore, integrated clinical decision support, for instance in the form of drug interactions, is not available in all systems.

For most clinicians the current daily workflow does not contain any moments for reflection and analysis of recorded information, which lessens the utilization of the full potential of an EHR. It is therefore necessary to create time to take advantage of these electronic tools. In the development and selection of an appropriate EHR, it is important to consider the ability of the systems to provide chairside decision support.

4. To enable data mining for research and improved patient care:

A well-designed EHR provides an opportunity for easy retrieval of data for the purposes of research and, consequently, better patient care. Furthermore, EHRs can facilitate communication between different EHR systems and offer plenty opportunities for multicenter trials, as well as co-care of patients by different health professionals in different settings.

A useful EHR system is designed to support clinical care; it should have a clean and simple visual design where each element clearly shows what should be done and the next steps in an intuitive manner; it should provide integrated decision support and store data in a form that makes for easy retrieval and analysis. Ultimately, EHR records, with appropriate security, should enable sharing of information among all care providers of the patient.

Selected Readings

American Society of Anesthesiologists. *ASA Physical Status Classification System.* http://www.asahq.org/Home/For-Members/Clinical-Information/ASA-Physical-Status-Classification-System. Accessed April 5, 2014.

Baum BJ. Inadequate training in the biological sciences and medicine for dental students. Impending crisis for dentistry. *J Am Dent Assoc.* 2007;138:16–25.

Bickley LS. *Bate's Guide to Physical Examination and History Taking.* 11th ed. Philadelphia, PA: Lippincott Williams and Wilkins; 2010.

Boland BJ, Wollan PC, Silverstein MD. Review of systems, physical examination, and routine tests for case-finding in ambulatory patients. *Am J Med Sci.* 1995;309:194–200.

Burris S. Dental discrimination against the HIV-infected: empirical data, law and public policy. *Yale J Regul.* 1996;13:1–104.

Findler M, Galili D, Meidan Z, et al. Dental treatment in very high risk patients with ischemic heart disease. *Oral Surg Oral Med Oral Pathol.* 1993;76:298–300.

Gary CJ, Glick M. Medical clearance: an issue of professional autonomy, not a crutch. *J Am Dent Assoc.* 2012;143(11):1180–1181.

Glick M. Did you take your medications? The dentist's role in helping patients adhere to their drug regimen. *J Am Dent Assoc.* 2006;137:1636–1638.

Glick M. Informed consent—a delicate balance. *J Am Dent Assoc.* 2006;137:1060–1062.

Glick M. *Medical Support System.* http://icemedicalsupport.com/. Accessed April 5, 2014.

Glick M. Rapid HIV testing in the dental setting. *J Am Dent Assoc.* 2005;136:1206–1208.

Glick M. Screening for traditional risk factors for cardiovascular disease: a review for oral healthcare providers. *J Am Dent Assoc.* 2002;133:291–300.

Glick M, Greenberg BL. The potential role of dentists in identifying patients' risk of experiencing coronary heart disease. *J Am Dent Assoc.* 2005;136:1541–1546.

Goodchild JH, Glick M. A different approach to medical risk assessment. *Endod Top.* 2003;4:1–8.

Gortzak RA, Abraham-Inpijn L, ter Horst G, Peters G. High blood pressure screening in the dental office: a survey among Dutch dentists. *Gen Dent.* 1993;41:246–251.

Hershey SE, Bayleran ED. Problem-oriented orthodontic record. *J Clin Orthod.* 1986;20:106–110.

Michota FA, Frost SD. The preoperative evaluation: use the history and physical rather than routine testing. *Cleve Clin J Med.* 2004;71:63–70.

Prause G, Ratzenhofer-Comenda B, Pierer G, et al. Can ASA grade or Goldman's cardiac risk index predict peri-operative mortality? A study of 16,227 patients. *Anaesthesia.* 1997;52:203–206.

Smeets EC, de Jong KJM, Abrahim-Inpijn L. Detecting the medically compromised dental patient in dentistry by means of the medical risk-related history. *Prev Med.* 1998;27:530–535.

Verdon ME, Siemens K. Yield of review of systems in a self-administered questionnaire. *J Am Board Fam Pract.* 1997;10(1):20–27.

World Health Organization. *International Statistical Classification of Diseases and Health Related Problems: The ICD-10.* 10th ed. Geneva, Switzerland: World Health Organization, WHO Press; 2005. http://www.who.int/classifications/icd/ICD-10_2nd_ed_volume2.pdf. Accessed April 5, 2014.

For the full reference lists, please go to http://www.pmph-usa.com/Burkets_Oral_Medicine.

CHAPTER 2

Overview of Clinical Research

Jane C. Atkinson, DDS
Dena Fischer, DDS, MSD, MS
Holli A. Hamilton, MD, MPH
Mary A. Cutting, MS, RAC

- ❑ DEFINITION OF CLINICAL RESEARCH
- ❑ STUDY DESIGNS
  Case Report and Case Series
  Cross-Sectional Studies
  Longitudinal Cohort Studies
  Randomized Controlled Trials
  Systematic Reviews
- ❑ EVIDENCE HIERARCHY
- ❑ ISSUES IN THE DESIGN, IMPLEMENTATION, AND INTERPRETATION OF CLINICAL RESEARCH
  Study Design

Sample Size
Selection of Controls
Study Bias
Outcome Assessment
Loss to Follow-Up and Retention
Analytical Issues
- ❑ ETHICAL CONSIDERATIONS AND REGULATORY REQUIREMENTS
- ❑ SAFETY MONITORING
  Safety Reporting
  Safety Oversight

Medicine, including oral medicine and traditional dentistry, is now taught and practiced to a greater or lesser extent using evidence-based practice.[1] This evidence base comes from clinical research. The purpose of this chapter is to provide a very brief overview of types of research involving human subjects and the features of good clinical research, including ethical and regulatory considerations. Those seeking additional information should read recent textbooks written about the topic.

DEFINITION OF CLINICAL RESEARCH

"Clinical research" can be defined broadly as patient-oriented research. This includes all studies in which investigators interact directly with subjects to collect research data and studies utilizing existing specimens from human subjects if the identity of the subject is known to at least one investigator.[2] If the codes identifying previously collected specimens or clinical data cannot be traced back to the subjects' identity, research using the specimens or data is usually not considered human subjects research.

Many types of studies are included under this definition of clinical research. Human subjects research includes studies of human disease mechanisms, natural history studies of disease, epidemiological studies, behavioral studies, studies of technologies used to diagnose human diseases, outcomes research, and health services research. If the study is testing an intervention as a treatment for disease, the study is a clinical trial. "Intervention" includes anything that can alter the course of a disease, such as a pharmaceutical agent, a medical device, a surgical technique, a behavioral intervention, or a public health program. Therefore, clinical trials are a subset of clinical research. Clinical research studies, whether interventional or observational, require approval by an institutional review board (IRB) and provision of informed consent by the research subjects if supported by US federal funds.

STUDY DESIGNS

Several types of designs are available to collect research information about individuals with diseases and conditions. The designs described below are commonly employed in clinical research.

Case Report and Case Series

A case report (singular) or case series (plural) is a description of one or several individuals with a disease or syndrome of interest. Examples include descriptions of the clinical course of a patient during a hospital stay, unusually shaped teeth in a child or children with a genetic syndrome, or an adult presenting with orofacial pain from an unusual source such as a metastatic tumor. The description should be complete enough for use by another clinician who may evaluate a similar case. If the study is a case series, the same diagnostic criteria should be used to group the cases together for a report.

Case series can be very valuable in the description of new diseases or conditions. A good example is the case series describing 63 cases of osteonecrosis of the jaw (ONJ) associated with the use of bisphosphonates.[3] An obvious limitation of this study design is the lack of a population of individuals without the disease or condition, or a "control" group. Other limits of a case series include the fact that most are performed retrospectively with data taken from existing clinical records. This introduces the potential for recall bias as the researchers are "looking back" at events and extracting record information, which is often a mixture of complete and incomplete facts. Also, the information is recorded for clinical care and not research purposes. Therefore, clinicians will use varying methods to evaluate patient outcomes, such as a nonhealing extraction site. If the patients were evaluated as part of a research study, the study team would use a predefined set of criteria to judge clinical outcomes and would collect a predefined set of information from the patients such as current and past medications.

Cross-Sectional Studies

Cross-sectional studies are employed frequently in clinical research. Research participants (also known as subjects) are evaluated at one time point and are not followed up over time, creating a dataset that is a "snapshot" of the condition under study. Prevalence studies use cross-sectional designs that involve describing the population under study, deriving a representative sample of that population, and defining the characteristics under study to establish the prevalence of a disease or condition in a population.[4] For example, the prevalence of oral human papillomavirus infection has been estimated through the National Health and Nutrition Examination

Survey (NHANES) 2009–2010. The NHANES study uses a statistically representative sample of the civilian non institutionalized US population.[5] Many factors must be considered when designing a cross-sectional prevalence study. First, it is not usually feasible to examine an entire population of individuals with a disease or condition. Therefore, the sample being examined should represent the entire population at risk and not only those most severely affected. In the example of ONJ, patients with small nonhealing affected sites that healed in two to three months without any intervention should be included as well as those with large lesions that persisted for months to represent the entire spectrum of the disease. Second, all research participants should be evaluated using the same, standardized methods (see the section "Outcome Assessment"). Prevalence studies for rare diseases usually require very large sample sizes and, therefore, may not be suitable for studies conducted at only one institution or when there are limited numbers of individuals with the disease of interest.[4]

Cross-sectional studies may also be utilized to draw associations between an exposure or risk factor and the presence of disease. Because research participants are evaluated at one time point, causal inferences cannot be drawn between the risk factor and disease, representing a major limitation of this study design. Using the example of periodontal disease and cardiovascular disease, the two conditions can occur together in a person because of a common underlying etiology, such as smoking, unhealthy personal habits, and/or limited access to the health care system.[6] Nevertheless, such cross-sectional designs have value in research, particularly to develop hypotheses for future studies. An initial association between a risk factor and presence of disease may be established in a cross-sectional study before consideration of a more resource-intensive study design in which risk factors for disease can be evaluated over time. When establishing initial associations using a cross-sectional design, the biologic plausibility between the risk factor(s) and disease and the strength of this association should be described.

Case-Control Studies

A case-control study is a type of observational retrospective study. The objective is to evaluate persons with the disease of interest (cases) and compare them with another group of persons with similar traits (controls) to determine whether certain exposures(such as being a current smoker) or characteristics are associated with the disease or lack of the disease. If the exposure is found more frequently in the cases, it is termed a "risk factor" for having the disease. Sometimes the exposure is found more frequently in the control group, suggesting that it might be a "protective factor" that helps protect against a disease. There are critical design issues that must be considered in a case-control study.[4] The exposure and disease in both cases and controls should be assessed in the same manner. Patients who have a severe disease may experience recall bias in that they remember more or over-report past exposures or symptoms than generally healthy controls because they are seeking an explanation for why they have a disease. The cases need to represent the entire population of those with the disease, and the controls must be selected from the same population as the cases. Finally, most experts recommend evaluating at least an equal number of controls as cases. Selection of controls for a case-control study can be difficult and can introduce bias into the study if not chosen carefully, as discussed at length in the literature.[7–9] A case-control study example performed across three dental practice-based research networks assessed risk factors for ONJ. ONJ cases were defined as having maxillary or mandibular exposed bone that clinically appeared necrotic, without regard to duration or size. For each case, three controls with no current or previous history of bone necrosis were selected from the same primary care practice where a case was diagnosed. Risk factors were ascertained in cases and controls, and the association between bisphosphonate use and ONJ was determined.[10]

Case-control studies are particularly beneficial when studying rare diseases. If the disease of interest is sufficiently rare, such as salivary gland cancers, it may be safe to assume that a sample of cases is representative of the entire population of those with the disease. Findings in case-control studies are typically reported in odds ratios, whereas cohort study findings are expressed in terms of relative risk. When interpreting the results of case-control studies, the strength of the association between the exposure and disease and the confidence interval of the association should be considered before making conclusions about the validity of the results. A finding of a "dose-response" (in which increasing levels of the exposure such as pack-years of smoking are associated with increasing rates of the disease or condition) increases the strength of the evidence.

Because of criticisms related to control selection in case-control studies, researchers may choose to utilize more than one control population when designing studies. In a classic example from the medical literature, the relation between estrogen use and endometrial cancer was established using a well-designed case-control study design and two control populations.[11]

Longitudinal Cohort Studies

Longitudinal cohort studies allow the opportunity to collect data over time. The purpose of this study design is to assess associations between an exposure or risk factor and subsequent development of disease or to determine outcomes of standard of care treatment. When performed prospectively to assess associations, a representative sample of the population of interest is assessed for an exposure at the beginning of the study, and then new cases of disease accrue during a period of follow-up evaluation. At the end of the study, the differences between those with and without the disease are evaluated. In some cases, a single population is observed over a period of time to observe the natural incidence of a condition or the natural history of a disease. For example, a study of Swedish adolescents estimated the incidence of temporomandibular muscle and joint disorder (TMJD) pain. All individuals aged 12–19 years in all Public Dental Service clinics in a Swedish county from 2000 to 2003 were followed over 3 years for development of TMJD pain.[12] Subjects with TMJD were evaluated for differences that distinguished them from subjects without TMJD. In this study, TMJD incidence was found to be greater in older children and girls. More frequently, research subjects may be selected for a particular exposure, along with a comparable group of controls, and both groups are followed up over time for development of disease.[13] An example of a longitudinal cohort study examining outcomes of treatment was a study of 264 implants placed in 51 individuals with ectodermal dysplasia who were followed to determine the incidence of implant failure.[14]

Cohort studies may also be retrospective, in which the exposure was captured in a standardized manner in the past, and disease status is determined at the time the study is initiated and subjects are followed. This study design assumes that the subject population (exposed and unexposed subjects) is representative of the general population, and exposure history is collected accurately. Definitions of disease outcome should be reliable and reproducible and held constant during the study duration. Standard criteria for determining the disease outcome should be applied to exposed and unexposed subjects to avoid bias. An important factor in longitudinal cohort studies is the ability to retain the cohort over time. Subjects who drop out of research studies may differ from those who remain and may introduce attrition biases into the population sample.

One significant advantage of well-conducted prospective cohort studies over other study designs is that the exposure is collected in a standardized fashion, and cases are incident (new cases). This design provides more information about the natural history of the disease, as well as direct estimates of incidence and relative risk.[4] Longitudinal cohort studies have the potential to initially or further establish the temporal relationship between exposure and disease and a dose response relationship, both of which increase the strength of the study conclusions.

Longitudinal studies by their nature are resource intensive, and large populations are often required to study rare diseases. Large sample sizes for rare diseases and long durations for chronic diseases may be required. Maintaining the use of consistent study methods, such as standardized collection of the exposure, and keeping subjects from dropping out of the study are continual challenges.

Randomized Controlled Trials

The purpose of randomized controlled trials (RCTs) is to determine whether a particular intervention is associated with a change in disease incidence or severity as determined by an outcome measure. An example of an outcome measure in an RCT testing an intervention for periodontal disease is reduction in pocket depth. RCTs provide the strongest evidence for the causal nature of a modifiable factor (such as inflammation in a periodontal pocket) and the effect that modifying the factor has on disease outcomes. Potential research subjects from a well-defined study population are assigned at random to receive or not receive the intervention(s) under study and then are observed for a specified time period for the occurrence of well-defined endpoints. One intervention may be compared to another intervention, "usual care", or placebo treatment. Large RCTs should not be undertaken until there is a substantial body of evidence suggesting that the intervention may be effective, but not so much evidence such that conducting the study would be considered unethical. In other words, there should be clinical equipoise before a study is launched.[15]

Clinical trials can be classified into four phases (phase I, II, III, or IV) or stages.[16] This stepwise approach reduces risks to people enrolled in the trial and allows investigators to determine potential effectiveness of a new treatment while minimizing time and costs. A phase I trial often is the "first-time in human" study, meaning trial participants are the first humans to receive the new drug. These studies are not randomized or blinded (masked). The primary goal is to evaluate the safety of the agent and determine a safe dose range for subsequent studies. A phase II trial tests the new drug in individuals who are randomized to different treatments, with goals of determining potential effectiveness and establishing a more complete safety profile. Feasibility of using the treatment also can be determined. The phase III trial enrolls hundreds or thousands of subjects and is sometimes called a "pivotal study." These trials are designed to enroll a much larger segment of the population with the disease, and results are used to gain drug approval from government agencies. Phase III trials should generate generalizable results and determine the *efficacy* of a treatment. Phase IV trials are post marketing studies to determine how well a treatment found to be efficacious in a phase III trial works in the community, and to assess any side effects associated with its long-term use. Studies designed to determine how well a treatment works in practice determine the *effectiveness* of a therapy.

A key component of RCTs is that subjects are assigned to one of the study arms at random to eliminate the potential for bias in treatment assignment. Certain forms of randomization that do not allow for random sequence generation, such as rolling dice, using hospital chart numbers, or using a birth date, are not acceptable randomization practices. Another important consideration is the random, concealed or "blinded" or "masked" allocation of treatment to ensure that any baseline differences in the treatment groups arise by chance alone. The random allocation process involves generating an unpredictable random sequence and then implementing the sequence in a way that conceals the interventions until subjects have been formally assigned to their groups.

Both randomization and concealment are necessary to avoid bias and maximize validity in RCTs, and reproducibility of the allocation order and the concealment process are necessary to maintain integrity of the research study. Other important features of high-quality RCTs include independent or "blind" assessment of research endpoints and data analysis based on the treatment assignment, also known as analysis by "intention to treat." Intention-to-treat analysis removes artifacts from the study that are caused by unequal attrition in the two study arms, or by treatment crossover.

There are three levels of concealing treatment (blinding or masking) in an RCT: (1) subjects are unaware of their study treatment group, (2) the investigators are unaware of the subject's study treatment group, and (3) the statistical analyses are conducted without knowledge of the groups' study treatment. Recent oral health RCTs that followed the strict principles of clinical trials were two phase III studies testing periodontal therapy as a treatment to prevent preterm birth[17] and to improve glycemic control.[18]

A limitation of the RCT study design is the concern about external validity, or the extent to which RCT results are applicable beyond the research study. In addition, RCTs are expensive because of the logistics involved in sampling, blinding, treating, and following hundreds of participants; in addition, extremely large sample sizes are required to study rare outcomes. Consequently, some research questions may be more appropriately addressed using other study designs.

Systematic Reviews

A systematic review is a structured process of comprehensively reviewing the literature focused on a research question in which inclusion and exclusion criteria for study selection are established *a priori*. The purpose of the systematic review is to determine the "state of the science" by objectively identifying, appraising, selecting, and synthesizing high-quality research evidence. Such reviews may also elucidate a paucity of high-quality evidence and, therefore, identify research questions to be addressed in future studies. Key principles of systematic reviews include the following[19]:

- Literature search: Develop a search strategy using multiple sources, checking of reference lists, hand-searching of key journals.
- Study selection: Develop criteria for inclusion and exclusion, eligibility checks by more than one reviewer, develop a strategy to resolve disagreements, keep a log of excluded studies with reasons for exclusion.
- Study quality assessment: Quality assessment by more than one observer, using established and standardized criteria for study quality assessment.
- Systematic extraction of data.
- Analysis, presentation, and interpretation of results: Address risk of bias (including the fact that negative studies are less likely to be published), consider strength of evidence, address limitations, consider implications for future research.

A meta-analysis pools data from different studies and treats them as one large study using statistical tools. Only high-quality evidence of a similar design, usually limited to RCTs, should be included in a meta-analysis. Observational studies are often limited by the effects of confounding and bias, therefore precluding their inclusion in pooled analyses.

EVIDENCE HIERARCHY

Clinical evidence is generated from a variety of study types. In general, evidence from literature that is classified as expert opinion, bench research with human samples that demonstrate biological plausibility, case reports, and case series is considered low-level evidence.[20] Higher level evidence (from lower to highest) is evidence from case-control studies, cohort studies, randomized controlled clinical trials, and systematic reviews/meta-analyses of clinical trials. However, consumers of medical literature should be cognizant of critical components of any research study when judging its value, and not accept that evidence is superior just because it ranks higher in traditional evidence pyramids. If a clinical trial is conducted poorly, its value is diminished and its conclusions may be meaningless. Critical elements of high-quality clinical research are discussed below.

Clinical research, regardless of its type, is a scientific study. Therefore, investigators must take care to conduct studies that minimize bias and maximize reproducibility. Many factors should be considered when evaluating clinical studies, including study design, sample size, subject selection, methods to ascertain disease and outcomes, ethical and human subjects concerns, and analytical approaches. Organizations such as the Cochrane Collaboration have developed sophisticated methods including systematic reviews to evaluate and synthesize the best literature to help develop practice guidelines that are based in evidence.[21] Other systems have been published to guide the evaluation of evidence by organizations developing guidelines.[22–25]

ISSUES IN THE DESIGN, IMPLEMENTATION, AND INTERPRETATION OF CLINICAL RESEARCH

Below are short descriptions of some of the features of clinical research to consider when reading the scientific literature. More complete descriptions of factors used to evaluate the quality of research are available in the *Cochrane Handbook for Systematic Reviews of Interventions*[21] or can be found as components of the GRADE system.[24,25]

Study Design

Investigators should employ a study design that is suitable for answering the clinical research question at hand. In general, an intervention should be tested in a clinical trial to assess whether it is an effective treatment for a disease. If an expert publishes a paper detailing the use of a new surgical approach to treat maxillary fractures of six

patients and declares the technique effective, a practitioner using evidence-based decision making should recognize that the paper does not provide sufficient evidence to declare the approach a success. This type of publication is a case series, and the expert's assertion of the effectiveness of the approach is termed "Expert Opinion." Assessing the efficacy of the new treatment approach requires that it be compared to either no treatment or the standard of care treatment in a controlled clinical trial, such as the clinical trials testing periodontal therapy as a means to prevent preterm birth[17] or to improve glycemic control in type 2 diabetes.[18]

Sample Size

Sample size is a critical issue in clinical trials. If the sample is too small, the findings on the efficacy of an intervention cannot be generalized to the population having the disease. This is particularly critical for phase III clinical trials that are designed to change clinical practice or impact public policy.

Many clinical studies suffer from small sample sizes, making it difficult to generalize study findings. Observational studies of select patient groups often make conclusions about the condition from small numbers of patients who are in active treatment in one medical center and who have the most severe disease. However, the patients evaluated in the study may not represent all patients in the general population. A single-center study does have value in generating new hypotheses for more research, but the studies need to be replicated in larger, more representative samples.[26] Studies of rare diseases can be difficult because few patients with the condition of interest are available for study. To overcome this problem, multicenter registries can be established that enroll and follow up subjects with a particular condition. Examples include the chromosome 22q11.2 deletion syndrome registry that has characterized the highly variable spectrum of the clinical consequences associated with this deletion in 906 affected individuals[27] and the international registry to assess safety of denosumab, an agent associated with ONJ.[13]

Case-control studies of dental disease (either caries or periodontal disease) must be large enough to make meaningful comparisons, especially given the complex, multifactorial etiologies of the diseases. Small sample size is often a reason why studies are excluded from evidence-based reviews.[28]

Selection of Controls

Another critical factor to consider when evaluating a case-control study is the selection of the control group. Are the controls drawn from the same population? Do they differ from patients with the disease of interest in many ways, or are they very similar?[7] Are equal numbers of cases and controls evaluated?[7]

Study Bias

Great care must be taken to avoid study bias. Methods to avoid bias in cohort studies include enrolling consecutive individuals reporting to a clinic with a disease of interest, or enrolling individuals randomly selected from an existing large population. Clinical trials should use randomization to assign subjects to the different treatment arms to avoid bias. Ideally, a clinical examiner collecting a study outcome should not know the group assignment of the subject being evaluated. This is best practice for both case-control studies and randomized clinical trials.

Another more complicated issue in clinical trials is the use of restrictive inclusion/exclusion criteria. To determine whether a new drug or a technique is effective for treating a disease, potential subjects with coexisting conditions may be excluded, or study participation may be limited to a particular age group. This creates a potential for study results to be only valid for a population similar to that enrolled in the trial, which may be a smaller subset of individuals with disease. An example of this problem is clinical trials testing therapies for non-Hodgkin's lymphoma (NHL). Although the majority of patients with NHL are older than 65 years, older adults were poorly represented in NHL RCTs.[29] Most RCTs testing caries preventive treatments studied children, although therapies are recommended for adults.[30]

Outcome Assessment

One challenge when conducting a clinical study is assessment of outcomes. Study outcomes or endpoints used in a clinical trial or study must provide reliable (consistent and repeatable) and valid signals to determine the efficacy of the intervention being tested or to reliably document disease prevalence and/or progression. The outcome must be reproducible, and there should be published evidence of its validity. For example, if the goal of a study is quantifying oral cancer pain, the investigator should use a validated instrument to collect pain measures appropriate for the population being studied. In this example, an appropriate instrument would be a pain scale that had been tested previously in a group that was similar culturally and had pain from the same origin, cancer. The methods for ascertainment of study outcomes also need to be standardized. In addition, examiners should be calibrated by having them each examine the same group of patients to measure their agreement with each other (interrater reliability) and to examine a set of patients repeatedly to measure their agreement with themselves (intrarater reliability).[31] Studies that include caries and periodontal disease changes as outcomes usually conduct yearly calibration sessions during which examiners are calibrated to a gold-standard examiner and compared numerically using percentage agreement or kappa scores.[17,32]

Loss to Follow-Up and Retention

Minimizing loss to follow-up is critical to study validity. There is no way to assure that a study is valid if loss to follow-up is not minimal, and when participant loss approaches the number included in study outcomes, any study conclusions are specious. Every effort should be made to avoid loss to follow-up. Both simple and sophisticated analytic methods are available to model missing data, but these cannot protect against bias created by subject loss. One can look at how participants lost to follow-up differ from those retained and undertake bootstrapping or other methods to impute missing data, but the truth lies somewhere between rigorous sensitivity analysis done by calculating results assuming that all those lost to follow-up were treatment failures and comparing them to results that assume all those lost to follow-up were treatment successes. Although neither is likely to be the complete truth, a range will be established though one will never know what happened to those lost from the study. From an ethical perspective, clinical research should always adhere to quality standards including minimizing loss to follow-up; to do otherwise is to disrespect the human subjects participating in the study and to squander resources.[33–35]

Thus, retention is a key issue in any well-designed and conducted study that involves subject follow-up. Pilot studies to test retention can be invaluable. Retention plans should be designed well in advance of study implementation. Many strategies can be used; however, it is not acceptable to take a wait-and-see attitude because the study could be undermined at the outset. Retention should be tracked carefully throughout the study and retention strategies improved during the study if they are found to be lacking.

Examples of retention strategies that can be considered when designing a study:

- Having a run-in period at the beginning of a study to eliminate those who will be lost or cannot comply.
- Obtaining reliable, complete subject contact information that may include alternate phone numbers, e-mail, and physical addresses.
- Obtaining names and contact information for designated family or friends who could be contacted for information on missing participants.
- Sending out communications such as newsletters and educational pieces that inform study participants of new findings in the field or progress of the study, as allowable.
- Sending out reminders such as birthday cards, text messages, phone messages, postcards, or letters.
- Having dedicated and professional study staff with low turnover to establish rapport with study participants.
- Employing outreach workers to find those who may be lost to follow-up.
- Having the data center follow-up individuals via phone or e-mail should they fail to respond to contacts made by the clinic or site. It is possible the participant has a personal reason for not continuing in the study.
- Reviewing death records and registries to account for those missing by demise.
- Reviewing public media to search for obituaries and accidents.
- Offering study visits during hours that accommodate clinical subjects; this may include evenings or weekends.
- Scheduling study visits with other necessary patient care to minimize the number of trips to the study site.

- Creating satellite clinics or sites near where patients are situated so that they are not required to travel as much. Venues for data collection may include visits to participants' homes, churches, schools, or worksites to allow study visits to be less disruptive to subjects' lives.
- Providing incentives that make it easier to participate in the study such as:
  - Child care
  - Paid transportation to the site
  - Remuneration for expenses as deemed appropriate by the IRBo

All these strategies should be presented to the IRB for their approval. They all must be agreed to by the participants as part of consent for participation, and to the extent possible, must protect participants' privacy. It is also important to obtain buy-in from all those who must cooperate for the strategy to be successful. Examples of those who must be engaged might include the board of education, ministry of health, other health care providers, or employers. With the exception of review of public information such as death registries or public media, subjects must provide consent for any strategy that involves contacting them to prevent privacy impingement. An engaged, informed, and interested study population is far more likely to be retained than one that is not.[34]

Analytical Issues

It is impossible in this limited space to discuss analytical issues fully. However, unless a study is fully hypothesis-generating and exploratory, the principal study hypothesis, sample size, power, and statistical analyses should be pre specified to protect against ad hoc analyses that attempt to milk provocative conclusions from the data. It is all too tempting to conduct analyses for which the study was not specifically designed; it is most unusual that convincing, robust conclusions can be drawn from such *a posteriori* analysis. Another grave threat to the validity of analysis is multiple comparisons or making too many comparisons for the study sample size. This will quickly undermine study power. Although many statistical corrections are available for multiple comparisons, there is no perfect method, and as such, this approach should be avoided unless necessary. Inappropriate use of statistical methods threatens the reproducibility of science.[36]

One should also predefine endpoints that will represent clinical significance in the study findings, independent of statistical significance. A common mistake is to conflate statistical significance with clinical significance. For example, an epidemiological study may result in a caries prevalence difference of 0.1 surfaces between sample groups. Because of a large sample size the difference may be statistically significant, but the clinical significance of the finding is open to question. The articulation of study analysis can be included in the protocol or in a separate statistical analysis plan depending on how complex and detailed the analysis will be.[37]

To improve the quality of randomized clinical trial reports, many journals require that investigators follow the principles articulated in the Consolidated Standards of Reporting Trials statement.[38] This statement includes a 25-item checklist and flow diagram that provides guidance for reporting results. Items that should be reported include the number of individuals screened for trial eligibility, the number of participants randomized overall and per treatment group, the number of study participants lost to follow-up, the number of those randomized whose results were analyzed, and the reasons for excluding participants' results from the final analysis.[38]

ETHICAL CONSIDERATIONS AND REGULATORY REQUIREMENTS

Regulatory requirements for research with human subjects vary according to the type of study conducted and the region or country in which the research is conducted. In the United States, starting an interventional clinical trial to test the safety and efficacy of an investigational new drug (IND) for disease treatment will require an IND application filed with the United States Food and Drug Administration (FDA) and approval from a local IRB. In the European Union (EU), the trial of an investigational drug may be started after a clinical trial authorization (CTA) dossier is authorized by a National Competent Authority and an Ethics Committee issues a positive opinion. The IND application or CTA dossier provides information about the properties of the drug and details of its manufacturing process, evidence of safety from preclinical (animal) studies, and plans for its clinical testing. For a simple observational study intended, for example, to identify the risk factors for a disease or condition, regulations for the protection of human subjects must be followed. These may vary with the region or country in which the research is conducted.

For any research study that involves human subjects, sponsors and investigators have an obligation to protect the participants, by weighing the foreseeable risks and anticipated benefits before initiating a study and by conducting the study with adequate rigor to produce scientifically valid results. The regulations and guidelines followed by clinical researchers today have their foundations in a variety of codes, resolutions, and guidelines adopted by national and international bodies, including the Nuremberg Code (1947),[39] the Declaration of Helsinki[40] (adopted in 1964 and amended several times through 2013), the Belmont Report prepared by the United States National Commission for the Protection of Human Subjects of Biomedical and Behavioral Research (1979),[41] the International Ethical Guidelines for Biomedical Research Involving Human Subjects published by the Council for International Organizations of Medical Sciences (released 1993, revised 2002),[42] and the E6 Good Clinical Practice guidelines developed by the International Conference on Harmonisation of Technical Requirements for Registration of Pharmaceuticals for Human Use (ICH).[43]

Beginning in 1990, the ICH brought together representatives of the regulatory bodies and industry representatives from the EU, Japan, and the United States. The mission of the ICH was to promote international harmonization of requirements, to streamline the process of conducting regulated clinical research in different countries. Providing a unified standard for technical requirements and acceptance of clinical data by the regulatory agencies of the participating jurisdictions was intended to facilitate the development and marketing pathway for new medical products. Topics covered by the ICH are categorized as Quality, Safety, Efficacy, and Multidisciplinary Guidelines, based on the criteria for approving new medicinal products. Guidelines in the Efficacy category deal with the design, conduct, safety, and reporting of clinical trials, and include the ICH Harmonised Tripartite Guideline for Good Clinical Practice[43] (ICH GCP E6), which was finalized in 1996. The Guideline defines Good Clinical Practice as "a standard for the design, conduct, performance, monitoring, auditing, recording, analyses, and reporting of clinical trials that provides assurance that the data and reported results are credible and accurate, and that the rights, integrity, and confidentiality of trial subjects are protected."

Section 2 of the ICH E6 document lists the thirteen principles of ICH GCP (Table 2-1), which emphasize ethical treatment of human subjects, sound science to justify and support a trial, and scientific rigor and quality in the conduct of the trial. Sections 3, 4, and 5 of the GCP document describe the responsibilities of the following entities involved in the conduct of a clinical trial:

- Independent ethics committee (IEC) or IRB defined as "an independent body constituted of medical professionals and non-medical members, whose responsibility it is to ensure the protection of the rights, safety and well-being of human subjects involved in a trial." The IEC or IRB is expected to review and approve the trial protocol and amendments, the means of obtaining and documenting informed consent, qualifications of the investigator, and so forth, and to conduct continuing review of the trial at least annually.
- Investigator, defined as "a person responsible for the conduct of the clinical trial at a trial site." The investigator "should be qualified by education, training, and experience to assume responsibility for the proper conduct of the trial." All individuals to whom the investigator delegates trial-related duties (e.g., associate investigators, study coordinators, and clinical research staff) are expected to be appropriately qualified and to follow GCP. Among the critical duties of the investigator are communication with the IEC/IRB, compliance with the protocol, accountability for the investigational product, proper conduct and documentation of the informed consent process, proper recording and reporting of trial data, and documentation and reporting of safety issues.
- Sponsor, defined as "an individual, company, institution, or organization which takes responsibility for the initiation, management, and/or financing of a clinical trial." The sponsor is responsible for establishing

TABLE 2-1 The Principles of Good Clinical Practice[43]
1. Clinical trials should be conducted in accordance with the ethical principles that have their origin in the Declaration of Helsinki and that are consistent with GCP and the applicable regulatory requirement(s).
2. Before a trial is initiated, foreseeable risks and inconveniences should be weighed against the anticipated benefit for the individual trial subject and society. A trial should be initiated and continued only if the anticipated benefits justify the risks.
3. The rights, safety, and well-being of the trial subjects are the most important considerations and should prevail over interests of science and society.
4. The available nonclinical and clinical information on an investigational product should be adequate to support the proposed clinical trial.
5. Clinical trials should be scientifically sound and described in a clear, detailed protocol.
6. A trial should be conducted in compliance with the protocol that has received prior institutional review board/independent ethics committee approval/favorable opinion.
7. The medical care given to, and medical decisions made on behalf of, subjects should always be the responsibility of a qualified physician or, when appropriate, of a qualified dentist.
8. Each individual involved in conducting a trial should be qualified by education, training, and experience to perform his or her respective task(s).
9. Freely given informed consent should be obtained from every subject prior to clinical trial participation.
10. All clinical trial information should be recorded, handled, and stored in a way that allows its accurate reporting, interpretation, and verification.
11. The confidentiality of records that could identify subjects should be protected, respecting the privacy and confidentiality rules in accordance with the applicable regulatory requirement(s).
12. Investigational products should be manufactured, handled, and stored in accordance with applicable good manufacturing practice. They should be used in accordance with the approved protocol.
13. Systems with procedures that assure the quality of every aspect of the trial should be implemented.

International Conference on Harmonisation Guideline for Good Clinical Practice E6(R1), 10 June 1996.

quality assurance and quality control systems, for using qualified individuals to design the trial, develop study documents, conduct the trial, manage the data, and provide safety oversight, for ensuring that adequate data are available to support use of an investigational product in the trial, for ensuring that an investigational product is manufactured in accordance with good manufacturing practice standards, labeled appropriately and maintained under appropriate conditions, for submitting applications for investigational product use and information on safety issues to the proper regulatory authorities, and for monitoring the trial to ensure that the rights and well-being of subjects are protected, that the trial data are accurate, complete, and verifiable, and that the trial is conducted in compliance with the protocol, with GCP, and with applicable regulatory requirements. Adherence to GCP is expected of all clinical research monitors and auditors appointed by the sponsor and all staff of contract research organizations to whom a sponsor transfers any study-related functions.

Sections 6 and 7 of the GCP guidelines outline the critical components of a clinical protocol and an Investigator's Brochure for an investigational product. Section 8 summarizes the minimum essential documents "which individually and collectively permit evaluation of the conduct of a trial and the quality of the data produced." The list includes documents to be generated before the trial begins, during the clinical conduct of the trial, and after completion or termination of the trial.

The importance of adhering to the principles of good clinical practice when conducting research with human subjects is widely recognized. While the ICH GCP standards were developed as guidelines, compliance with the ICH E6 GCP document is a legal requirement in some countries (e.g., Japan, Australia, Canada). In the EU, the ICH GCP is considered a scientific guideline, but legal requirements for following good clinical practice are implemented in Directive 2001/20/EC ("approximation of the laws, regulations and administrative provisions of the Member States relating to the implementation of good clinical practice in the conduct of clinical trials on medicinal products for human use") and Directive 2005/28/EC ("laying down principles and detailed guidelines for good clinical practice as regards investigational medicinal products for human use"). In addition, specific national laws apply within the EU member states (e.g., The Medicines for Human Use [Clinical Trials] Regulations 2004 and its amendments in the United Kingdom). In the United States, the FDA endorsed the ICH E6 GCP and published it as a guidance document, with the statement that it "represents the agency's current thinking on good clinical practices." While FDA guidance documents are not legally binding, the principles of good clinical practice and human subjects protection have been incorporated into law in various parts of the United States Code of Federal Regulations (e.g., 45 CFR part 46 on Protection of Human Subjects, which offers basic protections to human subjects involved in biomedical or behavioral research conducted or supported by federal departments and agencies, 21 CFR part 50 on Protection of Human Subjects and 21 CFR part 56 on IRBs, 21 CFR part 312 on IND Applications, 21 CFR part 314 on FDA approval to Market a New Drug, 21 CFR part 812 on Investigational Device Exemptions (IDE), 21 CFR part 814 on Premarket Approval of Medical Devices).

While the GCP guidance was developed for research using regulated investigational products (drugs, biologics, devices) in human subjects, the introduction to the ICH GCP guidance document states, "the principles established in this guidance may also be applied to other clinical investigations that may have an impact on the safety and well-being of human subjects." Similarly, the World Health Organization Handbook for Good Clinical Research Practice states: "To the extent possible, the principles of GCP should generally apply to all clinical research involving human subjects, and not just research involving pharmaceutical or other medical products...Although some principles of GCP may not apply to all types of research on human subjects, consideration of these principles is strongly encouraged wherever applicable as a means of ensuring the ethical, methodologically sound and accurate conduct of human subjects research."[44] Following the applicable parts of the GCP guidelines during the conduct of non-interventional studies provides a good starting point for complying with the variety of human subjects protection regulations that exist in countries around the world.

SAFETY MONITORING

Safety reporting and safety oversight constitute study safety monitoring. Such monitoring must accommodate the nature of the clinical research being conducted. It must never be overlooked that the goal of safety reporting and safety oversight is to protect the human subjects included in the research from the risks that are intrinsic to participating in the research. It is also important for those reading the literature to know what the risks of a new therapy, whether a drug, procedure, or approach, are in addition to the benefit. It is possible to do too little or too much with respect to safety reporting and safety oversight. A Goldilocks approach is needed: the design and procedures related to safety reporting and safety oversight must fit the study. To do otherwise is to create either too few processes to protect those participating in the research or to waste precious resources collecting unnecessary or duplicative data. This discussion will constitute a brief overview of safety monitoring; references are provided for further reading.

Safety Reporting

The requirements and processes of safety reporting are governed by multiple regulations, guidances, and policies. Currently, clinical research funded by the United States government must comply with safety reporting requirements specified by the Common Rule, 45 CFR 46,[45] and associated guidances and policies issued by the Office of Human Research Protections.[46] Studies governed by Food and Drug Law must comply with the requirements of the FDA.[47] There is overlap between some of the requirements as both have their basis in ICH guidance (see above). There are different regulations and guidances pertaining to studies that test biologics or drugs conducted under IND guidance,[48] studies that do not require an IND but include marketed products, and studies that test devices and materials. When designing the study, it is important to determine whether the study requires an IND under 21 CFR 312.2(a)[48] or IDE under 21 CFR 812.[49] Should an investigator be uncertain whether an IND or IDE is required, the appropriate agency can be contacted to obtain designation.[50–53]

Studies conducted under IND are required to collect "adverse events." Adverse events are any untoward medical occurrence associated with the use of the drug in humans, whether or not considered drug related (21 CFR 312.32 (a)). Adverse events can fall in certain special categories. Although adverse events are to be collected, certain of these special categories have specific reporting requirements. A very important category of adverse event is a "Serious Adverse Event." Reporting of these events captures information suggesting that a drug poses a significant threat to human subjects, and such reports require special scrutiny and attention. Serious adverse events are generally to be reported to the FDA and IRBs in an expedited fashion so that, if required, they can be acted upon quickly. Adverse events are considered serious if they result in any of the following outcomes:

- Death,
- An immediately life threatening adverse event,
- An inpatient hospitalization or prolongation of existing hospitalization,
- A persistent or significant incapacity or substantial disruption in the ability to conduct normal functions,
- A congenital anomaly or birth defect, or
- Any event that may not result in the above outcomes, but could jeopardize the patient or require medical or surgical intervention to prevent one of the above outcomes. (21 CFR 312.32(a).[48]

Other important safety definitions are "suspected adverse reaction," meaning that there is a "reasonable possibility" of a causal relationship between the drug and the adverse event (21 CFR 312.32(a)). "Unexpected" is another term applied to adverse events. For regulatory purposes, unexpected means that the event has not been observed with drug use previously (21 CFR 312.32(a)). For instance, other clinical studies testing the drug, whether published or unpublished, have not observed the event. IND sponsors and investigators working under IND are required to have specific knowledge of any adverse events, including their type and severity that have occurred with previous drug use so that they may recognize those events that require special focus, more detailed information, and expedited reported to the FDA and governing IRB.

The aforementioned safety reporting requirements are specific to drug and biologic studies under IND. For federally funded studies and studies under Food and Drug Law, there is a requirement to capture and report "Unanticipated Problems," following specific requirements and time frames. An unanticipated problem meets all the following criteria:

- "unexpected (in terms of nature, severity, or frequency) given (a) the research procedures that are described in the protocol-related documents, such as the IRB-approved research protocol and informed consent document; and (b) the characteristics of the subject population being studied;
- related or possibly related to participation in the research (possibly related means there is a reasonable possibility that the incident, experience, or outcome may have been caused by the procedures involved in the research); and
- suggests that the research places subjects or others at a greater risk of harm (including physical, psychological, economic, or social harm) than was previously known or recognized."

Unanticipated problems may or may not be either adverse events or serious adverse events. This definition can include events such as loss of subject privacy, or hazardous conditions, or risks related to participating in the research that are not related to a drug.

This is a very brief overview of safety reporting requirements; for those interested in more detail, see references listed below.

Safety Oversight

For studies of minimal risk, oversight by the principal investigator is often adequate. However, studies of greater risk and complexity may either benefit from or require different or independent safety oversight structures. Most familiar are Data and Safety Monitoring Boards (DSMBs) or Committees, groups of independent experts, usually convened by the sponsor, who oversee reports of study conduct, data quality, and safety information. DSMBs are usually governed by a charter which outlines how frequently meetings occur, what sorts of data will be reviewed, whether special meetings should be convened to address certain important or unexpected events, what are the rules of conduct, what constitutes a quorum, and what sorts of recommendations are expected. DSMBs are an important oversight mechanism in the protection of human subject safety. Relevant expertise independent of the study and its investigators are critical to the proper functioning of a DSMB. Thus, DSMBs must be carefully constituted and supported to perform effectively.[54]

This research was supported by the Extramural Research Program of the National Institutes of Health, National Institute of Dental and Craniofacial Research. The content of this publication is solely the responsibility of the authors and does not necessarily represent the official views of the National Institutes of Health.

Selected Readings

Bellera C, Praud D, Petit-Moneger A, et al. Barriers to inclusion of older adults in randomised controlled clinical trials on Non-Hodgkin's lymphoma: a systematic review. *Cancer Treat Rev.* 2013;39(7):812–817.

Berkman ND, Lohr KN, Ansari M, et al. *Methods Guide for Effectiveness and Comparative Effectiveness Reviews [Internet]. Agency for Healthcare Research and Quality (US).* http://www.ncbi.nlm.nih.gov/books/NBK174881/. Updated 2013. Accessed January 10, 2014.

DPTT Study Group, Engebretson S, Gelato M, Hyman L, et al. Design features of the Diabetes and Periodontal Therapy Trial (DPTT): a multicenter randomized single-masked clinical trial testing the effect of nonsurgical periodontal therapy on glycosylated hemoglobin (HbA1c) levels in subjects with type 2 diabetes and chronic periodontitis. *Contemp Clin Trials.* 2013;36(2):515–526.

Engebretson SP, Hyman LG, Michalowicz BS, et al. The effect of nonsurgical periodontal therapy on hemoglobin A1c levels in persons with type 2 diabetes and chronic periodontitis: a randomized clinical trial. *JAMA.* 2013;310(23):2523–2532.

Faggion CM Jr. The development of evidence-based guidelines in dentistry. *J Dent Educ.* 2013;77(2):124–136.

Norton WE, Funkhouser E, Makhija SK, et al. Concordance between clinical practice and published evidence: findings from the National Dental Practice-Based Research Network. *J Am Dent Assoc.* 2014;145(1):22–31.

US Department of Health and Human Services. *Guidance for Clinical Investigators, Sponsors, and IRBs. Investigational New Applications (INDs)—Determining Whether Human Research Studies Can Be Conducted Without an IND.* http://www.fda.gov/downloads/Drugs/GuidanceComplianceRegulatoryInformation/Guidances/UCM229175.pdf. Updated September 2013. Accessed July 2, 2014.

World Medical Association. *Declaration of Helsinki: Ethical Principles for Medical Research Involving Human Subjects*, amended October 2013. www.wma.net/en/30publications/10policies/b3/index.html, accessed July 2, 2014.

Xue F, Ma H, Stehman-Breen C, et al. Design and methods of a postmarketing pharmacoepidemiology study assessing long-term safety of Prolia(R) (denosumab) for the treatment of postmenopausal osteoporosis. *Pharmacoepidemiol Drug Saf.* 2013;22(10):1107–1114.

For the full reference lists, please go to http://www.pmph-usa.com/Burkets_Oral_Medicine.

CHAPTER 3

Pharmacotherapy

Mark Donaldson, BSP, PharmD

Jason H. Goodchild, DMD

Mark J. Wrobel, PharmD

PHARMACOTHERAPY FOR OROFACIAL BACTERIAL INFECTIONS

Many oral pathologies presenting to the dentist are inflammatory conditions associated with pain. A significant percentage of dental pain originates from acute and chronic infections, which necessitate operative intervention followed by analgesic therapy rather than an antibiotic. While clinical situations requiring antibiotic therapy may be limited, they typically include oral infections accompanied by elevated body temperature, pain, inflammation, and evidence of systemic involvement such as lymphadenopathy and trismus. This section will address the pharmacological management of orofacial bacterial infections, but does not specifically address caries or periodontal diseases.

Figure 3-1 introduces stepwise guidelines for antibiotic prescribing. Antibiotics are either required for *treatment* of an existing infection or *prevention* of a potential infection depending on the immunocompetency of the patient.

Systemic antimicrobials should only be prescribed where oral health care professionals know the most commonly

associated pathogens. Clinical effectiveness in treating an infection is based on correctly diagnosing the infecting microorganism(s) and choosing the most targeted and effective antibiotic. Ideally, bacteriologic assessment should be completed before treatment is started, however, certain conditions may prevent this from happening (i.e., an acutely ill patient cannot have antibiotic treatment delayed for the 48 hours or more that may be required to learn the results of bacteriologic tests). For this reason, the choice of antibiotic must be based empirically on the prescriber's knowledge of the usual causative microorganisms and the antibiotic(s) to which these organisms are normally susceptible.[1] Table 3-1 lists the most common pathogens associated with orofacial infections. In treating an acute orofacial infection, it is reasonable to start with an antibiotic to which the probable organisms (Gram-positive aerobes and intraoral anaerobes) are susceptible.

Narrow-spectrum antibiotics are effective against a specific family of Gram-positive or Gram-negative bacteria. *Extended-spectrum antibiotics* are often chemically modified narrow spectrum antibiotics that kill additional bacteria types, while *broad-spectrum antibiotics* affect both

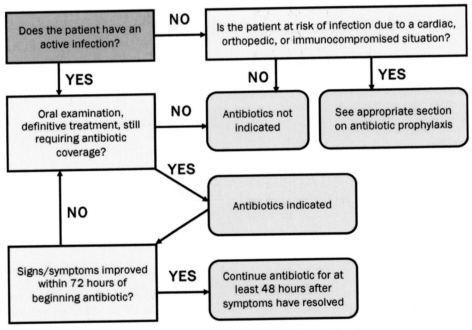

FIGURE 3-1 Stepwise guidelines when considering prescribing antibiotics.

TABLE 3-1 The Most Common Pathogens Associated With Orofacial Infections[142]

Suspected Pathogen	Commonality
Streptococcus	Most common
Actinomyces, Eubacterium, Leptotrichia	
Fusobacterium, Bacteroides, Prevotella, Porphyromonas	
Peptostreptococcus	
Lactobacillus	
Veillonella	Least common

TABLE 3-2   The Spectrum of Activity for the Most Commonly Used Antibiotics in Treating Orofacial Infections[143]

Narrow	Extended	Broad
Clindamycin, dicloxacillin, macrolides (erythromycin, clarithromycin, azithromycin), metronidazole, penicillin G, penicillin V	Cephalosporins (cephalexin, cefadroxil, cefaclor, cefuroxime), extended-spectrum penicillins (ampicillin, amoxicillin), fluoroquinolones (ciprofloxacin, levofloxacin, moxifloxacin)	Augmentin (amoxicillin plus clavulanate), sulfamethoxazole and trimethoprim, tetracyclines (tetracycline, doxycycline)

Gram-positive and Gram-negative bacteria. Table 3-2 categorizes the spectrum of activity for the most common antibiotics used to treat orofacial infections.

Penicillin VK (penicillin V potassium) is an ideal first-choice antibiotic for orofacial infections because it mainly targets Gram-positive aerobic and facultative bacteria, some anaerobes, and spirochetes. It is still considered the drug of choice for streptococcal infections. Penicillin causes bacterial lysis by interfering with the synthesis of peptidoglycan that is necessary for the formation of the bacterial cell wall. The "V" comes for the Latin word *vesco/vescar* meaning "eat." Penicillin G, the progenitor and gold ("G") standard for which this class of drugs derives its name, is typically given parenterally because it is unstable in the highly acidic stomach. Penicillin VK is the acid-stable formulation of penicillin G.

Penicillins are sometimes referred to as β-lactam antibiotics because their chemical structure contains a β-lactam ring. β-lactam antibiotics inhibit the formation of peptidoglycan cross-links in the bacterial cell wall, causing bacterial death via inhibition of cell wall synthesis. Cephalosporins such as cephalexin are also called β-lactam antibiotics based on their chemical structure, and therefore have a similar mechanism of action to penicillins. While all β-lactam antibiotics kill bacteria by the same mechanism of action, it is their individual chemical structures that determine their spectrum of activity. Ampicillin and amoxicillin are extended-spectrum penicillins, while the combination of antibiotics such as amoxicillin with the β-lactamase inhibitor clavulanate helps create a broad-spectrum antibiotic. β-lactamase is an enzyme some bacteria have developed to help resist the effects of β-lactam antibiotics.

Other narrow-spectrum antibiotics include metronidazole (a nitroimidazole antibiotic), clindamycin (a lincosamide antibiotic), and the macrolides, erythromycin, clarithromycin, and azithromycin. Metronidazole is only active against obligate anaerobic bacteria such as such as *Bacteroides, Campylobacter, Clostridium, Fusobacterium, Peptococcus, Peptostreptococcus, Prevotella*, and *Veillonella*, in which it interferes with nucleic acid synthesis causing microbial death. Clindamycin and the macrolide antibiotics inhibit bacterial protein synthesis by affecting the function of 30S or 50S ribosomal subunits. Thus, these antibiotics are largely bacteriostatic, not bactericidal. Clindamycin has better activity against most strains of *Staphylococcus aureus* than macrolides and is more active against Gram-positive and Gram-negative anaerobes; however, the macrolides are more effective against

Streptococcus pneumoniae as well as other typical (*Haemophilus influenzae* and *Moraxella catarrhalis*) and atypical (*Legionella pneumophila, Mycoplasma pneumonia, Chlamydophila pneumoniae*) upper respiratory tract pathogens.

The fluoroquinolones (e.g., ciprofloxacin, levofloxacin, moxifloxacin) are extended-spectrum antibiotics that act by interfering with bacterial nucleic acid synthesis. These antibiotics are not typically used as first-line agents for orofacial infections, though ciprofloxacin may have a role in treating susceptible species of *Pseudomonas*. Broad-spectrum agents such as sulfamethoxazole/trimethoprim and the tetracyclines (e.g., tetracycline, minocycline, doxycycline) are also rarely used first-line because of their potential to cause collateral damage (superinfection by resistant pathogens or selection of antibiotic resistance). All of these agents are less targeted in their microbial selection when compared to narrow-spectrum antibiotics. Sub-antibiotic doses of doxycycline have been used for periodontal disease, however, this activity is based on anti-inflammatory properties of the medication rather than antibacterial properties.[2] Typical adult and pediatric prescriptions for treatment of orofacial infections with all of these agents are listed in Table 3-3.

ANTIBIOTIC THERAPIES FOR IMMUNOCOMPROMISED PATIENTS

Numerous medical conditions are associated with suppression of the immune system either directly from an underlying disease (e.g., diabetes, cancer, organ transplantation) or from medications used to manage these diseases (e.g., cyclosporine, prednisone). A primary concern for an immunocompromised patient is the risk of poor healing and systemic spread of an orofacial infection. Therefore, consideration for appropriate antibiotics to treat an active dental infection is vital to enhance healing of an orofacial infection and to avoid a systemic infection. In addition to treatment of active infections, prophylactic antibiotics prior to invasive dental procedures have been suggested for patients who may be unable to mount an appropriate immune response.

In cases of patients with an underlying medical condition or who are receiving medical therapy that suppresses the immune system, the absolute neutrophil count (ANC) is an important marker for quantifying a patient's severity of immunosuppression. The ANC is calculated by multiplying the percentage of neutrophils plus bands

TABLE 3-3   Typical Prescriptions for the Most Commonly Used Antibiotics for Orofacial Infections

Generic Name (Brand Names)	Available Formulations	Usual Dosages	Notes
Amoxicillin (Amoxil, Trimox)	Capsule (250, 500 mg) Chewable tablet (125, 200, 250, 400 mg) Oral suspension (125, 200, 250, 400 mg/5 mL) Tablet (250, 500, 875 mg)	Adult: 250–500 mg q8h or 500–875 mg q12h Pediatric: 20–90 mg/kg/d divided q8–12h	Useful (with or without clavulanate) in combination with metronidazole in addition to scaling and root planing in the treatment of periodontitis associated with the presence of *Actinobacillus actinomycetemcomitans* (AA).[144]
Amoxicillin-clavulanate (Augmentin, Augmentin ES, Augmentin XR)	Chewable tablet (200-28.5, 400-57 mg) ER tablet (1000-62.5 mg) IR tablet (250-125, 500-125, 875-125 mg) Oral suspension (125-31.25, 200-28.5, 250-62.5, 400-57, 600-42.9 mg/5 mL)	Dosage based on amoxicillin content. Adult: IR tablets: 875 mg q12h; ER tablets: (not to be used in patients <40 kg): 2000 mg q12h Pediatric: 25–90 mg/kg/d divided q12h	For doses of 500 mg or 875 mg, 500 mg, or 875 mg tablets should be used because multiple smaller tablets would contain too much clavulanate. Especially useful in treating orofacial infections when beta-lactamase-producing *Staphylococci* or *Bacteroides* are present.
Azithromycin (Zithromax)	Oral suspension (100, 200 mg/ 5 mL) Tablet (250, 500 mg)	Adult: 500 mg day 1, then 250 mg once daily × 4 d Pediatric: 5–10 mg/kg once daily × 4 d	Use with caution in patients with a history of cardiovascular disease.[145]
Cephalexin (Keflex)	Capsule (250, 500, 750 mg) Oral suspension (125, 250 mg/5 mL)	Adult: 250–1000 mg q6–12h Pediatric: 25–100 mg/kg/d divided q6–8h	In patients with a history of severe reactions (urticaria, angioedema, bronchospasm, anaphylaxis), the rate of reactions to cephalexin in patients with a history of penicillin allergy is about 10%. For patients with a history of a less-than-severe reaction to cephalexin, the rate is closer to 0.1%.[146]
Ciprofloxacin[a] (Cipro, Cipro XR)	ER tablet (500, 1000 mg) IR tablet (100, 250, 500, 750 mg) Oral suspension (250, 500 mg/5 mL)	Adult: 250–750 mg q12h Pediatric[a]: 10–20 mg/kg q12h	
Clarithromycin (Biaxin, Biaxin XL)	ER tablet (500 mg) IR tablet (250, 500 mg) Oral suspension (125, 250 mg/5 mL)	Adult: IR tablets: 250–500 mg q12h; ER tablets (not for pediatric use): 1000 mg once a day Pediatric: 7.5 mg/kg q12h	Use with caution in patients with a history of cardiovascular disease.[147]
Clindamycin (Cleocin)	Capsule (75, 150, 300 mg) Oral solution (75 mg/5 mL)	Adult: 150–450 mg q6–8h Pediatric: 10 mg/kg q8h	About 1% of clindamycin users develop pseudomembranous colitis. Symptoms may occur 2–9 d after initiation of therapy; however, it has never occurred with the I-dose regimen of clindamycin used to prevent bacterial endocarditis and may not be any more frequent than other commonly used antibiotics.[148]
Doxycycline[b,c] (Periostat, Vibramycin)	Capsule (50, 75, 100, 150 mg) Oral suspension (25, 50 mg/5 mL) Tablet (20, 50, 75, 100 mg)	Adult: 100 mg q12h Pediatric: 2–4 mg/kg/d divided q12h	A specific formulation containing a subantimicrobial dosage is available for use as an adjunct to scaling and root planing or for subgingival application.
Erythromycin (E.E.S., EryPed, Ery-Tab)	Capsule (250 mg) Oral suspension (200, 400 mg/5mL) Tablet (250, 333, 400, 500 mg)	Adult: 250–500 mg q6h Pediatric: 7.5–12.5 mg/kg q6h	May want to consider an alternative macrolide in patients with underlying cardiac disease.[149]
Levofloxacin[a,c] (Levaquin)	Oral solution (125 mg/5 mL) Tablet (250, 500, 750 mg)	Adult: 250–750 mg once daily	
Metronidazole (Flagyl, Flagyl ER)	Capsule (375 mg) ER tablet (750 mg) IR tablet (250, 500 mg)	Adult: 500 mg q6–12h Pediatric: 30 mg/kg/d divided q6h	Key adverse event(s) related to dental treatment: unusual/metallic taste, glossitis, stomatitis, xerostomia (normal salivary flow resumes upon discontinuation), and furry tongue. Do not take with alcohol as a disulfiram-like reaction may occur.

TABLE 3-3   Typical Prescriptions for the Most Commonly Used Antibiotics for Orofacial Infections (*Continued*)

Generic Name (Brand Names)	Available Formulations	Usual Dosages	Notes
Moxifloxacin[a,c] (Avelox)	Tablet (400 mg)	Adults: 400 mg once daily	
Penicillin (Pen VK, Veetids)	Oral solution (125, 250 mg/5 mL) Tablet (250, 500 mg)	Adult: 250–500 mg q6–8h Pediatric: 25–50 mg/kg/d divided q6–8h	Also available as a suspension which may not be equivalent on a mg/mg basis to the tablets.
Tetracycline[b,c] (Sumycin)	Capsule (250, 500 mg)	Adult: 250–500 mg q6h Pediatric: 25–50 mg/kg/d divided q6h	

ER: extended-release; IR: immediate-release.

[a]Not recommended for routine use in children or adolescents <18 years old.

[b]Tetracyclines are not recommended for use during pregnancy or in children ≤8 years of age since they have been reported to cause enamel hypoplasia and permanent teeth discoloration.

[c]Take at least 2 hours before or 6 hours after the dose of a multivitamin that contains polyvalent cations (i.e., calcium, iron, magnesium, selenium, zinc).

TABLE 3-4   American Heart Association Antibiotic Regimens for Cardiac Prophylaxis[150]

Situation	Antibiotic	Single Dose 30–60 Min Prior to Procedure	
		Adults	Children
Able to take oral medication	Amoxicillin	2 g	50 mg/kg
Unable to take oral medication	Option 1: ampicillin	2 g IM or IV	50 mg/kg IM or IV
	Option 2: cefazolin or ceftriaxone	1 g IM or IV	50 mg/kg IM or IV
Allergic to penicillin but able to tolerate oral therapy	Option 1: cephalexin[a,b]	2 g	50 mg/kg
	Option 2: clindamycin	600 mg	20 mg/kg
	Option 3: azithromycin or clarithromycin	500 mg	15 mg/kg
Allergic to penicillin and unable to take oral medication	Option 1: cefazolin or ceftriaxone[b]	1 g IM or IV	50 mg/kg IM or IV
	Option 2: clindamycin	600 mg IM or IV	20 mg/kg IM or IV

IM, intramuscular; IV, intravenous.

[a]Or other first- or second-generation oral cephalosporin in equivalent adult or pediatric dosage.

[b]Cephalosporins should not be used in an individual with a history of anaphylaxis, angioedema, or urticaria with penicillins.

(immature neutrophils) with the absolute number of neutrophils from the total white blood cell (WBC) count. For example, if a patient had 2000/μL WBCs with 45% neutrophils and 5% bands, the patient's ANC is 1000/μL (2000/μL × 50%). An ANC < 500/μL represents a severe neutropenia with an increased incidence and severity of infection. It is important to recognize that although the ANC is a measure of immunosuppression due to disease, it is not a measure of the degree of immune compromise in patients whose immunosuppression is medication-induced.

Neutropenic Cancer Patients

Patients with cancer may be neutropenic from their chemotherapy treatment or their underlying cancer. Despite the lack of substantial scientific evidence, the National Cancer Institute recommends that the American Heart Association (AHA) regimen (Table 3-4) for prophylactic antibiotics be used for patients with indwelling venous access lines and an ANC between 1000 and 2000/μL before any invasive dental procedure.[3] Further consideration should be given to discussing more aggressive antibiotic therapy with the patient's oncologist in the presence of an orofacial infection.

The use of appropriate antibiotics for the treatment of an oral infection is particularly vital in immunocompromised cancer patients. The timing of dental treatment is complicated in patients being treated with cytotoxic cancer therapy since the definitive treatment (e.g., endodontic therapy, extraction) should be timed prior to chemotherapy-induced neutropenia or after the WBC counts return to an appropriate level. Clinical manifestations of an orofacial infection during chemotherapy-induced neutropenia are uncommon, which may be partly related to a decreased inflammatory response from deficient WBCs. Use of antibiotics and a delay of definitive dental treatment until WBC counts increase is a rational treatment plan for cancer patients with chemotherapy-associated neutropenia.

Topical antibiotics such as chlorhexidine 0.12% solution (swish and expectorate with 10 mL twice daily) are appropriate for localized gingival disease during neutropenia. The use of broad-spectrum antibiotics is appropriate for the treatment of active orofacial infections in neutropenic patients. The antibiotic can be changed to a narrower-spectrum agent based on appropriate susceptibility of bacterial isolates as identified through culture of draining pus. Outpatient cancer patients or patients without severe neutropenia may respond well to oral antibiotics such as penicillin VK, amoxicillin, clindamycin, azithromycin, tetracycline, or amoxicillin with clavulanate (Table 3-3).

Prophylactic Antibiotics in Immunocompromised Patients

The use of antibiotics prior to an invasive dental procedure has been suggested for a variety of immunocompromised conditions, including neutropenic cancer patients, patients with end-stage renal disease treated with hemodialysis, organ transplant patients, and poorly controlled diabetics. The evidence to support the practice of routine antibiotic prophylaxis prior to invasive dental procedures in these populations continues to evolve, however, and decisions to prescribe are often based on medicolegal concerns rather than evidence, which remains poor.[4,5] For these reasons, dental prescribers need to understand that the negative consequences of repeated antibiotic use, such as increased antibiotic resistance, costs, and potential allergic reactions, must always be weighed against the perceived benefit of infection prevention.[6]

To prevent rejection of transplanted organs, patients are routinely placed on immunosuppressive medications. These medications may include long-term prednisone, mycophenolate, cyclosporine, azathioprine, or others, which function by moderating the T-cell response of the patient to prevent graft rejection. An increased risk of infection is one side effect of these immunosuppressive medications. The use of antibiotic prophylaxis for invasive dental procedures in these patients is controversial. Discussion with the patient's transplant physician regarding the use of antibiotics is recommended. It is reasonable to use prophylactic antibiotics in the first few months after transplantation, when the patient has the highest risk of infection and acute graft rejection. Dosing of antibiotics recommended by the AHA for prevention of infective endocarditis is reasonable to recommend (Table 3-4). Since the incidence and severity of infection rises as the ANC falls below 1000/µL, patients with prolonged neutropenia are at higher risk of developing serious infectious complications.[7] In these high-risk patients as well as those with an obvious presence of infection, consideration for more aggressive antibiotic therapy should be given.[3]

ANTIBIOTIC PROPHYLAXIS AGAINST INFECTIVE ENDOCARDITIS AND PROSTHETIC JOINT INFECTIONS

Oral bacterial pathogens may be responsible for cases of infective endocarditis (IE) or late-prosthetic joint infections, yet it is unclear to what extent this results from dental office

procedures versus bacteremia from routine daily activities such as tooth brushing and chewing food. There is little evidence demonstrating that dental office procedures cause distant site infections,[8] therefore, the driving force behind the practice of antibiotic prophylaxis is the improbable yet possible devastating impact of a bacteremia-induced infection of a cardiac valve, prosthetic joint, or indwelling medical device.

Antibiotic prophylaxis in dentistry has been a subject of debate and controversy since 1955 when the AHA began developing recommendations for prophylactic antibiotics to prevent IE. These recommendations have set the standard of care for the past 60 years; however, there remains confusion surrounding which patients are at risk for distant site infections and which dental procedures and bacteria may be of greatest concern. Further complicating the issue is the ongoing emergence of resistant bacterial pathogens created by the indiscriminate use of antibiotics, the costs to the health-care system, the small risk of fatal allergic reactions, and reported low adherence rate on the part of physicians and dentists with respect to these guidelines.[4] Clearly what drives prophylactic antibiotic prescribing in dentistry is a combination of the AHA guidelines, long-standing belief, practice habits, and medicolegal considerations.

In the United States, there are antibiotic prophylaxis recommendations promulgated by the American Dental Association and medical specialty organizations (the AHA and the American Academy of Orthopaedic Surgeons) for two patient populations: those with specific cardiac abnormalities and those with orthopedic implants. Many other countries have ceased using antibiotic prophylaxis for infective endocarditis and prosthetic joint infections. This is due to a lack of prospective, randomized, placebo-controlled clinical trials that are needed to support definitive and evidence-based decision-making as to which dental procedures represent a significantly increased risk of distant site infection and which patients are at greatest risk. Also, the use of antibiotics in an attempt to prevent IE and orthopedic implant infections after dental procedures may contribute to the development of antibiotic resistance, which is a dire consequence for the population at large.

Patients With Cardiac Abnormalities

The latest AHA recommendations for the dental management of patients with cardiac abnormalities were published in 2007.[9] These guidelines define patients at risk for IE (Table 3-5), and the appropriate prophylactic antibiotic regimens (Table 3-4). The dental procedures most likely to put patients at risk include all dental procedures that involve manipulation of gingival tissue or the periapical region of teeth or perforation of the oral mucosa. Procedures and events that carry a low risk of IE for which prophylaxis is unnecessary can be seen in Table 3-6. The AHA does not recommend secondary antibiotic prophylaxis for patients with non-valvular cardiovascular devices (e.g., pacemaker) who are undergoing dental procedures.[10]

TABLE 3-5   Cardiac Conditions Associated With the Highest Risk of Endocarditis for Which Antibiotic Prophylaxis Is Recommended[150]

- Prosthetic cardiac valve.
- Previous infective endocarditis.
- Cardiac transplantation recipients who develop cardiac valvulopathy.
- Congenital heart disease (CHD)[a]:
  - Unrepaired cyanotic CHD, including palliative shunts and conduits.
  - Completely repaired congenital heart defect with prosthetic material or device, whether placed by surgery or by catheter intervention, during the first 6 m after the procedure.[b]
  - Repaired CHD with residual defects at the site or adjacent to the site of a prosthetic patch or prosthetic device (which inhibit endothelialization).

[a]Except for the conditions listed above, antibiotic prophylaxis is no longer recommended for any other form of CHD.
[b]Prophylaxis is recommended because endothelialization of prosthetic material occurs within 6 m after the procedure.

TABLE 3-6   Bacteremic Risks of Various Dental Procedures[12]

Incidence of Bacteremia	Dental Procedures
Higher[a]	• Dental extractions. • Periodontal procedures, including surgery, subgingival placement of antibiotic fibers/strips, scaling and root planing, probing, and recall maintenance. • Dental implant placement and replantation of avulsed teeth. • Endodontic (root canal) instrumentation or surgery only beyond the apex. • Initial placement of orthodontic bands but not brackets. • Intraligamentary and intraosseous local anesthetic injections. • Prophylactic cleaning of teeth or implants where bleeding is anticipated.
Lower[b]	• Restorative dentistry (operative and prosthodontic) with/without retraction cord.[c] • Local anesthetic injections (non-intraligamentary and non-intraosseous). • Intracanal endodontic treatment; post placement and buildup. • Placement of rubber dam. • Postoperative suture removal. • Placement of removable prosthodontic/orthodontic appliances. • Taking of oral impressions. • Fluoride treatments. • Taking of oral radiographs. • Orthodontic appliance adjustment.

[a]Prophylaxis should be considered for patients with total joint replacement who meet the criteria in Table 3-7. No other patients with orthopedic implants should be considered for antibiotic prophylaxis prior to dental treatment/procedures.
[b]Prophylaxis not indicated although clinical judgment may indicate antibiotic use in selected circumstances that may create significant bleeding.
[c]Includes restoration of carious (decayed) or missing teeth.

Patients With Prosthetic Joints

The latest guideline published by the American Dental Association (ADA) and American Academy of Orthopedic Surgeons (AAOS) for the dental management of at-risk orthopedic populations was published in 2013.[11] Unfortunately, these guidelines fall short in clearly delineating specific patient populations who may be at highest risk (Table 3-7) or dental procedures that may carry a higher bacteremic risk (Table 3-6) as outlined in the 2003 guidelines.[12] The new guideline states, "treatments and procedures applicable to the individual patient rely on mutual communication between patient, physician, dentist, and other healthcare practitioners." It proposes a shared decision-making tool designed to help the patient who has undergone an orthopedic procedure determine, with the assistance of his or her dentist or physician, whether taking an antibiotic prior to a dental procedure is prudent or necessary.[13] The final recommendations state that the practitioner might consider discontinuing the practice of routinely prescribing prophylactic antibiotics for patients with hip and knee prosthetic joint implants undergoing dental procedures since the evidence in support of this practice is limited.

If a practitioner wishes to prescribe an antibiotic to prevent late prosthetic joint infection (LPJI), the same antibiotic regimens supported by the AHA for cardiac indications (see Table 3-4) may be considered appropriate. Even if there are differences between the anatomy, microbiology, and possible pathogenesis of LPJI and IE, they do have in common the underlying mechanism of putative hematogenous spread from the mouth.

TABLE 3-7   Patients at Potential Increased Risk of Experiencing Hematogenous Total Joint Infection[12]

Patient Type	Condition Placing Patient at Risk
All patients during the first 2 y following joint replacement	• Not applicable
Immunocompromised or immunosuppressed patients	• Inflammatory arthropathies such as rheumatoid arthritis, systemic lupus erythematosus • Drug- or radiation-induced immunosuppression
Patients with comorbidities[a]	• Previous prosthetic joint infections • Malnourishment • Hemophilia • HIV infection • Type 1 diabetes • Malignancy

[a]Conditions shown for patients in this category are examples only; there may be additional conditions that place such patients at risk of experiencing hematogenous total joint infections.

Prophylactic Antibiotics in Hemodialysis Patients

Vascular access sites used for patients receiving hemodialysis are at increased risk of becoming infected. Treatment may require hospitalization, systemic antibiotics, and possible shunt removal. The most common infectious agents are Gram-positive bacteria, followed by Gram-negative and polymicrobial bacteria. Orofacial bacteria are infrequently the source of vascular access site infections. IE can result from vascular access infection, with up to 25% requiring heart valve replacement. The need for antibiotic prophylaxis for the prevention of shunt infections is controversial and there are no guidelines at this time.[14,15] A recent review suggests that for recipients of hemodialysis with arteriovenous shunts, prophylaxis is warranted at all times after implantation/revision, when dental procedures capable of inducing high-level bacteremia are planned.[16] Still, the AHA guidelines do not discuss whether antibiotic prophylaxis is recommended for hemodialysis shunts, and no well-designed clinical trials have been published in these patients to provide further guidance. Therefore, the best strategy is to consult with the patient's nephrologist to determine if prophylactic antibiotics are deemed necessary from their medical point of view.

PHARMACOTHERAPY FOR A COMMON OROFACIAL VIRAL INFECTION: ORAL HERPESVIRUS INFECTION

Herpes simplex virus 1 (HSV-1), the primary viral pathogen of oral infections, preferentially attacks neuronal tissues, but also attacks dermal and epidermal tissues. The virus enters through mucosal or skin surfaces, replicates rapidly in neurons, and usually establishes a latent infection in neuronal cell bodies. In oral infections, latency is established in the trigeminal ganglion, which can later affect the facial mucosa, including the mouth, nose, and eyes.[17] This viral reservoir allows for future reactivation (see reactivation

TABLE 3-8   Possible Triggers for Herpes Labialis Recurrence

Dental work/surgery	Fever
Sunlight/ultraviolet light	Dehydration
Emotional stress	Upper respiratory infection/ common cold
Menses/hormone changes	
Trauma (such as cut or crack on lip)	Temperature extremes
	Immunosuppression or
Lip tattoos or dermabrasion	weakened immune system

triggers, Table 3-8) where viral bodies are transported back to mucosal surfaces. Transmission requires direct contact with secretions containing virus. Salivary is the most common mode of transmission of HSV-1, although sexual, blood, and placental transmission are also possible. Many transmissions occur in childhood via nonsexual contact, including kissing or sharing eating utensils, lip balms, or towels.

Oral HSV-1 infections manifest in two different ways. The first is primary herpetic gingivostomatitis (HGS), which can affect the tongue, lips, gingivae, hard and soft palates, or buccal mucosa. Onset is usually between 6 months and 5 years of age or in the early 20s. Symptoms can range greatly from barely noticeable to severe, sometimes requiring hospitalization for dehydration due to inability to swallow because of pain.[18] The most common symptoms are fever, pain, and perioral/oral erythematous vesicles that eventually ulcerate. It is a self-limiting disease, but healing can take up to two weeks. The second and most common presentation (about 90% of HSV-1 orofacial infections[17]) is recurrent herpes labialis (RHL), which typically affects the border of the lip. Up to 60% of patients with RHL will experience prodromal symptoms that last a few hours at the site of reactivation. These symptoms may include pain, tingling, burning, tenderness, or itching.[18] Clusters of yellowish vesicles with or without an erythematous base appear at the reactivation site on the lip or vermilion border. These vesicles eventually ulcerate and crust over, with complete healing usually occurring in 7–10 days. In RHL, the location of each episode is usually the same.

Recurrent herpetic stomatitis is more rare than RHL but can be problematic for immunocompromised patients, including those with HIV/AIDS co-infection, patients undergoing transplants, radiotherapy, or chemotherapy, extensively malnourished patients, or patients with extensive burns.[18] An intraoral HSV-1 infection must be treated aggressively with systemic antiviral medications in these subgroups of patients to prevent significant morbidity and mortality. Figure 3-2 is a decision diagram for the treatment of RHL.

Oral Therapies for Oral and Perioral Herpes Infections

Oral nucleoside antiviral therapies (acyclovir, famciclovir, valacyclovir) are indicated in acute HGS. They are also more effective than topical therapies for the treatment of RHL. Dosing regimens for each of the three antivirals are in Table 3-9.

Literature detailing treatment of oral herpes infections with antivirals is sparse, especially in adult populations. Acyclovir suspension has been tested in young children with acute HGS and was shown to variably decrease the duration and severity of symptoms and reduce infectivity.[19] Famciclovir has been used successfully in the treatment of immuno-compromised patients with acute HGS, and is preferential

in older patients because of a simpler dosing schedule and definitive efficacy.[20] While there are no clinical trials testing valacyclovir in acute HGS, it is generally accepted as a plausible treatment alternative to famciclovir.[21,22]

There is evidence that oral antiviral therapies reduce RHL healing times to a greater extent than topical therapies,[23] though oral and topical therapies have not been tested head-to-head in a clinical trial. Significant differences in healing times between drug and placebo have been demonstrated in trials involving acyclovir,[24,25] famciclovir,[26,27] and valacyclovir.[28] In all trials, patients were treated within 12 hours of first experiencing prodromal symptoms. Given that all three oral therapies are now generic in the United States, it makes clinical sense to choose an antiviral with a low pill burden to improve adherence and efficacy. Both valacyclovir and famciclovir have one-day regimens that make RHL easy to treat while acyclovir must be taken multiple times daily for five days (see Table 3-9).[23]

Topical Therapies for Acute Recurrent Herpes Labialis

Some of the symptoms of RHL can be mitigated through the use of over-the-counter pain relievers and skin protectants. Protectants will help to moisturize the lesion and prevent painful cracking. Over-the-counter products to avoid

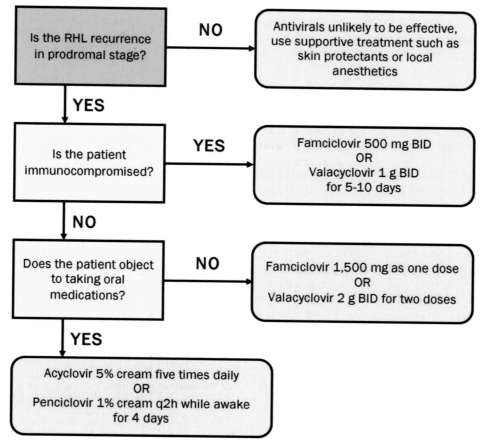

FIGURE 3-2 Stepwise guidelines for recurrent herpes labialis infection in adult patients.

TABLE 3-9   Prescription Systemic Antiviral Therapies for Oral Herpes Simplex Virus Infections

Generic Name	Acyclovir	Famciclovir	Valacyclovir
Brand name	Zovirax	Famvir	Valtrex
Dosage form	Capsule (200 mg) Oral suspension (200 mg/5 mL) Tablet (400, 800 mg)	Tablet (125, 250, 500 mg)	Tablet (500, 1000 mg)
HGS: child dose	15 mg/kg five times daily for 7 d (start within 72 h of symptoms, max single dose 200 mg)		
HGS: adult dose	400 mg tid or 200 mg five times daily for 7–10 d	500 mg tid for 7–10 d	1 g bid for 7–10 d
Recurrent episode of herpes labialis: dosing for adult[a]	400 mg tid or 200 mg five times daily for 5 d	1,500 mg as one dose	2 g bid for 1 d
Recurrent episode of herpes labialis: dosing for adult with HIV[a]	400 mg tid for 5–10 d or until clinical resolution occurs	500 mg bid for 5–10 d	1 g bid for 5–10 d
RHL prophylaxis: adult dose	400 mg bid (indefinite duration)		500 mg qd (indefinite duration)
Contraindications	Hypersensitivity to acyclovir or valacyclovir	Hypersensitivity to famciclovir	Hypersensitivity to acyclovir or valacyclovir
Precautions	Renal dysfunction or co-administration of nephrotoxic drugs		
Common side effects	Headache, nausea, abdominal pain, arthralgia, fatigue, pharyngitis, rash		
Rare but important side effects	Hematologic abnormalities, central nervous system side effects including seizure, confusion, and delirium		
Important drug interactions	Aminoglycosides, mycophenolate, probenecid, phenytoin	Digoxin, probenecid	Cimetidine, phenytoin, probenecid
Monitoring parameters	Serum creatinine, BUN, CBC/LFT if infection, anemia, or liver damage is suspected		

BUN, blood urea nitrogen; CBC, complete blood count; HGS, herpetic gingivostomatitis; HIV, human immunodeficiency virus; LFT, liver function test; RHL, recurrent herpes labialis.
[a]No evidence of efficacy if started beyond the prodrome stage.

include any product that has unproven efficacy or could be potentially damaging to the skin. Products of concern would be those that contain benzalkonium chloride (repeated use can dry out the skin) and salicylic acid (can erode the thin surface skin of the lip).[29]

Prescription nucleoside antiviral agents acyclovir and penciclovir have demonstrated efficacy in reducing healing times in RHL.[30,31] The cream formulation of acyclovir seems to perform better in trials, probably because of the ointment's poor skin penetration.[32] Acyclovir ointment can be used in immunocompromised patients. When compared in head-to-head trials, penciclovir seemed to outperform acyclovir.[33,34] However, the need to apply penciclovir about twice as often as acyclovir cream makes it a less convenient option for patients. A combination product containing 5% acyclovir and 1% hydrocortisone has been shown to reduce healing time and prevent ulcerative HSV-1 lesions from occurring to a greater extent than placebo and 5% acyclovir cream alone.[35]

Docosanol is a topical cream that can be bought without a prescription. It is active against HSV-1 and works by preventing the virus envelope from fusing with cells. The pivotal Phase III trial testing docosanol cream against a polyethylene glycol vehicle showed that docosanol reduces healing times if first applied during the prodrome stage.[36]

Dosage regimens for topical RHL treatments are in Table 3-10.

Prevention Strategies

One of the goals of RHL treatment, especially in those suffering from multiple outbreaks per year, is to decrease the number and severity of recurrences. Strategies to prevent recurrences of HSV-1 infection include basic avoidance of triggers (Table 3-8) when possible. While use of sunscreen has been shown to decrease the incidence of recurrence due to ultraviolet light,[37,38] these trials were performed under laboratory conditions and have not been verified in natural conditions.

In patients with regular recurrence and significant quality of life impairment as a result, the clinician may opt to use prophylactic drug therapy to reduce the recurrence rate. Oral acyclovir and valacyclovir have demonstrated efficacy in reducing RHL episodes in clinical trials.[39–41] A Cochrane review found that these two medications were also effective in RHL prevention in patients being treated for cancer, and that valacyclovir was no more effective than acyclovir.[42] Given that valacyclovir is a once-daily treatment and acyclovir is to be taken twice daily for prevention, valacyclovir may be the better choice for prevention, especially in patients

TABLE 3-10 Topical Antiviral Therapies for acute Herpes Labialis Infection			
Generic Name	Acyclovir	Penciclovir	Docosanol
Brand name	Zovirax	Denavir	Abreva
Rx only/OTC	Rx only	Rx only	OTC
Dosage form/route of administration	Cream (5%) Cream (5%) with hydrocortisone (1%) Ointment (5%)[a]	Cream (1%)	Cream (10%)
Dosing for adults and children ≥12 years old[b]	Cream: apply to lesion five times daily for 4 d	Apply to lesion every 2 h while awake for 4 d	Apply to lesion five times daily until lesion healed, up to 10 d
Contraindications	Hypersensitivity to acyclovir or valaclovir	Hypersensitivity to penciclovir or famciclovir	Hypersensitivity to docosanol
Common side effects	Pain, stinging, burning, redness at application site		

OTC, over-the-counter.

[a]Use of cream suggested over ointment because of lack of efficacy evidence.

[b]Needs to be started in the prodrome stage.

with low rates of medication adherence or who are on multiple concomitant medications.

PHARMACOTHERAPY FOR A COMMON OROFACIAL FUNGAL INFECTION: ORAL CANDIDIASIS

Over 150 species of *Candida* fungi exist, but *C. albicans* is most frequently detected commensal fungus of immunocompetent individuals, with colonization in up to 80% of healthy persons.[43] Conditions in the oral cavity must change in order to promote overgrowth and infection with *Candida*. Patients who are immunosuppressed through another condition (such as HIV/AIDS[44]), by medications (such as antibiotics[45] or inhaled corticosteroids[46]), or by a combination of both (such as cancer[47]) are at higher risk for development of primary oral candidiasis (POC). Other common risk factors include, but are not limited to: extremes of age (infants or elderly), diabetes mellitus, xerostomia, poor oral hygiene, chronic local irritation of oral mucosal membranes, and use of oral prostheses.[48]

POC can manifest several different ways, but the most common is acute pseudomembranous candidiasis (commonly called thrush). Pseudomembranous candidiasis has an extremely low mortality risk, but quality of life can be severely impaired by an infection. Patients will often complain of a burning mouth and trouble swallowing, eating, or tasting food, which can lead to unintended weight loss.[48] Acute atrophic or erythematous candidiasis is a common manifestation in HIV-infected patients,[44] and fungal angular cheilitis is a common problem in the young, old, and denture wearers.[48] Most infections will be limited to mucous membranes in the oral cavity, but there is a chance that the fungus could spread to the esophagus or the bloodstream in severely immunocompromised individuals.[48]

Treatment of Oral Candidiasis

Treatment of POC differs based on the severity of disease. For mild disease, the Infectious Diseases Society of America (IDSA) suggests topical treatment with either nystatin suspension or pastilles (no longer available in the United States) or clotrimazole troches (see Table 3-11 for topical therapy options).[49] There are no head-to-head trials of nystatin and clotrimazole for the treatment of POC. Since the latest version of the IDSA guidelines were released in 2009, the Food and Drug Administration (FDA) approved a once-daily miconazole buccal tablet, which was shown to be comparable to clotrimazole for the treatment of OC.[50] The advantage of the buccal tablet is that it is a once-daily treatment. The choice of topical agent should be based primarily on patient preference and product availability. Moderate-to-severe disease should be treated with systemic antifungals.

Triazole antifungal choices for POC include fluconazole, itraconazole, voriconazole, and posaconazole. Ketoconazole has fallen out of favor because of lower OC cure rates compared to fluconazole and concerns about drug-drug interactions and hepatotoxicity.[51] The IDSA lists fluconazole as the drug of choice in moderate-to-severe POC.[49] While efficacy between triazoles does not differ significantly, fluconazole and itraconazole solution have been shown to be superior to ketoconazole and itraconazole capsules in immunocompromised patients.[52-56] Itraconazole solution or posaconazole are first-choice agents for POC cases refractory to treatment with fluconazole (see Table 3-12). Amphotericin B oral suspension or voriconazole are last-line options for patients that fail itraconazole or posaconazole. If none of the oral options work, intravenous amphotericin B or a drug from the echinocandin class can be used. Continuous fluconazole is the drug of choice in prevention of POC in immunosuppressed patients.[49]

Treatment of Angular Cheilitis

Angular cheilitis has many different etiologies. Colonizing organisms such as β-hemolytic streptococci, *S. aureus* and *C. albicans* can develop into pathogens. If angular cheilitis does not have a bacterial or fungal origin, barrier creams such as petrolatum, zinc oxide, or lip balm can help protect

TABLE 3-11 Topical Prescription Medications for the Treatment of Oral Candidiasis

Generic Name	Clotrimazole	Miconazole	Nystatin
Brand name	Mycelex	Oravig	Mycostatin
Dosage form/route of administration	Troche (10 mg)	Tablet (50 mg)	Oral suspension (100,000 units/mL)
Usual adult dosage	10 mg troche dissolved in mouth five times daily for 7–14 d[a]	Apply one tablet to upper gum above incisor qd for 14 d	4–6 mL swished around in mouth for 1 min qid for 7–14 d[a]
Contraindications	None	Milk protein hypersensitivity	None
Precautions	Azole hypersensitivity	Azole hypersensitivity, hepatic impairment	Diabetes mellitus (contains sucrose), paraben hypersensitivity
Common side effects	Abdominal pain, nausea, diarrhea	Gingival pruritus, burning, or pain, toothache, nausea, vomiting, diarrhea, dysgeusia	Stomach upset
Rare but important side effects	Oral pruritus, elevated liver enzymes	Elevated hepatic enzymes	None
Important drug interactions	Tacrolimus	Cisapride, ranolazine, cilostazol	None
Monitoring parameters	Clinical cure	Clinical cure	Clinical cure

[a]use at least 48 hours after resolution.

TABLE 3-12 Systemic Prescription Medications for the Treatment of Oral Candidiasis

Clinical Use	First-line Agent	First-line If Refractory to Fluconazole	
Generic name	Fluconazole	Itraconazole	Posaconazole
Brand name	Diflucan	Sporanox	Noxafil
Dosage form/route of administration	Tablet (50, 100, 150, 200 mg) Oral suspension (10, 40 mg/mL)	Oral solution (10 mg/mL)	Oral suspension (200 mg/5 mL)
Usual adult dosage	200 mg on day 1, then 100 mg qd for 7–14 d	200 mg qd for 7–14 d	400 mg qd-bid for 7–14 d in refractory disease
Contraindications		Heart failure, ventricular dysfunction, pregnancy, co-administration with drug metabolized by CYP 3A4	Hypersensitivity to voriconazole
Precautions	Arrhythmias, hepatic disease, renal impairment, azole hypersensitivity	Ischemic heart disease, azole hypersensitivity, neutropenia	Arrhythmias, hepatic disease, azole hypersensitivity
Common side effects	Nausea, vomiting, headache, abdominal pain	Nausea, vomiting, diarrhea, headache, rash, fever	Arrhythmias, hypertension, hypotension, GI adverse events, rash, pruritus, hypokalemia, hyperglycemia, hypomagnesemia, hypocalcemia, blood dyscrasias
Rare but important side effects	Exfoliative skin disorders, hepatotoxicity, QT prolongation	QT prolongation, edema, hypertension, decreases in left ventricular function, elevated hepatic enzymes	Adrenal insufficiency, hepatic enzyme elevations, QT prolongation
Important drug interactions	Drugs metabolized through CYP 3A4 (weak inhibitor), CYP 2C9 (potent inhibitor), and CYP 2C19 (possible inhibitor)	Drugs metabolized through CYP 3A4 (potent inhibitor) and p-glycoprotein (may inhibit)	Ergot alkaloids, any drug that prolongs the QT interval, any drug that is metabolized through CYP 3A4 (potent inhibitor), any drug that is a p-glycoprotein inhibitor or is metabolized through p-glycoprotein (inhibitor)
Monitoring parameters	Serum creatinine and BUN, liver function tests	Liver function tests (long-term use)	Serum electrolytes

irritated skin. In the case of a fungal infection, topical nystatin or ketoconazole cream can be applied twice daily for sevendays. Nystatin also can be obtained with triamcinolone, a mild corticosteroid, to reduce inflammation. Bacterial angular cheilitis can be cured using mupirocin topical ointment three to four times daily.[48,57]

Denture Stomatitis

Dentures with soft liners are especially prone to fungal colonization because of leaching processes and the difficulty of manually cleaning the liner. Among denture wearers, the prevalence of denture stomatitis can be near 70%, and wearing dentures at night greatly increases the odds of developing a fungal infection.[58,59]

There is little evidence to suggest nystatin may be useful when applied to denture liners,[59] and topical nystatin has not demonstrated sustained clinical efficacy.[60] Even systemic antifungals such as fluconazole and itraconazole have incomplete efficacy in the treatment of denture stomatitis.[61] Overnight chlorhexidine and chlorine-based soaks have demonstrated efficacy,[59,62,63] but the American College of Prosthodontists does not recommend soaking dentures in sodium hypochlorite for longer than 10 minutes.[58]

Measures for the treatment of denture stomatitis should focus on oral hygiene (including manually cleaning dentures and using approved denture soaks) and removing dentures at night before bed. If a fungal infection is suspected, no treatment seems to work better than another; patient preference, product availability, and convenience (both cost and pill or drug burden) should all be taken into consideration. The infection should be treated two weeks beyond visible cure.

PHARMACOTHERAPY FOR ORAL LESIONS

Pharmacotherapy for Ulcerative Lesions

The main goal of treatment in active recurrent aphthous stomatitis (RAS) is to minimize symptoms while the patient waits for remission of intraoral ulcerations. While the disease is in remission, the goal is to reduce the frequency of recurrence. Basic management of an active ulcer can include antiseptics such as chlorhexidine and topical anesthetics such as lidocaine (see Table 3-17 for dosing).[64,65] For isolated recurrent ulceration, guidelines suggest topical corticosteroids applied twice daily for both RAS and Behçet disease (BD).[64,66] Resistant cases can be treated with higher-potency topical steroids (see Table 3-22), although most topical steroids are not formulated to adhere to mucosal surfaces in the oral cavity. Topical steroids should be used with caution in the oral cavity, as prolonged use can lead to oral candidiasis. For refractory or recurrent forms of ulcerative lesions, oral corticosteroids such as prednisone can be used, although long-term use of oral steroids can lead to serious adverse events (see Table 3-23). Other oral medications that have been useful in reducing ulceration recurrence include colchicine, pentoxifylline, azathioprine, thalidomide, and dapsone.[65] Isolated trials have demonstrated a benefit for injectable immunosuppressant medications, such as interferon alfa products, infliximab, and etanercept, in refractory BD.[66]

Pharmacotherapy for Oral Lichen Planus

Treatment of oral lichen planus (OLP) is aimed at symptom management, as the disease is difficult to treat. There is a lack of evidence for traditional OLP treatments, including topical and oral corticosteroids.[67] Intralesional steroid injections are not advised as they can cause mucosal atrophy and be quite painful.[68] There is some evidence to show topical pimecrolimus or tacrolimus might either be considered a first-line therapy or be useful in steroid-refractory cases,[69–72] but there is some concern that long-term use may be associated with malignancies. Oral immunosuppressants such as thalidomide, methotrexate, and mycophenolate have been used in OLP, but there is no evidence for their benefit outside of case reports.[73,74]

Therapy for Other Oral Lesions

Other vesiculobullous conditions with oral manifestations such as pemphigus vulgaris, bullous pemphigoid, and mucous membrane pemphigoid are usually managed with topical corticosteroids where possible. For refractory disease or to induce remission, combinations of oral corticosteroids and immunosuppressant medications such as azathioprine, dapsone, mycophenolate, or cyclophosphamide can be used.[75] There is no evidence to suggest one treatment is better than another.

PHARMACOTHERAPY FOR SALIVARY GLAND DISORDERS

Sialadenitis

Inflammation of salivary glands usually involves either the submandibular or parotid gland and is most commonly of bacterial origin. Predisposing factors to sialadenitis include older age, recent surgery and anesthetic use, salivary calculi, and anything that can slow or stop salivary flow including concomitant conditions (e.g., Sjögren's syndrome, sarcoidosis, dehydration), head or neck radiation chemotherapy, and medications (e.g., diuretics, opioids, radioactive iodine, anticholinergics).[76] For more details, see Chapter 10, "Salivary Gland Diseases." In community-acquired acute bacterial sialadenitis, the most common causative pathogen is *S. aureus*, which can be eradicated using an antibiotic with Gram-positive coverage such as amoxicillin with clavulanate or clindamycin (see Table 3-3).[77] Bacterial parotid sialadenitis is typically unilateral while viral presents most often bilaterally.[76] Most viral salivary gland infections manifest as viral parotitis with the most common cause being the mumps virus, Rubulavirus. Treatment of parotitis caused by mumps is usually supportive, with medications such as NSAIDs and acetaminophen being used to relieve pain and inflammation. Antiviral medications such as valacyclovir and acyclovir discussed earlier in this chapter would only be indicated in cases of HSV or cytomegalovirus infection.

Xerostomia

The mainstays of treatment of xerostomia involve palliative care such as sipping water, sucking on ice chips, and sugar-free lozenges, gums, and candies, which can stimulate saliva production. Non-prescription products include a wide variety of saliva substitutes in liquid and spray form that contain viscosity enhancers to increase retention time, electrolytes to mimic natural saliva, and flavoring agents for palatability. Though widely recommended and used, there is little evidence to show any saliva substitute is effective for xerostomia.[78] An oxygenated glycerol triester spray (Aquoral®) has been shown to be more beneficial than a water-based saliva substitute spray,[78,79] but it is prescription-only in the United States and costs a significant amount more than over-the-counter liquid and spray substitutes.

The treatment of choice for patients with xerostomia having residual salivary function is a sialagogue (see Table 3-25). Pilocarpine is a nonspecific cholinergic drug that primarily stimulates muscarinic receptors leading to increased secretion by exocrine glands. Cevimeline has a high affinity for muscarinic M3 receptors in salivary and lacrimal glands. Both drugs have proven efficacy in patients who have xerostomia due to Sjögren's syndrome or head-and-neck radiation treatment,[80–87] but because of its nonspecific receptor binding, pilocarpine has a higher incidence of side effects. Each drug has a carryover effect,[88] which suggests that patients may be able to have drug-free days, leading to fewer side effects and lower medication costs. In patients with a total loss of salivary gland function or tissue, such as those who have tissue loss due to radiation therapy, sialagogues will be of no use.

Sialorrhea and Drooling

Sialorrhea is the excess production of saliva while drooling is the spillage of normal saliva production from the anterior floor of the mouth.[89,90] Patients with neurological deficits, such as those with amyotrophic lateral sclerosis, Parkinson's disease, or cerebral palsy, often suffer from drooling. Other causes of drooling or sialorrhea can be drug-induced (clozapine[91]), oral or dental deformities, gastroesophageal reflux, nasal obstruction, and painful swallowing leading to pooling of saliva.

Traditional medications for the treatment of drooling target the reduction of saliva production using anticholinergic mechanisms. While they will reduce salivary output, they do not treat the underlying neuromuscular problems, so some patients may find the anticholinergic side effects outweigh the benefit of the drug. Additionally, the drying effect these medications have can lead to xerostomia, especially if the patient has a constant open mouth. Glycopyrrolate is the most common prescription medication for sialorrhea and drooling (see Table 3-26), with atropine sulfate, scopolamine, amitriptyline, and benztropine also being reported in the literature. OnabotulinumtoxinA (Botox®) injections into salivary glands with ultrasonic guidance have shown to be of some benefit in patients who have failed or are intolerant to anticholinergics.[89,90,92]

Prophylaxis for Radiation-Induced Xerostomia

Mucositis and xerostomia are acute side effects that are common during and after radiotherapy of the head and neck. Xerostomia often persists because the radiotherapy destroys salivary gland cells, leaving any residual salivary secretions more viscous. Amifostine is a radioprotective agent originally developed by the military that has indications for nephrotoxicity and xerostomia prophylaxis (Table 3-27). Amifostine reduces the incidence of both acute and chronic xerostomia in patients undergoing head and neck radiotherapy and has varying efficacy in reducing acute mucositis.[93–95] The use of amifostine has been associated with reduced incidence of tooth decay and loss.[96] Amifostine use does not seem to influence head-and-neck cancer control rates.[93–95]

PHARMACOTHERAPY FOR OROFACIAL PAIN

Orofacial pain typically results from two general pathologic mechanisms: (1) tissue injury and inflammation (*nociceptive pain*) or (2) a primary lesion or dysfunction of the nervous system (*neuropathic pain*). The first step in management of orofacial pain is to determine if the pain is primarily nociceptive or neuropathic or a combination of the two. This determination is critical for selecting medication(s) whose mechanisms of action will address the underlying pathophysiology (Figure 3-3). Although this determination is often straightforward in instances of acute pain such as toothache or mucosal pain with proximate physical findings (tenderness, signs of injury and inflammation), the determination can be more challenging when the pain is persistent without a clear local cause (e.g., myofascial pain, neuropathic pain). For additional information on this subject, see Chapter 12, "Orofacial Pain."

Pharmacotherapy for Nociceptive Orofacial Pain

There are three major etiologies of nociceptive orofacial pain: *odontogenic conditions* (e.g., pulpitis, apical periodontitis), *mucosal conditions* (e.g., ulcers, lichen planus, herpes simplex), and *musculoskeletal conditions* (e.g., myofascial pain, temporomandibular joint capsulitis, arthritis). With the exception of myofascial pain, these conditions result from an identifiable source of tissue injury and inflammation and nociceptor sensitization. Pain due to inflammation may also have an underlying infectious etiology; therefore, both anti-inflammatory analgesics and antimicrobial medications could be required (see **PHARMACOTHERAPY FOR OROFACIAL BACTERIAL INFECTIONS**).

While nociceptive orofacial pain can resolve spontaneously once the underlying cause (e.g., inflamed pulp, carious lesion, abscessed gingiva) is treated, a pharmacologic approach to pain management is the standard of care (Figure 3-3).[97] Based on current evidence, the drugs of choice to treat nociceptive orofacial pain are acetaminophen and non-steroidal anti-inflammatory drugs (NSAID). NSAIDs act by inhibiting cyclooxygenase (COX) enzymes responsible for the formation of prostaglandins that promote pain and inflammation.[98] Some commonly prescribed NSAIDs are included in Table 3-13. The synergistic effects of acetaminophen and an NSAID have been repeatedly shown to offer superior analgesic effects to either drug alone and they have a better side effect profile and less potential for abuse compared to opioids.[99] NSAIDs have also been shown to reduce postoperative nausea and vomiting by 30% compared to narcotics.[100] The most effective dose for the shortest period of time will provide the greatest pain relief balanced against patient safety. Strong familiarity with individual maximum recommended doses cannot be stressed enough.

For simplicity, practitioners could rely on the "2-4-24" (2 drugs, 4 doses, for 24 hours) mnemonic as the postoperative prescription of choice for acute nociceptive orofacial pain: a combination of ibuprofen 600 mg plus acetaminophen 1000 mg administered every 6 hours for 24 hours.[101] Due to the inflammatory process and the pharmacokinetics of these medications, routine dosing during the initial 24-hour postoperative period is required. If a patient is compliant with these four doses of two different medications, the majority of cases will not require any further analgesic medication beyond the first 24 hours. These doses can be administered every six hours either together or in a staggered fashion based on dentist and patient preference. The staggered approach is sometimes valuable for patients whom more frequent medication administration can be more psychologically beneficial following dental surgery. The key to success of this analgesic regimen is adherence; this will require patients setting alarms so that they do not miss the nighttime doses during the initial 24-hour postoperative period.

After the initial 24-hour postoperative period, patients can take pain medication solely on an "as needed" basis (either drug alone, or in combination). If patients still require routine pain medication after the initial 48 hours following the dental procedure despite excellent compliance, re-examination by the dental practitioner should be strongly encouraged.

Acetaminophen or a NSAID can also be given preoperatively to mitigate postoperative pain and postoperative

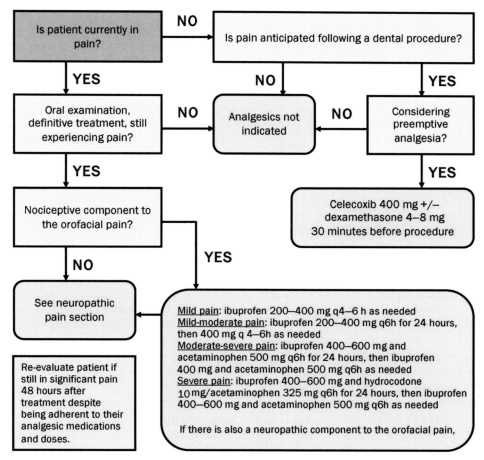

FIGURE 3-3 Stepwise guidelines for orofacial pain.

TABLE 3-13   Selected Non-Steroidal Anti-Inflammatory Drugs for Mild to Moderate Nociceptive Pain[151,152]

Generic Name	Celecoxib	Diclofenac	Ibuprofen	Naproxen	Naproxen Sodium
Brand name(s)	Celebrex	Voltaren	Motrin, Advil	Naprelan, Naprosyn	Aleve, Anaprox
Prescription status	Rx only	Rx only	Rx and OTC	Rx	Rx and OTC
Usual adult dosages[a]	200 mg q12h	50mg q12h	200–400 mg q4–6h	250 mg q6–8h or 500 mg q12h	275 mg q6–8h or 550 mg q12h
Maximum recommended daily dose	600 mg first day then 400 mg	200 mg	2400 mg	1250 mg first day, then 1000 mg	1375 mg first day, then 1100 mg
Notes	Less effective than full doses of naproxen or ibuprofen	Do not crush or chew	Available as OTC suspension (100 mg/5 mL)	Available as Rx suspension (125 mg/5 mL)	220 mg dose is available OTC

OTC, over-the-counter (nonprescription); Rx, prescription required for certain strengths.
[a]Based on 70 kg adult with normal hepatic and renal function.
Food decreases the rate of absorption and may delay the time to peak levels.
Use caution in allergy, renal or liver impairment, combination with anticoagulant or antiplatelet medications. Common side effects include dyspepsia, nausea, abdominal pain, headache, dizziness, somnolence, rash, elevated liver enzymes, constipation, fluid retention, peripheral edema, tinnitus, and ecchymosis.

pain medication requirements (*preemptive analgesia*).[102] This strategy could also include a glucocorticoid, such as dexamethasone 4 mg orally 30 minutes prior to the procedure.[103] A COX-2 selective NSAID such as celecoxib is ideal for preemptive analgesia as it will ameliorate the inflammatory response without prolonging bleeding or delaying wound healing compared to the non-selective NSAIDs.[104] The recommended dose is 400 mg administered orally 30 minutes prior to the procedure. For patients currently on an anticoagulant such as warfarin (Coumadin®), dabigatran (Pradaxa®), rivaroxaban (Xarelto®), or apixiban (Eliquis®), a COX-2 inhibitor such as celecoxib could replace the postoperative ibuprofen 600 mg prescription above as 200 mg given every 12 hours for the initial 24-hour postoperative period.

Since opioid-based analgesics are not anti-inflammatory agents, medications such as morphine, hydrocodone, and oxycodone are not considered drugs of choice in treating the three major categories of nociceptive orofacial pain. These medications should be reserved for the small percentage of dental patients with severe, uncontrolled orofacial and postoperative pain, and even then they are best prescribed as combination products which contain acetaminophen or a NSAID in addition to the narcotic moiety.[99]

Opioid-based analgesics used for orofacial pain share the common mechanism of agonist activity principally at the mu-opioid receptor, enhancing the effect of the endogenous pain-relieving chemicals dynorphin, enkephalin, and β-endorphin. Opioid-based analgesics have short half-lives and require repeat dosing (e.g., every four hours in the case of morphine); controlled-release formulations typically allow for twice-daily dosing with improved compliance and baseline pain relief for chronic pain (Table 3-14). Unlike NSAIDs, opioid-based analgesics do not have an analgesic ceiling, and increased pain relief can always be achieved by increasing doses. However, side effects are also

dose-dependent and can limit the maximum tolerated dose. Opioid-based analgesics are controlled substances due to high abuse potential.

Pharmacotherapy for Neuropathic Orofacial Pain

Treede et al. define neuropathic pain as "pain arising as a direct consequence of a lesion or disease affecting the somatosensory system."[105] Neuropathic orofacial pains include the classic cranial neuralgias (trigeminal and glossopharyngeal) and postherpetic neuralgia. Other forms of neuropathic orofacial pain include primary stomatodynia (burning mouth), phantom tooth pain (atypical odontalgia), and traumatic nerve injuries. Unlike nociceptive pain, neuropathic pain does not reflect actual tissue damage, but can be triggered by tissue injury and usually persists long after the injury has healed. The hallmark signs of neuropathic pain are mechanical hyperalgesia and allodynia, constant burning or paroxysmal shooting pain, and, less commonly, constant aching or pressure pain.[106] A minority of patients do not have pain as the primary manifestation of neuropathy but instead experience dysmorphic symptoms, paresthesia, and/or altered taste. Nociceptive pain can play a role in the initiation and maintenance of persistent neuropathic orofacial pain, and treatment may require analgesics (for nociceptive pain) alone or in combination with medications for neuropathic pain. Primary neuropathic pain can also have an inflammatory component, and effective management will require medications from multiple classes (e.g., anti-inflammatory medications, antibiotics).

Antidepressants and anticonvulsants are the mainstay of pharmacologic treatment for a variety of neuropathic pain syndromes, even though most are used off-label for these indications (Table 3-15). Combining an antidepressant and an anticonvulsant will produce a synergistic analgesic effect

TABLE 3-14 Opioid-Based Analgesics Commonly Used for Orofacial Pain[151,152]

Generic Name	Codeine	Hydrocodone	Morphine	Oxycodone	Tramadol
Available strengths with dosage forms	Oral solution (6 mg/mL) Tablet (15, 30, 60 mg)	ER capsule (10, 15, 20, 30, 40, 50 mg)	Biphasic ER capsule (30, 45, 60, 75, 90, 120 mg) ER capsule (10, 20, 30, 40, 50, 60, 70, 80, 100, 130, 150, 200 mg) ER tablet (15, 30, 60, 100, 200 mg) Oral solution (2, 4, 20 mg/mL) IR tablet (15, 30 mg)	Abuse-deterrent tablet (5, 7.5 mg) Capsule (5 mg) ER tablet (10, 15, 20, 30, 40, 60, 80 mg) IR tablet (5, 10, 15, 20, 30 mg) Oral solution (1, 20 mg/5 mL)	ER tablet (100, 200, 300 mg) Multiphase ER/IR capsule (100, 150, 200, 300 mg) ODT (50 mg) Tablet (50 mg)
Available in combination with APAP?	Yes	Yes	No	Yes	Yes
Available in combination with NSAID?	Yes (ASA)	Yes (ibuprofen)	No	Yes (ASA or ibuprofen)	No
Duration of action	4 h	ER: 12 h IR (combination products): 4 h	Biphasic ER: 24 h ER: 12 h All others: 8–12 h	ER: 12 h IR: 4 h	ER: 24 h IR: 6 h
Usual adult starting dosage	15–60 mg q4h	ER: 10 mg q12h IR (combination products): 5–10 mg q4–6h	Biphasic ER: 30 mg once daily ER: 15–30 mg q8–12h All others: 10–30 mg q4h	ER: 10 mg q12h IR: 5–15 mg q4–6h	ODT: 50 mg q4–6h Tablet: 50–100 mg q4–6h All others: 100 mg once daily
Notes	60 mg PO equivalent to 650 mg of ASA or APAP; 10% of people lack the enzyme (CYP 2D6) needed to make codeine active	The efficacy of the combination of hydrocodone and APAP is similar to that of codeine plus APAP; ER hydrocodone capsule not indicated for as-needed pain relief	Maximum dose of biphasic ER capsules is 1,600 mg due to renal toxicity of fumaric acid in the beads; chewing or crushing these beads can be fatal	Brands Oxecta and OxyContin have been reformulated to deter abuse of the drug by injection or snorting	Multiphase ER/IR capsules: 100 mg contains 25 mg IR and 75 mg ER, 200 mg contains 50 mg IR and 150 mg ER, 300 mg contains 50 mg IR and 250 mg ER

APAP, acetaminophen; ASA, aspirin; ER, extended-release; IR, immediate-release; ODT, orally disintegrating tablet.

TABLE 3-15 Commonly Used Medications for the Treatment of Neuropathic Pain Syndromes[151,152]

Generic Name (Brand Name)	Drug Class	Usual Daily Dosage for Neuropathic Pain	FDA-Approved Indications
Amitriptyline (Elavil)	TCA	25–100 mg qd (usually at bedtime)	Depression
Bupropion (Wellbutrin)	Oral antidepressant	IR: 100–150 mg qd–bid ER: 100–450 mg qd	Depression, seasonal affective disorder, smoking cessation
Carbamazepine (Carbatrol, Tegretol)	Anticonvulsant	400–800 mg divided bid	Bipolar disorder, epilepsy, trigeminal, or glossopharyngeal neuralgia
Desipramine (Norpramin)	TCA	Starting dose: 10–25 mg/d; usual effective dose: 50–150 mg/d	Depression
Desvenlafaxine (Khedezla, Pristiq)	SNRI	50 mg qd	Depression

(Continued)

TABLE 3-15 Commonly Used Medications for the Treatment of Neuropathic Pain Syndromes[151,152] (Continued)

Generic Name (Brand Name)	Drug Class	Usual Daily Dosage for Neuropathic Pain	FDA-Approved Indications
Duloxetine (Cymbalta)	SNRI	60 mg qd	Depression, diabetic neuropathy, fibromyalgia, generalized anxiety disorder, musculoskeletal pain, osteoarthritis
Gabapentin (Gralise, Horizant, Neurontin)	Anticonvulsant	IR: 1800–3600 mg divided tid ER: 1800 mg qd	Epilepsy, postherpetic neuralgia, restless legs syndrome, trigeminal neuralgia
Imipramine (Tofranil)	TCA	50–100 mg qd or in divided doses	Depression, enuresis in children
Milnacipran (Savella)	SNRI	50 mg bid	Fibromyalgia
Nortriptyline (Pamelor)	TCA	75 mg qd or in divided doses	Depression
Oxcarbazepine (Oxtellar, Trileptal)	Anticonvulsant	IR: 600–1,200 mg divided bid ER: 600–2400 mg qd	Partial seizures
Pregabalin (Lyrica)	Anticonvulsant	150–600 mg divided bid or tid	Epilepsy, fibromyalgia, neuropathic pain, postherpetic neuralgia
Venlafaxine (Effexor)	SNRI	IR: 75 mg qd or divided up to tid ER: 75–150 mg qd	Depression, generalized anxiety disorder, panic disorder, social anxiety disorder

ER, extended-release; FDA, United States Food and Drug Administration; IR, immediate-release; SNRI, serotonin-norepinephrine reuptake inhibitor; TCA, tricyclic antidepressant.

in neuropathic pain syndromes. It is interesting to note that while many medications used for nociceptive pain will be effective to a certain degree for neuropathic pain, the opposite is not true. There is limited to moderate evidence for the efficacy of anticonvulsants in orofacial pain disorders.[107]

Classic Cranial Neuralgias

While many oral health-care professionals will not prescribe the following agents, they could choose to make recommendations to the patient's medical practitioner or encounter patients who are taking them. Carbamazepine is FDA-approved for the treatment of pain due to trigeminal neuralgia. Oxcarbazepine, which is related to carbamazepine, has been shown to provide similar analgesia with fewer adverse effects and no need for drug level monitoring. Gabapentin is also FDA-approved for treatment of pain due to trigeminal neuralgia and several studies have shown that taking lower doses of gabapentin and morphine together provided better analgesia than taking either drug alone for trigeminal neuralgias.[108] Pregabalin, which is similar in structure to gabapentin, is approved for treatment of neuropathic pain associated with postherpetic neuralgia, diabetic peripheral neuropathy, and fibromyalgia. The dose of pregabalin can be titrated more rapidly than that of gabapentin, but because of some reports of euphoria, pregabalin is classified in the United States as a Schedule V controlled substance.[109]

While they are not first-line treatment and are primarily off-label, tricyclic antidepressants (TCA) such as amitriptyline, nortriptyline, and imipramine can relieve many types of neuropathic pain, including diabetic neuropathy,

postherpetic neuralgia, polyneuropathy, fibromyalgia, and nerve injury. The analgesic effects of these drugs are likely due to their inhibition of norepinephrine and serotonin reuptake. However, due to antagonism of cholinergic and histaminergic systems, side effects include sedation, urinary retention and hypotension. Selective serotonin reuptake inhibitors (SSRI) such as paroxetine and fluoxetine appear to be less effective than TCAs for treatment of neuropathic pain.[110] While as effective as TCAs for depression with fewer adverse effects, SSRIs do not possess analgesic properties.[111] Venlafaxine is a selective serotonin and norepinephrine reuptake inhibitor (SNRI) and has been shown to be effective in patients suffering from classic cranial neuralgias secondary to implant surgery.[112]

Ziconotide is a synthetic neuronal N-type calcium channel blocker administered intrathecally via a programmable microinfusion device for treatment of severe chronic pain refractory to other treatments. The drug has been effective, both as monotherapy and when added to standard therapy, for treatment of refractory severe chronic pain, including neuropathic pain. Severe psychiatric effects (paranoid reactions, psychosis) and central nervous system (CNS) toxicity (confusion, somnolence, unresponsiveness) can occur. Unlike opioids, ziconotide does not cause tolerance, dependence, or respiratory depression, and is not a controlled substance.[113]

Primary Stomatodynia

Burning mouth syndrome (stomatodynia) is associated with changes of a neuropathic nature the main location of which, peripheral or central, remains unknown. Functional magnetic resonance imaging studies suggest that stomatodynia patients have impaired brain network dynamics essential for descending inhibition, leading to diminished inhibitory control of sensory experience; as a consequence they may experience intraoral proprioception as burning pain.[114] Prior to making this diagnosis, it is important to rule out oral mucosal diseases, such as herpes simplex and aphthous stomatitis.[115] Other common conditions associated with mouth pain are psychiatric disorders, xerostomia (from drugs, connective tissue disease, or age), nutritional deficiencies (vitamins B_6 or B_{12}, iron, folate, zinc), and allergic contact stomatitis.[116]

If primary stomatodynia persists despite investigating and treating other common conditions associated with mouth pain (i.e. vitamin supplementation, zinc replacement, hormone replacement treatment and others), then topical drug treatment with capsaicin, clonazepam, lidocaine, benzydamine hydrochloride 0.15%, or aloe vera have been used with varying levels of success.

Treatment algorithms with systemic medications for stomatodynia continue to rank TCAs as first-line agents with either gabapentin or pregabalin as second choices (Table 3-15). Gabapentin or pregabalin are first-line agents in the elderly or when TCAs are contraindicated given their preferred side effect profile. Opioids are considered third-line agents.[114,116,117] Clonazepam and alpha-lipoic acid have demonstrated limited success in the treatment of stomatodynia. Clonazepam is a benzodiazepine and is started at 0.25 mg daily and increased by 0.25 mg weekly as needed. Doses of 3–6 mg daily (given in three divided doses) are common when treating burning mouth syndrome.[116] Alpha-lipoic acid can be used at doses ranging from 200–1800 mg daily. Most often it is given in the range of 200–600 mg daily in one or two divided doses. Doses higher than 600 mg daily are more likely to lead to adverse events (nausea, vomiting, vertigo).[117]

Other Neuropathic Face Pain

Other neuropathic pain in the facial region has been termed by the International Headache Society as persistent idiopathic facial pain and is subsequently described as persistent facial pain that does not have the characteristics of the cranial neuralgias and is not attributed to another disorder.[118] If a patient fails on the more traditional medications mentioned above, a trial-and-error approach can be attempted with other drugs that have been used for neuropathic pain, including but not limited to phenytoin, carbamazepine, clonazepam, valproate, phenothiazines, venlafaxine, mexiletine, and baclofen. Limited scientific evidence is available regarding these pharmacotherapy choices for neuropathic face pain and is based primarily on case reports in the literature.

Adjuvant Pharmacotherapy for Orofacial Pain

This category of medications includes four major classes of medication: the antidepressants and anticonvulsants described in Table 3-15 and the anxiolytics and muscle relaxants described in Table 3-16. Anticonvulsant and antidepressant classes generally affect conductance of ions that reduce neuronal excitability (Na, K, Ca, Cl). Anxiolytics and muscle relaxants are primarily centrally-acting agents (i.e., not at the neuromuscular junction). For most chronic orofacial pain conditions, the use of these medications is considered off-label, although there is considerable biomedical literature in support of their use.

Topical medications from several different drug classes can be very effective in providing local analgesia and can be mixed with mucosal adherent formulations for improved efficacy (Table 3-17). Scientific evidence from clinical trials is limited regarding these pharmacotherapy choices,[119] but nearly any drug that causes a local action can be formulated for topical use by a compounding pharmacy. There has been recent interest in using compounded topical gabapentin, antidepressants, NSAIDs, N-methyl-D-aspartate antagonists (dextromethorphan, memantine), opioids, and α_2-adrenergic agonists (clonidine), but standardized dosing guidelines are not yet available. Surgical approaches and the use of platelet-rich plasma have also been investigated for the treatment of neuropathic pain but these techniques are still experimental and cannot be recommended at this time.[120]

LOCAL ANESTHETICS
Injectables

Local anesthetics are the primary means of pain control during clinical dentistry. The first ester local anesthetics developed included procaine (Novocain®) and propoxycaine (Ravocaine®) in the early 1900s. These early formulations exhibited poor tissue diffusion, potent vasodilation, and were associated with frequent allergic reactions.[121,122] In the 1940's, lidocaine was introduced as the first amide-type local anesthetic with key improvements in speed of onset, duration of action, and reduced allergenicity.[123] Currently in the United States only amide-type local anesthetics are available for injection (see Table 3-24).

The mechanism of action of local anesthetics involves reversibly blocking the influx of sodium ions along the cell membrane, preventing the generation and conduction of nerve impulses.[122,124,125] In most patients, proper injection of local anesthetic quickly results in loss of pain sensation; however, sensations of temperature, touch, pressure, and motor function may only be modestly affected. This is explained by local anesthetics' preferential ability to block small nerve fibers more effectively compared to larger fibers (A-delta and C fibers are most susceptible to blockade).[125–127]

Structurally, injectable local anesthetics have three components: an aromatic moiety, an intermediate linkage, and a secondary or tertiary amine.[124,127] The aromatic portion is responsible for lipophilicity of the medication and can influence protein binding characteristics. The intermediate linkage defines the medication as either an ester or amide

TABLE 3-16 Anxiolytics and Muscle Relaxants as Adjuvant Pharmacotherapy for Neuropathic Orofacial Pain

Generic Name (Brand Name)	Drug Class	Usual Daily Dosage for Neuropathic Pain	FDA-Approved Indications
Baclofen (Lioresal)	SMR	5 mg tid, may increase 5 mg/dose every 3 d to a maximum of 80 mg/d	Muscle spasticity
Carisoprodol (Soma, Vanadom)	SMR	25–350 mg tid–qid	Muscle spasticity
Chlorzoxazone (Lorzone, Parafon Forte, Relax-DS)	SMR	500–750 mg tid–qid	Muscle spasticity
Clonazepam (Klonopin)	BZD	0.25 mg at bedtime for 1 w; increase dose by 0.25 mg every week (max dose: 1 mg tid)	Pain disorder, seizure disorder
Cyclobenzaprine (Amrix, Flexeril)	SMR	IR: 5–10 mg tid; ER: 15–30 mg qd	Muscle spasticity
Diazepam (Valium)	BZD	2–10 mg tid–qid	Anxiety, ethanol withdrawal, muscle spasticity, sedation induction, seizure disorders
Doxepin (Silenor, Sinequan)	TCA	10–50 mg at bedtime	Anxiety, depression, insomnia
Metaxalone (Skelaxin)	SMR	800 mg tid–qid	Muscle spasticity
Methocarbamol (Robaxin)	SMR	1.5 g qid for 2–3 d then decrease to 4–4.5 g/d in 3–6 divided doses	Muscle spasticity
Orphenadrine (Norflex)	SMR	100 mg bid	Muscle spasticity
Tizanidine (Zanaflex)	SMR	4–8 mg tid–qid	Muscle spasticity
Trazodone (Desyrel, Oleptro)	Antidepressant	50 mg tid	Depression

BZD, benzodiazepine; ER, extended-release; FDA, United States Food and Drug Administration; IR, immediate-release; SMR, skeletal muscle relaxant; TCA, tricyclic antidepressant.

TABLE 3-17 Topical Medications for Neuropathic Orofacial Pain

Generic Name (Brand Name)	Drug Class	Usual Daily Dosage for Neuropathic Pain
Benzocaine (Anbesol, Cepacol, Orajel, others)	Topical anesthetic	Lozenge: dissolve 1 lozenge slowly in mouth, may repeat every 2 h as needed. Topical gel: apply thin layer to affected area up to qid. Topical oral spray: apply 1 spray to affected area, then wait ≥1 min and expectorate; may repeat up to qid
Capsaicin (Capsicum, Capzasin, Qutenza, Zostrix)	Topical analgesic	Cream: apply tid–qid. Patch: apply to affected area up to tid–qid for 7 d. Patch may remain in place up to 8 h.
Clonidine (Catapres)	Antihypertensive, analgesic	Patch: 0.1 mg/24 h patch applied once weekly, if necessary, increase by 0.1 mg at 1 week intervals
Dexamethasone (Decadron, Dexasone)	Glucocorticoid (anti-inflammatory, immunosuppressive)	Oral solution: rinse and expectorate with 1 mg q4–6h as needed
Diphenhydramine (Benadryl, others)	Antihistamine	Oral solution: rinse and expectorate with 25 mg q4–6h as needed
Lidocaine (Lidoderm, Xylocaine)	Topical anesthetic	Cream/gel: apply a thin film to affected area bid–tid as needed. Oral solution: swish with 15 mL and expectorate q3–4h as needed. Patch: apply to painful area. Patch may remain in place up to 12 h in any 24-h period. No more than 1 patch should be used in a 24-h period.

and thusly determines the site of metabolism (ester anesthetics are hydrolyzed by pseudocholinesterases in the plasma, amide local anesthetics primarily undergo metabolism in the liver; the notable exceptions are articaine which is metabolized in both the plasma and liver, and prilocaine possibly in the kidneys).[122] The amine is hydrophilic and associated with the water solubility of the compound. Compounds that lack this portion are insoluble in water and are only useful topically.[128]

Although structurally related, four pharmacologic factors differentiate the available injectable anesthetic preparations.[127]

1. pKa (dissociation constant): defines the amount of charged and uncharged molecules at a given pH. Since only uncharged molecules of local anesthetic freely pass across cell membranes, pKa is important in determining onset of local anesthetic activity (e.g., the pKa of bupivacaine is higher than that of lidocaine accounting for a comparatively slower onset of action).[121,122,124]

2. Lipid solubility: defines the relative ease of local anesthetic molecules to pass across lipid cell membranes. The more local anesthetic that can cross a cell membrane, the more potent action.

3. Vasodilation: all local anesthetics cause vasodilation, thereby increasing blood flow to the site of injection. Some local anesthetics must be combined with a vasoconstrictor to be effective (e.g., lidocaine and articaine), whereas others exhibit less vasodilatory effect and are effective as plain solutions (e.g., prilocaine, mepivacaine).

4. Protein binding: helps to determine how long the local anesthetic molecule binds to receptor sites at the cell membrane. The ability of molecules to bind to receptors helps to dictate the duration of local anesthetic activity (e.g., bupivacaine = articaine > mepivacaine > lidocaine > prilocaine).[127]

Topicals

The use of topical local anesthetic preparations is indicated for the relief of pain on mucous membranes of the nose, mouth, and throat.[125] Preparations of benzocaine, dyclonine, lidocaine, prilocaine, and tetracaine are commonly used and may be supplied as aqueous solutions, suspensions, gels, sprays, or lozenges. Onset is rapid, generally occurring within two to five minutes.[122] Benzocaine and tetracaine topical anesthetics and prilocaine injectable local anesthetic have been associated with the development of drug-induced methemoglobinemia. Patients with diagnosed congenital methemoglobinemia should not take benzocaine, tetracaine, or prilocaine.

Practitioners should be aware that systemic absorption of topical local anesthetics occurs across mucous membranes, especially of the throat. As a result, over use or misuse of topical local anesthetics caries risk of toxic systemic effects (e.g., methemoglobinemia). A eutectic mixture of lidocaine and prilocaine (EMLA®) is also available but not recommended on mucous membranes because of the increased risk of systemic absorption.[125]

Vasoconstrictors

Vasoconstrictors are added to local anesthetic preparations to retard the systemic absorption of the drug and also increase the depth of the anesthetic effect.[121,122,124] Currently there are only two vasoconstrictors being used in local anesthetic preparations: epinephrine as 1:50,000, 1:100,000, or 1:200,000 concentrations; and levonordefrin as 1:20,000 concentration. Norepinephrine is no longer available because of its increased potential for adverse cardiac consequences (e.g., hypertension followed by rebound bradycardia).[129,130] Levonordefrin is close in structure to norepinephrine but its effects on blood pressure, pulse, and vasoconstriction are similar to those of epinephrine. Levonordefrin 1:20,000 should be considered equipotent to epinephrine 1:100,000.[122,130]

METHODS OF SEDATION

It is estimated that as many as 75% of adults in the United States experience some degree of dental fear ranging from mild to severe. Anesthesia and sedation services for dental outpatients are commonly indicated for the management of this type of fear, anxiety, and phobia. Dentists may provide various forms of sedation depending on education, insurance costs, competency, equipment, and state regulations. The levels of sedation are described in Table 3-18.[131] This section will focus primarily on current pharmacotherapy of minimal and moderate oral and inhalational sedation as defined in the ADA guidelines. Deep sedation and general anesthesia are not covered because the majority of general dentists have not pursued the advanced training necessary to utilize these modalities.

Inhalational Sedation With Nitrous Oxide-Oxygen

Nitrous oxide (N_2O) is an inorganic inhalation agent that is colorless, odorless to sweet smelling, and nonirritating to the tissues. Once inhaled and dissolved in the bloodstream it does not combine with hemoglobin and does not undergo biotransformation. Because of N_2O's low solubility, it is eliminated rapidly from the body via expiration, which is precisely the reverse process of uptake and distribution. It is considered the safest medication in the dental armamentarium as there has never been a reported death caused by N_2O-oxygen sedation in a dental office while dentists performed dental procedures with N_2O-oxygen as the sole sedative administered by means of an appropriately installed and maintained delivery system.[132]

In dentistry, N_2O-oxygen sedation is used for minimal sedation in adults and anecdotally may even provide pulpal anesthesia for pediatric patients in lieu of local anesthetics. Since N_2O-oxygen has only minor anesthetic properties, it

TABLE 3-18   Levels of Sedation[131]

Level of Sedation	Definition
Minimal sedation	A minimally depressed level of consciousness, produced by a pharmacological method, which retains the patient's ability to independently and continuously maintain an airway and respond normally to tactile stimulation and verbal command. Although cognitive function and coordination may be modestly impaired, ventilator and cardiovascular functions are unaffected.
Moderate sedation	A drug-induced depression of consciousness during which patients respond purposefully to verbal commands, either alone or accompanied by light tactile stimulation. No interventions are required to maintain a patent airway, and spontaneous ventilation is adequate. Cardiovascular function is usually maintained.
Deep sedation	A drug-induced depression of consciousness during which patients cannot be easily aroused but respond purposefully following repeated or painful stimulation. The ability to independently maintain ventilator function may be impaired. Patients may require assistance in maintaining a patent airway, and spontaneous ventilation may be inadequate. Cardiovascular function is usually maintained.
General anesthesia	A drug-induced loss of consciousness during which patients are not arousable, even by painful stimulation. The ability to independently maintain ventilator function is often impaired. Patients often require assistance in maintaining a patent airway, and positive pressure ventilation may be required because of depressed spontaneous ventilation of drug-induced depression of neuromuscular function. Cardiovascular function may be impaired.

TABLE 3-19   Pharmacologic Characteristics of Selected Benzodiazepines

Drug	Lipid Solubility	Onset (min)	Half-life (h)	Clinical Duration of Action (h)	Site of Metabolism	Active Metabolite	Usual Dosing
Diazepam	High	30–60	>24	n/a	CYP 1A2, 2C8,2C19, 3A3-4	Yes	2–20 mg/d
Lorazepam	Moderate	60–120	10–20	4	Hepatic glucuronidation	No	2–4 mg
Midazolam	High	IM: 0 PO: 15–30	1.5–5	1	CYP 3A3-5	No	0.25–0.75 mg/kg
Triazolam	High	15–30	1.5–2.5	2	CYP 3A4-7	No	0.125–0.5 mg

IM, intramuscular route; PO, oral route.

should always be used with local anesthesia. Some patients (hyper-responders) may begin to feel relaxed at very low concentrations (15%–20%), while others may require concentrations in excess of 50% (hypo-responders). Since the clinical endpoint is patient comfort in order to receive dental care, the patient should respond appropriately to verbal commands, vital signs should be stable, and there should be no loss of consciousness or protective reflexes (independent breathing). The majority of patients typically reach this state at levels between 20%–50%. The term "nitrous oxide sedation" is a misnomer and should always be referred to as "nitrous oxide-oxygen sedation" since these two gases must be given in combination. The most important fail-safe employed by all manufacturers of N_2O machines is to insure that during gas delivery to patients, N_2O concentrations never exceed 70% (700,000 ppm). This insures that the patient will always be receiving at least 30% oxygen, which is significantly more than what is available in ambient air.

Oral Pharmacotherapy for Minimal and Moderate Sedation

For those patients in whom N_2O-oxygen sedation is contraindicated, ineffective, or not available, the next safest form of sedation is oral or enteral sedation.[133] The benzodiazepines and their newer derivatives are the most widely used classes of drugs for minimal and moderate sedation. Their efficacy is equivalent to or greater than any of the other classes of sedatives and they are safer than chloral hydrate or barbiturates (phenobarbital, methohexital). Benzodiazepines enhance the primary inhibitory neurotransmitter, gamma-aminobutyric acid (GABA) at the $GABA_A$ receptor in the central nervous system. When benzodiazepines bind the $GABA_A$ receptor, the effect of rendering the neuron less responsive to excitatory stimuli is augmented. No effect is produced if GABA is not present; benzodiazepines can only potentiate the body's endogenous GABA. This pharmacology is the reason for the relative safety of benzodiazepines versus chloral hydrate or the barbiturates, which can render a response independently of GABA. Therefore, high doses of these agents may be lethal but death following overdose of benzodiazepines alone is extremely rare.[132] Table 3-19 illustrates some of the unique characteristics of the most frequently used benzodiazepines for adult oral sedation in the dental office.

The interaction between the different benzodiazepines and the different alpha receptors on the $GABA_A$ receptor complex result in their differing degrees of anxiolysis, sedation, muscle relaxation, amnesia, and anti-seizure activity. Nonselective receptor binding also results in similar adverse effect profiles between drugs in this class, which include cognitive impairment, residual daytime sedation, rebound insomnia, and the risk of abuse. Non-benzodiazepine sedatives selectively interact with only the α1 subunit of the GABA$_A$ receptor complex, reducing their potential to cause cognitive impairment and abuse. Though chemically distinct from benzodiazepines, their sedation effects and clinical profiles are indistinguishable from benzodiazepines. Furthermore, their effects can be reversed using the benzodiazepine antagonist, flumazenil. Table 3-20 illustrates some of the unique pharmacologic characteristics of the non-benzodiazepine sedatives.

Another sedative medication, ramelteon, is a melatonin MT1 and MT2 receptor agonist. It has high selectivity and affinity for both melatonin receptors and an onset of action of approximately 30 minutes, making it useful for treating patients who have difficulty with sleep onset. Ramelteon is available as 8 mg tablets and is not a controlled substance. The unique and targeted mechanism of action of this drug also limits its adverse side effect potential or "hangover" effect often found with other sedatives. Ramelteon has no measurable affinity for the GABA receptor complex, dopamine, or opiate receptors. It does not offer the benefit of anterograde amnesia found with benzodiazepines or other non-benzodiazepine agents, and its action cannot be reversed by flumazenil.[134,135]

While antihistamines are primarily used to manage allergic symptoms and reactions, they are also marketed as sedative-hypnotics. The sedative effect of these agents is not as strong as a benzodiazepine, but they may be excellent alternatives for selected patients because they have a very limited abuse potential and many people are already familiar with their effects from prior self-medication. Antihistamines have minimal effect on cardiovascular or respiratory function, and as they are considered safe during pregnancy, may be used in patients when pregnancy status is unknown. Only promethazine has a black box warning contraindicating its use in children less than 2 years of age due to increased risk for fatal respiratory depression. Table 3-21 illustrates some of the pharmacologic characteristics of the antihistamines.

PRECAUTIONS IN PREGNANT OR LACTATING WOMEN
Pharmacotherapy and Pregnant Women

Up to 20% of clinically recognized pregnancies at less than 20 weeks of gestation will undergo spontaneous abortion, with 80% of these occurring in the first 12 weeks of gestation.[136,137] While there is a general belief that any drug exposure during pregnancy poses a risk to the fetus, one early publication estimated that only 2%–3% of birth defects are thought to be caused by medications taken during pregnancy and the majority of birth defects have an unknown cause.[138] A more recent study showed that 96% of women use some form of non-prescribed or prescribed medication during pregnancy thus, despite the concern, women are exposed to a large number of substances during pregnancy either intentionally or inadvertently.[139] For the health-care professional, the challenge is to know which drugs may be safe and which medications to avoid.

The greatest teratogenic risk to the fetus is from three to eight weeks after conception. Placental transport is established at about the fifth week of embryonic life. Stopping a medication at week 10 because of teratogenic concerns does not substantially reduce the risk of malformation. In addition, the concept of a "placental barrier" is a misnomer; any drug or chemical substance administered to the mother is

TABLE 3-20	Pharmacologic Characteristics of Non-Benzodiazepine Sedatives					
Drug	Onset (min)	Time to Peak Plasma Level (h)	Half-life (h)	Clinical Duration of Action (h)	Site of Metabolism	Usual Dosing
Eszopiclone	<30	1	6	6	CYP 3A4, 2E1	2–3 mg
Zaleplon	30	1	1	4–5	Aldehyde oxidase, CYP 3A4	10–20 mg
Zolpidem	<30	1.6	2.5	6–8	CYP 3A4	10 mg
Zopiclone^a	30–60	<2	6	6–8	CYP 3A4, 2C8	7.5–15 mg

^{a}Not available in the United States

TABLE 3-21	Pharmacologic Characteristics of Selected Antihistamines					
Drug	Onset (min)	Time to Peak Plasma Level (h)	Half-life (h)	Clinical Duration of Action (h)	Site of Metabolism	Usual Dosing
Dimenhydrinate	30–60	2	6	<10	CYP 2D6	50–100 mg
Diphenhydramine	30–60	2	9	<10	CYP 2D6	25–50 mg
Hydroxyzine	15–30	<2	20	12	CYP 2D6	50–100 mg
Promethazine	20	4	9	4–6	CYP 2D6	25–50 mg

TABLE 3-22 Relative Potencies of Selected Topical Corticosteroids

Clobetasol	Most potent
Fluocinonide	
Triamcinolone[a]	↑
Fluocinolone	
Hydrocortisone acetate[b]	Least potent

[a]Formulation available specifically designed for oral mucosa.
[b]Available without a prescription.

TABLE 3-23 Serious Adverse Effects of Oral Medications Used for Intraoral Lesions

Drug or Drug Class	Possible Serious Adverse Effects
Corticosteroids	Fractures, hypercorticism, infection, adrenal suppression, cardiovascular events, hyperglycemia
Dapsone	Hemolysis, anemia, methemoglobinemia
Colchicine	Serious gastrointestinal side effects, bone marrow suppression, rhabdomyolysis
Thalidomide	Human teratogenesis, deep venous thrombosis, peripheral neuropathies
Azathioprine	Severe leukopenia, thrombocytopenia, macrocytic anemia, bone marrow suppression, pancytopenia

TABLE 3-24 Properties of Available[a] Local Anesthetics

Formulation	Anesthetic (mg)[b]	Vasoconstrictor (mg)[b,c]	Adult Maximum dose (absolute maximum)[d]	Maximum Number of Carpules[d]	Elimination Half-life (min)[e]	Pregnancy Risk Category
4% articaine/1:100,000 epinephrine	72	0.018	3.3 mg/lb (500 mg)	6.9	27 (hepatic 108)	C
4% articaine/1:200,000 epinephrine		0.009				
0.5% bupivacaine/1:200,000 epinephrine	9	0.009	0.6 mg/lb (90 mg)	10	210	C
2% lidocaine/1:50,000 epinephrine	36	0.036	3.3 mg/lb (500 mg)	5.5	96	B
2% lidocaine/1:100,000 epinephrine		0.018		13.8		
2% lidocaine		0	2.0 mg/lb (300 mg)	8.3		
2% mepivacaine/1:20,000 levonordefrin	36	0.09	2.6 mg/lb (400 mg)	11.1	114	C
3% mepivacaine	54	0		7.4		
4% prilocaine/1:200,000 epinephrine	72	0.009	4.0 mg/lb (600 mg)	8.3	96	B
4% prilocaine		0				

[a]In the United States.
[b]Per 1.8 mL carpule.
[c]Maximum dose of epinephrine is commonly considered to be 0.2 mg for healthy adults. The dose should be reduced to 0.04 mg for compromised patients.
[d]The adult maximum dose is expressed as a weight-based calculation (mg/lb). The absolute maximum dose noted in parentheses is the maximum recommended dose for individuals weighing at least 150 pounds. For smaller individuals (<150 lb), practitioners should rely on the weight-based calculation of local anesthetic doses.
[e]Assumes normal hepatic and renal function. Patients with compromised hepatic and/or renal function may have different rates of drug clearance. Additionally, patients taking cytochrome P450 1A2 isoenzyme inhibitors may have longer half-lives of local anesthetics.

TABLE 3-25 Prescription Medications for the Treatment of Xerostomia

Generic Name	Pilocarpine	Cevimeline
Brand name	Salagen	Evoxac
Dosage form	Tablet (5, 7.5 mg)	Capsule (30 mg)
Usual adult dosage	5 mg tid (may be titrated up to a maximum dose of 10 mg tid as needed, use lowest effective dose)	30 mg tid
Contraindications	Uncontrolled asthma, angle closure glaucoma, iritis	
Precautions	Controlled asthma or chronic obstructive pulmonary disease, history of cardiac disease including arrhythmias, angina, or myocardial infarction, history of biliary disease or gallstones, history of kidney stones, hepatic insufficiency (pilocarpine).	
Common side effects	Sweating (very frequent with pilocarpine, up to 68%), flushing, dizziness, rhinitis, nausea, chills, weakness, increased urinary frequency, headache.	
Rare but important side effects	Bronchospasm, sinus tachycardia, premature ventricular contractions, atrioventricular block, biliary contractions.	
Important drug interactions	Anticholinergic drugs (negate actions of each drug); beta-blockers (possible conduction disturbances); CYP 3A4 inhibitors or inducers (cevimeline is a substrate of CYP 3A4).	
Monitoring parameters	Monitor for side effects that may lead to discontinuation.	

TABLE 3-26 Prescription Medications for the Treatment of Sialorrhea/Drooling

Generic Name	Glycopyrrolate	Atropine Sulfate
Brand name	Robinul/Robinul Forte	Isopto Atropine
Dosage form	Tablet (1, 2 mg)	Ophthalmic drop (1%)
Usual adult dosage	1–2 mg bid–tid (use lowest effective dose) OR 1 mg 30–60 min prior to dental procedure	1 drop under the tongue as needed for drooling or before dental procedure (use with caution, can cause rapid xerostomia)
Contraindications	GI obstruction or motility problems, ulcerative colitis, ileus, glaucoma, prostatic enlargement, bladder or urinary tract obstruction.	
Precautions	Hepatic disease, renal disease, renal insufficiency, elderly, autonomic neuropathy, cardiac disease, cardiac arrhythmias, urinary retention.	
Common side effects	Vomiting, flushing, headache, constipation, nasal congestion and/or dryness, xerostomia, drowsiness, anhidrosis.	
Rare but important side effects	Sinus tachycardia, cardiac dysrhythmia, bradyarrhythmia, hyperthermia (especially in hot weather), seizure.	
Important drug interactions	Digoxin (increased concentrations); potassium salts (GI irritation); GI motility agents (would impair mechanism of action); anticholinergic drugs (additive effects).	
Monitoring parameters	Monitor for side effects that may lead to discontinuation.	

GI, gastrointestinal.

TABLE 3-27 Amifostine for Xerostomia Prophylaxis in Patients Undergoing Head-and-Neck Cancer Radiotherapy

Brand Name	Ethyol
Dosage form	Powder for injection (500 mg/vial)
Usual adult dosage	200 mg/m^2 as a 3-min IV infusion starting 15–30 min before radiotherapy
Contraindications	Hypersensitivity to aminothiol compounds, antihypertensive medications that cannot be interrupted 24 hours before administration of amifostine
Precautions	Cardiovascular/cerebrovascular conditions, hypotension, dehydration, hypocalcemia; must be adequately hydrated prior to administration
Common side effects	Diarrhea, nausea/vomiting, hypotension

(Continued)

TABLE 3-27 Amifostine for Xerostomia Prophylaxis in Patients Undergoing Head-and-Neck Cancer Radiotherapy (*Continued*)	
Brand Name	**Ethyol**
Rare but important side effects	Hypocalcemia, anaphylactoid reactions, dermatologic reactions, arrhythmias, reversible loss of consciousness
Important drug interactions	Antihypertensive agents or any drug that can lower blood pressure (potentiate hypotension)
Monitoring parameters	Blood pressure (every 3–5 min while giving infusion and after infusion), observe patient for signs of anaphylaxis, serum calcium in patients at risk of hypocalcemia, nausea and vomiting (antiemetics given before infusion)

TABLE 3-28 Relative Safety of Commonly Used Medications in Dentistry and the Pregnant or Breastfeeding Patient[153,154]			
Medication	**Safe During Pregnancy?**	**FDA Pregnancy Category**	**Safe During Breastfeeding?**
Analgesics and Anti-inflammatory Agents			
Acetaminophen	Yes	B	Yes
Aspirin	Avoid	C/D	Avoid
Codeine	Use with caution	C	Yes
Dexamethasone	Avoid	C	Yes
Hydrocodone	Use with caution	C	Use with caution
Ibuprofen	Avoid in third trimester	C/D	Yes
Oxycodone	Use with caution	B	Use with caution
Prednisone	Avoid	C	Yes
Antibiotics and Antifungals			
Amoxicillin	Yes	B	Yes
Azithromycin	Yes	B	Yes
Cephalexin	Yes	B	Yes
Chlorhexidine (topical)	Yes	B	Yes
Clarithromycin	Use with caution	C	Use with caution
Clindamycin	Yes	B	Yes
Clotrimazole (topical)	Yes	B	Yes
Doxycycline	Avoid	D	Avoid
Erythromycin	Yes	B	Use with caution
Fluconazole	Yes (single-dose regimens)	C/D	Yes
Metronidazole	Yes	B	Avoid
Nystatin	Yes	C	Yes
Penicillin	Yes	B	Yes
Terconazole (topical)	Yes	B	Yes
Tetracycline	Avoid	D	Avoid
Topical and Local Anesthetics			
Articaine	Use with caution	C	Use with caution
Benzocaine (topical)	Avoid	C	Use with caution
Bupivacaine	Use with caution	C	Yes
Dyclonine (topical)	Yes	C	Yes
Lidocaine (+/- epinephrine)	Yes	B	Yes
Lidocaine (topical)	Yes	B	Yes
Mepivacaine (+/- levonordefrin)	Use with caution	C	Yes
Prilocaine	Yes	B	Yes
Tetracaine (topical)	Avoid	C	Use with caution

TABLE 3-28 Relative Safety of Commonly Used Medications in Dentistry and the Pregnant or Breastfeeding Patient[153,154] (Continued)

Medication	Safe During Pregnancy?	FDA Pregnancy Category	Safe During Breastfeeding?
Sedatives			
Benzodiazepines	Avoid	D/X	Avoid
Zaleplon	Use with caution	C	Use with caution
Zolpidem	Use with caution	C	Yes
Emergency Medications			
Albuterol	Yes	C	Yes
Diphenhydramine	Yes	B	Avoid
Epinephrine	Use with caution	C	Yes
Flumazenil	Use with caution	C	Use with caution
Naloxone	Use with caution	C	Use with caution
Nitroglycerin	Use with caution	C	Use with caution

TABLE 3-29 The FDA's Pregnancy Category Definitions[155–157]

Pregnancy Category	Definition
A	Controlled studies in women fail to demonstrate a risk to the fetus in the first trimester (and there is no evidence of risk in later trimesters), and the possibility of fetal harm appears remote.
B	Either animal reproduction studies have not demonstrated a fetal risk but there are no controlled studies in pregnant women or animal reproduction studies have shown an adverse effect (other than a decrease in fertility) that was not confirmed in controlled studies in women in the first trimester (and there is no evidence of risk in later trimesters).
C	Either studies in animals have revealed adverse effects on the fetus (teratogenic, embryocidal, or other) and there are no controlled studies in women or studies in women and animals are not available. Drugs should be given only if the potential benefit justifies the potential risk to the fetus.
D	There is positive evidence of human fetal risk, but the benefits of use in pregnant women may be acceptable despite the risk (for example, if the drug is needed in a life-threatening situation or for a serious disease for which safer drugs cannot be used or are ineffective).
X	Studies in animals or human beings have demonstrated fetal abnormalities or there is evidence of fetal risk based on human experience, or both, and the risk of the use of the drug in pregnant women clearly outweighs any possible benefit. The drug is contraindicated in women who are or may become pregnant.

able to cross the placenta to some extent unless it is destroyed or altered during passage, or its molecular size and low lipid solubility limit placental transfer.

When considering the use of drugs for patients who are either pregnant, trying to conceive, or in whom pregnancy status is unknown, the dental practitioner prescribes a relatively small group of medications. Dentists should therefore be familiar with the risks and benefits of five main groups of medications and their relative safety in this critical population: (1) analgesics and anti-inflammatories; (2) antibiotics; (3) local anesthetics; (4) sedatives; and (5) emergency medications (Table 3-28). It is important to note that ibuprofen is representative of all NSAIDs in this table. The full adult dose and duration of antibiotics should be prescribed to pregnant women. Serious infections should be treated aggressively. The use of higher-dose regimens should be employed (e.g., cephalexin 500 mg three times a day rather than 250 mg three times a day), as they are cleared faster due to the increase in glomerular filtration rate in pregnancy. When considering combination products, the safety with respect to

either pregnancy or breastfeeding depends on the drug with greater risk. In a pregnant woman, prescribing oxycodone with acetaminophen would be done with caution, since the oxycodone moiety carries a higher risk. Finally, in an emergency situation, if the benefits to the mother exceed the risk to the fetus and a medication needs to be administered, it should always be administered, regardless of the FDA's pregnancy risk factor definitions (see Table 3-29).

Pharmacotherapy and Lactating Women

Breastfeeding percentages in the U.S. during the early postpartum period, at 6 months, and 12 months were found to be 81.9%, 60.6%, and 34.1%, respectively.[140] Many new mothers are told they must stop breastfeeding or "pump and discard" if they are taking certain medications, however, in the majority of cases, this counseling may be incorrect on the part of the oral health-care provider based on his or her limited education about breastfeeding and medications. Many of the studies about milk secretion and synthesis have been carried out in animals and there are considerable differences in the composition of milk in different species. Therefore, taking medications while breastfeeding represents a challenge for both patients and prescribers.

For most medications, the infant is exposed to a much higher concentration during pregnancy than during lactation; therefore, if a drug is considered acceptable during pregnancy, it is usually reasonable to continue it during breastfeeding.[141] There are exceptions, however, and the most important factors are the concentration of drug in the infant's blood and the effects that this might have. Table 3-28 summarizes the key clinical considerations for medications and breastfeeding when considering the same five groups of medications described above. Ibuprofen is again representative of all NSAIDs. COX-2 selective inhibitors should be avoided, as few data is available. Doses of aspirin > 100 mg should be avoided because of the risk of platelet dysfunction and Reye's syndrome. For antibiotics during breastfeeding, they may cause diarrhea in a breastfeeding infant due to altered bowel flora. If the infant develops a fever, take into account maternal antibiotic treatment.

Selected Readings

Baddour LM, Epstein AE, Erickson CC, et al. A summary of the update on cardiovascular implantable electronic device infections and their management: a scientific statement from the American Heart Association. J Am Dent Assoc. 2011;142(2):159–165.

Carlson ER. Diagnosis and management of salivary gland infections. Oral Maxillofac Surg Clin North Am. 2009;21(3):293–312.

Cernik C, Gallina K, Brodell RT. The treatment of herpes simplex infections: an evidence-based review. Arch Intern Med. 2008;168(11):1137–1144.

Chaparro LE, Wiffen PJ, Moore RA, Gilron I. Combination pharmacotherapy for the treatment of neuropathic pain in adults. Cochrane Database Syst Rev. 2012;7:CD008943.

Donaldson M, Donaldson D, Quarnstrom FC. Nitrous oxide–oxygen administration: when safety features no longer are safe. J Am Dent Assoc. 2012;143(2):134–143.

Donaldson M, Goodchild JH. Pregnancy, breast-feeding and drugs used in dentistry. J Am Dent Assoc. 2012;143(8):858–871.

Donaldson M, Goodchild JH. Appropriate analgesic prescribing for the general dentist. Gen Dent. 2010;58(4):291–297.

Drugs for pain. Treat Guidel Med Lett. 2013;11(128):31–42.

Goodchild JH, Donaldson M. Appropriate antibiotic prescribing for the general dentist. Gen Dent. 2009;57(6):626–634.

Malamed SF. Handbook of Local Anesthesia. 6th ed. St. Louis, MO: Elsevier Mosby; 2013:2–24.

Moore PA, Hersh EV. Combining ibuprofen and acetaminophen for acute pain management after third-molar extractions: translating clinical research to dental practice. J Am Dent Assoc. 2013;144(8):898–908.

Moore PA, Hersh EV. Local anesthetics: pharmacology and toxicity. Dent Clin North Am. 2010;54(4):587–599.

Pappas PG, Kauffman CA, Andes D, et al. Clinical practice guidelines for the management of candidiasis: 2009 update by the Infectious Diseases Society of America. Clin Infect Dis. 2009;48(5):503–535.

Rethman MP, Watters W 3rd, Abt E, et al. The American Academy of Orthopaedic Surgeons and the American Dental Association clinical practice guideline on the prevention of orthopaedic implant infection in patients undergoing dental procedures. J Bone Joint Surg Am. 2013;95(8):745–747.

Wilson W, Taubert KA, Gewitz M, et al. Prevention of infective endocarditis: guidelines from the American Heart Association: a guideline from the American Heart Association Rheumatic Fever, Endocarditis and Kawasaki Disease Committee, Council on Cardiovascular Disease in the Young, and the Council on Clinical Cardiology, Council on Cardiovascular Surgery and Anesthesia, and the Quality of Care and Outcomes Research Interdisciplinary Working Group. J Am Dent Assoc. 2008;139(suppl 1):3S–24S.

For the full reference lists, please go to http://www.pmph-usa.com/Burkets_Oral_Medicine.

CHAPTER 4

Ulcerative, Vesicular, and Bullous Lesions

Sook Bin Woo, DMD, MMSc, FDS RCSEd
Martin S. Greenberg, DDS, FDS RCSEd

Many ulcerative or vesiculobullous disease of the mouth have a similar clinical appearance. The oral mucosa is thin, and even slight trauma leads to rupture of vesicles and bullae forming eroded, red areas; fibrin forms over the erosion and an ulcer develops. As such, vesiculo-bullous lesions that have a characteristic appearance on the skin (such as tense blisters of bullous pemphigoid [BP]) have a somewhat nonspecific appearance on the oral mucosa.

Taking a careful and detailed history often provides as much information as the clinical examination and guides the clinician during the clinical examination. Four pieces of information in particular help the clinician rapidly categorize a patient's disease and simplify the diagnosis: the length of time the lesions have been present (acute or chronic lesions), a history of similar lesions (primary or recurrent

disease), the number of lesions present (single or multiple), and the location of lesions. In this chapter, the diseases are grouped according to the information just described. This information serves as a good starting point for students who are just learning to diagnose these disorders, as well as for experienced clinicians who are aware of the potential diagnostic pitfalls.

A complete review of systems should be obtained for each patient, including questions regarding the presence of skin, eye, genital, and rectal lesions as well as the presence of symptoms such as fever, joint pains, and muscle weakness to name a few. The clinical examination should include a thorough inspection of the exposed skin surfaces. Some knowledge of basic dermatology is helpful because many disorders occurring on the oral mucosa may also affect the skin.

Dermatologic lesions are classified according to their clinical appearance and include the following frequently used terms that are also applicable in the oral mucosa:

1. *Macules.* These are lesions that are flush with the adjacent mucosa and that are noticeable because of their difference in color from normal skin or mucosa. They may be red due to increased vascularity or inflammation, or pigmented due to the presence of melanin, hemosiderin, and foreign materials (including the breakdown products of medications). A good example in the oral cavity is the melanotic macule.
2. *Papules.* These are lesions raised above the skin or mucosal surface that are smaller than 1.0 cm in diameter (some use 0.5 cm for oral mucosal lesions). They may be slightly domed or flat-topped. Papules are seen in a wide variety of diseases, such as the yellow-white papules of pseudomembranous candidiasis.
3. *Plaques.* These are raised lesions that are greater than 1 cm in diameter; they are essentially large papules.
4. *Nodules.* These lesions are present within the dermis or mucosa. The lesions may also protrude above the skin or mucosa forming a characteristic dome-shaped structure. A good example of an oral mucosal nodule is the irritation fibroma.
5. *Vesicles.* These are small blisters containing clear fluid that are less than 1 cm in diameter.
6. *Bullae.* These are elevated blisters containing clear fluid that are greater than 1 cm in diameter (some use 0.5 cm for oral lesions).
7. *Erosions.* These are red lesions often caused by the rupture of vesicles or bullae, or trauma and are generally moist on the skin. However, they may also result from thinning or atrophy of the epithelium in inflammatory diseases such as lichen planus. These should not be mistaken for ulcers that are covered with fibrin and are yellow although erosions may develop into ulcers.
8. *Pustules.* These are blisters containing purulent material and appear yellow.
9. *Ulcers.* These are well-circumscribed, sometimes depressed lesions with an epithelial defect that is covered by a fibrin clot, resulting in a yellow-white appearance. A good example is an aphthous ulcer.
10. *Purpura.* These are reddish to purple discolorations caused by blood from vessels leaking into the connective tissue. These lesions do not blanch when pressure is applied and are classified by size as petechiae (less than 0.3 cm), purpura (0.4–0.9 cm), or ecchymoses (greater than 1 cm).

The first section of this chapter describes acute multiple lesions that tend to occur only as a single episode; the second portion covers recurring oral mucosal lesions; the third portion presents conditions characterized by chronic, continuous multiple lesions, and the final section describes diseases that present with single lesions. It is hoped that classifying the disorders in this way will help the clinician avoid the common diagnostic problem of confusing viral infections with recurrent oral conditions, such as recurrent aphthous stomatitis (RAS), or disorders that present as chronic progressive disease, such as pemphigus and pemphigoid.

THE PATIENT WITH ACUTE MULTIPLE LESIONS

The major diseases that cause acute multiple oral ulcers include viral and bacterial stomatitis, allergic and hypersensitivity reactions (particularly erythema multiforme and contact allergic stomatitis), and lesions caused by medications (such as cancer chemotherapy) (see Chapter 18, "Hematologic Diseases").

Herpes Simplex Virus Infection
Etiology and Pathogenesis

The Herpesviridae family of viruses contains eight different viruses that are pathogenic in humans with one affecting simians (Table 4-1). This chapter discusses only herpes simplex virus (HSV)-1, varicella-zoster virus (VZV), and cytomegalovirus (CMV) infections in detail because they cause oral ulcers. Epstein-Barr virus (EBV) rarely is associated with mucocutaneous ulcers in immunocompromised and immunosenescent patients; this is discussed in the differential diagnosis of "Traumatic Ulcerative Granuloma" below. Herpesviruses have a common structure: an internal core containing the viral genome, an icosahedral nucleocapsid, the tegument, and an outer lipid envelope containing viral glycoproteins on its surface that are derived from host cellular membranes.[1] Nonetheless, each of the herpesviruses is distinct.

HSV-1, an α-herpesvirus, is a ubiquitous virus, and 65% of adults in the United States older than age 70 are seropositive for it.[2] In general, infections above the waist are caused by HSV-1 and those below the waist by HSV-2, although with changing sexual practices, it is not uncommon to culture HSV-2 from oral lesions and vice versa.[3] The primary infection, which occurs on initial contact with the virus, is acquired by inoculation of the mucosa, skin, and eye with infected secretions. The virus then travels along the sensory nerve axons and establishes chronic, latent infection in the sensory ganglion (such as the trigeminal ganglion).[4] Extraneuronal latency (i.e., HSV remaining latent in cells other than neurons such as the epithelium) may play a role in recurrent lesions of the lips.[5] Recurrent HSV results when HSV reactivates at latent sites and travels centripetally to the mucosa or the skin, where it is directly cytopathic to epithelial cells, causing recrudescent HSV infection in the form of localized vesicles or ulcers.[6]

The most common sites of infection are the oral and genital mucosa and the eye. HSV infection of the cornea (keratitis) is a major cause of blindness in the world. HSV-1 or -2 may cause herpes whitlow, an infection of the fingers when virus is inoculated into the fingers through a break in the skin (Figure 4-1). This was a common occupational hazard (including within the dental profession) before the

Type of Human Herpesvirus (HHV)	Primary Infection	Recrudescent Lesions in Healthy Hosts	Recrudescent Lesions in Immunocompromised Hosts
Herpes simplex virus 1 (HHV-1)	Gingivostomatitis, keratoconjunctivitis, genital and skin lesions	Herpes labialis ("cold sores" "fever blisters"), intraoral ulcers, keratoconjunctivitis, genital and skin lesions	Ulcers at any mucocutaneous site, usually large and persistent; disseminated infection
Herpes simplex virus 2 (HHV-2)	Genital and skin lesions, gingivostomatitis, keratoconjunctivitis, neonatal infections, aseptic meningitis	Genital and skin lesions gingivostomatitis, aseptic meningitis	Ulcers at any mucocutaneous site, usually large and persistent; disseminated infection
Varicella-zoster virus (HHV-3)	Varicella (chicken pox)	Zoster (shingles)	Disseminated infection
Cytomegalovirus (HHV-4)	Infectious mononucleosis, hepatitis, congenital disease		Retinitis, gastroenteritis hepatitis, severe oral ulcers
Epstein-Barr virus (HHV-5)	Infectious mononucleosis-like, hepatitis, encephalitis		Hairy leukoplakia, lymphoproliferative disorders, mucocutaneous ulcers
HHV-6	Roseola infantum, otitis media, encephalitis		Fever, bone marrow suppression
HHV-7	Roseola infantum		
HHV-8	Infectious mononucleosis-like, febrile exanthema		Kaposi sarcoma, lymphoproliferative disorders, bone marrow suppression

TABLE 4-1   Herpesviridae That Are Pathogenic in Humans

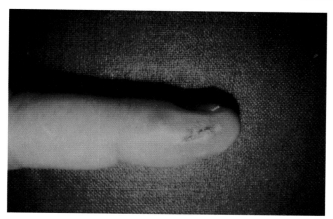

FIGURE 4-1   Primary herpetic whitlow on the finger of a dentist.

widespread use of gloves.[7,8] Other HSV-1 infections include herpes gladiatorum (infections of the skin spread through the sport of wrestling),[9] herpes encephalitis, HSV esophagitis, HSV pneumonia and neonatal and disseminated infection.[6]

HSV is an important etiologic agent in erythema multiforme, which is discussed below.[10,11] HSV has been recovered in the endoneurial fluid of 77% of patients with Bell palsy.[12] Treatment with antiviral therapy resulted in better outcomes, further supporting the concept of HSV involvement in the pathogenesis of Bell palsy.[13] However, VZV has also been strongly implicated in the development of Bell palsy.[13a]

Clinical Manifestations

Primary Gingivostomatitis

The majority of primary HSV-1 infections are subclinical and generally occur in children and teenagers, and young adults.[6,13,13b] There is a one- to three-day viral prodrome of fever, loss of appetite, malaise, and myalgia that may also be accompanied by headache and nausea. Oral pain leads to poor oral intake, and patients may require hospitalization for hydration. The disease is self-limiting in otherwise normal patients and resolves within 10–14 days, typical for a viral illness.

Oral Findings

Within a few days of the prodrome, erythema and clusters of vesicles and/or ulcers appear on the keratinized mucosa of the hard palatal mucosa, attached gingiva and dorsum of the tongue, and the nonkeratinized mucosa of the buccal and labial mucosa, ventral tongue, and soft palate (Figure 4-2 and Figure 4-3). Vesicles break rapidly down to form ulcers that are usually 1–5 mm and coalesce to form larger ulcers with scalloped borders and marked surrounding erythema. The gingiva is often erythematous, and the mouth is extremely painful, causing difficulty with eating. Pharyngitis causes swallowing difficulties. Primary HSV infection in adults follows a similar pattern.[14]

Recrudescent Oral HSV Infection

Reactivation of HSV may lead to asymptomatic shedding of HSV, in the saliva and other secretions, an important risk factor for transmission; it may also cause ulcers to form. Asymptomatic shedding of HSV is not associated with systemic signs and symptoms and occurs in 8%–10% of patients following dental treatment.[15] The term *recrudescent HSV* should be used to refer to the actual ulcerations caused by reactivated virus. Fever, ultraviolet radiation, trauma, stress, and menstruation are important triggers for reactivation of HSV.

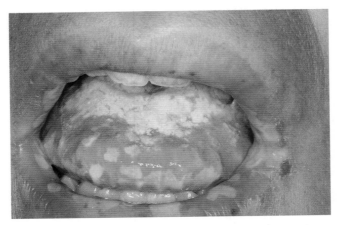

FIGURE 4-2 Primary herpetic gingivostomatitis with extensive involvement of the keratinized tissues of the tongue dorsum and non-keratinized tissues of the ventral tongue and labial mucosa. Courtesy of Dr. Nathaniel Treister, Boston, MA.

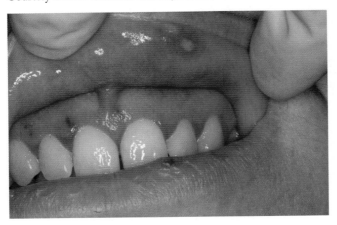

FIGURE 4-3 Primary herpetic gingivostomatitis with mild presentation: erythematous maxillary anterior gingiva with erythema and ulcer on upper labial mucosa, and crusted lesion on lower lip.

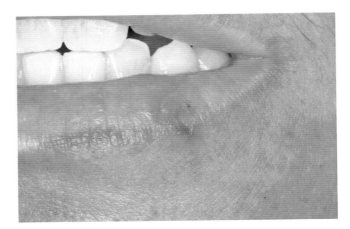

FIGURE 4-4 Clustered vesicles of recrudescent herpes labialis on vermilion.

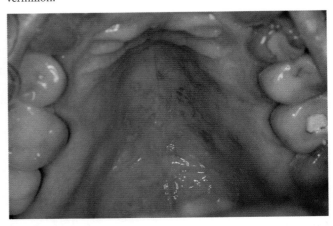

FIGURE 4-5 Recrudescent intraoral herpes simplex virus infection in an immunocompetent patient with clusters of small coalescent ulcers on the keratinized palatal mucosa.

Recrudescent HSV on the lips is called recurrent herpes labialis (RHL) and occurs in 20%–40% of the young adult population.[16,17] These are associated with a prodrome of itching, tingling, or burning approximately 50% of the time, followed in succession by the appearance of papules, vesicles, ulcers, crusting, and then resolution of lesions (Figure 4-4).[18] Pain is generally present only within the first two days. There is a suggestion that patients who do not experience a prodrome develop lesions from extraneural latent HSV within the epithelium and these lesions are less responsive to topical therapy.[19]

Recrudescent intraoral HSV (RIH) in the immunocompetent host occurs chiefly on the keratinized mucosa of the hard palatal mucosa, attached gingiva, and dorsum of the tongue[20] They present as 1–5 mm single or clustered painful ulcers with a bright erythematous border (Figure 4-5). One common presentation is the complaint of pain in the gingiva one to two days after a scaling and prophylaxis or other dental treatment. Lesions appear as 1–5 mm painful vesicles but more often ulcers on the marginal gingiva.

HSV in Immunocompromised Patients

In immunocompromised patients (such as those undergoing chemotherapy, who have undergone organ transplantation, or who have acquired immune deficiency syndrome [AIDS]), RIH infection may occur at any site intraorally and may form ulcers that may be several centimeters in size and may last several weeks or months if undiagnosed and untreated (Figure 4-6 and Figure 4-7).[21,22] In one study, 50% of patients with leukemia and 15% of patients who had undergone renal transplantation developed RIH infections.[23] Single RIH ulcers are clinically indistinguishable from recurrent aphthous ulcers if they occur on a nonkeratinized site.[24] These ulcers are painful and similar to those seen in immunocompetent patients except that they may be larger and often occur on nonkeratinized sites. They appear slightly depressed with raised borders. The presence of 1–2 mm vesicles or satellite ulcers at the edges of the main ulcer is a helpful sign.

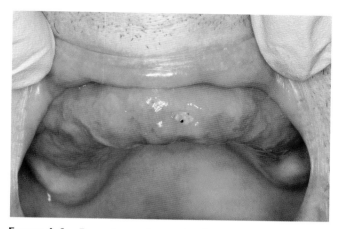

FIGURE 4-6 Recrudescent herpes simplex virus infection of the maxillary alveolar ridge mucosa in a patient with lymphoma.

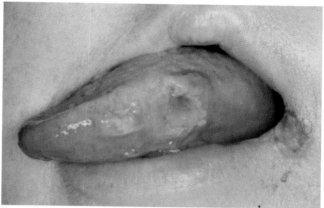

FIGURE 4-7 Recrudescent herpes simplex virus infection of the lateral tongue and oral commissure in a patient with leukemia post-allogenic transplantation.

If undiagnosed and left untreated, RIH infection may disseminate to other sites and cause severe infections in the immunocompromised population.[25] This is a particular problem in patients undergoing hematopoietic stem cell transplantation, where reactivation of HSV occurs in approximately 70% of patients.[26,27]

Differential Diagnosis

Coxsackievirus (CV) infections (especially hand–foot-and–mouth [HFM] disease) may present with widespread ulcerations of the oral cavity mimicking primary herpetic gingivostomatitis, but ulcers are generally not clustered and generalized gingival inflammation usually is not present. A viral culture or a cytology smear (see laboratory tests below) identifies HSV.

RIH infection in immunocompetent patients on the gingiva may resemble a localized area of necrotizing ulcerative gingivitis (NUG; see below), but there is usually a precipitating cause, such as fever or dental treatment. Cultures are positive for HSV, and lesions of NUG are widespread and diffuse rather than localized, as is often seen in RIH.

Traumatic ulcers on the palatal mucosa (such as from pizza burns) may resemble RIH.

RIH infection in immunocompromised hosts may occur at any intraoral site and can be differentiated from aphthous ulcers when necessary with a cytology specimen or culture.

In the immunocompromised population, ulcers secondary to CMV infection, fungal infection, and neutropenia must also be considered. Differentiation between these entities is accomplished by biopsy, culture, and blood tests.

Erythema multiforme, often triggered by a prior HSV infection may appear as multiple, coalescent ulcers (see below).

Laboratory Diagnosis

HSV isolation by cell culture is the gold standard test for the diagnosis since it grows readily in tissue culture. A single swab of the oral ulcers is performed. The advantage of a culture is that it has high sensitivity and specificity and allows for amplification of virions, subtyping, and testing for sensitivity to antiviral drugs. The disadvantage is that it needs specialized equipment, is expensive, is dependent on proper transport of the culture, and may take up to several days for a final result. Furthermore, healing lesions with low viral load will not be positive. HSV that reactivates in the saliva (asymptomatic shedding) will also grow in culture and may lead to a false positive result.

More recently, polymerase chain reaction (PCR) from swabs has been shown to detect HSV antigen three to four times more often than culture[28]; real-time PCR has also been shown to be highly sensitive and specific.[28a] However, PCR testing is expensive and detects DNA and not whole infectious particles, so a positive PCR test for HSV does not always equate with active infection. Nevertheless, it is a highly sensitive test.

HSV can be identified from scrapings from the base of lesions (especially vesicles) smeared onto glass slides. These can be stained with Wright, Giemsa (Tzanck preparation), or Papanicolaou stain to demonstrate the characteristic multinucleated giant cells or intranuclear inclusions as seen on histopathology (see below). However, this does not distinguish between HSV and VZV. A similar smear preparation can be used for the direct fluorescent antigen detection test using a monoclonal antibody against HSV conjugated to a fluorescent compound. Direct fluorescent antigen testing is more accurate than routine cytology.

Primary HSV infection is associated with elevated immunoglobulin (Ig)M titers that occur within days, followed several weeks later by permanent IgG titers (seroconversion) that indicate previous infection but confer no protection against reactivation. Recurrent infection is associated with a rise in IgG antibody titer in acute and convalescent sera, but a fourfold rise (a criterion that indicates active infection) is seen in only 5% of patients. The assay for HSV IgM is not particularly reliable for diagnostic purposes, and overall, the use of serology alone to diagnose recurrent infection is not advised.

HSV lesions are not generally biopsied because the clinical appearance and history are characteristic, and infection is readily confirmed with a culture or cytology specimen when necessary. However, if a scraping or biopsy is obtained, it will show the presence of multinucleated giant epithelial cells at the edge of the ulcer. The nuclei exhibit typical molding and have a ground-glass appearance (Figure 4-8). Since intact epithelium is necessary for the diagnosis, a biopsy for a lesion suspicious for HSV must always include epithelium adjacent to the ulcer or there may be a false negative result.

Management
Primary HSV Infection

Management is directed toward pain control, supportive care, and definitive treatment (Table 4-2). In the past, healthy patients with primary herpetic gingivostomatitis were treated only with hydration and supportive measures. However, since the acyclovir family of drugs is inexpensive, safe, and readily available, it is appropriate to treat even primary infections definitively because it reduces viral shedding and infectivity.

Acyclovir inhibits viral replication and is activated by virally produced thymidine kinase. As such, it has little activity against nonvirally infected cells.[29] The use of acyclovir at 15 mg/kg five times a day in children reduces the duration of fever, reduces HSV shedding, halts the progress of lesions, improves oral intake, and reduces the incidence of hospital admissions.[30] Valacyclovir, a prodrug of acyclovir, has three to five times the bioavailability of acyclovir and, together with famciclovir, is now widely used.[29]

Recrudescent HSV

RHL can often be suppressed by reducing tissue damage, such as using sunscreen.[31] Although RHL is self-limiting, the use of topical antiviral medications reduces shedding, infectivity, pain, and the size and duration of lesions. Topical antiviral medications such as 5% acyclovir cream,[32,33] 1% penciclovir cream,[34,35] and 10% docosanol cream are efficacious[36,37] if applied five to eight times a day at the first prodrome or sign of a lesion. Systemic therapy with valacyclovir (2 g every 12 hours for one day) or famciclovir (1500 mg single dose) are both effective in treating active lesions of RHL.[37a] For intraoral lesions, treatment is with 500–1000 mg valacyclovir three times a day or 400–800 mg of acyclovir for 7–10 days. Suppression of HSV infection in patients who develop frequent episodes, large lesions, or erythema multiforme is effected with variable doses of acyclovir, valacyclovir, and famciclovir.[37a,38–42] Similar suppressive regimens can be used for patients susceptible to recrudescent HSV after dental procedures.[43]

HSV in Immunocompromised Patients

In general, HSV infections in immunocompromised hosts should be treated with systemic antivirals to prevent dissemination to other sites (e.g., HSV esophagitis) or systemically. The primary pathogen for herpes encephalitis and herpes pneumonitis is HSV-1. For patients undergoing

TABLE 4-2 Pain Management and Supportive Care Measures
Pain Management
2% viscous lidocaine (swish and spit out 5 mL 4–5 times/d)
Liquid diphenhydramine (swish and spit out 5 mL 4–5 times/d)
Combination of viscous lidocaine, diphenhydramine, and a covering agent (such as Kaopectate™ or Maalox™) in 1:1:1 ratio
0.1% dyclonine hydrochloride
Benzydamine
Systemic analgesia
Supportive Care
Hydration
Ice chips or popsicles
Soft bland diet
Antipyretics such as ibuprofen as needed (avoid aspirin products)[a]

[a]The use of aspirin products in children who have a viral illness (especially varicella infection, influenza, or coxsackievirus infection) has been associated with Reye syndrome, a potentially fatal condition characterized by fatty degeneration of the liver and encephalopathy.

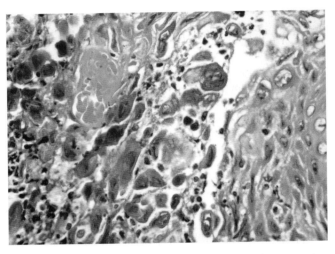

FIGURE 4-8 Biopsy of a herpes simplex virus ulcer demonstrating large epithelial cells with multiple ground-glass nuclei.

hematopoietic cell transplantation, antiviral therapy such as acyclovir or valacyclovir at suppressive doses should be initiated for all patients who are HSV seropositive (acyclovir 400 mg three times a day or 500 mg valacyclovir twice a day).[26,44] Acyclovir-resistant HSV is most frequently seen in this group of patients, where the virally derived thymidine kinase that activates acyclovir is mutated. In such cases, foscarnet or cidofovir is effective. The dosage of the acyclovir family of drugs should be adjusted for age and renal health.

A number of vaccines and new therapies against HSV are currently under development.[45,45a]

Varicella-Zoster Virus Infection
Etiology and Pathogenesis

Primary infection with varicella zoster virus (VZV), an α-herpesvirus, leads to varicella (chicken pox). As with all herpesviruses, the virus then becomes latent, usually in the dorsal root ganglia or ganglia of the cranial nerves.[46] Reactivation produces herpes zoster infection (HZI), commonly called shingles. The incidence of HZI increases with age and the degree of immunosuppression.[47] There are 1.5 to 3 cases of HZI per 1000 subjects; this increases to 10 per 1000 in those older than the age of 75 years.[48] Therefore, it is not uncommon to see HZI in the elderly, in patients undergoing cancer chemotherapy, in patients on chronic immunosuppressive drug therapy (such as those who have received organ transplants), and in patients with AIDS.[47,49] As with HSV, this virus is cytopathic to the epithelial cells of the skin and mucosa, causing blisters and ulcers. Transmission is usually by the respiratory route, with an incubation period of two to three weeks.[50]

Postherpetic neuralgia, a morbid sequela of HZI, is a neuropathy resulting from peripheral and central nervous system injury and altered central nervous system processing.[51]

Clinical Findings

Primary VZV infection generally occurs in the first two decades of life. The disease begins with a low-grade fever, malaise, and the development of an intensely pruritic, maculopapular rash, followed by vesicles that have been described as "dewdrop-like." These vesicles turn cloudy and pustular, burst, and scab, with the crusts falling off after one to two weeks. Lesions begin on the trunk and face and spread centrifugally. Central nervous system involvement may result in cerebellar ataxia and encephalitis. Other complications of varicella include pneumonia, myocarditis, and hepatitis.[50]

Immunocompromised hosts usually experience more severe disease with more blisters, a protracted course, and, not infrequently, involvement of the lungs, central nervous system, and liver; there is a significantly higher mortality rate.[52] Secondary bacterial infection by gram-positive cocci may have severe septic consequences.

HZI of the skin (shingles) occurs in adults and starts with a prodrome of deep, aching, or burning pain. There is usually little to no fever or lymphadenopathy. This is followed within two to four days by the appearance of crops of vesicles in a dermatomal or "zosteriform" pattern. This pattern describes the unilateral, linear, and clustered distribution of the vesicles, ulcers, and scabs in a dermatome supplied by one nerve. Thoracic/lumbar dermatomes are the most frequently involved, followed by the craniofacial area.[47] Lesions heal within two to four weeks, often with scarring and hypopigmentation. Occasionally, HZI may occur without the appearance of dermatomal lesions (zoster sine eruptione or zoster sine herpete), which makes the diagnosis of this condition challenging; these patients often present with facial palsy. In fact, VZV has been detected in up to 20% of patients with Bell palsy.[13a] A serious and occasional side effect of HZI is acute retinal necrosis.[49]

One of the most important complications of HZI is postherpetic neuralgia, defined as pain that lingers for 120 days[51,53] after the onset of the acute rash (see Chapter 12). In patients older than age 50, up to 70% developed postherpetic neuralgia and up to 50% have debilitating pain, usually of a sharp, stabbing, burning or gnawing nature lasting more than one month.[49,54] Some unfortunate patients experience pain for years.[51] Predisposing factors include older age, prodromal pain, and more severe clinical disease during the acute rash phase.[55,56]

Immunocompromised patients often experience more severe VZI that may appear atypical, be bilateral, and involve multiple dermatomes; retinitis, pneumonitis, and encephalitis have been reported as complications in this patient population. On rare occasions, HZI may involve not just the dorsal root ganglion but also the anterior horn cells, leading to paralysis.[49]

Oral Manifestations

Primary VZV infection presents as acute-onset ulcerations in the mouth that often pale in clinical significance when compared with the skin lesions.

In recurrent VZV infection, the ophthalmic division of the trigeminal (V) nerve is the cranial nerve most often affected (herpes zoster ophthalmicus); corneal involvement may lead to blindness.[49] Involvement of this nerve (V) leads to lesions on the upper eyelid, forehead, and scalp with V_1; midface and upper lip with V_2; and lower face and lower lip with V_3 (Figure 4-9). With the involvement of V_2, patients experience a prodrome of pain, burning, and tenderness, usually on the palate on one side. This is followed several days later by the appearance of painful, clustered 1–5 mm ulcers (rarely vesicles, which break down quickly) on the hard palatal mucosa or even buccal gingiva, in a distinctive unilateral distribution (Figure 4-10). Ulcers often coalesce to form larger ulcers with a scalloped border similar to those of HSV. These ulcers heal within 10–14 days, and postherpetic neuralgia in the oral cavity is uncommon. Involvement of V_3 results in blisters and ulcers on the mandibular gingiva and tongue.

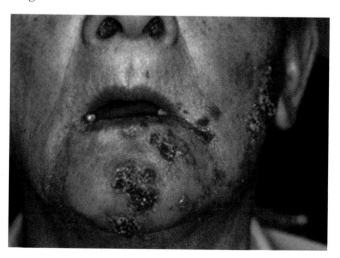

FIGURE 4-9 Facial lesions of herpes zoster involving the third division of the trigeminal nerve.

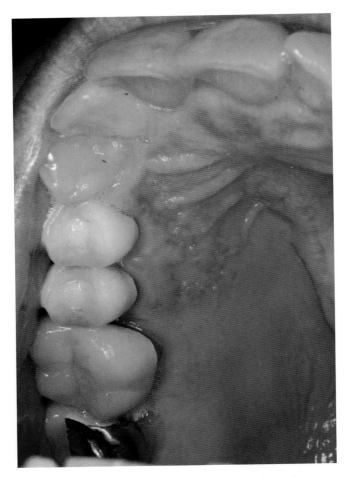

FIGURE 4-10 Palatal lesions of herpes zoster involving the second division of the trigeminal nerve; note unilateral distribution.

An uncommon complication of HZI involving the geniculate ganglion is Ramsay Hunt syndrome. Patients develop Bell palsy, vesicles of the external ear, and loss of taste sensation in the anterior two-thirds of the tongue.[50] HZI has been reported to cause resorption and exfoliation of teeth and osteonecrosis of the jawbones, especially in patients with human immunodeficiency virus (HIV) disease.[57–60,60a]

Differential Diagnosis

The pain that is often experienced in the prodrome before the onset of vesicles and ulcers may lead to an incorrect diagnosis of pulpitis, leading to unnecessary dental treatment such as endodontic therapy.

HSV infection appears in a similar fashion and if mild and localized to one side may be mistaken for HZI; cultures differentiate between the two. Other blistering/ulcerative conditions such as pemphigus or pemphigoid are chronic and/or progressive diseases that do not present unilaterally.

In severe cases of localized necrosis of the soft tissues and bone, acute necrotizing ulcerative periodontitis (NUP) should be considered, particularly in the HIV population. Coinfection with CMV is often noted in immunocompromised patients.[61] Medication- (such as bisphosphonate) and radiation-induced osteonecrosis of the jaws will have a history of exposure to bisphosphonate and radiation, respectively, and often is precipitated by dentoalveolar trauma in the absence of clustered ulcers.

In this age of bioterrorism, clinicians should be familiar with the signs of infection with vaccinia (smallpox virus), which presents with characteristic skin blisters and pustules.

Laboratory Findings

As with HSV infection, an oral swab for viral isolation using cell culture is still the best way to confirm a diagnosis of VZV infection, although VZV is more fastidious and difficult to culture. A simple smear stained with a standard laboratory stain would reveal the presence of multinucleated epithelial cells, but this does not distinguish between HSV and VZV. Direct fluorescent antibody testing using a smear has greater sensitivity.[62] This test uses a smear obtained by scraping the lesion and staining it with antibody against VZV conjugated to a fluorescent compound. The use of PCR and real-time PCR to detect viral antigen is expensive and highly sensitive, but the presence of VZV antigen does not always equate with active infection.[63,60a,28a]

After primary infection, the patient seroconverts and IgG against VZV is detectable in the serum, although this is not protective against future recrudescence. HZI causes a transient rise in IgM and an increase in levels of IgG, but these are not reliable for diagnostic purposes.[64]

Biopsy is usually not required and not the diagnostic test of choice since the clinical presentation is usually characteristic. If one should be performed, tissue should always include the intact epithelium adjacent to the ulcer since that is where the cytopathic effect in epithelium is best seen. VZV and HZI are cytopathic to the epithelial cells and result in the formation of multinucleated epithelial cells with viral inclusions, similar to and indistinguishable from HSV infection.

In HZI, there is inflammation of peripheral nerves leading to demyelination and wallerian degeneration, as well as degeneration of the dorsal horn cells of the spinal cord.[51]

Management

As with HSV infection, management of oral lesions of varicella and HZI is directed toward pain control (particularly, the prevention of postherpetic neuralgia), supportive care, and hydration (see Table 4-2), and definitive treatment to minimize the risk for dissemination, particularly in immunocompromised patients. Aspirin use, especially in children with VZV infection or influenza, may be associated with the development of Reye syndrome, which is potentially fatal, and is contraindicated; ibuprofen is the preferred analgesic.[65]

Treatment of primary VZV infection includes the use of acyclovir (800 mg five times a day).[66,67] This reduces infectivity, severity of lesions, and hospitalization for complications. However, acyclovir has poor bioavailability. Valacyclovir (1000 mg three times a day) or famciclovir (500 mg three times a day) for seven days is effective in treating HZI and should be started within 72 hours of disease onset.[54,55] These drugs also reduce the incidence of postherpetic neuralgia compared with acyclovir.

The first line of treatment for postherpetic neuralgia is gabapentin,[68] 5% lidocaine patch,[69] and 0.025%–0.8% topical capsaicin, and the second line of treatment is with opioid analgesics and tricyclic antidepressants.[53] The use of corticosteroids and antiviral therapy together in an attempt to reduce postherpetic neuralgia has not proved effective, although early treatment with famciclovir or valacyclovir may prevent it.[51,56,70] Other modalities of treatment have been reviewed.[51] Case reports suggest that botulinum toxin may provide relief.[71] For a more detailed description of management of postherpetic neuralgia, see Chapter 12, "Orofacial Pain."

A live, attenuated vaccine for the prevention of VZV infection has been shown to reduce the incidence of varicella outbreaks.[72] Vaccination of older adults with this vaccine causes an increase in antibody levels, boosts cell-specific immunity, and reduces the incidence and/or severity of subsequent HZI and postherpetic neuralgia.[73,74,74a]

Cytomegalovirus Infection
Etiology and Pathogenesis

Cytomegalovirus (CMV) is a β-herpesvirus, and 60%–70% of the adult population has been exposed.[75] Primary infection may be asymptomatic or cause an infectious mononucleosis–like disease. Manifestations of infection and disease are most evident in the immunocompromised population, such as patients who have received organ transplants or those who have AIDS. It is the most common cause of pneumonia within the first 120 days after hematopoietic stem cell transplantation.[76] Once exposed to CMV, this virus establishes latency within the connective tissue cells, such as the endothelium of blood vessels, mononuclear cells, and white blood cells.[77] CMV within endothelial cells may contribute to vascular inflammation, vascular occlusion, and end-organ damage.[78] Transmission is by direct transfer of infected white blood cells through intimate contact and through blood products.[77] In organ transplant recipients, CMV in the donor organ leads to CMV infection in the recipient.[79] There is growing evidence that CMV infection is associated with Guillain–Barré syndrome, as well as with polyradiculopathy and myopathy in patients with AIDS.[80,81]

A recent study on mucocutaneous CMV infection (mostly perianal) revealed that CMV infection of mucocutaneous sites was usually part of a polymicrobial infection with HSV or VZV.[82] The authors suggest that CMV in such cases is not the pathogenic agent for these ulcers since the presence of those two α-herpesviruses alone could account for the ulceration and tissue damage. These authors also noted that CMV was often found in nonlesional skin.

Clinical Findings

Primary CMV infection presents similarly to infectious mononucleosis with marked lymphocytosis; 20% of patients with infectious mononucleosis–like symptoms have CMV rather than EBV infection.[83] Unlike the more common EBV-associated infectious mononucleosis, there is fever but little lymphadenopathy or splenomegaly.[77] Serious complications include meningoencephalitis, myocarditis, and thrombocytopenia.

Approximately 90% of patients with AIDS have circulating antibodies against CMV.[84] In these patients, CMV tends to involve the eye (CMV retinitis that may result in blindness if untreated), gastrointestinal tract (CMV enteritis), and mucocutaneous sites, especially perianal and perigenital areas.

Oral Manifestations

CMV infection in the mouth in the immunocompromised patient tends to present as a single large ulcer and less often as multiple ulcers (Figure 4-11). They are usually painful and may have been present for weeks or months. Any site may be involved. Up to one-third of such ulcers are coinfected with other viruses of the herpes family, especially HSV and VZV.[85,86]

There have been occasional reports of mandibular osteomyelitis and tooth exfoliation associated with CMV and VZV infection.[61,87] Both viruses are associated with vasculopathy and thrombosis, which may be the underlying etiopathogenesis.[58,60,88]

Differential Diagnosis

As indicated earlier, CMV is often seen in association with HSV or VZV infections and, in such situations, may be a bystander rather than pathogenic. Therefore, evaluation for these other two viruses is essential for single or multiple ulcers in the immunocompromised population. In patients with HIV/AIDS, infections with mycobacteria, fungi, and other organisms must be ruled out.

Single ulcers present for weeks or months should be evaluated for squamous cell carcinoma or other malignancies. Since patients who develop such ulcers caused by opportunistic pathogens are often immunocompromised, one should have a high index of suspicion for a malignancy.

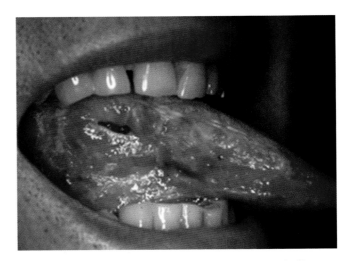

FIGURE 4-11 Cytomegalovirus ulcer on a background of hairy leukoplakia in a patient with AIDS.

Benign or malignant salivary gland tumors or soft tissue tumors may also become secondarily ulcerated from trauma. Single ulcers on the tongue may also represent traumatic ulcerative granuloma (see below).

Laboratory Tests

CMV infections of the oral cavity presenting as ulcers tend to be deep with viral particles residing in endothelial cells and tissue monocytes. As such, a culture of an ulcer infected by CMV is unlikely to be positive unless there is shedding of CMV from the ulcer surface. Furthermore, CMV is difficult to grow in culture, but may be performed using "shell vials" in which CMV is detected through the use of monoclonal antibodies.[89] Monitoring of systemic infection by CMV viral load and antigenemia through PCR using drawn blood or dried blood spots has become increasing important especially in the immunocompromised patient population.[89a] CMV matrix protein PP65 is also often found in neutrophils, and these can be assayed.[77] Antibody titers against CMV are unreliable for the diagnosis of active infection.

Biopsy for microscopic examination and/or to obtain tissue for culture is the test of choice for identification of CMV in oral ulcers.[86] CMV infection produces large intranuclear inclusions within endothelial cells and monocytes in the connective tissue, with an associated nonspecific chronic inflammation.[90] The use of immunohistochemical staining helps identify CMV if there are only a few infected cells. A biopsy has the advantage of also ruling out any of the other differential diagnoses discussed. It is important to make sure that the biopsy includes normal epithelium because if the ulcer is coinfected with HSV or VZV, these would be identified on the biopsy in the intact epithelium adjacent to the ulcer.

Management

As with all ulcerative lesions, pain is managed with topical anesthetics and systemic analgesics as needed, with appropriate dietary modifications and good hydration (see Table 4-2). CMV infection is treated with ganciclovir, valganciclovir (a valine ester and oral prodrug of ganciclovir with approximately 10-fold bioavailability of ganciclovir), foscarnet, or cidofovir; newer drugs include maribavir and letermovir.[90a] A CMV vaccine is currently under development.[90b]

Coxsackievirus Infection

Coxsackie (CV), a ribonucleic acid (RNA) virus, is a member of the genus *Enterovirus* and family Picornaviridae and has features in common with poliovirus; most are type A (CVA), and some type B (CVB).[91,92] More than 90% of infections caused by the nonpolio enteroviruses are either asymptomatic or result in nonspecific febrile illness. The viruses replicate first in the mouth and then extensively in the lower gastrointestinal tract, where they shed. Transmission is therefore primarily by the fecal-oral route, although some shedding occurs in the upper respiratory tract.

CVA infection is implicated in paralytic disease, a cold-like illness, and upper respiratory tract infection that is usually febrile, and pleurodynia.[91] CVB (in particular CVB4) infection is associated with the development of aseptic meningitis, sometimes complicated by encephalitis, carditis, and disseminated neonatal infection.[93] Enteroviruses have been implicated in the pathogenesis of type 1 insulin-dependent diabetes mellitus.[91,13b] One theory suggests direct destruction of the pancreatic islets by the virus, whereas another focuses on the viral infection triggering an autoimmune destruction of islet cells because of similarity between viral and islet cell antigens. CVB4 has also been implicated in the pathogenesis of primary Sjögren syndrome. Although enteroviral capsid protein VP1 was identified in the salivary gland samples of patients with primary but not secondary Sjögren syndrome, these studies were also refuted.[94,95,60a]

In the oral cavity, CV infections lead to three disease entities: HFM disease, herpangina, and lymphonodular pharyngitis.

HFM Disease

CVA16 and enterovirus (EV) 71 are the most common cause of this vesicular exanthem, although CVA4–7, CVA9, CVA10, CVA24, CVB2, and CVB5, as well as echovirus 18, have also been implicated.[91] EV 71 (closely related to CVA16) has been seen in large outbreaks in Southeast Asia. HFM disease, as with many CV infections, including herpangina, tends to be seasonal (usually summer), occurs in epidemic clusters, and has high transmission rates. Atypical HFM disease exhibits widespread oral and skin involvement and onychomadesis (separation of the nail plate from the nail bed) and is caused by CVA6.[95a]

While comparing cases of HFM disease caused by EV71 with those caused by CVA16, EV71 is much more likely to be associated with severe central nervous system disease (such as meningitis and brainstem encephalitis), paralysis, pulmonary edema, and death.[96] In one study of patients with HFM disease and herpangina, 83% of cases were caused by EV71 and only 8% by CVA or CVB.[97] In another study of EV71 infections, 87% of cases manifested with HFM disease and 13% with herpangina.[98]

Clinical Findings

HFM disease usually afflicts children younger than 10 years in summer. Patients have a low-grade fever and sore mouth; 75%–100% of patients have a skin rash, especially on the hands and feet (dorsa, palms, and soles) and 30% on the buttocks.[99,100] The rash is first red and macular and then becomes vesicular.

Oral Manifestations

Patients are febrile and complain of a sore mouth and throat. Lesions begin as erythematous macules that become vesicles and quickly break down to ulcers. Lesions are usually located on the tongue, hard and soft palate, and buccal mucosa but can present on any oral mucosal surface.[99,100]

Herpangina

The word *herpangina* derives from *herpes*, meaning "vesicular eruption," and *angina*, meaning "inflammation of the throat." CVA (serotypes 1–10, 16, and 22) are the most common viruses isolated from this disease.[91,101] But CVB1–5,[91,102] echoviruses, and EV71 have also been identified in this condition.[96]

Clinical Findings

As with all CV infections, children younger than 10 years are usually afflicted, and outbreaks usually occur in epidemics in summer. Patients develop fever, headache, and myalgia that usually last only one to three days.

Oral Manifestations

The first oral symptoms of herpangina are sore throat and pain on swallowing. There may be erythema of the oropharynx, soft palate, and tonsillar pillars. Small vesicles form, but these rapidly break down to 2–4 mm ulcers and these persist for 5 to 10 days (Figure 4-12).[91]

Lymphonodular pharyngitis is considered a variant of herpangina[91] and is associated with CVA10. Patients report a sore throat, but rather than presenting with vesicles that break down to ulcers, patients develop diffuse small nodules in the oropharynx.[103]

Differential Diagnosis

Lesions of both HFM disease and herpangina may resemble primary herpetic gingivostomatitis. However, lesions on the palms and soles are typical for HFM disease, and ulcers in the posterior oral cavity are typical for herpangina. Bright red and painful gingiva also characterizes primary HSV infection, and this is uncommon in CV infections. Chicken pox presents with generalized vesicular skin lesions, but ulcers are not prominent in the oral cavity; patients also appear more ill. Infectious mononucleosis (primary EBV infection) may also present with sore throat and purulent exudates, but serology distinguishes this from CV infections.

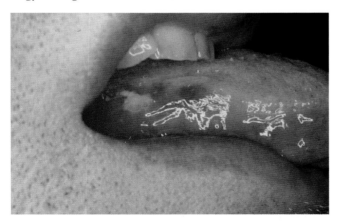

FIGURE 4-12 A cluster of ulcers on the tongue of a patient with herpangina. The patient also had lesions of the palate and posterior pharyngeal wall.

Streptococcal infections of the throat generally do not produce vesicles or ulcers seen in HFM disease or herpangina but rather a purulent exudate, although both may appear similar, cultures distinguish between the two.

Laboratory Tests

CVB infections may be diagnosed by culture (usually from the throat or feces), but only CVA9 and CVA16 grow readily and CVA is best identified by inoculation into newborn mice. Serum IgM to CVB can be detected early on but is not serotype-specific. Typing is mainly by molecular techniques or monoclonal antibodies.[92,92a]

Diagnosis is usually made on clinical findings, and culture and biopsies are rarely necessary for diagnosis. Nevertheless, skin biopsies of HFM disease and herpangina show intraepidermal vesicles with a mixed lymphocytic and neutrophilic infiltrate, degeneration of epidermal cells, and dermal edema. Eosinophilic nuclear inclusions and intracytoplasmic picornavirus particles are seen in the surrounding dermal vessels.[104,105] Biopsy of lymphonodular pharyngitis shows hyperplastic lymphoid nodules.

Management

CV infections are self-limiting (unless complications arise or the patient is immunocompromised), and management is directed toward control of fever and mouth pain, supportive care, and limiting contact with others to prevent spread of the infection. Effective antiviral agents for CV are not available.

Necrotizing Ulcerative Gingivitis and Necrotizing Ulcerative Periodontitis

NUG, formerly known as acute necrotizing ulcerative gingivitis (ANUG), and its more severe counterpart, NUP, were reclassified in 1999 by the American Academy of Periodontics under the category of "Necrotizing Periodontal Disease."[106] These are acute ulcerative-inflammatory conditions of the gingiva and periodontium, respectively, that are associated with polymicrobial infection. During World War I, NUG was dubbed "trench mouth" since it was frequent among the soldiers in the trenches. NUG and NUP have strong associations with immune suppression (especially AIDS), debilitation, smoking, stress, poor oral hygiene, local trauma, and contaminated food supply. Diabetes may also be a risk factor.[107] It is unclear if NUG is a forerunner of NUP, but they are often seen in patients with AIDS. Both NUP and noma thrive in communities characterized by a large low-socioeconomic class and extreme poverty.[108,109]

Etiology and Pathogenesis

The more important and constant of the microbes involved include *Treponema* species, *Prevotella intermedia*, *Fusobacterium nucleatum*, *Peptostreptococcus micros*, *Porphyromonas gingivalis*, *Selenomonas* species, and *Campylobacter*.[110–112] In patients with HIV, candida and herpesvirus are also commonly present.[112a] Since some of these fusospirochetal organisms are common in the periodontal tissues, many believe that it is the permissive environment of an immunocompromised host that allows these microbes to proliferate. The tissue destruction is most probably a result of the production of endotoxins and/or immunologic activation and subsequent destruction of the gingiva and adjacent tissues. In addition, patients show reduced neutrophil chemotaxis and phagocytosis, resulting in poor control of infection.[110] Some have identified herpesviruses within the crevicular fluid,[111] but such viruses shed readily in oral secretions, particularly in areas where there is tissue destruction and therefore may be nonpathogenic bystanders.

If there is underlying systemic illness, NUG and NUP can spread rapidly from the gingiva to the periodontium and into the soft tissues, giving rise to cancrum oris, noma, or orofacial gangrene. This is particularly devastating in children who are malnourished and live in poverty and is seen not infrequently in Africa. *Fusobacterium necrophorum* is likely to play an important role in the progression of NUP to cancrum oris because this organism produces a dermonecrotic toxin, hemolysin, leukotoxin, and proteolytic enzymes, all leading to extensive tissue destruction.[111] It may also stimulate the growth of *P. intermedia*.

Clinical Findings

NUG and NUP may or may not be associated with fever and malaise, although submandibular lymphadenopathy is usually present. This may be more prominent in patients with an underlying immunodeficiency.

However, noma is generally accompanied by fluctuating fever, marked anemia, high white cell count, general debilitation, and a recent history of some other systemic illness, such as measles.[109]

Oral Manifestations

NUG has a rapid and acute onset. The first symptoms include excessive salivation, a metallic taste, and sensitivity of the gingiva. This rapidly develops into extremely painful and erythematous gingiva with scattered punched-out ulcerations, usually on the interdental papillae, although any part

of the marginal gingiva may be affected (Figure 4-13). There is accompanying malodor, and there may be gingival bleeding. Because of the pain associated with the gingivitis, there is usually abundant buildup of dental plaque around the teeth because it may be too painful to perform effective oral hygiene.

Patients who are immunocompromised and neutropenic are prone to developing such lesions (Figure 4-14). In patients with AIDS, the prevalence of NUP is approximately 6% and is strongly predictive of a CD4 count less than 200 cell/mm³.[113] In this population, these areas may lead to osteonecrosis or necrosis of the soft tissues (Figure 4-15).[114]

In patients who have severe immunodeficiency or are malnourished, NUG and NUP may progress to noma (Figure 4-16). The overlying skin becomes discolored, and perforation of the skin ensues. The orofacial lesions

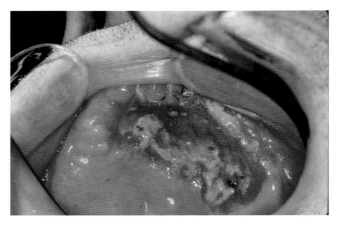

FIGURE 4-14 Fusospirochetal palatal lesions in a neutropenic patient.

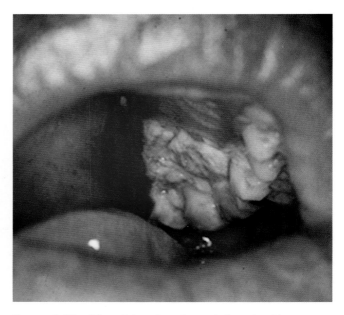

FIGURE 4-15 Necrotizing ulcerative periodontitis with osteonecrosis in a patient with AIDS.

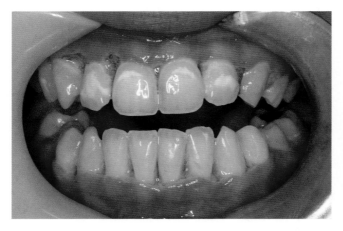

FIGURE 4-13 Necrotizing ulcerative gingivitis with typical punched out, necrotic and ulcerated interdental papillae. (Courtesy of Dr. Hani Mawardi, Boston, MA.)

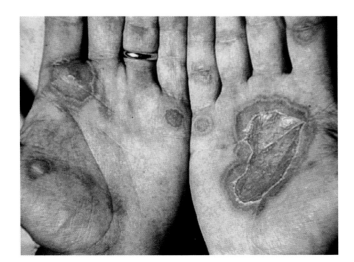

FIGURE 4-16 Erythema multiforme with target lesions of the skin of the hand.

are cone shaped, with the base of the cone within the oral cavity and the tip at the skin aspect. There is sloughing of the oral mucosa followed by sequestration of the exposed, necrotic bone and teeth. Without treatment, the mortality rate is 70%–90%.[111]

Differential Diagnosis

The acute onset of erythematous and ulcerated gingiva of NUG may suggest a diagnosis of primary herpetic gingivostomatitis, and this is readily ruled out with a culture. Desquamative gingivitis (caused by lichen planus, mucous membrane pemphigoid [MMP], pemphigus vulgaris [PV], and hypersensitivity reactions) may present primarily on the gingiva, with no skin findings. However, these conditions are not of acute onset but rather chronic and/or progressive over months and years and are characterized by inflammation rather than necrosis.

Neutropenic ulcers in patients on cancer chemotherapy may appear similar, leading to extensive ulceration and necrosis of the marginal gingiva and other mucosal surfaces.

Single large necrotic ulcers of noma suggest deep fungal infections or infections with the herpes family of viruses, especially in immunocompromised patients. Squamous cell carcinoma is also a consideration in this group of patients.

Laboratory Testing

Secretions from the gingival sulcus grow mixed flora but in particular will be culture positive for *Treponema species*, *Prevotella intermedia*, *Fusobacterium nucleatum*, and other bacteria as indicated above. Necrotizing gingival lesions may also be caused by microbes other than fusospirochetes, such as *Pseudomonas aeruginosa*.[115]

A biopsy is usually not helpful in making a diagnosis, although biopsies may be performed to rule out some other conditions that may have a similar clinical presentation. The

lesions demonstrate ulceration, extensive necrosis, leukocytoclasia, histiocytic vasculitis with luminal fibrin clots, and a prominent infiltrate of lymphocytes. More than half of the cases in patients who were HIV positive were immunoreactive for HIV p24 within focal histiocytes, whereas EBV RNA was identified in 1 (6%) of 17 cases.[116]

Management

This is directed toward supportive care and pain control (see Table 4-2), definitive treatment, and identification of underlying predisposing factors. In patients who are malnourished, nutritional rehabilitation is essential to halt the progress of gingival lesions to noma.

Definitive treatment of NUG and NUP consists of gentle debridement to remove as much of the debris and plaque as possible; this is best accomplished with topical anesthesia during the first few visits. The use of chlorhexidine digluconate mouthrinse led to resolution in >90% of cases.[117] Patients with more extensive disease and/or systemic symptoms may require antibiotics active against gram-negative anaerobes, such as β-lactams.[114] Interestingly, metronidazole, which has little activity against spirochetes, also is effective, suggesting that resolution can occur without treatment of the entire microbial complex.[117a]

Once the acutely painful episodes have resolved, scaling and root planing to completely remove all residual plaque and calculus are indicated. Periodontal surgery may be necessary to correct gingival and periodontal defects. It may be appropriate to test the patient for HIV or other immunosuppressive conditions, such as blood dyscrasia.

Cases of noma need aggressive treatment with nutritional supplementation, antibiotics, and tissue debridement. Nevertheless, survivors exhibit significant disfigurement and functional impairment from tissue loss and scarring.[111]

Erythema Multiforme

Erythema multiforme (EM) is an acute, self-limited, inflammatory mucocutaneous disease that manifests on the skin and often oral mucosa, although other mucosal surfaces, such as the genitalia, may also be involved.[118–120] It represents a hypersensitivity reaction to infectious agents (majority of cases) or medications.[134] There is still controversy over how best to classify EM. In general, EM is classified as EM minor if there is less than 10% of skin involvement and there is minimal to no mucous membrane involvement, whereas EM major has more extensive but still characteristic skin involvement, with the oral mucosa and other mucous membranes affected.[118,119] However, there is likely a subset of EM that affects the oral mucosa only without skin involvement. Historically, fulminant forms of EM were labeled Stevens–Johnson syndrome (SJS) and toxic epidermal necrolysis (TEN [Lyell disease]). However, more recent data suggest that EM is etiopathogenetically distinct from those two latter conditions, and they are discussed separately below.

Etiology and Pathogenesis

EM is a hypersensitivity reaction, and the most common inciting factors are infection, particularly with HSV, myco-plasma and Chlamydia pneumonia.[120a,120b] Drug reactions to NSAIDS, anticonvulsants, or other drugs play a smaller role.[118,119] Cases of oral EM precipitated by benzoic acid, a food preservative, have been reported.[120,121]

Studies show that recurrent EM is associated with HSV infection in 65%–70% of cases, both by history of HSV infection one to three weeks before onset of EM, sero-positivity for HSV antibodies, and identification of HSV antigens.[122–124] Some cases had concurrent RHL.[124] Using PCR techniques, HSV gene products have been identified in 71%–81% of cases of recurrent EM.[10,11] For nonrecurrent EM, this falls to 27%.[11] It is postulated that HSV antigens incite a T cell–mediated delayed-type hypersensitivity reaction that generates interferon-γ, with the amplified immune system recruiting more T cells to the area. Cytotoxic T cells, natural killer cells, and/or cytokines destroy the epithelial cells.[120] More recently, it has been suggested that CD34+ cells, Langerhans cell precursors, carry fragments of HSV DNA to the skin where it incites EM.[124a,124b]

Clinical Findings

EM generally affects those between ages 20 and 40 years, with 20% occurring in children.[118] Patients with recurrent EM have an average of six episodes a year (range 2–24), with a mean duration of 9.5 years; remission occurred in 20% of cases.[124] Episodes usually last several weeks.[118,119] There may be a prodrome of fever, malaise, headache, sore throat, rhinorrhea, and cough.[118] These symptoms suggest a viral (especially respiratory tract) infection, and this is not sur-prising since infectious agents are known to trigger EM.

Skin lesions appear rapidly over a few days and begin as red macules that become papular, starting primarily in the hands and moving centripetally toward the trunk in a symmetric distribution. The most common sites of involve-ment are the upper extremities, face, and neck.[118] The skin lesions may take several forms—hence the term *multiforme*. The classic skin lesion consists of a central blister or necrosis with concentric rings of variable color around it called typ-ical "target" or "iris" lesion that is pathognomonic of EM; variants are called "atypical target" lesions (Figure 4-16). The skin may feel itchy and burnt. Postinflammatory hyperpig-mentation is common in dark-skinned individuals and may be worsened by sun exposure.[118]

Oral Findings

The oral findings in EM range from mild erythema and erosion to large painful ulcerations (Figures 4-17 and 4-18).[118] When severe, ulcers may be large and confluent, causing difficulty in eating, drinking, and swallowing, and patients with severe EM may drool blood-tinged saliva. Extensive lip involvement with inflammation, ulceration, and crusting is common (Figures 4-19).

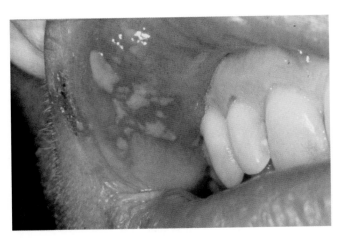

FIGURE 4-17 Intraoral erythema multiforme with coalescent aphthous-like ulcers and erythema of the buccal mucosa

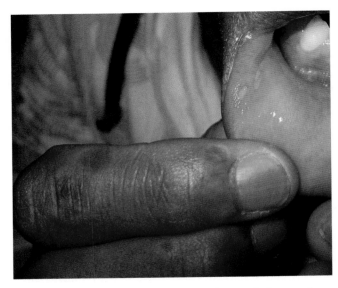

FIGURE 4-18 Erythema multiforme with target lesions on the skin of the fingers and intraoral ulcers. Courtesy of Dr. Adam Lipworth, Boston, MA.

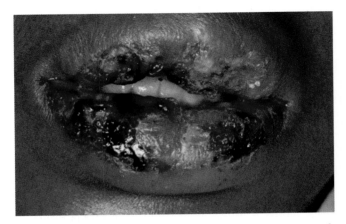

FIGURE 4-19 Erythema multiforme with hemorrhagic crusts of the lips.

Oral lesions are present in 23%–70% of patients with recurrent EM.[122–125,125a] The most commonly affected sites are the lips (36%), buccal mucosa (31%), tongue (22%), and labial mucosa (19%).[125] Genital and ocular sites are affected in 25 and 17% of cases, respectively.[124]

The concept of pure oral EM is controversial and not universally accepted since some dermatologists believe that the characteristic appearance and distribution of skin lesions are the sine qua non for the diagnosis of EM.[118] Nevertheless, cases of oral EM without skin involvement have been reported. Intraoral lesions take the form of irregular bullae, erosions, or ulcers surrounded by extensive erythema. Crusting and bleeding of the lips are common, but not always present.[126,–129]

Differential Diagnosis

Primary HSV gingivostomatitis with its viral prodrome and erosions and ulcerations may resemble oral EM, but these lesions are culture positive for HSV and do not usually present with the typical skin rash. Oral ulcers of HSV are usually smaller and well circumscribed, whereas EM lesions are larger and irregular. Autoimmune vesiculobullous disease such as pemphigus and pemphigoid may have oral ulcers and skin lesions, although skin lesions are bullous in nature and not maculopapular, without the centripetal progression seen in EM. They are chronic, slowly progressive diseases that usually persist for months, whereas EM heals within weeks.

Hemorrhagic crusts on the lips are seen in paraneoplastic pemphigus (PNPP) (associated with malignancies, see below) and SJS (often drug-induced, see below). The latter may be difficult to distinguish from EM.

Recurrent oral EM in the absence of skin findings may be confused with recurrent aphthous ulcers (see below), but aphthous ulcers present as discrete ovoid or round ulcers, whereas ulcers of EM are more diffuse and irregular with marked erythema.

Laboratory Findings

The diagnosis is made primarily on clinical findings and a recent history of recrudescent HSV infection. IgG and IgM levels are not a reliable test for recrudescence or asymptomatic reactivation although they may be suggestive.

Early cutaneous lesions show lymphocytes and histiocytes in the superficial dermis around superficial dermal vessels. This is followed by hydropic degeneration of basal cells, keratinocyte apoptosis and necrosis, subepithelial bulla formation, and a lymphocytic infiltrate.[130] Leukocyte exocytosis is also usually noted. Similar changes are seen in the biopsies of patients with oral EM.[131]

Management

Mild oral EM can be managed with systemic or topical analgesics for pain and supportive care since the disease is self-limiting and resolves within a few weeks. More severe cases are usually managed with systemic corticosteroids although patients often worsen on discontinuation of steroid therapy. Topical steroids may also help resolve lesions. Cases suspected of having HSV-associated EM should be treated with antiviral medications. Treatment with acyclovir at the first sign of disease in recurrent EM controls disease in approximately half of patients.[124] Other treatment modalities include dapsone, hydroxychloroquin, mycophenolate mofetil, azathioprine, colchicines, methotrexate, and intravenous immunoglobulin.[131a]

Continuous acyclovir at 400 mg twice a day prevents development of EM in most patients with HSV-associated disease, whereas EM not related to HSV responded well to azathioprine (100–150 mg/d).[124] Other studies have also shown good suppression of recurrent HSV-associated EM using 500 mg of valacyclovir twice a day or 250 mg of famciclovir twice daily.[42,132,132a] Dapsone (100–150 mg/d) and antimalarials are partially successful in suppressing recurrent outbreaks but may be associated with significant side effects.[124]

Stevens-Johnson Syndrome and Toxic Epidermal Necrolysis

Studies done within the last 10 to 15 years now support the concept that Stevens-Johnson Syndrome (SJS) is a less severe variant of Toxic Epidermal Necrolysis (TEN) and separate clinically and etiopathogenetically from EM. Although all three are hypersensitivity reactions and give rise to oral bullae, erosions, ulcers, and crusted lips, the skin lesions of SJS and TEN are different from EM. They are more severe and tend to arise on the chest rather than the extremities on erythematous and purpuric macules; these lesions are called "atypical targets." SJS is much more likely to be associated with medication use and *Mycoplasma pneumoniae* infection (especially in children) and rarely with HSV infection, whereas EM is much more likely to be associated with HSV infection.[133,136,136a]; some cases of Mycoplasma pneumonia are associated with EM.[120a] The more common inciting drugs include antibacterial sulfonamides, penicillin, anticonvulsants, and NSAIDs in children,[136b,136c] and allopurinol, oxicams, and nevirapine in adults.[137,136c] In Han Chinese, development of SJS/TEN to the aromatic anticonvulsants such as carbamazepine, phenytoin, and lamotrigine is highly associated with HLA-B*1502[137a]; other alleles associated with such reactions have also been identified.[137b]

The mucosal surfaces of the eye, genitalia, and mouth are almost always severely affected by SJS/TEN, always with skin involvement. The typical oral manifestation is extensive oral ulceration with hemorrhagic crusts on the vermilion and oral and other mucosal surfaces (Figure 4-20 and Figure 4-21). These lesions resemble oral lesions of PNPP, which are long-standing and associated with malignancy (see below) as well as EM.

Histopathologically, most of the disease is localized in the epidermis, presumably this being the site where the drug or its metabolite is bound, with less inflammation in the dermis

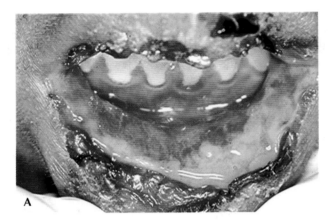

FIGURE 4-20 Stevens–Johnson syndrome. Lips and labial mucosa (A), skin (B), and penile (C) lesions in a 17-year-old male with Stevens–Johnson syndrome.

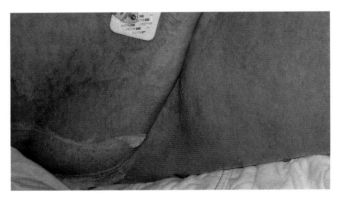

FIGURE 4-21 Toxic epidermal necrolysis with necrolysis or peeling of the epidermis. Courtesy of Dr. Adam Lipworth, Boston, MA.

as is usually seen in EM. The primary cytokine involved is tumor necrosis factor (TNF)-α.

Because of the severity of this condition, treatment is generally with intensive supportive care because of loss of skin barrier, intravenous immunoglobulin, systemic steroids, cyclosporine, plasmapheresis, cyclophosphamide, and TNF-αinhibitor[138,139,139a]

Plasma Cell Stomatitis and Oral Hypersensitivity Reactions

Etiology and Pathogenesis

This is a group of conditions that have protean manifestations. Oral hypersensitivity reactions may take the following forms:

1. Acute onset of ulcers such as in oral EM (discussed above)
2. Red and white reticulated lesions of a lichenoid hypersensitivity reaction (discussed in Chapter 5, "Pigmented Lesions of the Oral Mucosa")
3. Fixed drug eruption

4. Marked erosions and erythema especially on the gingiva with or without ulceration called plasma cell stomatitis (PCS).
5. Swelling of the lips/angioedema (see Chapter 20, "Immunologic Diseases")
6. Oral allergy syndrome that presents mainly with symptoms of itching with or without swelling of the oral structures and oropharynx

This discussion concentrates on lesions of PCS. PCS generally causes erythema and less often ulcers, but is included here for completeness.

PCS is a hypersensitivity reaction that was first described in the late 1960s and early 1970s and was likely a contact stomatitis to a component of chewing gum.[140] Since then, sporadic cases have continued to be reported, and these are all likely caused by a sensitizing contactant, whether or not the contactant is identified. These include khat (*Catha edulis*),[141] components of toothpaste,[141a] mint candies,[142] and household cleaners.[143] Sometimes, the terms *mucous membrane plasmacytosis* and *plasma cell orificial mucositis* are used because there may be involvement of the upper respiratory tract.[144] Because of the intense plasma cell infiltration, it is believed that this is a B cell–mediated disorder, with T cells augmenting the response. Some believe that this is caused by components of plaque bacteria, although this is not a universally accepted concept.[145]

Clinical Findings

PCS occurs within days of exposure to the contactant, with most signs and symptoms limited to the oral cavity. Some lesions may affect the periorificial tissues or the oropharynx, leading to upper airway symptoms of hoarseness, dysphagia, and mild airway obstruction.[144] Endoscopy may reveal erythematous and thickened mucosa, often with a cobblestoning pattern from the edema. An obvious allergen/contactant is not always identified.[144,146]

Oral Manifestations

PCS occurs within a few days of exposure. It presents as brightly erythematous macular areas of the oral cavity, almost always involving the marginal and attached gingiva or alveolar mucosa and often involving other soft tissues, such as the maxillary and mandibular sulcus or buccal mucosa (Figure 4-22). Ulcers may be present, and there may be epithelial sloughing and desquamation. The gingiva may also be swollen and edematous. Patients may complain of pain and sensitivity and bleeding of the gingiva on brushing. Angular cheilitis with fissuring and dry atrophic lips have been reported.[140,147]

Some cases reported as PCS consisted of a very localized area of erythematous gingiva, usually around a single tooth and measuring usually <1 cm.[145] Interestingly, two adults in this series also demonstrated plasma cell balanitis. It is

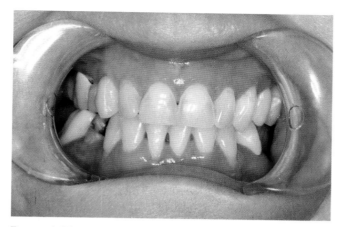

FIGURE 4-22 Plasma cell gingivitis presenting as desquamative gingivitis.

unclear if this represented classic PCS since most cases of PCS tend to be diffuse.

Differential Diagnosis

The differential diagnosis for PCS includes any of the desquamative gingivitis, such as erythematous/erosive lichen planus, and the autoimmune vesiculobullous disorders, such as MMP and PV. The lesions will become chronic if the patient continues to be exposed to an undetected allergen. A biopsy for both routine histology and direct immunofluorescence (DIF) studies to rule out MMP and PV is necessary to make the diagnosis.

Another condition that PCS can mimic is pubertal or pregnancy-induced gingivitis and plaque-associated gingivitis. The difference in the histopathology is in the density of plasma cells since nonspecific gingivitis generally is also associated with a plasma cell infiltrate. The clinical appearance of diffuse red gingiva with a history of a topical agent helps make the diagnosis. Some previous cases reported as PCS may constitute such plaque-associated and pubertal gingivitis.[145] Chronic granulomatous gingivitis caused by components of polishing agents such as pumice also often present with sensitive or painful erythematous gingiva. A biopsy will show the presence of particulate matters in the gingival connective tissue.

Mouth-breathers often present with erythematous and sometimes edematous gingiva, usually around the upper anterior teeth. A good history and correlation with the histopathologic findings help differentiate this from PCS.

Erythematous candidiasis may present with marked gingival erythema without the usual white curdy papules of "thrush" or pseudomembranous candidiasis. *Candida* may also secondarily infect an area of PCS.

Fixed drug eruptions are rare in the oral cavity, but there have been cases presenting as acute ulcers on the vermilion after exposure to drug such as levocetirizine, an antihistamine, resolution on withdrawal, and reulceration on rechallenge.[148]

PCS should not be confused with a direct toxic irritation of the tissues such as from strongly flavored foods and dentifrices.[149] This would occur in any individual and does not represent a hypersensitivity reaction because ulcers are caused by the noxious and caustic nature of the chemical causing a mucosal burn.

Laboratory Findings

Patch testing to identify an allergen may be helpful. A biopsy is the most useful diagnostic test for this condition.

A biopsy of the gingiva in PCS shows parakeratosis, epithelial hyperplasia, neutrophilic exocytosis, and numerous spongiotic pustules in the absence of *Candida*.[140,150] The most significant finding is dense sheets of plasma cells in the lamina propria; many dilated capillaries lie close to the surface, accounting for the marked erythema. Eosinophils are not seen usually.[144] Immunoperoxidase stains will invariably show the plasma cell infiltrate to be polyclonal, typical for a reactive/inflammatory process, and not monoclonal, which typifies neoplastic lesions.[71]

Management

PCS is self-limiting and will generally, but not always, regress if the contactant is identified and removed. Nevertheless, pain control and anti-inflammatory agents may be helpful during the healing process (see Table 4-2). Topical steroids may help reduce inflammation and speed healing (see Chapter 3).[151] Some lesions have resolved with intralesional triamcinolone injections, although the gingiva is a particularly difficult location for such injections.[152] Cases have also responded well to prednisone.[146] Gingivectomies may be needed to recontour lesions that are long-standing and more fibrotic. One case showed improvement with 2% fusidic acid.[153]

THE PATIENT WITH RECURRING ORAL ULCERS

Recurring oral ulcers are among the most common problems seen by clinicians who manage diseases of the oral mucosa. There are several diseases that should be included in the differential diagnosis of a patient who presents with a history of recurring ulcers of the mouth, including RAS (recurrent aphthous stomatitis), Behçet syndrome, recrudescent HSV infection, and recurrent oral EM. HSV infection and EM were discussed earlier in this chapter.

Recurrent Aphthous Stomatitis

RAS is a common disorder characterized by recurring ulcers confined to the oral mucosa in patients with no other signs of systemic disease. Hematologic deficiencies, immune disorders, and connective tissue diseases may cause oral aphthous-like ulcers clinically similar to RAS. These ulcers resolve when the underlying systemic condition resolves.

RAS affects approximately 20% of the general population, but when specific ethnic or socioeconomic groups are studied, the incidence ranges from 5% to 50%.[154] RAS is classified according to clinical characteristics: minor ulcers, major ulcers (Sutton disease, periadenitis mucosa necrotica recurrens), and herpetiform ulcers (Table 4-3). There are cases in which a clear distinction between minor and major ulcers is blurred, particularly in patients who experience severe discomfort from continuous episodes of ulcers. These lesions have been referred to as "severe" minor ulcers.

Etiology and Pathogenesis

It was once assumed that RAS was a form of recurrent HSV infection, and there are still clinicians who mistakenly call RAS "herpes." Many studies done during the past 40 years have confirmed that RAS is not caused by HSV.[155] This distinction is particularly important at a time when there is specific effective antiviral therapy available for HSV that is ineffective for RAS. "Herpes" is an anxiety-producing word, suggesting a sexually transmitted disease among many lay persons, and its use should be avoided when it does not apply. There have been theories suggesting a link between RAS and a number of other microbial agents, including oral streptococci, *Helicobacter pylori*, VZV, CMV, and human herpesvirus (HHV)-6 and HHV-7, but there are presently no conclusive data linking RAS to a specific microorganism.

The major factors presently linked to RAS include genetic factors, hematologic or immunologic abnormalities, and local factors, such as trauma and smoking. There is increasing evidence linking local immune dysfunction to RAS, although the specific defect remains unknown. During the past 30 years, research has suggested a relationship between RAS and lymphocytotoxicity, antibody-dependent cell-mediated cytotoxicity, defects in lymphocyte cell subpopulations, and an alteration in the CD4 to CD8 lymphocyte ratio.[156]

More recent research has centered on dysfunction of the mucosal cytokine network. The work of Buno and colleagues suggests that an abnormal mucosal cytokine cascade in RAS patients leads to an exaggerated cell-mediated immune response, resulting in localized ulceration of the mucosa.[157]

The best documented factor is heredity. Miller and colleagues studied 1,303 children from 530 families and demonstrated an increased susceptibility to RAS among children of RAS-positive parents.[158] A study by Ship showed that patients with RAS-positive parents had a 90% chance of developing RAS, whereas patients with no RAS-positive parents had a 20% chance of developing the lesions.[159] Further evidence for the inherited nature of this disorder results from studies in which genetically specific human leukocyte antigens (HLAs) have been identified in patients with RAS, particularly in certain ethnic groups.[160] There have been

recent studies by Bazrafshani and colleagues linking minor RAS to genetic factors associated with immune function, particularly genes controlling release of the proinflammatory cytokines interleukin (IL)-1B and IL-6.[161] A unified model of etiology postulates that triggers such as stress, or hormonal changes trigger a cascade of proinflammatory cytokines directed against oral mucosa.[161a]

Hematologic deficiency, particularly of serum iron, folate, or vitamin B$_{12}$, appears to be an etiologic factor in 5%–10% patients with aphthous-like ulcers although these sometimes occur on keratinized mucosa (Figure 4-23).[162] Studies of RAS populations from the United Kingdom show a higher level of nutritional deficiency than studies performed in the United States. Aphthous-like ulcers may also be seen in celiac disease.

It was initially reported in the 1960s that there is a negative correlation between RAS and a history of smoking, and many clinicians have reported that RAS is exacerbated when patients stop smoking. A study measuring a nicotine metabolite present in the blood of smokers confirmed that the incidence of RAS is significantly lower among smokers.[164]

The nicotine metabolites are believed to decrease levels of proinflammatory cytokines and increase anti-inflammatory cytokines.

Other factors that have been reported associated with RAS include anxiety, periods of psychological stress, localized trauma to the mucosa, menstruation, upper respiratory infections, and food allergy.

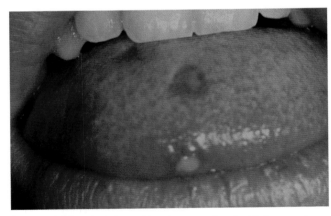

FIGURE 4-23 Aphthous-like ulcer associated with iron deficiency anemia; notice unusual location of ulcer on the keratinized mucosa of the tongue dorsum; ulcers resolved when iron deficiency anemia was treated.

TABLE 4-3	Types of RAS
Type of RAS	Clinical Findings
Minor	Most common (80%), <1.0 cm, lasting 7–14 days, no scarring
Major	>1.0 cm, lasting weeks, often with scarring
Herpetiform	<1.0 cm, >10 ulcers, dispersed widely over mucosa
Severe	Same as minor, but ulcers present continuously

Oral Findings

The first episodes of RAS most frequently begin during the second decade of life. The lesions are confined to the oral mucosa and begin with prodromal burning or the sensation of a small bump in the mucosa from 2 to 48 hours before an ulcer appears. During this initial period, a localized area of erythema develops. Within hours, a small white papule forms, ulcerates, and gradually enlarges over the next 48–72 hours. The individual lesions are round, symmetric, and shallow (similar to viral ulcers), but no tissue tags are present from ruptured vesicles, which helps distinguish RAS from diseases that start as vesicles, such as pemphigus, and pemphigoid. Multiple lesions are often present, but the number, size, and frequency vary considerably (Figures 4-24 through 4-27). The buccal and labial mucosae are most commonly involved. Lesions rarely occur on the heavily keratinized palatal mucosa or gingiva. In mild RAS, the lesions reach a size of 0.3–1.0 cm and begin healing within a few days. Healing without scarring is usually complete in 10–14 days.

Most patients with RAS have between one and six lesions at each episode and experience several episodes a year. The disease is an annoyance for the majority of patients with mild RAS, but it can be painfully disabling for patients with severe RAS and RAS major. Patients with major ulcers develop deep lesions that are larger than 1 cm in diameter and last for weeks to months. In the most severe cases, large portions of the oral mucosa may be covered with large deep ulcers that can become confluent, and are extremely painful, interfering with speech and eating. These patients may require hospitalization for intravenous feeding and treatment with systemic corticosteroids. The lesions may last for months and sometimes be misdiagnosed as squamous cell carcinoma, granulomatous disease, or blistering disease. The lesions heal slowly and leave scars that may result in decreased mobility of the uvula and tongue.

The least common variant of RAS is the herpetiform type, which tends to occur in adults. The patient presents with more than 10 small punctate ulcers, measuring <5 mm, scattered over large portions of the oral mucosa.

Differential Diagnosis

RAS is the most common cause of recurring oral ulcers and is essentially diagnosed by exclusion of other diseases. A detailed history and examination by a knowledgeable clinician should distinguish RAS from primary acute lesions such as viral stomatitis or erythema EM, from chronic multiple lesions such as pemphigus or pemphigoid, as well as from other conditions associated with recurring ulcers, such as RIH, connective tissue disease, drug reactions, and other dermatologic disorders. The history should include obtaining symptoms of HIV, connective tissue disease such as lupus erythematosus, gastrointestinal complaints suggestive of inflammatory bowel disease, and associated skin, eye, genital, or rectal lesions (Figures 4-27 and 4-28).

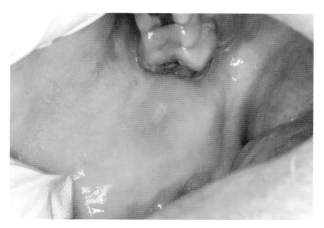

FIGURE 4-24 Recurrent aphthous stomatitis (minor) of the buccal mucosa.

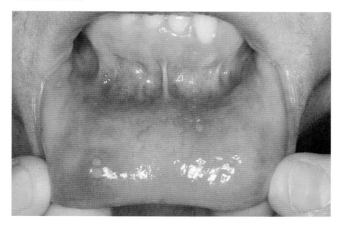

FIGURE 4-25 Recurrent aphthous stomatitis (minor) of the lower labial mucosa presenting with several ulcers.

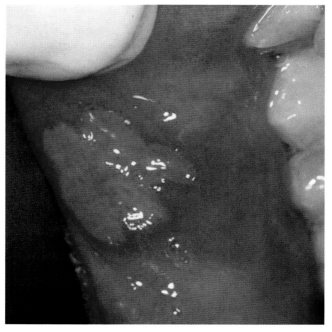

FIGURE 4-26 Recurrent aphthous stomatitis (major) of the buccal mucosa.

Laboratory Findings

Laboratory investigation should be ordered when patients do not follow the usual pattern of RAS, for example, when episodes of RAS become more severe, begin past the age of 40, or are accompanied by other signs and symptoms. Biopsies are only indicated when it is necessary to exclude other diseases, particularly granulomatous diseases such as Crohn disease, sarcoidosis, or blistering diseases such as pemphigus or pemphigoid.

Patients with severe minor aphthae or major aphthous ulcers should be investigated for systemic disorders, including connective tissue diseases and hematologic abnormalities, such as reduced levels of serum iron, folate, vitamin B12, and ferritin.[163] Patients with abnormalities in these values should be referred to an internist for further management. HIV-infected patients, particularly those with CD4 counts below 100/mm^3, may develop major aphthous ulcers, and, occasionally, such oral ulcers are the presenting sign of AIDS.[164a]

Biopsies reveal only a superficial ulcer covered by a fibrinous exudate with granulation tissue at the base and a mixed acute and chronic inflammatory infiltrate. Studies of early lesions of RAS demonstrate an infiltration of large granular lymphocytes and helper-induced CD4 lymphocytes with focal degeneration of basal cells. The appearance of the ulcer is associated with the appearance of cytotoxic suppressor lymphocytes.[80,89,165]

Management

Management is tailored to the severity of the disease. In mild cases with two or three small lesions, use of a protective emollient such as Orabase™ often alleviates pain and facilitates healing. Pain relief of minor lesions can be effected with a topical anesthetic agent such as benzocaine or lidocaine. In more severe cases, the use of a high-potency topical steroid preparation, such as fluocinonide, betamethasone, or clobetasol, placed directly on the lesion, shortens healing time and reduces the size of the ulcers. The effectiveness of the topical steroid is partially based on good instruction and patient compliance regarding proper use. The steroid gel should be applied directly to the lesion after meals and at bedtime two to three times a day or mixed with an adhesive such as Orabase™ prior to application. Larger lesions can be treated by placing a gauze sponge containing the topical steroid on the ulcer and leaving it in place for 15–30 minutes to allow for longer contact of the medication. Other topical preparations that have been shown to decrease the healing time of RAS lesions include amlexanox paste and a topical tetracycline or doxycycline, which can be used either as a mouthrinse or applied as a paste directly to the lesions[164b] Intralesional steroid injections can be used to treat large indolent major RAS lesions. It should be emphasized that no available topical therapy reduces the frequency of new lesions.

When patients with major aphthae or severe cases of multiple minor aphthae do not improve sufficiently with topical therapy, use of systemic therapy should be considered. Drugs that have been reported to reduce the number of ulcers in selected cases of major aphthae include colchicine, pentoxifylline, dapsone, short bursts of systemic steroids, and thalidomide.[166–170] Each of these drugs has the potential for side effects, and the clinician must weigh the potential benefits versus the risks.

Thalidomide, a drug originally marketed as a nonaddicting hypnotic in the 1950s, was withdrawn from the market in the early 1960s due to its association with multiple, severe, deforming, and life-threatening birth defects. Further investigation demonstrated that thalidomide has significant anti-inflammatory and immunomodulatory properties and is useful in treating a number of diseases, including erythema nodosum leprosum, discoid lupus erythematosus, graft-vs-host disease, multiple myeloma, and Behçet disease.[41] The drug has also been shown to reduce both the incidence and severity of major RAS in both HIV-positive and HIV-negative patients. The use of thalidomide for RAS should be reserved for management of severe major RAS where other less toxic therapies, including high-potency topical steroids, colchicine, and pentoxifylline, have failed to control the disease. Thalidomide must be used with extreme caution

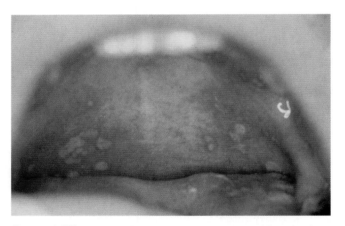

FIGURE 4-27 Herpetiform aphthous stomatitis with multiple <5 mm ulcers of palatal mucosa.

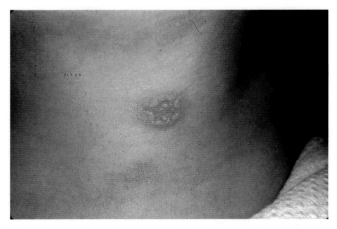

FIGURE 4-28 Early skin lesion of pemphigus vulgaris.

in women during childbearing years owing to the potential for severe life-threatening and deforming birth defects. All clinicians prescribing thalidomide in the United States must be registered in the REMS (Risk Evaluation Mitigation Strategy) program for thalidomide and patients receiving the drug must be thoroughly counseled regarding effective birth control methods that must be used whenever thalidomide is prescribed. For example, two methods of birth control must be used, and the patient must have a pregnancy test monthly. Other side effects of thalidomide include peripheral neuropathy, gastrointestinal complaints, drowsiness and deep vein thrombosis. Monitoring patients taking long-term thalidomide for the development of peripheral neuropathy with periodic nerve conduction studies is also recommended.

Behçet Disease (Behçet Syndrome)

Behçet's disease (BD) was initially described by the Turkish dermatologist Hulusi Behçet as a triad of symptoms including recurring oral ulcers, recurring genital ulcers, and eye involvement. BD is now understood to be a multisystem disorder with many possible manifestations. The highest incidence of BD has been reported in eastern Asia, the Middle East, and the eastern Mediterranean, particularly Turkey and Japan, where BD is a leading cause of blindness in young males; however, cases have been reported worldwide, including Europe and North America. BD is more severe in younger patients and patients with eye and GI involvement.[170a]

Etiology and Pathogenesis

BD is a systemic vasculitis characterized by hyperactivity of neutrophils with enhanced chemotaxis and elevated proinflammatory cytokines IL-8 and IL-17, with TNF-α playing a major role in the pathogenesis.[170b] The HLA-B51 genotype is most frequently linked to BD, especially in patients with severe forms of the disease in Asia.

Clinical Manifestations

The highest incidence of BD is in young adults between the ages of 25 and 40, with the oral mucosa as the most common site of involvement. The genital area is the second most common site of involvement and presents as ulcers of the scrotum and penis in males and ulcers of the labia in females. The eye lesions consist of uveitis, retinal vasculitis, vascular occlusion, optic atrophy, and conjunctivitis. Blindness is a common complication of the disease, and periodic evaluation by an ophthalmologist is necessary.[172–174]

Systemic involvement occurs in over half of patients with BD. Skin lesions resembling erythema nodosum or large pustular lesions occur in over 50% of patients with BD. These lesions may be precipitated by trauma, and it is common for patients with BD to have a cutaneous hyperreactivity to intracutaneous injection or a needlestick (pathergy). Arthritis occurs in greater than 40% of patients and most frequently affects the knees, ankles, wrists, and elbows. The affected joint may be red and swollen, as in

rheumatoid arthritis, but involvement of small joints of the hand does not occur, and permanent disability does not result.[175]

In some patients, central nervous system involvement is the most distressing component of the disease. This may include brainstem syndrome, involvement of the cranial nerves, or neurologic degeneration resembling multiple sclerosis that can be visualized by magnetic resonance imaging of the brain.[176] Other reported signs of BD include thrombophlebitis, intestinal ulceration, venous thrombosis, and renal, cardiac, and pulmonary disease. Both pulmonary involvement and cardiac involvement are believed to be secondary to vasculitis. Involvement of large vessels is life threatening because of the risk of arterial occlusion or aneurysms.

BD in children, which most frequently presents between the ages of 9 and 10 years, has similar manifestations to the adult form of the disease, but oral ulcers are a more common presenting sign in children, whereas uveitis is less common. Oral lesions are the presenting symptom in more than 95% of children with BD. A variant of BD, characterized by mouth and genital ulcers with inflamed cartilage, is associated with relapsing polychondritis.[177]

Oral Findings

The most common site of involvement of BD is the oral mucosa. Recurring oral ulcers appear in more than 90% of patients; these lesions cannot be distinguished either clinically or histologically from RAS (Figure 4-29). Some patients experience mild recurring oral lesions; others have deep, large, scarring lesions characteristic of major RAS. These lesions may appear anywhere on the oral or pharyngeal mucosa.

Differential Diagnosis

Because the signs and symptoms of BD overlap with those of several other diseases, particularly the connective tissue diseases, it has been difficult to develop criteria that meet with universal agreement. The most recent collaborative study developed the following diagnostic criteria based on a point system where 4 or more points is strongly associated

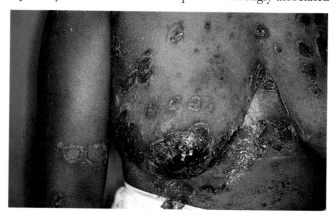

FIGURE 4-29 Extensive involvement of the skin in a patient with pemphigus vulgaris

with BD: oral, ocular, and genital lesions score 2 points each, while skin lesions, and neurologic and vascular manifestations score 1 point each. Positive pathergy test is an optional test but also scores 1 if positive.[178]

Laboratory Findings

BD is a clinical diagnosis based up the criteria described above. Laboratory tests are used to rule out other diseases, such as connective tissue (e.g., lupus erythematosus) and hematologic diseases causing severe neutropenia.

Management

The management of BD depends on the severity and the sites of involvement. Patients with sight-threatening eye involvement or central nervous system lesions require more aggressive therapy with drugs, with a higher potential for serious side effects. Azathioprine and other immunosuppressive drugs combined with prednisone have been shown to reduce ocular disease as well as oral and genital involvement.[179] Pentoxifylline, which has fewer side effects than immunosuppressive drugs or systemic steroids, has also been reported to be effective in decreasing disease activity, particularly of oral and genital lesions.[180,181] Dapsone, colchicine, and thalidomide have also been used effectively to treat mucosal lesions of BD.[182,183] Therapy with monoclonal antibodies such as infliximab and etanercept are playing an increasing role in therapy of BD particularly in patients who do not respond to anti-inflammatory and immunosuppressive drugs.[184,185]

THE PATIENT WITH CHRONIC MULTIPLE ULCERS

Patients with chronic multiple oral lesions, continuously present, for weeks to months are frequently misdiagnosed since their lesions are often confused with recurring oral mucosal disorders such as RAS and recrudescent HSV. The clinician can avoid misdiagnosis by carefully questioning the patient on the initial visit regarding the natural history of the lesions. In recurring disorders such as severe RAS, the patient may experience continual new episodes of ulceration of the oral mucosa, but individual lesions heal and new ones form. In the category of disease described in this section, the same lesions are present for weeks to months often expanding in size

The major diseases in this group are PV, pemphigus vegetans, BP (bullous pemphigoid), MMP, linear IgA disease (LAD), and erosive lichen planus. Lichen planus is discussed in Chapter 5, "Red and White Lesions of the Oral Mucosa." HSV infections in immunocompromised patients are discussed earlier in this chapter.

Pemphigus

Pemphigus includes a group of autoimmune, potentially life-threatening diseases that cause blisters and erosions of the skin and mucous membranes, characterized by intra-epithelial acantholysis. The predisposition to develop the

autoantibodies that cause pemphigus is genetically determined, but the triggering mechanism that initiates the immune response is unknown

Desmoglein 1 (DSG1), a glucoprotein adhesion molecule, is primarily found in the skin, whereas desmoglein 3 (DSG3) is chiefly detected in mucosal epithelium and individuals genetically susceptible to pemphigus harbor desmoglein reactive B and T cells.[185a] The immune reaction against these glycoproteins causes a loss of cell-to-cell adhesion, resulting in the separation of cells and the formation of intraepithelial bullae.[186]

The major variants of pemphigus are PV, pemphigus foliaceus, PNPP, and IgA pemphigus. Pemphigus vegetans is a variant of PV, and pemphigus erythematosus is a variant of pemphigus foliaceus. Pemphigus foliaceus is present in the endemic form referred to as "fogo selvagem" in rural areas of Brazil, possibly related to an insect bite. In pemphigus foliaceus, the blister occurs in the superficial granular cell layer, whereas in PV, the lesion is deeper, just above the basal cell layer. Mucosal involvement is not a feature of the foliaceus and erythematous forms of the disease, where the antibodies are only directed against DSG1. D-penicillamine and captopril may induce pemphigus, usually of the foliaceus or erythematosus rather than the vulgaris type. Discontinuation of the offending drug frequently results in spontaneous recovery.

IgA pemphigus is a rare form of pemphigus with deposition of IgA instead of IgG on surface epithelial cells with two subtypes, subcorneal pustular dermatosis and intraepithelial neutrophilic IgA dermatosis, sometimes reacting against desmocollin. It is unclear if this form of pemphigus affects the mucosa.

Pemphigus Vulgaris
Etiology and Pathogenesis

Pemphigus vulgaris (PV) is the most common form of pemphigus, accounting for more than 80% of cases. The underlying mechanism responsible for causing the intraepithelial lesion of PV is the binding of IgG autoantibodies to DSG3, a transmembrane glycoprotein adhesion molecule present on desmosomes. The loss of this glycoprotein results in loss of cell-to-cell adhesion resulting in intra-epithelial blisters. Patients with PV mainly involving the mucosa have antibodies primarily against DSG3, but patients with PV involving both the skin and mucosa will have antibodies against both DSG3 and DSG1.[187] Evidence for the relationship of the IgG autoantibodies to PV lesion formation includes studies demonstrating the formation of blisters on the skin of mice after passive transfer of IgG from patients with PV. There are 0.1–0.5 cases reported each year per 100,000 persons, with the highest incidence occurring in the fifth and sixth decades of life, although rare cases have been reported in children. PV occurs more frequently among Ashkenazi Jews. PV is strongly associated with increased frequency of HLA DRB*0402 in Ashkenazi Jews and HLA DQB*0503 in other ethnic races.

PV has been reported coexisting with other autoimmune diseases, particularly myasthenia gravis. Patients with thymoma also have a higher incidence of PV. Several cases of pemphigus have been reported in patients with other autoimmune disorders or those with neoplasms such as lymphoma. Death occurs most frequently in elderly patients and in patients requiring high doses of corticosteroids who develop infections and bacterial septicemia, most notably from *Staphylococcus aureus.*

Clinical Manifestations

The classic lesion of PV is a thin-walled bulla arising on otherwise normal skin or mucosa. The bulla rapidly breaks but continues to extend peripherally, eventually leaving large areas denuded of skin (Figures 4-28 and 4-29). A characteristic sign of the disease may be obtained by applying pressure to an intact bulla. In patients with PV, the bulla enlarges by extending to an apparently normal surface. Another characteristic sign of the disease is that pressure to an apparently normal area results in the formation of a new lesion. This phenomenon, called the Nikolsky sign, results from the upper layer of the skin pulling away from the basal layer. The Nikolsky sign is most frequently associated with pemphigus but may also occur in other blistering disorders. Some patients with pemphigus develop acute fulminating disease, but, in most cases, the disease develops more slowly, usually taking months to develop to its fullest extent.

Any mucosal and skin surface may be involved, and in severe cases, the conjunctival, pharyngeal, and laryngeal mucosa may be involved, along with extensive skin lesions. Patients with oral lesions of pemphigus may also have esophageal lesions, and if esophageal symptoms are present, endoscopic examination should be performed to determine the severity of the lesions.

Oral Findings

Up to 80%–90% of patients with PV develop oral lesions sometime during the course of the disease, and in 60% of cases, the oral lesions are the first sign. The oral lesions may begin as the classic bulla on a noninflamed base; more frequently, the clinician sees shallow irregular erosions and ulcers because the bullae rapidly break. A thin layer of epithelium peels away in an irregular pattern, leaving a denuded base (Figures 4-30 and 4-31). The edges of the lesion continue to extend peripherally over a period of weeks until they involve large portions of the oral mucosa. Most commonly, the lesions start on the buccal mucosa, often in areas of trauma along the occlusal plane. The palatal mucosa and gingiva are other common sites of involvement.

It is common for the oral lesions to be present for months before the skin lesions appear. If treatment is instituted during this time, the disease is easier to control. Frequently, however, the initial diagnosis is missed, and the lesions are misdiagnosed as HSV infection or candidiasis. The average time from the disease onset to diagnosis may often take over five months, and coexisting candidiasis may mask the typical clinical picture of the pemphigus lesions. There is a small subgroup of pemphigus patients whose disease remains confined

to the oral mucosa. These patients often have negative results on indirect and direct immuno-fluorescence testing.

Differential Diagnosis

If an accurate history and examination is performed, the clinician should be able to distinguish the lesions of pemphigus from those caused by acute viral infections or EM because of the acute nature of the latter diseases. It is also important for the clinician to distinguish pemphigus lesions from RAS. RAS lesions may be severe, but individual lesions heal and recur. In pemphigus, the same lesions continue to extend peripherally over a period of weeks to months. Lesions of PV are not round and symmetric like RAS lesions but are shallow and irregular and often have detached epithelium at the periphery. In early stages of the disease, the sliding away of the oral epithelium resembles skin peeling after a severe sunburn. In some cases, the lesions may start on the gingiva as desquamative gingivitis. It should be remembered that desquamative gingivitis is not a diagnosis in itself; these lesions must be biopsied to distinguish PV from subepithelial blistering diseases such as mucous membrane pemphigoid.

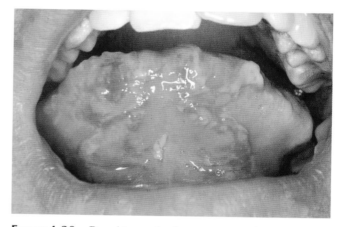

FIGURE 4-30 Pemphigus vulgaris presenting as shallow, irregular red erosions of the ventral tongue with ulcers and tissue tags.

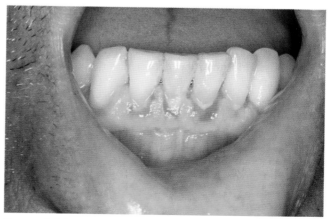

FIGURE 4-31 Pemphigus vulgaris presenting as erosions of the gingiva.

Laboratory Findings and Pathology

PV is diagnosed by biopsy and biopsies are best done on intact vesicles and bullae less than 24 hours old. However, because intact lesions are rare on the oral mucosa, the biopsy specimen should be taken from the advancing edge of the lesion, where areas of characteristic suprabasilar acantholysis may be observed by the pathologist. Specimens taken from the center of a denuded area are nonspecific histologically. Sometimes more than one biopsy is necessary before the correct diagnosis is rendered.

The separation of cells, called acantholysis, takes place in the lower layers of the stratum spinosum (Figure 4-32). Electron microscopic observations show the earliest epithelial changes as a loss of intercellular cement substance; this is followed by a widening of intercellular spaces, destruction of desmosomes, and, finally, cellular degeneration. This progressive acantholysis results in the classic suprabasilar bulla, which involves increasingly greater areas of epithelium, resulting in a loss of large areas of skin and mucosa.

A second biopsy, to be studied by direct immunofluorescence (DIF), should be performed whenever PV is included in the differential diagnosis. This study is best performed on a biopsy specimen that is obtained from clinically normal-appearing perilesional mucosa or skin, which should be placed in Michel's transport medium. In the laboratory, fluorescein-labeled antihuman immunoglobulins are placed over the patient's tissue specimen. In cases of PV, the technique will detect IgG bound to the surface of the keratinocytes (Figure 4-33).

Indirect immunofluorescent (IIF) antibody tests performed on a patient's serum are helpful in distinguishing PV from pemphigoid and other chronic oral lesions and in following the progress of patients during treatment of pemphigus. In this technique, serum from a patient with a bullous disease is placed over a prepared slide of a mucosal structure (usually monkey esophagus), and autoantibodies present in the serum will bind to the target antigen in the mucosa. The slide is then overlaid with fluorescein-tagged antihuman gammaglobulin. Patients with PV demonstrate antibodies against intercellular substances detected with the fluorescent microscope. The titer of the antibody has been related to the level of clinical disease and may be repeated periodically during treatment to determine disease activity. An enzyme-linked immunosorbent assay (ELISA) can distinguish anti-DSG1 antibodies from anti-DSG3 in serum samples.[187a,188] The ELISA test results combined with results from direct and IIF are the most accurate method to confirm a diagnosis of PV. The ELISA can distinguish PV from pemphigus foliaceus and may be helpful in determining disease activity and prognosis.[189]

Management

An important aspect of patient management is early diagnosis, when lower doses of medication can be used for

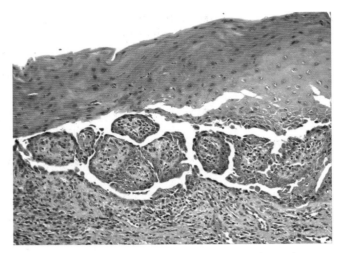

FIGURE 4-32 Photomicrograph of pemphigus vulgaris showing suprabasilar bulla with acantholysis.

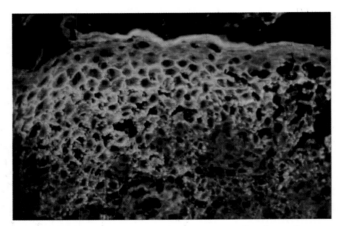

FIGURE 4-33 Direct immunofluorescence study of pemphigus vulgaris showing intercellular deposition of IgG.

shorter periods of time to control the disease. Management varies according to several factors, including the severity of the disease and the speed at which the disease progresses.

The mainstay of treatment remains high doses of systemic corticosteroids, usually given in dosages of 1–2 mg/kg/d. When substantial doses of steroids must be used for long periods, adjuvant therapy is recommended to reduce the steroid dose and their potential serious complications. The most commonly used adjuvants are immunosuppressive drugs such as mycophenolate mofetil, azathioprine, cyclophosphamide, and cyclophosphamide pulse therapy.[187b] Prednisone is used initially to bring the disease under control, and once this is achieved, the dose of prednisone is decreased to the lowest possible maintenance levels. Patients with only oral involvement also may need lower doses of prednisone for shorter periods, so the clinician should weigh the potential benefits of adding adjuvant therapy against the risks of long-term immunosuppression, such as blood dyscrasias and an increased risk of malignancy.

There is no one accepted treatment for PV confined to the mouth, but one five-year follow-up study of the treatment of oral PV showed no additional benefit of adding cyclophosphamide or cyclosporine to prednisone versus prednisone alone. Most studies of PV of the skin show a decreased mortality rate when adjuvant therapy is given along with prednisone.[190] The need for systemic steroids may be lowered further in cases of oral PV by combining topical with systemic steroid therapy, either by allowing the prednisone tablets to dissolve slowly in the mouth before swallowing or by using high-potency topical steroid creams. Dapsone has been shown to be effective.[191] Recalcitrant cases are treated with rituximab and intravenous immunoglobulins.[192] Rituximab is presently being used and evaluated as a first line treatment although some studies demonstrated a high rate of infection.[192a,193–195]

Paraneoplastic pemphigus

PNPP is a severe blistering disease that is a multiorgan disease associated with an underlying neoplasm, most frequently non-Hodgkin lymphoma, chronic lymphocytic leukemia, or thymoma. Castleman disease and Waldenström macroglobulinemia are also associated with cases of PNPP. This condition is also referred to as paraneoplastic autoimmune multiorgan syndrome because of the involvement of other systems such as the lungs in particular, and the variable skin findings, namely, pemphigus, pemphigoid, EM-like, graft-vs-host disease-like and lichen planus-like. The damage to the epithelium in PNPP is due to antibodies to desmogleins, plakins and an α-macroglobulin-like-protein.[195a]

Clinical Findings

Patients with PNPP develop severe blistering and erosions of the mucous membranes and skin. The onset of the disease is often rapid, and oral and conjunctival lesions are both common and often severe. These lesions may resemble the inflammatory lesions of a drug reaction, lichen planus, or EM, as well as the blisters seen in pemphigus (Figure 4-34).[195b] Lesions of the palms and soles are suggestive of PNPP.[196] In severe cases, the lesions may mimic TEN and often also involve the respiratory epithelium. Unlike EM or TEN, the lesions of PNPP continue to progress over weeks to months. Progressive pulmonary involvement occurs in up to 40% of patients with PNPP.[197]

Oral Manifestations

Oral ulcers and erythema are the most common manifestation of PNPP, and the oral disease is frequently extensive and painful. The lesions are frequently inflamed and necrotic, with large erosions covering the lips, tongue, and soft palate (Figure 4-35). Hemorrhagic crusts on the lips are characteristic.

Laboratory Findings

Histopathology of lesions of PNPP includes changes suggestive of EM, lichen planus, pemphigoid, and pemphigus. There is inflammation at the dermal–epidermal junction and keratinocyte necrosis in addition to the characteristic acantholysis seen in PV. DIF studies show deposition of IgG along the basement membrane similar to pemphigoid, as well as on the keratinocyte surface forming a lattice pattern similar to PV. IIF demonstrates antibodies that not only bind to epithelium but to liver, heart, and bladder tissue as well.[197a]

Management

Patients with PNPP secondary to localized tumors such as Castleman disease improve with the surgical removal of the tumor. Patients with PNPP resulting from lymphoma, however, have a poor prognosis and usually die within two years from a combination of the underlying disease, respiratory failure, and extensive mucocutaneous involvement.

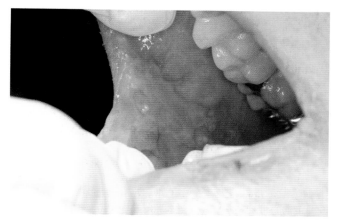

FIGURE 4-34 Extensive lesions of the buccal mucosa in a patient with paraneoplastic pemphigus.

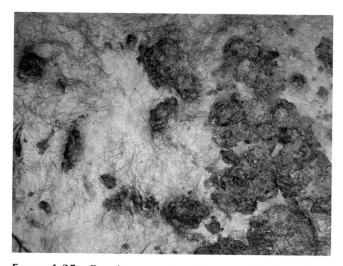

FIGURE 4-35 Pemphigus vegetans with vegetative lesions of the skin. Courtesy of Dr. Adam Lipworth, Boston, MA.

Use of a combination of prednisone, immunosuppressive drug therapy may help control the severity of the skin lesions, but oral, conjunctival, and pulmonary disease is frequently resistant to treatment. Rituximab and intravenous immunoglobulins can be helpful in these cases. High-potency topical steroid therapy, topical tacrolimus, and intralesional steroid injection can be helpful in reducing the severity of oral mucosal lesions.

Pemphigus Vegetans

Pemphigus vegetans, which accounts for 1%–2% of pemphigus cases, is a relatively benign variant of PV because the patient demonstrates the ability to heal the denuded areas. Two forms of pemphigus vegetans are recognized: the Neumann type and the Hallopeau type. The Neumann type is more common, and the early lesions are similar to those seen in PV, with large bullae and denuded areas. Attempts at healing result in vegetations of hyperplastic granulation tissue (Figure 4-35). In the Hallopeau type, which is milder, pustules, not bullae, are the initial lesions. These pustules are followed by verrucous hyperkeratotic vegetations.

Biopsy results of the early lesions of pemphigus vegetans show suprabasilar acantholysis. In older lesions, hyperkeratosis and pseudoepitheliomatous hyperplasia become prominent. DIF and IIF studies show changes identical to those seen in PV.

Oral Findings

Oral lesions are common in both forms of pemphigus vegetans and may be the initial sign of disease.[198] Gingival lesions may be lace-like ulcers with a purulent surface on a red base or have a granular or cobblestone appearance. Oral lesions that are associated with inflammatory bowel disease and resemble pemphigus vegetans clinically are referred to as pyostomatitis vegetans.[199]

Management

Treatment is the same as that for PV.

Subepithelial Bullous Dermatoses

Subepithelial bullous dermatoses are a group of mucocutaneous blistering diseases that are characterized by an autoimmune reaction that weakens a structural component of the basement membrane zone. The diseases in this group include BP, MMP, LAD, epidermolysis bullosa acquisita (EBA), and chronic bullous dermatosis of childhood. There is a significant overlap among these diseases, and the diagnosis is based on clinical manifestations combined with routine histopathology and molecular biology that identify the specific antigen. When one of these diseases is included in the differential diagnosis, a biopsy for DIF should be obtained. Research into pathologic mechanisms is defining the specific antigens in the basement membrane complex involved in triggering the autoantibody response. Subsets of patients diagnosed with a subepithelial bullous disease have been found to have an increased risk of an underlying malignancy, and a thorough workup should be considered during the initial phases of management.

Bullous Pemphigoid
Etiology and Pathogenesis

Bullous pemphigoid (BP), which is the most common of the subepithelial blistering diseases, occurs chiefly in adults older than the age of 60 years; it is self-limited and may last from a few months to five years. BP may be a cause of death in older debilitated individuals.[200] BP has occasionally been reported in conjunction with other diseases, particularly multiple sclerosis and malignancy, or drug therapy, particularly with diuretics.[201] A thorough evaluation for an underlying malignancy is recommended for patients with severe or recalcitrant BP.[201a]

BP is an autoimmune disease caused by the binding of autoantibodies to specific antigens found in the lamina lucida region of the basement membrane on the hemidesmosomes of epithelial basal cells. These antigens are glycoproteins referred to as BP antigens, BP 180 and BP 230.[202] Binding of antibody to antigen activates both leukocytes and complement, causing localized damage to the basement membrane, resulting in vesicle formation in the subepithelial region.

Clinical Manifestations

The characteristic skin lesion of BP is a tense blister on an inflamed base accompanied by urticarial plaques that chiefly involve the scalp, abdomen, extremities, axilla, and groin (Figure 4-36). Pruritus is a common feature of the skin lesions, which may initially present The disease is self-limiting but can last for months to years without therapy. Patients with BP may experience one episode or recurrent bouts of lesions. Unlike pemphigus, BP is rarely life threatening since the bullae do not continue to extend at the periphery to form large denuded areas, although death from sepsis or cardiovascular disease secondary to long-term

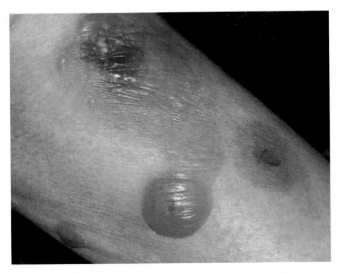

FIGURE 4-36 Bullous pemphigoid resulting in tense skin blisters. Courtesy of Dr. Adam Lipworth, Boston, MA

steroid use has been reported to be high in groups of sick elderly patients.[203]

Oral Findings

Oral involvement occurs in 10%–20% of BP patients.[203a] The oral lesions of BP are smaller, form more slowly, and are less painful than those seen in PV; the often extensive labial involvement seen in PV is not present. Desquamative gingivitis has also been reported as the most common oral manifestation of BP, and the gingival lesions may be the only site of oral involvement. The gingival lesions consist of generalized edema, inflammation, and desquamation with localized areas of discrete vesicle formation. The oral lesions are clinically and histologically indistinguishable from oral lesions of MMP, but early remission of BP is more common.

Differential Diagnosis

Oral diseases that appear clinically similar to BP are the erosive form of lichen planus, PV, and the other subepithelial bullous dermatoses. The erosive and ulcerative forms of LP frequently exhibit white Wickham striae at the periphery (see Chapter 5), along with ulcerations and erosions. PV usually has more extensive erosion of mucosa as well as skin involvement, and the lesions do not have the inflammation associated with MMP. The other subepithelial bullous dermatoses (described below) appear clinically similar to MMP and can only be distinguished by immunofluorescent and molecular techniques.

Laboratory Findings

Routine histology of a biopsy specimen demonstrates separation of the epithelium from the connective tissue at the basement membrane zone and an inflammatory infiltrate that is usually rich in eosinophils, particularly in skin biopsies.

DIF study of a biopsy specimen taken from perilesional inflamed tissue demonstrates deposition of IgG and C3 bound in a linear band to the basement membrane. IIF study of serum obtained from patients with BP demonstrates IgG antibodies bound to the epidermal aspect using the salt-split skin technique (see below). The salt-split skin test is particularly useful in distinguishing BP from EBA that has IgG antibodies localized to the dermal side of the salt-split skin (floor of the blister). Circulating autoantibodies against pemphigoid antigens BP 180 and BP 230 can be detected in serum samples using ELISA and are useful in both diagnosis and monitoring disease activity.[203b]

Management

Patients with localized oral lesions of BP may be treated with high-potency topical steroids, such as clobetasol or betamethasone, whereas patients with more extensive disease require use of systemic corticosteroids alone or combined with immunosuppressive drugs such as azathioprine, cyclophosphamide, mycophenolate, or rituximab.[203c] Patients with moderate levels of disease may minimize the use of systemic steroids by the use of dapsone or tetracycline, doxycycline, or minocycline, which may be combined with niacinamide.[204]

Mucous Membrane Pemphigoid MMP (Cicatricial Pemphigoid)

Etiology and Pathogenesis

Mucous membrane (MMP) is a chronic autoimmune subepithelial disease that primarily affects the mucous membranes of patients older than the age of 50 years, resulting in mucosal blistering, ulceration, and subsequent scarring in some organs. The disease occurs twice as frequently in women. The primary lesion of MMP occurs when autoantibodies directed against proteins in the basement membrane zone, acting with complement (C3), cause a subepithelial split and subsequent vesicle formation. Antibodies against basement membrane antigens have been identified in cases of MMP.[205] The antigens are most frequently present in the lamina lucida portion of the basement membrane, but the lamina densa may be the primary site of involvement in some cases. Subsets of MMP have been identified by the technique of immunofluorescent staining of skin that has been split at the basement membrane zone with the use of 1M sodium chloride prior to DIF (the "salt-split skin" technique).[206] The majority of cases of MMP demonstrate IgG directed against antigens on the epidermal side of the salt-split skin, which have been identified as BP Ag2 (BP180). However, cases of MMP have also been identified where the antigen is present on the dermal side of the split. This latter antigen has been identified as laminin-332 (previously referred to as epiligrin and laminin 5), an adhesion molecule that is a component of the anchoring filaments of the basement membrane.[206,207,207a] MMP associated with laminin-332 has been reported to carry a higher risk of association with an underlying malignancy, but the evidence for this is not conclusive. Further research is required regarding the possible association of pemphigoid with malignancy, and clinicians should consider a referral to rule out a possible underlying malignancy in newly diagnosed MMP patients.[208] Drugs such as clonidine, D-penicillamine, and L-DOPA have been reported as triggers for MMP.[208a]

Clinical Manifestations

MMP generally affects patients older than the age of 50 and is twice as common in women than in men. Lesions of MMP may involve any mucosal surface, but the oral mucosa is involved in more than 80% of cases, rarely with scarring. The conjunctiva is the second most common site of involvement and can lead to scarring and adhesions developing between the bulbar and palpebral conjunctiva called symblepharon (Figure 4-37). Corneal damage is common, and progressive scarring leads to blindness in close to 15% of patients. Lesions may also affect the genital mucosa, causing pain and sexual dysfunction. Laryngeal involvement causes pain, hoarseness, difficulty in breathing and may lead to death due to asphyxiation. Esophageal involvement may

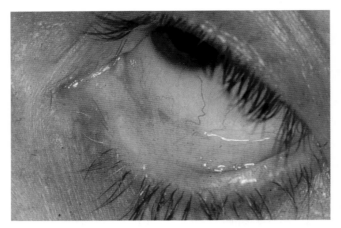

FIGURE 4-37 Mucous membrane pemphigoid of the conjunctiva with symblepharon formation.

cause dysphagia, which can lead to debilitation and death. Skin lesions, usually of the head and neck region, are present in 20%–30% of patients. HLA DQB*0301 is significantly increased in patients with widespread lesions.

Oral Findings

Oral lesions occur in more than 90% of patients with MMP. Desquamative gingivitis is the most common manifestation and may be the only manifestation of the disease appearing bright red (Figure 4-38 and Figure 4-39). Since these desquamative lesions resemble the lesions of erosive lichen planus and PV, all cases of desquamative gingivitis should be biopsied and studied with both routine histology and DIF for definitive diagnosis. Lesions may present as intact vesicles of the gingival or other mucosal surfaces, but more frequently they appear as nonspecific-appearing erythema and erosions (Figure 4-40). Unlike ocular pemphigoid, oral MMP rarely results in scarring.

Laboratory Findings

Patients with suspected MMP should have biopsy specimens taken for both routine and DIF studies. The specimen for routine histology and DIF should be taken from the edge of an ulcer, vesicle, or erythema and tissue. Histopathology reveals subepithelial clefting with preservation of basal cells and variable inflammation (Figure 4-41). Using the DIF technique (see "Laboratory Tests" under "PV" for description), biopsy specimens taken from MMP patients demonstrate positive immunofluorescence for IgG, C3 and sometimes IgA in the basement membrane zone in 50%–80% of patients (Figure 4-42). Using the salt-split skin technique, immunoreactants usually localize to the roof of the split (see above). Only 10% of MMP patients demonstrate positive IIF for circulating antibasement membrane zone antibodies. The conclusions of an international consensus conference published in 2002 concluded that both routine histology and DIF are essential when MMP is suspected.[208]

Management

Management of MMP depends on the severity of symptoms and site of involvement. When the lesions are confined to

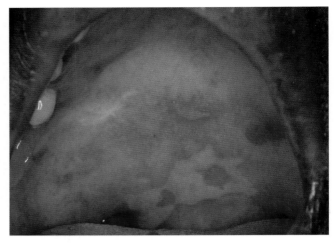

FIGURE 4-38 Palatal lesions of mucous membrane pemphigoid.

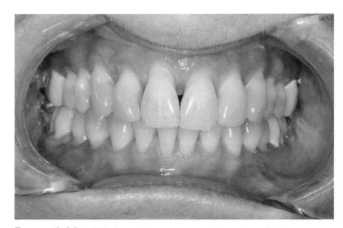

FIGURE 4-39 Moderate desquamative gingivitis of mucous membrane pemphigoid.

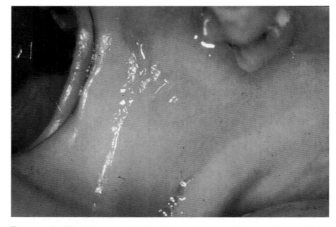

FIGURE 4-40 Intact vesicle of buccal mucosa in a patient with mucous membrane pemphigoid.

the oral mucosa, use of systemic corticosteroids should only be considered for short periods for severe outbreaks until steroid-sparing therapy can be instituted. Unlike PV, MMP

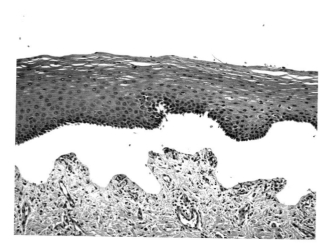

FIGURE 4-41 Photomicrograph of mucous membrane pemphigoid showing intact basal cells and subepithelial bulla.

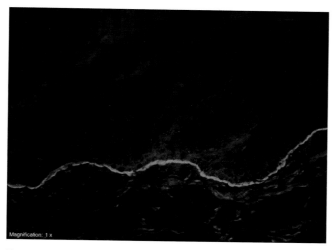

FIGURE 4-42 Direct immunofluorescence study of mucous membrane pemphigoid showing positive IgG deposition in the basement membrane zone.

is rarely a fatal disease, and long-term use of systemic steroids for oral lesion involvement alone is seldom indicated.

Patients with mild oral disease may be treated with topical and intralesional steroids. Desquamative gingivitis can often be managed with topical steroids in a soft dental splint that covers the gingiva, although the clinician using topical steroids over large areas of mucosa must closely monitor the patient for side effects such as candidiasis and effects of systemic absorption (Figure 4-43). When topical or intralesional therapy is not successful, use of a tetracycline, such as doxycycline or minocycline is often helpful in controlling desquamative gingivitis and other oral lesions. When there are severe oral lesions, conjunctival or laryngeal involvement, dapsone therapy is recommended as the next choice before considering long-term systemic steroids, immunosuppressive drug therapy or rituximab.[209,210] Since dapsone causes hemolysis and methemoglobinemia, glucose-6-phosphate dehydrogenase deficiency must be ruled out, and the patient's hemoglobin must be closely monitored. Another rare side

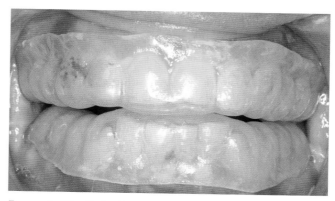

FIGURE 4-43 Soft splint used to hold topical steroids to treat desquamative gingivitis.

effect of dapsone is dapsone hypersensitivity syndrome, an idiosyncratic disorder characterized by fever, lymphadenopathy, skin eruptions, and occasional liver involvement. Patients resistant to dapsone should be treated with a combination of systemic corticosteroids and immunosuppressive drugs such as cyclophosphamide, particularly when there is risk of blindness from conjunctival involvement or significant laryngeal or esophageal damage. High-dose intravenous immunoglobulin therapy and rituximab has been shown in several series of cases to be effective adjuvant therapy in patients resistant to less conventional therapy.[203a,210a] The most effective therapy for severe MMP confined to the mouth has not been established due to lack of large clinical studies.[210b]

LAD and Chronic Bullous Disease of Childhood

Etiology and Pathogenesis

LAD is a subepithelial disease characterized by the deposition of mostly IgA rather than IgG in the basement membrane. LAD occurs most frequently in children below the age of 10 (known as chronic bullous disease of childhood [CBDC]) and adults older than 60 (Chen 2013). The clinical manifestations may resemble either dermatitis herpetiformis or pemphigoid. The cause of the majority of cases is unknown, but some reported cases have been drug-induced (drugs such as vancomycin, amiodarone, and nonsteroidal anti-inflammatory agents) or associated with systemic diseases, including hematologic malignancies, ulcerative colitis, or connective tissue diseases, such as dermatomyositis.[211,211a] The target antigens associated with a majority of cases of LAD are BP 180, BP 230, and LAD 285. Patients with CBDC often show an increased frequency of HLA-B8.[212,213]

Clinical Manifestations

The skin lesions of LAD are characterized by annular pruritic papules and blisters, giving a "cluster of jewels" appearance. In children, the skin of the lower abdomen, genitalia, and perineum are involved, whereas in adults, the disease affects the trunk and limbs. Ocular findings are frequently seen in adults and children.

Oral Findings

Oral lesions are common in LAD and may be seen in up to 70% of patients. These lesions are clinically indistinguishable from the oral lesions of MMP, with blisters, erosions and ulcers of the mucosa frequently accompanied by desquamative gingivitis.[214,214a,214b]

Laboratory Findings

Routine histology demonstrates subepithelial clefting similar to MMP, but DIF study will show linear deposition of IgA and occasionally, IgG and C3. Neutrophils are a prominent feature within the blister. IIF is usually negative, but when positive, it will demonstrate circulating IgA antibodies against a basement membrane antigen.[215] Some investigators believe that there is insufficient evidence to separate mucosal LAD from MMP if there is linear deposition of IgA (mucosal-dominant LAD), while others accept that there may be forms of MMP that bind IgA in a linear fashion at the basement membrane zone, and that LAD must present with skin lesions.[208]

Management

As with any subepithelial blistering disease, the clinician should consider the possibility of an underlying drug reaction or malignancy.

The oral lesions of LAD do not respond as well as MMP to either topical or systemic steroid therapy alone. Dapsone and sulfapyridine are often effective when topical steroids alone are insufficient.[216] More severe cases may require a combination of systemic corticosteroids and immunosuppressive drug therapy such as mycophenolate mofetil and some antibiotics such as trimethoprim/sulfamethoxazole are effective when used in combination with prednisone. Some cases of LAD and CBDC exhibit spontaneous remission.

Epidermolysis Bullosa Acquisita

Patients with EBA have IgG autoantibodies directed against type VII collagen, a component of the anchoring fibrils of the basement membrane. There are two forms of EBA: the classic form, which results in a lesion of the basement membrane with little inflammation, or the inflammatory form, which includes a significant infiltration of neutrophils.[203a]

Clinical Manifestations

The clinical course of EBA can resemble BP or MMP with widespread skin lesions or primary involvement of the oral mucosa, genital mucosa, conjunctiva, and larynx. Oral lesions present as erythema, erosion, ulcers and desquamative gingivitis.

Management

The treatment is similar as described for MMP and LAD, with therapy depending on the extent and severity of the clinical lesions. The classic form of the disease tends to

be resistant to treatment, whereas the inflammatory form often responds well to dapsone. Some patients with an inadequate response to dapsone have obtained remission by combining it with colchicine. Systemic corticosteroids, immunosuppressive drugs, rituximab, or intravenous immunoglobulin may be required to control the lesions in severe widespread EBA.

THE PATIENT WITH SINGLE ULCERS

The most common cause of single ulcers on the oral mucosa is trauma. The diagnosis is usually based on the history and physical findings. However, squamous cell carcinoma is always in the differential diagnosis for a nonhealing ulcer. As such, all ulcers present for two to four weeks with little evidence of healing should be biopsied to rule out squamous cell carcinoma or other pathology, and in the immunocompromised patients, deep fungal or viral infection. Oral cancer is discussed in detail in Chapter 8 "Oral and Oropharyngeal Cancer."

Infections that may cause a chronic oral ulcer include CMV ulcers (see above); mycobacterial infections (including atypical mycobacterial infections); the endemic mycoses such as histoplasmosis, blastomycosis, and coccidioidomycosis; nonendemic invasive fungal infections such as mucormycosis, aspergillosis, and cryptococcosis; and parasitic infections such as leishmaniasis. These are described detail in Chapter 22, "Infectious Diseases."

Traumatic Injuries Causing Solitary Ulcerations
Etiology and Pathogenesis

Single mucosal ulcers may be caused by direct physical/mechanical, thermal, or chemical trauma to the mucosa or even vascular compromise, causing tissue damage and ulceration. Acute bite injuries, an example of direct physical/mechanical trauma, occur often in the oral mucosa and may be particularly severe if this occurs when the mucosa is numb after local anesthesia has been given for dental procedures. Traumatic injuries may also result from malocclusion, ill-fitting dental prostheses, overzealous toothbrushing and flossing, self-injurious habits, and oral piercings.[217,218]

Thermal injuries including electrical burns are infrequently seen in children who inadvertently chew on electrical wiring. More commonly, thermal burns occur on the palatal mucosa from ingesting hot foods and beverages (such as hot pizza or coffee).[219] The use of a microwave oven to reheat foods often results in differential heating so that cheese and pastry fillings may be overheated compared with other parts of the food, leading to burns.[220] An iatrogenic cause of thermal injury is from a heated dental instrument inadvertently contacting the mucosa. The burn is usually more serious if the mucosa has been anesthetized and there is prolonged contact.[218,221]

Chemical trauma is caused by patients or dentists placing noxious and caustic substances directly on the mucosa either as a therapeutic measure or unintentionally.[222] Sucking on or chewing medications formulated to be swallowed (such as aspirin or oral bisphosphonates) may also lead to severe oral ulcers.[223,224225226] Mouthwashes or other over-the-counter oral care products with high alcoholic content, hydrogen peroxide, or phenols used too frequently or undiluted can cause mucosal ulcerations.[227,227a]Some over-the-counter medications for treating aphthous ulcers contain high concentrations of silver nitrate, phenols, or sulfuric acid and should be used with caution. Ulcers have also resulted in the use of denture cleansers as an oral rinse.[228] Prolonged contact of methacrylate monomer on the mucosa may also lead to necrosis of the mucosa. Necrosis of the bone and mucosa has been reported from chemicals used in endodontics if these are pushed past the apices of teeth.[229,229a]

Vascular compromise leads to oral ulcers and two main patterns are identified. One is a condition known as necrotizing sialometaplasia where there is local infarction of the salivary gland tissue leading to overlying ulceration, exfoliation of the necrotic tissue, and healing. Many etiologies have been identified including vasoconstrictors, sustained pressure and bulimia and the most common location for this condition is the hard palatal mucosa although any location that contains salivary glands may be affected.[229b,229c] Another is systemic vasculitis, where inflammation of vessels leads to thrombosis and infarction. Tongue necrosis is a particularly well-documented aspect of giant cell (temporal) arteritis.[229d]

Oral Findings

These present as acute ulcerations and necrosis of the mucosa with a clear antecedent history of injury (Figure 4-44). The extent of the ulceration depends on the agent involved and the site depends on the activity involved.

Electrical burns in particular are caused by high heat, are generally fairly extensive, involve the lips, and are generally seen in young children and toddlers.[217] The initial lesions are charred and dry-appearing. However, after a few days, this charred crust sloughs, and there may be excessive bleeding when the underlying vital structures are exposed.

Burns from hot foods and beverages are generally small and localized to the hard palatal mucosa or lips and are usually seen in teenagers and adults (Figure 4-45). The area usually presents as an area of tenderness and erythema that develops into ulcers within hours of the injury. It may take several days to heal depending on the extent of the injury.

Ulcers from vascular compromise such as necrotizing sialometaplasia and vasculitic lesions last for weeks and months.

Differential Diagnosis

Careful history taking and identification of the causative agent clinch the diagnosis. However, in all cases, patients should be carefully monitored to ensure that a secondary infection does not develop, particularly involving opportunistic agents such as HSV or *Candida*.

Laboratory Testing

None is required if there is a clear history of injury to the site. Culture may be needed if the areas do not heal well or if suppuration develops, suggesting a secondary bacterial infection. A biopsy should be performed if the ulcer does not heal within a few weeks. If leakage of an endodontic filler is suspected, periapical films should be taken.

Biopsy is not necessary if the etiology is obvious. However, if a biopsy is done, the mucosa will show ulceration with acute and chronic inflammation. The epithelium adjacent to the ulcer shows varying degrees of coagulation and necrosis.[230] Care must be taken to rule out the presence of infectious agents that may secondarily infect the site (such as HSV on the hard palatal mucosa).

Biopsies of necrotizing sialometaplasia show distinct stages of infarction of mucous glands to metaplasia of ducts to healing. For a diagnosis of giant cell arteritis, patients must fulfill three of the five criteria as set out by the American College of Rheumatology: age over 50, recent onset of localized headache, temporal artery tenderness or decreased temporal artery pulse, raised erythrocyte sedimentation rate greater than or equal to 50 mm/h, and positive temporal artery biopsy.[230a]

Management

Smaller lesions caused by less severe thermal or chemical injury heal on their own once the irritant is removed. Pain

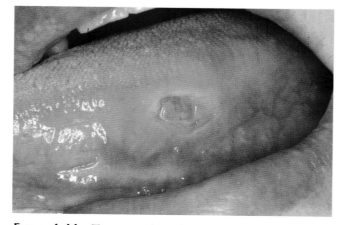

FIGURE 4-44   Traumatic ulcer of the lateral tongue, healing.

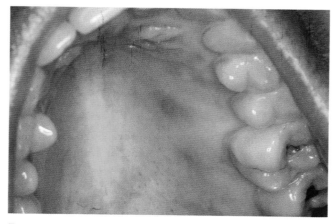

FIGURE 4-45   Ulcer from hot pizza burn on the palatal mucosa.

control can be achieved with topical anesthetics (such as viscous lidocaine). Topical steroids or intra-lesional steroid injections may be useful.[220,221] Avoidance of reinjury is also important, and this may be effected by counseling patients regarding the avoidance of use of caustic substances and the correct use of medications. Dentists also should be more aware of taking protective measures when using caustic substances and heated instruments.

Electrical burns are generally deep and more extensive, and healing often results in scarring and contracture. If the corners of the mouth are involved, microstomia may result. Children benefit from the use of microstomia prevention devices during this healing period, although surgical correction may still be required to restore function and esthetics. Antibiotics may be necessary to prevent a secondary infection since these burns often take several weeks to heal.[217,230b]

Necrotizing sialometaplasia heals on its own while ulcers of vasculitic origin will generally require treatment with systemic corticosteroids.

Traumatic Ulcerative Granuloma (Eosinophilic Ulcer of Tongue)
Etiology and Pathogenesis

This ulcerative condition of the oral cavity is considered traumatic in nature, although less than 50% of patients recall a history of trauma. These lesions have been experimentally induced in animals by inflicting crush injury on the tongue, the most common site of these lesions.[231] It is likely that the penetrating nature of the inflammation results in myositis that leads to chronicity. As such, other acute or chronic ulcerative conditions left untreated may become deep and penetrating. Similar lesions are seen on the ventral tongue in infants caused by the tongue rasping against newly erupted primary incisors, a condition known as Riga–Fede disease.[232] Patients with familial dysautonomia and other conditions, such as Riley–Day syndrome and Lesch–Nyhan syndrome, who have congenital incapacity to sense pain often also develop similar ulcerative and necrotic ulcers because they are unaware of the self-inflicted injury.[233]

Clinical Manifestations

There is a bimodal age distribution with one group in the first two years of life, where lesions are associated with erupting primary dentition.[232,233a] The second group is in adults in the fifth and sixth decades.[234]

Oral Findings

In children, the ulcers are always on the anterior ventral or dorsal tongue associated with erupting mandibular or maxillary incisors, respectively.[232] The tongue is the site of involvement in approximately 60% of adult cases, usually on the posterior and lateral aspects.[232,234,234a]

An ulcer develops that may not be painful in two-thirds of cases and may persist for months. A history of trauma is elicited in only 20%–50% of cases. The ulcer generally appears cleanly punched out, with surrounding erythema and keratosis if present for weeks or months (Figures 4-46 and 4-47). They range from 0.5 cm to several centimeters in size. The surrounding tissue is usually indurated. Other sites that may be involved include the buccal mucosa and labial mucosa, floor of the mouth, and vestibule, all sites where there is abundant underlying skeletal muscle. Five percent are multifocal, and recurrences are not uncommon. In some cases, the lesions present as an ulcerated mass on the lateral tongue.[235,236]

Differential Diagnosis

In children, the diagnosis is usually obvious because of the presence of newly erupted dentition and the location of the ulcers.

The long duration of these lesions, presence of induration, lack of pain, and lack of surrounding erythema readily distinguish them from RAS, although major aphthous ulcers are often associated with scarring and induration, and may develop into traumatic ulcerative granuloma. The presence

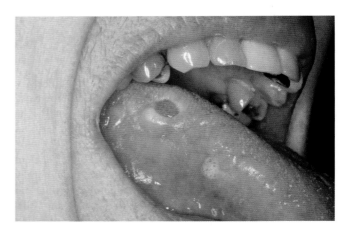

FIGURE 4-46 Traumatic ulcerative granuloma of the tongue, a typical site; note the surrounding keratosis.

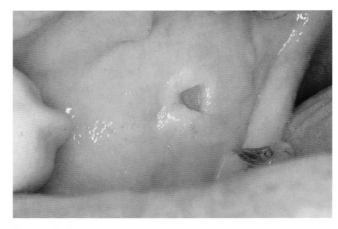

FIGURE 4-47 Traumatic ulcerative granuloma of the buccal mucosa; not the depressed appearance of the ulcer and surrounding keratosis.

of a single, chronic, painless ulcer with induration raises the suspicion for squamous cell carcinoma (especially if it is on the tongue), salivary gland malignancy or lymphoma. Rare cases that had been diagnosed as traumatic ulcerative granuloma have subsequently been shown to represent CD30+ T-cell lymphomas.[237,237a] An infectious etiology should also be considered, especially deep fungal or CMV infection, particularly in immunocompromised hosts. Another entity, EBV-associated mucocutaneous ulcers may appear similar and also contain CD30+ cells; these have been reported in immunocompromised and immunosenescent (elderly) patients.[237b]

Laboratory Findings

A biopsy is almost always needed to make the diagnosis and to rule out other conditions. Excision of the lesion often results in complete resolution of the ulcer.

The mucosa is ulcerated, but unlike an aphthous ulcer, the inflammation is deeply penetrating, with chronic inflammatory cells infiltrating the underlying skeletal fibers. There is muscle degeneration associated with variable numbers of eosinophils and mononuclear histiocyte-like cells.[232,234] Immunoperoxidase staining may be required to rule out a lymphoma, especially the CD30+ type.

Management

A careful history is important to rule out continued trauma to the site, although this is sometimes difficult to elicit and sometimes to prevent, especially if trauma occurs during sleep. Intralesional steroid injections performed over a few weeks will often resolve these lesions. Wound debridement also often leads to complete resolution, although up to one-third of cases recur. The use of a nightguard on the lower teeth may help reduce nighttime trauma.

Infections Causing Solitary Ulcers

Viral infections such as CMV and EBV of the herpes family may cause single ulcers that last for weeks or months in the immunocompromised or immunosenescent patient (see above). The deep mycoses (except for mucormycosis in patients with diabetes mellitus) were uncommon causes of oral lesions prior to HIV infection, myelosuppressive cancer chemotherapy, and immunosuppressive drug therapy. The dentist must consider this group of diseases in the differential diagnosis whenever isolated ulcerative oral lesions develop in known or suspected immunosuppressed patients. If there is reactive epithelial hyperplasia to the organism, lesions may appear as fungating masses resembling squamous cell carcinoma. Biopsy of suspected lesions, accompanied by a request for appropriate stains, is necessary for early diagnosis. Newer molecular-based diagnostic tests are also available. Please see Chapter 22 for a detailed discussion of such infections.

Selected Readings

Akintoye SO, Greenberg MS. Recurrent aphthous stomatitis. *Dent Clin North Am.* 2005;49:31–47.

Chan LS, Ahmed AR, Anhalt GJ, et al. The first international consensus on mucous membrane pemphigoid: definition, diagnostic criteria, pathogenic factors, medical treatment, and prognostic indicators. *Arch Dermatol.* 2002;138:370–379.

Ciarrocca KN, Greenberg MS. A retrospective study of the management of oral mucous membrane pemphigoid with dapsone. *Oral Surg Oral Med Oral Pathol Oral Radiol Endod.* 1999;88:159–163.

Corey L. Herpes simplex virus. In: Mandell GL, Bennett JE, Dolin R, eds. *Mandell, Douglas and Bennett's Principles and Practice of Infectious Diseases.* 6th ed. Philadelphia, PA: Elsevier, Churchill, Livingstone; 2005:1762–1780.

Farthing P, Bagan JV, Scully C. Mucosal disease series. Number IV. Erythema multiforme. *Oral Dis.* 2005;11:261–267.

Flaitz CM, Nichols CM, Hicks MJ. Herpesviridae-associated persistent mucocutaneous ulcers in acquired immunodeficiency syndrome. A clinicopathologic study. *Oral Surg Oral Med Oral Pathol Oral Radiol Endod.* 1996;81:433–441.

Gnann JW Jr, Whitley RJ. Clinical practice. Herpes zoster. *N Engl J Med.* 2002;347:340–346.

Greenberg MS, Friedman H, Cohen SG, et al. A comparative study of herpes simplex infections in renal transplant and leukemic patients. *J Infect Dis.* 1987;156:280–287.

Harman KE, Albert S, Black MM. Guidelines for the management of pemphigus vulgaris. *Br J Dermatol.* 2003;149:926–937.

Jones AC, Gulley ML, Freedman PD. Necrotizing ulcerative stomatitis in human immunodeficiency virus-seropositive individuals: a review of the histopathologic, immunohistochemical, and virologic characteristics of 18 cases. *Oral Surg Oral Med Oral Pathol Oral Radiol Endod.* 2000;89:323–332.

Oxman MN, Levin MJ, Johnson GR, et al. A vaccine to prevent herpes zoster and postherpetic neuralgia in older adults. *N Engl J Med.* 2005;352:2271–2284.

Sami N, Yeh SW, Ahmed AR. Blistering diseases in the elderly: diagnosis and treatment. *Dermatol Clin.* 2004;22:73–86.

Williams PM, Conklin RJ. Erythema multiforme: a review and contrast from Stevens-Johnson syndrome/toxic epidermal necrolysis. *Dent Clin North Am.* 2005;49:67–76, viii.

Woo SB, Lee SF. Oral recrudescent herpes simplex virus infection. *Oral Surg Oral Med Oral Pathol Oral Radiol Endod.* 1997;83:239–243.

Yancey KB, Egan CA. Pemphigoid: clinical, histologic, immunopathologic, and therapeutic considerations. *JAMA.* 2000;284:350–356.

Yazici H, Yurdakul S, Hamuryudan V. Behçet's syndrome. *Curr Opin Rheumatol.* 1999;1:53–57.

For the full reference lists, please go to http://www.pmph-usa.com/Burkets_Oral_Medicine.

CHAPTER 5

Red and White Lesions of the Oral Mucosa

Mats Jontell, DDS, PhD, FDS, RCSEd

Palle Holmstrup DDS, PhD, DrOdont

- ❐ RED AND WHITE TISSUE REACTIONS
- ❐ INFECTIOUS DISEASES
  Oral Candidiasis
  Hairy Leukoplakia
- ❐ PREMALIGNANT LESIONS
  Oral Leukoplakia and Erythroplakia
  Oral Submucous Fibrosis
- ❐ IMMUNOPATHOLOGIC DISEASES
  Oral Lichen Planus
  Drug-Induced Lichenoid Reactions
  Lichenoid Reactions of Graft-versus-Host Disease
  Lupus Erythematosus

- ❐ ALLERGIC REACTIONS
  Lichenoid Contact Reactions
  Reactions to Dentifrice and Chlorhexidine
- ❐ TOXIC REACTIONS
  Reactions to Smokeless Tobacco
  Smoker's Palate
- ❐ REACTIONS TO MECHANICAL TRAUMA
  Morsicatio
- ❐ OTHER RED AND WHITE LESIONS
  Benign Migratory Glossitis (Geographic Tongue)
  Leukoedema
  White Sponge Nevus
  Hairy Tongue

RED AND WHITE TISSUE REACTIONS

Oral mucosal lesions may be classified according to different characteristics. This chapter describes disorders of the oral mucosa that clinically appear red and/or white.

A white appearance of the oral mucosa may be caused by a variety of factors. The oral epithelium may be stimulated to an increased production of keratin (hyperkeratosis, Composition 1) or an abnormal but benign thickening of stratum spinosum (acanthosis, Composition 2). Intra- (Composition 3) and extracellular accumulation of fluid in the epithelium may also result in clinical whitening. Microbes, particularly fungi, can produce whitish pseudomembranes consisting of sloughed epithelial cells, fungal mycelium, and neutrophils, which are loosely attached to the oral mucosa (Composition 4).

A red lesion of the oral mucosa may develop as the result of atrophic epithelium (Composition 5), characterized by a reduction in the number of epithelial cells (Composition 6) or increased vascularization that is dilatation of vessels and/or proliferation of vessels.

Later in the chapter, Composition 7 and 8 describe the immune pathogenesis of oral lichen planus (OLP) and lichenoid contact reactions (LCRs).

Oral mucosal lesions also present with different tissue textures as reticular, plaque-like, papular, or pseudomembranous, which affect the clinical appearance of the lesions.

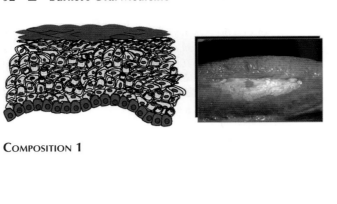

COMPOSITION 1

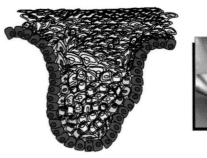

COMPOSITION 2

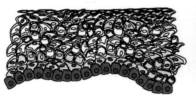
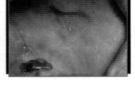

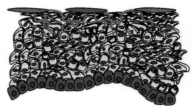
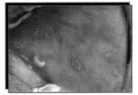

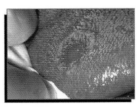

COMPOSITION 3

COMPOSITION 4

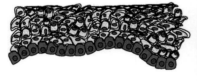
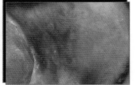

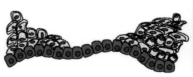
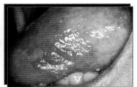

COMPOSITION 5

COMPOSITION 6

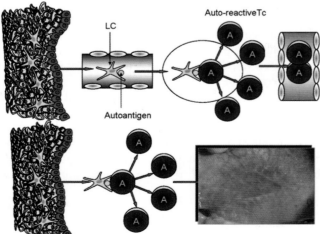

COMPOSITION 7

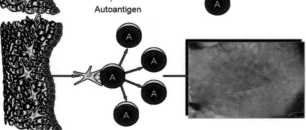
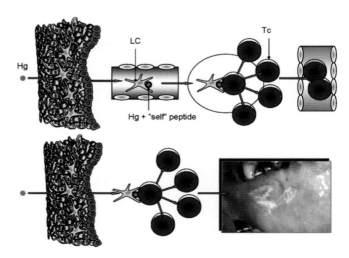

COMPOSITION 8

INFECTIOUS DISEASES

Oral Candidiasis

Oral candidiasis is the most prevalent opportunistic infection affecting the oral mucosa. In the vast majority of cases, the lesions are caused by *Candida albicans*. The pathogenesis is not fully understood, but a number of predisposing factors have been shown to convert *C. albicans* from the normal commensal flora (saprophytic stage) to a pathogenic organism (parasitic stage). *C. albicans* is usually a weak pathogen, and candidiasis is said to affect the very young, the very old, and the very sick.[1] Most candidal infections only affect mucosal linings, but rare systemic manifestations may have a fatal course.

Oral candidiasis is divided into primary and secondary infections (Table 5-1).[1] The primary infections are restricted to the oral and perioral sites, whereas secondary infections are accompanied by systemic mucocutaneous manifestations.

Etiology and Pathogenesis

C. albicans, *C. tropicalis*, and *C. glabrata* comprise together over 80% of the species isolated from human candidal infections.[1] To invade the mucosal lining, the microorganisms must adhere to the epithelial surface; therefore, candidal strains with better adhesion potential are more virulent than strains with poorer adhesion ability. The yeasts' penetration of the epithelial cells is facilitated by their production of lipases, and for the yeasts to remain within the epithelium, they must overcome constant desquamation of surface epithelial cells.

There is an apparent association between oral candidiasis and the influence of local and general predisposing factors. The local predisposing factors (Table 5-2) are able to promote growth of the yeast or to affect the immune response of the oral mucosa. General predisposing factors are often related to an individual's immune status and endocrine status (see Table 5-2). Drugs as well as diseases, which suppress the adaptive or the innate immune system can affect the susceptibility of the mucosal lining. Pseudomembranous candidiasis is also associated with fungal infections in young children, who neither have a fully developed immune system nor a fully developed oral microflora.

Denture stomatitis, angular cheilitis, and median rhomboid glossitis are referred to as *Candida*-associated infections as bacteria may also cause these infections.[2]

Epidemiology

The prevalence of candidal strains, as part of the commensal oral flora, shows large geographic variations, but an average figure of 35% has been calculated from several studies.[3] Candidal strains are more frequently isolated from women. A seasonal variation has been observed, with an increase during summer months. Hospitalized patients have a higher prevalence of the yeasts.[4] In healthy individuals, blood group O and non-secretion of blood group antigens are separate and cumulative risk factors for oral carriage of *C. albicans*.[5] In complete denture-wearers, the prevalence of denture stomatitis has been reported variously from 11%–67%.[6]

Clinical Findings

Pseudomembranous Candidiasis

The acute form of pseudomembranous candidiasis (thrush) is grouped with the primary oral candidiasis (see Table 5-1) and is recognized as the classic candidal infection (Figure 5-1). The infection predominantly affects patients taking antibiotics, immunosuppressant drugs, or having a disease that suppresses the immune system.

TABLE 5-1	Classification of Oral Candidiasis
Primary Oral Candidiasis	**Secondary Oral Candidiasis**
Acute	Familial chronic mucocutaneous candidiasis
Pseudomembranous	Diffuse chronic mucocutaneous candidiasis
Erythematous	Candidiasis endocrinopathy syndrome
	Familial mucocutaneous candidiasis
Chronic	Severe combined immunodeficiency
Pseudomembranous	DiGeorge syndrome
Erythematous	Chronic granulomatous disease
Plaque-like	Acquired immune deficiency syndrome (AIDS)
Nodular	
Candida-associated lesions	
Denture stomatitis Angular cheilitis Median rhomboid glossitis	

TABLE 5-2	Predisposing Factors for Oral Candidiasis and Candida-Associated Lesions
Local	
Denture wearing	
Smoking	
Atopic constitution	
Inhalation steroids	
Topical steroids	
Hyperkeratosis	
Imbalance of the oral microflora	
Quality and quantity of saliva	
General	
Immunosuppressive diseases	
Impaired health status	
Immunosuppressive drugs	
Chemotherapy	
Endocrine disorders	
Hematinic deficiencies	

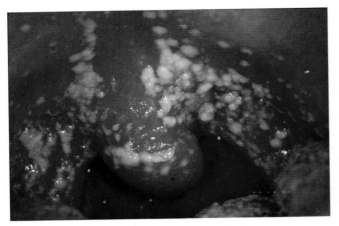

Figure 5-1 Pseudomembranous candidiasis during the immunosuppressive phase following heart transplantation.

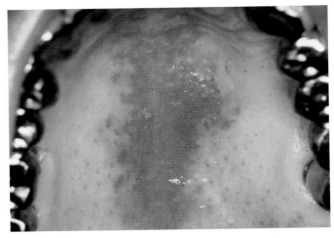

Figure 5-2 Erythematous candidasis caused by inhalation steroids.

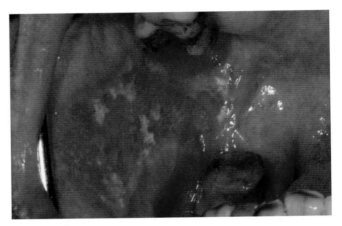

Figure 5-3 Chronic plaque-type candidiasis.

The infection typically presents with loosely attached membranes comprising fungal organisms and cellular debris, which leaves an inflamed, sometimes bleeding area if the pseudomembrane is removed. Less pronounced infections sometimes have clinical features that are difficult to discriminate from food debris like egg and yoghurt. The clinical presentations of acute and chronic pseudomembranous candidiasis are indistinguishable.[7] The chronic form may emerge as the result of human immunodeficiency virus (HIV) infections as patients with this disease may be affected by a pseudomembranous candidal infection for a long period of time. Patients treated with steroid inhalers may also show pseudomembranous lesions of a chronic nature. Patients infrequently report symptoms from their lesions, although some discomfort may be experienced from the presence of the pseudomembranes.

Erythematous Candidiasis

The erythematous form of candidiasis was previously referred to as atrophic oral candidiasis.[2] However, an erythematous surface may not just reflect atrophy but can also be explained by increased vascularization. The lesion has a diffuse border (Figure 5-2), which helps distinguish it from erythroplakia, which usually has a sharper demarcation and often appears as a slightly submerged lesion. Erythematous candidiasis may be considered a successor to pseudomembranous candidiasis but may also emerge *de novo*.[1] No quantitative differences exist between isolates of *C. albicans* from individuals with healthy oral mucosa and from patients with erythematous candidiasis.[8] The infection is predominantly seen in the palate and the dorsum of the tongue of patients who are using inhalation steroids. Other predisposing factors that can cause erythematous candidiasis are smoking and treatment with broad-spectrum antibiotics. The acute and chronic forms present with identical clinical features.

Chronic Plaque-Type and Nodular Candidiasis

The chronic plaque type of oral candidiasis replaces the older term, *candidal leukoplakia*. A white irremovable plaque characterizes the typical clinical presentation, which may be indistinguishable from oral leukoplakia (Figure 5-3).

A positive correlation between oral candidiasis and moderate to severe epithelial dysplasia has been observed,[9] and both the chronic plaque-type and the nodular type of oral candidiasis (Figure 5-4) have been associated with malignant transformation, but the possible role of yeasts in oral carcinogenesis is unclear.[10] It has been hypothesized that it may act through its capacity to catalyze nitrosamine production.[11]

Denture Stomatitis

The most prevalent site for denture stomatitis is the denture-bearing palatal mucosa (Figure 5-5). It is unusual for the mandibular mucosa to be involved. Denture stomatitis is classified into three different types.[12] Type I is limited to minor erythematous sites caused by trauma from the denture. Type II affects a major part of the denture-covered mucosa.

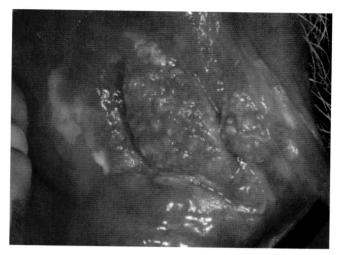

FIGURE 5-4 Chronic nodular candidiasis in the left retrocommissural area.

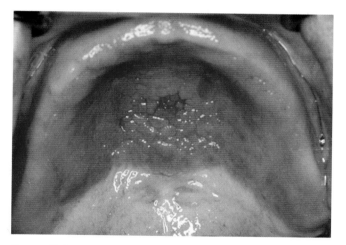

FIGURE 5-5 Denture stomatitis type III with a granular mucosa in the central part of the palate.

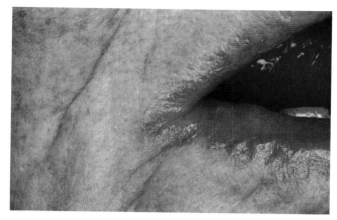

FIGURE 5-6 Angular cheilitis.

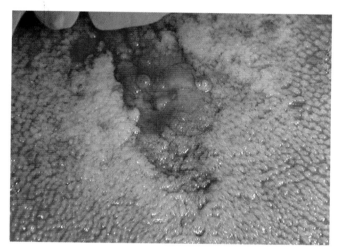

FIGURE 5-7 Median rhomboid glossitis.

In addition to the features of type II, type III has a granular mucosa. The denture serves as a vehicle that accumulates sloughed epithelial cells and protects the microorganisms from physical influences such as salivary flow. The microflora is complex and may, in addition to *C. albicans* contain bacteria from several genera, such as *Streptococcus-*, *Veillonella-*, *Lactobacillus-*, *Prevotella-* (formerly *Bacteroides*), and *Actinomyces-strains*.[13] It is not known to what extent these bacteria participate in the pathogenesis of denture stomatitis.

Angular Cheilitis

Angular cheilitis presents as infected fissures of the commissures of the mouth, often surrounded by erythema (Figure 5-6).[14,15] The lesions are frequently coinfected with both *Candida albicans* and *Staphylococcus aureus*. VitaminB$_{12}$ deficiency, iron deficiencies, and loss of vertical dimension have been associated with this disorder. Atopy has also been associated with the formation of angular cheilitis.[16] Dry skin may promote the development of fissures in the commissures,

allowing invasion by the microorganisms. Thirty percent of patients with denture stomatitis also have angular cheilitis, but this infection is only seen in 10% of denture-wearing patients without denture stomatitis.[17]

Median Rhomboid Glossitis

Median rhomboid glossitis is clinically characterized by an erythematous lesion in the center of the posterior part of the dorsum of the tongue (Figure 5-7).[18] As the name indicates, the lesion has an oval configuration. This area of erythema results from atrophy of the filiform papillae and the surface may be lobulated. The etiology is not fully clarified, but the lesion frequently shows a mixed bacterial/fungal microflora. Biopsies yield candidal hyphae in more than 85% of the lesions.[19] Smokers and denture-wearers have an increased risk of developing median rhomboid glossitis as well as patients using inhalation steroids. Sometimes a concurrent erythematous lesion may be observed in the palatal mucosa (kissing lesions). Median rhomboid glossitis is asymptomatic, and management is restricted to a reduction of predisposing factors. The lesion does not entail any increased risk for malignant transformation.

Oral Candidiasis Associated with HIV

More than 90% of acquired immune deficiency syndrome (AIDS) patients have had oral candidiasis during the course of their HIV infection, and the infection is considered a portent of AIDS development (Figure 5-8). The most common types of oral candidiasis in conjunction with HIV are pseudomembranous candidiasis, erythematous candidiasis, angular cheilitis, and chronic plaque-like candidiasis. As a result of the highly active antiretroviral therapy (HAART), the prevalence of oral candidiasis has decreased substantially. Oral candidiasis associated with HIV infection is presented in more detail in Chapter 22, "Infectious Diseases."

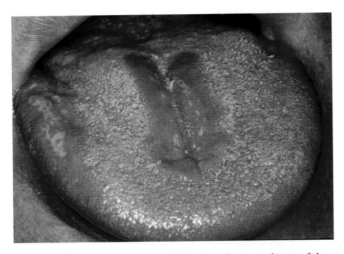

FIGURE 5-8 Erythematous candidiasis at the central part of the tongue in an AIDS patient. Hairy leukoplakia can be seen at the right lateral border.

Clinical Manifestations

Secondary oral candidiasis (see Table 5-1) is accompanied by systemic mucocutaneous candidiasis and other immune deficiencies.[20] Chronic mucocutaneous candidiasis (CMC) embraces a heterogeneous group of disorders, which, in addition to oral candidiasis, also affect the skin, typically the nail bed and other mucosal linings, such as the genital mucosa.[21] The face and scalp may be involved, and granulomatous masses can be seen at these sites. Approximately 90% of the patients with CMC also present with oral candidiasis. The oral manifestations may involve the tongue, and white plaque-like lesions are seen in conjunction with fissures. CMC can occur as part of endocrine disorders, including hyperparathyroidism and Addison's disease. Impaired phagocytic function by neutrophilic granulocytes and macrophages caused by myeloperoxidase deficiency have also been associated with CMC. Chediak-Higashi syndrome, an inherited disease with a reduced and impaired number of neutrophilic granulocytes, lends further support to the role of the phagocytic system in candidal infections as these patients frequently develop candidiasis. Severe combined immunodeficiency (SCID) syndrome is characterized by a defect in the function of the cell-mediated arm of the immune system. Patients with this disorder frequently contract disseminated candidal infections. Thymoma is a neoplasm of thymic epithelial cells that also entails systemic candidiasis. Thus, both the native and adaptive immune systems are critical to prevent development of systemic mucocutaneous candidiasis.

Diagnosis and Laboratory Findings

The presence of candidal microorganisms as a member of the commensal flora complicates the discrimination of the normal state from infection. It is imperative that both clinical findings and laboratory data (Table 5-3) are balanced in order

TABLE 5-3	*Candida* Isolation in the Clinic and Quantification from Oral Samples		
Method	**Main Steps**	**Advantages**	**Disadvantages**
Smear	Scraping, smearing directly onto slide	Simple and quick	Low sensitivity
Swab	Taken by rubbing cotton-tipped swabs over lesional tissue	Relatively simple	Selecting sampling sites critical
Imprint culture	Sterile plastic foam pads dipped into Sabouraud (Sab) broth, placed on lesion for 60 s; pad pressed on Sab agar plate and incubated; colony-counter used	Sensitive and reliable; can discriminate between infected and carrier states	Reading above 50 CFU/cm² can be inaccurate; selection of sites difficult if no clinical signs present
Impression culture	Maxillary and mandibular alginate impressions; casting in agar fortified with Sab broth; incubation	Useful to determine relative distributions of the yeasts on oral surfaces	Useful mostly as a research tool
Salivary culture	Patient expectorates 2 mL saliva into sterile container; vibration; culture on Sab agar by spiral plating; counting	As useful as imprint culture	Considerable chairside time; not useful for xerostomics; cannot identify site of infection
Oral rinse	Subject rinses for 60 s with PBS at pH 7.2, 0.1 M, and returns it to the original container; concentrated by centrifugation; cultured and counted as in previous methods	Comparable in sensitivity with imprint method; better results if CFU >50/cm²; simple method	Recommended for surveillance cultures in the absence of focal lesions; cannot identify site of infection

PBS, phosphate-buffered saline.
Source: Adapted from Sitheeque and Samaranayake.[10]

to arrive at a correct diagnosis. Sometimes antifungal treatment has to be initiated to assist in the diagnostic process.

Smear from the infected area comprising epithelial cells, creates opportunities for detection of the yeasts. The material is fixed in isopropyl alcohol and air-dried before staining with periodic acid–Schiff (PAS). The detection of yeast organisms in the form of hyphae- or pseudohyphae-like structures is usually considered a sign of infection although these structures have also been identified in normal oral mucosa.[22] This technique is particularly useful when pseudomembranous oral candidiasis and angular cheilitis are suspected. To increase the sensitivity, a second scrape can be transferred to a transport medium followed by cultivation on Sabouraud agar. To discriminate between different candidal species, an additional examination can be performed on Pagano-Levin agar. Imprint culture technique can also be used where sterile plastic foam pads (2.5 × 2.5 cm) are submerged in Sabouraud broth and placed on the infected surface for 60 seconds. The pad is then firmly pressed onto Sabouraud agar, which will be cultivated at 37°C. The result is expressed as colony forming units per cubic millimeter (CFU/mm²). This method is a valuable adjunct in the diagnostic process of erythematous candidiasis and denture stomatitis as these infections consist of fairly homogeneous erythematous lesions. Salivary culture techniques are primarily used in parallel with other diagnostic methods to obtain an adequate quantification of candidal organisms. Patients who display clinical signs of oral candidiasis usually have more than 400 CFU/mL.[23]

In chronic plaque-type and nodular candidiasis, cultivation techniques have to be supplemented by a histopathologic examination. This examination is primarily performed to identify the presence of epithelial dysplasia and to identify invading candidal organisms by PAS staining. However, for the latter, there is a definitive risk of false-negative results.

Management

Treatment for fungal infections, which usually include antifungal regimens, will not always be successful unless the clinician addresses predisposing factors that may cause recurrence. Local factors are often easy to identify but sometimes not possible to reduce or eradicate. Antifungal drugs have a primary role in such cases. In smokers, cessation of the habit may result in disappearance of the infection even without antifungal treatment (Figure 5-9A and B). The most commonly used antifungal drugs belong to the groups of polyenes or azoles (Table 5-4). Polyenes such as nystatin and amphotericin B are usually the first choices in treatment of primary oral candidiasis and are both well tolerated. Polyenes are not absorbed from the gastrointestinal tract and are not associated with development of resistance.[24] They exert the action through a negative effect on the production of ergosterol, which is critical for the yeast's cell membrane integrity. Polyenes can also affect the adherence of the fungi.[25]

Whenever possible, elimination or reduction of predisposing factors should always be the first goal for treatment of

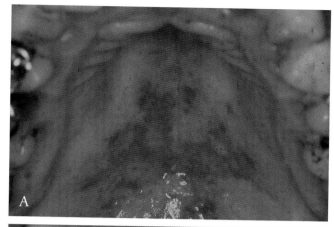

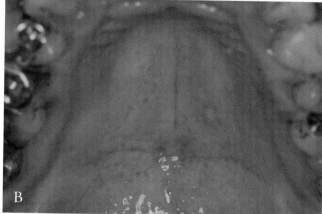

FIGURE 5-9 A, Smoking-induced erythematous candidiasis in the palatal mucosa. B, Clinical appearance after cessation of smoking.

denture stomatitis as well as other opportunistic infections. This involves improved denture hygiene and a recommendation not to use the denture while sleeping. The denture hygiene is important to remove nutrients, including desquamated epithelial cells, which may serve as a source of nitrogen, which is essential for the growth of the yeasts. Denture cleaning also disturbs the maturity of a microbial environment established under the denture. As porosities in the denture can harbor microorganisms, which may not be removed by physical cleaning, the denture should be stored in antimicrobial solutions during the night. Different solutions, including alkaline peroxides, alkaline hypochlorites, acids, disinfectants, and enzymes, have been suggested.[14] The latter seems to be most effective against candidal strains. Chlorhexidine may also be used but can discolor the denture and also counteracts the effect of nystatin.

Type III denture stomatitis may be treated with surgical excision in an attempt to eradicate microorganisms present in the deeper fissures of the granular tissue. If this is not sufficient, continuous treatment with topical antifungal drugs should be considered. Patients with no symptoms are rarely motivated for treatment, and the infection often persists

TABLE 5-4	Antifungal Agents Used in the Treatment of Oral Candidiasis		
Drug	**Form**	**Dosage**	**Comments**
Amphotericin B	Lozenge, 10 mg	Slowly dissolved in mouth 3–4 × /d after meals for 2 wk minimum	Negligible absorption from gastrointestinal tract. When given IV for deep mycoses may cause thrombophlebitis, anorexia, nausea, vomiting, fever, headache, weight loss, anemia, hypokalemia, nephrotoxicity, hypotension, arrhythmias, etc.
	Oral suspension, 100 mg/mL	Placed in the mouth after food and retained near lesions 4 × /d for 2 wk	
Nystatin	Cream	Apply to affected area 3–4 × /d	Negligible absorption from gastrointestinal tract. Nausea and vomiting with high doses.
	Pastille, 100,000 U	Dissolve 1 pastille slowly after meals 4 × /d, usually for 7 d	
	Oral suspension, 100,000 U	Apply after meals 4 × /d, usually for 7 d, and continue use for several days after postclinical healing	
Clotrimazole	Cream	Apply to the affected area 2–3 times daily for 3–4 wk	Mild local effects. Also has antistaphylococcal activity.
	Solution	5 mL 3–4 times daily for 2 wk minimum	
Miconazole	Oral gel	Apply to the affected area 3–4 times daily	Occasional mild local reactions. Also has antibacterial activity. Theoretically the best antifungal to treat angular cheilitis. Interacts with anticoagulants (warfarin), terfenadine, cisapride, and astemizole. Avoid in pregnancy and liver disease.
	Cream	Apply twice per day and continue for 10–14 d after the lesion heals	
Ketoconazole	Tablets	200–400-mg tablets taken once or twice daily with food for 2 wk	May cause nausea, vomiting, rashes, pruritus, and liver damage. Interacts with anticoagulants, terfenadine, cisapride, and astemizole. Contraindicated in pregnancy and liver disease.
Fluconazole	Capsules	50–100 mg capsules once daily for 2–3 wk	Interacts with anticoagulants, terfenadine, cisapride, and astemizole. Contraindicated in pregnancy and liver and renal disease. May cause nausea, diarrhea, headache, rash, liver dysfunction.
Itraconazole	Capsules	100 mg capsules daily taken immediately after meals for 2 wk	Interacts with terfenadine, cisapride, and astemizole. Contraindicated in pregnancy and liver disease. May cause nausea, neuropathy, rash.

IV, intravenously.
Source: Adapted from Ellepola and Samaranayake.[26]

without the patients being aware of its presence. However, the chronic inflammation may result in increased resorption of the denture-bearing bone.

Topical treatment with azoles such as miconazole is the treatment of choice for angular cheilitis[27] often infected by both *S. aureus* and candidal strains. This drug has a biostatic effect on *S. aureus* in addition to the fungistatic effect. Retapamulin can be used as a complement to the antifungal drugs. If angular cheilitis comprises an erythema surrounding the fissure, a mild steroid ointment may be required to suppress the inflammation. To prevent recurrences, patients have to apply a moisturizing cream, which may prevent new fissure formation.[28]

Systemic azoles may be used for deeply seated primary candidiasis, such as chronic hyperplastic candidiasis, denture stomatitis, and median rhomboid glossitis with a granular appearance, and for therapy-resistant infections, mostly related to compliance failure. There are several disadvantages with the use of azoles. They are known to interact with warfarin, leading to an increased bleeding propensity. This adverse effect may also be present with topical application as the azoles are fully or partly resorbed from the gastrointestinal tract. Development of resistance is particularly compelling for fluconazole in individuals with HIV disease.[29] In such cases, ketoconazole and itraconazole have been recommended as alternatives. However, cross-resistance has been reported between fluconazole on the one hand and ketoconazole, miconazole, and itraconazole on the other. The azoles are also used in the treatment of secondary oral candidiasis associated with systemic predisposing factors and for systemic candidiasis.

Prognosis of oral candidiasis is good when predisposing factors associated with the infection are reduced or eliminated. Persistent chronic plaque-type and nodular candidiasis have been suggested to be associated with an increased risk for malignant transformation compared with leukoplakia, not infected by candidal strains.[11,30] Patients with primary candidiasis are also at risk if systemic predisposing factors arise emerge. For example, patients with severe immunosuppression as seen in conjunction with leukemia and AIDS may encounter disseminating candidiasis with a fatal course.[31]

Oral Hairy Leukoplakia

Oral hairy leukoplakia (OHL) is the second most common HIV-associated oral mucosal lesion. HL has been used as a marker of disease activity since the lesion is associated with low CD4+ T-lymphocyte counts.[32,33] The lesion is not pathognomonic for HIV disease since other states of immune deficiencies, such as caused by immunosuppressive drugs and cancer chemotherapy, have also been associated with OHL.[34–36] Rarely, individuals with a normal immune system may present with OHL.[37,38]

Etiology and Pathogenesis

Oral hairy leukoplakia is strongly associated with Epstein-Barr virus (EBV) and with low levels of CD4+ T lymphocytes. Antiviral medication, which prevents EBV replication, is curative[39] and lends further support to EBV as an etiologic factor. There is also a correlation between EBV replication and a decrease in the number of CD1a+ Langerhans' cells, which, together with T lymphocytes, are important cell populations in the cellular immune defense of the oral mucosa.[40]

Epidemiology

The prevalence figures for OHL depend on the type of population investigated. Prior to the HAART era, the prevalence was 25%,[41] a figure that has decreased considerably after the introduction of more effective antiretroviral therapies. In patients who develop AIDS, the prevalence may be as high as 80%.[42] The prevalence in children is lower compared with adults and has been reported to be in the range of 2%.[43] The condition is more frequently encountered in men, but the reason for this predisposition is not known. A correlation between smoking and OHL has also been observed.[44]

Clinical Findings

Oral hairy leukoplakia is frequently encountered on the lateral borders of the tongue (Figure 5-10) but may also be observed on the dorsum and in the buccal mucosa.[45,46] The typical clinical appearance is vertical white folds oriented as a palisade along the borders of the tongue. The lesions may also be seen as white and somewhat elevated plaque, which cannot be scraped off. Oral hairy leukoplakia is asymptomatic,[47] although symptoms may be present when the lesion is superinfected with candidal strains. As OHL may present in different clinical forms, it is important to always consider

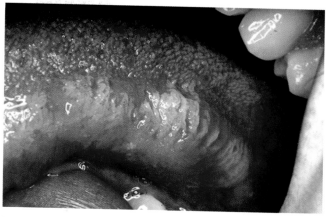

FIGURE 5-10 Hairy leukoplakia at the left lateral border of the tongue in an AIDS patient.

TABLE 5-5	Features of the Diagnosis of Oral Hairy Leukoplakia
Provisional diagnosis Characteristic gross appearance, with or without responsiveness to antifungal therapy	
Presumptive diagnosis Light microscopy of histologic sections revealing hyperkeratosis, koilocytosis, acanthosis, and absence of inflammatory cell infiltrate or light microscopy of cytologic preparations demonstrating nuclear beading and chromatin margination	
Definitive diagnosis In situ hybridization of histologic or cytologic specimens revealing positive staining for EBV DNA or electron microscopy of histologic or cytologic specimens showing herpesvirus-like particles	

DNA, deoxyribonucleic acid; EBV, Epstein-Barr virus.
Source: Adapted from Triantos et al.[45]

this mucosal lesion whenever the border of the tongue is affected by white lesions, particularly in immunocompromised patients.

Diagnosis

A diagnosis of OHL is usually based on clinical characteristics, but histopathologic examination and detection of EBV can be performed to confirm the clinical diagnosis (Table 5-5). It may most easily be confused with chronic trauma to the lateral borders of the tongue.

Pathology

The histopathology of OHL is characterized by hyperkeratosis often with a chevron-pattern surface and acanthosis.[45] Hairy projections are common, which is reflected in the name given to this disorder. Koilocytosis, with edematous epithelial cells and pyknotic nuclei, is also a characteristic histopathologic feature. The complex chromatin arrangements may mirror EBV replication in the nuclei of koilocytic epithelial cells. Candidal hyphae surrounded by polymorphonuclear granulocytes are also a common feature. The number of immunostained Langerhans' cells is considerably reduced.[48] Mild subepithelial inflammation may also be observed. EBV can be detected by *in situ* hybridization or by immunohistochemistry. Exfoliative cytology may be of value and can serve as an adjunct to biopsy.[45]

Management

Oral hairy leukoplakia can be treated successfully with antiviral medication,[39] but this is not often indicated as this disorder is not associated with adverse symptoms. In addition, the disorder has also been reported to show spontaneous regression. HL is not related to increased risk of malignant transformation. Medication with HAART has reduced the number of HL to a few percent in HIV-infected patients.

PREMALIGNANT DISORDERS

Oral Leukoplakia and Erythroplakia

Etiology and Pathogenesis

The development of oral leukoplakia and erythroplakia as premalignant lesions involves different genetic events. This notion is supported by the fact that markers of genetic defects are differently expressed in different leukoplakias and erythroplakias.[49–51] Activation of oncogenes and deletion and injuries to suppressor genes and genes responsible for DNA repair will all contribute to a defective functioning of the genome that governs cell division. Following a series of mutations, a malignant transformation may occur. For example, carcinogens such as tobacco may induce hyperkeratinization, with the potential to revert following cessation, but at some stage, mutations will lead to an unrestrained proliferation and cell division.

Epidemiology

The prevalence of oral leukoplakia varies among scientific studies. A comprehensive global review points at a prevalence of 2.6%.[52] Most oral leukoplakias are seen in patients beyond the age of 50 and infrequently encountered below the age of 30. In population studies, leukoplakias are more common in men,[53] but a slight majority for women has been found in some studies.[54,55]

Oral erythroplakia is not as common as oral leukoplakia, and the prevalence has been estimated to be in the range of 0.02%–0.1%.[56] The gender distribution is reported to be equal.

Clinical Findings

Oral leukoplakia is defined as a white plaque of questionable risk having excluded (other) known diseases or disorders that carry no increased risk for cancer.[57] This disorder can be further divided into a homogeneous and a nonhomogeneous type. The typical homogeneous leukoplakia is clinically characterized as a white, often well-demarcated plaque with an identical reaction pattern throughout the entire lesion (Figure 5-11). The surface texture can vary from a smooth and

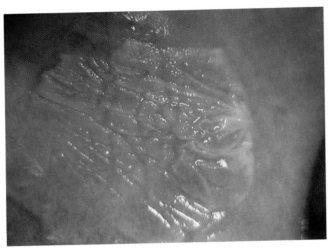

FIGURE 5-11 A homogeneous leukoplakia at the left buccal mucosa.

thin to a leathery appearance with surface fissures sometimes referred to as "cracked mud." The demarcation is usually distinct, which is different from an OLP lesion, where the white components have a more diffuse transition to the normal oral mucosa. Another difference between these two lesions is the lack of a peripheral erythematous zone in homogeneous oral leukoplakia. The lesions are asymptomatic in most patients.

The nonhomogeneous type of oral leukoplakia may have white patches or plaques intermingled with red elements (Figure 5-12A). Due to the combined appearance of white and red areas, the nonhomogeneous oral leukoplakia has also been called erythroleukoplakia and speckled leukoplakia. The clinical manifestation of the white component may vary from large white verrucous areas to small nodular structures. If the surface texture is homogeneous but contains verrucous, papillary (nodular), or exophytic components, the leukoplakia is also regarded as nonhomogeneous. Both homogeneous and nonhomogeneous leukoplakias may be encountered in all sites of the oral mucosa.

Oral leukoplakias, where the white component is dominated by papillary projections, similar to oral papillomas, are referred to as verrucous or verruciform leukoplakias.[58] Oral leukoplakias with this clinical appearance but with a more aggressive proliferation pattern and high recurrence rate are designated as proliferative verrucous leukoplakia (PVL) (Figure 5-13).[59] This lesion may start as a homogeneous leukoplakia but over time develop a verrucous appearance containing various degrees of dysplasia. PVL is usually encountered in older women, and the lower gingiva is a predilection site.[60] The malignant potential is very high, and verrucous carcinoma or squamous cell carcinoma may be present at the primary examination. As the reaction pattern is similar to what is seen in oral papillomas, the PVL has been suspected to have a viral etiology, although no such association has been confirmed.[61]

Oral leukoplakia may be found at all sites of the oral mucosa. Nonsmokers have a higher percentage of leukoplakias

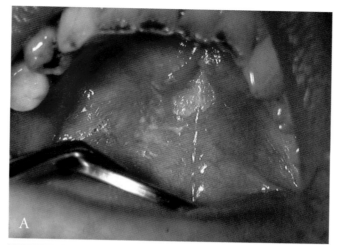

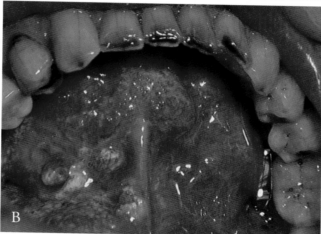

FIGURE 5-12 A, A nonhomogeneous leukoplakia in a heavy smoker. The left part of the lesion has a speckled appearance. B, The patient did not attend the follow-up visits for 3 years and developed a squamous cell carcinoma.

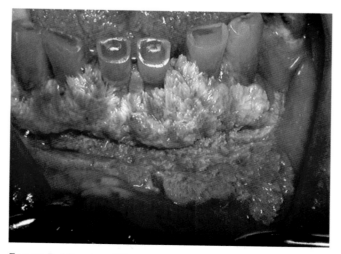

FIGURE 5-13 A proliferative verrucous leukoplakia in an 80-year-old woman.

at the border of the tongue compared with smokers.[54] The floor of the mouth and the lateral borders of the tongue have been considered high-risk sites for malignant transformation (Figure 5-12B). These sites have also been found to have a higher frequency of loss of heterozygosity compared with low-risk sites.[50] However, the distinction between high- and low-risk sites has been questioned leaving the size of the lesion and the homogenous/non-homogenous pattern being decisive characteristics for the prognosis.[55,62]

Oral erythroplakia has not been studied as extensively as oral leukoplakia, presumably because it is less common.[56] Erythroplakia is defined as a red lesion of the oral mucosa that excludes other known pathologies (Figure 5-14). The lesion comprises an eroded somewhat submerged red lesion that is frequently observed with a distinct demarcation against the normal-appearing mucosa. Clinically, erythroplakia is different from erythematous OLP as the latter has a more diffuse border and is surrounded by white reticular or papular structures. Erythroplakia is usually asymptomatic, although some patients may experience a burning sensation in conjunction with food intake.

A special form of erythroplakia has been reported that is related to reverse smoking of *chutta*, predominantly practiced in India.[63] The lesion comprises well-demarcated red areas in conjunction with white papular tissue structures. Ulcerations and depigmented areas may also be a part of this particular form of oral lesion.

Diagnosis

The diagnostic procedure of oral leukoplakia and erythroplakia is identical.[57,64] The provisional diagnosis is based on the clinical observation of a white or red patch that is not explained by a definable cause, such as trauma. If trauma is suspected, the cause, such as a sharp tooth or restoration, should be eliminated. If healing does not occur in two weeks, a tissue biopsy is essential to rule out malignancy.

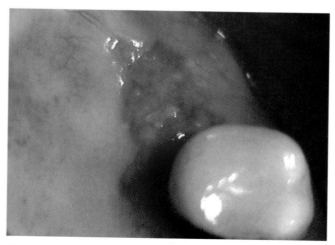

FIGURE 5-14 Erythroplakia at the alveolar ridge. The patient later developed a squamous cell carcinoma.

Pathology

The biopsy should include representative tissue of different clinical patterns. Hyperkeratosis without any other features of a definable diagnosis is compatible with homogeneous oral leukoplakia. If the histopathologic examination leads to another definable lesion, the definitive diagnosis will be changed accordingly. However, there is no uniform depiction of an oral leukoplakia and the histopathologic features of the epithelium may include hyperkeratosis, atrophy, and hyperplasia with or without dysplasia. When dysplasia is present, it may vary from mild to severe. Dysplasia may be found in homogeneous leukoplakias but is much more frequently encountered in nonhomogeneous leukoplakias[55,65-67] and in erythroplakias.[68] Epithelial dysplasia is defined in general terms as a precancerous lesion of stratified squamous epithelium characterized by cellular atypia and loss of normal maturation short of carcinoma in situ (Figure 5-15). Carcinoma *in situ* is defined as a lesion in which the full thickness of squamous epithelium shows the cellular features of carcinoma without stromal invasion.[69] A more detailed description of epithelial dysplasia is presented in Table 5-6. The prevalence of dysplasia in oral leukoplakias varies from 1%–30%, presumably due to various lifestyle factors involved and due to subjectivity in the histopathologic evaluation. The majority of erythroplakias display an atrophic epithelium with dysplastic features.[68] The significance of epithelial dysplasia for future development has been questioned.[70,71]

Management

Oral leukoplakia is a lesion with an increased risk of malignant transformation, which has great implications for the management of this oral mucosal disorder (Figure 5-16). Since alcohol and smoking are well-established risk factors for the development of oral squamous cell carcinomas, measures should be taken to influence the patients to discontinue such

TABLE 5-6	Criteria Used for Diagnosis of Epithelial Dysplasia
Loss of polarity of basal cells	
The presence of more than one layer of cells having a basaloid appearance	
Increased nuclear-cytoplasmic ratio	
Drop-shaped rete ridges	
Irregular epithelial stratification	
Increased number of mitotic figures	
Mitotic figures that are abnormal in form	
The presence of mitotic figures in the superficial half of the epithelium	
Cellular and nuclear pleomorphism	
Nuclear hyperchromatism	
Enlarged nuclei	
Loss of intercellular adherence	
Keratinization of single cells or cell groups in the prickle cell layer	

Source: Adapted from Pindborg et al.[69]

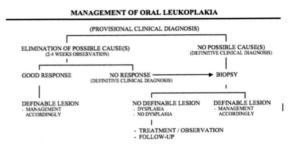

FIGURE 5-16 Management of oral leukoplakia/erythroplakia. Adapted from van der Waal I et al.[64]

habits. Cold-knife surgical excision, as well as laser surgery, is widely used to eradicate leukoplakias and erythroplakias but will not prevent all premalignant lesions from malignant development.[72-74] On the contrary, surgery has been strongly questioned as squamous cell carcinomas are almost equally prevalent in patients subjected and not subjected to surgery.[55] This may be explained by genetic defects even in clinically normal mucosa surrounding the removed lesion and is supported by a concept referred to as field cancerization.[75] Field cancerization is caused by simultaneous genetic instabilities in the epithelium of several extralesional sites that may lead to squamous cell carcinomas. However, in the absence of evidenced-based treatment strategies for oral leukoplakias, surgery will remain the treatment of choice for oral leukoplakias and erythroplakias. Such a treatment regimen is supported by the fact that serial sections of the total lesion after surgical removal has shown that as much as 7% of the lesions contained frank squamous cell carcinomas, which is not revealed by an incisional biopsy.[70]

Malignant transformation of oral leukoplakias has been reported in the range of 1%–20% over 1 to 30 years.[62,76,77]

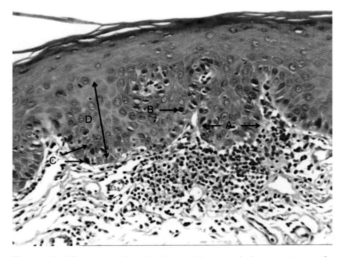

FIGURE 5-15 An oral epithelium with several characteristics of dysplasia (see Table 5-6).

According to the available European epidemiologic data, the incidence has been calculated not to exceed 1% per year.[78] Sixteen to sixty-two percent of oral carcinomas have been reported to be associated with leukoplakia at the time of the diagnosis,[79–81] and in an Indian house-to-house survey, 80% of oral cancers were reported to be preceded by oral precancerous disorders.[82] Until biomarkers are developed, management of oral leukoplakias and erythroplakias has to rely on traditional clinical and histopathologic criteria. Homogeneous oral leukoplakias are associated with a decreased risk for malignant transformation than nonhomogeneous leukoplakias and erythroplakias, and lesions not exceeding 200 mm² appear to have a better prognosis than larger lesions[55].

No consensus has been reached regarding management and follow-up of oral leukoplakias and erythroplakias. A general recommendation is to reexamine the premalignant site irrespective of surgical excision every three months for the first year. If the lesion does not relapse or change in reaction pattern, the follow-up intervals may be extended to once every six months. New biopsies should be taken if new clinical features emerge. Following five years of no relapse, self-examination may be a reasonable approach.

Oral Submucous Fibrosis

Oral submucous fibrosis is a chronic disease affecting the oral mucosa, as well as the pharynx and the upper two-thirds of the esophagus.[84] There is substantial evidence that lends support to a critical role of areca nuts in the etiology behind oral submucous fibrosis.[85]

Etiology and Pathogenesis

There is dose dependence between areca quid chewing habit and the development of this oral mucosal disorder. Areca nuts contain alkaloids, of which are coline seems to be a primary etiologic factor.[86] Arecoline has the capacity to modulate matrix metalloproteinases, lysyl oxidases, and collagenases, all affecting the metabolism of collagen, which leads to an increased fibrosis.[87] During the development of fibrosis, a decrease in the water-retaining proteoglycans will occur in favor of an increased collagen type I production. There is also evidence of a genetic predisposition of importance for the etiology behind oral submucous fibrosis. Polymorphism of the gene, which is coding for tumor necrosis factor α (TNF-α), has been reported to promote the development of the disorder.[88] Fibroblasts are stimulated by TNF-α, thereby participating in the development of fibrosis.[89] Aberrations of other cytokines of importance are transforming growth factor β and interferon-γ, which may lead to increased production and decreased degradation of collagen.

Epidemiology

Areca nut–derived products are commonly used by several hundred million individuals in the southern parts of Asia.[90] Regional variations exist regarding the preference of the areca nut use, which also accounts for variation in the oral sites affected. Oral complications are most commonly observed on the lips, buccal mucosa, retromolar area, and soft palatal mucosa.[91] The habit of chewing betel quid, containing fresh, dried, or cured areca nut, and flavoring ingredients is widespread in India, Pakistan, Bangladesh, and Sri Lanka and in immigrants coming from these regions.[92] Tobacco is often used in conjunction with betel quid. The habit is more common among women in some geographic areas, which is also reflected in the gender distribution of oral submucous fibrosis.

The global incidence of oral submucous fibrosis is estimated at 2.5 million individuals.[93] The prevalence in Indian populations is 5% for women and 2% for men.[90] Individuals in less than 20 years old seem to be affected more commonly by oral submucous fibrosis than individuals in other age groups. This is reflected in the advertisement of areca nut products, which is directed against younger age groups.

Clinical Findings

The first signs of oral submucous fibrosis are erythematous lesions, sometimes in conjunction with petechiae, pigmentations, and vesicles. These initial lesions are followed by a paler mucosa, which may comprise white marbling (Figure 5-17). The most prominent clinical characteristics will appear later in the course of the disease and include fibrotic bands located beneath an atrophic epithelium. Increased fibrosis eventually leads to loss of resilience, which interferes with speech, tongue mobility, and a decreased ability to open the mouth. The atrophic epithelium may cause a smarting sensation and inability to eat hot and spicy food. More than 25% of the patients also exhibit oral leukoplakias.[94]

Diagnosis

The diagnosis of oral submucous fibrosis is based on the clinical characteristics and on the patient's report of a habit

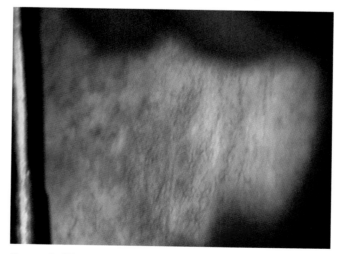

FIGURE 5-17 A patient with submucous fibrosis with restricted ability to open her mouth. The buccal mucosa has a marbling appearance.

of betel chewing. An international consensus has been reached where at least one of the following characteristics should be present[95]:

- Palpable fibrous bands
- Mucosal texture feels tough and leathery
- Blanching of mucosa together with histopathologic features consistent with oral submucous fibrosis (atrophic epithelium with loss of rete ridges and juxta-epithelial hyalinization of lamina propria)

Pathology

The early histopathologic characteristics for oral submucous fibrosis are fine fibrils of collagen, edema, hypertrophic fibroblasts, dilated and congested blood vessels, and an infiltration of neutrophilic and eosinophilic granulocytes.[96] This picture is followed by a down-regulation of fibroblasts, epithelial atrophy, and loss of rete pegs, and early signs of hyalinization occur in concert with an infiltration of inflammatory cells.[83] Epithelial dysplasia in oral submucous fibrosis tissues appeared to vary from 7%–26% depending on the study population.[97–99]

Management

Products derived from areca nuts are carcinogenic, regardless of concomitant use of tobacco products. Thus, treatment of oral submucous fibrosis should be focused on cessation of the chewing habits.[98] If this is successfully implemented, early lesions have a good prognosis as they may regress.[94] A plethora of treatment strategies have been tried, such as topical and systemic steroids, supplement of vitamins and nutrients, repeated dilatation with physical devices, and surgery. None of these treatments have reached general acceptance and the long-term results are dubious.

Malignant transformation of oral submucous fibrosis has been estimated in the range of 7%–13% and the incidence over a 10-year period at approximately 8%.[99]

IMMUNOPATHOLOGIC DISEASES

Lichenoid Reactions

Lichenoid reactions represent a family of lesions with different etiologies with a common clinical and histologic appearance.[100] Neither clinical nor histopathologic features enable discrimination between different lichenoid reactions but may be used to distinguish lichenoid reactions from other pathologic conditions of the oral mucosa. Oral lichenoid reactions include the following disorders:

- Oral lichen planus
- Lichenoid contact reactions
- Lichenoid drug eruptions
- Lichenoid reactions of graft-versus-host disease (GVHD)

Oral LCRs are included in the section below where allergic reactions are discussed since these lesions represent a delayed hypersensitivity reaction to constituents derived from dental materials or flavoring agents in for foods and other ingested substances.

Oral Lichen Planus
Etiology and Pathogensis

The etiology of OLP is not known.[100] During many years, it has become evident that the immune system has a primary role in the development of this disease.[101] This is supported by the histopathologic characteristics of a subepithelial band–formed infiltrate dominated by T lymphocytes[102] and macrophages and the degeneration of basal cells known as liquefaction degeneration (Figure 5-18). These features can be interpreted as an expression of the cell-mediated arm of the immune system being involved in the pathogenesis of OLP through T-lymphocyte cytotoxicity directed against antigens expressed by the basal cell layer.

Autoreactive T lymphocytes may be of primary importance for the development of OLP (Composition 7). These cells cannot discriminate between inherent molecules of the body and foreign antigens. Activation of the autoreactive T lymphocyte is a process that may arise in other parts of the body than the oral mucosa and may not even occur in concert with the onset of the mucosal lesion. Most likely, it is not one single peptide that has the potential to evoke the inflammatory response but several depending on the specificity of the autoreactive T lymphocyte. The conclusion that follows from this reasoning is that it is complicated to identify a single etiologic factor behind OLP. Other factors, such as stress, may also be of importance to establish this inflammatory process. It is not unusual that patients report that they have been exposed to negative social events months before the onset of the disease. Altogether, this makes the etiology behind OLP a multifactorial process comprising events that may take place at different time points and therefore difficult to investigate.

During recent years, an association between OLP and hepatitis C virus (HCV) has been described in populations from Japan and some Mediterranean countries. This association has not been observed in northern European countries or the United States. Furthermore, no clear association has been reported from Arabic countries,[103] with a very high HCV prevalence. It has been postulated that the association may be related to a genetic variability between countries. This is in part supported by the observation that specific alleles of the major histocompatibilty complex, such as HLA-DR6, are more prevalent in Italian patients with HCV-related OLP. However, no comprehensive explanation has been provided regarding the association between OLP and HCV.

Epidemiology

In the literature, different prevalence figures for OLP have been reported and vary from 0.5%–2.2%.[104–109] These figures may represent an underestimation as minor lesions may easily be overlooked. Among referred patients, the proportion of women is higher than that of men, but this may not be the case in the general population. The mean age at the time of diagnosis is approximately 55 years.

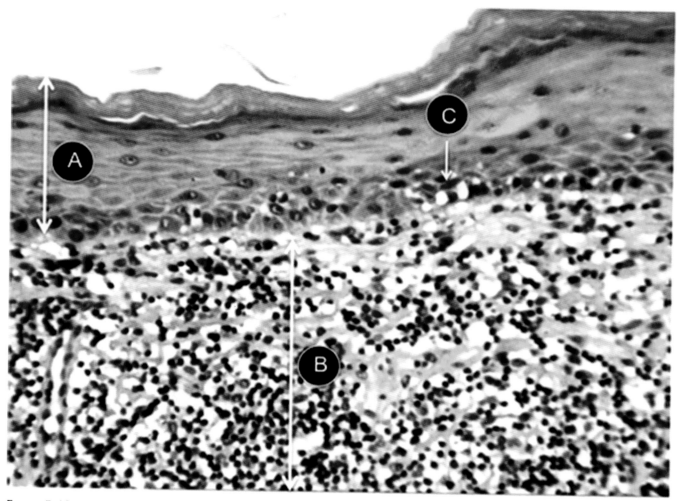

FIGURE 5-18 Lichenoid reaction with a subepithelial infiltrate of inflammatory cells and liquefaction degeneration in the basal cell layer.

Clinical Findings

OLP may contain both red and white elements and provide, together with the different textures, the basis for the clinical classification of this disorder. The white and red components of the lesion can be a part of the following clinical types[106]:

- Reticular
- Papular
- Plaque-like
- Bullous
- Erythematous
- Ulcerative

To establish a clinical diagnosis of OLP, reticular or papular textures have to be present.[110] If, in addition, plaque-like, bullous, erythematous, or ulcerative areas are present, the OLP lesion is designated accordingly. OLP confined to the gingiva may be entirely erythematous, with no reticular or papular elements present, and this type of lesion has to be confirmed by a biopsy.

The explanation of the different clinical manifestations of OLP is presumably related to the magnitude of the subepithelial inflammation. A mild degree of inflammation may provoke the epithelium to produce hyperkeratosis, whereas more intense inflammation will lead to partial or complete deterioration of the epithelium, histopathologically perceived as atrophy, erosion, or ulceration. This corroborates with the fact that most erythematous and ulcerative lesions are surrounded by white reticular or papular structures. An inflammatory gradient may be formed where the central part comprises an intense inflammatory process, whereas the periphery is less affected and the epithelial cells are able to respond with hyperkeratosis.

The reticular form of OLP is characterized by fine white lines or striae (Figure 5-19). The striae may form a network but can also show annular (circular) patterns. The striae often display a peripheral erythematous zone, which reflects a subepithelial inflammation. Although reticular OLP may be encountered in all regions of the oral mucosa, most frequently this form is observed bilaterally in the buccal mucosa

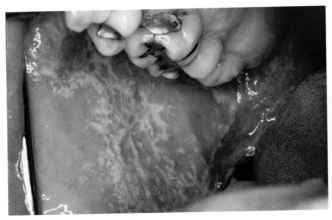

FIGURE 5-19 A reticular form of oral lichen planus.

and rarely on the mucosal side of the lips. Reticular OLP can sometimes be observed at the vermilion border.

The papular type of OLP is usually present in the initial phase of the disease (Figure 5-20).[106,107] It is clinically characterized by small white dots, which in most occasions intermingle with the reticular form. Sometimes the papular elements merge with striae as part of the natural course.

Plaque-type OLP shows a homogeneous well-demarcated white plaque that occurs in conjunction with striae (Figure 5-21). Plaque-type lesions may clinically be very similar to homogeneous oral leukoplakias. The difference between these two mucosal disorders is the presence of reticular or papular structures in the case of plaque-like OLP. The form is most often encountered in smokers,[107,109] and following cessation, the plaque may disappear and convert into the reticular type of OLP. Some scientific reports lend support to the premise that plaque-like OLP is overrepresented among OLP lesions transforming into oral squamous cell carcinomas.[111]

Typically, the reticular, papular, and plaque-like forms of OLP are asymptomatic, although the patient may experience a

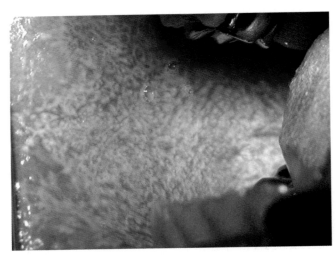

FIGURE 5-20 Papular oral lichen planus with dense cover of papules. In the upper left corner, the lesion has started to form a more reticular structure.

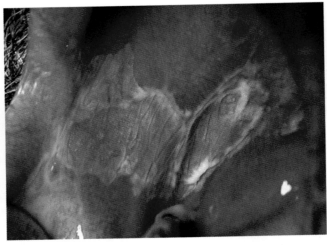

FIGURE 5-21 A plaque-like oral lichen planus with a plaque in the anterior part. In the posterior part, the lesion has features that are compatible with the reticular form.

feeling of roughness. The bullous form is very unusual but may appear as bullous structures surrounded by a reticular network.

Erythematous (atrophic) OLP is characterized by a homogeneous red area. When this type of OLP is present in the buccal mucosa or in the palate, striae are frequently seen in the periphery of the lesion. Some patients may display erythematous OLP exclusively affecting attached gingiva (Figure 5-22A).[112] This form of lesion may occur without any papules or striae and presents as desquamative gingivitis. Therefore, erythematous OLP may require a histopathologic examination in order to arrive at a correct diagnosis.

Ulcerative lesions are the most disabling form of OLP (Figure 5-23A). Clinically, the fibrin-coated ulcers are surrounded by an erythematous zone with white striae in the periphery.[113] This appearance may reflect a gradient of the intensity of subepithelial inflammation that is most prominent at the center of the lesion. As for the erythematous form of OLP, the affected patient complains of a smarting sensation in conjunction with food intake.

Clinical Manifestation

Cutaneous lesions may be encountered in approximately 15% of patients with OLP.[114] The classic appearance of skin lesions consists of pruritic erythematous to violaceous papules that are flat topped. The predilection sites are the trunk and flexor surfaces of arms and legs (Figure 5-24). The papules may be discrete or coalesce to form plaques. The patients report relief following intense scratching of the lesions, but trauma may aggravate the disease, which is referred to as a Koebner phenomenon. This phenomenon may also be of relevance for OLP, which is continuously exposed to physical trauma during mastication and tooth brushing.

The most frequent extra-oral mucosal site involved is the genital mucosa. Close to 20% of women presenting with OLP also have genital involvement.[114] Symptoms including burning, pain, vaginal discharge, and dyspareunia

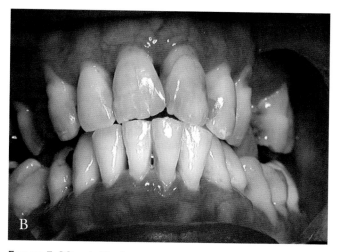

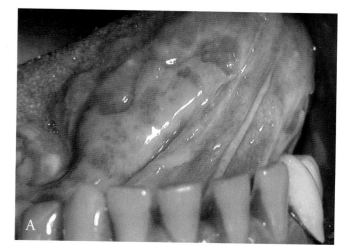

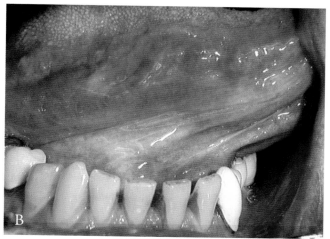

FIGURE 5-22 A, Erythematous oral lichen planus. B, Improvement of the lesion following optimal oral hygiene.

FIGURE 5-23 A, Ulcerative oral lichen planus. B, Complete epithelialization following 3 weeks of treatment with 0.025% clobetasol propionate gel, twice daily.

are frequently noted in patients with the erythematous or ulcerative forms of the disease. No relationship seems to exist between the degree of severity in the oral and genital sites. Genital lichen planus has been reported in males, but the association with OLP is not as frequent as for women. Esophageal lichen planus has been described to occur simultaneously with OLP in some patients, the main complaint being dysphagia.[114]

Diagnosis

Papules or reticular components have to be present in order to establish a correct clinical diagnosis. These pathognomonic components may exist together with plaque-like, erythematous, bullous, or ulcerative lesions. In patients with gingival erythematous lesions, it may be difficult to find striae or papules. A biopsy is usually required for an accurate diagnosis of this type of OLP. It is important that the biopsy is taken as far as possible from the gingival pocket to avoid inflammatory changes due to periodontal disease.

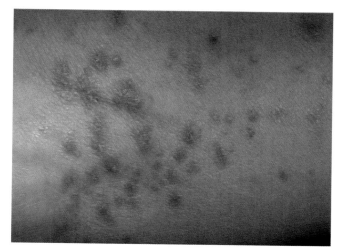

FIGURE 5-24 Cutaneous lichen planus on the flexor side of the fore arm.

OLP can often be separated from LCRs to dental materials, which are most often detected on the buccal mucosa and the lateral borders of the tongue. OLP, on the other hand, usually displays a more general involvement.[115]

Oral lichenoid drug eruptions[116] have the same clinical and histopathologic characteristics as OLP. The patient's disease history may give some indication as to which drug is involved, but OLP may not start when the drug was first introduced. Withdrawal of the drug and rechallenge are the most reliable ways to diagnose lichenoid drug eruptions but may not be possible to carry out.

Oral GVHD has the same clinical appearance as OLP, but the lesion is usually more generalized. The lichenoid reactions are frequently seen simultaneously with other characteristics, such as xerostomia and the presence of localized skin involvement and liver dysfunction, even if an oral lichenoid reaction may emerge as the only clinical sign of GVHD.

Oral mucosal lesions that do not belong to the group of lichenoid reactions may sometimes comprise a differential diagnostic problem. Discoid lupus erythematosus (DLE) shows white radiating striae sometimes resembling those of OLP. The striae present in DLE are typically more prominent, with a more marked hyperkeratinization, and the striae may abruptly terminate against a sharp demarcation (Figure 5-25). Histopathologic criteria for lupus erythematosus (LE) have been reported to discriminate against OLP with a sensitivity of 92% and a specificity of 96%.[117] Direct immunofluorescence for immunoglobulin IgM on biopsies of the clinically normal oral mucosa (lupus band test) may also be used, although they are only positive in less than 50% of

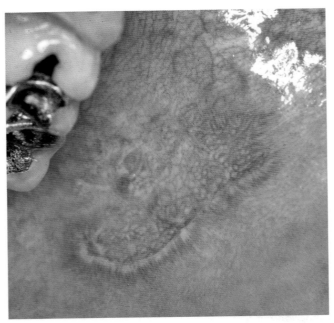

Figure 5-25 Discoid lupus erythematous of the left buccal mucosa.

the systemic lupus erythematosus (SLE) cases.[118] Plaque-like OLP is discriminated from homogeneous oral leukoplakia as the latter is not featured with papular or reticular elements.

Erythematous OLP of the gingiva exhibits a similar clinical presentation as mucous membrane pemphigoid. In pemphigoid lesions, the epithelium is easily detached from the connective tissue by a probe or a gentle searing force (Nikolsky's phenomenon). A biopsy for routine histology and direct immunofluorescence are required for an accurate differential diagnosis. Ulcerating conditions such as erythema multiforme and adverse reactions to nonsteroidal anti-inflammatory drugs (NSAIDs) may be difficult to distinguish from ulcerative OLP. The former lesions, however, do not typically appear with reticular or papular elements in the periphery of the ulcerations.

Pathology

To differentiate between the four types of lichenoid reactions, that is, OLP, LCR, lichenoid drug eruptions, and lichenoid reactions related to GVHD, a histopathologic examination is of modest diagnostic value. The reason is that the four lesions display the same histopathologic features. Undoubtedly, histopathology is a valuable tool when lichenoid reactions are to be discriminated from other mucosal lesions. The necessity of a biopsy to arrive at an accurate diagnosis of OLP has been discussed, but explicit guidelines have not been universally approved. When the diagnosis is uncertain, biopsies should always be taken.

The histopathologic features of OLP are (1) areas of hyperparakeratosis or hyperorthokeratosis, often with a thickening of the granular cell layer and a saw-toothed appearance to the rete pegs, and (2) "liquefaction degeneration," or necrosis of the basal cell layer; (3) an eosinophilic band may be seen just beneath the basement membrane and contain fibrin covering the lamina propria. A dense subepithelial band–shaped infiltrate of lymphocytes and macrophages is also characteristic of the disease (see Figure 5-18). Deposition of antibodies and complement can be observed but is not pathognomonic for OLP; therefore, this technique is not routinely used.

Management

Since the etiology behind OLP is unknown, basic conditions for development of preventive therapies are lacking. Thus, all current treatment strategies are aiming at reducing or eliminating symptoms. Several topical drugs have been suggested, including steroids, calcineurin inhibitors (cyclosporine and tacrolimus[119]), retinoids, and ultraviolet phototherapy.[104] Among these, topical steroids are widely used and accepted as the primary treatment of choice (Figure 5-23b). Some reports have advocated very potent steroids as clobetasol propionate in favor of intermediate steroids such as triamcinolone acetonide. However, no randomized clinical trials exist where different formulas, strengths, and classes of topically applied steroids have been compared. Topical application of cyclosporine, tacrolimus, and retinoids has been suggested as a second-line therapy for OLP. Cyclosporine has been reported to be less effective than clobetasol propionate and not significantly better than 1% triamcinolone paste. No adverse effects related to these two drugs have been reported except for a temporary burning sensation following the use of cyclosporine.[120] In a comparison of topical application of clobetasol and cyclosporine, the former has been found to be more effective in inducing clinical improvement, but the two drugs have comparable effects on symptoms. Clobetasol was found to give less stable results than cyclosporine when therapy ended and was ascribed a higher incidence of side effects, but none of these were severe enough to require discontinuation of therapy. Topical tacrolimus 0.1% ointment has been reported to have a better initial therapeutic response than triamcinolone acetonide 0.1% ointment.[121] However, this drug has been labeled with the US Food and Drug Administration's Black Box Warning: "Possibility of increased risk of malignancy (squamous cell carcinoma and lymphoma) in patients using topical tacrolimus/pimecrolimus for cutaneous psoriasis. These agents should be used in limited circumstances, and patients made aware of these concerns."[122] In conclusion, topical steroids should be used as the primary therapeutic choice for symptomatic OLP. Cyclosporine may be considered a second choice, although the efficacy has been questioned. Tacrolimus should only be used by experts when symptomatic OLP lesions are recalcitrant to topical steroids.

Topical steroids are preferably used as a mouth rinse or a gel. These formulas are often easier for the patient to administer than a paste. Although no systematic studies have compared different frequencies of application, a reasonable approach may be to apply the drug two to three times a day during three weeks followed by tapering during the following nine weeks until a maintenance dose of two to three times a week is reached. There are no consistent results that lend support to decreased levels of endogenous cortisol. However, patients are likely to experience transient suppression of the hypothalamic-pituitary-adrenal (HPA) axis and should not swallow but to "swish and spit out."

Relapses are common, and the general approach should be to use steroids at the lowest level to keep the patient free of symptoms. This approach necessitates an individual amendment of the steroid therapy to each patient. When potent topical steroids are used, a fungal infection may emerge, and a parallel treatment with antifungal drugs may be necessary when the number of applications exceeds once a day and antifungal treatment itself may result in significant improvement of symptoms and clinical features. Since half of OLP lesions exhibit candidal infection, antifungal treatment may be used before treatment with steroids.

Although topical steroids are usually able to keep OLP patients free of symptoms, systemic steroids are justified to control symptoms from recalcitrant lesions. One milligram per kilogram daily for seven days has been suggested, followed by a reduction of 10 mg each subsequent day.[114] A maintenance dose with topical steroids may be commenced during the tapering of the systemic steroids.

Erythematous OLP of the gingiva constitutes a therapeutic challenge. To be successful, it is critical to remove both sub- and supragingival plaque and calculus (Figure 5-22B).[123] If a microbial plaque–induced gingivitis is present, it seems to work in concert with gingival lichen planus and make the latter more resistant to pharmacologic treatment. Thus, oral hygiene should be optimized prior to the beginning of steroid treatment. Once the hygiene treatment is complete, some patients experience a decrease in or even elimination of symptoms and steroid treatment is no longer justified. If symptoms persist, steroid gels in prefabricated plastic trays may be used for 30 minutes at each application to increase the concentration of steroids in the gingival tissue.

As part of OLP lesions, ulcerative areas may be found in close contact with dental materials similar to what is observed in LCRs. The difference is the extension of the LCR, which is limited to such contacts. When symptomatic ulcerations of this kind are present as part of the OLP lesion, replacement of the dental material, usually amalgams, may convert a symptomatic to a non-symptomatic lesion.[115]

OLP is considered to be a premalignant disorder (Figure 5-26). Premalignant disorders entail an increased risk of malignant transformation at some site of the oral mucosa, not necessarily associated with a preexisting lesion. It is widely accepted that patients with OLP are predisposed to develop oral carcinomas, although it should be emphasized that the risk is low and presumably does not exceed an incidence of 0.2% per year.[104] It may be ambiguous to relate the increased risk to patients with a definite type of OLP lesions. In some studies, plaque-like lesions have been overrepresented, but ulcerative lesions are also suspected to be associated with malignant

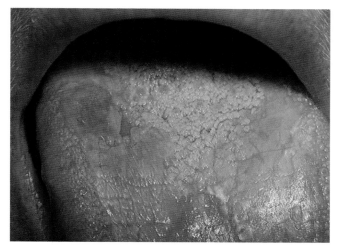

FIGURE 5-26 A squamous cell carcinoma developed in a plaque-like oral lichen planus.

transformation.[111] Albeit the risk for patients with OLP to contract oral squamous cell carcinomas is low, a minimum of annual monitoring has been suggested in conjunction with routine dental examination by the general dental practitioner.[110] For patients with symptomatic OLP, examination for malignancies will be a part of the evaluation of symptomatic treatment. In countries with limited health-care resources, it may be difficult to conduct annual monitoring, but at the time of diagnosis, patients need to be properly educated on the subject of the malignant potential of OLP.

Drug-Induced Lichenoid Reactions

Etiology and Pathogenesis

The mechanisms behind drug-induced lichenoid reactions (DILRs) are poorly understood.[116,124] As the clinical and histopathologic appearances resemble a delayed hypersensitivity reaction, it has been hypothesized that drugs or their metabolites, with the capacity to act as haptens, trigger a lichenoid reaction. Penicillin, gold, NSAID, and sulfonamides are examples of drugs that have been related to the development of DILRs.[125,126] Penicillin and gold may bind directly to self-proteins, which will be presented by antigen-presenting cells (APCs) and perceived as foreign by specific T lymphocytes, similar to a delayed hypersensitivity reaction. Drugs such as sulfonamides haptenate self-proteins indirectly, through formation of reactive metabolites, which will covalently bind to proteins present in the oral mucosa. It has been postulated that DILRs may result from poor drug metabolism because of genetic variation of the major cytochrome P-450 enzymes.[127,128]

Epidemiology

No prevalence figures are available for DILRs; most likely, DILRs are unusual and constitute a minority of the cases diagnosed as OLP.

Clinical Findings

Our knowledge about oral DILRs is limited and primarily based on case reports. It has been suggested that DILRs are predominantly unilateral and present with an ulcerative reaction pattern.[128] These characteristics are far from consistent and not useful to discriminate between OLP and DILRs (Figure 5-27A). At present, these two conditions should be considered clinically indistinguishable.[116]

Clinical Manifestations

Lichenoid drug eruptions appear similar to cutaneous lichen planus and may be severely pruritic (see Clinical Manifestations of OLP).

Diagnosis

Although diagnostic testing methods exist, they are in general of limited clinical value. One major problem that affects the use of diagnostic tests for drug hypersensitivity

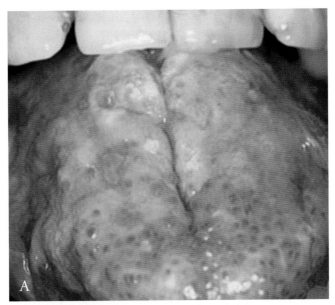

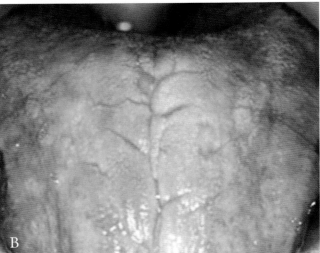

FIGURE 5-27 A, Drug-induced lichenoid reaction following 1 month of medication with a cholestyramine-containing drug. B, Three weeks following withdrawal of the drug.

is that the immune pathogenesis for most drugs, except for penicillin and gold, is virtually unknown. To be clinically classified as a DILR, the oral lesions should comprise a white reticulum or papules. These characteristics may be observed concurrently with erythematous and ulcerative lesions. DILRs are often a diagnostic challenge as the condition has been associated with a large number of drugs (Table 5-7). A correct diagnosis is easier to establish when a patient develops DILR after starting a new drug (see Figure 5-27). For practical reasons, it is difficult to conduct withdrawal unless a patient has a severe symptomatic case.

A DILR may not develop for several months after a new drug is started. It may also take several weeks before DILRs disappear following withdrawal.[116]

TABLE 5-7	Drug-Related Lichenoid Reactions
ACE inhibitors	
Allopurinol	
Amiphenazole	
Antimalarials	
Barbiturates	
BCG vaccine	
Captopril	
Carbamazepine	
Carbimazole	
Chloral hydrate	
Chloroquine	
Chlorpropamide	
Cholera vaccine	
Cinnarizine	
Clofibrate	
Colchicine	
Dapsone	
Dipyridamole	
Ethionamide	
Flunarizine	
Gaunoclor	
Gold	
Griseofulvin	
Hepatitis B vaccine	
Hydroxychloroquine	
Interferon-alpha	
Ketoconazole	
Labetalol	
Levamisole	
Lincomycin	
Lithium	
Lorazepam	
Mepacrine	
Mercury	
Metformin	
Methyldopa	
Metronidazole	
Niridazole	
NSAIDs	
Oral contraceptives	
Oxprenolol	
Para-aminosalicylate	
Penicillamine	
Penicillins	
Phenindione	
Phenothiazines	
Phenylbutazones	
Phenytoin	
Piroxicam	
Practolol	
Prazosin	
Procainamide	
Propranolol	
Propylthiouracil	
Protease inhibitors	
Prothionamide	
Quinidine	
Quinine	
Rifampicin	
Streptomycin	
Sulfonamide	
Tetracycline	
Tocainide	
Tolbutamide	
Triprolidine	

ACE, angiotensin-converting enzyme; BCG, bacille Calmette-Guérin; NSAIDs, nonsteroidal anti-inflammatory drugs.
Source: Adapted from Scully and Bagan.[124]

Management

DILRs are not usually seen in conjunction with severe life-threatening reactions such as toxic epidermal necrolysis. Discontinuance of the drug and symptomatic treatment with topical steroids are often sufficient. The patient should be properly educated about the responsible drug to prevent future DILRs.

Lichenoid Reactions of GVHD
Etiology and Pathogenesis

The major cause of GVHD is allogeneic hematopoietic cell transplantation, even if an autologous transplantation may also entail GVHD.[129,130] In GVHD, it is the transplanted immunocompetent tissue that attempts to reject the tissue of the host.[131] As the first step, conditioning of the host by chemotherapy and radiation will generate host cell damage, release of cytokines, and up-regulation of adhesion and major histocompatibility complex (MHC) molecules, which all facilitate recognition of alloantigens by donor T lymphocytes. A second step comprises an interaction between the recipient's APCs and the donor's T lymphocytes, which will perceive the histocompatibility antigens, expressed by APCs as foreign. This interaction may, in fact, be considered as the donor T lymphocytes recognizing the recipient's APCs as self-APCs expressing nonself-peptides. This interaction resembles the interaction between autoreactive T lymphocytes and APCs, hypothesized to play a role in the development of OLP. In a third step, the inflammatory cascade that follows the APC–T-lymphocyte reaction will stimulate proliferation of stromal cells, resulting in clinical features compatible with a lichenoid reaction.

Epidemiology

Chronic GVHD occurs in 15%–50% of patients who survive three months after transplantation and varies in incidence from 33% of HLA-identical sibling transplants to 64% of unrelated donor transplants. The risk for GVHD increases with the age of the marrow recipient.[130] Chronic GVHD is defined as occurring more than 100 days post-HCT, most commonly as a transition from acute GVHD. In 20%–30% of the patients, chronic GVHD may occur de novo.

Clinical Findings

Oral lichenoid reactions as part of GVHD may be seen both in acute and chronic GVHD, although the latter are more often associated with typical lichenoid features. The clinical lichenoid reaction patterns are indistinguishable from what is seen in patients with OLP, that is, reticulum, erythema, and ulcerations, but lichenoid reactions associated with GVHD are typically associated with a more widespread involvement of the oral mucosa (Figure 5-28).

Clinical Manifestations

The skin lesions often present with pruritic maculopapular and morbilliform rash, primarily affecting the palms and soles. violaceous scaly papules and plaques may progress to a generalized erythroderma, bulla formation, and, in severe cases, a toxic epidermal necrolysis–like epidermal desquamation.[129]

Diagnosis

The presence of systemic GVHD facilitates the diagnosis of oral mucosal changes of chronic oral GVHD. However, the oral cavity may, in some instances, be the primary or even the only site of chronic GVHD involvement. The lichenoid

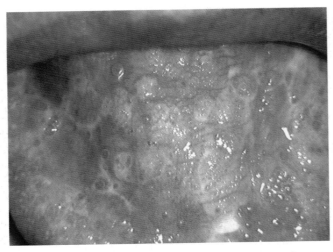

FIGURE 5-28 Lichenoid reaction in association with graft-versus-host disease following bone marrow transplantation.

eruptions are important in the diagnostic process of oral GVHD and have the highest positive predictive value of all reaction patterns.[131] It is not possible to distinguish between OLP and oral GVHD based on clinical and histopathologic features.

Management

The same treatment strategy as for OLP may be used for chronic oral GVHD, that is, topical steroid preparations, such as fluocinonide and clobetasol gel. Opportunistic infections such as candidiasis should always be considered in immunosuppressed patients. The development of secondary malignancies has been recognized as a potentially serious complication of GVHD. Patients with a history of oral GVHD should therefore be examined for oral malignancies as part of the medical follow-up procedure.

Lupus Erythematosus
Etiology and Pathogenesis

Lupus Erythematosus (LE) represents the classic prototype of an autoimmune disease involving immune complexes. Both the natural and the adaptive parts of the immune system are participating, with the latter involving both B and T lymphocytes.[132,133] Environmental factors are of importance as sun exposure, drugs, chemical substances, and hormones which all have been reported to aggravate the disease. A genetic predisposition is supported by an elevated risk for siblings to develop LE and by an increased disease concordance in monozygotic twins. More than 80 different drugs have been associated with the onset of SLE, including hydralazine, methyldopa, chlorpromazine, isoniazid, quinidine, and procainamide.[134]

Epidemiology

SLE predominantly affects women of reproductive age, and the prevalence decreases during the menopause. In the interval of 20–40 years, as much as 80% has been reported to be women.[135] This predominance has lent support to an involvement of hormones in the pathogenesis of LE as well as the fact that the disease can be precipitated by hormonal drugs. There are large variations in the distribution of the disease between different ethnic groups. In the United Kingdom, the prevalence of SLE among Asian individuals is 40 per 100,000; for Caucasians, it is 20 per 100,000 individuals.

Clinical Findings

The oral lesions observed in SLE and discoid lupus erythematosus (DLE) are similar in their characteristics, both clinically and histopathologically.[136] The typical clinical lesion comprises white striae with a radiating orientation, and these may sharply terminate toward the center of the lesions, which has a more erythematous appearance (see Figure 5-25). However, several clinical manifestations of oral LE exist. The most affected sites are the gingiva, buccal mucosa, tongue, and palate. Lesions in the palatal mucosa can be dominated by erythematous lesions, and white structures may not be observed (Figure 5-29). Oral mucosa lesions compatible with LE may be the first sign of the disease. Approximately 20% of the patients with LE have been reported to display oral lesions, although the figures vary from 9% to 45%.[137]

Clinical Manifestations

The classic categorization of LE into SLE and DLE has during recent years been supplemented with acute cutaneous lupus erythematosus and subacute cutaneous lupus erythematosus.[138–140] SLE may also occur in concert with other rheumatologic diseases such as secondary Sjögren's syndrome and mixed connective tissue disease. SLE diagnosis requires that four or more of the diagnostic criteria displayed in Table 5-8 should be present at each time point of the disease. The typical DLE diagnosis comprises well-demarcatedcutaneous lesions with round or oval erythematous plaques with scales

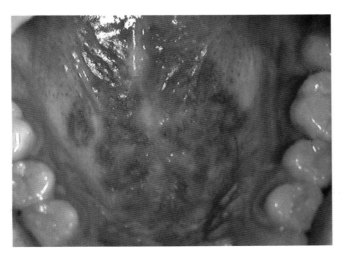

FIGURE 5-29 Lupus lesion in the palatal mucosa in a patient with systemic lupus erythematosus.

TABLE 5-8	American College of Rheumatology Criteria for Systemic Lupus Erythematosus*

1. Malar rash
2. Discoid lesions
3. Photosensitivity
4. Presence of oral ulcers
5. Nonerosive arthritis of two joints or more
6. Serositis
7. Renal disorder
8. Neurologic disorder (seizures or psychosis)
9. Hematologic disorder (hemolytic anemia, leukopenia, lymphopenia, or thrombocytopenia)
10. Immunologic disorder (anti-DNA, anti-SM, or antiphospholipid antibodies)

DNA, deoxyribonucleic acid.
A revised version has been published 1997 but the 1982 version seems to be the most widely used.
Source: Adapted from Tan *et al.*[140]
*Systemic lupus erythematosus diagnosis with 4 or more of 11 criteria present at any time.

and follicular plugging. These lesions may form butterfly-like rashes over the cheeks and nose known as malar rash.

Laboratory Findings

Antinuclear antibodies are frequently found in patients with SLE and can be used to indicate a systemic involvement, but patients with other rheumatologic diseases, such as Sjögren's syndrome and rheumatoid arthritis, may be positive as well. Moderate to high titers of anti-DNA and anti-Smith antibodies are almost pathognomonic of SLE.

Pathology

The clinical picture of LE varies, which also is reflected in the histopathology. The most common histopathologic features of LE are (1) hyperkeratosis with keratotic plugs, (2) atrophy of the rete processes, (3) deep inflammatory infiltrate, (4) edema in the lamina propria, and (5) thick patchy or continuous PAS-positive juxta-epithelial deposits.[118]

Diagnosis

Oral mucosal lesions seen in conjunction with different types of LE are clinically and histopathologically indistinguishable. Liquefaction degeneration may also be present, which may result in diagnostic problems in relation to OLP. The criteria mentioned above were tested among clinically atypical cases of DLE and the other groups of mucosal lesions, with a sensitivity of 92% and a specificity of 96% against both OLP and leukoplakia for the presence of two or more of the five criteria.[117] Direct immunohistochemistry is conducted to reveal granular deposition of IgM, IgG, IgA, and C3 (lupus band test).[118] The extralesional oral mucosa in SLE patients has a positive reaction to IgM in 45% of the cases in combination with variable deposits of IgG, IgA, and C3. DLE is accompanied by a positive antibody reaction in as little as 3% of the patients.

Management

Regarding treatment of oral mucosal LE lesions, no randomized clinical trials have been conducted. The oral lesions may respond to systematic treatment used to alleviate the disease and have to be evaluated first. When symptomatic intraoral lesions are present, topical steroids should be considered (Table 5-9). To obtain relief of symptoms, potent topical steroids such as clobetasol propionate gel 0.05%, betamethasone dipropionate 0.05%, or fluticasone propionate spray 50 µg aqueous solution are usually required. The treatment may begin with applications two to three times a day followed by a tapering during the next six to nine weeks. The overall objective is to use a minimum of steroids to obtain relief. Immunosuppressive drugs used to treat LE may precipitate opportunistic fungal and viral infections. Opportunistic oral infections can also originate the immunologic defects, which are part of the pathogenesis. Another complication of the drugs used in treatment of LE is mucosal ulceration caused by frequent exploitation of NSAIDs.

TABLE 5-9   Topical Therapy for Oral Lesions of Lupus Erythematosus

Topical Steroid Therapy*	Directions for Use†
0.05% fluocinonide gel	Place on affected area(s) 2 × /d for 2 wk
0.05% clobetasol gel	Place on affected area(s) 2 × /d for 2 wk
Dexamethasone elixir (0.5 mg/mL)	Swish and spit 10 mL 4 × /d for 2 wk
Triamcinolone acetonide 5 mg/mL	Intralesional injection
Topical antifungal therapy, 10 mg clotrimazole troches	Dissolve in mouth 5 × /d for 10 d
Nystatin suspension (100,000 U/mL)	Swish and spit 5 mL 4 × /day for 10 d
Chlorhexidine rinse (0.12%)	Swish and spit 10 mL 2 × /day until lesions resolve

Source: Adapted from Brennan et al.[141]
*Fungal infections are a side effect of topical steroids. †If lesions do not respond appropriately to topical steroids in 2 wk, consider systemic therapy such as antimalarials, steroids, thalidomide, clofazimine, and methotrexate.

Oral mucosal lesions often mirror the disease activity. They may regress spontaneously but can also persist for months or even years.

ALLERGIC REACTIONS

Lichenoid Contact Reactions

LCRs are considered due to a delayed hypersensitivity reaction to constituents derived from dental materials. The majority of patients are patch test positive to mercury (Hg), which lends support to LCR being an allergic reaction. Although Hg is usually considered the primary etiologic factor, other amalgam constituents may also initiate LCR.

Etiology and Pathogenesis

The pathogenesis of LCR is not fully elucidated, but based on the knowledge of delayed hypersensitivity, most likely the following will occur (Composition 8). Hg cannot be recognized by the immune system as the T-cell receptor (TCR), expressed by the T lymphocytes, is primarily limited to the identification of peptides. However, Hg ions are highly reactive and may bind to self-proteins of the oral epithelium, which will induce transformation changes of the protein. This assembly between Hg and protein will be perceived as nonself, and following pinocytosis by APCs, such as the Langerhans' cells of the oral epithelium, these cells will degrade the protein complex to oligopeptides. The activated APCs will mature through the migration to regional lymph nodes and start to express the Hg-containing peptides together with class II molecules on the cell surface. Class II molecules represent a subset of glycoproteins derived from the MHC, which is critical for the APC–T-lymphocyte interaction. The process of antigen presentation is therefore considered to be class II molecule restricted. Within the lymph node, an interaction between the assembly of class II molecule–Hg-containing peptide on the APC and the TCR expressed on the antigen-specific T lymphocyte will occur. This interaction is known as the first signal in the antigen-presenting process. The second signal comprises further cellular interactions, which is decisive for the clonal expansion of the Hg peptide–specific T lymphocytes to take place. These cells will migrate into the bloodstream to reach and patrol all peripheral tissues of the body. At this state, the patient is considered to be sensitized against Hg.

Once the oral mucosa of a sensitized individual is re-exposed to Hg, the Langerhans' cells in the oral epithelium are able to present peptide-conjugated Hg to the peripheral T lymphocytes with an appropriate TCR. Thus, in a sensitized individual, the Langerhans' cells are able to fulfill their mission in situ and do not have to migrate to the regional lymph node to encounter an appropriate T lymphocyte. The interaction between the cells instigates a cytokine production, which will lead to an attraction of inflammatory cells necessary to mount a local immune response in the Hg-exposed oral mucosa and eventually also lead to healing once Hg exposure is eliminated. The cytokine profile produced is most likely responsible for the stimulation of inherent cells of the oral mucosa, which gives rise to the clinical reaction pattern of LCR.

Epidemiology

No prevalence figures for LCR have been reported in the literature. The gender distribution seems to be different from OLP, with a higher proportion of women among patients affected by LCR. No significant differences regarding general diseases, drugs, or history of allergy between the LCR and OLP have been reported.

Clinical Findings

Oral LCRs are considered to be a type of delayed hypersensitivity reaction to constituents derived from dental materials, predominantly amalgam fillings.[142–144] Clinically, LCRs display the same reaction patterns as seen in OLP, that is, reticulum, papules, plaque, erythema, and ulcers (Figure 5-32A). The most apparent clinical difference between OLP and LCR is the extension of the lesions. The majority of LCRs are confined to sites that are regularly in contact with dental materials, such as the buccal mucosa and the border of the tongue. Lesions are hardly ever observed in sites as the gingiva, palatal mucosa, floor of the mouth, or dorsum of the tongue.[115,142] Most LCRs are non-symptomatic, but when erythematous or ulcerative lesions are present, the patient may experience discomfort from spicy and warm food constituents. The duration with which the material is in contact with the oral mucosa has a decisive influence on the development of LCR. The clinical implication of this is that some lesions, especially those on the lateral border of the tongue with high mobility, may extend somewhat beyond the direct contact of dental material.

Lichenoid reactions in contact with composites have been observed on the mucosal side of both the upper and lower lips.[145] The majority of this type of LCR resolve following treatment with chlorhexidine. Further studies have to be conducted to substantiate a true lichenoid nature of these lesions.

Diagnosis

The diagnosis is primarily based on the topical relationship to dental materials.[115] OLP may display similar clinical characteristics, and replacement of the culprit dental material may assist to discriminate between LCR and OLP (Figure 5-32B). However, OLP may also improve following the replacement but to a lesser extent compared to LCR.[115,146,147] The patch test is of minor clinical significance as a substantial number of patients with LCR will test negative to relevant test compounds, although the lesions will resolve following replacement of the dental material.[115,146] Histopathology will not be of any assistance in the discrimination between OLP and LCR.

Management

Replacement of dental materials in direct contact with LCR will result in cure or considerable improvement in at least 90% of the cases (Figure 5-32B).[115] Most lesions should be expected to heal within one to two months. There is no need for replacement of restorative materials that are not in direct contact with the LCR. Healing does not seem to depend on what type of dental material is used for replacement. Although a malignant potential of LCR has been suggested, no prospective studies have been conducted to support this hypothesis.[148]

Reactions to Dentifrice and Chlorhexidine

Delayed hypersensitivity reactions to toothpastes (Figure 5-30) and mouthwashes have been reported, but such reactions are rare.[149–153] The compounds responsible for the allergic

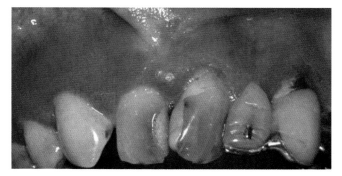

FIGURE 5-30 An erythematous attached gingiva in a patient allergic to dentifrice.

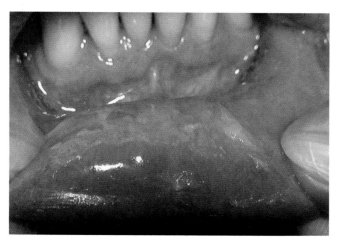

FIGURE 5-31 Dentifrices-related desquamation of the oral epithelium at the mucosal side of the lower lip.

reactions may include flavor additives such as carvone and cinnamon or preservatives. These flavoring constituents may also be used in chewing gum and produce similar forms of gingivostomatitis. The clinical manifestations include fiery red edematous gingiva, which may include both ulcerations and white lesions. Similar lesions may involve other sites, such as the labial, buccal, and tongue mucosae. The clinical manifestations are characteristic and form the basis of the diagnosis, which is supported by healing of the lesions after withdrawal of the allergen-containing agent. Dentifrice may also cause a disturbed desquamation, which clinically can be observed as thin veils of keratin (Figure 5-31).

TOXIC REACTIONS

Reactions to Smokeless Tobacco

Smokeless tobacco represents a nonhomogeneous group of compounds used with different intraoral application methods. Three different geographic areas are of special interest: South Asia, the United States, and Scandinavia. In India, tobacco is often used in combination with betel leaf, sliced areca nut, and powdered slaked lime, which increases the toxicity of the compound. There is a definitive association between this form of smokeless tobacco and oral cancer (see oral submucous fibrosis).

Smokeless tobacco in the United States and Scandinavia can be divided into three different groups: chewing tobacco, moist snuff, and dry snuff.[154] All three are different regarding composition, manufacturing procedures, and type of consumers. In Scandinavia, moist snuff is the most popular compound but different in the manufacturing process from moist snuff used in the United States.[155] The latter contains higher concentrations of tobacco-specific nitrosamines and nitrite. This compound has reached an increased attractiveness in favor of dry snuff.

The clinical picture varies in relation to the type, brand, frequency, and duration of use of moist snuff.[156–159] In its mildest form, the lesion may just be noted as wrinkles at the site of application,

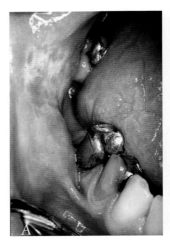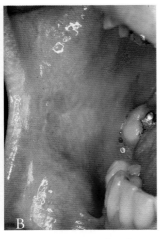

FIGURE 5-32 A, Lichenoid contact reaction associated with an amalgam crown. B, Improvement following replacement with a porcelain crown.

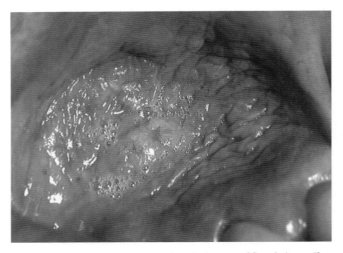

FIGURE 5-33 Lesion associated with the use of Swedish snuff.

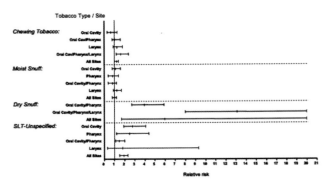

FIGURE 5-34 Summary relative rish for oral cancer and related sites according to SLT product type. Adapted from.[161]

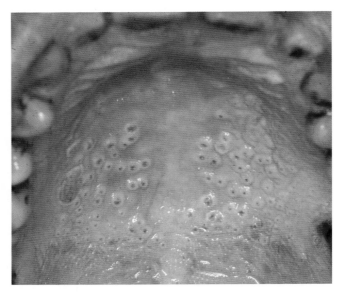

FIGURE 5-35 Smoker's palate with pronounced orifices of the accessory salivary glands.

whereas high consumers may display a white and leathery lesion (Figure 5-33), which sometimes contains ulcerations. Hyperkeratinization, acanthosis, and epithelial vacuolizations are common histopathologic features together with different degrees of subepithelial inflammation. Gingival retractions are the most common adverse reaction seen in conjunction with a smokeless tobacco habit. These retractions are irreversible, whereas the mucosal lesion usually regresses within a couple of months. Oral mucosal lesions are less frequently observed in association with chewing tobacco compared with moist snuff.

There is a distinct difference between lesions caused by smokeless tobacco and oral leukoplakia with respect to the presence of epithelial dysplasia, which is more frequently found in the latter. Furthermore, the degree of dysplasia is also of a milder nature. The carcinogenic potential of smokeless tobacco has been a subject of considerable debate, and no global consensus has been reached. However, it is undisputable that smokeless tobacco products contain nitrosamines, polycyclic hydrocarbons, aldehydes, heavy metals, and

polonium 210, which all have a potential to cause harm.[160,161] Some studies conclude that there is a higher risk of oral cancer and pancreas cancer, results that have not been confirmed by others. The World Health Organization International Agency for Research on Cancer established in its report from 2004 that "overall, there is sufficient evidence that smokeless tobacco causes oral cancer and pancreatic cancer in humans, and sufficient evidence of carcinogenicity from animal studies." In a recent comprehensive review, it is concluded that the use of moist snuff and chewing tobacco imposes minimal risks for cancers of the oral cavity and other upper respiratory sites, with relative risks ranging from 0.6 to 1.7 (Figure 5-34). The use of dry snuff imposes higher risks, ranging from 4 to 13, and the risks from smokeless tobacco, unspecified as to type, are intermediate, from 1.5 to 2.8.[160]

Smoker's Palate

The most common effects of smoking are presented clinically as dark brown pigmentations of the oral mucosa (smoker's melanosis) and as white leathered lesions of the palate, usually referred to as nicotine stomatitis or smoker's palate. In smoker's palate, an erythematous irritation is initially seen, and this lesion is followed by a whitish palatal mucosa reflecting a hyperkeratosis (Figure 5-35). As part of this lesion, red dots can be observed representing orifices of accessory salivary glands, which can be enlarged and display metaplasia. Histopathologically, smoker's palate is characterized by hyperkeratosis, acanthosis, and a mild sub epithelial inflammation.

The prevalence of smoker's palate has been reported in the range of 0.1%–2.5%.[162–164] Smoker's palate is more prevalent in men and is a common clinical feature in high consumers of pipe tobacco and cigarettes and among individuals who practice inverse smoking.[165] The etiology is probably more related to the high temperature rather that the chemical composition of the smoke, although there is a synergistic effect of the two.[166]

REACTIONS TO MECHANICAL TRAUMA

Morsicatio

Morsicatio is instigated by habitual chewing (Figure 5-36). This parafunctional behavior is done unconsciously and is therefore difficult to bring to an end. Morsicatio is most frequently seen in the buccal and lip mucosa and never encountered in areas that are not possible to traumatize by habitual chewing. Typically, morsicatio does not entail ulcerations but encompasses an asymptomatic shredded area. In cases of more extensive destruction of oral tissues by habitual chewing, a psychiatric disorder should be suspected. The prevalence has been reported to be in the range of 1.12%–0.5%.[167–169] Morsicatio is three times more common among women.

Morsicatio has a very typical clinical appearance, and the diagnosis is relatively easy to establish, with one exception. If the lesion affects the borders of the tongue, it may mimic hairy leukoplakia. This also has bearing for the histopathologic picture, which is characterized by hyperkeratosis and

acanthosis. A careful disease history will assist in the discrimination between the two conditions. The management is limited to assurance, and the patient should be informed about the parafunctional behavior. The condition does not involve any negative corollary.

Frictional Hyperkeratosis

Oral frictional hyperkeratosis is typically clinically characterized by a white lesion without any red elements. The lesion is observed in areas of the oral mucosa subjected to increased friction caused by, for example, food intake (Figure 5-37).

Etiology and Pathogenesis

Frictional hyperkeratosis is observed in areas subjected to increased abrasion, which stimulates the epithelium to respond with an increased production of keratin. The reaction can be regarded as a physiologic response to minor trauma. Smoking and alcohol consumption have been reported as predisposing factors. Thus, the development of frictional hyperkeratosis is facilitated when the oral mucosa is exposed to these factors.

Epidemiology

In population studies, the prevalence has been reported to be in the range of 2%–7%. Predisposing factors such as smoking and alcohol will increase the prevalence, and frictional hyperkeratosis is the most common mucosal lesion in individuals with these habits.

Clinical Findings

Frictional hyperkeratosis is often seen in edentulous areas of the alveolar ridge but may also be observed in other parts of the oral mucosa exposed to increased friction or trauma. The lesion is asymptomatic but can cause anxiety to the patient as it can be perceived as a malignant or premalignant lesion. Differential diagnosis against homogeneous leukoplakia is

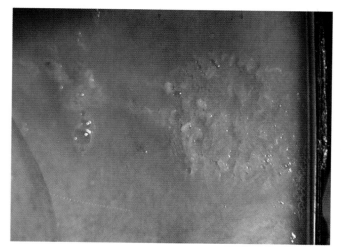

FIGURE 5-36 Morsicatio of the retrocommissural area of the left buccal mucosa.

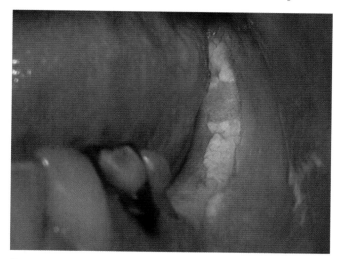

FIGURE 5-37 Frictional keratosis of the edentulous alveolar ridge.

clinically based on a combination of features such as the affected site and a more diffuse demarcation.

Diagnosis

For most lesions, the diagnosis can be established based on clinical features. As frictional hyperkeratosis does not carry any symptoms and is caused by comparatively common habits, it may be difficult to relate the lesions to increased friction. If the diagnosis is doubtful, biopsy is mandatory to exclude premalignant lesions. The histopathologic picture is characterized by hyperkeratosis without dysplasia and no or mild subepithelial inflammation. The ultimate way to differentiate between frictional keratosis and leukoplakia is to reduce or eliminate predisposing factors and await remedy.

Management

No surgical intervention is indicated. Information about the nonmalignant nature of the lesions and attempts to reduce predisposing factors are sufficient.

OTHER RED AND WHITE LESIONS

Benign Migratory Glossitis (Geographic Tongue)

Geographic tongue is an annular lesion affecting the dorsum and margin of the tongue. The lesion is also known as erythema migrans. The typical clinical presentation comprises a white, yellow, or gray slightly elevated peripheral zone (Figure 5-38).

Etiology and Pathogenesis

Although geographic tongue is one of the most prevalent oral mucosal lesions, there are virtually no studies available with the objective to elucidate the etiology behind this disorder. Heredity has been reported, suggesting the involvement of genetic factors in the etiology.

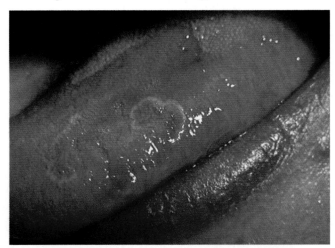

FIGURE 5-38 Geographic tongue with newly developed lesions on an erythematous area that has just started to recover from a previous lesion.

Epidemiology

The prevalence for geographic tongue varies considerably between different investigations, which may reflect not only geographic differences but also patient selection procedures and diagnostic criteria. The most frequently reported prevalence is in the range of 1%–2.5%.[170] The gender distribution appears to be equal.

Clinical Findings

Geographic tongue is circumferentially migrating and leaves an erythematous area behind, reflecting atrophy of the filiform papillae. The peripheral zone disappears after some time, and healing of the depapillated and erythematous area starts. The lesion may commence at different starting points, the peripheral zones fuse, and the typical clinical features of a geographic tongue emerge. Depending on the activity of the lesion, the clinical appearance may vary from single to multiple lesions occupying the entire dorsum of the tongue. Disappearance of the peripheral zone may indicate that the mucosa is recovering. Geographic tongue is characterized by periods of exacerbation and remission with different durations over time. The disorder is usually non-symptomatic, but some patients are experiencing a smarting sensation. In these cases, a parafunctional habit, revealed by indentations at the lateral border of the tongue, may be a contributing factor to the symptoms. Patients often report that their lesions are aggravating during periods of stress. Geographic tongue and fissured tongue may be observed simultaneously. Most likely, fissured tongue should be interpreted as an end stage of geographic tongue in some patients (Figure 5-39).[171]

A geographic appearance can be observed at other sites of the oral mucosa than on the dorsum of the tongue and then is denoted geographic stomatitis.[172–175] The information about geographic stomatitis is sparse and relies on case reports. A similar clinical presentation as for geographic stomatitis may be seen as part of Reiter's disease. This disease is characterized by arthritis, uveitis or conjunctivitis, and urethritis. Reiter's disease is considered to be a reaction that originates from a gastroenteral or urogenital infection.[176,177]

Clinical Manifestations

An increased prevalence of geographic tongue has been observed in patients with generalized pustular psoriasis.[178,179] In psoriasis in general, no such association has been revealed.[180] No studies have demonstrated that patients with geographic tongue are at increased risk of acquiring psoriasis. An atopic constitution has also been associated with geographic tongue, but this was not confirmed by a recently conducted study in the United States.[181] In this study, a negative relationship with smoking was revealed.

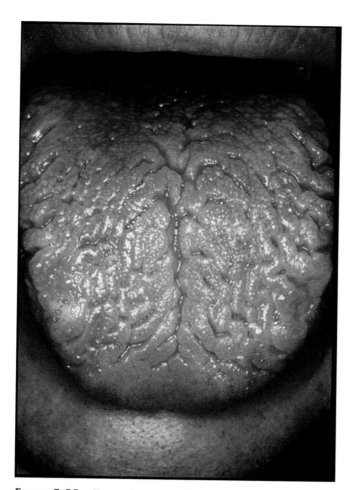

FIGURE 5-39 Fissured tongue with minor geographic lesions.

Diagnosis

The clinical features of this mucosal disorder are quite characteristic, and histopathologic confirmation is rarely needed. If biopsy is considered, it should involve the peripheral zone to capture the lesion's typical histopathologic features. These include parakeratosis, acanthosis, subepithelial inflammation of T lymphocytes, and transepithelial migrating neutrophilic granulocytes. These cells may be a part of microabscesses formed near the surface, similar to those found in pustular psoriasis (Munro's microabscesses).[182]

Management

As the etiology is unknown, no causal treatment strategy is available. Symptoms are rarely present, and the management is confined to proper information about the disorder's benign character. When symptoms are reported, topical anesthetics may be used to obtain temporary relief. Other suggested treatment strategies include antihistamines, anxiolytic drugs, or steroids, but none of these has been systematically evaluated.

Geographic tongue may regress, but it is not possible to predict when and to which patient this may happen. The prevalence of the disease seems to decrease with age, which supports spontaneous regression over time.

Leukoedema
Etiology and Pathogenesis

The etiology of leukoedema is not clear.

Epidemiology

The prevalence of leukoedema in Caucasians has been estimated at 50%.[183] The lesion is even more prevalent in the black population. The distribution between genders has been found to be equal.

Clinical Findings

Leukoedema is a white and veil-like alteration of the oral mucosa that is merely considered a normal variant. The condition is often encountered bilaterally in the buccal mucosa (Figure 5-41) and sometimes at the borders of the tongue. Leukoedema is less clinically evident after stretching the mucosa but reappears after this manipulation is discontinued. In more pronounced cases, leukoedema is accompanied by mucosal folds. The condition is asymptomatic and has no malignant potential.

Diagnosis

The clinical features of leukoedema are quite different from oral keratosis, such as leukoplakia, as the demarcation is diffuse and gentle stretching results in a temporary disappearance. The histopathology is characterized by parakeratosis and acanthosis together with intracellular edema in epithelial cells of stratum spinosum.

Management

There is no demand for treatment as the condition is nonsymptomatic and has no complications, including premalignant features.

White Sponge Nevus
Etiology and Pathogenesis

White sponge nevus is initiated following mutations in those genes that are coding for epithelial keratin of the types K4 and K13.[184] In K4-deficient mice, epithelial disturbances have been reported that are compatible with white sponge nevus.[185]

Epidemiology

White sponge nevus has been listed as a rare disorder by the National Institutes of Health, which implicates a prevalence below 1 in 200,000. In a population study of 181,338 males between 18 and 22 years of age, two cases of white sponge nevus were identified.[186] The clinical appearance usually commences during adolescence, and the gender distribution has been reported to be equal.

Clinical Findings

White sponge nevus is an autosomal dominant disorder with high penetrans. The typical clinical appearance is a white lesion with an elevated and irregular surface comprising fissures or plaque formations (Figure 5-40). The most affected sites are the buccal mucosa, but the lesion may also be encountered in other areas of the oral cavity covered by parakeratinized or non-keratinized epithelium. The disorder may also involve extraoral sites, such as the esophagus and anogenital mucosa. Although the lesion does not entail any symptoms, it may cause dysphagia when the esophagus is involved.[187]

Diagnosis

White sponge nevus may constitute a differential diagnostic problem as this disorder may be taken for other oral dyskeratoses, for example, oral leukoplakia and plaque-type candidiasis. The hallmark microscopic feature of this disorder is pronounced intracellular edema of the superficial epithelial cells, predominantly located within the stratus spinosum. Cells with pyknotic nuclei are present, and these cells may imitate koilocytosis observed in viral infections. Deep fissures in the non-dysplastic epithelium may reach just above the basal layer, but the lower portions of the epithelium are not involved. No or just mild infiltrations may be seen in the subepithelial tissue.

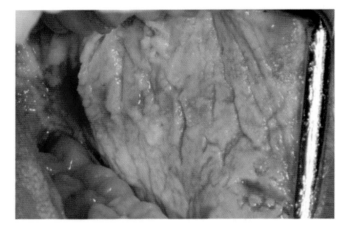

FIGURE 5-40   White sponge nevus.

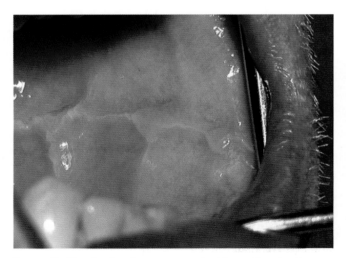

FIGURE 5-41   Leukoedema associated with parafunctional behavior.

Management

White sponge nevus does not entail any symptoms, and no treatment is therefore required. Systemic antibiotics have been used in an attempt to resolve the disorder, but with non-consistent results. When a positive effect is obtained, the recurrence rate is considerable. White sponge nevus is a totally benign condition.

Hairy Tongue
Etiology and Pathogenesis

The etiology of hairy tongue is unknown in most cases.[188] A number of predisposing factors have been related to this disorder, such as neglected oral hygiene, a shift in the microflora, antibiotics and immunosuppressive drugs, oral candidiasis, excessive alcohol consumption, oral inactivity, and therapeutic radiation. The impact of ignored oral hygiene and oral inactivity is supported by the high prevalence of hairy tongue in hospitalized patients, who are not able to carry out their own oral hygiene. Hairy tongue is also associated with smoking habits.[189]

Epidemiology

The reported prevalence varies between different geographic areas, diagnostic criteria, and the frequencies of predisposing factors. In studies from the United States and Scandinavia, the prevalence of hairy tongue is reported below 1%.[162]

Clinical Findings

Hairy tongue is characterized by an impaired desquamation of the filiform papilla, which leads to the hairy-like clinical appearance (Figure 5-42). The elongated papillae have to reach lengths in excess of 3 mm to be classified as "hairy," although lengths of more than just 15 mm have been reported in hairy tongue.[189] The lesion is commonly found in the posterior one-third of the tongue but may involve the entire dorsum. Hairy tongue may adopt colors from white to black depending on food constituents and the composition of the oral microflora. Patients with this disorder may

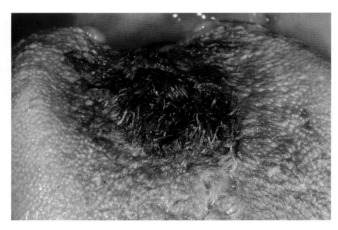

FIGURE 5-42   Hairy tongue.

experience both physical discomfort and esthetic embarrassment related to the lengths of the filiform papillae.

Diagnosis

The diagnosis is based on the clinical appearance, and microbiologic examinations do not give any further guidance.

Management

The treatment of hairy tongue is focused on reduction or elimination of predisposing factors and removal of the elongated filiform papillae. The patients should be instructed on how to use devices developed to scrape the tongue. The use of food constituents with an abrasive effect may also be used to prevent recurrences. Attempts have been made with tretinoin, but this treatment has not reached any widespread acceptance. Patients should be informed about the benign and noncontagious nature of hairy tongue.

Selected Readings

Brennan MT, Valerin MA, Napenas JJ, et al. Oral manifestations of patients with lupus erythematosus. *Dent Clin North Am.* 2005;49:127–141, ix.

Chattopadhyay A, Caplan DJ, Slade GD, et al. Incidence of oral candidiasis and oral hairy leukoplakia in HIV-infected adults in North Carolina. *Oral Surg Oral Med Oral Pathol Oral Radiol Endod.* 2005;99:39–47.

Holmstrup P, Vedtofte P, Reibel J, et al. Long-term treatment outcome of oral premalignant lesions. *Oral Oncol.* 2006:42(5):461–474.

Issa Y, Brunton PA, Glenny AM, et al. Healing of oral lichenoid lesions after replacing amalgam restorations: a systematic review. *Oral Surg Oral Med Oral Pathol Oral Radiol Endod.* 2004;98:553–565.

Lodi G, Carrozzo M, Furness S, Thongprasom K. Interventions for treating oral lichen planus: a systematic review. *Br J Dermatol.* 2012;166(5):938–947.

Mays JW, Fassil H, Edwards DA, et al. Oral chronic graft-versus-host disease: current pathogenesis, therapy, and research. *Oral Dis.* 2013;19(4):327–346.

Reichart PA, Philipsen HP. Oral erythroplakia—a review. *Oral Oncol.* 2005;41:551–561.

Rice PJ, Hamburger J. Oral lichenoid drug eruptions: their recognition and management. *Dent Update.* 2002;29(9):442–447.

Rodu B, Jansson C. Smokeless tobacco and oral cancer: a review of the risks and determinants. *Crit Rev Oral Biol Med.* 2004;15:252–263.

Samaranayake LP, Keung Leung W, Jin L. Oral mucosal fungal infections. *Periodontol 2000.* 2009;49:39–59.

Shulman J, Carpenter W. Prevalence and risk factors associated with geographic tongue among US adults. *Oral Dis.* 2006;12:381–386.

Terrinoni A, Rugg EL, Lane EB, et al. A novel mutation in the keratin 13 gene causing oral white sponge nevus. *J Dent Res.* 2001;80:919–923.

Thongprasom K, Prapinjumrune C, Carrozzo M. Novel therapies for oral lichen planus. *J Oral Pathol Med.* 2013;42(10):721–727. doi: 10.1111/jop.12083.

van der Waal I. Potentially malignant disorders of the oral and oropharyngeal mucosa; present concepts of management. *Oral Oncol.* 2010;46(6):423–425.

For the full reference lists, please go to http://www.pmph-usa.com/Burkets_Oral_Medicine.

CHAPTER 6

Pigmented Lesions of the Oral Mucosa

Alfredo Aguirre, DDS, MS
Faizan Alawi, DDS
Jose Luis Tapia, DDS, MS

❏ ENDOGENOUS PIGMENTATION
❏ FOCAL MELANOCYTIC PIGMENTATION
  Freckle/Ephelis
  Oral/Labial Melanotic Macule
  Oral Melanoacanthoma
  Melanocytic Nevus
  Malignant Melanoma
❏ MULTIFOCAL/DIFFUSE PIGMENTATION
  Physiologic Pigmentation
  Drug-Induced Melanosis
  Smoker's Melanosis
  Postinflammatory (Inflammatory) Hyperpigmentation
  Melasma (Chloasma)
❏ MELANOSIS ASSOCIATED WITH SYSTEMIC OR GENETIC DISEASE
  Hypoadrenocorticism (Adrenal Insufficiency or Addison's Disease)
  Cushing's Syndrome/Cushing's Disease
  Hyperthyroidism (Graves' Disease)
  Primary Biliary Cirrhosis
  Vitamin B_{12} (Cobalamin) Deficiency
  Peutz–Jeghers Syndrome
  Café au Lait Pigmentation
  HIV/AIDS-Associated Melanosis

❏ IDIOPATHIC PIGMENTATION
  Laugier–Hunziker Pigmentation
❏ TREATMENT OF MUCOCUTANEOUS MELANOSIS
❏ DEPIGMENTATION
  Vitiligo
❏ HEMOGLOBIN AND IRON-ASSOCIATED PIGMENTATION
  Ecchymosis
  Purpura/Petechiae
  Hemochromatosis
❏ EXOGENOUS PIGMENTATION
  Amalgam Tattoo
  Graphite Tattoos
  Ornamental Tattoos
  Medicinal Metal-Induced Pigmentation
  Heavy Metal Pigmentation
  Drug-Induced Pigmentation
  Hairy Tongue
❏ SUMMARY

Healthy oral soft tissues present a typical pink to red hue with slight topographical variations of color. This chromatic range is due to the interaction of a number of tissues that compose the mucosal lining, for example, the presence or absence of keratin on the surface epithelium, the quantity, superficial or deep location of blood vessels in the subjacent stroma, the existence of lobules of adipocytes, and the absence of melanin pigmentation in the basal cell layer of the epithelium.[1] Although oral and perioral pigmentation may be physiologic in nature, particularly in individuals with dark skin complexion, in the course of disease, the oral mucosa and perioral tissues can assume a variety of discolorations, including brown, blue, gray, and black.[2] Such color changes are often attributed to the deposition, production, or increased accumulation of various endogenous or exogenous pigmented substances. However, although an area may appear pigmented, the discoloration may not be related to

TABLE 6-1   Common Causes of Endogenous Oral and Perioral Discoloration

Source	Etiology	Examples of Associated Lesion, Condition, or Disease
Vascular	Developmental, hamartomatous, neoplastic, genetic, autoimmune	Varix, hemangioma, lymphangioma, angiosarcoma, Kaposi's sarcoma, hereditary hemorrhagic telangiectasia, CREST syndrome
Extravasated hemorrhage, hemosiderin	Trauma, idiopathic, genetic, inflammatory, autoimmune	Hematoma, ecchymosis, purpura, petechiae, vasculitis, hemochromatosis
Melanin	Physiologic, developmental, idiopathic, neoplastic, reactive, drugs, hormones, genetic, autoimmune, infectious	Melanotic macule, ephelis, actinic lentigo, melanocytic nevus, malignant melanoma, physiologic pigmentation, chloroquine-induced pigmentation, lichen planus pigmentosus, Laugier–Hunziker pigmentation, smoker's melanosis, oral submucous fibrosis, Peutz–Jeghers disease, adrenal insufficiency, Cushing's syndrome, HIV/AIDS
Bilirubin	Trauma, alcohol, infection, neoplasia, genetic, autoimmune	Jaundice

TABLE 6-2   Sources of Exogenous Oral and Perioral Pigmentation

Source	Etiology	Examples of Associated Lesion, Condition, or Disease
Metal	Iatrogenic, medications, environment	Amalgam tattoo, chrysiasis, black tongue, heavy-metal pigmentation
Graphite/ink	Trauma, factitious, tribal customs	Graphite tattoo
Bacteria	Poor oral hygiene, antibiotics	Hairy tongue
Drug complexes	Medications	Minocycline-induced pigment
Plant derivatives	Factitious, tribal customs	Ornamental tattoo, orange mouth

TABLE 6-3   Miscellaneous Lesions That May Be Associated With Oral Mucosal Discoloration

Lesion	Color
Pyogenic granuloma	Red, blue
Peripheral ossifying fibroma	Red, blue
Peripheral giant cell granuloma	Red, blue
Mucocele	Blue
Mucoepidermoid carcinoma	Blue
Acinic cell carcinoma	Blue
Lymphoma	Blue, purple
Vascular leiomyoma	Red, blue
Metastatic cancer	Red, blue
Fordyce granule	Yellow
Lipoma	Yellow
Granular cell tumor	Yellow

actual pigment but rather to the deposition or accumulation of organic or inorganic substances, including various metals and drug metabolites.

Hemoglobin, hemosiderin, and melanin represent the most common endogenous sources of mucosal color change (Table 6-1). A submucosal collection of hemoglobin or hemosiderin, produced by extravasation and/or lysis of red blood cells, may impart a red, blue, or brown ephemeral appearance to the oral mucosa. Melanin, which is synthesized by melanocytes and nevus cells, may appear brown, blue, or black, depending on the amount of melanin and its spatial location within the tissue (i.e., superficial vs. deep).[3]

Exogenous pigmentations are usually associated with traumatic or iatrogenic events that result in the deposition of foreign material directly into the mucosal tissues (Table 6-2).[4] In some cases, the substances may be ingested, absorbed, and distributed hematogenously into connective tissues, particularly in areas subject to chronic inflammation, such as the gingiva. In other instances, these ingested substances can actually stimulate melanin production, thus precipitating the color change. Chromogenic bacteria can also produce oral pigmentation, usually resulting in discoloration of the dorsal tongue. Certain foods, drinks, and confectionaries can also result in exogenous pigmentation. However, in most cases, the discoloration can be easily reversed.

The manifestation of oral pigmentation is quite variable, ranging from a solitary macule to large patches and broad, diffuse tumefactions. The specific hue, duration, location, number, distribution, size, and shape of the pigmented lesion(s) may also be of diagnostic importance.[5] Moreover, to obtain an accurate diagnosis, thorough social, family, medical, and dental histories are required, and various diagnostic procedures (e.g., colonoscopy) and laboratory tests, including biopsy, may be necessary. Thus, an understanding of the various disorders and substances that can contribute to oral and perioral pigmentation is essential for the appropriate evaluation, diagnosis, and management of the patient.

Lesions that are associated with mucosal discoloration but are vascular in origin, including developmental, hamartomatous, and neoplastic lesions (e.g., hemangioma, lymphangioma, angiosarcoma, Kaposi's sarcoma), are described elsewhere in this textbook and thus are excluded from the current discussion. However, it should be noted that these entities are frequently considered in the differential diagnosis of both macular and mass-forming pigmented lesions. Table 6-3 lists additional lesions that may be associated

ENDOGENOUS PIGMENTATION

Melanin is found universally in nature.[6,7] Melanin is the pigment derivative of tyrosine and is synthesized by melanocytes, which typically reside in the basal cell layer of the epithelium. Investigations into normal melanocyte homeostasis have yielded the discovery that keratinocytes actually control melanocytic growth.[8] Yet the mechanisms by which melanocytes are stimulated to undergo cell division remain poorly understood. Their presence in the skin is thought to protect against the damaging effects of actinic irradiation. They also act as scavengers in protecting against various cytotoxic intermediates.[9] The role of melanocytes in oral epithelium is not clear.

In general, native melanocytes are not commonly observed in routine biopsies of oral mucosal epithelium, unless the specimens are derived from individuals of non-Caucasoid descent. Oral melanocytic pigmentation in a Caucasian individual is almost always considered pathologic in origin, although the pathology or pigment in and of itself may be of no significant clinical consequence.

Melanin is synthesized within specialized structures known as melanosomes. Melanin is actually composed of eumelanin, which is a brown-black pigment, and pheomelanin, which has a red-yellow color.[6] The term *melanosis* is frequently used to describe diffuse hyperpigmentation.

with oral mucosal discoloration. Each of these lesions is also discussed in more detail elsewhere in this textbook.

Overproduction of melanin may be caused by a variety of mechanisms, the most common of which is related to increased sun exposure. However, intraorally, hyperpigmentation is more commonly a consequence of physiologic or idiopathic sources, neoplasia, medication or oral contraceptive use, high serum concentrations of pituitary adrenocorticotropic hormone (ACTH), postinflammatory changes, and genetic or autoimmune disease. Therefore, the presence or absence of systemic signs and symptoms, including cutaneous hyperpigmentation, is of great importance to elucidate the cause of oral pigmentation. However, if the etiology of the pigmentation cannot be clinically ascertained, a tissue biopsy is warranted for definitive diagnosis. This is critical because malignant melanoma may present with a deceptively benign clinical appearance.

In addition to biopsy and histologic study, various laboratory and clinical tests, including diascopy, radiography, and blood tests, may be necessary for definitive diagnosis of oral pigmentation.[10] Dermascopy, also known as epiluminescence microscopy, is another increasingly employed clinical test that can be useful in the diagnosis of melanocytic lesions.[11,12] Although current instrumentation is designed primarily for the study of cutaneous pigmentation, several studies have described the use of dermascopy in the evaluation of labial and anterior lingual pigmentation.[13,14] Briefly, this noninvasive technique is performed through the use of a handheld surface microscope using incident light and oil immersion.[14] A more advanced method makes use of binocular stereo

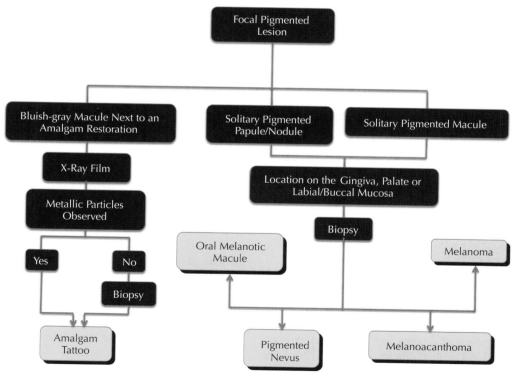

FIGURE 6-1   Focal pigmented lesions. Algorithm illustrating clinical procedures needed to segregate and diagnose common focal pigmented lesions.

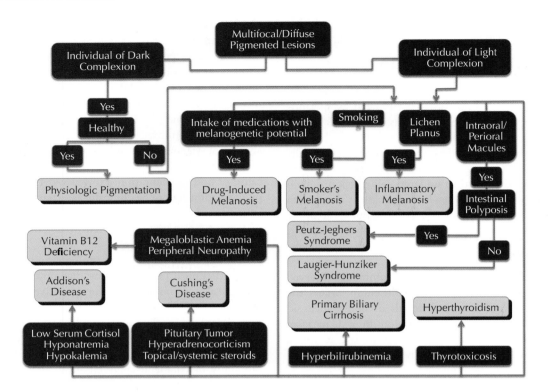

Figure 6-2 Multifocal and diffuse pigmented lesions. Algorithm illustrating the clinical presentation of pigmented lesions with accompanying habits, endoscopic features, and systemic/laboratory findings that allow their segregation.

microscopes with or without the assistance of digital technology and imaging software. This diagnostic technique has been shown to be effective in discriminating melanocytic from nonmelanocytic lesions and benign versus malignant melanocytic processes.[11] Some studies have clearly demonstrated the benefits of dermascopy training programs in increasing proper use of the technique and accuracy of diagnosis.[12] Since prospective and controlled studies detailing the predictive value and efficacy of dermascopic diagnosis of oral pigmentation have not been performed, the practitioner should be wary of its use in common clinical dental practice.

In summary, melanin pigmentation may be physiologic or pathologic, and it clinically presents with focal, multifocal, or diffuse patterns. Figure 6-1 and Figure 6-2 show algorithms that can assist the clinician to associate these patterns with selected pigmented conditions.

FOCAL MELANOCYTIC PIGMENTATION

Freckle/Ephelis

The cutaneous freckle, or ephelis, is a commonly occurring, asymptomatic, small (1–3 mm), well-circumscribed, tan- or brown-colored macule that is often seen on the sun-exposed regions of the facial and perioral skin (Figure 6-3).[15] Ephelides are most commonly observed in light-skinned individuals and are quite prevalent in red- or light blond–haired individuals.[16] Freckles are thought to be developmental in origin.

Polymorphisms in the *MC1R* gene are strongly associated with the development of childhood freckles.[16] Another putative freckles-predisposition gene has also been mapped to chromosome 4q32–q34.[17]

Ephelides are usually more abundant in number and darker in intensity during childhood and adolescence. Freckles tend to become darker during periods of prolonged sun exposure (spring, summer) and less intense during the autumn and winter months. Yet the increase in pigmentation is solely related to an increase in melanin production without a concomitant increase in the number of melanocytes. With increasing age, the number of ephelides and color intensity tends to diminish. In general, no therapeutic intervention is required.

Oral/Labial Melanotic Macule
Etiology and Pathogenesis

The melanotic macule is a unique, benign, pigmented lesion that has no known dermal counterpart.[18,19] Melanotic macules are the most common oral lesions of melanocytic origin. In one large-scale retrospective study, melanotic macules made up over 85% of all solitary melanocytic lesions diagnosed in a single oral pathology laboratory.[20] Although the etiology remains elusive, trauma has been postulated to play a role. Sun exposure is not a precipitating factor.[19]

Clinical Features

Melanotic macules develop more frequently in females, usually in the lower lip (labial melanotic macule) and gingiva.

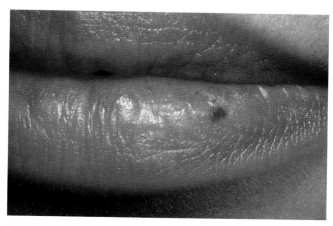

Figure 6-3 Ephelis of the lower vermilion border. Brown pigmented macule with circumscribed borders on the left lower vermilion border.

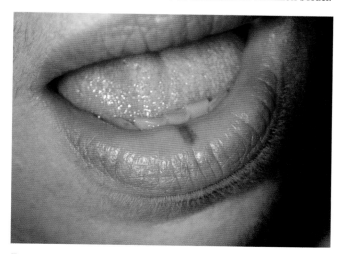

Figure 6-4 Melanotic macule of the lower labial mucosa. (Courtesy of Dr. John Fantasia, North Shore-LIJ Health System, LIJMC, New Hyde Park, New York.)

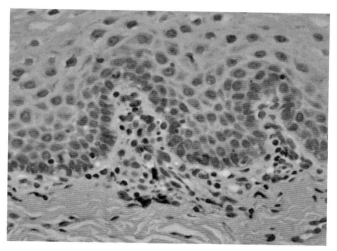

Figure 6-5 Melanotic macule exhibiting increased melanin pigmentation within the basal cell layer and melanin incontinence (hematoxylin–eosin stain, ×400). (Courtesy of Dr. John Fantasia, North Shore-LIJ Health System, LIJMC, New Hyde Park, New York.)

A macular lesion that, histologically, exhibits increased numbers of melanocytes should not be diagnosed as a melanotic macule but rather as melanocytic hyperplasia. A recent report highlighted the importance in making this distinction.[22] The report described a case of malignant melanoma of the palate arising in a patient who, years earlier, had a benign "melanotic macule" removed from the same region. A retrospective review of the original biopsy, which had initially been diagnosed as a melanotic macule, in fact revealed evidence of melanocytic hyperplasia. Thus, this case illustrates the need to be wary of such lesions and that their biologic potential remains unclear inasmuch as oral melanocytic hyperplasia may potentially herald the development of malignant melanoma.[22]

Differential Diagnosis

The differential diagnosis may include melanocytic nevus, malignant melanoma, amalgam tattoo, and focal ecchymosis. If such pigmented lesions are present after a two-week period, ecchymosis can usually be ruled out, and a biopsy specimen should be obtained to secure a definitive diagnosis. Since oral mucosal malignant melanomas have no defining clinical characteristics, a biopsy of any persistent solitary pigmented lesion is always warranted.

Oral Melanoacanthoma
Etiology and Pathogenesis

Oral melanoacanthoma is another unusual, benign, melanocytic lesion that is unique to the mucosal tissues.[23] Oral melanoacanthoma is an innocuous melanocytic lesion that may spontaneously resolve, with or without surgical intervention.[23–25] Although the term *melanoacanthoma* may imply a neoplastic process, the oral lesion is actually reactive in nature. Most patients report a rapid onset; and acute trauma or a

However, any mucosal site may be affected. Although the lesion may develop at any age, it generally tends to present in adulthood. Congenital melanotic macules have also been described occurring primarily in the tongue.[21] Overall, melanotic macules tend to be small (<1 cm), well circumscribed, oval or irregular in outline, and often uniformly pigmented (Figure 6-4). Once the lesion reaches a certain size, it does not tend to enlarge further. Unlike an ephelis, a melanotic macule does not become darker with continued sun exposure. Overall, the oral melanotic macule is a relatively innocuous lesion, does not represent a melanocytic proliferation, and does not generally recur following surgical removal.

Pathology

Microscopically, melanotic macules are characterized by the presence of abundant melanin pigment in the basal cell layer without an associated increase in the number of melanocytes (Figure 6-5).[18,19] The pigmentation is often accentuated at the tips of the rete pegs, and melanin incontinence into the subjacent lamina propria is commonly encountered.

history of chronic irritation usually precedes the development of the lesion. A biopsy is always warranted to confirm the diagnosis, but once established, no further treatment is required. The biopsy procedure itself may lead to spontaneous regression of the lesion. The underlying source of the irritation should be eliminated to minimize recurrence.

Clinical Features

Oral melanoacanthoma usually presents as a rapidly enlarging, ill-defined, darkly pigmented macular or plaque-like lesion, and mostly develop in black females.[23,25] Although lesions may present over a wide age range, the majority occur between the third and fourth decades of life. Typically, melanoacanthoma presents as a solitary lesion; however, bilateral and multifocal lesions have been reported.[26,27]

Oral melanoacanthomas are generally asymptomatic; however, pain has been reported.[24] Although any mucosal surface may be involved, close to 50% of melanoacanthomas arise on the buccal mucosa.[28] The size of the lesion is variable, ranging from small and localized to large, diffuse areas of involvement, measuring several centimeters in diameter. The borders are typically irregular in appearance, and the pigmentation may or may not be uniform (Figure 6-6).

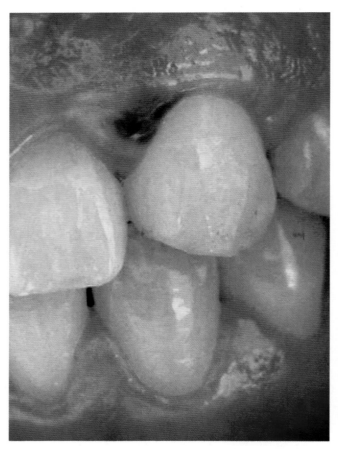

FIGURE 6-6 Melanoacanthoma. Pigmented macule on the attached and marginal gingiva displaying irregular borders. (Reprinted with permission from Quintessence International.[27])

Although there is a recognized cutaneous melanoacanthoma,[29] it is clear that the similarities with oral melanoacanthoma lie solely in the nomenclature. Cutaneous melanoacanthoma represents a pigmented variant of seborrheic keratosis and typically occurs in older Caucasian patients. Dermatosis papulosa nigra is a relatively common facial condition that typically manifests in older black patients, often female, and represents multiple pigmented seborrheic keratoses.[30] These small papules are often identified in the malar and preauricular regions of the face.

Pathology

Microscopically, oral melanoacanthomas are characterized by a proliferation of benign, dendritic melanocytes throughout the full thickness of an acanthotic and spongiotic epithelium (Figure 6-7).[25] A mild lymphocytic infiltrate with exocytosis is also characteristic. Occasional eosinophils may be observed.

Diagnosis

Because oral melanoacanthoma may resemble other melanocytic lesions, such as pigmented nevus, melanotic macule, and melanoma, a biopsy is warranted to obtain a definitive diagnosis.

Melanocytic Nevus
Etiology and Pathogenesis

Melanocytic nevi include a diverse group of clinically and/or microscopically distinct lesions.[31,32] Unlike ephelides and melanotic macules, which result from an increase in melanin pigment synthesis, nevi arise as a consequence of melanocytic growth and proliferation.[33] In the oral cavity, the intramucosal nevus is most frequently observed, followed by the common blue nevus.[34,35] Compound nevi

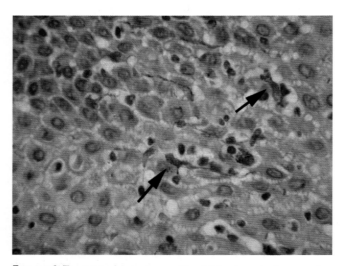

FIGURE 6-7 Melanoacanthoma. Dendritic-shaped, pigmented melanocytes (*arrows*) are noted throughout the full thickness of a spongiotic and acanthotic epithelium (hematoxylin–eosin stain; ×400 original magnification).

are less common, and the junctional nevus and combined nevus (a nevus composed of two different cell types) are infrequently identified. Rare reports of congenital nevus, Spitz nevus, balloon cell nevus, and the cellular, epithelioid, and plaque-type variants of blue nevus have also been described.[36–41] However, the list of morphologically distinct nevi continues to expand.

Relatively little is known about the pathogenesis of the various melanocytic nevi. In fact, there is still debate as to whether "nevus cells" are a distinct cell type derived from the neural crest or if they are simply a unique or immature form of melanocyte.[6,33] Nonetheless, the lesional nevus cells are cytologically and biologically distinct from the melanocytes that colonize the basal cell layer of the epidermis and oral epithelium. Although native melanocytes tend to have a dendritic morphology, most nevic cells tend to be round, ovoid, or spindle shaped.[42] Additional differences include the tendency for nevus cells to closely approximate one another, if not aggregate in clusters, and their ability to migrate into and/or within the submucosal tissues.[9]

In general, both genetic and environmental factors are thought to play a role in nevogenesis.[31,33] The effect of sun exposure on the development of cutaneous nevi is well recognized. However, there are also age- and location-dependent differences in the presentation, number, and distribution of nevi. Although most melanocytic nevi are acquired, some may present as congenital lesions (including in the oral cavity). Moreover, there are several examples of increased nevus susceptibility in various inherited diseases, thus confirming the role of genetics. Familial atypical multiple mole melanoma syndrome is characterized by the formation of histologically atypical nevi[43]; epithelioid blue nevus may be associated with the Carney complex[44]; markedly increased numbers of common nevi are characteristic in patients with Turner's syndrome[45] and Noonan's syndrome[46]; and congenital nevi are typical of neurocutaneous melanosis.[47] Thus, these findings also bring to question whether nevi are true benign neoplasms or hamartomatous or developmental in nature, as they have been historically characterized. A recent study by Pollock et al. demonstrated that up to 90% of dermal melanocytic nevi exhibit somatic, activating mutations in the *BRAF* oncogene.[48] Mutations in the *HRAS* and *NRAS* oncogenes have also been identified.[49,50] This lends further credence to the notion that melanocytic nevi are neoplastic. Currently, it is unknown whether oral melanocytic nevi also harbor any of these same mutations.

Clinical Features

Cutaneous nevi are a common occurrence. The average Caucasian adult patient may have several nevi; some individuals may have dozens.[31,32] The total number of nevi tends to be higher in males than females. In contrast, oral melanocytic nevi are rare, typically present as solitary lesions, and may be more common in females.

Oral melanocytic nevi have no distinguishing clinical characteristics.[33] Lesions are usually asymptomatic and often present as a small (<1 cm), solitary, brown or blue, well-circumscribed nodule or macule (Figure 6-8). Up to 15% of oral nevi may not exhibit any evidence of clinical pigmentation.[33] Once the lesion reaches a given size, its growth tends to cease and may remain static indefinitely. In rare cases, multifocal lesions have been described.[51] Although some studies suggest a greater prevalence of oral nevi in black patients, other studies have not identified any significant racial predilection. Oral nevi may develop at any age; however, most are identified in patients over the age of 30. The hard palate represents the most common site, followed by the buccal and labial mucosae and gingiva.

Pathology

In the evolutionary stages of an intramucosal (or intradermal) nevus, the nevus cells initially maintain their localization to the basal layer, residing at the junction of the epithelium and the basement membrane and underlying connective tissue (Figure 6-9).[33,42] These junctional nevi are usually small (<5 mm), macular or nonpalpable, and tan to brown in appearance. Over time, the clustered melanocytes are thought to proliferate down into the connective tissue, often in the form of variably sized nests of relatively small, rounded cells. Nonetheless, some nevus cells are still seen at the epithelial–connective tissue interface. Such nevi often assume a dome-shaped appearance and are referred to as compound nevi. As the lesion further matures, the nevus cells completely lose their association with the epithelial layer and become confined to the submucosal tissue, often with an associated decrease in the amount of pigmentation.[33] At this point, the lesion is given the designation of intramucosal nevus and, clinically, may appear brown or tan or even resemble the color of the surrounding mucosa.

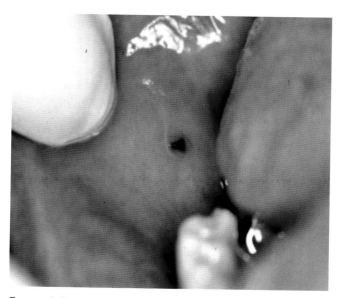

FIGURE 6-8   Intramucosal nevus of the right buccal mucosa.

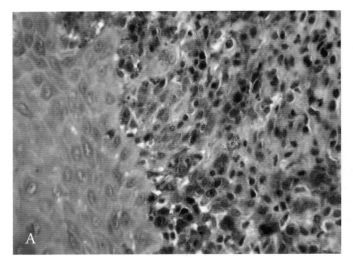
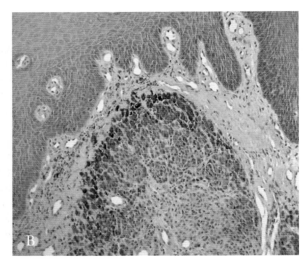

FIGURE 6-9 (A) Compound nevus: Nevus cells are located at the junction of the epithelium and connective tissue and within the submucosal tissue. The cells are variably pigmented (hematoxylin–eosin stain; ×400 original magnification). (B) Intramucosal nevus: The nevus cells are located within the lamina propria, with no evidence of any junctional component. The superficial melanocytes are heavily pigmented. Melanin is less evident in the remaining cells (hematoxylin–eosin stain; ×100 original magnification).

Unlike intramucosal nevi, blue nevi are not derived from the basal layer melanocytes. Blue nevi are characterized by a variety of microscopic appearances.[37,39,41] The "common" blue nevus, which is the most frequent histologic variant seen in the oral cavity, is characterized by an intramucosal proliferation of pigment-laden, spindle-shaped melanocytes. The blue nevus is described as such because the melanocytes may reside deep in the connective tissue and the overlying blood vessels often dampen the brown coloration of melanin, which may yield a blue tint. The less frequently occurring cellular blue nevus is characterized by a submucosal proliferation of both spindle-shaped and larger, round- or ovoid-shaped melanocytes. It should be noted that histologic differentiation of the two forms is not purely semantic. Although the common blue nevus usually has an innocuous clinical course, the cellular blue nevus may behave more aggressively and exhibit a greater rate of recurrence.[52] Rare reports of malignant transformation have also been associated with the cellular cutaneous variant. To date, transformation of an oral nevus has not been well documented in the literature. Nonetheless, it is advised that all oral nevi, regardless of histologic type, be completely removed as they may still represent a potential precursor of malignant melanoma.[9,31,53]

Diagnosis

Biopsy is necessary for diagnostic confirmation of an oral melanocytic nevus since the clinical diagnosis includes a variety of other focally pigmented lesions, including malignant melanoma. Various vascular phenomena may also be considered in the differential diagnosis. Complete but conservative surgical excision is the treatment of choice for oral lesions. Recurrence has only rarely been reported. Laser and intense pulse light therapies have been used successfully for the treatment of cutaneous nevi.[54] However, their value in the treatment of oral nevi is unknown.

Malignant Melanoma
Etiology and Pathogenesis

Malignant melanoma is the least common but most deadly of all primary skin cancers. Similar to other malignancies, extrinsic and intrinsic factors play a role in the pathogenesis of melanoma. A history of multiple episodes of acute sun exposure, especially at a young age; immunosuppression; the presence of multiple cutaneous nevi; and a family history of melanoma are all known risk factors for the development of cutaneous melanoma.[31,55] Melanoma-prone families have a high incidence of germline mutations in the tumor suppressor genes, $CDKNA2/p16^{INK4a}$ or, less commonly, $CDK4$.[43,56] Similar to melanocytic nevi, melanomas also frequently exhibit mutations in the $BRAF$, $HRAS$, and $NRAS$ proto-oncogenes.[47,57] Other recurrent molecular findings, including $MC1R$ polymorphisms and alterations or loss of PTEN function, have also been described.[58,59] This suggests that several distinct genetic changes are required for the molecular evolution of melanoma.

Clinical Features

Cutaneous melanoma is most common among white populations that live in the sunbelt regions of the world.[60] However, mortality rates are higher in blacks and Hispanics. Epidemiologic studies suggest that the incidence is increasing in patients, especially males older than 45 years.[60] In contrast, the incidence is decreasing in patients younger than 40 years. Overall, there is a male predilection, but melanoma is one of the most commonly occurring cancers in women of child-bearing age.[61] However, there is no significantly increased incidence of melanoma in pregnancy, and there is no difference in survival rates between pregnant and non pregnant women with the disease.[61,62]

Melanomas may develop either de novo or, much less commonly, arise from an existing melanocytic nevus.[31,55] On the facial skin, the malar region is a common site for melanoma since this area is subject to significant solar exposure. In general, the clinical characteristics of cutaneous melanoma are best described by the ABCDE criteria: asymmetry, irregular borders, color variegation, diameter greater than 6 mm, and evolution or surface elevation.[63] These criteria are very useful (although not absolute[64]) in differentiating cutaneous melanoma from other focally, pigmented melanocytic lesions.

There are four main clinicopathologic subtypes of melanoma. These include superficial spreading melanoma, lentigo maligna melanoma, acral lentiginous melanoma, and nodular melanoma.[55] In the first three subtypes, the initial growth is characterized by radial extension of the tumor cells (radial growth phase). In this pattern, the melanocytic tumor cells spread laterally and therefore superficially. These lesions have a good prognosis if they are detected early and treated before the appearance of nodular lesions, which indicates invasion into the deeper connective tissue (i.e., a vertical growth phase). The development of nodularity in a previously macular lesion is often an ominous sign.[63]

Melanomas may present with a wide array of histologic and cytologic patterns, and clinical prognosis directly correlates with a number of different microscopic findings. The prognosis of melanoma can be ascertained by Breslow's tumor thickness criteria or Clark's level of invasion. Surface ulceration, vascular or lymphatic invasion, neurotropism, high mitotic index, and absence of lymphocytes infiltrating the tumor are all associated with a poor prognosis.[9,31,55] In addition, various clinical parameters, including tumor site, age of the patient (>60 years), gender (male), and regional or distant metastasis, also are predictive of poor prognosis. The five-year survival rate of patients with metastatic melanoma is less than 15%.[55]

Increased awareness of the epidemiologic and biologic properties of cutaneous melanoma is necessary for the clinical practitioner. However, a discussion of cutaneous malignant melanoma has little bearing on the clinical, histologic, demographic, and biologic profiles associated with primary mucosal malignant melanoma. In brief, mucosal melanomas are very distinct neoplasms.[65–69]

Primary mucosal melanomas comprise less than 1% of all melanomas. The majority develop in the head and neck, most in the sinonasal tract and oral cavity.[65,70] The prevalence of oral melanoma appears to be higher among black-skinned and Japanese people than among other populations.[65,69] The tumor presents more frequently in males than females. Unlike the cutaneous variant, which has distinct and well-recognized risk factors associated with its development, the etiology of oral melanoma remains unknown. *BRAF* mutations are rarely observed in mucosal melanomas.[57,66,67]

Oral melanoma may develop at any age, but most present over the age of 50.[68,69,71] Any mucosal site may be affected; however, the palate represents the single most common site of involvement.[68,71,72] The maxillary gingiva/alveolar crest is the second most frequent site.[71,73] Oral melanomas have no distinctive clinical appearance. They may be macular, plaque-like or mass-forming, well circumscribed or irregular, and exhibit focal or diffuse areas of brown, blue, or black pigmentation (Figure 6-10). Up to one-third of oral melanomas may exhibit little or no clinical evidence of pigmentation (amelanosis).[68,74] In some cases, oral melanomas may present with what appear to be multifocal areas of pigmentation. This phenomenon is often explained by the fact that some tumors may exhibit both melanotic and amelanotic areas.[68,69]

Additional signs and symptoms that may be associated with oral melanoma are nonspecific and similar to those observed with other malignancies. Ulceration, pain, tooth mobility or spontaneous exfoliation, root resorption, bone loss, and paresthesia/anesthesia may be evident. However, in some patients, the tumors may be completely asymptomatic.[70] Thus, the clinical differential diagnosis may be quite

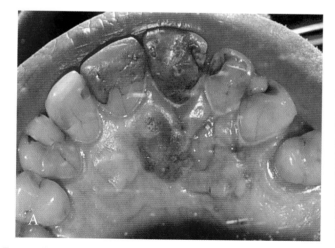
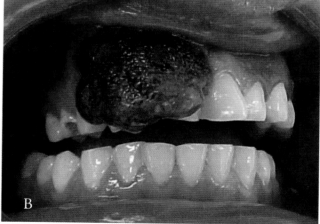

FIGURE 6-10 (A) Malignant melanoma exhibiting macular involvement of the anterior hard palate. (Courtesy of Dr. Guy DiTursi, VA Medical Center-Buffalo, Buffalo, New York). (B) Malignant melanoma presenting as a mass on the maxillary gingiva. (Courtesy of Dr. Rocio Fernandez, National Autonomous University of Mexico, Mexico City, Mexico.)

extensive and could include melanocytic nevus, oral melanotic macule, and amalgam tattoo, as well as various vascular lesions and other soft tissue neoplasms. It is for this reason that a biopsy of any persistent solitary pigmented lesion is always warranted.[75]

Oral mucosal malignant melanoma is associated with a very poor prognosis. Studies have demonstrated five-year survival rates of 15%–40%.[69,70,76] The palate shows the worst prognosis compared to other intraoral sites.[77] Regional lymphatic metastases are frequently identified and contribute to the poor survival rates.[78] Less than 10% of patients with distant metastases survive after five years.[69] The 10-year-survival rate is 0%.[79]

Pathology

Microscopically, oral mucosal melanomas (like cutaneous melanomas) may exhibit a radial or a vertical pattern of growth. The radial or superficial spreading pattern is often seen in macular lesions; clusters of pleomorphic melanocytes exhibiting nuclear atypia and hyperchromatism proliferate within the basal cell region of the epithelium, and many of the neoplastic cells invade the overlying epithelium (pagetoid spread) as well as the superficial submucosa (Figure 6-11).[4] Once vertical growth into the connective tissue is established, the lesions may become clinically tumefactive.

Owing to its rare occurrence, even most renowned clinical cancer centers do not have a large enough cohort of cases to reliably and significantly correlate the histologic findings with prognosis.[69] Thus, apart from tumor thickness greater than 5 mm and the presence of lymphovascular invasion, many of the histologic parameters, including the Breslow classification and Clark's level of invasion, that impart a poor prognosis for cutaneous melanoma generally do not apply to oral melanoma.[4,9,68,72]

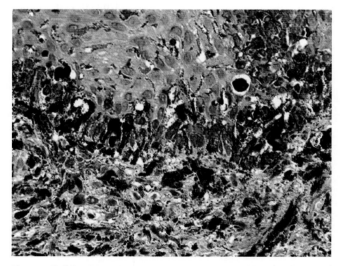

FIGURE 6-11 Heavily pigmented malignant melanoma exhibiting primarily a radial growth phase with pagetoid spread of tumor cells (hematoxylin–eosin stain; ×400 original magnification). (Photomicrograph courtesy of Dr. Julien Ghannoum.)

Diagnosis

One of the main clinical and microscopic challenges in diagnosing oral melanoma is determining whether the lesion is a primary neoplasm or a metastasis from a distant site. This is not a semantic distinction since confirming the primary site will dictate the patient's clinical stage and the type of therapy he or she will undergo. A history of a previous melanoma, sparing of the palate and gingiva, amelanosis, and microscopic features, such as a lack of junctional activity and pagetoid spread, are findings that may be more suggestive of a metastatic tumor.[9]

Management

For primary oral melanomas, ablative surgery with wide margins remains the treatment of choice.[4,69,80] Adjuvant radiation therapy may also be necessary.[76] However, as the sole therapeutic modality, it remains unclear whether radiation therapy is beneficial for the treatment of oral mucosal melanoma.[74,80] Computed tomography and magnetic resonance imaging studies should be undertaken to explore metastases to the regional lymph nodes.[4] A variety of chemotherapeutic and immunotherapeutic strategies are often used if metastases are identified or for palliation.[81–83]

Melanoma is one of the most immunogenic cancers, and currently, there are several clinical immunotherapeutic trials being conducted to test the effects of various antitumor vaccines.[81] Adjuvant interferon-α-2B therapy has already been approved for the treatment of primary cutaneous melanomas greater than 4 mm in thickness.[81] Unusual side effects of chemotherapy and immunotherapy may include the onset of autoimmunity.[84–86] The appearance of autoantibodies and clinical manifestations of autoimmune disease, including vitiligo, have been associated with statistically significant improvements in overall survival rates for patients with cutaneous melanoma.[85,86] The discovery of KIT and BRAF mutations and the development of novel immunotherapeutic agents that specifically target and inhibit these oncogenic pathways have provided new alternative treatments.[87]

MULTIFOCAL/DIFFUSE PIGMENTATION

Physiologic Pigmentation

Physiologic pigmentation is the most common multifocal or diffuse oral mucosal pigmentation (Table 6-4). Dark-complexioned individuals, including blacks, Asians, and Latinos, frequently show patchy to generalized hyperpigmentation of the oral mucosal tissues.[10] Although in many patients, the pigment is restricted to the gingiva, melanosis of other mucosal surfaces is not uncommon (Figure 6-12). The pigment is typically first observed during childhood and does not develop de novo in the adult. The sudden or gradual onset of diffuse mucosal pigmentation in adulthood, even in darker-skinned patients, should alert the clinician to consider a pathological genesis. A differential diagnosis

TABLE 6-4	Etiology of Multifocal, Diffuse, or Generalized Mucocutaneous Melanosis
Physiologic pigmentation	
Laugier–Hunziker pigmentation	
Postinflammatory hyperpigmentation	
Drug induced	
Hormone induced	
Adrenal insufficiency	
Cushing's syndrome/Cushing's disease	
Hyperthyroidism	
Primary biliary cirrhosis	
Hemochromatosis (early stages)	
Genetic disease	
Vitamin B_{12} deficiency	
HIV/AIDS (late stages)	
Malignant melanoma	

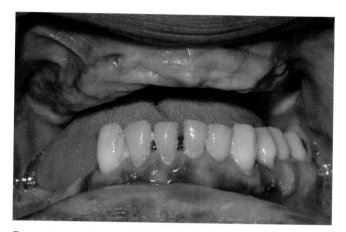

FIGURE 6-12 Physiologic pigmentation of the maxillary and mandibular gingiva. Note the patchy distribution of the pigment. (Courtesy of Dr. Christine Chu, Private Practice, New York, New York.)

may include idiopathic, drug-induced, or smoking-induced melanosis (discussed below). Hyperpigmentation associated with endocrinopathic and other systemic disease should also be considered. A thorough history and laboratory tests are necessary to obtain a precise diagnosis.

Microscopically, physiologic pigmentation is characterized by the presence of increased amounts of melanin pigment within the basal cell layer. This pigmentation is considered a variation of normal. Nonetheless, the appearance of brown to black discoloration, even intraorally, can be esthetically displeasing to some patients. Thus, surgical intervention may be necessary. Gingivectomy and laser therapy have been used to remove pigmented oral mucosa.[88,89] Cryosurgery has also been reported to effectively remove oral pigmentation.[90,91] However, with all these modalities, the pigmentation may eventually recur. The cause of the repigmentation remains unclear.

Drug-Induced Melanosis
Etiology and Pathogenesis

Medications may induce a variety of different forms of mucocutaneous pigmentation, including melanosis. Pigmentation that is caused by the soft tissue deposition of drug metabolites or complexes and pigment associated with deposition of lipofuscin or iron are discussed later in this chapter.

The chief drugs implicated in drug-induced melanosis are the antimalarials, including chloroquine, hydroxychloroquine, and quinacrine (Figure 6-13).[92–97] In the Western world, these medications are typically used for the treatment of autoimmune disease. Other common classes of medications that induce melanosis include the phenothiazines, such as chlorpromazine, oral contraceptives, and cytotoxic medications such as cyclophosphamide and busulfan.[98–105]

Table 6-5 lists selected known melanin-inducing medications.

Clinical Features

It has been estimated that 10%–20% of all cases of acquired melanocytic pigmentation may be drug induced.[97] Intraorally, the pigment can be diffuse yet localized to one mucosal surface, often the hard palate, or it can be multifocal and involve multiple surfaces. Some drugs may even be associated with a specific pattern of pigmentation.[93] Much like other forms of diffuse pigmentation, the lesions are flat and without any evidence of nodularity or swelling. Sun exposure may exacerbate cutaneous drug-induced pigmentation.[97]

Pathology

Microscopically, there is usually evidence of basilar hyperpigmentation and melanin incontinence without a concomitant increase in the number of melanocytes. Although the mechanisms by which melanin synthesis is increased remain unknown, one theory is that the drugs or drug metabolites stimulate melanogenesis. Alternatively, some drugs,

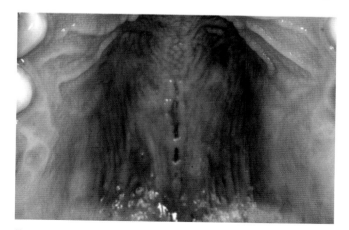

FIGURE 6-13 Drug-induced pigmentation of the palate in a patient who was taking quinacrine for the treatment of discoid lupus erythematosus. (Reprinted from Lerman et al.,[94] with permission from Elsevier.)

TABLE 6-5	Medications Associated With Mucocutaneous Pigmentation
Amiodarone	
Amodiaquine	
Azidothymidine	
Bleomycin	
Chloroquine	
Chlorpromazine	
Clofazimine	
Gold	
Hydroxychloroquine	
Hydroxyurea	
Imatinib	
Imipramine	
Ketoconazole	
Mepacrine	
Methacycline	
Methyldopa	
Minocycline	
Premarin	
Quinacrine	
Quinidine	

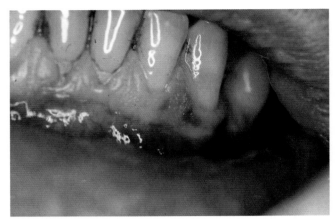

FIGURE 6-14   Smoker's melanosis. The attached mandibular left gingiva shows pigmented macules on the side where the patient places the cigarette to smoke.

including chloroquine and chlorpromazine, have been shown to physically bind melanin.[106] This complexation of melanin and drugs within melanocytes may contribute to the adverse mucocutaneous effects.

Diagnosis

If the onset of the melanosis can be chronologically and accurately associated with the use of a specific medication (frequently within several weeks or months before development of the pigmentation), then no further intervention is warranted. In most cases, the discoloration tends to fade within a few months after the drug is discontinued.[93,97] However, pigmentation associated with hormone therapy may tend to persist for longer periods of time, despite discontinuation of the medications.[104]

A differential diagnosis includes other causes of diffuse mucosal pigmentation. Laboratory tests may be necessary to rule out an underlying endocrinopathy.

Smoker's Melanosis

Diffuse melanosis of the anterior vestibular maxillary and mandibular gingivae, buccal mucosa, lateral tongue, palate, and floor of the mouth is occasionally seen among cigarette smokers.[107,108] Most smokers (including heavy smokers) usually fail to show such changes. However, in certain individuals, melanin synthesis may be stimulated by tobacco smoke products. Indeed, among dark-skinned individuals who normally exhibit physiologic pigmentation, smoking

stimulates a further increase in oral pigmentation.[109] The pigmented areas are brown, flat, and irregular; some are even geographic or map-like in configuration (Figure 6-14).

The mechanism by which smoking induces the pigmentation remains unknown. Smokeless tobacco (snuff) does not appear to be associated with an increase in oral melanosis.[110,111] Thus, it is possible that one or more of the chemical compounds incorporated within cigarettes, rather than the actual tobacco, may be causative. Another possibility is that the heat of the smoke may stimulate the pigmentation. However, passive smoking in children may result in increased gingival pigmentation.[112]

Epidemiologic studies suggest that oral melanosis increases prominently during the first year of smoking.[110] A reduction in smoking may lead to fading of the pigmentation.[113,114] Histologically, basilar melanosis and melanin incontinence are observed. Unlike other smoking-related oral conditions, smoker's melanosis is not a preneoplastic condition.[114]

Alcohol has also been associated with increased oral pigmentation.[113,115,116] In alcoholics, the posterior regions of the mouth, including the soft palate, tend to be more frequently pigmented than other areas. It has been suggested that alcoholic melanosis may be associated with a higher risk of cancers of the upper aerodigestive tract.[116]

Diffuse or patchy melanotic pigmentation is also associated with oral submucous fibrosis.[115] Unlike smoker's melanosis, oral submucous fibrosis is a preneoplastic condition caused by habitual chewing of areca (betel) nut. This custom is common in some East Asian cultures. In addition to the melanosis, increased fibrosis of the oral soft tissues is characteristically present.

Postinflammatory (Inflammatory) Hyperpigmentation

Postinflammatory hyperpigmentation is a well-recognized phenomenon that tends to develop more commonly in dark-complexioned individuals.[117] Most cases present as either focal or diffuse pigmentation in areas that were subjected to previous injury or inflammation.[118] The acne-prone face is a relatively common site for this phenomenon.[117] Although unusual, postinflammatory pigmentation may also develop in the oral cavity.[119,120] In rare cases, the mucosa overlying a nonmelanocytic malignancy may become pigmented.[121]

Oral pigmentation has also been described in patients with lichen planus (lichen planus pigmentosus).[122] This phenomenon has been described in various races, including Caucasians (Figure 6-15). In addition to the typical microscopic features associated with lichen planus, there is also evidence of basilar hyperpigmentation and melanin incontinence. Upon resolution of the lichenoid lesion, in most cases, the pigmentation eventually does subside. Although it may be mere semantics, it is unclear whether lichen planus–associated pigmentation should be appropriately characterized as postinflammatory or inflammatory pigmentation. In addition, spontaneous postsurgical healing pigmentation of palatal donor sites for free gingival grafts has been reported.[123]

Melasma (Chloasma)

Melasma is a relatively common, acquired symmetric melanosis that typically develops on sun-exposed areas of the skin and frequently on the face.[124] More than five million people in the United States have this condition.[125] The forehead, cheeks, upper lips, and chin are the most commonly affected areas (Figure 6-16). There is a distinct female predilection, and most cases arise in darker-skinned individuals. Unlike other forms of diffuse melanosis, melasma tends to evolve rather rapidly over a period of a few weeks.[124,126]

The term *melasma* has been used to describe any form of generalized facial hyperpigmentation, including those related to postinflammatory changes and medication use. However, the term is most appropriately used to describe the pigmentary changes associated with sun exposure and

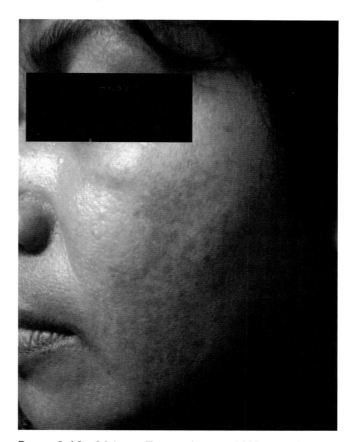

FIGURE 6-16   Melasma. Forty-eight-year-old Hispanic female with patchy pigmentation on the left side of her face that developed during her first pregnancy 15 years earlier.

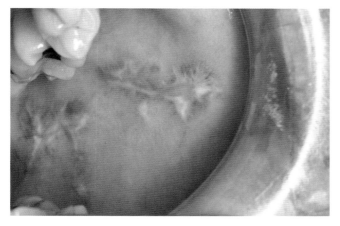

FIGURE 6-15   Lichen planus–associated pigment. Classic-appearing Wickham's striae and surrounding pigmentation are seen in this Caucasian patient with biopsy-proven lichen planus. (Courtesy of Dr. Carl Allen, The Ohio State University, Columbus, Ohio.)

hormonal factors, including pregnancy and contraceptive hormones.[127] Both pregnancy and use of oral contraceptives have also been associated with oral mucosal melanosis.[104,126] Rare cases of idiopathic melasma have also been described in females and, much less commonly, males.[128,129] In most cases, it is the combination of estrogen and progesterone that induces the pigment. Estrogen replacement therapy alone, without progesterone, does not precipitate melasma.[124,126] In idiopathic cases, significantly elevated levels of luteinizing hormone have been identified in both sexes, with associated decreases in serum estradiol (in women)[128] and testosterone (in males).[129] Despite the existence of evidence on the hormonal pathogenesis of melasma, the available data are conflicting and perhaps due to the varied genetic background of the populations studied.[125] In view of recent research studies, it appears to be that hormones may play a role in some patients' melasma but the association is weaker than previously believed.[8,9,130] Various thyroid abnormalities, including hypothyroidism, may also play a role in the pathogenesis of pregnancy- and nonpregnancy-associated melasma.[127,131]

A biopsy typically reveals basilar melanosis with no increase in the number of melanocytes. However, the melanocytes that are present may be larger than those in the adjacent normally pigmented areas.[132] Melasma may spontaneously resolve after parturition, cessation of the exogenous hormones, or regulation of endogenous sex hormone levels. A successful therapeutic approach for the treatment of melasma consists in the topical administration of a triple combination product (4% hydroquinone, 0.05% tretinoin, and 0.01% fluocinolone acetonide) along with photoprotection (SPF 30 sunscreen).[133]

MELANOSIS ASSOCIATED WITH SYSTEMIC OR GENETIC DISEASE

Hypoadrenocorticism (Adrenal Insufficiency or Addison's Disease)

Etiology and Pathogenesis

Hypoadrenocorticism is a potentially life-threatening disease, as much for its systemic complications as its under-diagnosis.[134] A variety of etiologies may precipitate adrenal insufficiency.[135] In adults, autoimmune disease represents one of the most common causes where the majority of patients show the presence of circulating autoantibodies to steroidogenic enzyme 21-hydroxylase.[136–138] However, infectious agents, neoplasia, trauma, certain medications, and iatrogenic causes may lead to adrenal destruction or an impairment of endogenous steroid production. In rare cases, adrenal insufficiency may also be a consequence of genetic disease.[139–141] Regardless of etiology, the end result is essentially the same; that is, a decrease in endogenous corticosteroid levels.

As steroid levels decrease, there is a compensatory activation of ACTH secretion from the anterior pituitary gland.[135] ACTH then acts on the adrenal cortex to stimulate steroid production and ACTH secretion stops.

If low steroid levels persist, there is a loss of feedback inhibition, resulting in persistent secretion of ACTH into the serum. Concurrently, the serum levels of α-melanocyte-stimulating hormone (α-MSH) also increase. At the molecular level, this is explained by the fact that the precursor proopiomelanocortin gene contains the sequences of both the ACTH and α-MSH genes.[142] During processing of the progenitor hormone, the ACTH and α-MSH genes may be cleaved independently of one another, thus creating two distinct hormones. However, the α-MSH sequence is actually contained within a portion of the ACTH gene; in fact, the first 13 amino acids of the ACTH hormone are identical to α-MSH.[142] Upon cellular processing of the ACTH messenger ribonucleic acid transcript, the sequence containing the α-MSH gene is cleaved and is further processed into its own secretable form. Apart from the wide array of tissues and organs that these hormones act upon, both α-MSH and ACTH are also thought to have stimulatory effects on melanocytes.[142] However, the exact mechanism by which melanin synthesis increases remains unclear.

Clinical Features

Weakness, poorly defined fatigue, and depression are some of the typical presenting signs of the illness. However, in some patients, the first sign of disease may be mucocutaneous hyperpigmentation.[135] Generalized bronzing of the skin and diffuse but patchy melanosis of the oral mucosa are hallmarks of hypoadrenocorticism. Any oral surface may be affected. In some patients, oral melanosis may be the first manifestation of their adrenal disease (Figure 6-17).[143] Diffuse hyperpigmentation is more commonly associated with chronic rather than acute-onset disease.

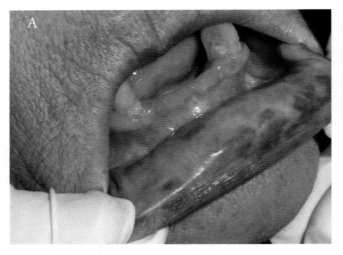
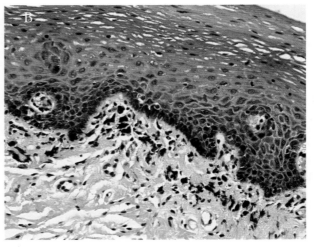

FIGURE 6-17 (A) Addison's disease. Patchy brown pigmentations in the labial mucosa of an individual with Addison's disease. (Courtesy of Dr. Jose Castillo, School of Dentistry, University Mayor, Santiago, Chile.) (B) Addison's disease. Prominent melanin pigmentation in the basal cell layer and melanin incontinentia in the papillary and reticular lamina propria (hematoxylin–eosin stain; ×400 original magnification). (Courtesy of Dr. Benjamin Martinez, School of Dentistry, University Mayor, Santiago, Chile.)

Diagnosis

The diagnosis of oral addisonian pigmentation requires a clinicopathologic correlation. Endocrinopathic disease should be suspected whenever oral melanosis is accompanied by cutaneous bronzing. An oral biopsy typically shows increased melanin in the basal cell layer with melanin incontinence. Thus, the differential diagnosis includes other causes of diffuse pigmentation, including physiologic and drug-induced pigmentation. Laboratory tests, including the evaluation of serum cortisol and electrolyte levels, are necessary to make a diagnosis of addisonian hyperpigmentation. Serum cortisol levels of less than 100 nmol/L at 9:00 a.m. is a diagnostic of deficiency.[138] Hyponatremia and hyperkalemia are frequently associated with adrenal insufficiency.[135] Treatment consists of exogenous steroid replacement therapy with glucocorticoids and mineralocorticoids. There is evidence supporting the use of adrenal androgens such as dehydroepiandrosterone to improve the quality of life of patients with Addison's disease.[138] With appropriate therapy, the pigmentation will eventually resolve.

Cushing's Syndrome/Cushing's Disease
Etiology and Pathogenesis

Cushing's syndrome develops as a consequence of prolonged exposure to relatively high concentrations of endogenous or exogenous corticosteroids.[144] Most cases are iatrogenic in origin and associated with poorly controlled or unmonitored use of topical or systemic steroids. Cushing's syndrome may also arise as a result of various endogenous etiologies, including an activating pituitary tumor (Cushing's disease) and a primary, activating, adrenal pathology (hyperadrenocorticism), as well as ectopic secretion of corticosteroids, ACTH, or corticotropin-releasing hormone by various neoplasms, including small cell carcinoma of the lung.[144–146] Recently, Cushing's syndrome has been described in patients with activating, germline mutations in the ACTH receptor.[147]

Clinical Features

Overall, Cushing's syndrome is more prevalent in female patients.[148] However, prepubertal onset is more commonly seen in boys.[149] Apart from the wide array of systemic complications, including weight gain and the characteristic "moon facies," diffuse mucocutaneous pigmentation may be seen in a subset of patients, specifically those whose pathology cis associated with increased ACTH secretion. Thus, in most cases, the affected patients have a primary pituitary neoplasm.[144] The pattern of oral pigmentation is essentially identical to that seen in patients with adrenal insufficiency.

Diagnosis

Three main tests are used for the diagnosis of Cushing's syndrome: low-dose dexamethasone suppression test, midnight plasma cortisol, and 24-hour urinary free cortisol.[148] The pigmentation often resolves following appropriate surgical, radiation, or drug therapy for the specific source of the endocrinopathy. Pasireotide (a somatostatin analog) has been approved for the treatment of Cushing's syndrome.[150,151]

Hyperthyroidism (Graves' Disease)

Melanosis is a common consequence of hyperthyroidism (Graves' disease), especially in dark-skinned individuals. Studies suggest that at least 40% of black patients with thyrotoxicosis may present with mucocutaneous hyperpigmentation.[152,153] In contrast, melanosis is very rarely observed in Caucasian patients with the disease. The pigmentation tends to resolve following treatment of the thyroid abnormality.[153] The mechanism by which excessive thyroid activity stimulates melanin synthesis remains unclear.

Primary Biliary Cirrhosis

Diffuse mucocutaneous hyperpigmentation may be one of the earliest manifestations of primary biliary cirrhosis.[154] Up to 47% of patients with this condition develop diffuse melanosis.[155] This uncommon disease is of unknown etiology, although it is thought to be autoimmune in nature as evidenced by the presence of antimitochondrial antibodies.[155] Primary biliary cirrhosis develops mainly in middle-aged women. The disease results from damage to small intrahepatic bile ducts. The mechanism by which melanosis develops is unknown.

Primary biliary cirrhosis may also be a source of generalized nonmelanocytic mucocutaneous discoloration.[154,156] Jaundice is usually an end-stage complication of primary biliary cirrhosis.[156] However, jaundice may also be associated with a variety of other etiologies, including liver cirrhosis, hepatitis, neoplasia, gallstones, congenital disorders, and infection. Jaundice is caused by excessive levels of serum bilirubin (a breakdown product of hemoglobin). Hyperbilirubinemia often induces a yellowish discoloration of the skin, eyes, and mucous membranes. Treatment of the underlying disease will lead to resolution of jaundice. A differential diagnosis should include carotenemia (excessive β-carotene levels) and lycopenemia (excessive lycopene, a compound found within tomatoes and other fruits and vegetables).[157,158] However, the oral mucosal tissues are not affected in either of these latter conditions.

Vitamin B$_{12}$ (Cobalamin) Deficiency

Vitamin B$_{12}$ deficiency may be associated with a variety of systemic manifestations, including megaloblastic anemia, various neurologic signs and symptoms, and various cutaneous and oral manifestations, including a generalized burning sensation, erythema, and atrophy of the mucosal tissue.[159,160] Diffuse mucocutaneous hyperpigmentation is a rare, and poorly recognized, complication of vitamin B$_{12}$ deficiency.[161–164] This hyperpigmentation is reminiscent of Addison's disease.[165] The mechanisms by which melanosis develops are unknown. However, the pigmentation resolves following restoration of vitamin B$_{12}$ levels.[162,163]

Peutz–Jeghers Syndrome

Peutz–Jeghers syndrome is an autosomal dominant disease that is associated with mutations in the *STK11/LKB1* tumor suppressor gene.[166] Clinical manifestations include intestinal polyposis, cancer susceptibility, and multiple, small, pigmented macules of the lips, perioral skin, hands, and feet (Figure 6-18 and Figure 6-19). The macules may resemble ephelides, usually measuring <0.5 cm in diameter. However, the intensity of the macular pigment is not influenced by sun exposure. Although uncommon, similar-appearing lesions may also develop on the anterior tongue and buccal and labial mucosae. The lip and perioral pigmentation is highly distinctive, although not pathognomonic for this disease (see Laugier–Hunziker pigmentation).[167] Histologically, these lesions show increased basilar melanin without an increase in the number of melanocytes. The medical management for

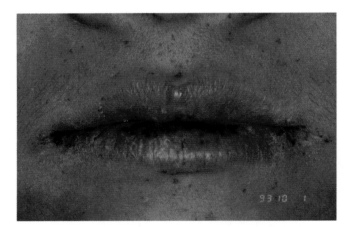

FIGURE 6-18 Multiple small macules and patches with a perioral distribution in an 11-year-old male with Peutz–Jeghers syndrome. (Courtesy of Dr. Mario E. Ramos, Private practice, Midland Park, NJ.)

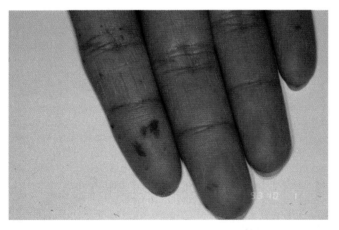

FIGURE 6-19 Multiple pigmented macules on the fingertips in in an 11-year-old male with Peutz–Jeghers syndrome. (Courtesy of Dr. Mario E. Ramos, Private practice, Midland Park, NJ.)

Peutz–Jeghers syndrome consists in surveillance and treatment of hamartomatous polyps.[168]

Other genetic diseases associated with a triad of gastrointestinal disease, cancer susceptibility, and mucocutaneous pigmented macules among other findings include Cowden syndrome (and the allelic Bannayan–Riley–Ruvalcaba and Lhermitte–Duclos syndromes) and Cronkhite–Canada syndrome.[169,170]

Café au Lait Pigmentation

Solitary, idiopathic café au lait ("coffee with milk") spots are occasionally observed in the general population, but multiple café au lait spots are often indicative of an underlying genetic disorder.[171] Café au lait pigmentation may be identified in a number of different genetic diseases, including neurofibromatosis type I, McCune–Albright syndrome, and Noonan's syndrome (Table 6-6).[172–192] Café au lait spots typically present as tan- or brown-colored, irregularly shaped macules of variable size. They may occur anywhere on the skin, although unusual, examples of similar-appearing oral macular pigmentation have been described in some patients.[174,193]

Neurofibromatosis type I is an autosomal dominant disease caused by a mutation or a deletion of the NF1 gene localized in chromosome 17.[194] Neurofibromatosis type I is associated with the development of multiple neurofibromas

TABLE 6-6	Diseases Commonly Associated With Café au Lait Pigmentation
Ataxia-telangiectasia	
Familial café au lait spots	
Familial cavernous malformation	
Fanconi's anemia	
Hereditary nonpolyposis colorectal cancer	
Idiopathic epilepsy	
Johanson–Blizzard syndrome	
McCune–Albright syndrome	
Microcephalic osteodysplastic primordial dwarfism	
Neurofibromatosis type 1	
Neurofibromatosis type 1/Noonan's syndrome	
Neurofibromatosis type 2	
Nijmegen breakage syndrome	
Noonan's syndrome	
Ring chromosome 7 syndrome	
Ring chromosome 11 syndrome	
Ring chromosome 12 syndrome	
Ring chromosome 15 syndrome	
Ring chromosome 17 syndrome	
Russell–Silver syndrome	
Tuberous sclerosis	
Turcot's syndrome	

of various histologic subtypes.[195] In addition, the size, number, and age at onset of the cutaneous café au lait spots are of diagnostic importance for this disease. Axillary and/or inguinal freckling (Crowe's sign) and pigmented lesions of the iris (Lisch nodules) are also highly characteristic of neurofibromatosis type I.[195]

McCune–Albright syndrome and the genetically and phenotypically similar Mazabraud disease[196] are sporadically occurring diseases that are characterized by polyostotic fibrous dysplasia, various endocrinopathies (McCune–Albright), and soft tissue myxomas (Mazabraud disease). In some patients, Addison's disease or Cushing's syndrome may be a potential consequence of McCune–Albright syndrome.[135,182] The café au lait spots in McCune–Albright syndrome appear distinct from those associated with neurofibromatosis. The borders of the pigmented macules are irregularly outlined, whereas in neurofibromatosis, the borders are typically smooth.[197]

Noonan's syndrome and the allelic LEOPARD syndrome (multiple lentigines, electrocardiographic-conduction abnormalities, ocular hypertelorism, pulmonary stenosis, abnormal genitalia, retardation of growth, and sensorineural deafness) are autosomal dominant disorders that, among other findings, are also associated with pigmented mucocutaneous macules and multiple melanocytic nevi.[174,198] The classic-appearing café au lait spots are more characteristically seen in patients with the Noonan's phenotype. The LEOPARD phenotype is typically associated with numerous, small, freckle-like macules often involving the facial skin.

Microscopically, when compared with adjacent uninvolved skin, genetic café au lait spots exhibit basilar melanosis without a concomitant increase in the number of melanocytes.[197] The melanocytes that are present demonstrate giant melanosomes (macromelanosomes) that may be visible under light microscopy.[199] In contrast, when compared with similar-appearing lesions in otherwise normal patients, genetic café au lait spots do exhibit increased numbers of melanocytes.[197]

The pathogenesis of genetic café au lait pigmentation remains elusive. It is unclear how the gene mutations that give rise to the various genetic diseases stimulate melanin production. A recent study suggests that the colocalization of neurofibromin (the neurofibromatosis type 1 gene) and amyloid precursor protein in melanosomes may be important for the development of the pigmented lesions in neurofibromatosis patients.[200]

HIV/AIDS-Associated Melanosis

Diffuse or multifocal mucocutaneous pigmentation has been frequently described in HIV-seropositive patients.[201–206] The pigmentation may be related to intake of various medications, including antifungal and antiretroviral drugs,[205,207] or as a result of adrenocortical destruction by virulent infectious organisms.[208] However, melanosis has also been identified in some patients, including newly diagnosed patients, with no history of adrenocortical disease or medication intake.

In these patients, the cause of the hyperpigmentation is undetermined.

Recent studies suggest that melanosis may be an actual, potentially late-stage, clinical manifestation of HIV/AIDS.[201,203,204,209] Goldstein et al. demonstrated a significant correlation between mucocutaneous pigment and CD4 counts cells/μLf200.[209] Studies have also shown that the immune dysregulation associated with HIV/AIDS leads to increased secretion of α-MSH from the anterior pituitary gland, which may also stimulate increased melanin synthesis.[210]

HIV/AIDS patients may present with a history of progressive hyperpigmentation of the skin, nails, and mucous membranes. The pigmentation resembles most of the other forms of diffuse melanosis. The buccal mucosa is the most frequently affected site, but the gingiva, palate, and tongue may also be involved.[211] Like all diffuse melanoses, HIV-associated pigmentation is microscopically characterized by basilar melanin pigment, with incontinence into the underlying submucosa.

IDIOPATHIC PIGMENTATION

Laugier–Hunziker Pigmentation

Etiology and Pathogenesis

Laugier–Hunziker pigmentation (also known as Laugier–Hunziker syndrome) was initially described as an acquired, idiopathic, macular hyperpigmentation of the oral mucosal tissues, specifically involving the lips and buccal mucosae.[212] Subsequent reports detailed involvement of other oral mucosal surfaces, as well as pigmentation of the esophageal, genital, and conjunctival mucosae and the acral surfaces.[213–216] Up to 60% of affected patients also may have nail involvement, usually in the form of longitudinal melanotic streaks and without any evidence of dystrophic change.[217] The fingernails are more commonly affected than the toenails.

A relatively limited number of cases have been reported in the literature. This suggests that either this form of pigmentation is exceedingly rare or it is poorly recognized and thus, underreported. Laugier–Hunziker pigmentation is typically identified in adult patients, with relatively equal sex predilection. This condition more commonly develops in Caucasian or light-skinned individuals. Nonetheless, it remains unclear whether this represents a distinct racial predilection or simply an example of clinician bias in the interpretation of the pigmentation.

No systemic abnormalities have been identified in any affected individuals. As a result, some investigators have suggested changing the name of this unusual condition to mucocutaneous lentiginosis of Laugier and Hunziker,[215] idiopathic lenticular mucocutaneous pigmentation,[218] or acquired dermal melanocytosis.[219] Nonetheless, a recent report of Laugier–Hunziker pigmentation occurring in a mother and three of her adult children does suggest the possibility of a genetic predisposition.[213]

Clinical and Microscopic Features

Patients typically present with multiple, discrete, irregularly shaped brown or dark brown oral macules (Figure 6-20). Individual macules are usually no more than 5 mm in diameter.[167] In rare instances, the lesions may coalesce to produce a diffuse area of involvement.[216] Increased melanin pigmentation in the basal cell layer without an increase in the number of melanocytes and melanin incontinentia in the superficial lamina propria are characteristic of this syndrome.[220]

Diagnosis

A differential diagnosis may include physiologic, drug- or heavy metal–induced pigmentation, endocrinopathic disease, and Peutz–Jeghers syndrome.[167] Thus, it is critical to confirm a lack of other systemic signs or symptoms associated with the pigmentation, including gastrointestinal bleeding. If all other potential sources for the pigmentation are ruled out, the clinician may consider the diagnosis of Laugier–Hunziker pigmentation. Hence, in most cases, this is a diagnosis of exclusion.[214,215] Despite the close resemblance of the labial pigmentation to that observed in Peutz–Jeghers syndrome, *STK11/LKB1* gene mutations have not been identified in patients with Laugier–Hunziker pigmentation.[167]

Management

The pigmentation may be esthetically unpleasing, but it is otherwise innocuous. Although treatment is generally not indicated, laser and cryotherapy have been used with some success.[221,222] A biopsy shows findings similar to those seen in other forms of diffuse pigmentation.[214]

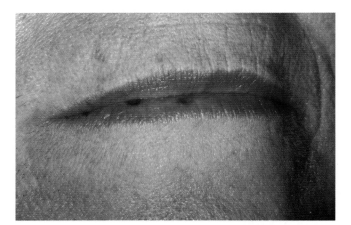

FIGURE 6-20 Laugier–Hunziker pigmentation. Multiple pigmented macules are observed in this healthy female who underwent colonoscopy and laboratory studies that ruled out Peutz–Jeghers syndrome and Addison's disease. This multifocal pattern of pigmentation is reminiscent of Peutz–Jeghers syndrome.

TREATMENT OF MUCOCUTANEOUS MELANOSIS

In general, focally pigmented lesions warrant removal, for both diagnostic and therapeutic purposes. However, apart from those cases associated with neoplasia, surgical intervention is less of an option for the treatment of multifocal or diffuse pigmentation. Drug-induced melanosis and other examples of exogenously stimulated generalized pigmentation may spontaneously subside after withdrawal of the offending substance. In other cases, the discoloration may be persistent, if not permanent. In such cases, the cosmetic disfigurement may result in significant social, psychological, and emotional stress.

Different thickness flap, gingivectomy, cryotherapy, electrosurgery, bur abrasion, and scraping with a scalpel have been successfully used to treat gingival pigmentation.[223,224] Laser therapy has also proven to be an effective modality for use in the treatment of bothersome oral pigmentation.[89,128] However, the beneficial effects may only be temporary, with recurrence of at least partial pigmentation in upward of 20% of treated patients.[89] Various types of lasers have been used, including superpulsed CO_2,[89] Q-switched Nd-YAG,[221] and Q-switched alexandrite lasers.[222]

Perioral and facial pigmentation are more challenging to treat since skin type may dictate the occurrence of postoperative complications, including postinflammatory hyperpigmentation.[225] Although laser[226] and cryotherapy[227] have been used to successfully treat such cases, experimental forms of phototherapy have also been employed, including intense pulsed light[228] and fractional photothermolysis.[229] However, first-line therapy remains the application of topical medications, that is, bleaching creams.[225] Although single agents such as azelaic acid or hydroquinone have been used, more commonly, dual- or triple-combination therapy is recommended. A combination of 4% hydroquinone (0.05%) retinoic acid (0.01%) fluocinolone acetonide has proven to be effective in greater than 90% of patients.[230] However, the majority of patients undergoing such therapy may experience immunologic sensitivity or other treatment-related adverse events, including the development of exogenous ochronosis.[231–233]

Exogenous ochronosis is a form of intense cutaneous hyperpigmentation with or without atrophic striae and coarsening of the skin or formation of numerous coalesced, black papules. This phenomenon is more commonly observed in black individuals, usually female, who have undergone long-term bleaching therapy. The intense color changes develop in the areas where the cream was applied (frequently on the face) and are related to the accumulation of a yellow-brown pigmented substance (not melanin) in the dermis.[231] This pigmentation may be permanent. Q-switched Nd: YAG laser therapy appears to be effective in reducing the dyschromia associated with exogenous ochronosis.[234]

Finally, there are several substances, including novel tyrosinase inhibitors[235] that have demonstrable skin-lightening effects in animal models. However, these chemicals remain largely experimental and have not yet been proven to be effective in humans.

DEPIGMENTATION

Vitiligo

Etiology and Pathogenesis

Vitiligo is a relatively common, acquired, autoimmune disease that is associated with hypomelanosis.[236–238] Vitiligo affects 0.5%–2.0% of the world population with no gender or racial preference.[239,240] Although the precise etiology remains unknown, autoimmunity, cytotoxicity, genetics, and alterations from metabolic or oxidative stress have been implicated in this condition where the end result is a destruction of the melanocytes.[241]

The pathogenesis of vitiligo is multifactorial, with both genetic and environmental factors playing a role in the development of this disease. A recent study has identified a single-nucleotide polymorphism in a vitiligo-susceptibility gene that is also associated with susceptibility to other autoimmune diseases, including diabetes type 1, systemic lupus erythematosus, and rheumatoid arthritis.[236,242] Additional putative vitiligo-susceptibility genes have been mapped to various other chromosomal regions.[238]

Clinical Features

The classification for vitiligo has been recently revised, and now this condition is segregated into nonsegmental vitiligo, segmental vitiligo, and unclassified/undetermined vitiligo. Multiple achromic patches with remitting-relapsing course are seen in nonsegmental vitiligo. Segmental vitiligo shows a characteristic dermatomeric distribution of the achromic patches with a rapid onset that is usually not progressive.[243]

The onset of vitiligo may occur at any age, but more frequently during the second and third decade of life.[241,244] The depigmentation is more apparent in patients who have a darker skin tone. Yet the disease actually occurs in all races. Vitiligo may also arise in patients undergoing immunotherapy for the treatment of malignant melanoma.[245] Studies suggest that this phenomenon may be associated with a better prognosis for this group of patients.[85]

Vitiligo rarely affects the intraoral mucosal tissues. However, hypomelanosis of the inner and outer surfaces of the lips and perioral skin may be seen in up to 20% of patients (Figure 6-21).[246]

Pathology

Microscopically, there is a destruction of melanocytes by antigen-specific T cells and complete loss of melanin pigmentation in the basal cell layer.[239] The use of histochemical stains such as Fontana-Masson will confirm the absence of melanin.

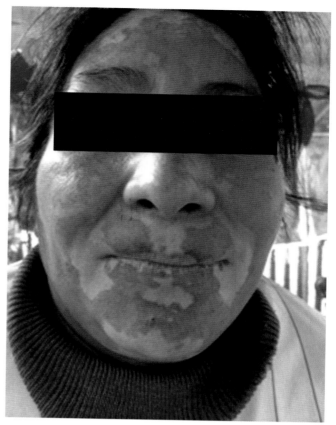

FIGURE 6-21 Forty-four-year-old Hispanic female presenting segmental vitiligo involving the forehead, face, and lips.

Management

In most cases, the objective of therapeutic intervention is to stimulate repigmentation. Topical corticosteroids, topical calcineurin inhibitors, ultraviolet B narrow band, and psoralen and ultraviolet A exposure have proven to be effective nonsurgical therapies.[243,247,248] In rare cases, small foci of normal pigmented skin may be contained within otherwise diffuse areas of hypomelanosis. Thus, to create a unified skin color, cutaneous bleaching may be considered.

From the standpoint of therapy, labial vitiligo is more resistant to the typical treatments used for cutaneous vitiligo. Due to a lack of hair follicles, the lips do not have a reservoir of melanocytes that can be stimulated to produce pigment.[246] Thus, surgical intervention may be the only option to achieve an esthetic result. Autologous epithelial grafts have been used successfully, with patients often reporting a more acceptable cosmetic appearance.[246,249] Split-thickness skin grafts have been reported as having the highest repigmentation success rate.[250] Punch grafting and micropigmentation (whereby an exogenous brown pigment is injected into the lip, much like a tattoo) have also been reported.[248,249] In rare instances, surgical intervention may stimulate spontaneous repigmentation of vitiligenous lesions elsewhere on the body.[248]

HEMOGLOBIN AND IRON-ASSOCIATED PIGMENTATION

Ecchymosis

Traumatic ecchymosis is common on the lips and face yet uncommon in the oral mucosa, except in cases related to blunt-force trauma and oral intubation.[251] Immediately following the traumatic event, erythrocyte extravasation into the connective tissue will appear as a bright red macule or as a swelling if a hematoma forms. The lesion will assume a brown discoloration within a few days, after the hemoglobin is degraded to hemosiderin. The differential diagnosis must include other focally pigmented lesions. If the patient recalls an episode of trauma, however, the lesion should be observed for two weeks, by which time it should resolve.

When multiple brown macules or swellings are observed and ecchymosis is included in the differential diagnosis, a hemorrhagic diathesis or coagulation disorder should be considered.[252] Patients taking anticoagulants may present with oral ecchymosis, particularly on the buccal mucosa or tongue, either of which can be traumatized while chewing. Ecchymoses of the oral mucosa may also be encountered in patients with liver cirrhosis, in patients with leukemia, and additionally, in patients with end-stage renal disease who are undergoing dialysis treatment.[253,254] Laboratory tests, including bleeding time, prothrombin time, partial thromboplastin time, and international normalization ratio, should be obtained in instances of spontaneous ecchymoses to explore defects in the coagulation pathways.

Purpura/Petechiae

Capillary hemorrhages will appear red initially and turn brown in a few days once the extravasated red cells have lysed and have been degraded to hemosiderin. The distinction between purpura and petechiae is essentially semantic and based solely on the size of the focal hemorrhages. Petechiae are typically characterized as being pinpoint or slightly larger than pinpoint and purpura as multiple, small 2–4 mm collections of extravasated blood.[252] The same precipitating events can elicit either clinical presentation.

Oral purpura/petechiae may develop as a consequence of trauma, viral, or systemic disease (Table 6-7).[252–266] Petechiae secondary to platelet deficiencies or aggregation disorders are usually not limited to the oral mucosa but may occur concomitantly on the skin. Viral disease is more commonly associated with oral rather than cutaneous petechiae. In most cases, the petechiae are identified on the soft palate, although any mucosal site may be affected. When trauma is suspected, the patient should be instructed to cease whatever activity may be contributing to the presence of the lesions. Within two weeks, the lesions should resolve. Failure to do so should arouse suspicion of a hemorrhagic diathesis, a persistent infectious disease, or other systemic disease, and appropriate laboratory investigations must be undertaken.

TABLE 6-7 Causes of Oral Purpura/Petechiae

Amyloidosis
Aplastic anemia
Bulimia
Chronic renal failure
Fellatio
Forceful coughing
Hemophilia
Henoch–Schönlein purpura
HIV/AIDS
Infectious mononucleosis
Leukemia
Liver cirrhosis
Nonspecific trauma
Oral intubation
Oral submucous fibrosis
Overexertion
Papular-purpuric "gloves and socks" syndrome
Streptococcal infection
Systemic lupus erythematosus
Thrombocytopenia
von Willebrand's disease

Hemochromatosis

Hemochromatosis is a chronic, progressive disease that is characterized by excessive iron deposition (usually in the form of hemosiderin) in the liver and other organs and tissues.[267,268] Idiopathic, neonatal, blood transfusion, and heritable forms of this disease are recognized. Complications of hemochromatosis may include liver cirrhosis, diabetes, anemia, heart failure, hypertension, and bronzing of the skin. Studies also suggest an increased incidence of cancer in patients with hemochromatosis.[269]

The cutaneous pigmentation is seen in over 90% of affected patients, regardless of the etiology of the disease.[268] The primary oral manifestation of hemochromatosis is a blue-gray to brown pigmentation affecting mainly the palate and gingiva.[270,271]

Early on in the course of disease, the pigmentation may be more commonly a result of basilar melanosis rather than iron-associated pigment.[268] Iron deposition within the adrenal cortex may lead to hypoadrenocorticism and ACTH hypersecretion, with the associated addisonian-type changes. In the later stages of hemochromatosis, the pigmentation is usually a result of hemosiderosis and melanosis.

A lower labial gland biopsy has been shown to be an easy and effective method for the diagnosis of hemochromatosis.[272,273] Increased melanin pigment may be seen in the basal cell layer, whereas golden or brown-colored hemosiderin can be seen diffusely scattered throughout the submucosal and salivary gland tissues. A Prussian blue stain will confirm the presence of iron. Since hemochromatosis can cause a number of serious complications, medical referral is necessary.

EXOGENOUS PIGMENTATION

Amalgam Tattoo

Etiology and Pathogenesis

The most common pigmented lesion in the oral mucosa is amalgam tattoo.[274] By definition, these are iatrogenic in origin and typically a consequence of the inadvertent deposition of amalgam restorative material into the submucosal tissue.

Clinical Features

Amalgam tattoos may be found in up to 1%–3% of the general population.[20,275] The lesions are typically small, asymptomatic, macular, and bluish gray or even black in appearance.[276] They may be found on any mucosal surface. However, the gingiva, alveolar mucosa, buccal mucosa, and floor of the mouth represent the most common sites.[274] The lesions are often found in the vicinity of teeth with large amalgam restorations or crowned teeth that probably had amalgams, around the apical region of endodontically treated teeth with retrograde restorations or obturated with silver points, and in areas in and around healed extraction sites (Figure 6-22).[277,278] Amalgam tattoo of the head and neck skin may occur in dentists and represents an occupational hazard resulting from failure to use facial protective barriers.[279]

Pathology

Microscopically, amalgam tattoos show a fine brown granular stippling of collagen fibers, with a particular affinity for vessel walls and nerve fibers (Figure 6-23) with little or no inflammation. In some cases, large aggregates of black material may be seen and could result in a foreign body–type giant cell granulomatous inflammation. However, a mild to moderate lymphocytic inflammatory infiltrate is more commonly seen.[274]

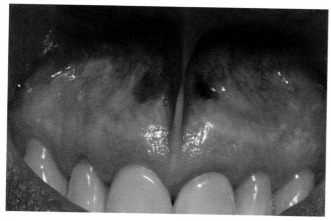

FIGURE 6-22   Amalgam tattoo of the maxillary alveolar mucosa. The pigment was associated with retrograde amalgam restorations.

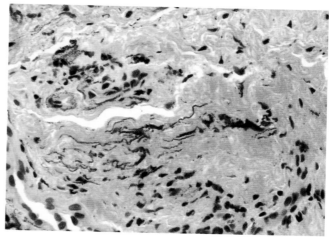

FIGURE 6-23   Amalgam tattoo. Spherules of restorative dental material (amalgam) are seen decorating collagen fibers. A characteristic perivascular distribution of the particles is observed (hematoxylin–eosin stain; ×400 original magnification).

Management

The amalgam particles are typically fine spherules that decorate collagen fibers. However, sometimes they are large enough to be identified on dental radiographs. In some patients, the focal argyrosis may compromise esthetics; thus, surgical removal may be warranted. A report on a two-stage surgical approach (subepithelial connective tissue graft followed by laser surgery) to eliminate an amalgam tattoo has yielded excellent results.[280] However, since amalgam tattoos are innocuous, their removal is not always necessary, particularly when they can be documented radiographically.[281] In the absence of radiographic evidence of amalgam, if the lesion is not in proximity to a restored tooth, or if the lesion suddenly appears, a biopsy is warranted. A typical differential diagnosis includes melanotic macule, nevus, and melanoma.

Pigmentation associated with other dental restorative materials has also been described.[282,283] Studies have demonstrated that metal components from almost all forms of cast alloy material can be detected in the adjacent tissues.[282] Titanium has been associated with pigmentation of the skin, specifically in areas around orthopedic implants.[284] Thus, it is conceivable that dental implants may also be a potential source of exogenous oral pigmentation.

Graphite Tattoos

Graphite tattoos are an unusual source of focal exogenous pigmentation. They are most commonly seen on the palate and gingiva and represent traumatic implantation of graphite particles from a pencil (Figure 6-24).[285] The lesions may be indistinguishable from amalgam tattoos, often presenting as a solitary gray or black macule. Since the traumatic event often occurs in childhood, many patients may not report a history of injury. Thus, a biopsy is often warranted. Microscopically, graphite particles resemble those of amalgam.

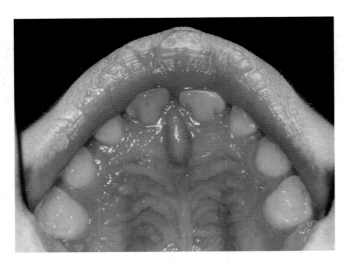

FIGURE 6-24 Graphite tattoo. Four-year-old male with a round bluish macule on the hard palate, posterior to the incisive papilla. The child fell down with a pencil in his mouth and punctured his palate.

When the graphite tattoo involves areas of cosmetic concern, removal of the lesion and a subsequent autogenous connective tissue graft provide a highly esthetic outcome.[285]

Ornamental Tattoos

Mucosal tattoos in the form of lettering or intricate artwork are becoming increasingly common phenomena. Amateur tattoo inks are permanent and consist of simple, carbon particles originating from a variety of sources, including burnt wood, plastic, or paper, and from a variety of inks, such as India ink, pen ink, and plant-derived matter.[286,287] Q-Switched laser therapy has been used successfully to remove tattoos of the oral mucosa.[288]

In certain tribal cultures, ornamental mucocutaneous tattooing is considered a rite of passage and esthetically pleasing.[289] In most cases, the pigment is plant derived. Female members of certain tribes are more likely to exhibit this form of exogenous pigmentation, usually in an effort to make themselves more attractive or desirable.

An unusual South African female tribal custom includes brushing the teeth and gums with a chewed root of the tree *Euclea natalensis*, with the belief that it promotes oral health.[290] This plant root contains naphthoquinones and other organic substances that have putative antibacterial properties.[291] Naphthoquinones are pigmented, and the mouths of root users are typically bright orange.[291] Unlike ornamental tattoos, this form of pigmentation is usually transient and reversible.

Medicinal Metal-Induced Pigmentation

Historically, a variety of metallic compounds have been used medicinally for the treatment of various systemic diseases. Fortunately, with the advent of methotrexate for the treatment of rheumatoid arthritis, gold therapy is in less demand.[292,293] Colloidal silver is another metal-based substance that has been historically touted for its beneficial health effects.[294] Although its medical use has been significantly curtailed, it has become widely available among patients using "complementary and alternative medicine therapies."[295,296] Gold and colloidal silver have both been associated with diffuse cutaneous pigmentation. Silver may cause a generalized blue-gray discoloration (argyria), whereas gold-induced pigment may appear blue-gray or purple (chrysiasis).[297,298] In both cases, the pigmentation may be persistent, if not permanent, even following discontinuation of the substance. Rare examples of diffuse oral argyria have been reported.[299] Chrysiasis does not involve the oral mucosal tissues since it is thought that exposure to ultraviolet light or other high-intensity light sources precipitate the pigmentation. However, oral lichenoid eruptions have been associated with systemic gold therapy.[300]

In contrast to the systemic therapies, metal salts remain a component of some topical medications and other substances that are used in clinical practice. Examples include silver nitrate and zinc oxide. Silver nitrate cautery has been used to treat recurrent aphthous stomatitis,[301] and zinc oxide is a common component of sunblock creams.[302] Both substances have been associated with focal mucocutaneous pigmentation. Using of zinc oxide containing sunblock in severely chaffed lips may result in the development of hyperpigmentation. The histological findings are similar to an amalgam tattoo. However, scanning electron microscopy and radiographic microanalysis unveil the presence of zinc in elastic fibers.[303] Medicinal silver-associated pigment appears as brown or black particulate matter dispersed throughout the connective tissue.[304] A clinicopathologic correlation is necessary since, clinically and microscopically, these forms of pigmentation may be difficult to differentiate from amalgam tattoos.

Generalized black pigmentation of the tongue has been attributed to the chewing of bismuth subsalicylate tablets, a commonly used antacid.[305] This phenomenon is unlike black hairy tongue, which is associated with elongation of the filiform papillae, hyperkeratosis, and superficial colonization of the tongue by bacteria. Black tongue induced by bismuth subsalicylate is caused by deposition of actual pigment (bismuth sulfide), without any other lingual changes.[278] Discontinuation of the antacid and cleansing of the tongue are curative. It should be noted that typical black hairy tongue may also be attributed to the use of bismuth subsalicylate.

Heavy Metal Pigmentation

Diffuse oral pigmentation may be associated with ingestion of heavy metals. Nowadays, this phenomenon is unusually encountered. Yet it remains an occupational and health hazard for some individuals who work in certain industrial plants and for those who live in the environment in and around these types of facilities.[306,307] Other relatively common environmental sources include paints, old plumbing, and seafood.

Lead, mercury, bismuth, and arsenic have all been shown to be deposited in oral tissue if ingested in sufficient quantities or over an extended period of time.[306–309] These ingested metal salts tend to extravasate from vessels in areas of chronic inflammation. Thus, in the oral cavity, the pigmentation is usually found along the free marginal gingiva, where it often dramatically outlines the gingival cuff. This metallic line usually has a gray to black appearance. In some patients, the oral pigmentation may be the first sign of heavy metal toxicity. Additional systemic signs and symptoms of heavy metal poisoning may include behavioral changes, neurologic disorders, intestinal pain, and sialorrhea. Diffuse mucocutaneous melanosis may also be observed in some affected individuals.[306]

Drug-Induced Pigmentation

Minocycline, which is a tetracycline derivative and frequently used in the treatment of acne, is a relatively common cause of drug-induced nonmelanin-associated oral pigmentation.[310,311] Similar to tetracycline, minocycline can cause pigmentation of developing teeth. However, most patients are prescribed minocycline in early adulthood. When taken chronically, minocycline metabolites may become incorporated into the normal bone. Thus, although the teeth may be normal in appearance, the surrounding bone may appear green, blue, or even black.[310] As a result, the palatal and alveolar mucosae may appear similarly and diffusely discolored. In addition, roots show a green color, whereas developing roots tend to be black.[312]

Minocycline can also induce actual pigmentation of the oral soft tissues, as well as the skin and nails. Minocycline-induced soft tissue pigmentation may appear gray, brown, or black. Often the pigmentation is patchy or diffuse in its presentation. Although a biopsy may reveal basilar melanosis, more commonly, aggregates of fine brown or golden particles are identified within the submucosal tissue.[311,312] The particles are often intracellular and contained within macrophages. Superficially, the submucosal pigment may resemble melanin and does actually stain with what is thought to be a melanin-specific (Fontana-Masson) histochemical stain.[312] However, an iron stain (Prussian blue) also highlights many of the same particles.[311] Thus, it is likely that the particulate substance represents an actual precipitated drug metabolite rather than true melanin.

The mucosal discoloration produced by minocycline often subsides within months after discontinuation of the medication.[312] Nowadays, acceptable esthetic outcomes are obtained even in severe cases of cutaneous pigmentation associated with minocycline intake when Alexandrite 755-nm laser therapy is used.[313] However, the bone pigment may persist for longer periods of time, if not indefinitely.

Methacycline, another tetracycline derivative that is no longer widely used in clinical practice, can also produce a similar form of pigmentation.[314]

Imatinib (a tyrosine kinase inhibitor used for the treatment of chronic myeloid leukemia) has the potential to induce mucosal pigmentation.[312,315,316]

Hairy Tongue

Hairy tongue is a relatively common condition of unknown etiology.[317] The change in oral flora associated with chronic antibiotic therapy may be causative in some patients. The discoloration involves the dorsal tongue, particularly the middle and posterior one-third. Rarely children are affected. The filiform papillae are elongated, sometimes markedly so, and have the appearance of fine hairs.[318] The hyperplastic papillae then become pigmented by the colonization of chromogenic bacteria, which can impart a variety of colors, including white, green, brown, or black (Figure 6-25). Various foods, drinks, and confectionaries can contribute to the diffuse discoloration. Smoking of tobacco or crack cocaine has been associated with black hairy tongue.[318,319] Rare examples of black hairy tongue have also been linked to the use of psychotropic medications.[320] Black hairy tongue has also been associated with other pharmacos such as tetracycline, linezolid, olanzapine, bismuth, and erlotinib.[321–323]

Black hairy tongue is so characteristic in its presentation that biopsy is not required, and a clinical diagnosis is usually appropriate. Microscopically, the filiform papillae can be seen as extremely elongated and hyperplastic with hyperkeratosis. Superficial microbial colonization of the papillae is a prominent feature. There are no additional pathologic findings in the remaining epithelium or in the connective tissue. Treatments consist of having the patient brush the tongue, or use a tongue scraper, and limit the ingestion of color-forming foods and drinks until the discoloration resolves. Since the cause is often undetermined, the condition may recur.

SUMMARY

Oral pigmentation may be focal, multifocal, or diffuse. The lesions may be blue, red, purple, brown, gray, or black. They may be macular or tumefactive. Importantly, some are localized harmless accumulations of melanin, hemosiderin, or exogenous metal; others are harbingers of systemic or genetic disease, and some can be associated with life-threatening

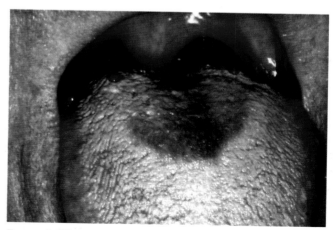

FIGURE 6-25 Hairy tongue. Elongated lingual filiform papillae displaying a gamut of colors ranging from white, to brown and black discoloration of the dorsum of the tongue.

medical conditions that require immediate intervention. The differential diagnosis for any given pigmented lesion can be quite extensive and can include examples of endogenous and exogenous pigmentation. Although biopsy is a helpful and necessary aid in the diagnosis of focally pigmented lesions, the more diffuse lesions will require a thorough history and laboratory studies to arrive at a definitive diagnosis.

Selected Readings

Abbasi NR, Shaw HM, Rigel DS, et al. Early diagnosis of cutaneous melanoma: revisiting the ABCD criteria. *JAMA.* 2004;292:2771–2776.

Alawi F. Pigmented lesions of the oral cavity: an update. *Dent Clin North Am.* 2013;57(4):699–710. doi: 10.1016/j.cden.2013.07.006.

Blignaut E, Patton LL, Nittayananta W, et al. (A3) HIV phenotypes, oral lesions, and management of HIV-related disease. *Adv Dent Res.* 2006;19:122–129.

Cabrera VP, Rodu B. Differential diagnosis of oral mucosal petechial hemorrhages. *Compendium.* 1991;12:418–422.

De Giorgi V, Massi D, Carli P. Dermoscopy in the management of pigmented lesions of the oral mucosa. *Oral Oncol.* 2003;39:534–535.

Dereure O. Drug-induced skin pigmentation. Epidemiology, diagnosis and treatment. *Am J Clin Dermatol.* 2001;2:253–262.

Hicks MJ, Flaitz CM. Oral mucosal melanoma: epidemiology and pathobiology. *Oral Oncol.* 2000;36:152–169.

Gaeta GM, Satriano RA, Baroni A. Oral pigmented lesions. *Clin Dermatol.* 2002;20(3):286–288.

Gondak RO, da Silva-Jorge R, Jorge J, et al. Oral pigmented lesions: clinicopathologic features and review of the literature. *Med Oral Patol Oral Cir Bucal.* 2012;17(6):e919–e924.

Meleti M, Vescovi P, Mooi WJ, van der Waal I. Pigmented lesions of the oral mucosa and perioral tissues: a flow-chart for the diagnosis and some recommendations for the management. *Oral Surg Oral Med Oral Pathol Oral Radiol Endod.* 2008;105(5):606–616. doi: 10.1016/j.tripleo.2007.07.047.

Muller S. Melanin-associated pigmented lesions of the oral mucosa: presentation, differential diagnosis, and treatment. *Dermatol Ther.* 2010;23(3):220–229. doi: 10.1111/j.1529–8019.2010.01319.x.

Shah KN. The diagnostic and clinical significance of cafe-au-lait macules. *Pediatr Clin North Am.* 2010;57(5):1131–1153. doi: 10.1016/j.pcl.2010.07.002.

Taieb A, Alomar A, Bohm M, et al. Guidelines for the management of vitiligo: the European Dermatology Forum consensus. *Br J Dermatol.* 2013;168:5–19. doi: 10.1111/j.1365–2133.2012.11197.x.

For the full reference lists, please go to http://www.pmph-usa.com/Burkets_Oral_Medicine.

CHAPTER 7

Benign Lesions of the Oral Cavity and the Jaws

A. Ross Kerr, DDS, MSD

K. C. Chan, DMD, MS, FRCD(C)

Joan A. Phelan, DDS

This chapter provides an overview of the clinical features, diagnosis, and management of nonmalignant growths and tumors of the oral cavity and the jaws. A variety of lesions of miscellaneous etiologies are discussed, many of which are not true neoplasms. If left untreated, some of the lesions discussed in this chapter can lead to extensive tissue destruction and deformity, whereas others may interfere with oral function. Regardless, one of the major clinical considerations in the management of these growths and tumors is to identify their benign nature and to distinguish them from potentially life-threatening malignant neoplasms. Identification can only be established with certainty by microscopic examination of excised tissue; therefore, biopsy is often an essential step in their diagnosis and management.

VARIANTS OF NORMAL

Structural variations of the oral cavity and the jaws are sometimes mistakenly identified as tumors, but they are usually easily recognized as being within the range of normal findings, and biopsy is rarely indicated. Examples of such structural variants are tori; localized nodular connective tissue thickening of the attached gingiva; enlarged papillae associated with the opening of Stensen's duct; Fordyce spots; and sublingual varicosities in older individuals.

Localized nodular enlargements (exostoses) of the cortical bone of the midline of the palate (torus palatinus), the lingual aspect of the mandible (torus mandibularis), and the buccal aspects of either jaws occur frequently,[1] and are considered to be normal structural variants (Figure 7-1). The lack of obvious irritants for most tori, and their negligible growth after an initial slow but steady period of development, also suggest that they are usually neither inflammatory hyperplasias nor neoplasms. Histologically, tori consist of layers of dense cortical bone covered by periosteum and a thin overlying layer of epithelium with minimal rete peg development. Tori may pose a mechanical problem in the construction of dentures; they are frequently traumatized as a result of their prominent position and thin epithelial covering, and the resulting ulcers are slow to heal. There have been reports of bisphosphonate-associated osteonecrosis involving tori.[2,3] Rarely, tori on the palate or lingual mandibular ridge may become sufficiently large to interfere with eating and speaking. Unless a torus is exceptionally large, its surgical removal (when dictated by mechanical concerns) is not a major procedure. Similar nodular growths or exostoses arise on the buccal aspect of the maxillary and mandibular alveolae and must be differentiated from bony enlargement secondary to bone diseases such as fibrous dysplasia or Paget's disease.

Unencapsulated lymphoid aggregates are normally present in the oral cavity located primarily on the soft palate, the posterolateral aspects of the tongue (Figure 7-2), the dorsum of the tongue, and the anterior tonsillar pillar. An increase in size as a result of benign (reactive) processes as well as lymphoid neoplasms may represent benign or follicular lymphoid hyperplasia. These may masquerade clinically as a malignancy. Histologic criteria based on architectural, cytologic, and immunologic features of the lymphoid aggregate have been described.[4,5]

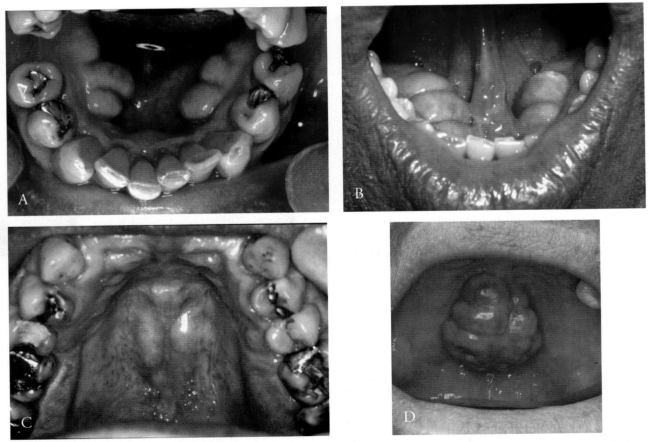

FIGURE 7-1   (A) Mandibular tori (tori mandibularis). (B) Mandibular tori. Note traumatic keratosis on the left side due to the large size of the tori. (C) Maxillary torus (torus palatinus). (D) Maxillary torus. Note the large size with a "pedunculated base."

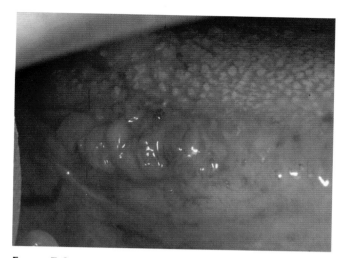

FIGURE 7-2 Right posterolateral tongue revealing a prominent foliate papilla region containing unencapsulated lymphoid aggregates. A similar presentation was seen on the left side.

BENIGN SOFT TISSUE LESIONS

Inflammatory/Reactive Hyperplasia of Soft Tissue

The term *inflammatory hyperplasia* is used to describe a large range of commonly occurring nodular growths of the oral mucosa that histologically represent inflamed fibrous and granulation tissue. The size of these reactive hyperplastic masses may be large or small, depending on the degree to which one or more of the components of the inflammatory reaction and healing response are exaggerated. Some are predominantly epithelial overgrowths with only scanty connective tissue stroma; others are fibromatous, with a thin epithelial covering, and may exhibit either angiomatous, desmoplastic (collagenous), or fibroblastic features. In many lesions, different sections may reveal examples of each of these histologic patterns. Like scar tissue, some inflammatory hyperplasias appear to mature and become less vascular (paler and less friable) and more collagenous (firmer and smaller) with time. Others appear to have a high proliferative ability for exophytic growth until they are excised. This variability of histologic appearance is reflected in the wide range of clinical characteristics exhibited by inflammatory hyperplasias.

The major etiologic factor for these lesions is generally assumed to be chronic trauma from ill-fitting dentures, calculus, overhanging dental restorations, acute or chronic tissue injury from biting, or fractured teeth. With some of these lesions (e.g., pregnancy epulis), the levels of circulating hormones play a role. The majority of lesions occur peripherally on the oral mucosal surface, where irritants are quite common and therefore are subject to continual masticatory trauma. Clinical appearance is swollen, distended, ulcerated, red to purple in color due to dilated blood vessels, and they exhibit acute and chronic inflammatory exudates and

localized abscesses. Erosion of the underlying cortical bone rarely occurs with peripheral inflammatory hyperplasias; if noted, there should be a strong suspicion that an aggressive process or even malignancy is involved. An excisional biopsy is indicated except when the procedure would produce marked deformity; in such a case, incisional biopsy to establish the diagnosis is mandatory. If the chronic irritant is eliminated when the lesion is excised, the majority of inflammatory hyperplasias will not recur, thus confirming the benign nature of these lesions.

Fibromas, Cowden Syndrome, Tuberous Sclerosis

Fibromas may occur as either pedunculated or sessile (broad-based) growths on any surface of the oral mucous membrane. They are also called traumatic or irritation fibromas (Figure 7-3).[6,7] The majority remain small, and lesions that are >1 cm in diameter are rare. The giant cell fibroma exhibits a somewhat nodular surface and is histologically distinguished from other fibromas by the presence of stellate-shaped and multinucleated cells in the connective tissue. The etiology of the giant cell fibroma is not known.

Multiple fibromas may indicate Cowden syndrome (multiple hamartoma and neoplasia syndrome) or tuberous sclerosis. Cowden syndrome is inherited as an autosomal dominant trait caused by mutations in the phosphatase and tensin homolog gene (PTEN) and for which clinical diagnostic criteria have been proposed.[8] Oral and perioral findings[9] include multiple papules on the lips and gingivae, papillomatosis (benign fibromatosis) of the buccal, palatal, faucial, and oropharyngeal mucosae often producing a "cobblestone" effect on these mucous membranes, and the tongue is also pebbly or fissured. Multiple papillomatous nodules (histologically inverted follicular keratoses or trichilemmomas) are often present on the perioral, periorbital, and perinasal skin, and the mucosal surface of the oropharynx often manifests a cobblestone effect

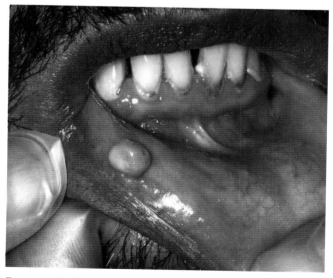

FIGURE 7-3 Irritation fibroma (traumatic fibroma). Patient reports a daily habit of biting this lesion for several months.

on these mucous membranes. Multiple papillomatous nodules are often present also on the pinnae of the ears and neck, accompanied by lipomas, hemangiomas, neuromas, vitiligo, café au lait spots, and acromelanosis elsewhere on the skin. A variety of neoplastic changes occur in the organs exhibiting hamartomatous lesions, particularly an increased rate of breast and thyroid carcinoma and gastrointestinal malignancy. Squamous cell carcinoma of the tongue and basal cell tumors of the perianal skin are also reported.

Tuberous sclerosis is an inherited disorder caused by mutations in the tuberous sclerosis complex (TSC1 or TSC2) genes that is characterized by seizures and mental retardation associated with hamartomatous glial proliferations and neuronal deformity in the central nervous system.[10] Fine wart-like lesions (adenoma sebaceum) occur in a butterfly distribution over the cheeks and forehead (Figure 7-4), and histologically similar lesions (vascular fibromas) have been described intraorally (Figure 7-4B).[11] Characteristic hypoplastic enamel defects (pitted enamel hypoplasia) occur in 40%–100% of those affected.[12] Rhabdomyoma of the heart and other hamartomas of the kidney, liver, adrenal glands, pancreas, and jaw are described. The neoplastic transformation of the glial proliferations constitutes the "internal malignancy" of this syndrome.

Fibrous Inflammatory Hyperplasias

The epulis fissuratum is a reactive inflammatory lesion associated with the periphery of ill-fitting dentures[13] that histologically resembles the fibroma. The growth is often split by the edge of the denture, resulting in a fissure, one part of the lesion lying under the denture and the other part lying between the lip or cheek and the outer denture surface (Figure 7-5). This lesion may extend the full length of one side of the denture. Many such hyperplastic growths will become less edematous and inflamed following the removal of the associated chronic irritant, but they rarely resolve entirely. In the preparation of the mouth to receive dentures, these lesions are excised to prevent further irritation and to ensure a soft tissue seal for the denture periphery.

Pulp polyps or chronic hyperplastic pulpitis represents an analogous condition. They occur when the pulpal connective tissue proliferates through a large pulpal exposure and fills the cavity in the tooth with a mushroom-shaped polyp that is connected by a stalk to the pulp chamber (Figure 7-6). Masticatory pressure may lead to keratinization of the epithelium covering these lesions. Pulp polyps contain few sensory nerve fibers and are remarkably insensitive. The crowns of teeth affected by pulp polyps are usually so badly destroyed by caries that endodontic treatment is not feasible.

Inflammatory papillary hyperplasia is a common lesion with a characteristic clinical appearance that develops on the central hard palate in response to chronic denture irritation in approximately 3%–4% of denture wearers.[14] Old and ill-fitting complete maxillary dentures appear to be the strongest stimuli, but the lesion is also seen under partial maxillary dentures. The exact pathogenesis is unclear, but this palatal

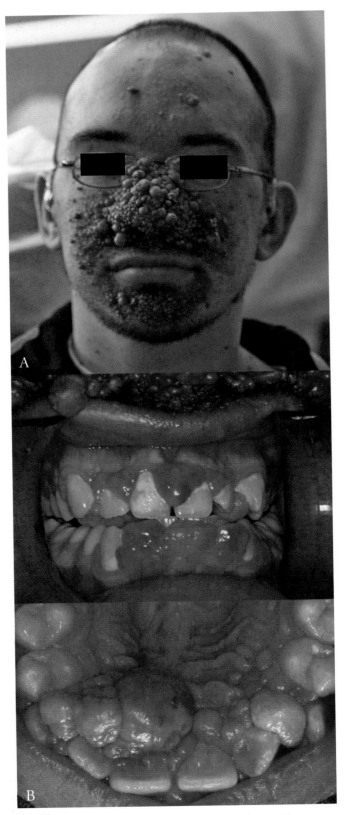

FIGURE 7-4 (A) Young male with tuberous sclerosis. There are extensive wart-like lesions (adenoma sebaceum) in a butterfly distribution over the face. (B) Same patient as in Figure 7-4A showing intraoral fibromas. Generalized hypoplastic pitted enamel changes are absent.

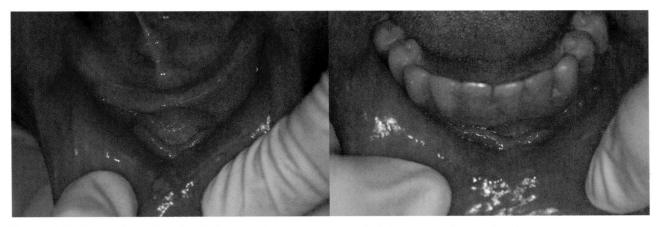

FIGURE 7-5 Fibrous hyperplasia (epulis fissuratum) secondary to a poorly fitting mandibular complete denture.

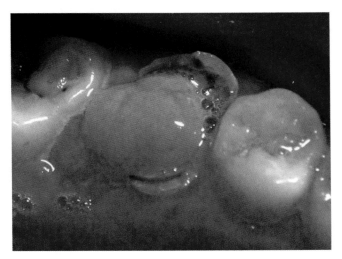

FIGURE 7-6 Pulp polyp (hyperplastic pulpitis) within a carious maxillary premolar.

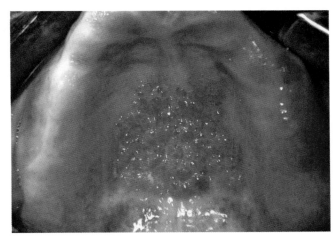

FIGURE 7-7 Papillary hyperplasia under a poorly fitting maxillary complete denture.

lesion is usually associated with denture stomatitis due to chronic candidal infection. The lesion may be red to scarlet with swollen and tightly packed projections resembling the surface of an overripe berry (Figure 7-7). Such lesions are friable, often bleed with minimal trauma, and may be covered with a thin whitish exudate. When the candidal infection is eliminated, either by removing the denture or by topical administration of an antifungal agent, the papillary surface becomes less erythematous than the rest of the palate and consists of tightly packed nodular projections. If tiny, the nodular projections may even pass unnoticed unless stroked with an instrument or disturbed by a jet of air. Histologic examination of these lesions demonstrates their exophytic nature, and neither epithelial invasion of the submucosa nor resorption of the palatine bone occurs. Mild cases may be treated successfully by topical or systemic antifungals alone,[15] otherwise, papillary hyperplasia is surgically excised or removed by electrocautery, cryosurgery, or laser surgery. The old denture or a palatal splint can be used as a postoperative surgical dressing, followed by fabrication of a new denture.[16]

Fibrous inflammatory hyperplasias have no malignant potential, and recurrence following excision is almost always a result of the failure to eliminate the source of chronic irritation. The occasional report of squamous cell carcinoma arising in an area of chronic denture irritation, however, underlines the fact that an oral growth, even that associated with an obvious chronic irritant, cannot be assumed to be benign until proven so by histologic study. Thus, whenever possible, all fibrous inflammatory hyperplasias of the oral cavity should be treated by local excision, with microscopic examination of the excised tissue.

Pyogenic Granuloma, Pregnancy Epulis, and Peripheral Ossifying or Cementifying Fibroma

Pyogenic granuloma is a hemorrhagic nodule that occurs most frequently on the gingiva (although it can occur on any surface) and that has a strong tendency to recur after simple excision if the associated irritant is not removed (Figure 7-8).[17] It may be difficult on occasion to identify the causative chronic irritation for these lesions, but their proximity to the gingival margin suggests that calculus,

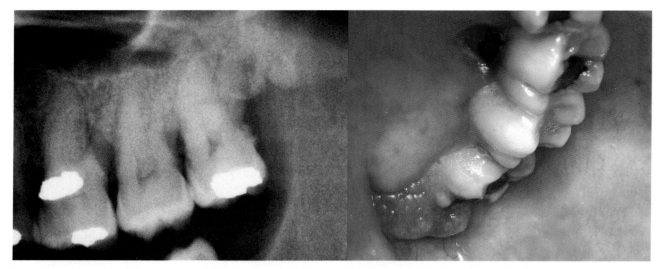

FIGURE 7-8   Pyogenic granuloma associated with a periodontal defect on the distal aspect of the maxillary left third molar. There is radiographic evidence of subgingival calculus, a likely etiologic factor.

food materials, and overhanging dental restoration margins are important irritants that should be eliminated when the lesion is excised. Their friable, hemorrhagic, and frequently ulcerated appearance correlates with their histologic structure. They are composed of proliferating endothelial tissue, much of which is canalized into a rich vascular network with minimal collagenous support. Neutrophils, as well as chronic inflammatory cells, are consistently present throughout the edematous stroma, with microabscess formation. Histologically, differentiation from a hemangioma is important. Despite the common name for the lesion, a frank discharge of pus is not present; when such a discharge occurs, it is likely a sinus tract from an underlying periodontal or periapical abscess, the opening of which is often marked by a nodule of granulation tissue (parulis).

Identical lesions with the same histologic structure occur in association with the florid gingivitis and periodontitis that may complicate pregnancy[18] and are referred to as pregnancy epulis or pregnancy tumor. The prevalence of pregnancy epulides increases toward the end of pregnancy (when levels of circulating estrogens are highest), and they tend to shrink after delivery (when there is a precipitous drop in circulating estrogens). This suggests that hormones play a role in the etiology of the lesion,[19] secondary to an increase in angiogenic factor expression and a reduction in the apoptosis of granulation tissue.[20] Similar to pregnancy gingivitis, these lesions do not occur in mouths that are kept scrupulously free of even minor gingival irritation, and local irritation is also clearly an important etiologic factor. Both pyogenic granulomas and pregnancy epulides may mature and become less vascular and more collagenous, gradually converting to fibrous epulides. Small isolated pregnancy tumors occurring in a mouth that is otherwise in excellent gingival health may sometimes be observed for resolution following delivery, but the size of the lesion or the presence of a generalized

pregnancy gingivitis or periodontitis supports the need for treatment during pregnancy.

The peripheral ossifying or cementifying fibroma is found exclusively on the gingiva; it does not arise in other oral mucosal locations. Clinically, it varies from pale pink to cherry red and is typically located in the interdental papilla region (Figure 7-9). This reactive proliferation is named because of the histologic evidence of calcifications that are seen in the context of a hypercellular fibroblastic stroma. Peripheral ossifying or cementifying fibromas occur in teenagers and young adults and are more common in women. The existence of these lesions indicates the need for a periodontal consultation, and treatment should include the elimination of subgingival irritants and gingival pockets throughout the mouth, as well as excision of the gingival growth.

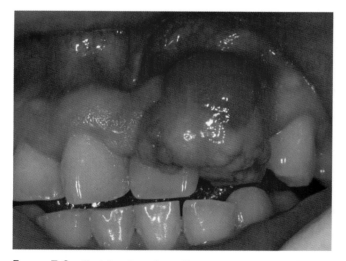

FIGURE 7-9   Peripheral ossifying fibroma in a teenage male associated with the maxillary buccal gingiva. The lesion was pedunculated.

Peripheral Giant Cell Granuloma

Giant cell granuloma occurs either as a peripheral exophytic lesion found exclusively on the gingiva or as a centrally located lesion within the jaw, skull, or facial bones (the central giant cell granuloma is described in the section that includes bone lesions). Peripheral giant cell granulomas are five times as common as the central lesions. Both peripheral and central lesions are histologically similar and are considered to be examples of benign inflammatory hyperplasia in which cells with fibroblastic, osteoblastic, and osteoclastic potential predominate.[21]

Nodular Fasciitis and Proliferative Myositis

Nodular fasciitis, a non-neoplastic connective tissue proliferation, usually occurs on the trunk or extremities of young adults. It appears as a rapidly growing nodule that histologically imitates a malignant mesenchymal neoplasm but that clinically behaves in a benign fashion. Oral nodular fasciitis occurs at all ages, with the majority during the fourth and fifth decades, with no gender predilection. The most common oral site is the buccal mucosa, most have an exophytic presentation, and growth rates are variable.[22] Nodular fasciitis has distinctive microscopic features that allow for the diagnosis, and the predominant cell type is the myofibroblast. The microscopic features of some of these lesions resemble a sarcoma, and this presents a diagnostic challenge for the pathologist. Proliferative myositis[23] and focal myositis[24] are lesions of skeletal muscle that have similar clinical features and are differentiated by histopathologic findings. Rare cases have been described in the tongue and in other neck and jaw muscles. Proliferative myositis is a reactive fibroblastic lesion that infiltrates around individual muscle fibers. Despite the nomenclature, these lesions do not show histologic signs of inflammation.

Gingival Enlargement

Gingival enlargement or overgrowth is usually caused by local inflammatory conditions such as poor oral hygiene, food impaction, or mouth breathing. Systemic conditions such as hormonal changes, drug therapy, or tumor infiltrates may also cause or contribute to the severity of gingival enlargement. Histologically, there are a number of explanations for gingival enlargement: hypertrophy (an increase in cell size), hyperplasia (an actual increase in cell number), edema, vascular engorgement, the presence of an inflammatory cell infiltrate, or an increase in dense fibrous connective tissue. One or more of these explanations may predominate depending on the underlying cause.

Inflammatory Gingival Enlargement

Inflammatory gingival enlargement occurs in sites of chronic suboptimal oral hygiene where there is accumulation of plaque, supragingival calculus formation, impaction of food, or the presence of aggravating factors such as orthodontic appliances, mouth breathing, hormonal changes, or other systemic diseases. The clinical diagnosis of inflammatory gingival enlargement is straightforward, with tissues exhibiting a glossy edematous bright red or purplish red color and a tendency to hemorrhage on slight provocation (Figure 7-10). A fetid odor may result from the decomposition of food debris and accumulation of bacteria. In long-standing cases of inflammatory enlargement, there may be an associated loss of periodontal attachment leading to periodontal disease.

Histologically, the exudative and proliferative features of chronic inflammation are seen: a preponderance of inflammatory cells, vascular engorgement, new capillary formation, and associated degenerative changes. Pseudopockets formed by gingival enlargement make the maintenance of good oral hygiene difficult, perpetuating a cycle of inflammation. Long-standing inflammatory gingival enlargement may demonstrate relatively firm, resilient, and pink gingivae that do not bleed readily nor demonstrate pitting edema following directly applied pressure with a periodontal probe. This is due to a greater fibrous component with an abundance of fibroblasts and collagen fibers.

Gingival inflammation affecting primarily the maxillary anterior region may be observed in mouth breathers.[25] Hormonal changes (such as during pregnancy or puberty) may exaggerate the local immune response to local factors and contribute to gingival enlargement.[26] The impaired collagen synthesis associated with vitamin C deficiency (scurvy) may also complicate inflammatory gingival enlargement.

Treatment of the inflammatory type of gingival enlargement begins with the establishment of excellent oral hygiene, together with the elimination of all local and/or systemic predisposing factors if possible. This includes a professional debridement (supragingival scaling or subgingival root planing) and prophylaxis, and correction of faulty restorations, carious lesions, or food impaction sites. Close follow-up after initial therapy is required to assess improvements in home care and tissue response that will dictate subsequent treatment options. For refractory cases, adjunctive topical or systemic antimicrobials or surgical options may be indicated. The successful treatment of gingival enlargement in mouth

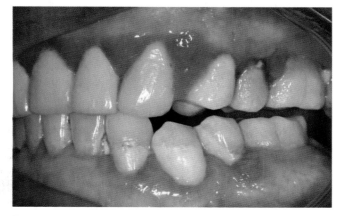

FIGURE 7-10 Inflammatory gingival enlargement secondary to local factors.

breathers depends primarily on the elimination of the habit. Patients should be referred to an otolaryngologist to determine if there is any obstruction of the upper air passages and/or to an orthodontist to assess the potential for treatment to permit the normal closure of the lips during sleep. A tissue biopsy should be considered whenever the cause is unclear, when there is a poor response to local therapy, or to rule out rare systemic diseases that may present with gingival enlargement (e.g., acute myelogenous leukemia).

Drug-Induced Gingival Enlargement

Drug-induced gingival enlargement is most commonly associated with the administration of anticonvulsants (principally phenytoin), cyclosporine, and calcium channel blocking agents. The extent of inflammation, fibrosis, and cellularity depends on the duration, dose, and identity of the drug; on the quality of oral hygiene; and on individual susceptibility that stems from genetic factors and environmental influences. These drugs likely exert their influence not by direct regulation of extracellular matrix metabolism or proliferation of gingival fibroblasts but due to the dysregulation of cytokines and growth factors.[27]

Phenytoin-induced gingival enlargement (Figure 7-11) is the most prevalent, affecting approximately 50% of patients who use the drug for longer than three months.[28] Although rare, gingival enlargement has also been reported in patients taking other anticonvulsants, namely valproic acid, phenobarbital, and vigabatrin.[28] The immunosuppressant agent cyclosporine causes gingival enlargement in 25%–30% of adults and, notably, in greater than 70% of children (Figure 7-12).[28] Nifedipine and diltiazem are responsible for most cases of calcium channel blocker–induced gingival enlargement, with a prevalence of approximately 5%–20%.[28] There are also reports of gingival enlargement following use of verapamil, felodipine, and amlodipine.

There is a characteristic clinical appearance of drug-induced gingival enlargement, although there is much variation predicted by various factors, principally

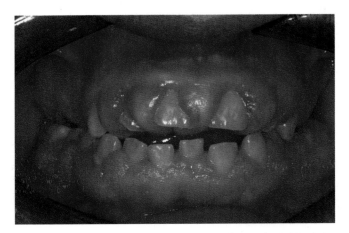

FIGURE 7-11   Gingival enlargement secondary to long-standing phenytoin use.

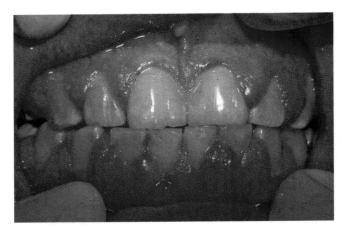

FIGURE 7-12   Gingival enlargement secondary to long-standing cyclosporine use.

plaque-associated gingival inflammation. After approximately one month of drug use, interdental papillae enlargement begins, usually in the anterior regions. The attached gingivae are generally involved, although the enlargement may become more extensive, leading to gingival disfigurement and associated esthetic and functional complications. There are reports that cyclosporine-induced enlargements are less fibrotic compared with those caused by phenytoin or calcium channel blockers.[27] The diagnosis is easily established based on the history of chronic drug use and the clinical appearance.

Prevention through optimal oral hygiene is essential to minimize the severity of enlargement. For patients treated for epilepsy, medications must be reviewed before orthodontic treatment is begun. There are several treatment options for drug-induced gingival enlargement. The most predictable treatment is either the withdrawal or change of medication. However, the control of the underlying medical condition necessitating the use of these medications is not always guaranteed following replacement with a new medication, and physicians may be reluctant to change the patient's regimen. There are, however, a variety of new-generation anticonvulsants, immunosuppressants, and antihypertensives available today. Tacrolimus is a new immunosuppressant that has been shown to be an effective replacement for cyclosporine and does not seem to cause gingival enlargement.[27] Nonsurgical treatments such as professional gingival debridement and topical or systemic antimicrobials may ameliorate gingival enlargement. There are equivocal reports supporting the efficacy of systemic antibiotics, most notably azithromycin to treat renal transplant patients with cyclosporine-induced enlargement.[29] A single randomized controlled trial demonstrated that folic acid supplementation before initiation of phenytoin led to a significant reduction in phenytoin-induced enlargement.[30] Surgical management is reserved for severe cases and usually does not provide long-term efficacy.[29] Conventional gingivectomy is the most commonly employed, although periodontal flap surgery may be indicated when osseous recontouring is needed, if there are mucogingival considerations, or in pediatric patients in whom tooth eruption is affected. Laser ablation gingivectomy may offer an advantage over conventional surgery since procedures are faster and there is improved hemostasis and more rapid healing.[29]

Hereditary Gingival Fibromatosis

Both autosomal dominant and autosomal recessive patterns of inheritance are recognized. Genetic heterogeneity and variable expressivity contribute to the difficulty encountered in assigning this diagnosis to a specific syndrome. Gingival fibromatosis without other syndrome-associated physical or mental abnormalities is not rare (Figure 7-13). A putative inherited mutation is in the *sos1* gene.[27] Enlargement may be present at birth or may become apparent only with the eruption of the deciduous or permanent dentitions. The most common problems associated with hereditary gingival fibromatosis are tooth migration, prolonged retention of the primary dentition, and diastemata. Enlargement may completely cover the crowns of the teeth, resulting in difficulty masticating or speaking and poor esthetics. Histologic features include proliferative fibrous overgrowth with a highly collagenized connective tissue stroma sparsely populated with fibroblasts and blood vessels.

Other Causes of Gingival Enlargement

Patients with acute myelogenous leukemia (principally acute monocytic [M4] or acute myelomonocytic [M5] leukemia) may present with gingival leukemic infiltrates (Figure 7-14).[31] Others include von Recklinghausen's neurofibromatosis (neurofibromatosis 1), Wegener's granulomatosis, sarcoidosis, Crohn's disease, primary amyloidosis, Kaposi's sarcoma, acromegaly, and lymphoma.

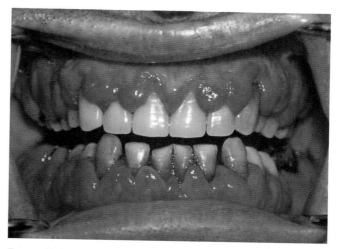

FIGURE 7-14 Gingival enlargement associated with acute myelogenous leukemia.

Benign Soft Tissue Tumors

Oral mucosal benign tumors comprise lesions that form from fibrous tissue, adipose tissue, nerve, and muscle. Benign proliferations of blood vessels and lymphatic vessels resemble neoplasms but do not have unlimited growth potential and therefore are more appropriately considered hamartomatous proliferations.

Epithelial Tumors

There are several benign oral epithelial virus–induced growths, principally those caused by the human papillomavirus (HPV).[32,33] Molecular biologic techniques (e.g., in situ hybridization, polymerase chain reaction) used to detect HPV[34,35] reveal that viral deoxyribonucleic acid (DNA) can be found in these lesions but may also be present in normal oral mucosa. There are more than 120 HPV strains, of which at least 25 have been detected in oral lesions. Much attention has been focused on the relationship between HPV and oropharyngeal carcinogenesis (see Chapter 8, "Oral and Oropharyngeal Cancer"). High-risk oncogenic HPV subtypes (predominantly HPV 16) are far more likely to be detected in cancers involving the oropharynx and tonsils compared with the oral cavity.[36,37]

Of the benign oral epithelial HPV–induced growths (Figure 7-15), viral papilloma (also called squamous papilloma) is relatively common. It usually occurs in the third to fifth decades, most commonly as an isolated small growth (<1 cm diameter) on the palate, ranging in color from pink to white, rugose (ridged or wrinkled), exophytic, and pedunculated. When these lesions occur on the surface of the lips, alveolar gingivae, or palate, they are well keratinized, and on nonkeratinized mucosal surfaces, they appear soft and pink/red. HPV DNA is detected in approximately 50% of squamous papillomas, predominantly HPV 6, followed by HPV 11.[33]

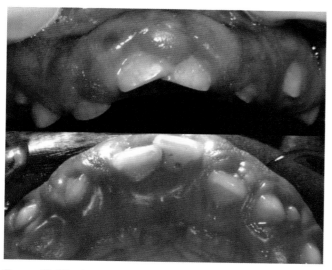

FIGURE 7-13 Hereditary gingival fibromatosis. Note the severity, with almost complete coverage of teeth in some locations.

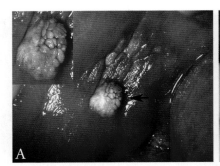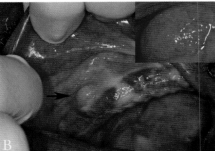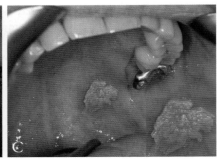

FIGURE 7-15 (A) Viral papilloma involving the right buccal mucosa. Note the papillary and highly keratinized surface, presumably related to the location (see inset). (B) Viral papilloma with a pebbled surface (inset) involving the right maxillary alveolar ridge. (C) Viral papilloma with a papillary surface (inset) involving the soft palate.

The common wart, verruca vulgaris, is generally found on the skin (sometimes in association with similar skin lesions, often on the fingers) and is caused by the cutaneous HPV subtypes 2 and 57. When involving the oral cavity, these warts are similar in appearance to viral papillomas and tend to involve the lips, gingivae, and hard palate. Oral papillomas and warts are clinically similar, and local excision is desirable. Care should be exercised when removing HPV-related oral lesions with electrocautery or laser as there exists the possibility of aerosolizing HPV particles. Although these lesions are probably infectious, a history of direct contact with another infected person is unusual, except in the case of multiple and often recurrent oral warts associated with sexual contact or maternal transmission, referred to as condyloma acuminatum (see Chapter 22, Infectious Diseases). HPV 6 and 11 are detected in these lesions.

Focal epithelial hyperplasia (Heck's disease), a condition characterized by numerous soft, well-circumscribed, flat, and sessile (i.e., nonpapillomatous) papules that are distributed throughout the oral mucosa, is endemic in some Eskimo and Native American communities but is rare in white people. Recent findings among Puerto Ricans and blacks suggest that further searches for this lesion may show it to be more widespread. Histologically, it is characterized by nondyskeratotic nodular acanthosis, which forms the basis of the papules, and a subepithelial lymphocytic infiltration. HPV DNA 13 and 32 are detected in 75%–100% of these lesions.[33]

Intraoral papillomatosis, often florid, is common in the HIV-infected population (Figure 7-16), particularly since the advent of highly active antiretroviral therapy (HAART).[38] Florid papillomatosis may also occur in patients with conditions such as ichthyosis hystrix (a congenitally acquired deforming skin papillomatosis) and Down syndrome.

Molluscum contagiosum is a dermatologic infection acquired by direct skin contact and characterized by clusters of tiny firm nodules that can be curetted from the skin. It is composed of clumps of proliferating epithelial cells with prominent eosinophilic inclusion bodies. This condition is not a neoplasm, but it is included here as one of the spectra of oral epithelial proliferations that result from viral infection. Both intraoral and labial lesions of molluscum

contagiosum have been reported,[39,40] principally in human immunodeficiency virus (HIV)-infected patients. It is caused by a poxvirus that infects the skin, where the virus replicates in the stratum spinosum, producing the characteristic and pathognomonic Cowdry type A inclusion bodies that are commonly associated with poxvirus infections.[41]

Keratoacanthoma[42,43] is a localized lesion that is typically found on sun-exposed skin, including the upper lip. The rapid growth of a keratoacanthoma may be quite frightening, to the point where it is often mistakenly diagnosed as squamous or basal cell carcinoma. These lesions appear fixed to the surrounding tissue (similar to some carcinomas), often grow rapidly, and are usually capped by thick keratin. Occasionally, the lesion matures, exfoliates, and heals spontaneously, but more frequently, block excision is required, and the diagnosis is established from microscopic evaluation. Epithelial tissue adjacent to the lesion is sharply demarcated from that of the lesion, which appears to lie in a cup-shaped depression. The proliferating epithelium constituting this lesion consists of masses of reasonably well-differentiated squamous cells that often produce keratin pearls and show little cellular atypia. The lesion's usual location on the upper lip (where squamous cell carcinoma of actinic etiology is rare, compared with the lower lip) should remind the clinician to consider keratoacanthoma in the differential diagnosis. Intraoral keratoacanthomas are rare.[44,45] Treatment of this lesion is conservative excision, although some believe that it is not clearly separable from squamous cell carcinoma and advocate wide excision to prevent recurrence.

Vascular Anomalies

Vascular anomalies cular anomalies have been classified using standardized terminology developed by the International Society for the Study of Vascular Anomalies.[46]

Hemangiomas

Hemangiomas of the head and neck are true neoplasms and appear a few weeks after birth and grow rapidly. They are characterized by endothelial cell hyperplasia and in most cases undergo involution, with residual telangiectatic, fatty, or scar tissue apparent in approximately 40%–50% of

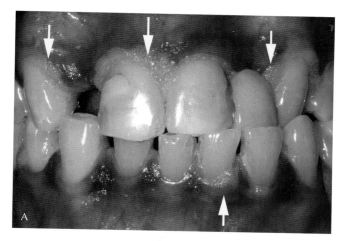

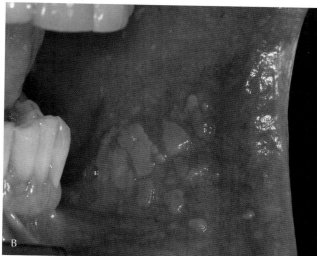

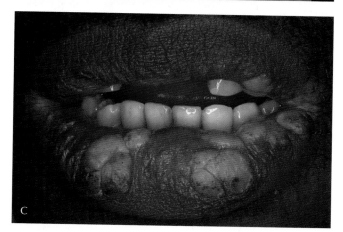

FIGURE 7-16 (A) HIV-associated florid papillomatosis involving free marginal gingivae. (B) HIV-associated florid papillomatosis involving buccal mucosa. Note coalescing papules, which are flat. (C) HIV-associated florid papillomatosis involving the lips.

patients.[47] They have been described in almost all head and neck locations in a variety of presentations: superficial and deep, small and large, most commonly as solitary lesions but also as multiple lesions. Small lesions may be clinically

indistinguishable from pyogenic granulomas and superficial venous varicosities. Capillary of caverneous hemangiomas involving any organ system are now classified as infantile hemangiomas; the former is superficial and the latter is deeper.

Vascular Malformations

Vascular malformations (Figure 7-17) are structural aberrations in components of the vascular apparatus and may be clinically apparent at birth, grow slowly proportional to the growth of the child (characterized by hypertrophy), and never involute. They may be classified depending on the vessel type involved or flow types: arterial and arteriovenous (high flow), capillary, or venous (low flow). Centrally located malformations must be distinguished from the many osteolytic tumors and cyst-like lesions that affect the jaws (see below). Arterial and arteriovenous malformations may first develop following hormonal changes (such as puberty), infections, or trauma, and, clinically, they may be firm, pulsatile, and warm. Venous malformations can sometimes appear first in early adulthood, and, clinically, they are soft and easily compressible.

Diascopy is the technique of applying pressure to a suspected vascular lesion to visualize the evacuation of coloration (Figure 7-18) and may facilitate the differentiation of a small vascular lesion from a pigmented lesion (see Chapter 6, Pigmented Lesions of the Oral Mucosa). Care should be taken in performing biopsies or excising all vascular lesions: (1) they have a tendency for uncontrolled hemorrhage and (2) the extent of the lesion is unknown since only a small portion may be evident in the mouth. Therefore, identification of the precise anatomic location and depth of tissue extent is warranted before treatment, particularly for

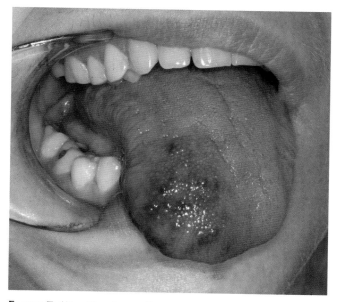

FIGURE 7-17 Vascular malformation involving the tongue, which developed two months before in a 25-year-old female.

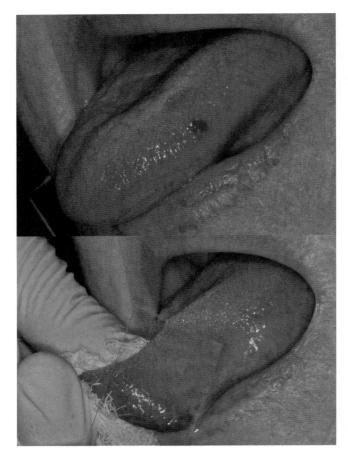

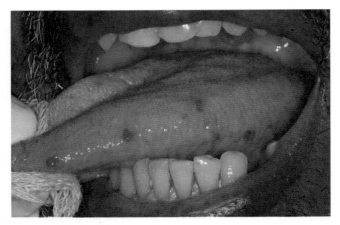

FIGURE 7-19 Osler-Wendu-Rendu syndrome (hereditary hemorrhagic telangiectasia). Note discrete multiple red papules associated with dilated vessels. Patient has similar papules distributed on his labial mucosae and finger tips.

FIGURE 7-18 Diascopy of a small capillary malformation on the lateral border of the tongue. Note blanching of the lesion.

the high-flow lesions. Angiography, computed tomography (CT), and magnetic resonance imaging (MRI) are all useful imaging techniques.[48] Treatment modalities (alone or in combination) depend on the type of vascular anomaly and include corticosteroids, propranolol, pulsed-dye laser therapy, sclerotherapy, superselective intra-arterial embolization (SIAE), radiotherapy, or surgical excision/ resection using electrocoagulation.[49]

Angiomatous Syndromes

A number of syndromes are associated with vascular malformations, including Osler-Weber-Rendu syndrome (hereditary hemorrhagic telangiectasia)[50] (Figure 7-19), blue rubber bleb nevus syndrome, Bannayan-Zonana syndrome, Sturge-Webersyndrome[51] (Figure 7-20), Klippel-Trénaunay syndrome, Servelle-Martorell syndrome, von Hippel-Lindau syndrome,[52] and Maffucci's syndrome.[53]

Lymphangioma

The term lymphangioma is a misnomer since it considered to be a lymphatic malformation similar to other vascular malformations.[46] It is characterized by an abnormal proliferation of lymphatic vessels. The most common extraoral

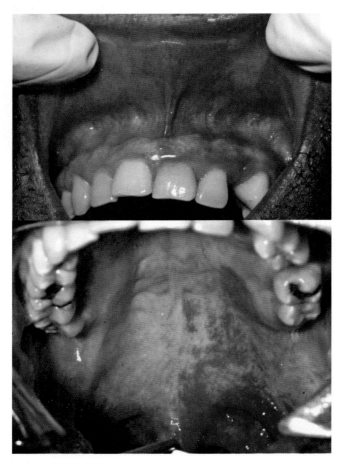

FIGURE 7-20 Sturge-Weber syndrome. Hypervascular changes are unilateral, which is consistent with a trigeminal nerve distribution, in this case following the second (maxillary) branch of the left trigeminal nerve.

and intraoral sites are the neck (predominantly in the posterior triangle) and tongue, respectively. The vast majority (80%–90%) of lymphangiomas arise within the first 2 years of life and are an important cause of congenital macroglossia.[54] Clinically, lymphangiomas are a slow-growing and painless soft tissue masses. This frequently presents without a clear anatomic outline, dissects tissue planes, and can be more extensive than anticipated. Intraosseous lymphangiomas have been reported.[55] Occasionally, they may undergo a rapid increase in size secondary to inflammation from an infection or hemorrhage from trauma. Large lymphangiomas may become life threatening if they compromise the airway or vital blood vessels,[56] and those spreading into and distending the neck are macrocystic and are referred to as cystic hygromas.

Differential diagnoses of lymphatic malformations of the tongue include infantile hemangioma or other vascular malformations, congenital hypothyroidism, mongolism, amyloidosis, neurofibromatosis, various storage diseases (e.g., Hurler's syndrome and glycogen storage disease), and primary muscular hypertrophy of the tongue, all of which may cause macroglossia. Abnormalities of the mucosa overlying a lymphatic malformation may give the appearance of a localized glossitis and may draw attention to the presence of a small lesion buried in the tongue. The typical oral lymphatic malformation has a racemose or pebbly surface.

The treatment of lymphatic malformations is dictated by their type, anatomic site, and extent of infiltration into surrounding structures.[49] Surgical excision is the most common, and sclerotherapy (with chemotherapeutic agents such as picabinil [OK-432] or ethanol) is also advocated. Recurrence of oral lymphangiomas has been reported, presumably because the lesion is interwoven between muscle fibers, preventing complete removal.

Glomus Tumor and Other Vascular Endothelial Growths. An unusual abnormality, glomus tumor[57] (glomangioma) develops as a small, painful, unencapsulated nodule. It represents a proliferation of the modified smooth muscle pericytic cells found in the characteristic type of peripheral arteriovenous anastomosis known as the glomus. In addition to having a distinctive histology, these lesions also may secrete various catecholamines. The glomus tumor is rare in the mouth but can occur around the carotid body, in the jugulotympanic region, and in the vagus nerve. Glomus tumors arising in the carotid bodies may produce neck masses and are referred to as chemodectomas or paragangliomas.

Neurogenic Lesions
Traumatic Neuroma

A traumatic neuroma is not a true tumor but a proliferation of nerve tissue that is caused by injury to a peripheral nerve.[58,59] Nerve tissue is encased in a sheath composed of Schwann cells and their fibers. When this sheath is disrupted, the nerve loses its framework. When a nerve and its sheath are damaged, the proximal end of the damaged nerve proliferates into a mass of nerve and Schwann cells mixed with dense fibrous scar tissue. In the oral cavity, injury to a nerve may occur from injection of local anesthesia, surgery,

or other sources of trauma.[60] Traumatic neuromas are often painful. The discomfort may range from pain on palpation to severe and constant pain. Most traumatic neuromas occur in adults. Traumatic neuromas in the oral cavity may occur in any location where a nerve is damaged; the mental foramen area is the most common location. The definitive diagnosis is made on the basis of a biopsy and microscopic examination. Traumatic neuromas are treated by surgical excision. Recurrence rates for neuromas are rare.

Oral Mucosal Neuromas and Multiple Endocrine Neoplasia Syndrome 2

Multiple endocrine neoplasia 2 (MEN 2) syndromes caused by inherited mutations in the RET proto-oncogene and characterized by tumors or hyperplasias of neuroendocrine tissues.[61] Patients with MEN 2B present with a characteristic phenotype that includes medullary thyroid carcinoma, pheochromocytoma, prominent corneal nerve fibers, a "Marfanoid" body habitus, enlarged lips, and neuromas on the eyelids and oral mucosal tissues. Identification of mucosal neuromas may precede other components of the syndrome. Management includes prophylactic total thyroidectomy, ideally before the age of 1 year.

Palisaded Encapsulated Neuroma

The palisaded encapsulated neuroma[62] is a benign tumor of the peripheral nerve that clinically and histologically resembles the neurofibroma and schwannoma. The lesions are solitary and found in older adults, a feature that distinguishes them from the neuromas in MEN syndrome. The palisaded encapsulated neuroma is a well-circumscribed partially encapsulated nodule composed of spindle-shaped cells exhibiting areas of nuclear palisading often admixed with axons. They contain Schwann cells, perineural cells, and axons and can be distinguished from neurofibromas and schwannomas both by their light microscopic appearance and by immunohistochemical stain that is positive for EMA and S-100.[63] The palisaded encapsulated neuroma is treated by conservative excision, and recurrence is rare.

Neurofibroma and Schwannoma

Neurofibroma and schwannoma (neurilemmoma) are benign tumors derived from the tissue that envelops nerves and includes Schwann cells and fibroblasts.[64,65] Although neurofibroma and schwannoma are distinct tumors microscopically, they are quite similar in their clinical presentation and behavior. The tongue is the most common intraoral location (Figure 7-21). Neurofibromas and schwannomas may occur at any age, without any sex predilection. Microscopic examination of a neurofibroma reveals a fairly well-delineated but diffuse proliferation of spindle-shaped Schwann cells. A schwannoma is encapsulated and exhibits varying amounts of two different microscopic patterns. One pattern consists of cells in a palisaded arrangement around eosinophilic areas and the other consists of less cellular spindle-shaped cells in a loose myxoid-appearing stroma. For these two lesions, light microscopic examination is generally sufficient to establish the diagnosis. The partial encapsulation of a palisaded encapsulated neuroma may resemble the schwannoma. Differences in immunohistochemical staining have been demonstrated and may be helpful in establishing the definitive diagnosis. The treatment for a neurofibroma or schwannoma is surgical excision. They generally do not recur.

Neurofibromatosis

Multiple neurofibromas occur in a genetically inherited disorder known as neurofibromatosis 1 (NF1) or von Recklinghausen's disease. This disease is transmitted as an autosomal dominant trait, and the *NF1* gene has been identified.[66] Oral neurofibromas are a common feature of the disease. The presence of numerous neurofibromas or a plexiform-type neurofibroma is pathognomonic of NF1.

Patients with NF1 are at increased risk of the development of malignant tumors, especially malignant peripheral nerve sheath tumor, leukemia, and rhabdomyosarcoma.[66–68]

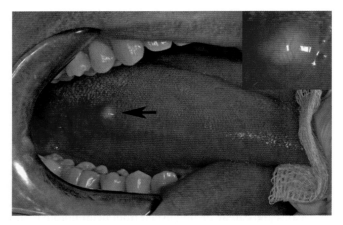

FIGURE 7-21 Neurogenic tumor involving the right lateral tongue.

Granular Cell Tumor

The granular cell tumor is a benign tumor composed of large cells with a granular cytoplasm. The pathogenesis of this tumor has not been established, but most evidence suggests that it arises from Schwann cells or their primitive mesenchymal precursors. The granular cell tumor most often occurs on the tongue (Figure 7-22A), followed by the buccal and labial mucosa. Other intraoral sites include the palate (Figure 7-22B), gingiva, and the floor of the mouth. The tumor appears as a painless, nonulcerated nodule. The majority of cases occur in adults with a female predilection. Immunocytochemical staining[69–71] reveals reactivity for S-100 protein and myelin. A report of a granular cell variant of the traumatic neuroma[72] supports further the neurogenic origin of this tumor, as do reports of granular cell tumors associated with neurofibromatosis.[73] Microscopic examination reveals large oval-shaped cells with a granular cytoplasm. The granular cells are found in the connective tissue. The overlying surface epithelium exhibits pseudoepitheliomatous hyperplasia, which is a benign proliferation of epithelium into the connective tissue. This tumor is treated by conservative surgical excision and does not recur.

The congenital epulis, or congenital epulis of the newborn, is a benign neoplasm composed of cells that closely resemble those seen in the granular cell tumor that occurs in adults. The ultrastructural and immunohistochemical features are different from the granular cell tumor that occurs in adults, confirming that this lesion is a completely separate entity. The neoplasm most likely arises from a primitive mesenchymal cell.[74] The congenital epulis is present at birth and presents as a smooth-surfaced, sessile, or pedunculated mass on the gingiva. It usually occurs on the anterior maxillary alveolar ridge and almost always occurs in girls. The congenital epulis is treated by surgical excision and does not recur. Occasionally, the tumors will regress without treatment.[75]

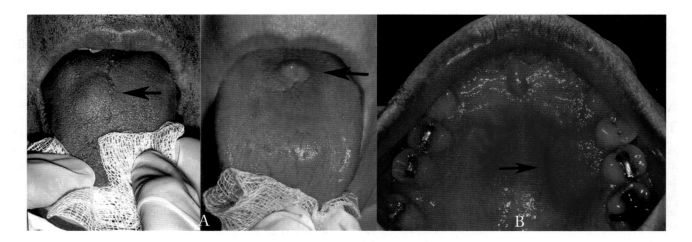

FIGURE 7-22 (A) Granular cell tumors of the tongue, the most common site for this benign lesion. (B) Granular cell tumor involving the palate, an unusual site.

Melanotic Neuroectodermal Tumor of Infancy

Melanotic neuroectodermal tumor of infancy is a benign neoplasm that occurs in young children and almost always occurs during the first year of life. Results of ultrastructural and immunocytochemical studies of this tumor are consistent with its origin from cells of the neural crest. The tumor most commonly occurs in the maxilla, followed by the skull, mandible, and brain. The tumor presents as a rapidly enlarging mass that destroys bone and may exhibit blue-black pigmentation. It has a high recurrence rate, and malignant transformation has been reported rarely. Histologically, the tumor is composed of collections of cells that resemble melanocytes admixed with smaller round cells and variable amounts of melanin. High levels of urinary vanillylmandelic acid are often found in patients with this tumor, and the levels tend to return to normal when the tumor is resected. Conservative surgical removal is usually adequate, but the behavior of this tumor is unpredictable.[76,77]

Lipoma

The lipoma is a benign tumor of mature fat cells.[78] When occurring in the superficial soft tissue, the lipoma appears as a yellowish mass with a thin surface of epithelium (Figure 7-23). Because of this thin epithelium, a delicate pattern of blood vessels is usually observed on the surface. Deeper lesions may not demonstrate this finding and therefore are not as easily identified clinically. The majority of oral lipomas are found on the buccal mucosa and tongue and occur in individuals over 40 years of age, without any sex predilection.

There are several microscopic variants of the lipoma. The classic description is of a well-delineated tumor composed of lobules of mature fat cells that are uniform in size and shape.

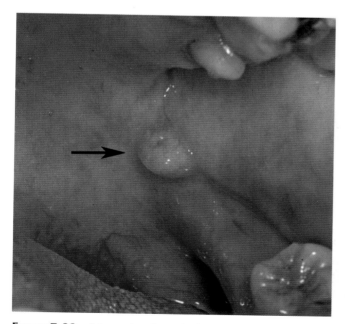

FIGURE 7-23 Lipoma involving the buccal mucosa. Note yellow color.

Those tumors with a significant fibrous connective tissue component are designated fibrolipoma, those with numerous small blood vessels angiolipoma, those with a mucoid background myxoid lipomas, and those with an admixture of uniform spindle cells spindle cell lipoma. The pleomorphic lipoma demonstrates spindle cells and bizarre, hyperchromatic giant cells and may be difficult for the pathologist to clearly distinguish from a pleomorphic liposarcoma. A lipoma that infiltrates among skeletal muscle bundles is called an intramuscular lipoma. It has been reported in the oral soft tissues but is rare.[79] The lipoma is treated by conservative surgical excision and generally does not recur. Intramuscular lipomas have a somewhat higher recurrence rate because they are more difficult to remove completely.

Tumors of Muscle

Tumors of muscle are extremely uncommon in the oral cavity. The rhabdomyoma, a benign tumor of striated muscle, has been reported to occur on the tongue. The vascular leiomyoma, a benign tumor of smooth muscle cell and vascular endothelium, occasionally occurs in the oral cavity. Treatment is local surgical excision, and recurrence is rare.[80]

BENIGN HARD TISSUE LESIONS

Benign Fibro-Osseous Lesions

Benign fibro-osseous lesion is a generic histologic designation for a diverse group of bone lesions that are named for the similarity of their histologic appearance. They are composed of cellular fibrous connective tissue admixed with either osteoid and bone trabeculae or rounded small to large calcified masses that have traditionally been described as cementoid material. Benign fibro-osseous lesions of the jaws include fibrous dysplasia, ossifying fibroma, and the cemento-osseous dysplasias. Radiographic correlation is critical for diagnosis.[81]

Fibrous Dysplasia

Fibrous dysplasia is a condition that is characterized by the replacement of bone with fibro-osseous tissue. The well-vascularized and cellular fibrous tissue contains trabeculae or spherules (small spheres) of poorly calcified non-lamellar bone that are formed by osseous metaplasia. Fibrous dysplasia starts in childhood, presenting with a slowly progressive enlargement of bone that generally slows or ceases with puberty.[82,83] The pathogenesis is related to GNAS (guanine nucleotide binding protein, alpha stimulating) gene mutation.[84,85] The most widely accepted theory is that fibrous dysplasia results from an abnormality in the development of bone-forming mesenchyme. Radiographically, fibrous dysplasia classically presents with a "ground glass" appearance and may have varying degrees of radiopacity and lucency depending on the amount of calcified material present. The abnormal bone merges with the adjacent normal bone. Plain film imaging and CT are useful in the diagnosis of fibrous dysplasia.[86,87]

Biopsy of involved bone reveals a tissue that is often described as "gritty" or "sandy." Several forms of fibrous dysplasia have been described.[81,82] The monostotic form, characterized by the involvement of a single bone, is the most common form. Polyostotic forms are characterized by the involvement of more than one bone and include different types: (1) craniofacial fibrous dysplasia, in which the maxilla and adjacent bones are involved; (2) Jaffe's type (or Jaffe-Lichtenstein type), in which there is multiple bone involvement along with an irregular macular melanin pigmentation of the skin (café au lait spots); and (3) rare cases in children (McCune-Albright syndrome or Albright's syndrome), in which there is severe, progressive bone involvement with café au lait skin pigmentation and precocious puberty. An elevation in serum alkaline phosphatase may be seen in patients with extensive polyostotic disease.[82] In most cases, once diagnosis has been confirmed, management is appropriate with superficial recontouring of the lesion or curettage of large radiolucent lesions.[88] Radiotherapy is contraindicated in the treatment of fibrous dysplasia. Radiotherapy administered in earlier decades of the 20th century may have played a role in the rare cases of malignant transformation to fibrosarcoma or osteogenic sarcoma. Attempts at treating advanced cases of the polyostotic form with calcitonin have not been successful.[89]

The clinical problems associated with fibrous dysplasia of bone are related to the site and extent of involvement. In the long bones, deformity and fractures are common complications that often lead to the initial diagnosis. In the jaws and other parts of the craniofacial skeleton, involvement of adjacent structures such as the cranial sinuses, cranial nerves, and ocular contents can lead to serious complications in addition to cosmetic and functional problems. Intracranial lesions arising from the cranial bones may produce seizures and electroencephalographic changes. Extension into and occlusion of the maxillary and ethmoid sinuses and mastoid air spaces are common.[90] Proptosis, diplopia, and interference with jaw function also often prompt surgical intervention.

Ossifying Fibroma

Ossifying fibroma is a slow-growing, well-circumscribed, benign tumor of bone that probably arises from cells of the periodontal ligament. Radiographically, it has a well-circumscribed margin that is confirmed by subsequent surgery (Figure 7-24). The cementifying fibroma has been reclassified under the category of ossifying fibroma.[91] The ossifying fibroma is a benign fibro-osseous lesion that is histologically composed of cellular fibrous connective tissue containing varying amounts of osteoid, rounded cementoid calcifications, and bone. This benign tumor occurs in the mandible more frequently than the maxilla. It is usually diagnosed in the third to fourth decades of age, with a female predilection. Treatment involves conservative surgical excision of the tumor. A variant of the ossifying fibroma is designated as juvenile ossifying fibroma that appears in younger individuals. This tumor exhibits more aggressive behavior and a greater propensity for recurrence.[91,92]

Cemento-Osseous Dysplasias

Three forms of this dysplastic process involving bone of the jaws are described: periapical cemento-osseous dysplasia, focal cemento-osseous dysplasia, and florid cemento-osseous dysplasia. Periapical and florid types are generally most appropriately diagnosed on the basis of the clinical and radiographic features. The focal type requires a biopsy to establish a definitive diagnosis. The etiology and pathogenesis of these conditions are unknown.[82] These lesions become more radiopaque with time; large calcified masses become a characteristic histologic feature.

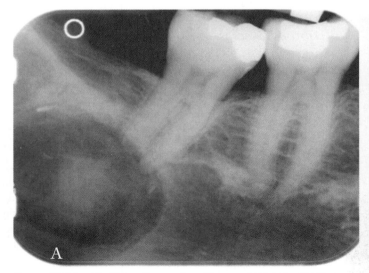
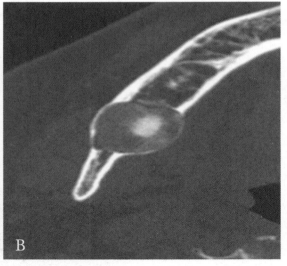

FIGURE 7-24   Ossifying fibroma in a 64-year-old female. (A) Periapical and (B) cropped axial CT bone window images show a well-circumscribed, mixed radiolucent-radiopaque entity of the posterior right mandible. The entity has concentric expansion and remodeled the overlying buccal and lingual cortices.

Periapical cemento-osseous dysplasia, previously called cementoma, occurs at the apical aspect of vital mandibular anterior teeth.[9394] It is most commonly reported in black women over age 40 years and begins with a radiolucent phase slowly increasing in radiodensity. The condition is asymptomatic and does not require treatment. Differential diagnosis includes dental pulp–related periapical inflammatory disease, and establishment of tooth vitality is critically important.

Focal cemento-osseous dysplasia differs from the periapical form since it occurs at the apical aspect of posterior teeth.[81] It is also reported to occur frequently in white women. Biopsy and histologic examination of the tissue are required to establish the diagnosis.

Florid cemento-osseous dysplasia presents as an exuberant form of cemento-osseous dysplasia, involving multiple quadrants of the maxilla and mandible.[95] Cystic changes similar to simple bone cysts may be seen in association with florid cemento-osseous dysplasia (Figure 7-25).[91,96] The calcified masses of the dysplastic bone do not resorb with the alveolar process in edentulous patients. In patients with tissue-borne removable dentures, secondary infection may occur from mucosal perforation and subsequent communication between the dysplastic bone and oral cavity.

Langerhans Cell Histiocytosis (Histiocytosis X)

Langerhans cell histiocytosis, formerly called histiocytosis X, comprises a group of conditions that are characterized histologically by a monoclonal proliferation of large mononuclear cells accompanied by a prominent eosinophil infiltrate. The mononuclear cells have been identified as Langerhans cells (the most peripheral cell of the immune system) by their immunologic staining characteristics and the presence of a cytoplasmic inclusion called the Birbeck granule.[97] Whether these conditions represent a neoplastic process or a non-neoplastic, immunologic, or reactive process remains controversial.

Historically, the clinical spectrum of Langerhans cell histiocytosis includes (1) single or multiple bone lesions with no visceral involvement (eosinophilic granuloma); (2) a chronic disseminated form that includes the classic Hand-Schüller-Christian triad of skull lesions, exophthalmos, and diabetes insipidus; and (3) an acute disseminated form (Letterer-Siwe disease) that affects multiple organs and has a poor prognosis. Each of these forms tends to affect patients at different ages, with the eosinophilic granuloma affecting older children and young adults, the chronic disseminated form affecting young children, and the acute disseminated form affecting infants and children under the age of 2 years.[98–101] Recently, the World Health Organization committee on histiocytic/reticulum cell proliferations and the Histiocyte Society revised the clinical classification of histiocytic disorders. Langerhans cell histiocytosis is currently classified by the clinical extent and severity of disease at diagnosis (Table 7-1).[102]

The single or multiple eosinophilic granulomas with no systemic or visceral involvement are the most common presentation. Both the maxilla and the mandible may be affected in Langerhans cell histiocytosis, both with and without systemic involvement. Early lesions present radiographically as well-defined, non-corticated radiolucencies. With time, the lesions enlarge and coalesce with one another, resulting in more bone destruction (Figure 7-26). Involvement

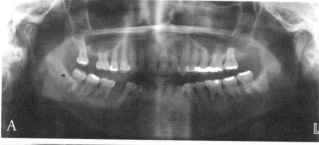

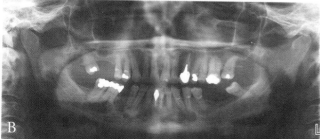

FIGURE 7-25 Florid cemento-osseous dysplasia (A) without and (B) with simple bone cyst association.

TABLE 7-1	Current Clinical Classification of Langerhans Cell Histiocytosis
Single organ system disease	
• Unifocal	
• Multifocal	
Multi-organ system disease	
• No organ dysfunction	
• Organ dysfunction	
○ Low-risk, excellent prognosis organs:	
■ Skin, bone, lymph node, pituitary	
○ High-risk, poor prognosis organs:	
■ Lung, liver, spleen, hematopoietic	

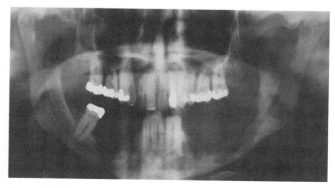

FIGURE 7-26 Langerhans cell histiocytosis. Multiple, well-defined, non-corticated radiolucencies have coalesced to give the appearance of diffuse mandibular bone destruction.

of the alveolar process may mimic periodontal disease, but Langerhans cell histiocytosis starts at the mid-root level.[103] The gingival soft tissues may also be involved, and this may resemble periapical or periodontal inflammatory disease.

The diagnosis of Langerhans cell histiocytosis is made by biopsy and histologic examination. The treatment varies, based on the clinical presentation of the disease. Solitary eosinophilic granuloma may be treated by surgical curettage. Low-dose radiation therapy has been used successfully for lesions that are multiple, less accessible, or persistent.[100] The older the patient with Langerhans cell histiocytosis and the less visceral involvement, the better the prognosis. Langerhans cell histiocytosis is a life-threatening disease in infants and very young children.

Giant Cell Lesions of Bone

Giant cell lesions include the peripheral giant cell granuloma (see soft tissue tumors above) and the central giant cell granuloma, aneurysmal bone cyst, and cherubism discussed here. These conditions are all non-neoplastic lesions that are characterized by a similar histologic appearance. Common to all of them is the presence of numerous multinucleated giant cells in a background of mesenchymal cells that contain round to ovoid nuclei. Extravasated red blood cells and hemosiderin deposits are commonly found in these lesions. The aneurysmal bone cyst contains varying-sized blood-filled spaces frequently admixed with trabeculae of bone. The bone lesions of cherubism are similar to those of the central giant cell granuloma.

Central Giant Cell Granuloma (Central Giant Cell Lesion)

Central giant cell granuloma occurs more frequently in the mandible than the maxilla, generally anterior to the first molar, and often crosses the midline. Most central giant cell granulomas are diagnosed before age 30 years. The radiographic features vary from small lesions mimicking periapical inflammatory disease to large, destructive, multilocular radiolucencies (Figure 7-27). Complaint of pain is an inconsistent feature of these lesions. Treatment usually involves conservative curettage. Other treatment modalities include systemic calcitonin, intralesional injections of corticosteroids, and subcutaneous α;-interferon injections. Recurrence rates ranging from 11% to 49% have been reported.[104–109]

The diagnosis of a central giant cell granuloma requires an evaluation for hyperparathyroidism (see also Chapter 23, Diabetes Mellitus and Endocrine Disorders).[107] Serum calcium, phosphorus, and alkaline phosphatase levels should be obtained prior to surgical removal of a giant cell granuloma, and if abnormal, parathyroid hormone (PTH) levels should be assessed. Lesions radiographically and histologically identical to the giant cell granuloma occur in primary and secondary hyperparathyroidism, and treatment of the lesion in these cases involves treatment of the hyperparathyroidism rather than treatment of the giant cell granuloma. Primary

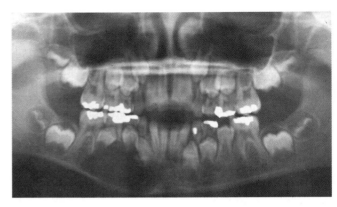

FIGURE 7-27 Giant cell granuloma. A panoramic radiograph of a giant cell granuloma in a child with a mixed dentition.

hyperparathyroidism is a result of uncontrolled PTH due to a parathyroid gland abnormality. Secondary hyperparathyroidism develops, usually in patients with chronic renal disease, due to an increase in PTH production in response to chronic low levels of serum calcium.

Aneurysmal Bone Cyst

The term *aneurysmal bone cyst* is a misnomer since this lesion is not a true cyst and exhibits no epithelial lining. It does contain varying-sized blood-filled spaces. The lesion occurs less frequently in the jaws than in the long bones and usually involves the mandible rather than the maxilla.[110–112] Tissue histologically consistent with aneurysmal bone cyst can be seen in association with other bone diseases, such as fibrous dysplasia. Consequently, aneurysmal bone cysts have been categorized as either primary, for those occurring alone, or secondary, for those occurring in association with another bone disease.[113] Primary aneurysmal bone cysts have been found to result from oncogenic activation of the *USP6* gene on chromosome 17p13.[114] Eighty percent of aneurysmal bone cysts occur in patients younger than 30 years of age; both sexes are equally affected.[110] The clinical signs and symptoms are nonspecific. Pain has been reported (however not consistently), and enlargement of the involved bone is common. The radiographic appearance varies from unilocular to multilocular (Figure 7-28). Treatment depends on the size of the lesions and includes curettage, enucleation, and resection. Recurrence is attributed to incomplete removal.[112]

Cherubism

Cherubism is a rare disease of children that is characterized by bilateral painless swellings (mandible and maxilla) that cause fullness of the cheeks; firm, protuberant, intraoral, alveolar masses; and missing or displaced teeth.[115–118] Submandibular lymphadenopathy is an early and constant feature that tends to subside after the age of 5 years and usually has regressed by the age of 12 years. Maxillary involvement can often produce a slightly upward turning of the child's eyes, revealing an abnormal amount of sclera beneath them. It was the upward "looking toward heaven" cast of the eyes combined

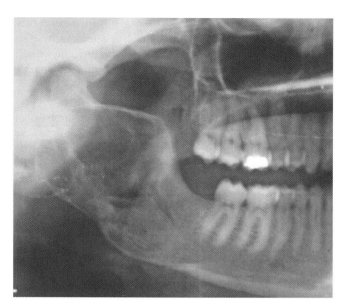

FIGURE 7-28   Aneurysmal bone cyst. An aneurysmal bone cyst presenting as a multilocular radiolucency in the angle of the mandible of a 31-year-old woman.

with the characteristic facial chubbiness of these children that prompted the term cherubism. Cherubism is inherited as an autosomal dominant trait, with a penetrance of nearly 100% in males and 50%–75% in females.[119] Genetic over-expression of SH3BP2 on chromosome 4p16 for the 3BP2 protein is the etiology.[91] Other patterns of inheritance and the occurrence of cherubism in association with other syndromes have been described.[118–120]

The clinical appearance may vary from barely discernible posterior swellings of a single jaw to a grotesque anterior and posterior expansion of both jaws, with concomitant difficulties in mastication, speech, swallowing, and respiration. Disease activity declines with advancing age. Radiographically, the lesions are multiple well-defined multilocular radiolucencies in the mandible and maxilla. They are irregular in size and usually cause marked destruction of the alveolar bone. Numerous displaced and unerupted teeth appear to be floating in radiolucent spaces. Serum calcium and phosphorus are within normal limits, but serum alkaline phosphatase may be elevated. Histologically, the lesions of cherubism resemble the central giant cell granuloma, but may exhibit eosinophilic deposits surrounding blood vessels throughout the lesion. A variety of treatments have been recommended: no active treatment and regular follow-up, extraction of teeth in the involved areas, surgical contouring of expanded lesions, or complete curettage. Long-term longitudinal investigations have reported that the childhood lesions become partially or completely resolved in the adult.[115,117]

Paget's Disease of Bone (Osteitis Deformans)

Paget's disease of bone is a chronic disease of the adult skeleton characterized by focal areas of excessive bone resorption followed by bone formation.[121–123] Histologically, the involved bone demonstrates prominent reversal lines that result from the resorption and deposition of bone. There is also replacement of the normal bone marrow by vascular fibrous connective tissue. Paget's disease of bone affects about 3% of the population over 45 years of age and is rare in patients younger than 40 years of age. Malignant transformation to osteosarcoma and giant cell tumor occurs in less than 1% of patients.[124–126] The etiology of Paget's disease is not well understood. The possibility of an infective viral etiology is suggested by the ultrastructural demonstration of intranuclear inclusions in the abnormal osteoclasts both in Paget's disease and in the cells of Paget's disease-associated osteosarcoma.[122,127,128] In recent years, genetic mutations affecting osteoclastogenesis, such as inactivation of TNFRSF11B for osteoprotegerin and mutation of SQSTM1 for the NFKappaB signaling pathway, have been found in some cases of Paget's disease of bone.[91]

Although some patients with Paget's disease have no symptoms, many experience considerable pain and deformity. The narrowing of skull foramina can cause ill-defined neuralgic pains, severe headache, dizziness, and deafness. The bony lesions of Paget's disease produce characteristic deformities of the skull, jaw, back, pelvis, and legs that are readily recognized both clinically and radiographically. Enlargement of the affected bone is common. Irregular overgrowth of the maxilla may lead to the facial appearance described as "leontiasis ossea," and edentulous patients may complain that their dentures no longer fit. Radiographically, there are patchy radiolucent and radiopaque changes that have been described as a "cotton wool" appearance.[123,126] Other radiographic findings of the jaw bones include loss of the lamina dura, root resorption, and hypercementosis. CT and Tc 99m diphosphonate bone scanning are used to define the extent of bone involvement.[121,123]

Craniofacial disorders, associated medical problems (e.g., cardiac failure, hypercalcemia), and the incidence of malignant transformation have encouraged the use of a variety of new treatments.[125,127] These agents include antibiotics (i.e., intravenous mithramycin, an effective inhibitor of osteoclastic activity), hormones of human and animal origin (high-dose glucocorticoids and porcine, salmon, and human calcitonin administered subcutaneously or by nasal spray or suppository), salts such as the diphosphonate etidronate (which effectively reduces bone resorption), and cytotoxic agents such as plicamycin and dactinomycin. Urinary levels of calcium and hydroxyproline (a measure of collagen metabolism) and serum alkaline phosphatase levels (a measure of osteoblastic activity) are useful for diagnosing Paget's disease and for monitoring bone resorption and deposition during treatment.

In addition to cosmetic issues, dental concerns include poor healing of dental extraction sites and excessive postsurgical bleeding from the highly vascular bone that is characteristic of this disease. Bone that exhibits unusually rapid change or enlargement suggests the possibility of malignant transformation. In view of the rarity of a giant cell tumor in the jaws except as a complication of Paget's disease,[129] the finding of this lesion in a patient who is older than 40 years of age should raise the possibility of previously undiagnosed Paget's disease.

Cysts of the Jaws and Adjacent Soft Tissues

Cysts are defined as fluid-filled epithelium-lined pathologic cavities. Odontogenic and non-odontogenic cysts occur in the oral soft tissues and in the maxilla and mandible. The cysts included here are those that are most common in the jaws and adjacent soft tissues.

Odontogenic Cysts
Radicular Cyst (Periapical Cyst)

A radicular cyst is a true cyst that occurs in association with the root of a nonvital tooth. It is the most commonly occurring cyst in the oral region.[130] An inflammatory response occurs in the periapical tissue, resulting in resorption of bone and formation of granulation tissue that is infiltrated by acute and chronic inflammatory cells. The epithelial lining for the radicular cyst is thought to develop as a result of proliferation of the rests of Malassez entrapped in the inflamed granulation tissue. Histologically, the radicular cyst appears as a squamous epithelium-lined cyst lumen surrounded by inflamed fibrous connective tissue. Most radicular cysts are asymptomatic and discovered on radiographic examination. They appear as well-circumscribed radiolucencies at the apex or lateral to a tooth root (Figure 7-29). The radicular cyst is treated by endodontic therapy, apicoectomy, or extraction and curettage of the periapical tissues. A residual cyst forms when the tooth is removed and all or part of a radicular cyst is left behind. Radiographically, the residual cyst appears as a well-circumscribed radiolucency located at the site of a previously extracted tooth. Either biopsy or excision of the lesion with histologic examination of the tissue is necessary

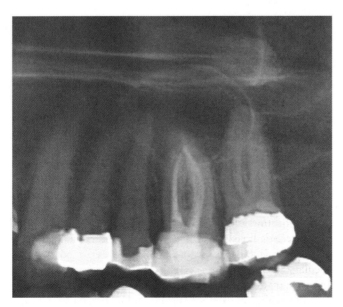

Figure 7-29 Radicular (periapical) cyst.

for diagnosis and the treatment is based on the diagnosis. The treatment of a residual cyst involves conservative surgical excision. The cyst does not recur since the tooth associated with the pathogenesis of the cyst has been removed.

Dentigerous Cyst (Follicular Cyst)

A dentigerous or follicular cyst is diagnosed on the basis of its very specific location. The dentigerous cyst forms around the crown of an unerupted or impacted tooth, which may be part of the regular dentition or a supernumerary tooth. The dentigerous cyst arises from the epithelium of the dental follicle and remains attached to the neck of the tooth, enclosing the crown within the cyst. The epithelial lining varies from cuboidal to squamous and from very thin to hyperplastic. Some unerupted teeth (e.g., third molars and canines) appear to be more susceptible than others to the development of such cysts. Dentigerous cysts have the potential for attaining a large size and also tend to resorb the roots of adjacent teeth.[131] Neoplastic changes such as plexiform ameloblastoma[132] and carcinoma[133,134] have been reported to occur within segments of the wall of dentigerous cysts. This potential for neoplastic change, infiltration beyond the cyst wall, and the occasional finding of other odontogenic tumors in association with a dentigerous cyst fully justify the need for histopathologic examination of all material derived from jaw cysts. The eruption cyst is the soft tissue analog of the dentigerous cyst; it presents clinically as a bluish gray swelling of the mucosa over an erupting tooth, most commonly first permanent molars and maxillary incisors. These are also referred to as eruption hematomas.[130] If any treatment is needed, excision of a wedge of the mucosa to expose the tooth crown is usually adequate.

Keratocystic Odontogenic Tumor (Odontogenic Keratocyst)

Since 2005, the World Health Organization has classified the odontogenic keratocyst as the keratocystic odontogenic tumor.[135,136] Reasons to consider this lesion as a cystic neoplasm include its aggressive clinical course, its tendency for recurrence, its association with certain genetic abnormalities and its occurrence in the Nevoid Basal Cell Carcinoma (Gorlin-Goltz) syndrome.[135,136] The keratocystic odontogenic tumor is characterized by its unique histologic appearance.[137–139] The lumen is lined by epithelium that is generally 8–10 cell layers thick and surfaced by parakeratin. The interface between the epithelium and connective tissue is devoid of rete ridges and the basal cell layer is palisaded and prominent. The parakeratin forms a wavy, corrugated surface. Budding of the cyst lining into the connective tissue is also described as a feature of this cystic neoplasm. The posterior mandible is the most common site of occurrence. However, the keratocystic odontogenic tumor may occur in any location in the maxilla or mandible. Radiographically, the keratocystic odontogenic tumor may present as a small, asymptomatic, unilocular radiolucency. However, larger, multilocular radiolucencies are common presentations of this cystic neoplasm (Figure 7-30).

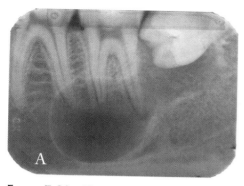
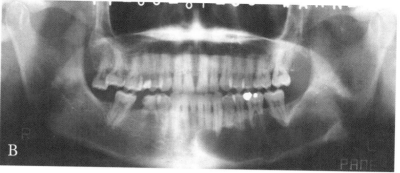

FIGURE 7-30 Keratocystic odontogenic tumor. (A) A keratocystic odontogenic tumor presenting as a well-circumscribed radiolucency mimicking a periapical inflammatory lesion. (B) A keratocystic odontogenic tumor presenting as a large radiolucency in the mandible.

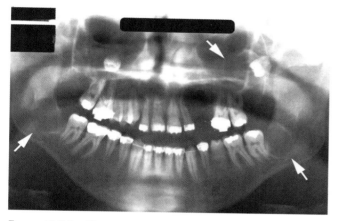

FIGURE 7-31 Keratocystic odontogenic tumor in Nevoid Basal Cell Carcinoma syndrome. The multiple radiolucencies seen in this patient with the syndrome are histologically shown to be keratocystic odontogenic tumors.

Complete removal of the keratocystic odontogenic tumor is necessary to prevent recurrence and may be difficult due to the thin, fragile nature of the cyst wall. Treatment ranges from decompression and enucleation to peripheral ostectomy and chemical cauterization to resection.[138]

The keratocystic odontogenic tumor can occur as an isolated cyst or as a component of the Nevoid Basal Cell Carcinoma syndrome (Figure 7-31). This syndrome is inherited as an autosomal dominant trait that exhibits high penetrance and variable expressivity. Mutation of the *PTCH1* gene on chromosome 9q22.3-31 has been shown to be the cause of the syndrome.[135,140] In addition to keratocystic odontogenic tumors (usually multiple), components of the syndrome include (among many others) basal cell carcinomas developing at an early age in non–sun exposed skin, mild hypertelorism, enlarged calvarium, calcification of the falx cerebri, and rib abnormalities.[140,141] Pitting of the soles and palms (local areas of undermaturation of the epithelial basal cells) is an additional finding in about half of the individuals affected by the syndrome. Despite the syndrome's name, multiple basal cell carcinomas occur in only 50% of cases. Appropriate

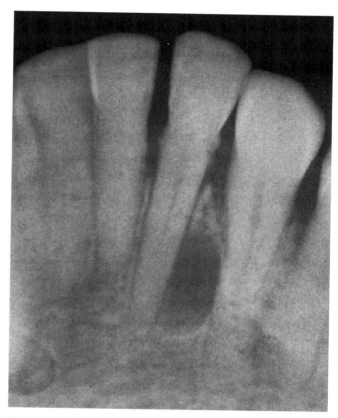

FIGURE 7-32 Lateral periodontal cyst. A lateral periodontal cyst presenting as a well-circumscribed radiolucency between the roots of a mandibular lateral and cuspid.

treatment for the keratocystic odontogenic tumors is simple curettage or marsupialization of the cysts.[142]

Lateral Periodontal Cyst (Botryoid Odontogenic Cyst). Although the lateral periodontal cyst has a distinct and characteristic histologic appearance, the cyst is named for its location.[143] It most often presents as an asymptomatic unilocular (rarely multilocular) radiolucency, lateral to the root of a vital mandibular cuspid or premolar tooth. (Figure 7-32). Histologically, the lateral periodontal cyst exhibits a very thin lining of stratified squamous epithelium with focal epithelial thickenings. The gingival cyst is the soft tissue analog of the lateral periodontal cyst. These cysts are treated by conservative surgical excision. A few cases of recurrence of lateral periodontal cysts have been reported.

Calcifying Odontogenic Cyst (Gorlin Cyst)

The calcifying odontogenic cyst is usually a nonaggressive cystic lesion lined by odontogenic epithelium that resembles that of the ameloblastoma, but with characteristic ghost cell keratinization.[144,145] It is usually a well-defined lesion that can present either as a unilocular or multilocular radiolucency. Calcifications are seen radiographically as radiopaque areas within a radiolucent lesion. Odontomas have been seen in association with calcifying odontogenic cysts.[146] A solid, noncystic variant histologically resembling the calcifying odontogenic cyst has been described. The calcifying odontogenic cyst is generally treated by surgical enucleation and usually does not recur. The solid variant has been reported to exhibit more aggressive behavior. Consequently, in recent years, the World Health Organization proposed renaming the cyst to calcifying cystic odontogenic tumor.[147]

Glandular Odontogenic Cyst (Sialo-Odontogenic Cyst)

Since 1987, the glandular odontogenic cyst has been recognized as a distinct developmental cyst of the jaws, bearing histologic resemblance to the botryoid odontogenic cyst and mucoepidermoid carcinoma.[148,149] Clinically, the glandular odontogenic cyst commonly affects middle-aged adults with no sex predilection. The anterior mandible is a frequent site of occurrence. Patients may be asymptomatic or have a painless jaw swelling at presentation. Radiographically, the glandular odontogenic cyst can manifest as a well-defined unilocular or multilocular radiolucency. Histologically, key diagnostic features of the cyst lining include eosinophilic cuboidal (hobnail) cells, clear cells, intraepithelial microcysts, and epithelial spheres.[149] The glandular odontogenic cyst is locally aggressive and tends to recur after surgery.

Buccal Bifurcation Cyst

The buccal bifurcation cyst is recognized as an inflammatory odontogenic cyst of the pediatric population.[150,151] Clinically, the cyst typically manifests as a swelling buccal to the furcation of the mandibular first or second molar. The cyst may also present bilaterally.[150,151] The affected tooth is vital, but may have a deep periodontal pocket. Radiographically, the buccal bifurcation cyst appears as a well-defined unilocular radiolucency centered on the furcation of the mandibular molar. An occlusal radiographic projection will show the cyst tipping the roots of the affected molar lingually (Figure 7-33).[150] Histologic features of the buccal bifurcation cyst consists of a non-specific, inflamed cyst lining. The buccal bifurcation cyst should not recur after curettage.

Non-Odontogenic Cysts

Nasopalatine Canal (Duct) Cyst

The nasopalatine canal (duct) cyst is derived from remnants of epithelium-lined vestigial oronasal duct tissue.[152,153] The cyst is located within the nasopalatine canal and presents as a unilocular radiolucency between the roots of vital maxillary central incisors (Figure 7-34). The cyst lining varies from squamous to respiratory (pseudostratified ciliated columnar) epithelium. Blood vessels and nerve tissue, contents of the nasopalatine canal, are frequently seen in the connective tissue wall of the cyst. The clinical evaluation involves differentiating this cyst from a normal nasopalatine foramen and a radicular cyst. The cyst of the incisive papilla is the soft tissue analog of the nasopalatine canal cyst. Both are treated by conservative excision and do not recur.

Nasoalveolar (Nasolabial) Cyst

The nasoalveolar cyst is a soft tissue cyst of uncertain pathogenesis with no alveolar bone involvement.[154,155] The cyst is observed in older adults, with a 4:1 female predilection. Clinically, the cyst presents as a swelling in the mucolabial fold. The cyst lining varies from squamous to respiratory

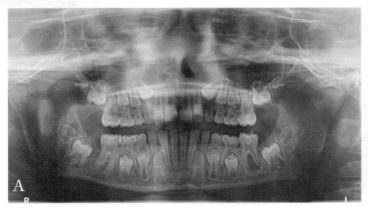
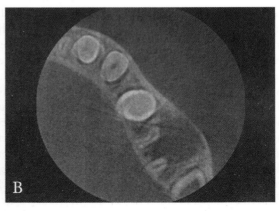

Figure 7-33 Buccal bifurcation cyst. (A) Panoramic and (B) axial cone beam CT images of a buccal bifurcation cyst associated with the mandibular left first molar. The cyst has tipped the molar roots to the lingual mandibular cortex.

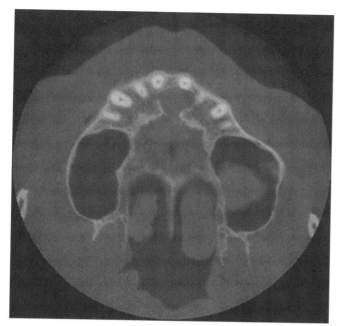

FIGURE 7-34 Nasopalatine canal (duct) cyst. Axial cone beam CT image shows a histologically proven nasopalatine canal (duct) cyst arising within the nasopalatine canal.

(pseudostratified ciliated columnar) epithelium. Treatment is surgical excision, and recurrence is rare.

Pseudocysts

Simple (Traumatic, Hemorrhagic) Bone Cyst

The simple bone cyst[156,157] is a pathologic cavity in bone that is not lined with epithelium. The cause is uncertain, although, traditionally, an association with trauma has been suggested. The lesion is found most often in young patients, with an equal distribution between males and females. The lesion presents radiographically as a well-defined radiolucency that characteristically demonstrates a scalloping pattern around the roots of teeth. The lesion is usually asymptomatic and discovered on routine radiographs. Surgical intervention reveals a void within the bone, and healing generally follows intervention.

Odontogenic Tumors

The classification of odontogenic tumors that is most commonly used divides these tumors into three categories based on the type of cell that forms the tumor: (1) epithelial, (2) mesenchymal, and (3) mixed epithelial and mesenchymal. Odontogenic tumors,[158,159] are derived from tooth-forming tissues, and the developmental stages of tooth formation are emulated in the various odontogenic tumors.

Epithelial Odontogenic Tumors
Ameloblastoma

The ameloblastoma is the best known of the epithelial odontogenic tumors. It is a slow-growing and locally aggressive

epithelial odontogenic tumor. The microscopic appearance of this tumor includes tumor cells resembling ameloblasts, with no formation of calcified material. The ameloblastoma is most commonly seen in the posterior mandible but may also arise in the maxilla and anterior aspect of the jaws. The radiographic appearance ranges from a unilocular to a multilocular radiolucency (Figure 7-35). Ameloblastomas are rare in children, with most cases occurring in patients between 20 and 50 years of age. Complete removal of the tumor is required to prevent recurrence; the plan for reconstruction often influences the extent of surgery. Rare examples of metastatic foci of an ameloblastoma in lungs or regional lymph nodes have been reported.[160–163]

Microscopically, all ameloblastomas show a fibrous stroma, with islands or masses of proliferating epithelium that resembles the odontogenic epithelium of the enamel organ (i.e., palisading of cells around proliferating nests of odontogenic epithelium in a pattern similar to ameloblasts). Follicular, plexiform, and acanthomatous histologic variants of this tumor show basal cells, stellate reticulum, and squamous metaplasia. These histologic variants show no correlation with either the clinical appearance of the lesion or its behavior, and variation may be seen between different sections of the same tumor. A unicystic variant of the ameloblastoma tends to occur during teenage years and has been reported to exhibit a less aggressive behavior. Fewer than 20% of unicystic ameloblastomas have been reported to recur after curettage, whereas over 75% of solid ameloblastomas will recur unless treated by resection.[163] Attempts have been made to marsupialize unicystic tumors. Recurrence is associated with incomplete removal of the tumor.

Adenomatoid Odontogenic Tumor

Adenomatoid odontogenic tumor (AOT) is a tumor of odontogenic epithelium that exhibits behavior very different from the ameloblastoma. This tumor is characterized histologically by a very distinct capsule surrounding the tumor and structures resembling ducts ("adenomatoid") within the epithelium.[164,165] Approximately 70% of AOTs occur in females younger than 20 years of age and 70% involve the anterior jaw.[164,165] Association with an impacted canine is common. This lesion rarely recurs even with conservative curettage.

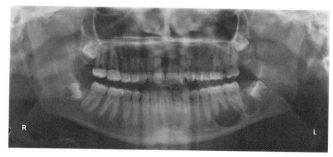

FIGURE 7-35 Ameloblastoma. Panoramic image shows a multilocular presentation of a histologically proven ameloblastoma.

Calcifying Epithelial Odontogenic Tumor (Pindborg Tumor)

The rare calcifying epithelial odontogenic tumor differs from other epithelial odontogenic tumors in that the epithelium does not resemble the epithelium of the tooth-forming apparatus. It is composed of sheets of polyhedral epithelial cells with very little stroma. The cells of this tumor may be quite pleomorphic, with large nuclei. Foci of hyalin amyloid material and calcifications exhibiting concentric rings are frequently seen in this tumor. It is important for the pathologist to recognize this distinctive tumor so that it is not misdiagnosed as a squamous carcinoma. The calcifying epithelial odontogenic tumor resembles an ameloblastoma; it is locally invasive and presents as a unilocular or multilocular swelling in the molar-ramus region.[166,167] Treatment is given by enucleation or local block excision; the recurrence rate is reported to be 20%.

Squamous Odontogenic Tumor

The squamous odontogenic tumor is a rare lesion composed of multiple islands of squamous epithelium.[168] The squamous epithelium does not exhibit the ameloblast-like features seen in the ameloblastoma. It is reported to occur equally within the maxilla and mandible. Radiographically, this tumor does not have distinctive features. The radiolucent area may resemble periodontal bone loss or periapical inflammatory disease. Conservative surgical excision is the treatment of choice for this tumor.

Mesenchymal Odontogenic Tumors

Odontogenic Myxoma

Myxomas are tumors composed of very loose cellular connective tissue containing little collagen and large amounts of an intercellular substance that is rich in acid mucopolysaccharide.

Myxomas are slow-growing and invasive tumors that can become very large and distend the maxilla or mandible. Since similar lesions are very rare in other bones and since some oral myxomas contain tiny epithelial remnants that resemble inactive odontogenic epithelium, tumors with this histologic appearance that occur in the jaw bone are assumed to be odontogenic in origin. This lesion usually consists of very small rounded and angular cells lying in an abundant mucoid stroma that is reminiscent of dental pulp. Characteristically, it appears radiographically as a unilocular or multilocular lesion and is clinically and radiographically indistinguishable from other lesions that present with a similar radiographic appearance (Figure 7-36). Treatment is similar to that recommended for ameloblastoma.[82,169]

Central Odontogenic Fibroma

The central odontogenic fibroma is a tumor composed of mature fibroblastic tissue admixed with nests and strands of odontogenic epithelium in varying amounts.[170] It is an uncommon, slow-growing, and nonaggressive lesion. These tumors are usually well-defined unilocular radiolucencies. They are generally small, yet they may cause root resorption. Treatment is conservative excision.[82,170]

Cementoblastoma

The cementoblastoma[171] is a cementum-producing lesion that is fused to the roots of a vital tooth (Figure 7-37). The tumor often occurs in young adults and is associated with a mandibular molar or premolar. Pain is a frequent complaint. Early in its development, this tumor presents as a periapical radiolucency that may be indistinguishable from a periapical inflammatory lesion. Later, the cementoblastoma demonstrates a pathognomonic appearance—a well-defined radiopaque mass surrounded by a radiolucent halo that

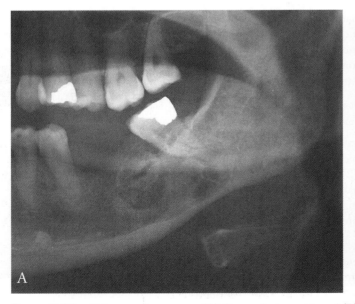
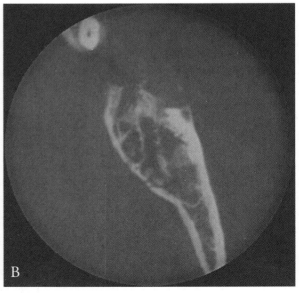

FIGURE 7-36 Odontogenic myxoma. (A) Cropped panoramic and (B) axial cone beam CT images show a well-defined multilocular radiolucency with long straight septa, characteristic of odontogenic myxoma.

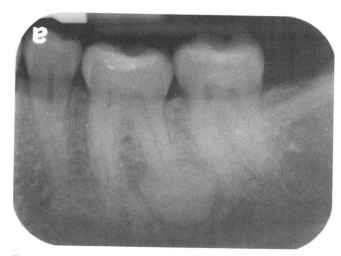

FIGURE 7-37 Cementoblastoma. Periapical image shows classic radiographic presentation of cementoblastoma fused to the root of the mandibular left first molar.

incorporates the root of the tooth. Treatment involves removing both the tooth and the attached cementoblastoma. The cementoblastoma does not recur.

Mixed Odontogenic Tumors
Ameloblastic Fibroma

The ameloblastic fibroma is a nonencapsulated tumor that is composed of mesenchymal tissue resembling dental papillae and small islands of odontogenic epithelium resembling dental lamina.[172] Most cases of this tumor are in patients under 20 years of age, particularly very young children, and congenital cases have been reported.[173] The most common location is the mandibular premolar and molar region. Radiographically, it presents as a radiolucency that may be well defined, poorly defined, unilocular, or multilocular. When tooth formation is associated with this tumor, the tumor is called an ameloblastic fibro-odontoma. The tumor is treated by surgical excision, and the recurrence rate is low.

Compound and Complex Odontomas

Compound and complex odontomas[172,174] are nonaggressive lesions that are more likely to be hamartomatous than neoplastic. Odontogenic cysts and other tumors may also be associated with odontomas. Most odontomas are identified in adolescents and young adults. The compound odontoma is most commonly seen in the anterior maxilla and the complex odontoma in the posterior mandible. A compound odontoma consists of a collection of numerous small teeth. Despite its designation as a hamartoma, the compound odontoma is considered the most common of the odontogenic tumors. It is usually diagnosed by the radiographic identification of multiple small tooth structures. The complex odontoma appears radiographically as a radiopaque mass. It consists of a mass of enamel, dentin, cementum, and pulp that does not morphologically resemble a tooth. Histologic examination

of the tissue is generally needed to establish the diagnosis. Treatment of the compound or complex odontoma requires surgical excision. These lesions are not expected to recur.

Benign Non-odontogenic Tumors of the Jaws
Osteomas/Gardner's Syndrome

Osteomas are benign tumors of bone that are composed of mature cancellous or cortical bone. They can form within the bone as a well-circumscribed radiopacity or on the surface of bone as either a sessile or polypoid bony-hard mass. Osteomas are asymptomatic and are generally undetected unless they are discovered on routine radiographic evaluation or cause facial asymmetry. Most are initially diagnosed in young adults. Maxillary and mandibular tori were described earlier in this chapter. Although they are histologically identical to osteomas, they do not have unlimited growth potential and are not considered neoplasms.[175–179]

The most significant feature of osteomas is the association with Gardner's syndrome. Gardner's syndrome is caused by mutations of the *APC* gene and inherited as an autosomal dominant trait with nearly 100% penetrance.[176] A specific gene mutation responsible for Gardner's syndrome has been identified. Adenomatous polyps of the colon develop in the second and third decades in individuals with Gardner's syndrome. These polyps ultimately exhibit malignant transformation to adenocarcinoma.[176] Patients with Gardner's syndrome develop multiple osteomas of the maxilla and mandible that precede the diagnosis of colonic polyps (Figure 7-38). Other components of Gardner's syndrome include supernumerary teeth, impacted teeth, skin cysts, and fibrous tumors of the skin.

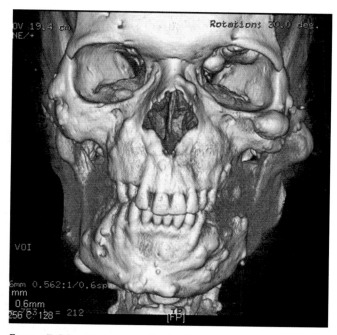

FIGURE 7-38 Osteomas in Gardner's syndrome. Three dimensional CT reconstructed image shows multiple craniofacial osteomas in a 30-year-old male diagnosed with Gardner's syndrome.

Osteoblastoma and Osteoid Osteoma

Osteoblastoma[180] and osteoid osteoma[181] occur much more commonly in other bones than the jaws. They are clinically, radiographically, and histologically very similar lesions. The size of the lesion is a distinguishing feature: the osteoblastoma is larger than 2 cm, and the osteoid osteoma is smaller than 2 cm. Pain is a presenting feature for both lesions. The pain associated with an osteoid osteoma responds to aspirin and other nonsteroidal anti-inflammatory drugs, whereas the pain associated with an osteoblastoma does not. Most lesions arise before age 30 years, and there is a higher prevalence in males. Radiographically, the osteoblastoma presents as a radiolucency that may be either well or poorly defined, with patchy areas of radiopacity within the lesion. The osteoid osteoma is more likely to present with a surrounding zone of sclerosis. Histologically, they both resemble the cementoblastoma but are not attached to a tooth. They are composed of sheets or irregular trabeculae of bone that exhibit prominent reversal lines. The bone is lined by osteoblast and osteoclast-like cells that contain multiple and large hyperchromatic nuclei. The central portion of the osteoid osteoma contains a concentration of nerve tissue. Careful evaluation of the radiograph and biopsy specimen by the pathologist is needed to distinguish them from an osteosarcoma. These tumors are generally treated by conservative excision.[182]

Chondroma and Chondromyxoid Fibroma

Cartilaginous tumors of the jaws are very rare. Any tumor-containing cartilage in the oral cavity and jaws must be evaluated very carefully by the pathologist to exclude malignancy. However, benign tumors of cartilage occurring in the jaws have been reported. The chondromyxoid fibroma is composed of spindle-shaped and stellate-shaped cells in a myxoid and cartilaginous stroma.[183] The major concern with cartilaginous tumors in the jaws is to ensure that the diagnosis is correct. Benign cartilaginous tumors are treated by conservative excision. Multiple chondromas are components of Ollier's disease (multiple enchondromas) and Maffucci's syndrome (multiple enchondromas with soft tissue hemangiomas).

Desmoplastic Fibroma

The desmoplastic fibroma of bone is a rare tumor that has been reported to occur in the jaws.[184–186] It is composed of uniform-appearing fibroblasts and abundant collagen fibers. The degree of cellularity may vary, but the cells of the desmoplastic fibroma do not show atypia and mitoses are not present. Most tumors have occurred in the mandible in patients under 30 years of age. Painless enlargement of the mandible with an associated unilocular radiolucency is the most common presentation. Radiographically, the tumor may be well or poorly defined and occasionally multilocular. This tumor can behave in an aggressive fashion; accordingly, treatment is based on the extent and rate of tumor growth.

Selected Readings

Abla O, Egeler RM, Weitzman S. Langerhans cell histiocytosis: Current concepts and treatments. *Cancer Treat Rev*. 2010;36:354–359.

Chiong C, Jayachandra S, D Eslick G, et al. A rare case of langerhans cell histiocytosis of the skull in an adult: a systematic review. *Rare Tumors*. 2013;5:e38.

Chowdhury S, Aggarwal A, Mittal N, Shah A. Brown tumor of hyperparathyroidism involving craniomaxillofacial region: a rare case report and literature review. *Minerva Stomatol*. 2013;62:343–348.

Dayan D, Nasrallah V, Vered M. Clinico-pathologic correlations of myofibroblastic tumors of the oral cavity: 1. Nodular fasciitis. *J Oral Pathol Med*. 2005;34:426–435.

Eversole R, Su L, ElMofty S. Benign fibro-osseous lesions of the craniofacial complex. A review. *Head Neck Pathol*. 2008;2:177–202.

Fakhry C, Gillison ML. Clinical implications of human papillomavirus in head and neck cancers. *J Clin Oncol*. 2006; 24:2606–2611.

Guerrissi JO. Giant cells mandibular lesion: surgical treatment with preservation of the dentition. *J Craniofac Surg*. 2013;24:1394–1396.

Guo YY, Zhang JY, Li XF, et al. PTCH1 gene mutations in keratocystic odontogenic tumors: a study of 43 Chinese patients and a systematic review. *PLoS One*. 2013;8:e77305.

Li TJ. The odontogenic keratocyst: a cyst, or a cystic neoplasm? *J Dent Res*. 2011;90:133–142.

Lowe LH, Marchant TC, Rivard DC, Scherbel AJ. Vascular malformations: classification and terminology the radiologist needs to know. *Semin Roentgenol*. 2012;47(2):106–117.

McDonald J, Bayrak-Toydemir P, Pyeritz RE. Hereditary hemorrhagic telangiectasia: an overview of diagnosis, management, and pathogenesis. *Genet Med*. 2011;13(7):607–616.

Mohanty S, Gulati U, Mediratta A, Ghosh S. Unilocular radiolucencies of anterior mandible in young patients: a 10 year retrospective study. *Natl J Maxillofac Surg*. 2013;4:66–72.

Moline J, Eng C. Multiple endocrine neoplasia type 2: an overview. *Genet Med*. 2011;13(9):755–764.

Northrup H, Krueger DA. Tuberous sclerosis complex diagnostic criteria update: recommendations of the 2012 international tuberous sclerosis complex consensus conference. *Pediatr Neurol*. 2013;49(4):243–254.

Pilarski R, Burt R, Kohlman W, et al. Cowden syndrome and the PTEN hamartoma tumor syndrome: systematic review and revised diagnostic criteria. *J Natl Cancer Inst*. 2013;105(21):1607–1616.

Premalatha BR, Patil S, Rao RS, et al. Odontogenic tumor markers - An overview. *J Int Oral Health*. 2013;5:59–69.

Rapp TB, Ward JP, Alaia MJ. Aneurysmal bone cyst. *J Am Acad Orthop Surg*. 2012;20:233–241.

Shankar YU, Misra SR, Vineet DA, Baskaran P. Paget disease of bone: a classic case report. *Contemp Clin Dent*. 2013;4:227–230.

Shi RR, Li XF, Zhang R, et al. GNAS mutational analysis in differentiating fibrous dysplasia and ossifying fibroma of the jaw. *Mod Pathol*. 2013;26:1023–1031.

Syrjanen S. Human papillomavirus infections and oral tumors. *Med Microbiol Immunol*. 2003;192(3):123–128.

Theos A, Korf BR. Pathophysiology of neurofibromatosis type 1. *Ann Intern Med*. 2006;144:842–849.

Wader J, Gajbi N. Neoplastic (solid) calcifying ghost cell tumor, intraosseous variant: report of a rare case and review of literature. *J Clin Diagn Res*. 2013;7:1999–2000.

For the full reference lists, please go to http://www.pmph-usa.com/Burkets_Oral_Medicine.

CHAPTER 8

Oral and Oropharyngeal Cancer

Joel Epstein DMD, MSD, FRCD(C), FDS RCSEd

Sharon Elad, DMD, MSc

❑ INTRODUCTION

❑ EPIDEMIOLOGY

❑ ORAL CANCER CLASSIFICATION

❑ SQUAMOUS CELL CARCINOMA
  Etiology and Risk Factors
  Pathogenesis
  Presenting Signs and Symptoms
  Diagnosis and Histopathology
  Staging of Oral Cancer—TNM System
  Diagnostic aids
  Imaging
  Acquisition of a Tissue Specimen
  Treatment

Prognosis
Prevention

❑ OTHER HEAD AND NECK CANCERS
  Malignant Tumors of the Salivary Glands
  Malignant Tumors of the Jaw
  Sarcomas of the Soft Tissues
  Metastases to the Head and Neck

❑ OTHER PATHOLOGIC CONDITIONS RELATED TO ORAL CANCER
  Nasopharyngeal Carcinoma
  Paraneoplastic Syndromes and Oral Cancer
  Head and Neck Malignant Disease in AIDS

❑ SUMMARY

INTRODUCTION

Oral cancer is a broad term that includes various malignant diagnoses that present in the oral tissues. Even though the management and prognosis may be different between types and stages of oral cancer, it always has a dramatic impact on the patient's life. The cancer and cancer therapy are associated with morbidities that may negatively affect the quality of life—from the time of diagnosis, during cancer therapy, in the immediate period after the cancer treatment, and continue throughout the life of the patient.

The older literature often combines oral cancer and oropharyngeal cancer (OPC) making the evaluation of epidemiology, pathogenesis, and outcomes difficult to assess as it is now recognized that oral and OPC must be evaluated individually.[1-3] To develop a uniform baseline for discussion, the anatomical domains need to be defined.[4] The oral cavity includes the lips, the labial and buccal mucosa, the anterior two-thirds of the tongue, the retromolar pad, the floor of the mouth, the gingiva, and the hard palate. The oropharynx includes the palatine and lingual tonsils, the

posterior one-third (base) of the tongue, the soft palate, and the posterior pharyngeal wall. See Figure 8-1.

This chapter will provide a general review of various types of oral and oropharyngeal malignant diseases, with a focus on the most common type, oral squamous cell carcinoma (OSCC). This chapter will also review other cancers in the

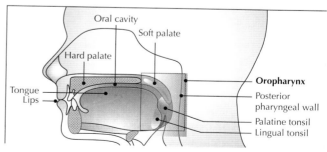

FIGURE 8-1 The oral cavity and oral pharynx. (From Cleveland, JL et al., The connection between human papillomavirus and oropharyngeal squamous cell carcinomas in the United States: Implications for dentistry, *J Am Dent Assoc.* 2011;142(8):917; used with permission © 2011 The American Dental Association.)

173

head and neck, including nasopharyngeal cancer (NPC), paraneoplastic syndromes, and head and neck malignant disease in AIDS.

This topic is highly relevant to all health-care professionals caring for patients during all phases of cancer treatment, including early detection and diagnosis, precancer treatment dental care and prevention, and managing oral and dental care for cancer survivors.

EPIDEMIOLOGY

Cancer of the oral cavity and pharynx affects 10.8 of every 100,000 individuals in the United States, based on the National Cancer Institute data, and 7.2 of every 100,000 individuals will have cancer in oral cancer.[5] The estimated new oral and pharyngeal cancer cases in the United States for 2013 were projected to be 41,380, which represents 2.5% of all estimated new cancer cases.[6] The same report estimated the number of death due to oral and pharyngeal cancers in the United States to be 7890 for 2013. Based on the most recent data, approximately 1.1% of the US population will be diagnosed with oral cavity and pharynx cancer at some point during their lifetime.[7] Based on the data from Surveillance, Epidemiology, and End Results program for 2003 to 2009 the 5-year survival in the United States was 62.2%.[7] This is a marked improvement in the relative survival when compared to 1950 to 1954, in which the relative survival was calculated to be 46%.[8] The US data indicates that the lifetime risk of being diagnosed with oral or pharyngeal cancer in males is 1.52% and in females 0.68%.[9] The statistics are similar throughout North America but vary throughout the world; in Hungary, the incidence is up to 21.1 cases per 100,000 population.[10]

In South and Southeast Asia, the prevalence of oral cancer is high. Oral cancer is ranked one of the sixth most frequent malignancies in Asia with nearly 274,300 new cases occur each year. Although an overall incidence rate of more than 10 per 100,000[11] has been reported, it may reach an annual incidence rate of as high as 21.4 per 100,000 individuals in some districts of India.[12,13]

Cultural habits, including betel quid chewing, alcohol consumption, and reverse smoking, as well as low socioeconomic status and low consumption of fruits and vegetables contribute to this high prevalence. The trend differs between countries in this region (increases in Pakistan and decreases in Philippines and Sri Lanka) and even between provinces of the same country (Thailand).[11]

The majority of oral cancers are squamous cell cancers. Other malignant diseases that can occur in the oral cavity include tumors of the salivary glands, lymph nodes, bone, and soft tissue.

Approximately 95% of oral cancer occur in people older than 40 years, with an average age at diagnosis of approximately 60 years.[14] However, OSCC at a young age and even in pediatric patients has attracted attention in the literature.[15,16]

The majority of oral cancers involve the lateral borders and base of the tongue.[5] The lips, gingiva, dorsal tongue, palate, and salivary glands are less common sites. Primary squamous cell carcinoma (SCC) of bone is rare; however, a tumor may develop from epithelial rests and from epithelium of odontogenic lesions, including cysts and benign lesions. Individuals who have had a previous cancer are at high risk of developing a second primary oral cancer.[17] African Americans in the United States have a lower risk of developing oral or pharyngeal cancer than Caucasians (9.6 vs. 11.2 per 100,000 population).[18]

Data published specifically for oropharyngeal carcinoma associated with human papilloma viruses (HPVs) showed increased incidence from 2000 to 2009, most of which is related to an increase in incidence in Caucasian males. In contrast, the incidence in black males at the same time decreased.[4] Analysis of tissues collected by national registries during the years 1984 to 2004 showed that increase in the population-level incidence of OPCs in the United States since 1984 is caused by HPV infection.[19,20] These reports document changing risk factors for OPC; nevertheless there is no evidence that detection of high-risk HPV can accurately predict the development of OPC in the oral cavity.[4]

Tumors of the salivary glands, the majority of which involve the parotid glands, represent less than 5% of all head and neck tumors. Approximately two-thirds of these are benign mixed tumors (pleomorphic adenomas). In order of decreasing frequency, the malignant salivary gland tumors are mucoepidermoid carcinoma, adenoid cystic carcinoma, adenocarcinoma, SCC, malignant pleomorphic adenoma, undifferentiated carcinoma, lymphoma, melanoma, and a mixed group of sarcomas. Malignant salivary gland tumors are more common in the submandibular, sublingual, and minor salivary glands than the parotid glands.[21]

ORAL CANCER CLASSIFICATION

Oral cancer nomenclature represents basically the histopathological characteristics of the lesion. To facilitate communication between health-care providers, a classification system was established by the World Health Organization (WHO). The classification system is updated from time to time based on advances in technology and outcome data.

According to the WHO classification of tumors, the morphology of the cells and the tissue architecture as seen in light microscopy is used to define the neoplasm, which may correlate with the biology and behavior of the cancer.

Three main publications within the WHO series of "Cancer Pathology and Genetics" refer to oral cancer, including cancer of the oral cavity and oropharynx, cancer of the salivary glands, and odontogenic tumors.[22–24] Tables 8-1 and 8-2 provide an overview of the WHO classification of malignancies of the oral cavity. Additional variants are continuously being reported in the literature.

TABLE 8-1   WHO Classification of Oral Cancer[23]
Epithelial cancer
Squamous cell carcinoma
Verrucous carcinoma
Basaloid squamous cell carcinoma
Papillary squamous cell carcinoma
Spindle cell carcinoma (sarcomatoid SCC)
Acantholytic squamous cell carcinoma
Adenosquamous carcinoma
Carcinoma cuniculatum
Lymphoepithelial carcinoma
Salivary gland cancer
Salivary gland carcinoma
Acinic cell carcinoma
Mucoepidermoid carcinoma
Adenoid cystic carcinoma
Polymorphous low-grade adenocarcinoma
Basal cell adenocarcinoma
Epithelial-myoepithelial carcinoma
Clear cell carcinoma, NOS
Cystadenocarcinoma
Mucinous adenocarcinoma
Oncocytic carcinoma
Salivary duct carcinoma
Myoepithelial carcinoma
Carcinoma ex pleomorphic adenoma
Salivary gland adenomas[a]
Soft tissue cancer[b]
Kaposi sarcoma
Hematolymphoid cancer
Diffuse large B-cell lymphoma
Mantle cell lymphoma
Follicular lymphoma
Extranodal marginal zone B-cell lymphoma of MALT type
Burkitt lymphoma
T-cell lymphoma
Extramedullary plasmacytoma
Langerhans cell hystiocytosis
Extramedullary myeloid sarcoma
Follicular dendritic cell sarcoma
Secondary tumors

Abbreviations: MALT, mucosa-associated lymphoid tissue; NOS, not otherwise specified; SCC, squamous cell carcinoma; WHO, World Health Organization.

[a]Salivary gland adenomas are basically benign tumors. However, some may be destructive or progress to cancer and therefore were included in the table. This includes pleomorphic adenoma, myoepithelioma, basal cell adenoma, Warthin's tumor, canalicular adenoma, duct papilloma, and cystadenoma.

[b]Additional soft tissue sarcomas that were reported in the literature include malignant melanoma, fibrosarcoma, malignant fibrous histiocytoma, liposarcoma, malignant peripheral nerve sheath tumor, angiosarcoma, leiomyosarcoma, and rhabdomyosarcoma.

TABLE 8-2   WHO Classification of Odontogenic Cancer[24]
Odontogenic carcinomas
Metastasizing (malignant) ameloblastoma
Ameloblastic carcinoma—primary type
Ameloblastic carcinoma—secondary type (dedifferentiated), intraosseous
Ameloblastic carcinoma—secondary type (dedifferentiated), peripheral
Primary intraosseous squamous cell carcinoma—solid type
Primary intraosseous squamous cell carcinoma derived from keratocystic odontogenic tumor
Primary intraosseous squamous cell carcinoma derived from odontogenic cysts
Clear cell odontogenic carcinoma
Ghost cell odontogenic carcinoma
Odontogenic sarcomas
Ameloblastoma fibrosarcoma
Ameloblastic fibrodentino- and fibro-odontosarcoma
Other tumors
Melanotic neuroectodermal tumor of infancy

Abbreviation: WHO, World Health Organization.

SQUAMOUS CELL CARCINOMA

Etiology and Risk Factors

The incidence of oral cancer is age related, which may reflect time for the accumulation of genetic changes and duration of exposure to initiators and promoters. These include chemical and physical irritants, viruses, and hormonal effects. In addition, decreased immunologic surveillance over time may be another explanation to the age relation, such as seen in individuals following solid organ and hematopoietic stem cell transplantations, individuals treated with chemotherapy, and HIV-infected individuals.

Tobacco and Alcohol

Tobacco products and alcohol are acknowledged risk factors for oral cancer.[2,14] Tobacco contains potent carcinogens, including nitrosamines, polycyclic aromatic hydrocarbons, nitrosodiethanolamine, nitrosoproline, and polonium. Tobacco smoke contains carbon monoxide, thiocyanate, hydrogen cyanide, nicotine, and metabolites of these constituents. Nicotine is a powerful and addicting drug. Epidemiologic studies have reported that up to 80% of oral cancer patients were smokers.[16] In addition to the risk of developing primary cancers, the risk of recurrent and second primary oral cancers is related to continuing smoking after cancer treatment. Among individuals who were observed for one year, 18% developed a recurrence or a second primary oral cancer, and those who continued to smoke had a 30% risk. The effect of smoking on cancer risk diminishes 5 to 10 years after quitting.

Most studies have focused on cigarette use; however, other forms of tobacco use have been associated with oral cancers. Benign hyperkeratosis and epithelial dysplasia have been documented after short-term use of smokeless tobacco products, and it is likely that chronic use is associated with an increasing incidence of malignant lesions.[14] The potential risk of oral cancer with cannabis is unclear as data are inconsistent.[25,26]

All forms of alcohol, including "hard" liquor, wine, and beer, have been implicated in the etiology of oral cancer. In some studies, beer and wine are associated with greater risk than hard liquor. Several studies identified subpopulations in which alcohol is not a risk factor for oral cancer, such as nonsmoking, nonbetel chewing subjects[27,28] or MTHFR TT genotype in Asians.[29] In contrast, other studies identified subpopulations at a higher risk for oral cancer following high-dose long-lasting exposure to alcohol, such as subjects with ADH1C*1/*2 in Caucasian,[30] ADH1C*1/*2 or ADHA1C*2/*2 in Asians,[31] and ALDH2*2 in Asians.[32] The combined effects of tobacco and alcohol result in a synergistic effect on the development of oral cancer.[33] The mechanisms by which alcohol and tobacco act synergistically may include dehydrating effects of alcohol on the mucosa, increasing mucosal permeability, and the effects of potential carcinogens in alcohol or tobacco. Various enzymatic pathways have been suggested as playing a role in the mechanism of the synergistic effect of smoking and alcohol on the oral mucosa.[32] Likewise, it was speculated that smoking and alcohol interaction may influence central nervous system activity.[32]

Betel (Areca) Nut

People with a betel quid chewing habit, with or without added tobacco, are at a higher risk to develop oral cancer. In parts of Asia where the use of betel nut mixed with lime to form a quid is widespread (e.g., India, Taiwan), the incidence of oral cancer is high and more commonly involves the buccal mucosa.[14] It was suggested that similar pattern may exist among immigrants originating from Asia.[34,35] Furthermore, substitutes for betel quid, such as gutkha and pan masala, are potential carcinogenic as well.[36]

Human Papilloma Virus

HPVs are DNA viruses that infect various epithelial surfaces.[3] There are more than 120 types of HPVs. HPV-16 and -18 are considered high-risk subtypes due to their association with malignant tumors.[4,37] HPV-16 alone is associated with about 85% to 95% of HPV-positive OPCs. The virus penetrates the host cell and integrates into the host cell genome where it can replicate. Malignant transformation occurs through the expression of two HPV viral oncogenes, E6 and E7.[38] There are many unanswered questions of the biology of HPV infection that include clearance versus persistence of virus, latency and carcinogenesis, site localization, recurrence, and second primary cancers.

HPV is transmitted by direct contact, primarily by means of vaginal, anal, and oral sex. Risk of developing HPV-positive OPC increases with increasing number of self-reported lifetime sexual partners (oral and vaginal), younger age at first sexual activity, and history of having a same-sex partner; in addition, the level of risk can vary according to tumor site.[4,39,40] It is important to note that these findings are related to oropharyngeal carcinoma, whereas HPV is not well defined as risk factor for oral cancer.

Nutritional Factors

Consumption of fruits and vegetables is associated with a reduced risk for oral cancer.[41,42] This may be due to the antioxidant vitamins C and E and flavonoids.[43] Elevated but inconsistent oral cancer risks have been observed for diets high in eggs and butter and for certain types of meats.[44]

Vitamin A may play a protective role in oral cancer.[14] This hypothesis is based on population studies of vitamin A deficiency where an association with the risk of SCC was observed and on studies of reduction in carcinogenesis in cultured head and neck SCC cell lines.[45,46] This hypothesis was supported by the fact that vitamin A may cause regression of premalignant leukoplakia.[47] Conversely, an epidemiologic study found no association between frequency of vitamin A supplement and head and neck cancer risk.[43]

A decreased risk of head and neck cancer was observed with long-term intake of vitamin C and with term intake of calcium supplement. However, dose-response trends were not observed.[43]

In recent years, vitamin D deficiency has also been associated with a plethora of pathologies. However, the association with oral cancer was only based on preliminary studies.[48,49]

Other Risk Factors

There is no evidence that denture use, denture irritation, irregular teeth or restorations, and chronic cheek-biting habits are related to oral cancer risk.[14,50,51] However, the role of local trauma in the development of oral cancer remains controversial.[52–54] It is possible that chronic trauma, in the presence of other risk factors and carcinogens, may promote the transformation of epithelial cells, as has been demonstrated in animal studies.

High alcohol content in mouthwashes has been implicated in oral cancer in the past. More recent studies suggest no significant trend in risk with increasing daily use; and no association between use of mouthwash containing alcohol and oral cancer risk has been found.[55,56] Confounding factors include smokers using mouthwash more frequently; thus, any correlation between regular use of high-alcohol mouthwash and oral cancer may be confounded by alcohol and tobacco use. Furthermore, the alcohol content of mouthwashes has been reduced, and increased use of nonalcohol-based mouthwash has been an ongoing trend.

In lip cancer, sun exposure, fair skin and a tendency to burn, pipe smoking, and alcohol are identified risk factors.[57]

Recurrent Herpes simplex virus of the lip has not been associated with increased cancer risk.

The suggested association between sideropenic anemia (Plummer–Vinson disease) and head and neck cancers appears to be more of limited significance in lesions arising in the postcricoid region of the hypopharynx. At the same time, it has been demonstrated that normal hemoglobin levels appear to be associated with improved locoregional control and overall cancer survival.[58]

Patients undergoing allogeneic hematologic stem cell transplantation (HSCT) are at an increased risk of developing secondary neoplasms, particularly leukemias and lymphomas, which may manifest in the oral tissues. Likewise OSCC has been reported up to a 20-fold increase in risk in these patient populations.[59-61] OSCC is documented after an extended period of immunosuppression posttransplantation and with similar molecular changes, as seen in nonmedically induced immunosuppression.[62,63] Oral cancer may behave more aggressively in patients posthematopoietic stem cell transplantation (HSCT) with chronic graft versus host disease and associated immunosuppression.[63,64] Other immunosuppressed patients show increased risk for oral cancer as well, such as patients after liver transplantation.[65] These cancers may be associated with HPV.[62]

Certain inherited cancer syndromes show increased risk for oral cancer.[66] For example, oral cancer is one of the cancers that are typical for Fanconi anemia patients. Fanconi anemia is usually diagnosed in an early age. With HSCT, the life expectancy of these patients is increased.[67] Cowden syndrome, xeroderma pigmentosum, and dyskeratosis congenita have also been reported in association with oral cancer.[68,69]

The WHO has listed several oral conditions as having the potential to transform into oral cancer, including lichen planus, leukoplakia, erythroplakia, actinic cheilitis, and submucous fibrosis.[70] It is clear that even within the umbrella of potentially malignant disorders, there is a spectrum of risks for the development of oral cancer. For example, the risk for oral cancer in erythroleukoplakia is higher than the risk for oral cancer in lichen planus. Even within a certain oral condition, there may be variable risk for transformation. For example, under the term "leukoplakia," proliferative verrucous leukoplakia is more aggressive and has a high risk of progression to SCC.[71]

Pathogenesis

Carcinogenesis is a genetic process that leads to a change in molecular function, cell morphology, and ultimately in cellular behavior. This process is not limited to the epithelium but involves a complex epithelial, connective tissue, and immune function interaction.

Major genes involved in OSCC include oncogenes and tumor suppressor genes (TSGs). Regulatory genetic molecules may be involved as well.[72] The genetic changes may be reflected in allelic loss or addition at chromosome regions corresponding to proto-oncogenes and TSGs, or epigenetic changes such as DNA methylation or histone deacetylation.

Extracellular enzymes, cell surface molecules, and immune function play a role in the development and spread of oral cancer; viruses and carcinogens are involved as well.

While the principle studies have been related to epithelial changes, some of the components listed above can comprise complex environment that suggests an epithelium–connective tissue theoretical model. For example, the interplay of the extracellular enzymes, cell surface molecules, growth factors, and immune system lead to epithelial–connective tissue interaction. According to this model, mucosal differentiation and maturation of epithelial cells represents an epithelial and connective tissue bidirectional process that may be involved in carcinogenesis.

Recently, a new model of carcinogenesis was suggested, which lead to the cancer stem cell (CSC) hypothesis.[73] According to this hypothesis, not all epithelial cells are capable of generating a tumor, and only long-surviving cells, such as stem cells, can undergo the summative oncogenic alterations required for carcinogenesis. Currently, there is lack of specific markers for identifying potential CSCs.

Oncogenes

Oncogenes may encode for growth factors, growth factor receptors, protein kinases, signal transducers, nuclear phosphoproteins, and transcription factors. Although proto-oncogenes increase cell growth and effect differentiation and are likely involved in carcinogenesis, few have been consistently reported in head and neck squamous cell carcinoma. Proto-oncogenes associated with head and neck squamous cell carcinoma include ras (rat sarcoma), cyclins, myc (myelocytomatosis), erb-b (erythroblastosis), bcl (B-cell lymphoma), int-2, CK8, CK19, and epidermal growth factor receptor (EGFR).[74,75] Each of these oncogenes families has several genes and isoforms with potential roles in the carcinogenesis. For example, the ras family has three genes (Hras, Kras, Nras), and it represents one of the most mutated oncogenes in human cancer, including oral cancer.[75]

Tumor Suppressor Genes

TSGs negatively regulate cell growth and differentiation. Functional loss of TSGs is common in carcinogenesis and in OSCC. Both copies of a TSG must be inactivated or lost for loss of function (the "two-hit" hypothesis). Chromosomes are numbered (1–23), and the arms of each chromosome are divided by the centromere into a short arm (designated P) and a long arm (designated Q). These TSGs have been associated with sites of chromosome abnormalities where loss of genetic nucleic segments has been reported to commonly involve chromosome arms 3p, 4q, 8p, 9p, 11q, 13q, and 17p. TSGs involved in head and neck squamous cell carcinoma are P53, Rb (retinoblastoma), and p16INK4A. Other candidates include FHIT (fragile histidine triad), APC (adenomatous polyposis coli), DOC1 VHL (gene for von Hippel–Lindau syndrome), and TGF-R-II (gene for transforming growth factor type II receptor).

Gene-Regulating Proteins

Part of the oncogenic gene regulation is performed by transcription factors. These transcription factors are proteins binding to DNA sequences to permit or inhibit co-binding to RNA polymerase, which in turn regulates the activation of the DNA segment respective gene. Transcription factors that were identified from oral tumors and their potential contribution to oral cancer are listed in Table 8-3.[76]

Loss of Heterozygosity

Loss of heterozygosity (LOH) or allelic loss has been studied in oral premalignant lesions and predicts the malignant risk of low-grade dysplastic oral epithelial lesions.[77–82] The importance of allelic loss has been shown in retrospective and cross-sectional study and confirmed in a prospective study of patents with dysplasia, where lesions with allelic loss at 3p, 9p, and 17p predict risk of progression to SCC, even in histologically benign or tissue with mild dysplasia.[83] This is of importance as the majority of potentially malignant oral lesions (hyperplasia, mild and moderate dysplasia) do not progress to cancer. Lesions that progress to SCC appear to differ genetically from nonprogressing lesions, even though they may not demonstrate different histomorphologic findings. Therefore, molecular analysis may become necessary in diagnosis. LOH on 3p and/or 9p is seen in virtually all progressing cases. LOH on 3p and/or 9p has a 3.8 times relative risk of developing SCC, and if additional sites of LOH are present (4q, 8p, 11q, 13q, or 17p), a 33-fold increase in risk of progression to cancer is seen. Accumulation of allelic loss is seen in progressing lesions, and the majority of progressing dysplasia have LOH on more than one arm (91% vs. 31% of nonprogressing dysplasia); 57% have loss on more than two arms (vs. 20% of dysplasia without progression). LOH on 4q, 8p, 11q, 13q, and 17p is common in severe dysplasia/carcinoma in situ or SCC.

Hypermethylation

The role of promoter hypermethylation of CpG islands is being investigated in OSCC as methylation of epigenetic DNA has been shown to result in a loss of function in some genes involved in cell cycle regulation and DNA repair that may lead to loss or change in TSGs involved in carcinogenesis.[84,85] Changes in DNA methylation of six genes and a significantly higher frequency of methylation in a number of TSGs, including cyclin A1 and p16 promoter sequences, have been seen. Mitochondrial DNA (mtDNA) content increases with oxidative damage as possible compensation to mitochondrial dysfunction. mtDNA, as assessed by polymerase chain reaction for specific mitochondrial genes, was shown to increase with severity of dysplasia and in SCC. These findings support the model of accumulation of genetic alterations as mucosal disease progresses from benign to dysplasia and potentially to SCC and the contention that mtDNA increases with histologic grade.

MicroRNA

MicroRNAs are small segments of nonencoding single-stranded RNAs that mediate gene expression at the posttranscriptional level by mRNA degradation or translational repression. Aberrant microRNA may disrupt the normal regulation and lead to malignancy. MicroRNAs function either as oncogenes or as tumor suppressors and were suggested to play a role in oral cancer.[86]

Extracellular Enzymes

Matrix metalloproteinase (MMP) 2 and tissue inhibitor of metalloproteinase play a role in cancer initiation and development. Others have also supported the prognostic significance of tissue inhibitors of MMP.

The development of malignant epithelial neoplasms is associated with disruption of cell-to-cell and cell-to-matrix adhesion. Syndecans are a family of heparin sulfate proteoglycan receptors that are thought to participate in both cell-to-cell

TABLE 8-3	List of Some Commonly Oncogenic Transcription Factors Associated With Oral Cancer[a]
OTF	Oncogenic potential in OSCC
AP-1	Overexpression, nuclear expression increased according to the degree of dysplasia, lymph node metastasis, increased transcriptional activity
NF-κB	Differential expression, activation, proliferation, malignant transformation, invasion
c-Myc	Overexpression, DNA amplification, DNA-binding activity, progression of oral cancer
STAT	Early overexpression and activated form of TF, active in OSCC
β-catenin	Nuclear overexpression, oral cancer progression, metastasis
Snail	Overexpression, activation, invasion, correlated with EMT
HIF1α	Overexpression, progression, expression correlates with poor prognosis, invasion
Mutated p53 (GOF)	Inactivated protein, GOF of mutant p53 propel mitosis by expressing cyclin A and cyclin B, GOF leads to shorter disease-free survival, prevention apoptosis after DNA damage, chemoresistance, disease progression

Abbreviations: EMT, epithelial–mesenchymal transition; GOF, gain-of-function; OSCC, oral squamous cell carcinoma; OTF, oncogenic transcription factors.
[a]Modified with permission from Yedida et al.[66]

and cell-to-matrix adhesion. A reduction of syndecan 1 correlated with histologic grade, tumor size, and mode of invasion.[14]

The initiation or progression of oral cancer may be associated with polymorphism of the *vascular endothelial growth factor (VEGF)* gene.[87] Connective tissue growth factor was suggested to effect the invasive and migratory abilities of OSCC cell lines.[88]

SCC mainly spreads by direct local extension and by regional extension, primarily via the lymphatics. Regional spread in the oral mucosa may occur by direct extension and possibly by submucosal spread and result in wide areas of involvement. Production of type I collagenase, heparanase, prostaglandin E_2, and interleukin-1 may affect the extracellular matrix, and motility of epithelial cells may allow invasion.[89,90] Changes in the basement membrane, such as the breakdown of laminin and collagen, occur with invasion. Understanding the biology of invasion by malignant cells may lead to additional approaches to diagnosis and management.

Cell Surface Changes

Changes in cell surface receptors and major histocompatibility class I and class II antigens have been reported and may indicate that immune surveillance and immune function may be affected in patients with oral cancer. Other cell surface changes include a loss of cytoplasmic membrane binding of lectins, which has been shown to correlate to the degree of cellular atypia.

Intercellular adhesion molecule (ICAM)-5 (telencephalin) is reported to be expressed only in the somatodendritic membrane of telencephalin neurons. ICAM-5 may play a role in tumorigenesis and perineural invasion. Alpha(v)beta6 integrin is frequently expressed in SCC and in leukoplakia that progress but not in lesions that did not progress, suggesting that this integrin could be associated with malignant transformation.

Additional cell surface markers are altered in neoplastic dedifferentiation; examples are the loss of ABO blood group antigens, β_2-microglobulin, and involucrin and a loss of reaction to pemphigus antisera.

Alterations in cell-bound immunoglobulins and circulating immune complexes are detectable, but the importance of these changes is unclear.

Immunosuppression

The development of malignant disease at a higher rate in immunosuppressed patients indicates the importance of an intact immune response. Mononuclear cell infiltration correlates with prognosis, and more aggressive disease is associated with limited inflammatory response. Total numbers of T cells may be decreased in patients with head and neck cancer, and the mixed lymphocyte reaction is reduced in some patients, and a diminished migration of macrophages has been demonstrated. Cluster of differentiation 8 lymphocytes (T suppressor cells) predominate in the infiltrate, suggesting that immunosuppression is associated with progression of disease. Langerhans' cells may be altered in neoplastic epithelium.[91,92] Further

understanding of immune function and the response to SCC may lead to the development of new therapies that modulate the immune response as is suggested by major therapeutic breakthroughs in other cancers such as malignant melanoma.

Viruses

The potential role of viruses in oral cancer is under continuing study. The interaction of viruses with other carcinogens and oncogenes may be an important mechanism of disease.

HPV is a documented risk factor for OPC.[93] It was also identified in oral cancer.[94] Current epidemiology show HPV much more commonly associated with OPC. However, as the change in risk factors with HPV continues to evolve, HPV-related lesions are increasingly reported at other head and neck sites including the oral cavity.[4,95] Up to 75% of OPC and 26% of oral SCC have been associated with high-risk HPV, showing a continuing trend to increasing HPV in SCC.[94,96] The most common HPV subtypes detected in OPC are HPV 16 and 18 (68% and 34%, respectively).[4,95,97] Other types of HPV detected in OSCC are HPV-6,11,31,33,35, and 56. Generally, HPV-associated OPC is histologically less differentiated than non-HPV-associated OPC and has better prognosis. No similar trend has been reported for oral cancer.[3]

Herpes simplex virus has been reported to produce a number of mutations in cells. A co-carcinogenic effect between Herpes simplex virus and chewing tobacco has been demonstrated in animal studies, but not in human studies. Smokers demonstrate higher antibody titers to Herpes simplex virus, suggesting reactivation. Neutralizing antibodies to Herpes simplex virus are present in the serum of patients with oral cancer at higher titers in those who have advanced cancer, and antibody response to Herpes simplex virus antigen is greater in patients than in controls. However, Herpes simplex virus has not been detected in human OSCC. If Herpes simplex virus plays any role in human OSCC, it would represent a "hit and run" effect, which leaves no evidence of its presence after its oncogenic effect and based on this may represent a coincidental finding.

Presenting Signs and Symptoms

Unfortunately, patients are most often identified after the development of symptoms associated with advanced stages of disease. Discomfort is the most common symptom that leads a patient to seek care and may be present at the time of diagnosis in up to 85% of patients.[14] Individuals may also present with an awareness of a mass in the mouth or neck. Dysphagia, odynophagia, otalgia, limited movement, oral bleeding, neck masses, and weight loss may occur with advanced disease. Loss of sensory function, especially when it is unilateral, is a red flag that may indicate neural involvement and requires that cancer be ruled out. Loss of function involving the tongue can affect speech, swallowing, and diet.

Possible tissue changes may include a red, white, or mixed red-and-white lesion; a change in the surface texture producing a smooth, granular, rough, or crusted lesion; or the presence of a mass or ulceration (Figures 8-2–8-6).

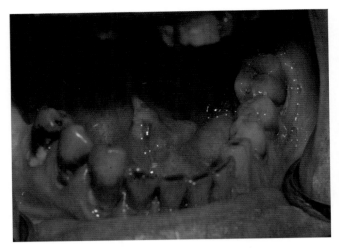

FIGURE 8-2 Nonindurated, nontender, asymptomatic red lesion (erythroplakia) involving the floor of the mouth, pathologic interpretation: squamous cell carcinoma.

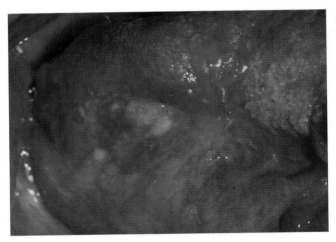

FIGURE 8-3 Irregular leukoplakia/erythroplakia on the right lateral tongue in the site of a previous T1N0MO cancer treated by surgical excision. Biopsy identified recurrent squamous cell carcinioma.

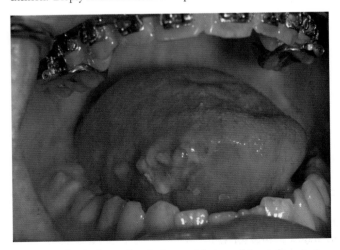

FIGURE 8-4 Indurated and ulcerated lesion of the right anterior tongue in a 15-year-old girl, persisting after removal of orthodontic appliances, proven to be squamous cell carcinoma on biopsy.

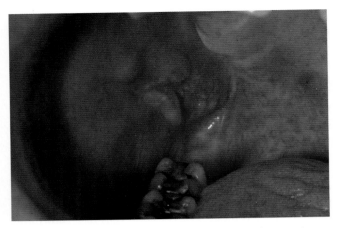

FIGURE 8-5 Nonpainful, irregular, indurated exophytic and ulcerated buccal mass histolpathology revealed squamous cell carcinoma.

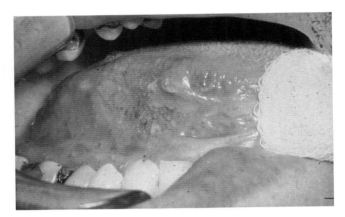

FIGURE 8-6 Eroded, erythroleukoplakic, indurated lesion in the right posterior third of the lateral border of tongue diagnosed as squamous cell carcinoma.

The lesion may be flat or elevated and may be minimally palpable or indurated. The high-risk sites for oral carcinoma include the lower lip, the anterior floor of the mouth, and the lateral borders of the tongue.

The clinical presentation may take a different shape in verrucous carcinoma, a subtype of OSCC with characteristic clinical findings. It can be described clinically as grainy, papillary, verruciform, fungating, or cauliflower-like. Verrucous carcinoma may develop from progression of proliferative verrucous leukoplakia and progress to carcinoma.[98–100]

Lymphatic spread of oral carcinoma most commonly involves the submandibular and digastric nodes, and the upper cervical nodes, but can also involve the remaining nodes of the cervical chain. The nodes most commonly involved are those that are on the same side as the primary tumor, although the closer the tumor is to the midline and the more posterior in the oral cavity or oropharynx, the more common are the involvement of the bilateral and contralateral nodes. Lymph node involvement may not occur in an orderly fashion. Lymph nodes associated with cancer become enlarged and firm to hard in texture, and with progression may become fixed and not mobile. The nodes are not tender unless they are associated with secondary infection or an inflammatory response is present, which may occur after a biopsy. The fixation of nodes to adjacent tissue due to invasion of cells through the capsule is a late occurrence and is evidence of aggressive disease. The fixation of the primary tumor to adjacent tissue overlying bone suggests the involvement of the periosteum and possible spread to bone. Spread of tumor is critical for prognosis and for selection of treatment. The understaging of nodes by cursory assessment or the overstaging of nodes following a biopsy, when an inflammatory component may be present, impacts the selection of treatment. Therefore, accurate node examination is needed before biopsy.

Diagnosis and Histopathology

The diagnosis is primarily based on histopathology. Within the epithelial tumors, SCC is the most prevalent oral malignancy. It has several subtypes based on histopathology (Table 8-1). Some of the variants may have unique clinical presentation.

For the diagnosis of OSCC, dysplasia involves the full thickness of the epithelium and the basement membrane is violated. Dysplasia describes a range of cellular abnormalities that includes changes in cell size and morphology, increased mitotic figures, hyperchromatism, nuclear size and nuclear-cytoplasmic ratio, and alteration in normal cellular orientation and maturation. Well-differentiated carcinoma retains some anatomic features of epithelial cells including the ability to produce keratin, whereas poorly differentiated carcinoma loses the anatomic pattern and function of epithelium. Tumors may be associated with a mixed inflammatory infiltrate. Inflammatory and reactive lesions can be difficult to differentiate from dysplasia, and the experience of the pathologist becomes important with the need for clinical reassessment and repeat investigation. Invasion of lymphatics, blood vessels, and perineural spaces is of critical importance but is difficult to determine.

Histologically, verrucous carcinoma is characterized by piling up of keratin on the surface, with downgrowth of club-shaped fingers of hyperplastic epithelium with a pushing front rather than infiltration into the connective tissue. Dysplasia may be mild. Usually, a dense infiltrate of lymphocytes and plasma cells is present. Verrucous carcinoma rarely spreads to lymph nodes and typically remains locally destructive.[101] The difficulty in diagnosis and treatment is due to benign histology or mild dysplastic change that may be seen despite progressive and recurrent disease.

The term "basaloid squamous carcinoma (BSC)" has been introduced for tumors of which the major portion is composed of solid growth of basaloid cells with small cystic spaces containing periodic acid–Schiff– and alcian blue–positive material. The histologic hallmark of the neoplasm is that of an OSCC in intimate relationship with a basaloid component. Immunohistochemical findings may be helpful in distinguishing BSC from the histopathologically similar tumors.[102] HPV-associated cancers of the oral cavity are more likely to have basaloid features.[103] BSC has a poorer prognosis than the conventional SCC.

Spindle cell carcinoma, also referred to as sarcomatoid SCC, is a rare variant of SCC. The histologic criteria of spindle cell carcinoma is dependent on the demonstration of epithelial changes ranging from prominent dysplasia to frank OSCC in conjunction with a dysplastic spindle cell element or evidence of direct transition of epithelial cells to dysplastic spindle cells. Osteoid-appearing material within the spindle cell component can be found.[104]

A few cases have been reported of adenoid SCCs of the oral mucosa. It is also known as acantholytic SCC. It is mostly seen in the skin and very rare in the oral cavity. The adenoid structure results from loss of cohesion of the epidermoid tumor cells. It may show pseudovascular morphology.[105]

Papillary SCC is an exophytic papillary lesion that shows epithelial dysplasia, possibly even carcinoma in situ, and relatively inconspicuous areas of invasive SCC and should be distinguished from verrucous carcinomas.[106]

Rare cases of carcinoma cuniculatum have been reported. Carcinoma cuniculatum is a rare variant of carcinomas usually involving the foot. Histologically, stratified squamous epithelium is observed with keratin-filled crypts but without cytologic features of malignancy.[107]

Intraoral sebaceous carcinoma probably represents a sebaceous-like differentiation. It is relatively rare. The differential diagnosis may be confused with mucoepidermoid carcinoma.[108]

While histopathology is the gold standard in diagnosis, it is a subjective assessment of tissue, with inter- and intrarater variability.[100,109] However, phenotypic changes appear following molecular changes, and it is possible that as molecular markers become available, they will provide additional information and may ultimately become the gold standard in diagnosis and even targets for therapy.[110]

Histopathology is important in the grading of the SCC. Grading refers to the degree of histopathologic derangement of the tissue architecture and difference of the cellular morphology as compared to normal tissue. The less-differentiated tumors receive the higher grading score on a scale of I to III or a scale of I to IV, with less differentiation at higher score. High grade cancer represents a more aggressive tumor.

Staging of Oral Cancer—TNM System

The American Joint Committee on Cancer (AJCC) has developed Tumor-Nodes-Metastasis (TNM) staging system of cancer, which reflects the prognosis, and is therefore determinants for the treatment strategy.[111] T is the size of the primary tumor, N indicates the presence of regional lymph nodes, and M indicates distant metastasis. The staging system for OSCC combines the T, N, and M to classify lesions as stages 1 through 4. The AJCC classification is principally a clinical description of the disease. Many clinicians combine an imaging-based assessment of the size, lymph nodes, and metastasis with the AJCC clinical staging.

There are separate TNM classifications for carcinoma of the lip and oral cavity (Table 8-4), cancer of the oropharynx (Table 8-4), and salivary gland carcinomas (Table 8-5). The classification uses the same principles with adjustment to the specific anatomical region. It is important that the site of the primary cancer from the oral cavity and oropharynx and lip be clearly separated in order that etiology and outcomes of SCC at each location can be assessed.

TABLE 8-4	Staging of oral cancer and oropharyngeal cancer	
	Staging of Oral Squamous Cell Carcinoma[a]	**Staging of Oropharyngeal Cancer**[a]
TX	Primary tumor cannot be assessed	Primary tumor cannot be assessed
T0	No evidence of primary tumor	No evidence of primary tumor
Tis	Carcinoma in situ	
T1	Tumor 2 cm or less in greatest dimension	Tumor 2 cm or less in greatest dimension without extraparenchymal extension[b]
T2	Tumor more than 2 cm but not more than 4 cm in greatest dimension	Tumor more than 2 cm but not more than 4 cm in greatest dimension without extraparenchymal extension
T3	Tumor more than 4 cm in greatest dimension	Tumor more than 4 cm in greatest dimension or extension to lingual surface of epiglottis
T4a	Moderately advanced local disease[b]	Moderately advanced local disease
	(lip) Tumor invades through cortical bone, inferior alveolar nerve, floor of mouth, or skin (chin or nose)	Tumor invades the larynx, extrinsic muscle of tongue, medial pterygoid, hard palate, or mandible[b]
	(oral cavity) Tumor invades through cortical bone, into deep/extrinsic muscle of tongue (genioglossus, hyoglossus, palatoglossus, and styloglossus), maxillary sinus, or skin of face	
T4b	Very advanced local disease	Very advanced local disease
	(lip and oral cavity) Tumor invades masticator space, pterygoid plates, or skull base, or encases internal carotid artery	Tumor invades lateral pterygoid muscle, pterygoid plates, lateral nasopharynx, or skull base, or encases carotid artery
NX	Regional lymph nodes cannot be assessed	Regional lymph nodes cannot be assessed
N0	No regional lymph node metastasis	No regional lymph node metastasis[c]
N1	Metastasis in a single ipsilateral lymph node, 3 cm or less in greatest dimension	Metastasis in a single ipsilateral lymph node, 3 cm or less in greatest dimension
N2	Metastasis in a single ipsilateral lymph node, more than 3 cm but not more than 6 cm in greatest dimension	Metastasis in a single ipsilateral lymph node, more than 3 cm but not more than 6 cm in greatest dimension
	In multiple ipsilateral lymph nodes, none more than 6 cm in greatest dimension	In multiple ipsilateral lymph nodes, none more than 6 cm in greatest dimension
	In bilateral or contralateral lymph nodes, none more than 6 cm in greatest dimension	In bilateral or contralateral lymph nodes, none more than 6 cm in greatest dimension
N2a	Metastasis in a single ipsilateral lymph node, more than 3 cm but not more than 6 cm in greatest dimension	Metastasis in a single ipsilateral lymph node, more than 3 cm but not more than 6 cm in greatest dimension
N2b	Metastasis in multiple ipsilateral lymph nodes, none more than 6 cm in greatest dimension	Metastasis in multiple ipsilateral lymph nodes, none more than 6 cm in greatest dimension
N2c	Metastasis in bilateral or contralateral lymph nodes, none more than 6 cm in greatest dimension	Metastasis in bilateral or contralateral lymph nodes, none more than 6 cm in greatest dimension
N3	Metastasis in a lymph node more than 6 cm in greatest dimension	Metastasis in a lymph node more than 6 cm in greatest dimension
M0	No distant metastasis	No distant metastasis
M1	Distant metastasis	Distant metastasis
Stage grouping		
Stage 0	Tis N0 M0	
Stage I	T1 N0 M0	
Stage II	T2 N0 M0	
Stage III	T3 N0 M0	
	T1 N1 M0	
	T2 N1 M0	
	T3 N1 M0	

TABLE 8-4	Staging of oral cancer and oropharyngeal cancer (*Continued*)	
	Staging of Oral Squamous Cell Carcinoma[a]	Staging of Oropharyngeal Cancer[a]
Stage IVA		T4a N0 M0
		T4a N1 M0
		T1 N2 M0
		T2 N2 M0
		T3 N2 M0
		T4a N2 M0
Stage IVB		Any T N3 M0
		T4b Any N M0
Stage IVC		Any T Any N M1

[a]Superficial erosion alone of bone/tooth socket by gingival primary is not sufficient to classify a tumor as T4.
[b]Mucosal extension to lingual surface of epiglottis from primary tumors of the base of the tongue and vallecula does not constitute invasion of larynx.
[c]Metastases at level VII are considered regional lymph node metastases.
Source: Adapted with permission from AJCC.[111]

TABLE 8-5	Staging of Salivary Gland Tumors	
TX	Primary tumor cannot be assessed	
T0	No evidence of primary tumor	
T1	Tumor 2 cm or less in greatest dimension without extraparenchymal extension[a]	
T2	Tumor more than 2 cm but not more than 4 cm in greatest dimension without extraparenchymal extension	
T3	Tumor more than 4 cm in greatest dimension and/or tumor having extraparenchymal extension	
T4a	Moderately advanced local disease[a]	
	Tumor invades skin, mandible, ear canal, and/or facial nerve	
T4b	Very advanced local disease	
	Tumor invades skull base and/or pterygoid plates and/or encases carotid artery	
NX	Regional lymph nodes cannot be assessed	
N0	No regional lymph node metastasis	
N1	Metastasis in a single ipsilateral lymph node, 3 cm or less in greatest dimension	
N2	Metastasis in a single ipsilateral lymph node, more than 3 cm but not more than 6 cm in greatest dimension	
	In multiple ipsilateral lymph nodes, none more than 6 cm in greatest dimension	
	In bilateral or contralateral lymph nodes, none more than 6 cm in greatest dimension	
N2a	Metastasis in a single ipsilateral lymph node, more than 3 cm but not more than 6 cm in greatest dimension	
N2b	Metastasis in multiple ipsilateral lymph nodes, none more than 6 cm in greatest dimension	
N2c	Metastasis in bilateral or contralateral lymph nodes, none more than 6 cm in greatest dimension	
N3	Metastasis in a lymph node more than 6 cm in greatest dimension	
M0	No distant metastasis	
M1	Distant metastasis	
Stage grouping		
Stage 0		Tis N0 M0
Stage I		T1 N0 M0
Stage II		T2 N0 M0
Stage III		T3 N0 M0
		T1 N1 M0
		T2 N1 M0
		T3 N1 M0

TABLE 8-5	Staging of Salivary Gland Tumors (*Continued*)
Stage IVA	T4a N0 M0
	T4a N1 M0
	T1 N2 M0
	T2 N2 M0
	T3 N2 M0
	T4a N2 M0
Stage IVB	Any T N3 M0
	T4b Any N M0
Stage IVC	Any T Any N M1

[a]Extraparenchymal extension is clinical or macroscopic evidence of invasion of soft tissues. Microscopic evidence alone does not constitute extraparenchymal extension for classification purposes.
Source: Reprinted with permission from AJCC.[111]

Diagnostic Aids

Early detection of potentially malignant and malignant lesions is a continuing goal. Patient history, thorough head and neck and intraoral examinations, is a prerequisite. The definitive test for diagnosis remains tissue biopsy. Several aids to the oral examination have been suggested in the past, including light technologies, vital tissue staining using toluidine blue (TB), and computer-assisted cytology of oral brush biopsy specimens.[112–114] Additional markers based on blood of saliva samples are also under investigation.[115]

Toluidine Blue

Vital staining with TB may be used as an adjunctive aid in assessing potentially malignant oral mucosal lesions. TB is a metachromatic dye, which has an affinity to bind with DNA. TB staining has been correlated with LOH profiles in tissue biopsies. TB can be applied directly to suspicious lesions or used as an oral rinse. The assessment of dye uptake depends on clinical judgment and experience (Figures 8-7 and 8-8). Positive retention of TB (particularly in areas of leukoplakia, erythroplakia, and uptake in a peripheral pattern of an ulcer) may indicate the need for biopsy or assist in identifying the site of biopsy. False-positive dye retention may occur in inflammatory and ulcerative lesions, but false-negative retention is uncommon. A return appointment in 14 days, providing time for inflammatory lesions to improve, may lead to a decrease in false-positive results. TB has been suggested as a diagnostic tool in potentially malignant oral lesions at risk of progressing to squamous cell cancer, where it may provide guidance for the selection for the biopsy site and accelerates the decision to biopsy. In postradiotherapy follow-up, the retention of TB may assist in distinguishing nonhealing ulcers and persistent or recurrent disease.

Currently, TB is cleared by the Food and Drug Administration (FDA) as an adjunctive marking aid in combination with a chemiluminescence light device, rather than to be marketed as a stand-alone diagnostic tool. The use of TB has been suggested by the Council on Scientifics affairs of the American Dental Association, in high-risk patients and

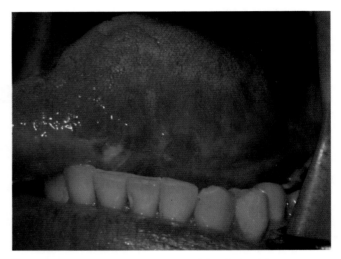

FIGURE 8-7 Asymptomatic erythroplakia-leukoplakia.

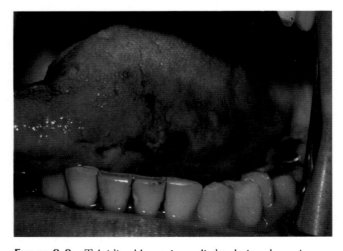

FIGURE 8-8 Toluidine blue stain applied to lesion shown in 8-7, with stain retained on the areas of erythroplakia. Subsequent biopsy diagnosed as squamous cell carcinoma. The more superior area of leukoplakia stained with toluidine blue also diagnosed as squamous cell carcinioma, and would likely not have been diagnosed without toluidine blue, which led to change in the surgical treatment to include this site in the resection.

high-risk clinical settings by experienced providers; however, there is no guidance as to the use of TB in the general practice setting due to lack of clinical studies in these settings.[114]

Visualization Adjunctive Tools

Chemiluminescent devices generate light based on chemical reactions. The suspected area of mucosa appears brighter. Other products generate fluorescent light using a LED source, sometimes combined with optical filtration of a viewfinder, to enhance natural tissue fluorescence. When using the fluorescence light, the suspected area shows loss of fluorescence, which appears dark. Oral cavity fluorescence, using blue light excitation, is thought to represent the tissue structure, metabolic activity, presence of hemoglobin, vessel dilatation, and possibly inflammation.[113] Localized modification in these factors may change the reflective features of the tissue.

These products are promoted to assist the practitioner in discovering mucosal abnormalities, specifically oral potentially malignant disorders and evaluate margins of resection site. There is no consensus regarding the sensitivity and specificity of these devices, and their ability to detect early disease. Nonetheless, fluorescence has been shown to provide evidence on lesion margins in patients with known malignant lesions.

There is an increasing interest in the use of confocal microscopy and optical coherent tomography systems to provide tissue diagnosis in real time, noninvasively, and in situ. Such diagnostic approach is available in dermatology and anticipated to be developed for oral mucosal application in the future. Other imaging modalities are being studied due to the need for improved detection and to assist in diagnosis and treatment.[116]

Cytology

Cytology of the oral mucosa is used to assess cellular morphology. The introduction of a brush designed to sample the entire thickness of the oral epithelium renewed interest in cytology for oral disease.

Originally, the cytobrush was combined with a computer-assisted analysis of the cytologic sample, assessing the cell morphology and keratinization. The final diagnosis was made by a pathologist based on the standard histomorphologic criteria. Further developments in cytology include molecular evaluation of exfoliated cells for molecular markers of dysplasia or carcinoma to improve the diagnostic and prognostic value.[117–121]

Molecular Analysis

Molecular markers obtained from tissue specimens have been suggested to assist with detection and evaluation of cancerous lesions including c-erbB2, Ki67/Mcm2, Cyclin D1, p53, COX-1 and 2, telomerase, loss of 3p or 9p, 8p, 4q, 11q, 13q, 17p.[76,122,123] Studies have also shown that biomarkers of OSCC are present in saliva.[124–129] Despite the potential of a number of new molecular approaches for cancer detection,

further study is needed as much of the current technology limits their implementation into routine clinical use.[130]

Microarray technology has enabled studies of potential biomarkers of protean types (methylation, mRNA, chromosomal insertion and deletion, miRNA, and protein biomarkers) that are specific to the OSCC state and to its metastasis. However, use in clinical practice is not possible at this time and continuing research and technical development is needed.[131]

Single-nucleotide polymorphisms are caused by a change in the genomic sequence in a single nucleotide. It may not necessarily lead to an amino acid alteration but may be a marker for disease predisposition. Genetic polymorphism is in its early stages of investigation for oral cancer.[132,133]

Imaging

Routine radiology, computed tomography (CT), nuclear scintiscanning, magnetic resonance imaging, and ultrasonography can provide evidence of bone involvement or can indicate the extent of some soft tissue lesions (Figures 8-9 to 8-15). The selection of the appropriate imaging modality is dependent on the type and location of the suspected tumor. Positron emission therapy using the radiolabeled glucose analog 18-fluorodeoxyglucose offers a functional imaging approach for the entire body.

Acquisition of a Tissue Specimen

In addition to standard surgical biopsy techniques, tissue can be acquired for histopathology by using fine-needle aspiration (FNA) or core needle biopsy (CNB). Open biopsy of enlarged lymph nodes is not recommended; in such cases, FNA biopsy should be considered. FNA/CNB also may aid in the evaluation of suspicious masses in other areas of the head and neck, including masses that involve salivary glands, tongue, and palate, or when there is contraindication for conventional biopsy (e.g., thrombocytopenia). Ultrasound may assist in guiding FNA/CNB.

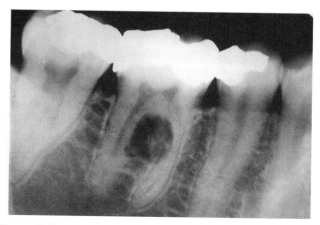

FIGURE 8-9 Periapical radiograph demonstrating bone destruction in the furcation of the first molar tooth and associated resorption of the root. A subsequent biopsy specimen demonstrated squamous cell carcinoma, which was diagnosed as a primary intra-alveolar lesion.

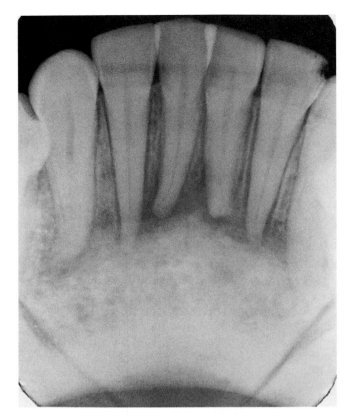

FIGURE 8-10 Periapical radiograph demonstrating an irregular radiolucency involving the bone of the apical region of the mandibular anterior teeth, without a change in root anatomy. The teeth tested vital. The radiographic finding was the first indication of involvement of the bony adenocarcinoma.

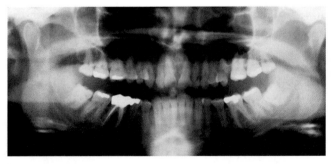

FIGURE 8-11 Panoramic radiograph taken at the time of diagnosis of adenocarcinoma.

Treatment

The principal objective of treatment is to cure the patient of cancer. The choice of treatment depends on cell type and degree of differentiation, the site and size of the primary lesion, lymph node status, the presence of local bone involvement, the ability to achieve adequate surgical margins, and the presence or absence of metastases. Treatment decisions are also impacted by appraisal of the ability to preserve oropharyngeal function, including speech, swallowing, and

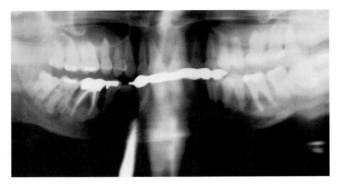

FIGURE 8-12 Massive bone destruction of the mandible, shown after 5 years of follow-up in a case of adenocarcinoma (see Figures 8-10 and 8-11) extending to the molar regions bilaterally. The anterior teeth had been lost due to progressive destruction of the anterior mandible and floor of the mouth.

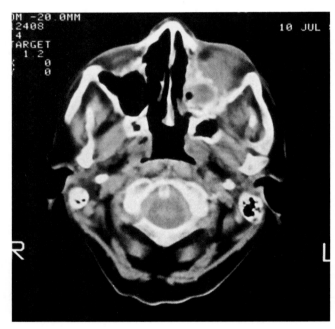

FIGURE 8-13 Computed tomographic scan demonstrating destruction of the medial wall of the antrum and opacification of the antrum. Additional views suggested that the opacification represented a tissue mass that was consistent with tumor.

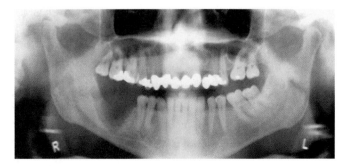

FIGURE 8-14 Panoramic radiograph showing bony destruction of the molar region of the right mandible due to invasion of contiguous tumor. Paresthesia of the right lip was present at the time of diagnosis.

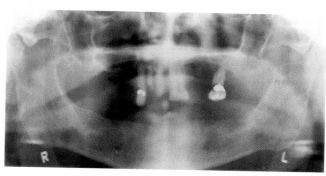

FIGURE 8-15 Panoramic radiograph demonstrating a destructive lesion of the right mandible overlying the mandibular canal. Anesthesia of the mandibular nerve and jaw pain were present. The bone biopsy specimen was consistent with metastatic colon carcinoma, which was subsequently diagnosed.

esthetics, as well as the medical and mental status of the patient. Furthermore, the support available to the patient throughout therapy, a thorough assessment of the potential complications of each therapy, the experience of the oncologist team, and the personal preferences and cooperation of the patient all influence the operative decisions. If the lesion is not cured by the initial therapy, the options for treatment may be limited, and the likelihood of cure is reduced.[134]

Surgery and radiation are used with curative intent in the treatment of oral cancer. Chemotherapy and targeted therapy are used together with the principal therapeutic modalities of radiation and surgery and is now considered the benchmark for management of advanced disease. Either surgery or radiation may be used for T1 and T2 lesions; however, combined radiation and chemotherapy with or without surgery is usually employed for more advanced disease.

Technical advances such as intensity-modulated radiotherapy (IMRT), newer faster forms of image-guided IMRT (image-guided radiotherapy [IGRT]), and proton beam therapy reduce the size of the high-dose field of irradiation and limit the exposure of adjacent vital structures, including the salivary glands. However, the total tissue volume that is exposed to lower doses increases. Due to poor cure rates in head and neck cancer, particularly at advanced stages of disease, more intensive treatment including hyperfractionation, combined chemoradiotherapy, and re-irradiation for recurrence of second primary cancers are utilized.

Surgery

Surgery is indicated for (1) early or localized oral cancer, (2) tumors involving bone, and when the side effects of surgery are expected to be less significant than those associated with radiation, (3) tumors that lack sensitivity to radiation, and (4) recurrent tumor in areas that have previously received radiotherapy. Surgery also may be used in palliative cases to reduce the bulk of the tumor and to promote drainage from a blocked cavity (e.g., antrum). Surgery may fail due to incomplete excision, tumor seeding in the wound, and tumor biology, including unrecognized lymphatic or hematogenous

spread, neural invasion, or perineural spread. Adequate surgical margins are required but may not be attainable due to the size and the location of the tumor and limited information on the molecular status of the margins.

Surgery results in a sacrifice of structure and associated postsurgery fibrosis, which may have important esthetic and functional considerations. In some cases with minimal bone involvement of the alveolar crest, a partial mandibulectomy may allow the continuity of the mandible to be maintained. However, in many cases, mandibulectomy and resection in continuity with the involved nodes are required. Surgical management of clinically positive cervical nodes is often completed at the time of primary surgery. Neck dissection can be used in salvage treatment of cancer that has recurred in the neck. Tumors with node involvement should be treated aggressively due to poorer prognosis that is seen with positive nodes. Management of the N0 neck remains a subject of discussion.[135,136]

Surgical excision of dysplastic and malignant lesions can be accomplished with laser therapy. Such therapy for these lesions is generally well tolerated and usually decreases the period of hospitalization and may have similar outcomes as traditional surgical interventions.[137] However, laser therapy has the disadvantage of limiting the assessment of the margins for histopathologic confirmation.

In respect to OPC and tongue base cancer, transoral robotic surgery has become a common practice with the potential advantage of application in less accessible sites.[138,139] Controlled clinical trials are needed to assess this technique's added value to the armamentarium of treatment approaches.

Additional advances in surgical management include new surgical approaches and new approaches to reconstruction, such as vascularized flaps, microvascular reconstruction, and neurologic anastomoses of free grafts.[140] Reconstruction with the use of osseointegrated implants offers the ability to provide stable prostheses and enhanced esthetic and functional results. The ability to place implants in irradiated bone has increased options for rehabilitation.

Radiation Therapy

Radiation therapy may be administered with intent to cure, as a single modality, as part of a combined radiation surgery and/or chemotherapy management, or for palliation.[134,141,142] Radiotherapy with intent to cure causes early and late toxicities. In palliative care, radiation may provide symptomatic relief from pain, bleeding, ulceration, and oropharyngeal obstruction. Hyperfractionation of radiation (usually twice-daily dosing) is one of the strategies to increase intensity of treatment to increase tumoricidal effects, which results in more severe acute effects. High-dose re-irradiation is offered in some centers as salvage treatment and may be considered in case of recurrent or second primary head and neck cancer, particularly when salvage surgery is not feasible.

Radiation kills cells by interaction with water molecules in the cells, producing charged molecules that interact with biochemical processes in the cells and by causing direct damage to DNA. The affected cells may die or remain incapable of division. Due to a greater potential for cell repair in normal tissue than in malignant cells and a greater susceptibility to radiation due to the higher growth fraction of cancer cells, a differential effect is achieved. To achieve therapeutic effects, radiation therapy is delivered in daily fractions for a planned number of days. The relatively hypoxic central tumor cells are less susceptible to radiotherapy but may become better oxygenated as peripheral cells are affected by radiation and thus become more susceptible to subsequent fractions of radiation. OSCCs are considered radiosensitive, and early lesions are highly curable. In general, the more differentiated the tumor, the less rapid will be the response to radiotherapy. Exophytic and well-oxygenated tumors are more radiosensitive, whereas large invasive tumors with small growth fractions are generally less responsive. OSCC that involves bone reduces the probability of response and cure with radiation alone. Small cervical metastases may be controlled with radiation therapy alone when included in the treated volume, although advanced cervical node involvement is better managed with combined therapy.

The biologic effect of radiation depends on the dose per fraction, the number of fractions per day, the total treatment time, the total dose of radiation, and the radiation used (e.g., electron, neutron, proton). Methods for representing the factors of dose, fraction size, and time of radiation with a single calculation using the time-dose fraction (TDF) and the nominal standard dose (NSD) calculations have been described.[143–148] When comparing studies of radiation effect and when describing the results of studies of cancer patients treated with radiotherapy, reporting the total dose is inadequate because of the importance of fraction size and the time of therapy (which are not available for comparison). The use of the TDF or the NSD will facilitate the understanding of the biologic effect. The tolerance of the vascular and connective tissues to radiation influences both the success of tumor control and the development of treatment complications. The late complications of radiotherapy are due to effects on vascular, connective, and slowly proliferating parenchymal tissues. Late effects are related to the number of fractions, fraction size, total dose, tissue type, and volume of tissue irradiated and if combined with chemotherapy. An increase in fraction size or a reduction in the number of fractions with the same total dose results in increased late complications, including tissue fibrosis and soft tissue and bone necrosis.

Radiation therapy has the advantage of treating the disease in situ and avoiding the need for the removal of tissue and may be the treatment of choice for many T1 and T2 tumors, particularly in the base of the tongue and oropharynx.[134] Radiation may be administered to a localized lesion by using implant techniques (brachytherapy) or to a region of the head and neck by using external beam radiation. External beam therapy can be provided in such a way as to protect adjacent uninvolved tissues, with enhanced effects by using smaller boost fields or by combining external beam and interstitial techniques. Innovations in radiation therapy include IMRT, using radiation beams of varying intensity, which provides the ability to conform the prescription dose to the shape of the target tissues in three dimensions, reducing the dose to surrounding normal tissues. During the optimization process, each beam is divided into small "beamlets" whose intensity can be varied so that the optimal dose and distribution are obtained. The resultant intensity profile of each beam is complex. Rapid dose gradients outside the target result in sparing of normal tissues. IMRT and other advanced beam therapies are ideally suited for head and neck malignancies given the proximity of these tumors to critical structures, including the brainstem, optic chiasm, and salivary glands. IMRT has been shown to have comparable disease control as standard radiotherapy in head and neck oncology, with reduced acute and late toxicity. Additional ability to modify dose and fields of radiation has been introduced with IGRT in which integrated CT guides changes in radiation throughout the course of treatment as treatment causes change in volume of tumor during treatment. Proton and neutron beam therapy results in rapid drop off of radiation that can be tailored to the ideal target, potentially reducing exposure of adjacent tissues on entry and exit from the planned target tissue.

The combination of radiotherapy with chemotherapy is a standard approach for management of advanced stage disease (Stage 3 and 4).[134] Combined chemotherapy and radiation therapy has increased cure rates but is associated with a concomitant increase in toxicity. Primary tumors of the posterior third of the tongue, oropharynx, and tonsillar pillar are best treated by external beam radiotherapy, with or without chemotherapy, while localized oral lesions will be treated primarily by surgery.

Combined radiotherapy and surgery combine the advantages and disadvantages of each modality. Advantages of radiotherapy include the potential to eradicate well-oxygenated tumor cells at the periphery of a tumor and to manage subclinical regional disease. Surgery may more readily manage tumor masses that may possess relatively radiation-resistant hypoxic cells and tumor that involves bone.

Often the combined treatment includes the three modalities—radiotherapy, surgery, and chemotherapy. Continuing study may shed a new light about the preferred combined treatment protocol. Parameters related to the radiotherapy (altered fractionation and employing different radiation sources), the surgery, and the chemotherapy (selection of agents and timing) are to be considered.

Radiation can be used preoperatively, postoperatively, or with a planned split-course approach, although there is controversy on the best approach. The advantages of preoperative radiation are the destruction of peripheral tumor cells, the potential control of subclinical disease, and the possibility of converting inoperable lesions into operable lesions. The disadvantages include delayed surgery and delayed postsurgical healing. The addition of chemotherapy following a combination of radiotherapy and surgery is used to treat cells that remain at the margin of resection and potential regional and systemic spread. Local control of the primary disease appears to be similar with preoperative or postoperative radiotherapy, but in some series, the incidence of metastases was lower in the postoperative group.

Radiation Sources

For treatment of superficial tumors, radiation with low penetration may be used. Low-kilovolt radiation (50–300 kV) can be used in the treatment of skin and lip lesions. Electron beam therapy provides superficial radiation and has largely replaced low-kilovolt x-ray machines because electrons produce a rapid dose buildup and falloff of dose; thus, the depth of penetration can be relatively controlled. Electrons are useful in providing radiation to skin lesions, parotid tumors, and cervical nodes. Deep-seated tumors may be treated with heavy-particle irradiation, such as neutron beam radiation, which is considered for salivary gland tumors and central nervous system malignancies.

Megavoltage radiation using cobalt 60 or the use of a linear accelerator of ≥4 MeV is reported to be skin and bone sparing. Linear accelerators are the basis of current technology in photon-based radiation therapy, the differing energies providing variable penetration due to its ability to vary the energy of the photons. Heavy-particle radiation therapy may have increased effect in salivary gland tumors and may be combined with gamma knife surgery for local disease with poor prognostic features.[148] Proton beam therapy is available at some centers, and use in head and neck cancer continues to be evaluated. Facilities with neutron beam capability are less common.[134]

Cancer Treatment Planning

The radiation treatment plan is determined by the tumor site and size, relation to vital structures, the volume to be radiated, radiation technology available, the number of treatment fractions, the total number of days of treatment, and the tolerance of the patient.[142] The dose to the eye, optic chiasm or spinal cord, salivary glands, alveolar bone, and soft tissue can be limited through the selection of the radiation source, field setup, and shielding and by moving the uninvolved tissue out of the field. The current approach to treatment with the greatest potential to spare high-dose irradiation to vital tissue adjacent to tumor includes IMRT, IGRT, and proton therapy. For repeated doses of radiation to be applied to the site of treatment, the patient and the area of treatment are immobilized, using various techniques and materials, including head holders; bandages; laser positioning, using head and neck "landmarks" or tattoos; and custom acrylic shells. Custom shells provide the best means of immobilization and positioning of patients that are critical in IMRT, IGRT, and proton beam therapy. These techniques may be combined with an oral device to position the mandible, allowing the

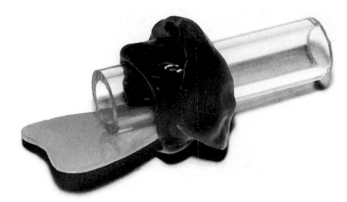

FIGURE 8-16 Tongue and mandibular positioning device. The tube is clear acrylic; the tongue deflector is acrylic but cut to shape and attached by baseplate wax that has been softened and formed to the dentition or residual alveolar ridge.

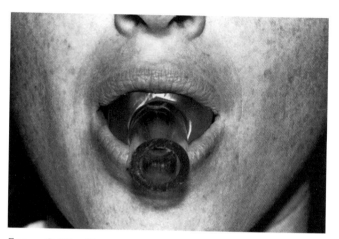

FIGURE 8-17 Tongue and mandibular positioning device placed intraorally. The wax impression and tube displace the soft tissue minimally to reduce the local irritation that can occur during irradiation.

maxilla or mandible to be moved into or out of the radiation field (Figures 8-16–8-18). The oral device can incorporate a tongue depressor to position the tongue in or out of the treatment field. This device can be made by using an acrylic tube around which wax is placed. Impressions in warmed baseplate wax can be readily accomplished with bite pressure. The tube serves as a handle and can facilitate respiration. The device can be left as wax or can be processed in acrylic.

Treatment planning requires localization of the tumor, and tumor margins can be marked with radiopaque gold seeds or lead wire or based on real-time CT such as incorporated into IGRT. If a shell is used, markings can be placed on the shell or by a marking on the skin (Figures 8-19–8-21). The three-dimensional contours of the radiation field as planned by computer modeling and alterations can be made as needed. IGRT provides accurate and ongoing tumor contours and margin delineation during radiotherapy.

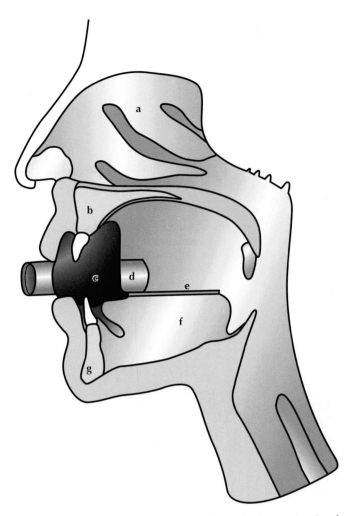

FIGURE 8-18 Schematic diagram of the positioning device placed intraorally. a, nasal cavity; b, upper alveolus; c, wax impression; d, acrylic tube; e, acrylic tongue depressor; f, tongue; g, lower alveolus.

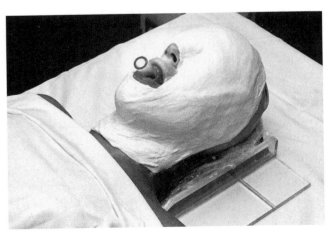

FIGURE 8-19 A patient positioned on a head support. An oral positioning device is in place, and plaster bandages have been placed to form an impression.

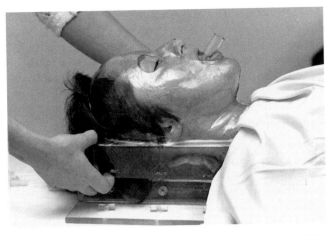

FIGURE 8-20 The acrylic shell is made following removal of the plaster impression. A plaster facial model is poured, and the shell is formed to the model by means of a vacuform technique. The shell and the oral positioning device are used to place the patient in a reproducible position on the machine. Mesh acrylic materials can now be directly adapted to the patients face.

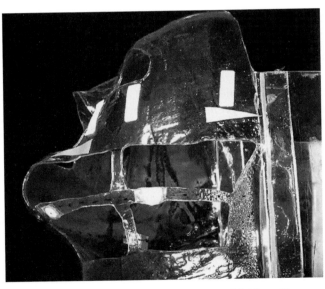

FIGURE 8-21 The final shell with cutouts and field markings and identification wedges prior to radiation treatment.

For most epithelial malignancies, radiation is commonly delivered in 180 to 220 cGy per fraction for six to seven weeks to a total dose of 6500 to 7500 cGy. Hyperfractionation protocols vary; commonly 100 to 150 cGy is delivered twice daily. Therapy can be accelerated to produce a total dose of 5000 cGy in three weeks. In IMRT, computer modeling drives multiple fields in an arc fashion with modulated intensity of the fields. The tumor dose is calculated at the crossover of the fields employed to yield tumoricidal doses in three dimensions conforming to the tumor and avoiding vital structures when possible. Modern radiation therapy is now using smaller margins around the tumor using elaborate treatment algorithms. Smaller number of fields were used in the past (Figure 8-22), which provide the model for modern multifield modulated therapy. More complex setups include boost fields and sequential-field setups to maximize therapeutic effects and reduce complications (Figures 8-23 and 8-24).

Brachytherapy

Interstitial and intracavitary implants may be used to treat primary cancers in the head and neck. Brachytherapy may be the primary treatment modality for localized tumors in the anterior two-thirds of the oral cavity, for boosted doses of radiation to a specific site, or for treatment following recurrence. The isotopes used include cesium, iridium, and gold. Directly implanted sources may be used to deliver radiation, or an afterloading technique may be used in which the radiation source is placed by using previously inserted catheters or guide tubes.

The frequency of tissue necrosis is related to the treated volume, fraction size and total dose of radiation therapy, the proximity of the radioactive implant to bone, and the

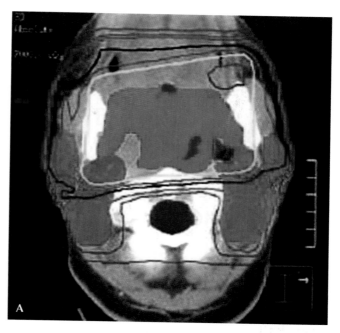

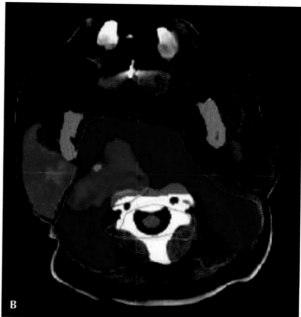

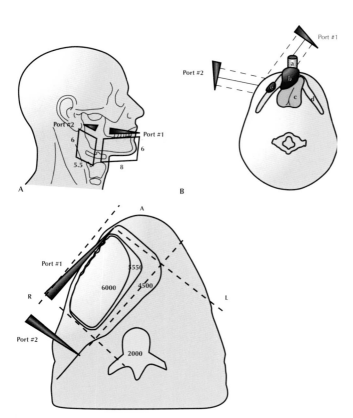

FIGURE 8-22 *A,* Treatment plan for external beam radiotherapy using a wedged-pair field set-up for squamous cell carcinoma involving the buccal mucosa adjacent to the mandible. The field size and wedges are shown. *B,* The positioning device was designed to displace the tongue laterally away from the high-dose volume, as demonstrated in this figure. a, acrylic tube; b, wax impression; c, tongue; d, mandible; e, tumor. *C,* Radiotherapy treatment plan with detailed representation of the field set-up and isodose calculations. IMRT provides multiple fields or "beamlets" allowing tissue contours to maximize radiation over the tumor and minimize dose to critical structures, but extends low dose radiation on a broader area.

FIGURE 8-23 *A,* Conventional radiation is delivered in few fields and may result in high-dose exposure across the region of exposure. Exposure to vital structures such as midbrain and optic nerves and salivary gland may be included in the high-dose volume. *B,* IMRT allows control of contours of radiation fields and allows tailoring of dose to enable high dose to tumor volumes and shaping of fields to result in reduced dose to vital tissues such as brain stem, optic nerves, and salivary gland.

presence of comorbid risk factors including dental status. Tissue deflectors can be made to deflect the tongue so that an implant designed to treat a cancer of the tongue does not expose adjacent alveolar bone. These devices can be fabricated by using a double layer of flexible mouthguard material or by

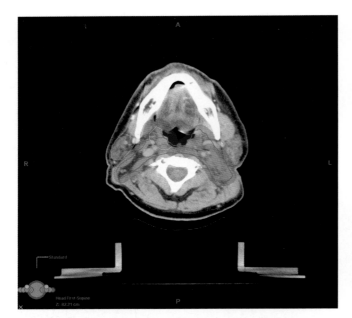

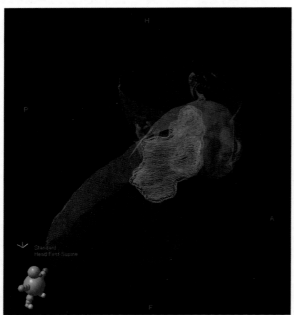

FIGURE 8-24 *A,* Two-dimensional representation of IMRT dosing to unilateral tumor, with minimal dose to salivary glands and spinal cord, with high treatment dose to tumor and parapharyngeal lymph nodes. *B,* Three-dimensional reconstruction of treatment fields using IMRT, where doses are contoured in three dimensions to maximize tumor dose and minimize dose to vital and uninvolved structures.

using heat-cured acrylic (Figure 8-25). Lead foil can be added to the surface of the deflector if needed. Similarly, devices can be made to keep radiation from superficial treatment of the lip from affecting the alveolar bone (Figure 8-26). Lead cutouts can be made and placed on the skin to isolate the lesion; these may be used in combination with an intraoral device that can shield the intraoral tissues (Figure 8-27).

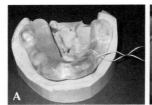
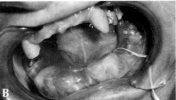

FIGURE 8-25 *A,* Tongue deflector, fabricated by using three thicknesses of vacuform vinyl on the side of the planned implant. The vinyl provides a smooth soft surface to displace the tongue away from the alveolus. *B,* The appliance in situ.

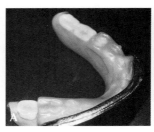
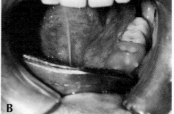

FIGURE 8-26 *A,* A denture that has been modified with a double thickness of lead shielding attached with baseplate wax. *B,* The modified appliance, shown in situ, prevents exposure of the alveolus to the radiation source.

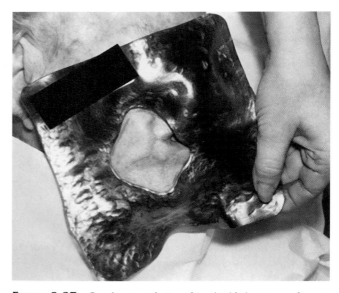

FIGURE 8-27 Lead cutout designed to shield the tissue adjacent to the tumor from radiation exposure.

Chemotherapy
Cytotoxic Chemotherapy

Chemotherapy may be used as induction therapy prior to local therapies, concurrent chemoradiotherapy (CCRT), and adjuvant chemotherapy after local treatment.[134,142] The common chemotherapy protocols are listed in Table 8-6.

The objective of induction chemotherapy is to promote initial tumor reduction and to provide early treatment of micrometastases due to the recognition that local control

TABLE 8-6	Current Chemotherapy Regimens for Locally Advanced Oral Cancer (Stages III–IVB)	
Patient Stage	**Chemotherapy Regimen**	**Comment**
For primary systemic therapy with concurrent radiation		
	Cisplatin 100 mg/m² IV on days 1, 22, and 43	
	Cisplatin 40–50 mg/m² IV weekly for 6–7 wk	
	Cetuximab 400 mg/m² IV loading dose 1 wk before the start of radiation therapy, then 250 mg/m² weekly	Premedicate with dexamethasone, diphenhydramine, and ranitidine
	Cisplatin 20 mg/m² IV on day 2 weekly for up to 7 wk plus paclitaxel 30 mg/m² IV on day 1 weekly for up to 7 wk	
	Cisplatin 20 mg/m²/d IV on days 1–4 and 22–25 plus 5-FU 1000 mg/m²/d by continuous IV infusion on days 1–4 and 22–25	
	5-FU 800 mg/m² by continuous IV infusion on days 1–5 given on the days of radiation plus hydroxyurea 1 g PO q12h (11 doses per cycle)	Chemotherapy and radiation given every other week for a total of 13 wk
	Carboplatin 70 mg/m²/d IV on days 1–4, 22–25, and 43–46 plus 5-FU 600 mg/m²/d by continuous IV infusion on days 1–4, 22–25, and 43–46	
	Carboplatin AUC 1.5 IV on day 1 weekly plus paclitaxel 45 mg/m² IV on day 1 weekly	
For patients receiving postoperative concurrent chemoradiation		
	Cisplatin 100 mg/m² IV on days 1, 22, and 43 (3, 4) or 40–50 mg/m² IV weekly for 6–7 wk	
For induction chemotherapy		
	Docetaxel 75 mg/m² IV on day 1 plus cisplatin 100 mg/m² IV on day 1 plus 5-FU 100 mg/m²/d by continuous IV infusion on days 1–4 every 3 wk for three cycles; then 3–8 wk later, carboplatin AUC 1.5 IV weekly for up to 7 wk during radiation therapy; then 6–12 wk later, pursue surgery if applicable	
	Docetaxel 75 mg/m² IV on day 1 plus cisplatin 75 mg/m² IV on day 1 plus 5-FU 750 mg/m²/d by continuous IV infusion on days 1–4 every 3 wk for four cycles; then 4–7 wk later, radiation	Surgical resection can be pursued before or after chemotherapy
	Paclitaxel 175 mg/m² IV on day 1 plus cisplatin 100 mg/m² IV on day 2 plus 5-FU 500 mg/m²/d by continuous IV infusion on days 2–6 every 3 wk for three cycles; then radiation with cisplatin 100 mg/m² IV on days 1, 22, and 43	

- Additional chemotherapy protocols, including cetuximab-based protocols, are in use for patients with metastatic (incurable) head and neck cancers.
- Modified from http://emedicine.medscape.com/article/2006216-overview; accessed March 19, 2014.

has improved with aggressive combined therapy, but distant failure due to metastatic disease has increased. The principal agents that have been studied alone or in combination in head and neck cancer are taxol and derivatives, platinum derivatives (cisplatin and carboplatin), 5-fluorouracil, and hydroxyurea, although hydroxyurea is rarely used in current protocols. Chemotherapy, particularly in combination with radiation therapy, is associated with potential local toxicities, such as mucositis; nausea, vomiting, and bone marrow suppression may also occur. The initial tumor response to chemotherapy prior to radiotherapy may predict tumor responsiveness to radiation. Induction chemotherapy has not yet become standard in treatment protocols; there is evidence of impressive response rates; however, survival benefit remains to be established.[150]

CCRT protocols are now the standard of care for stage 3 and 4 as primary therapy and for disease with poor prognostic findings following surgery including close margin and vascular invasion by tumor.[134,151] As CCRT has become more widely used, the morbidities associated with these therapies have become more pronounced.

Targeted Therapy

As with treatment of other malignancies, new target-directed chemotherapeutic agents are being studied as adjuncts or replacements for older agents. The EGFR antibody, cetuximab (Erbitux®, ImClone, New York, NY) has become the first new chemotherapeutic accepted by the FDA for head and neck SCC in decades. The role of EGFR modulators continue to be defined in head and neck SCC. Other EGFR inhibitors, including erlotinib (Tarceva™, OSI Pharmaceuticals, LLC, Northbrook, IL), are under investigation for head and neck squamous cell carcinoma.[152]

Combined Protocols

Cytotoxics and targeted therapy may be used in combination (Table 8-6). Research will continue and may include investigations into increasing the number of drugs used in combination, increasing the number of courses of chemotherapy provided, using modulators of chemotherapeutics, and modifying administration, such as by intermittent and continuous infusion. Throughout all studies, tumor site (oral vs. oropharynx), differentiation, and HPV status are now essential features that must be addressed due to differences in etiology, response to therapy, and prognosis.

Photodynamic Therapy

Photodynamic therapy applies light over a tissue that initially absorbed exogenous sensitizer. The sensitizing agent may be delivered systemically or topically and then after it selectively accumulates in target tissue. The subsequent light delivery to the target tissue results in cellular destruction. Due to the focused cellular destruction, the complications and disfigurement associated with this treatment are relatively small.[153] Although photodynamic therapy in oral cancer has some encouraging preliminary results, it is not accepted routine treatment.[154–159]

Gene Therapy

Gene therapy is being studied with the objective of reversing dysplasia in oral epithelial lesions. The modalities evaluated include suicide gene therapy, immunotherapy, oncolytic virus therapy, inhibition of tumor angiogenesis, gene deletion therapy, and antisense RNA.[160] Considering the high rate of mutation in p53 in oral cancer, gene therapy focused on *p53* gene, mostly with adenoviral vectors, shows promise. Additional target genes and vectors are currently being studied.[160] None of these approaches have reached conventional clinic care settings.

Immunotherapy

Immunotherapy offers the potential for additional approaches to management, alone or in combination with other therapies. Clinical practice guidelines for management of malignant melanoma and other cancers are forthcoming.[161–164] Based on an analysis of a gene expression profile in matched tumor and normal fibroblast cell lines, a number of proteins have been detected that might be potential targets for immunotherapy in individuals with head and neck cancer.[165] Cell lines studies and animal models support the introduction of immunotherapy for treatment of head and neck cancer.[166,167]

Prognosis

The most important predictors for survival of oral cancer are the presence of HPV and stage of disease at diagnosis.[168,169] Unfortunately, the majority of oral cancers continue to be diagnosed in advanced stages, after becoming symptomatic. Cancers positive for HPV, particularly type 16, have a better prognosis compared to HPV-negative tumors[170,171] This fact is now used to stratify the patient's risk; however, HPV testing must not be considered in isolation, as other causative factors, such as tobacco exposure may influence the staging.[172]

Additional prognostic indicators for oral cancer include the depth of penetration, perineural invasion, differentiation level, lymphocytic infiltrate at interface, status of surgical margins.[173,174] Molecular markers are being investigated.[130]

There is rarely a second chance for a cure as cure rates decline rapidly if the lesion is not successfully managed with initial therapy, and therefore, the initial approach to therapy is critical. Locoregional causes of death from head and neck cancer may be due to erosion of major vessels, erosion of the cranial base, nutritional compromise, cachexia, and secondary infection of the respiratory tract. Drinking profile (alcohol use) could affect cancer mortality.[175] The fact that the overall survival in younger patients is better than that of older patients suggests that the more complex medical backgrounds and comorbidities of older patients may lead to additional systemic complications and poorer outcomes.[176]

Prevention

Primary prevention has focused on tobacco as a major cause of upper aerodigestive tract cancers, and attention has been paid to strategies for tobacco cessation.[177–179] Diet has been studied in developing countries with evidence supporting fresh fruits and vegetables, but this has not been evident in the developed world. Likewise vitamin supplements have not been shown effective.[47] HPV, which, as mentioned previously, is associated OPC, is recognized as a sexually transmitted family of viruses. The dramatic increase in HPV-related OPCs leads to consideration for HPV preventive vaccination, and appeal for reduction in numbers of sexual partners and reduced oral-genital contact.[93,95,180]

Head and neck and oral examinations have been shown in a large trial in India to result in earlier identification of OSCC and to translate into improved survival compared with a control group.[181] These findings were confirmed in long-term follow-up in the same study population.[182] Furthermore, it is possible that this approach is cost-effective as shown in this high-risk patient population.[183] But it is unclear whether this approach would be successful in countries with a lower incidence rate of OSCC and a higher paid workforce.

A recent position paper by the US Preventive Services Task Force (USPSTF) noted that there is insufficient evidence to assess the balance of benefits and harms of screening for oral cancer in asymptomatic adults by nondental providers.[184] Although the USPSTF conclusion represents the available evidence in terms of cost-effective and risk benefit analysis, it challenges guidance from a public health perspective and specifically excluded dental providers in its recommendations. It is assumed that early detection based on a visual and tactile examination performed in the dental care setting will be associated with improved survival with reduced costs. Considering that oral cancer screening is an integral component of the overall routine comprehensive head and neck examination in the primary dental care setting (opportunistic screening), it is considered to be good practice.[114,185]

OTHER HEAD AND NECK CANCERS

Malignant Tumors of the Salivary Glands

Salivary gland tumors most commonly arise in the parotid glands, where the majority of tumors are benign. Malignant tumors of the salivary glands develop more commonly in the submandibular, sublingual, and minor salivary glands (approximately 40%, 70%–90%, and 45%–80% of salivary gland malignancies, respectively). The parotids may be the site of transformation in relatively small number of the cases (approximately 15%–35% of salivary gland malignancies). The cause of salivary gland tumors remains obscure, but ionizing radiation has been identified as a risk factor. Many chromosomal events and oncogenes are postulated in the pathogenesis of salivary gland cancer.[186]

Clinical Presentation and Diagnosis

Malignant salivary gland tumors most commonly present as a painless mass. When the mass is superficial or large, it may cause intraoral or extraoral asymmetry. When the mass is intraoral, it may be ulcerated. Neurologic involvement may lead to discomfort and numbness, and with parotid gland tumors, involvement of the facial nerve may cause facial paralysis. In the floor of the mouth, the salivary gland cancer may cause ankyloglossia.[187] Most small malignant lesions are clinically indistinguishable from benign lesions. The most common site of minor salivary gland cancer is the posterior hard palate, but other sites in the oral cavity or upper respiratory tract may be involved. Most salivary gland tumors spread by local infiltration, by perineural or hematogenous spread, and less commonly via lymphatics. The staging of salivary gland tumors is shown in Table 8-5.

Biopsy of masses in the major glands may be accomplished by FNA or CNB,[187,188] and diagnosis may be made without open biopsy. However, surgical biopsy may be necessary if FNA is not diagnostic. In masses involving minor glands, biopsy can be performed with routine techniques.

Treatment and Prognosis

Studies assessing treatment and prognosis are complicated by the large variety of histologic types, and the small numbers seen of salivary gland cancer subtypes. Therefore, treatment trials provide limited guidance. Surgery is the principal treatment of the primary tumor.[189] Despite the anticipated low proliferative index of many salivary gland cancers, radiotherapy at a high dose is effective and may be employed in malignant salivary gland tumors.[186] Postoperative radiation can contribute to cure and improved local control and is indicated for patients with residual disease following surgery, extensive perineural involvement, lymph node involvement, high-grade malignant disease, tumors with more than one local recurrence after surgery, inoperable tumors, or malignant lymphoma and for those who refuse surgery. Doses and fractionation similar to those used in the treatment of SCC are usually employed. Heavy-particle radiation sources (neutron beam and proton beam) have been shown to provide effective treatment for salivary gland tumors.[149]

Various single-agent chemotherapy protocols and combination protocols have been evaluated, but in general all are small studies, limiting conclusions.[21] Unlike with OSCC, chemotherapy does not seem to be effective for advanced or metastatic salivary gland diseases.[190] It is possible that the slow growth of salivary gland cancer could explain the overall poor results to date with chemotherapy protocols. Furthermore, advances in management may mirror those of breast cancer where subtypes of salivary gland cancer may be assessed by evaluation of cell surface markers including HER2-neu, EGFR, and other markers, to guides chemotherapy and targeted therapies.[21] Among the chemotherapeutics examined, limited benefit has been seen, while data on targeted agents is being evaluated alone or in combination with cytotoxic chemotherapy.[190]

The prognosis of salivary gland tumors is related to tumor type (histology and degree of differentiation) and stage of disease (tumor size, lymph node involvement, and extension of disease). Small tumors have favorable prognosis. The "4-cm" rule suggests that cancers that are less than 4 cm do well regardless of histological type or grade.[21,191] Acinic cell tumor, low-grade mucoepidermoid carcinoma, and mixed tumors have a high probability of cure with surgical management. Tumors with a poor prognosis include large tumors, adenocarcinoma, adenoid cystic carcinoma, high-grade mucoepidermoid carcinoma, poorly differentiated carcinoma, and SCC. Histologic findings that correlate with lymph node involvement include deep (>8 mm) and diffuse invasion of stromal tissue and invasion of lymphatics.

Malignant Tumors of the Jaw

Malignant lesions of the jaws may be of hematopoietic origin, such as lymphoma and multiple myeloma, or of bone origin, such as osteosarcoma, chondrosarcoma, and Ewing sarcoma. Metastases to the jaws should be considered during clinical evaluation of any cancer patient with a cancer history, particularly in breast, prostate, gastrointestinal, and renal carcinoma. The following section focuses on osteosarcoma, which is the most common bone-originating jaw malignancy.

Osteosarcoma

Osteosarcoma is a malignant tumor, characterized by the formation of bone or osteoid by tumor cells. Osteosarcomas of the jaws may develop in a broad range of ages but are more common in the third and fourth decade.[192] Osteosarcoma occurs slightly more often in the mandible than in the maxilla. Most osteosarcomas of the jaws are centrally located in the bone. Juxtacortical or parosteal location, a location adjacent to the outer surface of the cortical bone, is unusual. Osteosarcomas may also develop in a patient affected by Paget's disease or in a patient who has been irradiated either for a benign bone lesion or for adjacent soft tissue disease. The latent time period may vary widely.

Clinical Presentation and Diagnosis

The most common presenting finding of osteosarcomas of the jaws is mass (85%–95.5%).[193] Pain accompanies the swelling in approximately half of cases, and trigeminal sensory disturbances occur in about one-fifth of cases.[194] Additional symptoms associated with intraosseous location consist of mobile teeth, toothache, and nasal obstruction.

The radiographic appearance varies between radiopaque, radiolucent, and mixed. The border of the lesion is not well defined. The classic radiograph presentation of "sun ray appearance," in which the radiograph may show an opaque lesion, with bony trabeculae directed perpendicularly to the outer surface. This is observed in about 25% of cases. Over time, there is expansion and perforation of the cortical bone. The osteolytic type is far less characteristic and appears as an ill-defined radiolucency that causes expansion and destruction of the cortical bone. In the presence of teeth, a widening of the periodontal ligament may be observed even before changes can be noticed elsewhere in the bone. Root resorption may create a spiky shape to the apical third. Loss of follicular cortices of unerupted teeth is highly suggestive of malignancy. Widening of the mandibular canal is another ominous sign. Bone scintigraphy will show a positive uptake in tumor but is not diagnostic.

Histopathologically, proliferation of atypical osteoblasts is observed and irregular osteoid and bone formation is seen. A proliferation of anaplastic fibroblasts may be seen. Vascular clefts may be encountered, resulting in terms such as telangiectatic osteogenic sarcoma. Multinucleated giant cells may be scarce or abundant. Osteosarcomas of the jaws are, in general, better differentiated than similar tumors in the long bones. Even if the tumor largely consists of malignant-looking cartilage, the so-called chondroblastic type, it is still to be considered an osteosarcoma whenever osteoid and bone are present in the stroma. Low-grade osteosarcomas may be misdiagnosed as fibrous dysplasia or other benign fibro-osseous lesions. Osteosarcomas are usually graded according to histopathologic criteria in low-grade to high-grade malignancies.

Treatment and Prognosis

Treatment requires aggressive local surgery. Several authors report the use of (neo)adjuvant chemotherapy. Others report that the introduction of chemotherapy did not dramatically alter the prognosis of osteosarcoma of the jaw.[195]

Metastasis is usually via the bloodstream and often occurs within one to two years. Of the patients who die from osteosarcoma, most do so with uncontrolled local disease. The 5- and 10-year survival rates after treatment are approximately 60% to 70% and 50%, respectively.[195,196] Large tumors, higher grade, secondary osteosarcomas or recurrence were associated with decreased survival. Mandibular location and clear surgical margins were associated with improved survival.[152]

Sarcomas of the Soft Tissues

Soft tissue sarcomas of the oral cavity are rare and account for approximately 1% of all oral malignancies.[197,198] Subtypes include fibrosarcoma, malignant fibrous histiocytoma, liposarcoma, rhabdomyosarcoma, leiomyosarcoma, angiosarcoma, and alveolar soft part sarcoma. Soft tissue sarcoma usually presents as a slow- or rapid-growing swelling of the mucosa involving any part of the oral cavity. Treatment usually consists of surgery with adjuvant radiotherapy for those with high-grade tumors and/or positive margins following surgery.[199,200] The efficacy of adjuvant chemotherapy is poorly defined.

Metastases to the Head and Neck

Metastatic tumors to the oral region are uncommon and may occur in the oral soft tissues or in the jawbones. The most common primary sites for oral metastases are the lung, kidney, liver, and prostate for men, and breast, female genital organs, kidney, and colo-rectum for women.[201] Prostate and breast metastases were mainly concentrated in the jaws rather than the soft oral tissues.

The clinical presentation of metastasis to the jawbones includes swelling, pain, and paresthesia.[201] Metastases to the oral soft tissues may manifest as a submucosal mass or gingival mass;[202] ulceration is rare. Metastasis diagnosed at extraction site was reported as well and probably represent a late diagnosis of a pre-existing metastasis to the alveolar bone. Radiographic presentation is mainly radiolucent with poorly defined border, although radiopacities or mixed radiographic lesions may be seen in some cases.[201,203]

A diagnosis of oral metastasis is a poor prognostic indicator, and literature suggest an average seven-month survival time and the treatment is mainly supportive.[201]

OTHER PATHOLOGIC CONDITIONS RELATED TO ORAL CANCER

Nasopharyngeal Carcinoma

NPC presents a number of concerns to dental providers because patients may present with complaints that may mimic temporomandibular disorders (TMDs) or as neck masses.[204] The common clinical presentation of NPC is otalgia and neck mass. Common TMD signs and symptoms include pain and limited jaw opening. Symptoms that aid in differentiation of TMD and NPC may occur late or concurrently and include dysphagia, nasal stuffiness, nose bleed, neck mass, or cranial involvement.[205,206] Risk factors for NPC include Epstein–Barr virus infection, smoking, childhood consumption of salted fish and other preserved foods that are common in a Cantonese diet, and originating from southern China.

Long-term survival is approximately 50% because most patients are identified after the tumor that has spread regionally and with lymph node involvement. FNA can provide tissue diagnosis, and the sensitivity can be enhanced by DNA amplification (polymerase chain reaction) of the Epstein–Barr virus (EBV) genome, which is commonly associated with NPC but is rare in other head and neck cancers. Furthermore, rapid clearance of EBV DNA from plasma may be used as a marker for response to treatment.[207,208] HPV has been reported in NPC, although the clinical significance of this finding is not clear.[94,209]

Treatment requires radiation therapy and increasingly combined radiation therapy and chemotherapy.[206,210] The new radiotherapy techniques may reduce the risk for cancer treatment–related oral complications. Nevertheless, these oral complications are substantial and have great impact on the quality of life in these patients. Surgery may play a role in treatment of recurrent or metastatic disease.[204] Transoral robotic surgery is becoming more commonly used in early-stage NPC. Treatment options for small-volume recurrence include nasopharyngectomy, brachytherapy, radiosurgery, stereotactic radiation therapy, IMRT, or a combination of surgery and radiation therapy, with or without concurrent chemotherapy.[204] For palliative treatment of metastatic disease, radiotherapy and/or chemotherapy is advised.[204] Preliminary clinical data from NPC patients with advanced disease suggest that photodynamic therapy may be helpful, but it is not currently part of standard treatment paradigms.[211]

Paraneoplastic Syndromes and Oral Cancer

Oral cancer is reported in the literature in association with several syndromes or chronic diseases. These disorders are considered paraneoplastic because they accompany the malignant tumor but are not directly related to the cancerous mass, its invasion, or metastasis. The diagnosis of oral cancer may precede, develop simultaneously, or develop following the diagnosis of the paraneoplastic syndrome.

Within the group of endocrine paraneoplastic syndromes, oral cancer may be associated with inappropriate secretion of antidiuretic hormone, humoral hypercalcemia, hypercalcemia with leukocytosis, and autoimmune polyendocrinopathy-candidiasis-ectodermal dystrophy. Within the group of cutaneous paraneoplastic syndromes, oral cancer was associated with Bazex syndrome (acrokeratosis paraneoplastica), Sweet syndrome (acute febrile neutrophilic dermatosis), and paraneoplastic pemphigus.[212,213] Additional vascular, hematological, rheumatoid, and ocular syndromes were associated with oral cancer.[214]

Head and Neck Malignant Disease in AIDS

HIV infection that leads to immunosuppression increases the risk of the development of neoplastic disease.[215] Advances in the management of HIV infection have led to a reduction in the prevalence of manifestations of immunosuppression including oral findings, but if immunosuppression progresses, oral findings may develop. Improved management of HIV disease using combined antiretroviral therapy (CART) and newer agents has led to a dramatic decrease in the prevalence of oral manifestations. Rates of AIDS-defining cancers appeared to be stable across the last decade, except for non-Hodgkin lymphoma (NHL), which appeared to decrease.[216] There are conflicting data in regard to the reduced rate of Kaposi sarcoma (KS) and lymphoma.[217,218]

KS was the most common neoplastic disease of AIDS prior to CART therapy, occurring in up to 55% of homosexual males with AIDS and often representing the first sign of progression to AIDS or occurring during the course of the disease. KS is less common in patients with AIDS whose risk factor is not sexual transmission, suggesting that KS is associated with a sexually transmitted agent, which has been identified as human herpesvirus (HHV)-8. KS is a multicentric neoplastic proliferation of endothelial cells and can involve any oral site, but most frequently involves the attached mucosa of the palate, gingiva, and dorsum of the tongue. Lesions begin as blue purple or red purple flat discolorations that can progress to tissue masses that may ulcerate (Figures 8-28–8-29). The lesions do not blanch with pressure. Initial lesions are asymptomatic but can cause discomfort and interfere with speech, denture use, and eating when lesions progress. The differential diagnosis includes ecchymosis, vascular lesions, salivary gland tumor, and metastatic disease. Definitive diagnosis requires biopsy.

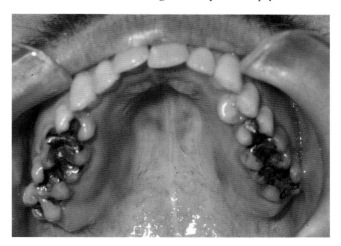

FIGURE 8-28 Bilateral involvement of the anterior and posterior hard palate with purple discolorations consistent with Kaposi sarcoma.

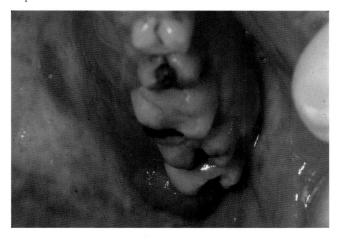

FIGURE 8-29 Palatal and gingival involvement by Kaposi sarcoma, with discoloration and enlargement and soft tissue mass on the maxillary tuberosity.

Intralesional chemotherapy for treatment of oral KS provides effective palliation.[219-223] Intralesional treatment with vinblastine and interferon has been reported. The lesions can be treated with the injection of vinblastine (0.2 mg/mL) under local anesthesia. The effect of treatment may continue for several weeks and may result in palliation for approximately four months (see Figure 8-30). Repeat injection can be completed with similar efficacy. KS is radiosensitive, and radiation can be palliative for regional disease. Fractionated radiotherapy (for a total dose of 25–30 Gy over 1–2 weeks) may be provided for oral KS. If KS progresses at multiple sites, systemic chemotherapy is needed. Additional approaches to management include drugs that reduce angiogenesis, antiviral agents for HHV-8 infection, and agents that block VEGF.

Certain lymphoma subtypes are more common in people with AIDS. NHL is considered an AIDS-defining entity, and this disease is currently the most common type of cancer in HIV-infected individuals in the United States and Europe.[224] NHL, most commonly of B-cell origin, not only may present with central nervous system involvement but also may present with head, neck, or oral lesions. Hodgkin disease is not considered an AIDS-defining malignancy; however, its incidence increased in HIV-infected individuals.[225] The lymphomas are aggressive and carry a poor prognosis. Treatment of lymphoma with chemotherapy for HIV patients on antiretroviral therapy may be challenging.

Oropharyngeal SCC has been reported in patients with HIV disease. In the era of CART, although HPV-related oral lesions are more prevalent, the prevalence of oral or OPCs in patients with HIV is suspected to increase.[226]

SUMMARY

New understanding about oral cancer has emerged in the last few years. This include information about the etiologic risk factors, current epidemiology, advances in treatment of the malignant disease, recommendations for prevention, and importance of surveillance for possible cancer recurrence or new second cancers. The role of the dental profession extends from detection and diagnosis of head and neck cancers throughout the cancer continuum of treatment and survivorship. Appropriate oral care requires an understanding of the disease and treatment and close communication with the oncology team.

Selected Readings

Asiaf A, Ahmad ST, Mohammad SO, Zargar MA. Review of the current knowledge on the epidemiology, pathogenesis, and prevention of human papillomavirus infection. *Eur J Cancer Prev.* 2014;23:206–224.

Blanchard P, Bourhis J, Lacas B, et al. Taxane-cisplatin-fluorouracil as induction chemotherapy in locally advanced head and neck cancers: an individual patient data meta-analysis of the meta-*analysis* of chemotherapy in head and neck cancer group. *J Clin Oncol.* 2013;31:2854–2860.

Cesarman E. Pathology of lymphoma in HIV. *Curr Opin Oncol.* 2013;25:487–494.

Chaturvedi AK, Anderson WF, Lortet-Tieulent J, et al. Worldwide trends in incidence rates for oral cavity and oropharyngeal cancers. *J Clin Oncol.* 2013;31:4550–4559.

Dogan S, Hedberg ML, Ferris RL, et al. Human papillomavirus and Epstein-Barr virus in nasopharyngeal carcinoma in a low-incidence population. *Head Neck.* 2014;36:511–516.

D'Souza G, Cullen K, Bowie J, et al. Differences in oral sexual behaviors by gender, age, and race explain observed differences in prevalence of oral human papillomavirus infection. *PLoS One.* 2014;9:e86023.

Edwards PC. Oral cancer screening for asymptomatic adults: do the United States Preventive Services Task Force draft guidelines miss the proverbial forest for the trees? *Oral Surg Oral Med Oral Pathol Oral Radiol.* 2013;116:131–134.

Fakhry C, D'Souza G. Discussing the diagnosis of HPV-OSCC: common questions and answers. *Oral Oncol.* 2013;49:863–871.

Gonzalez-Moles MA, Scully C, Ruiz-Avila I, Plaza-Campillo JJ. The cancer stem cell hypothesis applied to oral carcinoma. *Oral Oncol.* 2013;49:738–746.

Gotti D, Danesi M, Calabresi A, et al. Clinical characteristics, incidence, and risk factors of HIV-related Hodgkin lymphoma in the era of combination antiretroviral therapy. *AIDS Patient Care STDS.* 2013;27:259–265.

Jemal A, Simard EP, Dorell C, et al. Annual Report to the Nation on the Status of Cancer, 1975–2009, featuring the burden and trends in human papillomavirus(HPV)-associated cancers and HPV vaccination coverage levels. *J Natl Cancer Inst.* 2013;105:175–201.

Huang SH, O'Sullivan B. Oral cancer: current role of radiotherapy and chemotherapy. *Med Oral Patol Oral Cir Bucal.* 2013;18:e233-e240.

Kammerer PW, Koch FP, Santoro M, et al. Prospective, blinded comparison of cytology and DNA-image cytometry of brush biopsies for early detection of oral malignancy. *Oral Oncol.* 2013;49:420–426.

Karimi MY, Kapoor V, Sharma SC, Das SN. Genetic polymorphisms in FAS (CD95) and FAS ligand (CD178) promoters and risk of tobacco-related oral carcinoma: gene-gene interactions in high-risk Indians. *Cancer Invest.* 2013;31:1–6.

Kolokythas A, Bosman MJ, Pytynia KB, et al. A prototype tobacco-associated oral squamous cell carcinoma classifier using RNA from brush cytology. *J Oral Pathol Med.* 2013;42:663–669.

Krishna Rao SV, Mejia G, Roberts-Thomson K, Logan R. Epidemiology of oral cancer in Asia in the past decade—an update (2000–2012). *Asian Pac J Cancer Prev.* 2013;14:5567–5577.

Mishra R. Cell cycle-regulatory cyclins and their deregulation in oral cancer. *Oral Oncol.* 2013;49:475–481.

Maurer K, Eschrich K, Schellenberger W, et al. Oral brush biopsy analysis by MALDI-ToF mass spectrometry for early cancer diagnosis. *Oral Oncol.* 2013;49:152–156.

Mehrad M, Carpenter DH, Chernock RD, et al. Papillary squamous cell carcinoma of the head and neck: clinicopathologic and molecular features with special reference to human papillomavirus. *Am J Surg Pathol.* 2013;37:1349–1356.

Mirghani H, Amen F, Moreau F, et al. Human papilloma virus testing in oropharyngeal squamous cell carcinoma: what the clinician should know. *Oral Oncol.* 2014;50:1–9.

National Cancer Institute. *SEER Stat Fact Sheets: Oral Cavity and Pharynx Cancer.* http://seer.cancer.gov/statfacts/html/oralcav.html. Updated 2013. Accessed December 21, 2013.

Page DB, Postow MA, Callahan MK, et al. Immune modulation in cancer with antibodies. *Annu Rev Med.* 2014;65:185–202.

Paolini F, Massa S, Manni I, et al. Immunotherapy in new pre-clinical models of HPV-associated oral cancers. *Hum Vaccin Immunother.* 2013;9.

Paparella ML, Olvi LG, Brandizzi D, et al. Osteosarcoma of the jaw: an analysis of a series of 74 cases. *Histopathology.* 2013;63:551–557.

Park ES, Shum JW, Bui TG, et al. Robotic surgery: a new approach to tumors of the tongue base, oropharynx, and hypopharynx. *Oral Maxillofac Surg Clin North Am.* 2013;25:49–59, vi.

Petti S, Masood M, Messano GA, Scully C. Alcohol is not a risk factor for oral cancer in nonsmoking, betel quid non-chewing individuals. A meta-analysis update. *Ann Ig.* 2013;25:3–14.

Printz C. Highlights from the ASCO annual meeting. *Cancer.* 2013;119:3104–3105.

Richmon JD, Quon H, Gourin CG. The effect of transoral robotic surgery on short-term outcomes and cost of care after oropharyngeal cancer *surgery. Laryngoscope.* 2014;124(1):165–171.

Robbins HA, Shiels MS, Pfeiffer RM, Engels EA. Epidemiologic contributions to recent cancer trends among HIV-infected people in the United States. *AIDS.* 2014;28(6):881–890.

Sankaranarayanan R, Ramadas K, Thara S, et al. Long term effect of visual screening on oral cancer incidence and mortality in a randomized trial in Kerala, India. *Oral Oncol.* 2013;49:314–321.

Sciubba JJ, Helman JI. Current management strategies for verrucous hyperkeratosis and verrucous carcinoma. *Oral Maxillofac Surg Clin North Am.* 2013;25:77–82, vi.

SEER Cancer Statistics Review. *Cancer Statistics Review 1975–2010:* Introduction. Table 1. http://seer.cancer.gov/csr/1975_2010/results_merged/sect_01_overview.pdf. Updated 2013. Accessed December 21, 2013.

SEER Cancer Statistics Review. *Cancer Statistics Review 1975–2010:* Introduction. Table 1.4. *http://*seer.cancer.gov/csr/1975_2010/results_merged/sect_01_overview.pdf. Updated 2013. Accessed December 21, 2013.

SEER Cancer Statistics Review. *Cancer Statistics Review 1975–2010:* Introduction. Table 1.5. http://seer.cancer.gov/csr/1975_2010/results_merged/sect_01_overview.pdf. Updated *2013.* Accessed December 21, 2013.

SEER Cancer Statistics Review. *Cancer Statistics Review 1975–2010:* Introduction. Tables 1.17-8. http://seer.cancer.gov/csr/1975_2010/results_merged/sect_01_overview.pdf. Updated 2013. Accessed December 21, 2013.

SEER Cancer Statistics Review. *Cancer Statistics Review 1975–2010:* Introduction. Tables 1.6-7. http://seer.cancer.gov/csr/1975_2010/results_merged/sect_01_overview.pdf. Updated 2013. Accessed December 21, 2013.

Tahtali A, Hey C, Geissler C, et al. HPV status and overall survival of patients with oropharyngeal squamous cell carcinoma—a retrospective study of a German head and neck cancer center. *Anticancer Res.* 2013;33:3481–3485.

U.S. Preventive Services Task Force. *Screening for Oral Cancer.* http://www.uspreventiveservicestaskforce.org/uspstf/uspsoral.htm. Updated 2013. Accessed December 21, 2013.

Walline HM, Komarck C, McHugh JB, et al. High-risk human papillomavirus detection in oropharyngeal, nasopharyngeal, and oral cavity cancers: comparison of multiple methods. *JAMA Otolaryngol Head Neck Surg.* 2013;139:1320–1327.

Yanik EL, Tamburro K, Eron JJ, et al. Recent cancer incidence trends in an observational clinical cohort of HIV-infected patients in the US, 2000 to 2011. *Infect Agent Cancer.* 2013;8:18.

Yedida GR, Nagini S, Mishra R. The importance of oncogenic transcription factors for oral cancer pathogenesis and treatment. *Oral Surg Oral Med Oral Pathol Oral Radiol.* 2013;116:179–188.

For the full reference lists, please go to http://www.pmph-usa.com/Burkets_Oral_Medicine.

CHAPTER 9

Oral Complications of Nonsurgical Cancer Therapies: Diagnosis and Treatment

Douglas E. Peterson, DMD, PhD, FDS RCSEd

Siri Beier Jensen, DDS, PhD

❐ OVERVIEW
   Types of Cancer Therapies
   Epidemiology of Oral Complications of Cancer
      Therapies
❐ ORAL CARE PROTOCOLS FOR CHEMOTHER-
   APY AND HEAD AND NECK RADIATION
   PATIENTS
   Oral Care Precancer Treatment
   Implementation of Systematic Basic Oral Care
      Protocols for Oncology Patients
   Oral Decontamination
   Oral Hydration
❐ ORAL TOXICITY IN BOTH CHEMOTHERAPY
   AND HEAD/NECK RADIATION PATIENTS
   Oral Mucositis
   Oral Pain
   Oral Hemorrhage

❐ HIGH-DOSE CHEMOTHERAPY PATIENTS
   Hematopoietic Stem Cell Transplantation Patients
❐ TARGETED CANCER THERAPIES
   Oral Ulcerations/Stomatitis Induced by Targeted
      Cancer Therapies
❐ HEAD AND NECK RADIATION PATIENTS
   Acute and Late Oral Complications
❐ ONCOLOGY PATIENTS RECEIVING
   BONE-STABILIZING AGENTS

OVERVIEW

Oral complications from cancer therapies can often cause significant morbidity to the patient. The oral toxicity may cause disruption of cancer treatment compromising the prognosis and increase health-care costs. A wide range of oral complications of cancer therapies often appear concurrently, which may complicate diagnoses and management, for example, intense oral and pharyngeal pain induced by a combination of oral mucositis, oropharyngeal candidiasis, salivary gland hypofunction, and xerostomia frequently lead to dysphagia in cancer patients compromising nutritional intake.[1] Thus, oral complications of cancer therapies may severely impact

quality of life during cancer treatment or as late oral complications months or years following treatment.

Oral complications induced by cancer therapies result from a complex interplay among multiple factors and the recognition of the underlying mechanisms causing oral complications continues to develop. The current approach to minimize the incidence and severity of oral complications of cancer therapies is:

• The elimination of preexisting dental, periodontal, and mucosal infections in conjunction with regular oral assessment;
• The implementation of basic oral care protocols;

- The prompt diagnosis of emerging oral complications during and after cancer therapy with adequate alleviation and treatment.[2]

An interdisciplinary approach, including dental professionals, is required to work in close collaboration with the patient to regularly and by validated outcome measures to evaluate, prevent, and treat oral complications of cancer therapies.

This chapter addresses oral complications of nonsurgical cancer therapies and evidence-based clinical practice guidelines for management.

Types of Cancer Therapies

Design of cancer treatment protocols is based on a number of key considerations, beginning with histopathologic confirmation of type of malignancy. Additional components include staging (solid tumors), age and performance status of the patient, projected efficacy in relation to toxicity, and patient preferences.

Hematologic Malignancy Patients

Patients with hematologic disease (Figures 9-1 and 9-2) may be treated by moderate-to-high-dose chemotherapy, with or without hematopoietic stem cell transplantation (HSCT). As with head and neck cancer patients (see next section), factors influencing incidence and severity of oral complications across patients include extent of oral disease prior to cancer treatment, intensity of cancer therapy, genetically governed susceptibility to oral mucosal injury, and patient compliance with health professional recommendations regarding oral hygiene, diet, and related variables.

HSCT-related oral toxicities are additionally influenced by the degree of genetic disparity between donor and patient.

Acute and/or chronic graft-versus-host disease (GVHD) that results from immune-modulated injury to the patient's tissues can cause clinically significant oral disorders, including salivary gland and/or oral mucosal disease.

Head and Neck Cancer Patients

Depending on key variables such as staging, cancer treatment for a patient with solid head and neck cancer (e.g., oral, oropharyngeal, or laryngeal tumor) can consist of the following:

- Surgical excision
- Head and neck radiation, administered in fractionated or hyperfractionated doses five times/week for six to seven weeks for a total cumulative dose of approximately 6000–7000 cGy.
- Multimodality treatments that incorporate chemotherapy based on the following schema:

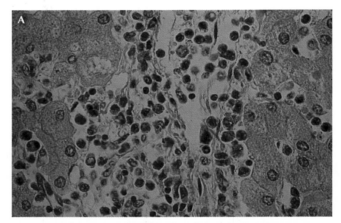

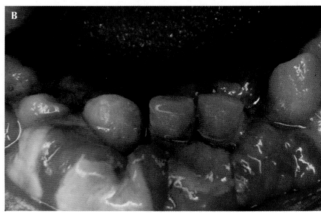

FIGURE 9-2 Acute leukemia can be considered "naturally metastatic" in that the neoplasm arises within the white blood cell progenitors produced in the bone marrow. Because of the systemic circulation of these cells, the disease is typically widespread by time of diagnosis. (A) Histopathology based on hepatic biopsy, demonstrating widespread infiltrate of the blast leukemic cells. (B) Gingival leukemic infiltrate in newly diagnosed acute myelogenous leukemia patient. Note the extensive gingival engorgement caused by the infiltrating leukemic cells. The resulting ischemia can contribute to development of tissue necrosis as well as opportunistic infection such as pseudomembranous candidiasis. (From Peterson[65] reprinted with permission from Quintessence Publishing.)

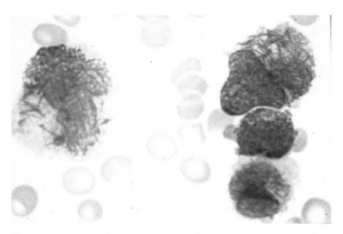

FIGURE 9-1 Peripheral blood smear from a patient with newly diagnosed acute myelogenous leukemia in blast crisis. The high-dose induction chemotherapy regimen that will be used to treat this patient is profoundly myelosuppressive and typically causes severe ulcerative oral mucositis for at least two weeks duration. The interface of profound myelosuppression with disruption in integrity of the oral mucosal barrier can result in risk for life-threatening bacteremia and/or sepsis. (From Peterson[65] reprinted with permission from Quintessence Publishing.)

- Neoadjuvant chemotherapy:
  - Administered prior to surgery, for purposes of debulking tumor
- Adjuvant chemotherapy:
  - Administered after surgery and prior to head and neck radiation
- Concurrent/ concomitant chemotherapy:
  - Administered in combination with head and neck radiation, typically on a weekly basis throughout the duration of the six to seven weeks of radiation

As with hematologic malignancy patients, factors influencing incidence and severity of oral complications in head and neck cancer patients include the extent of oral diseases prior to cancer treatment, intensity and anatomic location of cancer therapy, genetically governed susceptibility to oral mucosal injury and patient compliance with health professional recommendations regarding oral hygiene, diet, and related variables.

Patients Receiving Targeted Cancer Therapies

Use of targeted cancer therapies such as mammalian target of rapamycin (mTOR) inhibitors has increased in recent years.[3,4] These biologics are directed to molecular pathways that are unique to tumor cells, versus normal cells. Despite their targeting, however, side effects such as oral mucosal and dermal lesions can occur (see section on "Targeted Cancer Therapies").

Epidemiology of Oral Complications of Cancer Therapies

Types of oral complications vary in pattern, duration, and intensity for each individual patient and depending on the cancer therapy regimen and dose intensity: for example, cancer chemotherapy, head and neck radiation therapy, targeted cancer therapies, and HSCT.[5-8] The Oral Care Study Group and the Mucositis Study Group of the Multinational Association of Supportive Care in Cancer/International Society of Oral Oncology (MASCC/ISOO) have performed systematic reviews of the most common oral complications of cancer therapies and provided prevalence of oral mucositis,[9,10] oral pain,[11] oral fungal infection,[12] oral viral infection,[13] salivary gland hypofunction and xerostomia,[14] dysgeusia,[15] trismus,[16] dental disease,[17] osteoradionecrosis (ORN),[18] and bisphosphonate osteonecrosis[19] in relation to various regimens of cancer therapy (Table 9-1).

ORAL CARE PROTOCOLS FOR CHEMOTHERAPY AND HEAD AND NECK RADIATION PATIENTS

Oral Care Precancer Treatment

Elimination or stabilization of selected oral disease prior to the initiation of chemotherapy in head and neck cancer patients can prevent or mitigate subsequent acute oral toxicities such as infection of dental, dental pulpal, or periodontal

TABLE 9-1	Oral Toxicities in Cancer Patients
Complication	Weighted Prevalence
Bisphosphonate osteonecrosis	6.1% for all studies (mean)
	Studies with documented follow-up = 13.3%
	Studies with undocumented follow-up = 0.7%
	Epidemiological studies = 1.2%
Dysgeusia	CT only = 56.3% (mean)
	RT only = 66.5% (mean)
	Combined CT and RT = 76% (mean)
Oral fungal infection	Of clinical oral fungal infection (all oral candidiasis):
	Pretreatment = 7.5%
	During treatment = 39.1%
	Posttreatment = 32.6%
	Of oral candidiasis clinical infection by cancer treatment:
	During HNC RT = 37.4%
	During CT = 38%
Oral viral infection	In patients treated with CT for hematologic malignancies:
	Patients with oral ulcerations/sampling oral ulcerations = 49.8%
	Patients sampling oral ulcerations = 33.8%
	Patients sampling independently of the presence of oral ulcerations = 0%
	In patients treated with RT:
	Patients with RT only/sampling oral ulcerations = 0%
	Patients with RT and adjunctive CT/ sampling oral ulcerations = 43.2%
Dental disease	For dental caries in patients treated with cancer therapy:
	All studies = 28.1%
	CT only = 37.3%
	Post-RT = 24%
	Post-CT and post-RT = 21.4%
	Of severe gingivitis in patients undergoing CT = 20.3%
	Of dental infection/abscess in patients undergoing CT = 5.8%
Osteoradionecrosis	In conventional RT = 7.4%
	In IMRT = 5.2%
	In RT and CT = 6.8%
	In brachytherapy = 5.3%
Trismus	For conventional RT = 25.4%
	For IMRT = 5%
	For combined RT and CT = 30.7%
Oral pain[a]	VAS pain level (0–100) in HNC patients:
	Pretreatment = 12/100

(Continued)

TABLE 9-1   Oral Toxicities in Cancer Patients (*Continued*)

Complication	Weighted Prevalence
	Immediately posttreatment = 33/100
	1 mo posttreatment = 20/100
	EORTC QLQ-C30 pain level (0–100) in HNC patients:
	Pretreatment = 27/100
	3 mo posttreatment = 30/100
	6 mo posttreatment = 23/100
	12 mo posttreatment = 24/100
Salivary gland hypofunction and xerostomia	Of xerostomia in HNC patients by type of RT:
	All studies
	Pre-RT = 6%
	During RT = 93%
	1–3 mo post-RT = 74%
	3–6 mo post-RT = 79%
	6–12 mo post-RT = 83%
	1–2 y post-RT = 78%
	>2 y post-RT = 85%
	Conventional RT
	Pre-RT = 10%
	During RT = 81%
	1–3 mo post-RT = 71%
	3–6 mo post-RT = 83%
	6–12 mo post-RT = 72%
	1–2 y post-RT = 84%
	>2 y post-RT = 91%
	IMRT
	Pre-RT =12%
	During RT = 100%
	1–3 mo post-RT = 89%
	3–6 mo post-RT = 73%
	6–12 mo post-RT = 90%
	1–2 y post-RT = 66%
	>2 y post-RT = 68%

Abbreviations: CT, chemotherapy; EORTC QLQ-C30, European Organisation for Research and Treatment of Cancer Quality of Life Questionnaire C30; HNC, head and neck cancer; IMRT, intensity-modulated radiation therapy; MASCC/ISOO, Multinational Association of Supportive Care in Cancer/International Society of Oral Oncology; RT, radiation therapy; VAS, visual analog scale.

[a]Pain is common in patients with HNCs and is reported by approximately half of patients before cancer therapy, by 81% during therapy, by 70% at the end of therapy, and by 36% at 6 months posttreatment.

Source: Modified from NCI PDQ website: Oral complications of chemotherapy/head & neck radiation. **http://www.cancer.gov/cancertopics/pdq/supportivecare/oralcomplications/HealthProfessional/page1.**

origin. Decision making regarding this medically necessary precancer treatment oral care is illustrated in Figure 9-3.

Implementation of Systematic Basic Oral Care Protocols for Oncology Patients

Oral care interventions are pertinent to all cancer patients to prevent and reduce the incidence and severity of oral complications and promote oral comfort during and following cancer therapies.

Development and implementation of oral care protocols should be interdisciplinary (nurse, physician, dentist, dental hygienist, dietician, pharmacist, and others as relevant) and include education of the patient, family, and healthcare professionals. The protocols should be focused on regularly scheduled oral assessment and decontamination to reduce the risk of infection, oral moisturization to reduce the risk of friction and trauma-induced oral mucosal injury, and pain management to promote oral comfort and avoid dose reduction and interruption of cancer treatment.[2]

Oral Decontamination

Toothbrushing two to three times a day with a soft, nylon-bristled toothbrush (with regular replacement of the toothbrush) is recommended.[2,9] The bristles can be softened in warm water if oral hygiene procedures become discomforting or can be modified to an ultrasoft toothbrush to ensure continued mechanical oral decontamination for as long as possible during cancer treatment. Toothbrushing should be supplemented by dental flossing once daily with instruction on atraumatic technique. Fluoridated toothpaste should be used, supplemented by high-concentration prescription of fluoride regimens if the patient's ability to perform oral care is compromised or if increased risk of dental caries due to salivary gland hypofunction (e.g., 5000 ppm fluoride toothpaste or 1% neutral sodium fluoride gel in a dental tray for five minutes before bedtime. The dental tray should overlap the gingival margins of the teeth and still avoid unnecessary contact with the gingiva). Toothpastes containing sodium dodecyl/laureth sulfate (surfactant) and mint flavor should be avoided if it causes soreness of the oral mucosa. Antiseptic mouthwashes such as 0.12% chlorhexidine gluconate may be administered as a supplement to toothbrushing depending on the manifestation of periodontal disease or if toothbrushing is no longer possible due to oral pain.[2,20] Professional mechanical bacterial plaque removal should be performed before the patient begins rinsing with chlorhexidine gluconate.[21]

Oral Hydration

Alleviation of xerostomia comprises gustatory, masticatory, or pharmacologic stimulation of residual salivary gland secretory capacity or regular and frequent sipping and topical application to the oral cavity of water, bland rinses, or saliva substitutes (e.g., mouthwash, spray, or gel).[22] Lubrication of

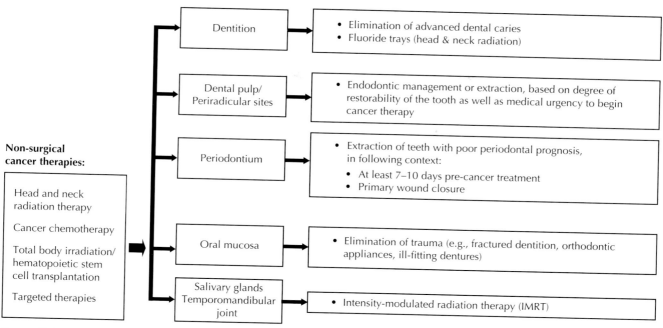

FIGURE 9-3 Precancer treatment oral care.

lips should be incorporated to prevent crusting and ulceration of the prolabium.

The use of bland rinses, for example 0.9% saline rinse or sodium bicarbonate solution (1 teaspoon salt, 1 teaspoon baking soda in 1 L of water) is recommended in cancer therapy populations for decontamination, moisturization, neutralization of pH and for promoting oral comfort.[2] Saline and sodium bicarbonate rinses are harmless to the oral cavity and can thus be performed several times each day as needed.

Evidence-based clinical practice guidelines for management of salivary gland hypofunction and xerostomia are described in detail in Chapter 10, "Salivary Gland Diseases."

ORAL TOXICITY IN BOTH CHEMOTHERAPY AND HEAD/NECK RADIATION PATIENTS

Cancer patients can be at high risk for oral complications secondary to their cancer treatment (For clinical management of oral complications, see Figure 9-4). Incidence and severity are governed by a number of cancer treatment variables, as described below.

Oral Mucositis

Oral mucositis can have a significant clinical and economic consequence in oncology practice (Figure 9-5). The pain associated with the lesion can be so severe that hospitalization of the patient is needed to support the nutritional intake and other daily functions. The pain can also cause dose reduction in future cycles of chemotherapy, thus compromising optimal delivery of the chemotherapy regimen.

Despite the prominence of oral pain in the clinical setting, however, there has been limited investigative research into the neuropathology component of the lesion. Mucosal injury in neutropenic cancer patients can be source of systemic infection, with the resultant morbidity and, in selected patients, mortality. Oral mucositis can thus cause clinically and economically adverse impacts.

The current five phase pathobiologic model of oral mucositis is complex and involves both epithelium and submucosa (Figure 9-6).[23] Incidence of oral mucositis in patients receiving high-dose chemotherapy is approximately 40%. Evidence-based guidelines for oral mucositis are based in supportive care.[9] There is only one U.S. Food & Drug Administration-approved biologic for prevention of oral mucositis (see the section "HSCT Patients").

Oral Pain

The level of oral pain should be scored on a systematic basis, using a validated pain ladder.[11,24]

Pain management by patient-controlled analgesia with morphine in HSCT or transdermal fentanyl in conventional and high-dose chemotherapy with or without total body irradiation, 2% morphine mouthwash in head and neck radiation therapy, or 0.5% doxepin mouthwash (patient population not specified) have been recommended or suggested depending on the level of evidence as interventions to treat pain due to oral mucositis.[25] Management of pain from oral mucositis during head and neck radiation typically begins with nonsteroidal

Management strategy

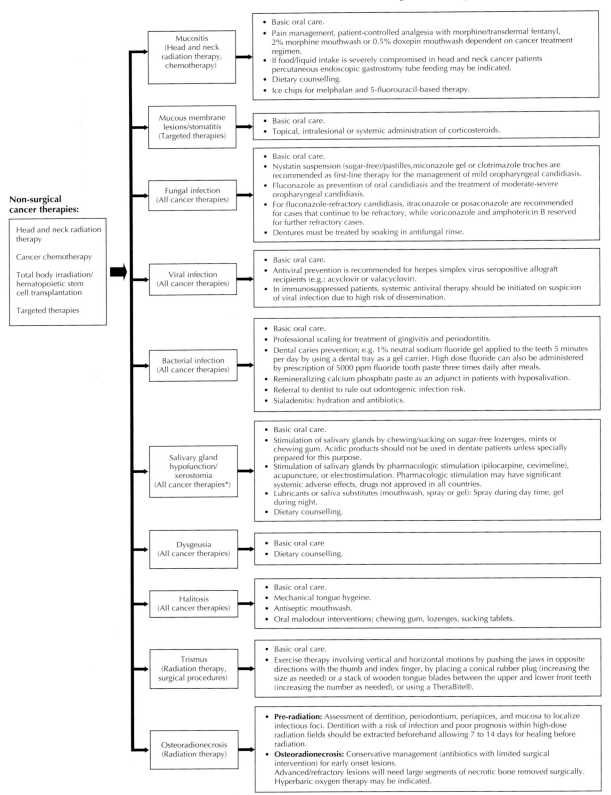

FIGURE 9-4 Clinical management of oral complications of nonsurgical cancer therapies.
*For example, radiation therapy, including radioactive iodine for thyroid cancer and total body irradiation for the treatment of hematological malignancy.

anti-inflammatory drugs (NSAIDs) since generally there is not an increased risk of hemorrhage and this can be combined with opioids as the severity of oral mucositis and pain increases.[26]

Depending on severity of mucositis, topical anesthetic rinses can be used to allow for continuity of oral care and food intake with the precaution that the patient is carefully

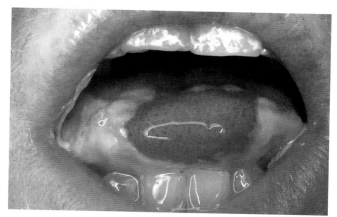

FIGURE 9-5 Oral mucositis in breast cancer patient receiving high-dose chemotherapy. The extensive pseudomembranous lesions can significantly impair normal oral function and represent a portal of entry for severe systemic infection. (From Peterson[65] reprinted with permission from Quintessence Publishing.)

informed to avoid mechanical trauma and burns in the anesthetized mucosal areas.[11]

Oral Hemorrhage

Compromised basic oral care increases the risk of oral infection (gingivitis, periodontitis, oral candidiasis), which increases the risk of oral hemorrhage. Hemorrhage may also be caused by cancer treatment–induced thrombocytopenia in patients receiving high-dose chemotherapy or undergoing HSCT.

Hemorrhage can be controlled with adequate periodontal and antifungal treatment. However, if prolonged hemorrhage occurs, periodontal treatment should be discontinued and the oncologist/hematologist consulted. Further management of oral hemorrhage includes the use of vasoconstrictors, clot-forming agents, and tissue protectants.[27]

HIGH-DOSE CHEMOTHERAPY PATIENTS

Chemotherapy can be used in a variety of primary or adjunctive oncology settings (Table 9-2). In addition to oral mucositis, oral infection arising from pre-existing high-risk oral lesions can occur in association with chemotherapy-induced myelosuppression (Table 9-3). Unlike head and

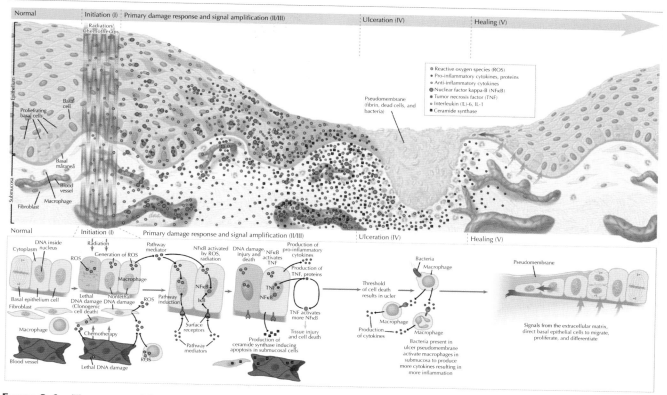

FIGURE 9-6 The conceptual framework for oral mucositis pathobiology consists of five stages, ranging from initial injury with hours of exposure to high-dose cancer therapy to eventual healing approximately two to four weeks after cessation of that treatment. Although the illustration depicts an orderly and sequential mechanistic process, the likely course of molecular and cellular events is more likely dysregulated and biologically confounded. (From Sonis.[23])

neck radiation patients, however, long-term effects of high-dose chemotherapy on the oral tissues are rare.

Patients may develop pseudomembranous candidiasis during periods of bone marrow suppression (Table 9-4). Contributing factors may also include compromised oral hygiene during periods of oral mucositis as well as salivary hypofunction induced by medications used to support the care of the patients (e.g., antiemetics). Clinical diagnosis can often be established based on history and examination, although the assessment may be confounded by the concurrent presentation of chemotherapy-induced oral mucositis as noted above. Topical oral antifungal therapy with nystatin rinses or clotrimazole troches can be considered for management (Table 9-5). Resolution of the lesion typically occurs in the setting of bone marrow recovery and reestablishment of optimal oral care.

TABLE 9-2	Chemotherapy Treatments for Oral Cancer
Neoadjuvant (debulk): Sole use prior to surgery (e.g., 5 days 5-fluorouracil: mucositis)	
Adjuvant (curative): Use after surgery/before RT (e.g., 5 days 5-fluorouracil: mucositis)	
Concurrent/concomitant (synergistic): Combination with RT (e.g., head and neck radiation therapy + weekly cisplatin)	

Abbreviation: RT, radiation therapy.
Source: From Peterson[65] reprinted with permission from Quintessence Publishing.

TABLE 9-3	High-Risk Oral Lesions in the Myelosuppressed Cancer Patient
Advanced and/or symptomatic dental caries	
Periapical pathoses symptomatic within past 90 d	
Severe periodontal disease for which prognosis of dentition is poor	
Mucosal lesions secondary to trauma from prosthetic or orthodontic appliances	

Source: From Peterson[65] reprinted with permission from Quintessence Publishing.

TABLE 9-4	Candidiasis
Risk Factors:	
Myelosuppression	
Mucosal injury	
Salivary compromise	
Antibiotics	
Steroids	
Increased length of hospital stay	
Diagnosis:	
History	
Assessment of risk factors	
Examination	
Culture as needed	
Treatment:	
Nonmedicated oral rinse	
Topical antifungal (systemic therapy if indicated)	
Removal of dentures	

Source: From Peterson[65] reprinted with permission from Quintessence Publishing.

The periodontium may infrequently be a site of acute infectious flare during profound myelosuppression (Figure 9-7). These lesions are rarely encountered in oncology practice. When they do occur, however, the infection may

TABLE 9-5	Topical Therapies for Oropharyngeal Candidiasis (7–14 days)
Clotrimazole troche (10 mg)	
Four to five times per day	
Nystatin oral suspension (100,000 U/mL)	
5 mL four times per day	
Nystatin pastilles (200,000 U)	
Four to five times per day	
Fluconazole solution (e.g., 10 mg)	
Swish and expectorate three times per day	
Amphotericin B oral suspension (100 mg/mL)	
1 ml, four times per day	

Source: From Lerman et al.[66] reprinted with permission from Dental Clinics of North America.

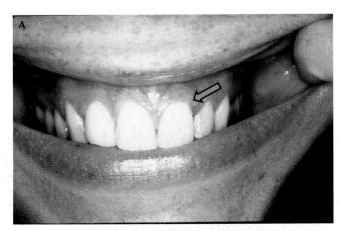

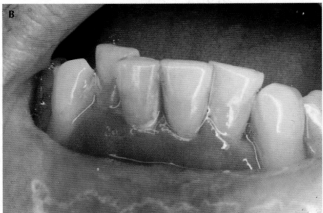

FIGURE 9-7 (A) Acute periodontal infection (arrow) in a neutropenic cancer patient with <500/mm³. Classic inflammatory signs including erythema and purulence are not clinically prominent due to suppression of neutrophil number and function. (B) Acute periodontal infection in a chemotherapy cancer patient with <1000 neutrophils/mm³. Classic inflammatory signs are more evident due to a more robust neutrophil response. (From Peterson[65] reprinted with permission from Quintessence Publishing.)

not be readily detectable due to the impaired inflammatory response in the setting of profound neutropenia. Treatment usually consists of supervised oral hygiene (e.g., 3% hydrogen peroxide or 0.12% chlorhexidine digluconate rinses) and consideration of a broad range of antimicrobial therapy if clinical presentation so indicates.

Hematopoietic Stem Cell Transplantation Patients

HSCT patients are at risk for development of a wide range of oral toxicities (Table 9-6). Incidence and severity are directly influenced by many key variables. For example, the patient undergoing HSCT will typically receive conditioning regimen containing chemotherapy at a high-dose or reduced intensity level. As with chemotherapeutic regimens in the non-HSCT setting, risk for infection increases as the depth and duration of myelosuppression increase. An additional key factor is degree of genetic homology between the donor and recipient. Chapter 21, "Transplantation Medicine," provides further detail regarding these risk factors.

Infections in HSCT patients can be of viral, bacterial, and/or fungal origin.

Oral Viral Infection

Oral viral infection caused by reactivation of herpes simplex virus (HSV) does not commonly occur in contemporary oncology practice, since prevention by thymidine kinase inhibitors such as acyclovir, valacyclovir, or their derivatives are highly effective. Pretransplant serologic testing for carrier status of HSV is important in identifying which patients

TABLE 9-6   Oral Complications of Hematopoietic Stem Cell Transplantation

Transplant Phase	Oral Complication
Phase I: Preconditioning	Oral infections: dental caries, endodontic infections, periodontal disease (gingivitis, periodontitis), mucosal infections (i.e., viral, fungal, bacterial)
	Gingival leukemic infiltrates
	Metastatic cancer
	Oral bleeding
	Oral ulceration: aphthous ulcers, erythema multiforme
	Temporomandibular dysfunction
Phase II: Conditioning Neutropenic Phase	Oropharyngeal mucositis
	Oral infections: mucosal infections (i.e., viral, fungal, bacterial), periodontal infections
	Hemorrhage
	Xerostomia and salivary gland hypofunction
	Taste dysfunction
	Neurotoxicity: dental pain, muscle tremor (e.g., jaws, tongue)
	Temporomandibular dysfunction: jaw pain, headache, joint pain
Phase III: Engraftment Hematopoietic Recovery	Oral infections: mucosal infections (i.e., viral, fungal, bacterial)
	Acute GVHD
	Xerostomia and salivary gland hypofunction
	Hemorrhage
	Neurotoxicity: dental pain, muscle tremor (e.g., jaws, tongue)
	Temporomandibular dysfunction: jaw pain, headache, joint pain
	Granulomas/papillomas
Phase IV: Immune Reconstitution Late Posttransplant	Oral infections: mucosal infections (i.e., viral, fungal, bacterial)
	Chronic GVHD
	Dental/skeletal growth and development alterations (pediatric patients)
	Xerostomia and salivary gland hypofunction
	Relapse-related oral lesions
	Second malignancies
Phase V: Long-term Survival	Relapse or second malignancies
	Dental/skeletal growth and development alterations

Abbreviation: GVHD, graft-versus-host disease.
Source: Reprinted from: NCI PDQ website: Oral complications of chemotherapy/head and neck radiation. http://www.cancer. gov/cancertopics/pdq/supportivecare/oralcomplications/Patient.

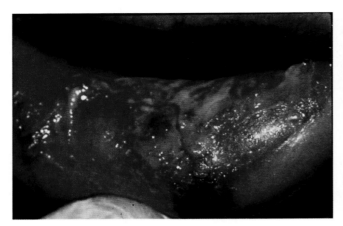

FIGURE 9-8 Reactivated herpes simplex virus in an immunocompromised hematopoietic cell transplant patient can be extensive and fatal. The compromised mucosal and circulating immune defenses result in a rapidly progressing, painful, and sometimes fatal systemic viral infection. Fortunately, antiviral prophylaxis or treatment with thymidine kinase inhibitors such as acyclovir or its derivatives is highly efficacious. Drug-resistant herpes simplex is an infrequent occurrence. (Photo courtesy of Dr. M. M. Schubert. From Peterson[65] reprinted with permission from Quintessence Publishing.)

may benefit from the viral prophylactic regimen. HSV titers greater than or equal to 1:16 are often used clinically as the indicator for the initiation of the prophylactic regimen.

The infection (Figure 9-8), when it does occur, can co-develop in the setting of oral mucositis and/or acute GVHD[27]; this in turn not only confounds the diagnostic process but also intensifies the severity of the mucosal injury.

As with all infections in this population, early diagnosis is essential to initiate a prompt, directed treatment. Viral culturing remains the gold standard. Other types of testing such as direct immunofluorescence, immunoassay, and shell vial testing may be useful in the context of producing more rapid results.

Oral Candidiasis

Pseudomembranous candidiasis, as with high-dose chemotherapy patients who did not undergo stem cell rescue, can occur in settings of compromised mucosal and salivary defenses (Figure 9-9). Other types of fungal infection can also occur including lesions caused by *Aspergillus*, *Mucormycosis*, and *Rhizopus* spp. Culturing and biopsy of these latter lesions are essential for diagnosis in that the lesions may mimic clinical appearance of nonyeast toxicities in HSCT patients.

Additional detailed information regarding prevention of infectious complications among these patients is provided in the 2009 guideline report by Tomblyn et al.[28] The reader is also referred to Chapter 21 for more detailed discussion of these lesions as well as preventive and management of oral toxicity unique to the HSCT patient population.

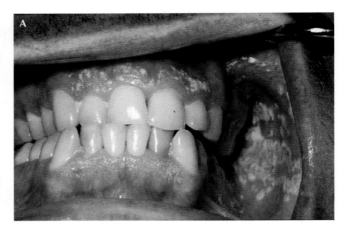

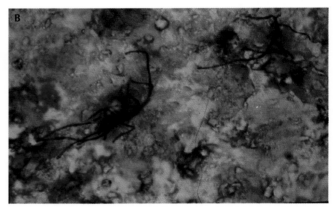

FIGURE 9-9 Pseudomembranous candidiasis can occur in oncology patients secondary to myelosuppression and/or compromised salivary defense mechanisms. From Peterson[65] reprinted with permission from Quintessence Publishing. (A) Clinically documented pseudomembranous candidiasis in an allogeneic hematopoietic cell transplant patient with chronic graft-versus-host-disease (GVHD) involving the major salivary glands. The resultant compromised salivary flow and composition (e.g., lactoferrin, salivary IgA, transferrin, and mucins) can lead to this and opportunistic infections. (B) Cytologic smear demonstrating the dimorphic candidal organism and hyphae.

TARGETED CANCER THERAPIES

Oral Ulcerations/Stomatitis Induced by Targeted Cancer Therapies

Targeted cancer therapies include monoclonal antibodies and small-molecule drugs interfering with specific extra- and intracellular pathways required for tumor progression (Table 9-7). Such pathways include inhibition of growth factor receptors involved in cancer cell proliferation and angiogenesis, by intracellular delivery of small molecules toxic to cancer cells, by inducing apoptosis of cancer cells, or by triggering an immune response resulting in the destruction specifically of cancer cells. They are increasingly being used to treat cancers such as, renal cell carcinoma, non–small cell lung cancer, breast cancer, colorectal cancer, squamous cell carcinoma of the head and

TABLE 9-7	Examples of Targeted Cancer Therapies Potentially Causing Oral Ulceration/Stomatitis	
Drug Class	Targeted Agent	Example/s of Treatment Indications
mTOR inhibitor	temsirolimus	Kidney cancer
Tyrosine kinase inhibitor	erlotinib	Pancreatic and non–small cell lung cancer
Tyrosine & kinase inhibitor	sunitinib	Kidney cancer, gastrointestinal stromal tumor
Tyrosine kinase inhibitor	sorafenib	Kidney, liver and thyroid cancer
Vascular endothelial growth factor A-inhibitor	bevacizumab	Colorectal, lung, breast, glioblastoma, kidney and ovarian cancer

Abbreviation: mTOR, mammalian target of rapamycin.
Source: Adapted from references.[66,31]

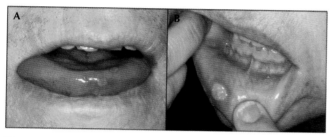

FIGURE 9-10 Selected mammalian target of rapamycin (mTOR) inhibitors used for treatment of cancer have caused oral mucosal lesions that clinically are uniquely distinct from oral mucositis caused by conventional cancer therapies such as chemotherapy and head and neck radiation (From Pilotte et al.[32]). The oral lesions caused by targeted therapies resemble recurrent aphthous ulceration clinically and often respond to topical, intralesional or systemic corticosteroid management. This clinical phenotype is thus quite different from the traditional model of oral mucositis. Further research regarding pathobiology and optimal clinical management including prevention is needed.

neck, non-Hodgkin's lymphoma, and leukemia. Oral mucosal toxicity is a relatively frequent adverse effect of selected molecularly targeted cancer therapies, here among the mammalian target of rapamycin (mTOR) inhibitors.[3,4,29–31]

The clinical manifestation of mTOR inhibitor-induced oral toxicity resembles aphthous stomatitis and is distinct from conventional oral mucositis (Figure 9-10). It may cause the need of dose reductions of cancer treatment or delay treatment due to pain. The lesions typically appear within a few days after administration of the first cycle of the drug (a mean of 10 days has been reported (range of 4–25 days) and resolve in approximately one week.[30] It is a characteristic that the prevalence and severity are less pronounced during following cycles of targeted cancer therapy. The lesions are characterized by painful, distinct, ovoid, superficial, well-demarcated ulcerations with a central gray area surrounded by an erythematous halo and are localized on the movable oral/oropharyngeal mucosa while not manifest on the keratinized mucosa of the hard palate, gingiva, or dorsum of the tongue. The pathogenesis may be similar to aphthous stomatitis.[29,31]

Patients who develop oral mucosal ulcerations from molecularly targeted cancer therapies may be more prone to develop acneiform dermatitis and nonspecific cutaneous rashes.[3,29]

Among mucosal adverse effects, diarrhea has been the most frequently reported in a meta-analysis of selected targeted cancer therapies (i.e., vascular endothelial growth factor [VEGF] inhibitor bevacizumab, epidermal growth factor [EGF] tyrosine kinase inhibitors gefitinib and erlotinib, the dual tyrosine kinase inhibitor lapatinib [interferes with HER2/neu and EGF receptors], multitargeted receptor tyrosine kinase inhibitor sorafenib and sunitinib, and trastuzumab, which interferes with HER2/neu receptors).[8]

Furthermore, patients treated by sunitinib (multitargeted receptor tyrosine kinase inhibitor) regimens have been found to have a higher risk of all-grade xerostomia.[8] The clinical management strategy of mTOR inhibitor-associated stomatitis is empirically based on drugs that have been used for the prevention and treatment of aphthous stomatitis and includes topical, intralesional, or systemic corticosteroid therapy depending on the severity of the oral lesions.[30,32]

HEAD AND NECK RADIATION PATIENTS

Acute and Late Oral Complications

Oral Mucositis

Oral mucositis induced by radiation therapy is the consequence of a complex cascade of biological events involving the epithelium and the submucosa.[33,34] The extent of oral mucosal damage is strongly related to the radiation dose, volume of irradiated mucosa, and fractionation regimen and is characterized by mucosal atrophy and erythema followed by ulceration and subsequent healing after completing cancer therapy. Oral mucositis is primarily affecting the buccal mucosa, lateral margins and ventral surface of the tongue, soft palate, floor of the mouth, and lips. The ulcerations are commonly colonized with bacteria contributing to the mucositis development.[34] The first clinical signs of oral mucositis in radiation therapy are erythema, epithelial sloughing, and oral discomfort presenting by the end of the first week (days 7–14) of a conventional 2 Gy/day, five times a week radiation regimen. Ulceration will typically become clinically evident during the second week of radiation, and increase in severity in the subsequent weeks of radiation treatment. The lesions will then usually resolve during the four weeks following cessation of the cancer treatment. Oral mucositis results in severe pain and the patient often requires systemic narcotics for pain relief. Oral mucositis also negatively affects nutrition, oral hygiene, and quality of life. In general, the oral lesions will heal within two to four weeks after radiation; however, some patients will develop late radiation effects of the oral mucosa characterized by epithelial atrophy, telangiectasia, loss of deeper capillary vessels, and fibrosis of the submucosa leaving the oral mucosa permanently prone to infection, in particular oral candidiasis, and mechanical trauma (Figure 9-11).

Management of oral mucositis includes oral pain control, basic oral care, prevention and treatment of infection, and nutritional support; see details of basic oral care in the

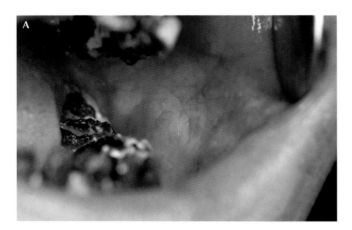

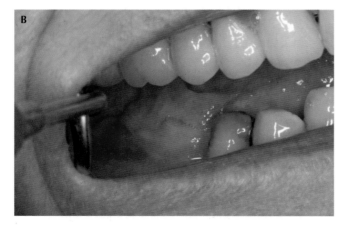

FIGURE 9-11 Late mucosal radiation sequelae. (A) Dryness, telangiectasia, and fibrosis of the left buccal mucosa with pronounced soreness. Conventional radiation therapy one year previously for oral cancer. The unstimulated whole saliva flow rate is 0.04 mL/min and the stimulated whole saliva flow rate is 0.16 mL/min. The patient also has rampant caries due to hyposalivation and impaired oral hygiene (complicated by oral pain and trismus). (B) Chronic ulceration of the right margin of the tongue as late radiation sequelae. Intensity-modulated radiation therapy two years previously for tonsil cancer on the right side. The patient's mandibular denture had to be adjusted to reduce mechanical friction in the area.

section "Implementation of Systematic Basic Oral Care Protocols for Oncology Patients."[2]

The evidence-based clinical practice guidelines for the prevention and treatment of oral mucositis have been reviewed by the Mucositis Study Group, MASCC/ISOO.[2,25,35–44] The results were incorporated into recommendations or suggestions at three levels: (1) *in favor* of interventions for oral mucositis, (2) *against* interventions for oral mucositis, or (3) no guideline possible due to insufficient or conflicting evidence.

The MASCC/ISOO oral mucositis clinical management guidelines represented by recommendations or suggestions *in favor* of interventions directed to head and neck radiation patients include oral care protocols,[2] low-level laser therapy (wavelength around 632.8 nm),[41] benzydamine hydrochloride (in patients receiving moderate dose radiation therapy, i.e., up to 50 Gy),[39] systemic zinc supplements,[43] and 2% morphine mouthwash or 0.5% doxepin mouthwash to reduce pain from oral mucositis.[25]

The MASCC/ISOO oral mucositis clinical management guidelines recommend *avoiding* sucralfate mouthwash for the prevention and treatment of oral mucositis in head and neck radiation patients.[25] Neither iseganan mouthwash nor polymyxin/tobramycin/amphotericin B lozenges/paste and bacitracin/clotrimazole/gentamicin lozenges are recommended to prevent oral mucositis in head and neck radiation patients.[25]

MASCC/ISOO oral mucositis clinical management guideline suggestions of interventions *not to be used* to prevent oral mucositis in head and neck radiation patients include chlorhexidine mouthwash (however, chlorhexidine may be used on the indication of reducing oral microbial load if insufficient oral hygiene),[2] misoprostol mouthwash,[39] and systemic pilocarpine.[44]

Salivary Gland Hypofunction and Xerostomia

Radiation therapy may induce salivary gland hypofunction (decreased saliva secretion) and xerostomia (a subjective feeling of oral dryness), that is, radiation therapy in head and neck cancer involving the salivary glands within the radiation field, total body irradiation in hematopoietic stem cell transplantation, and radioactive iodine in thyroid cancer.[12] Irradiation of salivary glands in head and neck cancer patients results in a substantial decline in saliva secretion within the first week of radiation therapy with a continuous reduction that may reach scarcely measurable saliva secretion by the sixth week of treatment. A further decline may be noted up to three months after completion of radiation therapy (Figure 9-12). However, salivary glands may have the potential to gradually recover within one to two years if gland-sparing radiation regimens have been applied, for example, intensity-modulated radiation therapy, and if it has been achievable to keep the radiation dose to the gland tissue below thresholds of ~26 Gy to the parotid gland and ~39 Gy to the submandibular gland.[45,46]

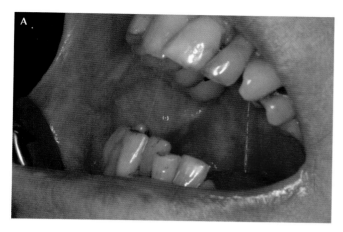

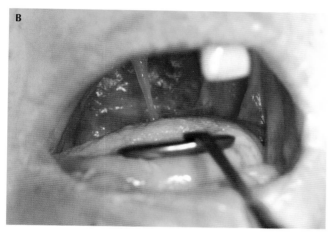

FIGURE 9-12 Hyposalivation and viscous saliva following radiation therapy. (A) Unilaterally irradiated for tonsil cancer two years previously, unstimulated whole saliva flow rate 0.01 mL/min, stimulated whole saliva flow rate 0.23 mL/min, the saliva is thick and sticky, which is a hallmark of salivary gland dysfunction during and after radiation therapy. (B) Intensity-modulated radiation therapy for cancer of the left maxillary sinus, unstimulated whole saliva flow rate 0 mL/min, stimulated whole saliva flow rate 0.20 mL/min. The saliva is extremely thick and sticky and crusts of dried saliva constituents are seen at the back of the oropharynx causing immense discomfort to the patient.

Xerostomia is the most common late adverse effect of radiation therapy in head and neck cancer patients with an immense negative impact on quality of life affecting general comfort and oral functions of speech, taste, and chewing/swallowing, which may further result in inadequate food intake and difficulties with social interaction. Thus, to ease coping mechanisms, it is of great importance to the patient to be informed of the expected acute and late salivary gland physiologic changes and the timeline of late radiation sequelae, in particular to prepare the patient of the further deterioration of salivary gland function initially after end of cancer therapy.

Management of salivary gland hypofunction and xerostomia is symptomatic by the stimulation of a residual salivary gland secretory capacity or by the use of water, bland rinses or saliva substitutes,[22] see the section on oral hydration. For evidence-based clinical practice guidelines for management of salivary gland hypofunction and xerostomia, see Chapter 10, "Salivary Gland Diseases." Furthermore, salivary gland hypofunction implies a high risk of dental caries, attrition, abrasion, and erosion (Figure 9-13); oral candidiasis (Figure 9-14); and increased mucosal sensitivity and risk for mucosa/mucosal trauma (Figure 9-11).

Oropharyngeal Candidiasis

Oral and oropharyngeal candidiasis is common in head and neck radiation patients with a prevalence of oral candidiasis of 37% during treatment.[12] The most common cause of oral candidiasis is *Candida albicans* with clinical presentations as (1) erythematous candidiasis manifest as red inflamed areas of the mucosa, (2) pseudomembranous candidiasis (thrush) manifest as removable white curd-like pseudomembranes, (3) chronic hyperplastic candidiasis manifest as hyperkeratotic white patches, which cannot be removed, (4) angular cheilitis manifest as erythema, fissuring, and ulceration of the labial commissures (Figure 9-14).[47–49] Oral candidiasis is often associated with a burning mucosal sensation and taste changes (e.g., metallic taste).[50,51] During radiation therapy, manifestations of erythematous and pseudomembranous candidiasis are common. They should be considered within the differential diagnosis of oral mucositis or as a comorbidity contributing to the symptom profile of oral mucosal injury.

In general, topical agents are considered preferable to systemic agents due to lower risk of side effects and drug interactions; however, compliance can be compromised with the administration of topical agents several times a day during active cancer treatment compared to once-a-day administration of systemic agents. Also, recent studies present an inconsistent picture of the efficacy of topical agents in patients receiving cancer therapy.[12] Additional considerations of antifungal treatment decision making in the head and neck cancer radiation population are salivary gland dysfunction and oral mucositis/chronic mucosal radiation sequelae, since the administration of antifungal treatment as troches/pastilles require saliva to dissolve and can be traumatic to a vulnerable oral mucosa. Systemic agents may be limited by their side effects and drug interactions while the emergence of resistant species is also an important concern, in particular for antifungal prophylaxis.[12] For further details on oral candidiasis and management guidelines, see Chapter 5.

Oral Bacterial Infections

Irradiated head and neck cancer patients are prone to oral mucosal infection/gingivitis due to salivary gland hypofunction, trismus, oral mucositis/chronic mucosal radiation sequelae, oral pain, and compromised oral

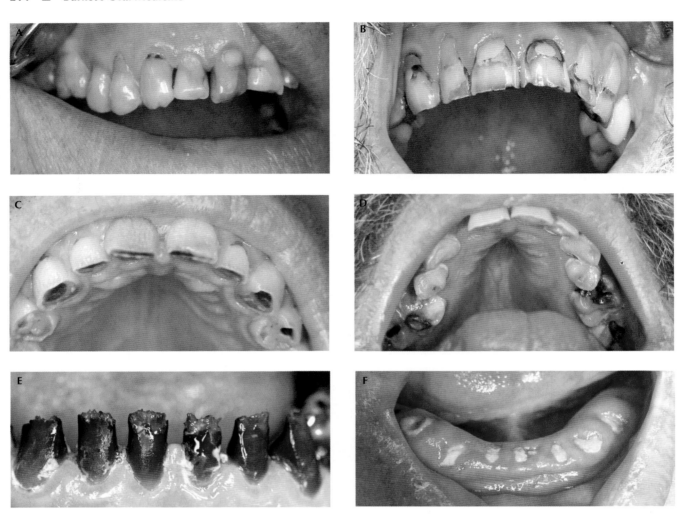

Figure 9-13 Characteristic clinical manifestations of dental caries, attrition, abrasion, and erosion in patients with radiation-induced hyposalivation. (A–B) Dental caries along the cervical area of the incisors and canines. This type of lesion often spreads circumferentially in the cervical area of the tooth and may result in amputation of the tooth crown if profound carious lesions develop. (C–D) Generalized demineralization (less translucent and whitish color of the teeth) with rapid and pronounced attrition/abrasion/erosion of the incisal, occlusal, and palatinal surfaces of the teeth. (E) Complete loss of enamel and extensive demineralization of the dentine with heavy brown discoloration of the teeth. Notice the localization to the lower anterior teeth which are normally least prone to dental caries. (F) Complete carious destruction of the tooth crowns. The roots have been treated endodontically and left in the jaw to avoid surgical intervention and prevent osteoradionecrosis. Also note the dry lips.

hygiene. Also dental caries is a disease of infectious character, and head and neck cancer patients are at high risk of rampant caries.[17,52] Bacterial infections involving the bone, for example, periodontal infection and periapical infection, increase the risk of ORN (see section Osteoradionecrosis).[17,53,54]

Thus, prevention of oral bacterial infection is directed toward reducing the microflora, and dental caries should be managed by supplemental administration of high-dose fluoride; see the section "Oral Decontamination".[2,55] In irradiated head and neck cancer patients suffering from salivary gland hypofunction, the major salivary glands may become acutely infected (bacterial sialadenitis) due to retrograde bacterial colonization through the gland ducts.[54]

Oral and Perioral Viral Infections

The risk of oral and perioral reactivation or de novo viral infections is low in head and neck cancer radiation patients. Herpes simplex virus infection is the most common viral infection followed by other Herpesviridae; for example, varicella zoster virus, Epstein-Barr virus, and cytomegalovirus.[13] There is a significant increase in prevalence if treated with combined chemotherapy and radiation therapy.[13]

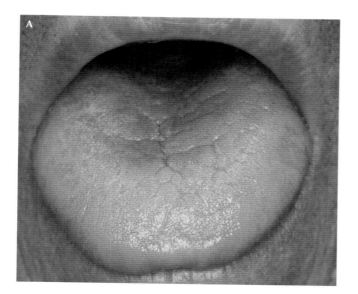

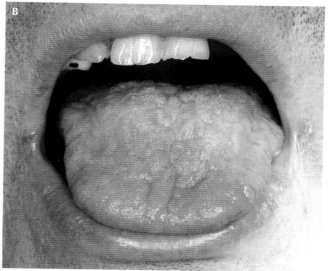

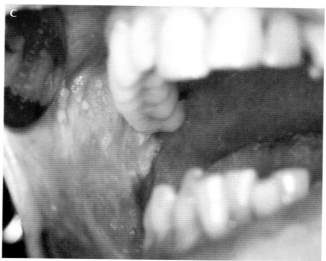

FIGURE 9-14 Oral candidiasis following radiation therapy. For all the patients shown periodic acid-Schiff (PAS) stained smear tests are positive for Candida blastospores and hyphae. Furthermore, all the patients have radiation-induced hyposalivation and xerostomia. (A) Erythematous candidiasis. The dorsum of the tongue is depapillated, fissured, and with slight central erythema. The patient describes a stinging sensation from the tongue. (B) Erythematous candidiasis and angular cheilitis caused by *Candida albicans*. The dorsum of the tongue is depapillated, fissured, and erythematous and the corners of the mouth are erythematous, fissured, and ulcerated. The patient describes a burning sensation from the tongue. (C) Recurrent pseudomembranous candidiasis two years after radiation therapy for tonsil cancer. The oral mucosa is erythematous and covered with white plaques that can be scraped off. The patient suffered from significant dysphagia which resolved when prophylactic antifungal treatment was established.

For further details on viral infections and management guidelines, see Chapter 22, "Infectious Diseases."

Dysgeusia (Taste Alterations)

Dysgeusia often occurs with head and neck radiation therapy and chemotherapy and can appear as hypogeusia (decreased taste sensation), dysgeusia (distorted taste sensation; e.g., bitter, metallic, sour, salty, or unpleasant) or hypergeusia (increased taste sensation).[15] Dysgeusia may onset within the first week of head and neck radiation due to a direct toxic effect on

taste cells further aggravated by salivary gland hypofunction, oral infections, compromised oral hygiene, drug intake, zinc deficiency, gastrointestinal reflux or as sequelae from cancer surgery and may not resolve until months after cancer treatment.[56] Some patients may experience permanent dysgeusia.[15]

Halitosis

Halitosis (oral malodor) may be due to compromised oral hygiene during cancer therapy.[57] Further aggravating oral factors can be accumulation of food debris, oral mucositis, oral candidiasis, periodontal infection, salivary gland hypofunction, or tumor growth/tissue necrosis. Systemic causes of halitosis can be gastrointestinal disease, hepatic disease, renal disease, or upper airway/lung infections. Halitosis can be reduced by comprehensive basic oral care procedures with emphasis on mechanical tongue hygiene, supplemented by antiseptic mouthwashes and oral malodor interventions.[58]

Trismus

Trismus (restricted mouth opening) is frequent in head and neck radiation patients and may severely impact food intake, speech, and compromise oral hygiene. Radiation therapy can induce fibrosis of the temporomandibular joint and oral soft tissues depending on the inclusion in the radiation field, and this can be further aggravated by tumor growth into the temporomandibular joint/masticatory muscles and surgical procedures. Radiation-induced trismus can onset from the end of radiation therapy or any time (e.g., years) following cancer therapy. The appearance and severity are rather unpredictable, and thus, it is of outmost importance with prevention by daily exercise therapy in a lifelong perspective; however, the evidence base for this is inconclusive.[16,59] After head and neck radiation, mouth opening has been reported to decrease by 18% on average compared to before cancer treatment.[60]

Osteoradionecrosis[61]

ORN is defined as "necrosis of bone due to obstruction of its blood supply." Patients who have received high-dose radiation therapy to the head and neck are at lifelong risk of ORN, the risk being directly related to the radiation dose to the bone, with an overall risk of approximately 15% (Figure 9-15).[18] ORN most frequently involves the mandible compared with the maxilla. Clinical manifestations include pain, sensory disturbances, infection, and fistulas.

Management of ORN is based on prevention that begins with a comprehensive oral and dental care before radiation therapy and a close follow-up postradiation. If smaller lesions form, management is conservative with limited surgical intervention and antibiotics, whereas advanced or treatment refractory lesions need large segments of necrotic bone removed. Hyperbaric oxygen therapy is commonly recommended to prevent ORN, but clinical efficacy is inconclusive.[18]

ONCOLOGY PATIENTS RECEIVING BONE-STABILIZING AGENTS

Patients with skeletal metastatic disease (e.g., multiple myeloma) may benefit from the use of bone-stabilizing agents (Figures 9-16 and 9-17).[62] There are three different classes of these agents, all designed to reduce of skeletal bone fracture:

- Bisphosphonates
- Denosumab
- Antiangiogenics

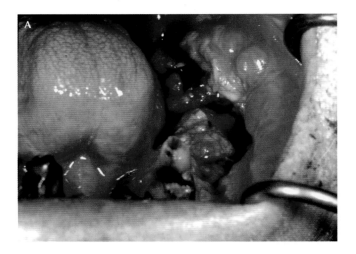

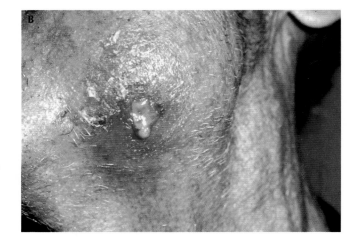

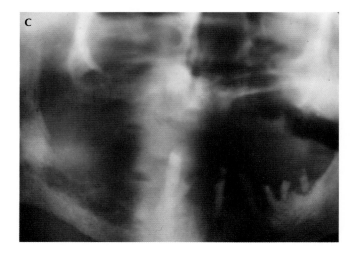

FIGURE 9-15 Osteoradionecrosis of the left mandible. (A) Root tips were present several months after completion of high-dose external beam radiation to the left mandible. (B) Facial skin lesion exhibiting purulent drainage. (C) Panoramic radiograph demonstrating findings consistent with extensive left mandibular bone destruction. (Photos courtesy of L. Assael.)

Agent	Action	Medical Use
Bisphosphonates Alendronate Risedronate Pamidronate Zoledronic Acid	Osteoclast inhibitor via mevalonate pathway	Osteoporosis Bone metastasis Multiple myeloma Antitumor
Denosumab	RANK-RANKL pathway inhibitor	Osteoporosis Bone metastasis
Antiangiogenics Bevacizumab Sunitinib Sorafenib	VEGF inhibitors	Advanced tumors

FIGURE 9-16 Therapeutic approaches for bone stabilization. (Courtesy of C. Migliorati.)

Bisphosphonates	Denosumab
Pyrophosphate analogue Osteoclast Inhibitor through the mevalonate pathway	Human monoclonal antibody against RANK-ligand that inhibits osteoclasts by blocking RANK receptors
Incorporate in the skeleton and remains for years	Will be active for 4 to 6 months but does not incorporate in the skeleton
4mg infusion every 4 weeks Acute phase reaction	120mg subcutaneous injection every 4 weeks No acute phase reaction
Causes MRONJ	Causes MRONJ

FIGURE 9-17 Key differences between bisphosphonates and denosumab as used in oncology practice. (Courtesy of C. Migliorati.)

Medication-related osteonecrosis of the jaw (MRONJ) can develop in a small subset of these patients (Figures 9-18 and 9-19).[19,63] Despite differences in mechanism of action across these three classes, risk for development of MRONJ is comparable (approximately 1%–2%) in the oncology population. The lesion has been classically characterized by the following three criteria:

• Exposed oral bone where gingival or alveolar mucosa normally occurs
• No history of head and neck radiation
• Lasting for more than eight weeks.

It is important to note, however, that clinically exposed oral bone may not be evident in the early stage of MRONJ.

Although actual incidence in the clinical setting is low, resolution of the lesion can be protracted and associated with considerable oral morbidity in some patients. Patients about to be placed on a long-term protocol of one of these agents should undergo oral evaluation and dental treatment of lesions that may contribute to the risk of developing MRONJ in the future. Examples of such preexisting oral lesions include advanced dental caries, moderate to severe periodontal disease, and periradicular lesions. These lesions should ideally be eliminated prior to the initiation of the bone-stabilizing regimen.

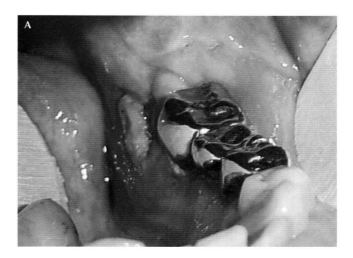
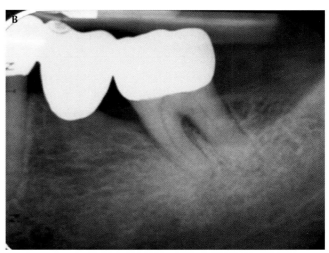

FIGURE 9-18 Osteonecrosis of the jaw in cancer patient receiving bone-stabilizing agents. (A) Exposed bone on lingual aspect of posterior left mandible. (B) Periapical radiograph demonstrating evidence of diffuse osseous destruction. (Photos courtesy of C. Migliorati.)

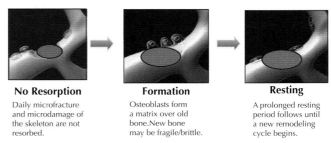

No Resorption
Daily microfracture and microdamage of the skeleton are not resorbed.

Formation
Osteoblasts form a matrix over old bone.New bone may be fragile/brittle.

Resting
A prolonged resting period follows until a new remodeling cycle begins.

Suppression of normal bone turnover

FIGURE 9-19 Inhibition of bone remodeling by bisphosphonates. (Courtesy of C. Migliorati.)

Treatment for MRONJ, if it does occur, depends on staging of the lesion (Figure 9-20).[64] Current literature

Category	Criteria
At risk	Clinically normal, asymptomatic patients who have received antiresorptive therapy
Stage 0	No clinical evidence of exposed bone, but presence of non-specific symptoms or clinical and/or radiographic abnormalities
Stage 1	Exposed and necrotic bone in patients who are asymptomatic and have no evidence of infection
Stage 2	Exposed and necrotic bone associated with pain and/or signs of infection in the region of bone exposure with or without purulent drainage
Stage 3	Exposed and necrotic bone in patients with pain, infection, and at least one of the following: exposure and necrosis extending beyond the local alveolar tissues; radiographic evidence of osteolysis extending to the inferior mandibular border or the maxillary sinus floor; pathologic fracture; oro-antral, oro-nasal or oro-cutaneous communication

FIGURE 9-20 Am Assoc Oral Maxillofac Surg staging criteria for osteonecrosis of the jaw. (Courtesy of C. Migliorati.)

For the full reference lists, please go to http://www.pmph-usa.com/Burkets_Oral_Medicine.

suggests that conservative, nonaggressive therapy may be most beneficial in management of early stage MRONJ. As with any dental intervention, it is essential that thorough discussion and informed consent documentation be performed with the patient prior to initiating the MRONJ management (Figure 9-21).

Patients with MRONJ should be managed by professionals with experience in managing such lesions.
Use of systemic antibiotics is recommended for patients with active infection and or clinical paresthesia.
Home oral hygiene maintenance is essential; utilize oral rinses with chlorhexidine as needed.
Conservative protocol, with periodic clinical evaluation of the progress of disease in MRONJ stages 1 & 2
Pain management as needed
Surgical intervention in advanced cases (stage 3 AAOMS) and in non-responding lesions

FIGURE 9-21 Treatment of medication-related osteonecrosis of the jaw, based in part on reference 64. (Courtesy of C. Migliorati.)

CHAPTER 10

Salivary Gland Diseases

Leah M. Bowers, DMD
Philip C. Fox, DDS, FDS, RCSEd
Michael T. Brennan, DDS, MHS, FDS, RCSEd

The most common presenting complaints of a patient with salivary gland disease are oral dryness (xerostomia) or a glandular swelling or mass. This chapter discusses how to evaluate a patient with these and other signs and symptoms suggestive of salivary gland disease, including clinical examination techniques and imaging modalities. Specific diseases and disorders of the salivary glands are introduced as well as management options for xerostomia and sialorrhea.

SALIVARY GLAND ANATOMY AND PHYSIOLOGY

Saliva is produced by the three major paired salivary glands (the parotid, submandibular, and sublingual glands) and numerous minor salivary glands distributed throughout the mouth and extending into the tracheobronchial tree (Figures 10-1). It is

estimated that there are also between 600 and 1000 minor salivary glands named for the sites which they occupy (i.e., labial, buccal, lingual, palatal, retromolar). In addition, there are three sets of minor salivary glands of the tongue: the glands of Weber, found along the border of the lateral tongue; the glands of von Ebner, surrounding the circumvallate papillae, and the glands of Blandin and Nuhn, also known as the anterior lingual glands, found in the anterior ventral tongue. Mucoceles may arise in the glands of Blandin and Nuhn, highlighting their distinctive anatomic location.

The major salivary glands can also be classified based on the dominant saliva-producing acinar cell type: serous, mucous, or a mix of serous and mucous cells. Serous cells produce a more watery, enzyme-rich saliva, while mucous cells secrete a more viscous fluid with plentiful salivary

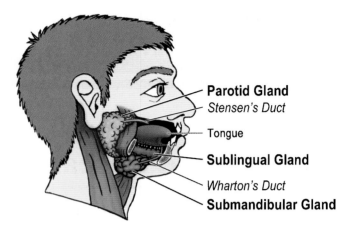

Parotid Gland
Stensen's Duct

Tongue

Sublingual Gland

Wharton's Duct
Submandibular Gland

FIGURE 10-1 Diagrammatic representation of a salivary gland acinus-duct unit.

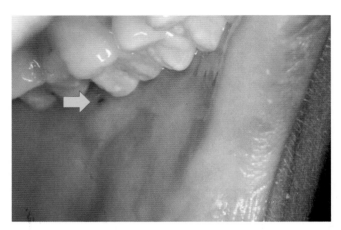

FIGURE 10-2 Opening of Stensen's duct on the left buccal mucosa.

glycoproteins known as mucins. The parotid gland is composed primarily of serous cells; those of the submandibular gland are a mix of mucous and serous types, while those of the sublingual and minor salivary glands are of the mucous type. The glands of Weber are mucous-secreting glands, the glands of von Ebner are purely serous, and the glands of Blandin and Nuhn are mixed mucous and serous glands.

Parotid saliva is secreted through Stensen's ducts, the orifices of which are visible on the buccal mucosa in the vicinity of the maxillary first or second molar (Figure 10-2). Submandibular gland saliva is secreted through the submandibular duct (Wharton's duct), which drains saliva from each submandibular gland and exits at the sublingual caruncles on either side of the lingual frenulum (Figure 10-3). Sublingual saliva may enter the floor of the mouth directly via the short, independent ducts of Rivinus. One or more of these ductules may converge to form the major duct of the sublingual salivary gland (also known as Bartholin's duct), which opens into the submandibular duct. The minor glands secrete their mucinous product onto the mucosa through short ducts.

Histologically, the major salivary glands are composed of acinar (secretory cells) and ductal cells arranged like a cluster of grapes on a stem. The clustered acinar cells (the "grapes") make up the secretory end pieces, while the ductal cells (the "stems") form an extensively branching system that modifies and transports the saliva from the acini into the oral cavity. There are three types of ductal cells: intercalated, striated, and interlobular (Figure 10-4).

Whole saliva (WS; the mixed fluid contents of the oral cavity) is a hypotonic fluid relative to blood plasma and is composed of secretions from the major and minor salivary glands. It is composed of greater than 99% water and less than 1% proteins and salts. WS may also contain variable amounts of gingival crevicular fluid, microorganisms, food debris, exfoliated mucosal cells, and mucus. The exact composition of WS follows a circadian rhythm: at night and in the resting state, the submandibular and sublingual glands are the main contributors with some saliva also being produced

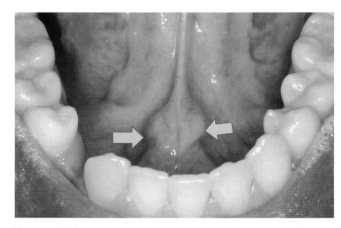

FIGURE 10-3 Opening of Wharton's duct on the floor of mouth.

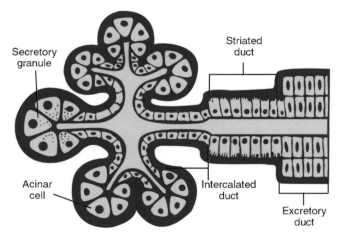

Secretory granule

Striated duct

Acinar cell

Intercalated duct

Excretory duct

FIGURE 10-4 Diagrammatic representation of salivary gland acini and ducts.

by the minor salivary glands.[1] Techniques designed to collect saliva solely from an individual parotid gland or glands or the submandibular glands will produce a purer sample of saliva without the numerous contaminants found in WS. Upon stimulation, the parotid and submandibular glands are responsible for the majority of saliva production with minor gland secretions accounting for less than 10% of the saliva. Stimulation of salivation occurs between 10% and 20% of the day, with the amount of time dependent on habit and dietary preferences.

Normal daily production of WS ranges from 0.5 to1.5 L. Production of saliva involves initial water transport from the serum into the terminal portion of the acinar cell followed by selective reabsorption of sodium and chloride and the secretion of potassium and bicarbonate to produce a hypotonic solution.[2] Upon stimulation of the salivary flow rate, sodium, chloride, and bicarbonate concentrations increase, and potassium decreases via an ion exchange mechanism in the ductal system. Salivary protein secretion, mostly from the acinar cells, results in a protein-rich hypotonic fluid.[2] Salivary proteins are numerous and serve a variety of functions including digestion (e.g., α-amylase, lipase, proteinases, DNase, and RNase) and protection (immunoglobulins, lysozyme, lactoferrin, lactoperoxidase, mucins).

The secretion of salivary fluid and salivary proteins is controlled by both the sympathetic and the parasympathetic subsystems of the autonomic nervous system.[3] The dominant stimulus for fluid secretion is via muscarinic-cholinergic receptors, which release acetylcholine, inducing the secretion of saliva by acinar cells in the end pieces of the salivary gland ductal tree. Stimulus for salivary protein secretion is via sympathetic β-adrenergic receptors that release noradrenaline.

Both electrolyte concentrations and volume of saliva may be influenced by a number of factors including circadian rhythm, various stimuli, and number of functional secretory units. Factors that may increase salivary flow include taste and olfactory stimuli, mechanical stimulation, pain, pregnancy-related hormonal changes, aggression, and sympathomimetic and parasympathomimetic drugs. Menopause-related hormonal changes, stress, anti adrenergic, and anticholinergic drugs will decrease salivary flow rate.[4] A loss of acini, seen in a number of clinical conditions, particularly the autoimmune exocrinopathy Sjögren's syndrome (SS), results in a decreased production of saliva.

The question as to whether salivary flow diminishes with normal aging has been the subject of much debate; many studies suggest age-related changes in either volume or salivary constituents, while others have found no related changes. These studies, however, defy comparison since the methodologies differ.[5] Postmortem histologic studies show that with aging, parenchymal tissue of the salivary glands undergo replacement with fat, connective tissue, and oncocytes. In addition, acinar atrophy, ductal dilatation, and inflammatory infiltration have been observed with aging in normal subjects.[6]

It is generally accepted that in healthy, non medicated adults, salivary production remains stable with age despite the loss of acinar cells. To explain this phenomenon, it is hypothesized that a secretory reserve capacity exists.[7] Disease, surgery, radiotherapy, and chemotherapy tax this reserve capacity, resulting in compromised function.[8] A gradual, age-related loss of this reserve capacity may explain the greater magnitude of effect from conditions adversely affecting saliva production in older individuals compared to their younger counterparts.

DIAGNOSIS OF THE PATIENT WITH SALIVARY GLAND DISEASE

The most common presentation of salivary gland disease is *xerostomia* denoting a subjective complaint of dry mouth. *Hyposalivation* refers to a quantified reduced salivary flow rate and may or may not be accompanied by xerostomia. Similarly, xerostomia may or may not be associated with hyposalivation and can be a result of, for example, a change in salivary composition to a greater mucous content. *Hypersalivation* (ptyalism) refers to an increase in production of saliva and/or a decrease in oral clearance of saliva. *Salivary gland dysfunction* is commonly used to indicate decreased salivary flow or another quantifiable alteration in salivary performance.

Since individuals with salivary gland dysfunction may be at risk of a variety of oral and systemic complications due to alterations in normal salivary performance, a thorough objective examination to identify the basis of their condition is warranted. Since salivary gland dysfunction may be the result of a systemic disorder, early recognition and accurate diagnosis may be of great benefit to an individual's general health and well-being. Once the presence of salivary gland dysfunction has been established, appropriate treatment should be implemented with follow-up as necessary.

Since the causes of xerostomia and salivary gland dysfunction are numerous, a systematic approach to establish diagnosis and appropriate treatment is necessary. Patients should be queried regarding the duration of their complaint, whether the condition is progressive or intermittent, possible circadian association and severity which may suggest salivary gland hypofunction. An initial evaluation should also include a detailed evaluation of associated symptoms, a past and present medical history, a head/neck/oral examination, and an assessment of salivary function involving quantification of unstimulated and stimulated salivary flow. Further techniques that may be indicated are analysis of salivary constituents, salivary imaging, biopsy, and clinical laboratory assessment. These are described below in greater detail. Patients should also be questioned concerning dryness at other body sites, especially the eyes and other mucosal surfaces.

Causes of salivary gland hypofunction include xerogenic medications (including many antidepressants, anticholinergics, antispasmodics, antihistamines, antihypertensives, sedatives, diuretics, and bronchodilators[9]) and other agents (e.g., caffeine, alcohol, cigarette smoking), irradiation to the head and neck (i.e., external and internal beam radiation therapy), systemic disease (e.g., diabetes mellitus), salivary gland masses, psychological conditions (e.g., depression, anxiety),

TABLE 10-1	**Partial List of Differential Diagnoses for Salivary Gland Hypofunction**
Autoimmune	Chronic graft-versus-host disease Sjögren's syndrome
Developmental	Salivary gland aplasia
Iatrogenic	External beam radiation Internal beam radiation Postsurgical (adenectomy, ductal ligation) Botox injection
Inflammatory	IgG4-related disease (Küttner tumor; Mikulicz's disease)
Infectious	Viral: CMV, HIV, hepatitis C Granulomatous: Tuberculosis
Medication-associated	
Neoplastic	Benign and malignant salivary gland tumors
Nonneoplastic	Sialolithiasis
Systemic	Anorexia nervosa, diabetes mellitus, chronic alcoholism, sarcoidosis

Abbreviation: CMV, cytomegalovirus.

malnutrition (e.g., bulimia, dehydration), autoimmune disease (e.g., SS), and other unspecified or undiagnosed conditions.[9] A partial list of differential diagnosis for salivary gland hypofunction is outlined in Table 10-1.

Symptoms of Salivary Gland Dysfunction

Symptoms of salivary gland hypofunction are related to decreased fluid in the oral cavity and this may have an effect on mucosal hydration and oral functions. Patients may complain of dryness of all the oral mucosal surfaces, including the lips and throat, and difficulty chewing, swallowing, and speaking. Other associated complaints may include oral pain, an oral burning sensation, chronic sore throat and pain with swallowing. The mucosa may be sensitive to spicy or coarse foods, limiting the patient's enjoyment of meals, which may compromise nutrition.[10–12] Often, patients experiencing chronic salivary gland hypofunction will carry water with them at all times and sip frequently to relieve their oral dryness.

Unfortunately, the general complaint of oral dryness is not correlated well with decreased salivary function, although specific symptoms may be.[13] For example, although complaints of oral dryness at night or on awakening have not been found to be associated reliably with reduced salivary function, the complaints of oral dryness while eating, the need to sip liquids to swallow food, or difficulties in swallowing dry food have all been highly correlated with measurable decreases in secretory capacity. These complaints focus on oral activities (swallowing and eating) that rely on stimulated salivary function.

Past and Present Medical History

Collection of the past and present medical history may reveal medical conditions or medications known to be associated with salivary gland dysfunction leading to a direct diagnosis (e.g., a patient who has received radiotherapy for a head and neck malignancy or an individual taking a tricyclic antidepressant). More than 400 drugs with xerogenic potential have been identified including antidepressants, anticholinergics, antispasmodics, antihistamines, antihypertensives, sedatives, and bronchodilators,[9] and therefore a complete history of all medications being taken (including over-the-counter medications, supplements, and herbal preparations) is critical. Often the temporal association of symptom onset with the treatment is a valuable clue. When the history does not suggest an obvious diagnosis, further exploration of the symptomatic complaint should be undertaken. A patient's report of eye, throat, nasal, skin, or vaginal dryness, in addition to xerostomia, may be a significant indication of a systemic condition, such as SS.[14]

Clinical Examination

Signs of salivary gland hypofunction may affect several areas of the oral cavity and mouth. The lips are often dry with cracking, peeling, and atrophy. The buccal mucosa may be pale and corrugated. The dorsal tongue may appear smooth due to a loss of papillation and erythematous or may appear fissured. Due to the absence of the buffering capacity supplied by saliva, there is often an increase in erosive lesions and dental caries. The carious lesions often affect the root surfaces and the cusp tips of teeth: areas usually resistant to decay. The decay may be progressive even in the presence of good oral hygiene and recurrent decay is common. An increased accumulation of food debris and plaque may occur in interproximal areas due to the lack of cleansing saliva flow. Patients with xerostomia may have increased plaque indices and bleeding on probing scores.[15]

Two additional indications of oral dryness are the "lipstick" and "tongue blade" signs. In the former, the presence of lipstick or shed epithelial cells on the labial surfaces of the anterior maxillary teeth is indicative of reduced saliva; saliva would normally wet the mucosa and aid in cleansing the teeth. A positive "tongue blade" sign results when a tongue blade, pressed gently and then lifted away from the buccal mucosa, adheres to the tissue. Both signs suggest that the mucosa is not sufficiently moisturized by saliva.

Candidiasis is often associated with salivary gland dysfunction, and many stigmata of an oral colonization may be present. The erythematous form of candidiasis, appearing as red patches on the mucosa, is more prevalent than the more familiar white, curd-like pseudomembranous (thrush) form (Figure 10-5). Angular cheilitis, seen as persistent cracking or fissuring of the oral commissures, is also common.

Salivary gland dysfunction can also be associated with enlargement of the salivary glands. Since salivary gland

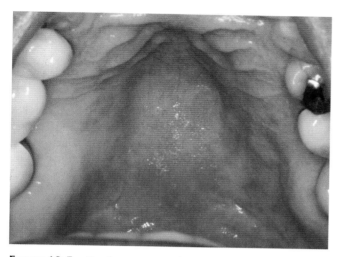

FIGURE 10-5 Erythematous candidiasis of the hard palate in a patient with salivary gland hypofunction.

enlargement can be associated with a variety of inflammatory, infectious, or neoplastic and other conditions, the etiology of the enlargement must be established.[16] Examination of the normal salivary gland by inspection and palpation should be painless and without detection of a mass or masses. Enlarged glands that are painful on palpation are indicative of infection, acute inflammation, or tumor. The consistency of the gland should be slightly rubbery but not hard. Neoplasms, either benign or malignant, of the salivary glands usually present as painless masses but may also present with dull pain suggestive of an inflammation-based process.

The major salivary glands should also be palpated to determine whether saliva can be expressed via the main excretory ducts. Normally, saliva can be expressed from each major gland orifice by gently compressing the glands and by drawing pressure toward the orifice. The expressed saliva should be colorless and transparent, watery, and copious. Viscous or scant secretions suggest chronically reduced function. A cloudy exudate may be a sign of bacterial infection, although some patients with very low salivary function will have hazy, flocculated secretions that are sterile. In these cases, there may be mucoid accretions and clumped epithelial cells, which result in a cloudy appearance. The exudate should be cultured if it does not appear clinically normal, particularly in the case of an enlarged gland.

Major Salivary Glands

The parotid glands, the largest of the salivary glands, are positioned on the lateral aspect of the face overlying the posterior surface of the mandible, anteroinferiorly to the auricle. Traditionally, the gland has thought to have a superficial and deep lobe based on the course of the facial nerve as it traverses the gland. Most benign tumors of the parotid gland are located within the superficial lobe and therefore are amenable to resection by superficial parotidectomy. However, it is not uncommon to discover that masses thought to be confined to the superficial lobe in fact extend into the deep lobe.

Because of its relationship to the parotid gland, it is important to document function of the facial nerve when evaluating parotid masses. Facial nerve paralysis is usually indicative of malignancy. Rarely, infection or rapidly growing benign tumors may cause facial nerve paralysis. Other findings suggesting malignancy include multiple masses, a fixed mass with invasion of surrounding tissue, and the presence of cervical lymphadenopathy.

Bilateral parotid gland masses are usually due to lymphadenopathy, Warthin's tumors, lymphoepithelial cysts (LECs) and enlarged lymph nodes in the setting of HIV, SS, or rarely other salivary gland tumors such as the acinic cell adenocarcinoma. Multiple painless masses within a single parotid gland may be due to Warthin's tumors, lymph nodes, metastatic disease, and other benign and malignant tumors.

The submandibular gland is a horseshoe-shaped structure located in the submandibular triangle of the neck and is bordered superiorly by the inferior border of the mandible and inferiorly by the anterior and posterior bellies of the digastric muscle. The sublingual glands are paired glands lying on opposite sides of the lingual frenulum, superior to the mylohyoid muscle. Tumors in the submandibular or sublingual glands usually present as painless, solitary, slow-growing mobile masses. Bimanual palpation, with one hand intraorally on the floor of the mouth and the other extraorally below the mandible, is necessary to evaluate the glands adequately. Tumors of the minor salivary glands are usually smooth masses located most commonly on the hard or soft palate but may present anywhere minor salivary glands are present.

Salivary gland neoplasms arise most commonly in the parotid glands followed by the submandibular, sublingual, and minor salivary glands. Generally speaking, the relative proportion of malignant neoplasms is greater the smaller the gland: that is, a neoplasm in the parotid gland is statistically more likely to be benign than one arising in a minor salivary gland.

Certain clinical signs and symptoms are more likely to be present in a malignant neoplasm of the salivary glands. These include ulceration of the overlying mucosa, fixation of the mass to deeper tissue planes, induration, invasion, and cervical lymphadenopathy. Additional clinical findings such as otalgia, dysphagia, odynophagia, trismus, paresthesia, a history of cancer, or cachexia may further raise suspicion.[17]

Other lesions may mimic the presentation of salivary gland tumors. Inflammatory diseases, infections, and nutritional deficiencies may present as diffuse glandular enlargement (usually of the parotid gland). Patients who are seropositive for HIV may develop cystic lymphoepithelial lesions (LELs) that may be confused with tumors.[18] Both melanoma and squamous cell carcinoma can metastasize to the parotid gland and appear similar to a primary salivary tumor.[19] Chronic sialadenitis in the submandibular glands can commonly be confused with a tumor.

Sialometry

Salivary flow rates provide essential information for diagnostic and research purposes, and therefore, gland function should be determined by objective measurement techniques. Salivary flow rates can be calculated from the individual major salivary glands or from a mixed sample of the oral fluids termed whole saliva (WS).

Since unstimulated salivary gland function is the predominant state, this greatly influences overall oral comfort and protection of the oral cavity. Normal subjects are found to complain of a dry mouth when unstimulated whole salivary flow is reduced 40%–50%.[20] Examination of stimulated salivary flow can allow for assessment of the relative functional capacity of the salivary glands and help determine whether sialagogues are likely to be beneficial. Therefore, it is important to assess both unstimulated and stimulated salivary flow when investigating a complaint of xerostomia.

The main methods of WS collection include the draining, suction, spitting, and absorbent (sponge) methods.[21] The latter two are used most often. In the spitting method, the patient allows saliva to accumulate in the mouth and then expectorates into a pre-weighed tube, usually once every 60 seconds for 5–15 minutes. The absorbent method uses a pre-weighed gauze sponge placed in the patient's mouth for a predetermined amount of time.[22] To ensure an unstimulated sample, the patient is instructed to refrain from eating, drinking, smoking, chewing gum, and oral hygiene practices or any other oral stimulation for at least 90 minutes prior to the test session. Excessive movement and talking is discouraged during the testing period.

For a general assessment of salivary function, unstimulated WS collection is recommended. It is quick and easy to perform, accurate and reproducible, and does not require expensive or labor-intensive equipment.[23] Ideally, dentists would determine baseline values for unstimulated WS output at an initial examination allowing for later comparisons if patients begin to complain of oral dryness or present with other signs and symptoms of salivary dysfunction.

If a stimulated WS collection is desired, a standardized method of stimulation should also be employed. Chewing an unflavored gum base or an inert material such as paraffin wax or a rubber band at a controlled rate (usually 60 times per minute which can be paced using a metronome) is a reliable and reproducible means of inducing saliva secretion. For research investigations, 2% citric acid may be placed on the tongue at 30-second intervals.

Flow rates are determined gravimetrically in milliliters per minute per gland, assuming that the specific gravity of saliva is 1 (i.e., 1 mL of saliva is equivalent to 1 g). Samples to be retained for compositional analysis should be collected on ice and frozen until tested.[24] Flow rates are affected by many factors. Patient position, hydration, diurnal and seasonal variation, and time since stimulation can all affect salivary flow. Regardless of the technique chosen for saliva collection, it is critical to use a well-defined, standardized, and clearly documented procedure. This allows for meaningful comparisons between individuals for study purposes and for repeat measures in an individual over time.

Individual parotid gland saliva collection is performed by using Carlson-Crittenden collectors or a modified Lashley cup.[25] Collectors are placed over the Stensen's duct orifices and are held in place with gentle suction. Collection of saliva from the submandibular and sublingual glands may be accomplished using custom-made collectors such as the Wolff collector placed over the opening of the Wharton's duct at the floor of the mouth.[26] Saliva from individual submandibular and sublingual glands is collected with an aspirating device[27] or an alginate-held collector called a segregator.[28]

Collection of saliva from the individual major salivary glands has the advantage of allowing for assessment of individual gland function, which is not contaminated with food debris and microorganisms. However, these techniques may be tedious and require custom-made collection devices.[26] Collection and sialochemistry of saliva collected from individual glands may reveal changes such as selective hyposecretion of the submandibular/sublingual salivary glands and changes in electrolytes and proteins (enzymes) observed in SS, reflecting the effect of autoimmune attack on the secretory cells in individual salivary glands.[23]

It is difficult to determine an absolute "normal" value for salivary output due to great interindividual variability and consequently a large range of normal values.[29] However, using the collection methods described earlier, most experts agree that unstimulated WS flow rates of <0.1 mL/min and stimulated WS flow rates of <0.7 mL/min are abnormally low and indicative of marked salivary gland hypofunction. It is important to recognize, however, that higher levels of output do not guarantee that function is normal. Indeed, they may represent marked hypofunction for some individuals. These stated values represent a lower limit of normal and should serve only as a guide for the clinician.

Sialochemistry

When investigating a complaint of salivary gland dysfunction, it is important to recognize that changes in salivary composition may be as important as a reduction in salivary output in some cases. Therefore, the demonstration of seemingly adequate salivary flow alone is not a guarantee of normal salivary gland function. Numerous changes in salivary chemistries have been described with a variety of salivary gland disorders.[30–32] However, most reported alterations are related to reduced gland function rather than a specific disorder. Therefore, most salivary constituent changes are nonspecific diagnostically and have minimal utility in determining the cause of the salivary gland dysfunction.

Normal saliva is a colorless, transparent fluid with a slightly acidic pH ranging between 6 and 7. It is composed of approximately 99% water with contributions of inorganic ions of Na^+, Cl^-, Ca^{2+}, K^+, HCO^{3-}, H^2PO^{4-}, F^-, I^-, and Mg^{2+} and thiocyanate. The bicarbonate ions serve as a buffering agent, while the presence of calcium and phosphate neutralize acids detrimental to tooth structure as well as contributing to remineralization of the tooth surface. The organic components of saliva include urea, ammonia, uric acid, glucose, cholesterol, fatty acids, lipids, amino acids, steroid hormones, and proteins. Many of the constituent proteins such as mucins, amylases, agglutinins, lactoferrin, and secretory IgA play a role in protection of the oral tissues.[33]

Salivary Diagnostics

Saliva has been shown to be an important medium for diagnosis and monitoring of a number of systemic conditions.[34–36] It is now used routinely to diagnose viral infections[37] and determine blood alcohol[38] and hormone levels[39,40] and to screen for drugs of abuse.[41] The use of saliva in diagnostics has many advantages over blood including relative ease of collection with no requirement for special equipment or training, non invasiveness, and cost-effectiveness for screening of large populations.[33]

Established tests for the detection of antibodies to HIV-1 and HIV-2 in saliva, such as the Food and Drug Administration [FDA]-approved OraQuick ADVANCE Rapid HIV-1/2 Antibody Test (OraSure Technologies, Bethlehem, PA), provide for rapid, convenient, and relatively inexpensive screening.[42] Additional saliva-based assays are available to detect and quantify specific periodontal disease-associated bacteria and high-risk human papilloma virus (MyPerioPath, Oral DNA Labs, Brentwood, TN).

Saliva-based assays for early detection and diagnosis of cancer are in development. Currently, research into the presence of tumor markers in saliva for oral cancers and precancers and variation in the salivary microbiome

associated with other cancers shows promise.[42,43] In addition, research is ongoing involving detection of known saliva-based markers for myocardial infarction and for new markers for SS in patients with sicca symptoms (dry eyes, dry mouth).[42]

With respect to genomic medicine or "personalized medicine," sialochemistry may play an increasingly important role in the early detection, monitoring, and progression of systemic and oral diseases. We are likely to see the increased utilization of saliva as a diagnostic fluid, and consequently, dentists will have greater involvement in the identification and monitoring of certain non oral disorders.[33]

Salivary Gland Imaging

The choice of imaging modality of the salivary glands is dependent on the clinical presentation. Depending on the technique used, imaging can provide information on salivary function, anatomic alterations, and space-occupying lesions within the glands. The following describes specific techniques as they relate to the diagnosis of salivary gland disorders. This section discusses plain film radiography, sialography, ultrasonography (US), radionuclide imaging, magnetic resonance imaging (MRI), and computed and positron emission tomography (PET) (Table 10-2). Advances in imaging techniques have resulted in a shift from a reliance on plain films and sialograms to nearly sole usage of computed tomography (CT), MRI, and US.[44]

Plain Film Radiography

Plain film radiography often serves as the initial imaging modality for evaluation of the major salivary glands due to its availability; however, its clinical value is limited and superior imagining techniques may be available depending on the clinical scenario. It is useful particularly for the visualization of radiopaque sialoliths and the evaluation of bony

TABLE 10-2 Salivary Gland Imaging Modalities: Indications, Advantages, and Disadvantages

Imaging Modality	Indications	Advantages	Disadvantages
Plain film	Sialolith	Readily available	Prone to anatomic overlap; Radiolucent stones not visualized
Sialography	Sialoliths; Abnormalities of ductal system	Visualizes ductal anatomy/ blockage	Invasive; Requires iodine-containing dye; No quantification; Contraindicated in active infection
Ultrasonography	Mass detection; Biopsy guidance	Noninvasive; Cost-effective	No visualization of deep parotid; No quantification of function; Observer variability
Radionuclide imaging (scintigraphy)	Salivary gland function	Quantification of function Noninvasive	Lengthy procedure; High cost; Radiation exposure; No morphologic data
Computed tomography	Inflammatory conditions Calcified structures Bony erosion	Differentiates osseous structures from soft tissue	No quantification; Requires dye injection; Radiation exposure
Magnetic resonance imaging	Neoplastic processes	Superior soft tissue resolution No radiation exposure	Contraindicated with ferromagnetic materials, pacemakers
Positron emission tomography	Salivary gland functional alterations and inflammation	Highly sensitive to metabolic activity	Radiation exposure; No morphologic information; High cost; Lengthy procedure

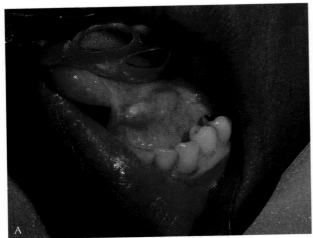
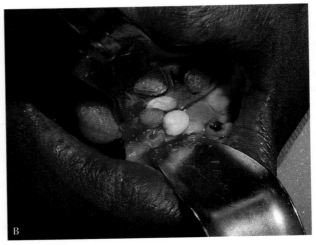

FIGURE 10-6   (A) Sialolith within the left submandibular gland duct. (Courtesy of Dr. Michael D. Turner, New York University.) (B) Surgical exploration of a sialolith within the left submandibular duct. (Courtesy of Dr. Michael D. Turner, New York University.)

destruction associated with malignant neoplasms and it can provide a background for interpretation of the sialogram.

Since the salivary glands are located relatively superficially, radiographic images may be obtained using standard dental radiographic techniques. Symptoms suggestive of salivary gland obstruction (acute swelling of the gland and pain; sialoliths—Figure 10-6A and Figure 10-6B) warrant plain film radiography of the major salivary glands to detect calcified blockages. Panoramic or lateral oblique and anteroposterior (AP) projections are used to visualize the parotid glands. However, anatomic structures may overlap in panoramic views obscuring the appearance of a stone. A standard occlusal film can be placed intraorally adjacent to the parotid duct to visualize a stone close to the gland orifice but will not capture the entire parotid gland. Sialoliths obstructing the submandibular gland may be visualized by panoramic, occlusal, or lateral oblique views.

Smaller stones or poorly calcified sialoliths may not be visible on plain films. If a stone is not evident with plain film radiography but clinical evaluation and history are suggestive of salivary gland obstruction, additional imaging (generally with sialography) may be necessary.

Sialography

Sialography allows for the radiographic visualization of the parotid and submandibular salivary glands and ducts following retrograde instillation of soluble contrast material into Stensen's or Wharton's ducts (Figure 10-7). The ducts of the sublingual glands are too small for reliable injection of contrast medium.[44]

Sialography is the recommended method for evaluating intrinsic and acquired abnormalities of the ductal system (e.g., ductal stricture, obstruction, dilatation, and ruptures) and for identifying and localizing sialoliths because it provides the clearest visualization of the branching ducts and acinar end pieces. Normally, as the submandibular gland duct traverses

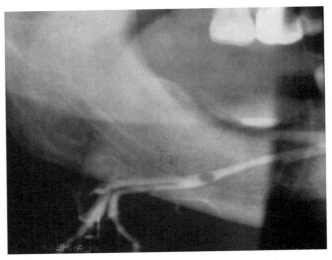

FIGURE 10-7   A sialogram of the submandibular gland demonstrating an uncalcified sialolith in Wharton's duct, which can be visualized where the submandibular duct overlies the inferior alveolar canal. (Courtesy of Dr. Elisa Mozaffari, University of Pennsylvania.)

the parenchyma, it demonstrates an abrupt transition in ductal diameter while the parotid gland duct diameter shows a more gradual decrease. The normal ductal architecture has a "leafless tree" appearance (see Figure 10-7).

When a patient presents with a history of rapid-onset, painful swelling of a single gland (typically brought on by eating), sialography is the indicated imaging technique. Radiopaque sialoliths may appear as voids. Focal collections of contrast medium within the gland (sialectasis or abnormal salivary ductal dilation) are seen in the cases of sialadenitis and SS. Sialography may also be a valuable tool in pre-surgical planning for removal of salivary masses. Radiographic views for sialography include panoramic, lateral oblique, AP, and "puffed-cheek" AP views.

Oil- and water-based contrast media (both containing iodine and therefore contraindicated in patients with iodine sensitivity) are available. Oil-based contrast material is not diluted by saliva or absorbed across the mucosa, which allows for maximum opacification of the ductal and acinar structures. However, if extravasation into the glandular tissue occurs, the residual contrast material will remain at the site and may interfere with subsequent CT images. Inflammatory responses and even the formation of granulomas have been reported following sialography using oil-based contrast.[45,46] In addition, injection of oil-based contrast media requires more pressure because of its viscosity and may be more painful for the patient.

Water-based dyes are soluble in saliva and can diffuse into the glandular tissue, which can result in decreased radiographic density and poor visualization of peripheral ducts compared with oil-based contrast. Therefore high-viscosity water-soluble contrast agents that allow better visualization of the ductal structures are preferable.

Following the sialographic procedure, the patient should be instructed to massage the gland and/or to suck on lemon drops to promote the flow of saliva and contrast material out of the gland. A postprocedure radiograph is performed after approximately one hour. If a substantial amount of contrast material remains in the salivary gland, follow-up visits should be scheduled until the contrast material elutes or is fully resorbed. Incomplete clearing can be due to obstruction of salivary outflow, extraductal or extravasated contrast medium, collection of contrast material in abscess cavities, or impaired secretory function.

Digital subtraction sialography (DSS), whereby the image taken before contrast is injected is "subtracted" from the image taken after injection, continues to be the standard technique for high-resolution imaging of the extraglandular and intraglandular salivary ductal system.[47] It is considered to be the first choice in diagnostic imaging for the detection of subtle anatomical ductal changes[48,49] and is helpful in suspected cases of calculi or ductal stricture. DSS provides enhanced contrast resolution and therefore permits the detection of small stones. Functional information can also be obtained after sialagogue administration.

Clinical indications for performing DSS are an acute swelling or palpable mass in the submandibular or parotid regions or gradual or chronic enlargement of a salivary gland where sialolithiasis or sialadenitis is suspected.[49] The principle weaknesses of DSS are that it is invasive (since it requires ductal cannulation), uses contrast and ionizing radiation, and has a high incidence of technical failure.[50]

Two contraindications to sialography are active infection and allergy to contrast media. Sialography performed during active infection may further irritate and potentially rupture the already inflamed gland. In addition, the injection of contrast material might force bacteria throughout the ductal structure and worsen an infection. The iodine in the contrast media may induce an allergic reaction and can also interfere with thyroid function tests and with thyroid cancer evaluation by nuclear medicine if these are done concurrently.

Ultrasonography

US is particularly useful in the assessment of superficial masses of the parotid and submandibular glands. It is relatively inexpensive, widely available, safe, and can be used to delineate superficial salivary gland lesions as precisely as CT and MRI.[50] High-frequency US provides excellent resolution and characterization of tissue without exposure to radiation.[50] Due to its many advantages, US is becoming the method of choice for the initial evaluation of the salivary glands, especially in children and pregnant women,[44] particularly when evaluating for suspected sialolithiasis and salivary gland abscesses.[50] US can be used to distinguish focal from diffuse disease, assess adjacent vascular structures and vascularity, distinguish solid from cystic lesions, guide fine-needle aspiration biopsy (FNAB), and perform nodal staging.[44] It can also correctly differentiate malignant lesions from benign lesions in 90% of cases, distinguish glandular from extraglandular masses with an accuracy of 98%, and confirm the clinical suspicion of a mass.[51] Therefore, US may be employed as an initial imaging technique to guide the clinician in determining whether further imaging is required.[50] Additional characterization of tumors can then be accomplished using cross-sectional imaging techniques such as CT or MRI.[44]

Due to their superficial locations, the parotid and submandibular glands are easily visualized by US (Figure 10-8), although the deep portion of the parotid gland is difficult to assess because of the overlying mandibular ramus.[52,53] Although US cannot directly visualize the facial nerve, it can suggest its position by accurate identification of intraglandular vessels within the parotid. Superficial lesions, particularly in the parotid and the submandibular glands, may also be amenable to core biopsy or fine-needle aspiration cytology (FNAC) under US guidance.

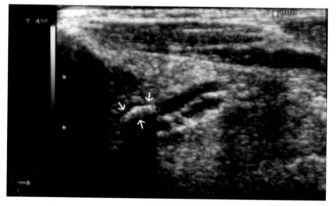

Figure 10-8 Ultrasound of a salivary gland. A sialolith within the left submandibular gland is visualized (arrows).

Recent studies have evaluated sonographic diagnostic criteria for SS.[54] It has been proposed that salivary gland ultrasonography (SGUS) may be used in addition to or in place of the minor salivary gland biopsy (MSGB) as a part of the diagnostic criteria for SS.[55] SGUS may also represent a promising tool for earlier disease detection and for monitoring disease activity and progression in established SS patients. In addition, SGUS has been shown to be effective in identifying SS patients with changes indicative of lymphoma development.[56]

Radionuclide Salivary Imaging

Scintigraphy with technetium (Tc) 99m pertechnetate is a dynamic and minimally invasive diagnostic test to assess salivary gland function and to determine abnormalities in gland uptake and excretion.[57] Scintigraphy provides quantitative information on the functional capabilities of the glands (Figure 10-9).[58] It can estimate the severity of salivary gland involvement and functional disorders, which may not be accurately reflected by morphological damage.[59] In addition to being noninvasive, scintigraphy has the advantages that it is easy to perform, reproducible, and generally well tolerated by the patient.[59]

Technetium is a pure gamma ray–emitting radionuclide that is taken up by the salivary glands (following intravenous injection), transported through the glands, and then secreted into the oral cavity. The parotid and submandibular glands are visualized distinctly, as well as the thyroid gland, which binds and retains Tc. Both uptake and secretory phases can be recognized on the scans. Uptake of Tc 99m by a salivary gland indicates that there is functional epithelial tissue present. The Tc 99m scan has been shown to correlate well with salivary output[60] and serves as a measurement of fluid movement in the salivary acinar cells.[61]

Scintigraphy is indicated for the evaluation of patients when sialography is contraindicated or cannot be performed (i.e., in cases of acute gland infection or iodine allergy) or when the major duct cannot be cannulated successfully. It has also been used to aid in the diagnosis of ductal obstruction, sialolithiasis, gland aplasia, Bell's palsy, and SS.

Salivary gland scintigraphy (SGS) has been proposed as a valid and noninvasive alternative approach to functional evaluation of salivary gland involvement in xerostomic patients. Scintigraphy can provide information on both parenchyma and excretion of all major salivary glands after a single intravenous injection: a distinct advantage over other imaging techniques.[62] In addition, an abnormal SGS result is accepted by the American–European consensus group as a criterion for the diagnosis of SS.[62] SGS results also correlate with saliva production, sialography, and focus score (FS) in the MSGB.[62]

A normal scintigraphic time-activity curve may be separated into three phases: flow, concentration, and washout. The flow phase is about 15–20 seconds in duration and

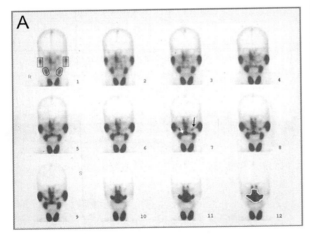 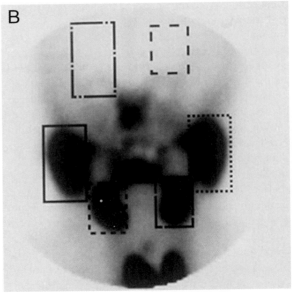

FIGURE 10-9 (A, left) Technetium 99m pertechnetate radionuclide image (scintigram) of the major salivary glands. This sequential salivary scintigram is an anterior Water's projection of an individual with normal salivary function. The four major glands are outlined in frame 1 as regions of interest for further analyses. In frame 7, the dark arrow denotes Stensen's duct and the white arrow Wharton's duct, both emptying into the oral cavity. A secretagogue, usually citric acid, is placed in the oral cavity between frames 9 and 10, inducing a rapid emptying of the salivary glands. In frame 12, 10 minutes following application of the secretagogue, tracer is absent in the salivary glands and concentrated in the oral cavity, which is outlined. (Courtesy of Dr. Frederick Vivino, University of Pennsylvania.) (B, right) A single frame of a salivary scintigram demonstrating significant uptake in both parotid and submandibular glands (four lower windows) with excretion into the oral cavity. The two upper windows represent background activity from the blood flow, which is subtracted from the four regions of interest to determine specific salivary activity. (Courtesy of Dr. Frederick Vivino, University of Pennsylvania.)

represents the time immediately following radionuclide injection when the isotope is equilibrating in the blood and accumulating in the salivary gland at a submaximal rate. The concentration (or uptake) phase represents the accumulation of Tc 99m pertechnetate in the gland through active transport. With normal salivary function, the radionuclide will be secreted and tracer activity should be apparent in the oral cavity without stimulation after 10–15 minutes. Approximately 15 minutes after administration, tracer concentration begins to increase in the oral cavity and decrease in the salivary glands. A normal image will demonstrate symmetric uptake of Tc 99m by both the parotid and the submandibular glands. The sublingual glands cannot be distinguished reliably.

In the excretory or washout phase, the patient is given a lemon drop, or citric acid is applied to the tongue to stimulate secretion. Normal clearing of Tc 99m should be prompt, uniform, and symmetric. Activity remaining in the salivary glands after stimulation is suggestive of obstruction, certain tumors, or inflammation.

With notable exceptions, neoplasms arising within the salivary glands do not concentrate Tc 99m. The exceptions are Warthin's tumor and oncocytomas which arise from ductal tissue. These neoplasms retain Tc 99m because they do not communicate with the ductal system and will appear as areas of increased activity on static images.[63] This becomes apparent during the washout phase when the glandular signal decreases following stimulation while activity is retained in the tumor. In contrast, other salivary tumors may appear as voids or areas of decreased activity on scintigram.

Several rating scales are used for the evaluation of salivary scintigrams; however, no standard rating method presently exists.[64] Current approaches to functional assessment include visual interpretation, time-activity curve analysis, and numeric indices. Most radiologists interpret Tc 99m scans by visual inspection and clinical judgment. A semi quantitative method exists in which Tc 99m uptake and secretion are calculated by computer analysis of user-defined regions of interest.

One widely used classification scheme proposed by Schall et al.[65,66] uses visual interpretation and relies upon the intensity of uptake and activity of the salivary gland after administration of an excretory stimulus. This scheme involves assignment of one of four grades: grade 1 representing no impairment and grade 4 being the total absence of uptake and glandular activity. This classification scheme is subjective, and borderline results may present an interpretive challenge. However, this scheme is currently considered the standard method for salivary scintigram interpretation.[62]

CT and CBCT

CT is considered the gold standard in the evaluation of inflammatory diseases of the salivary glands. Landmark adjacent structures such as the retromandibular vein, carotid artery, and deep lymph nodes can also be identified on CT.

CT is especially useful in the evaluation of acute inflammatory processes since it is able to depict mandibular cortical bone erosion and destruction, cutaneous changes, and submandibular duct calculi. Since calcified structures are well visualized by CT, this modality is especially useful for the evaluation of inflammatory conditions that are associated with sialoliths. In addition, bony erosion due to malignant processes and sclerosis can be visualized using CT.[50] Since CT can define the characteristic hypervascular wall seen in abscesses and can provide definition of cystic walls, it is possible to distinguish fluid-filled masses (i.e., cyst) from abscesses.

CT images of salivary glands should be obtained by using continuous fine cuts through the involved gland. Axial-plane cuts should include the superior aspect of the salivary glands, continuing to the hyoid bone and visualizing potentially enlarged lymph nodes in the suprahyoid neck region. Nonenhanced and contrast-enhanced CT images are obtained routinely (Figure 10-10). The initial nonenhanced scans are reviewed for the presence of sialoliths, masses, glandular enlargement or asymmetry, nodal involvement, and loss of tissue planes. Glandular damage from chronic disease often alters the density of the salivary glands and makes the identification of masses more difficult; contrast-enhanced images are more defined and will therefore accentuate pathology. Tumors, abscesses, and inflamed lymph nodes will show abnormal enhancement when compared with normal structures. Enhanced CT can also help in staging malignant disease of the salivary glands and in assessing lymphadenopathy of the pharynx and neck. Coronal and sagittal reconstructions can be used in the evaluation of perineural spread.[67]

Conventional CT can be combined with sialography to examine salivary gland ductal systems and detect sialoliths; however, conventional CT sialography requires the use of

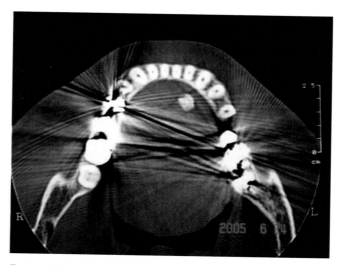

FIGURE 10-10 Sialolith of the left submandibular duct, on axial computed tomography. (Courtesy of Dr. Michael D. Turner, New York University.)

intravenous atropine to minimize early runoff of contrast and impaired ductal opacification caused by prolonged scan time. This problem can be overcome with ultrafast CT imaging techniques.[68] In addition, ultrafast CT is indicated for patients who are unable to lie still long enough for adequate MRI (e.g., pediatric, geriatric, claustrophobic, and mentally or physically challenged patients)and for patients for whom MRI is contraindicated.

CT maintains several advantages over MRI: it is less costly and more readily available.[50] CT can also be used in patients in whom MRI is contraindicated such as in those with certain pacemakers or implants. Dental restorations may interfere with CT imaging and may require repositioning the patient to a semi axial position. Additional disadvantages of CT include radiation exposure and the administration of iodine-containing contrast media for enhancement.

Cone Beam CT

Cone beam CT (CBCT) is increasingly being employed in dentomaxillofacial imaging since it provides high spatial resolution of osseous structures at a lower dose of radiation than conventional CT.[50] Using a cone-shaped x-ray beam and two-dimensional detectors, the CBCT scanner collects volume data by means of a single rotation taking 9–40 seconds. CBCT sialography provides several advantages over conventional sialography including three-dimensional reconstruction and allowing for manipulation of image rotation, slice thickness, and generation of various cross-sectional slices. These advantages are particularly valuable in cases of complex anatomy.[67] Overall, CBCT sialography appears to offer an improvement in imaging of the salivary gland ductal system over conventional sialography.

Magnetic Resonance Imaging

MRI provides superior soft tissue resolution over CT and is particularly advantageous in staging oral cavity malignancies involving the floor of the mouth and complex disease processes involving multiple anatomic spaces.[69]

MRI has become the imaging modality of choice for preoperative evaluation of salivary gland tumors because of its excellent ability to differentiate soft tissues and availability of multiplanar imaging (Figure 10-11).[70] MRI allows for not only localization of a lesion but also the assessment of extracranial extent. It also provides a higher degree of accuracy in assessing perineural and intracranial spread of malignancies.[44] Using contrast-enhanced MRI, detection of early perineural invasion or a mildly enlarged nerve is possible: a great advantage over CT. MRI has also proven to be valuable in the detection of postoperative recurrences.[44] In addition, MRI is particularly useful in the assessment of disorders that mimic parotid swelling such as hypertrophy of the muscles of mastication.[50]

MRI is further preferred for salivary gland imaging because patients are not exposed to radiation, no intravenous contrast media are required routinely, and it is less prone to artifact from dental restoration than CT. The utility of MRI has been enhanced by combining it with sialography.[71,72] This allows a much finer evaluation of ductal alterations and any filling defects. MRI is contraindicated for patients with cardiac pacemakers, automatic cardioverter defibrillators, or ferromagnetic metallic implants. Patients who cannot maintain a still position or those with claustrophobia may have difficulty tolerating the MRI procedure.

MRI may also be useful in detection of parotid gland changes associated with undiagnosed SS.[73] Changes on MRI that can be associated with SS in the parotid are described as having an inhomogeneous internal pattern in both T1- and T2-weighted images; appearing as a "salt-and-pepper" or "honeycomb-like" appearance.[74] Head and neck MRI can also be a useful tool for the detection of central nervous system involvement in SS. Several recent cases have reported MRI-detected trigeminal nerve disturbance resulting in the diagnosis of SS.

Recently, new MRI techniques, such as dynamic contrast-enhanced MRI (DCE-MRI), diffusion-weighted MRI, and proton MRI spectroscopy, have shown promising results in the differentiation between benign and malignant salivary gland tumors. For example, malignant salivary gland tumors can be differentiated from pleomorphic adenomas but not from Warthin's tumors using DCE-MRI.[44]

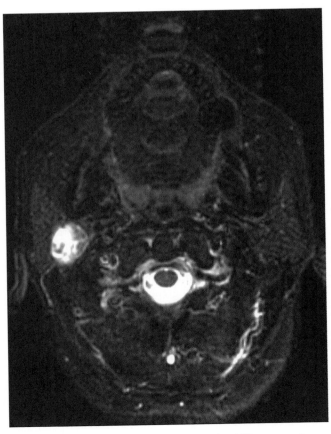

FIGURE 10-11 MRI image of a salivary gland. The opaque image in the right parotid gland is a pleomorphic adenoma.

Positron Emission Tomography

PET has been used recently for evaluation of the salivary glands. Preliminary reports suggest that it may be useful for measuring regional salivary gland function and recognizing inflammatory changes.[75] PET has also been shown to be of use in the incidental detection of salivary gland tumors, but does not reliably differentiate benign from malignant neoplasms.[50] A combination of SGS and fluorodeoxyglucose (FDG) PET is favored for the differentiation of various parotid gland tumors over nondiagnostic needle aspiration.[76]

18F-FDG PET/CT is a powerful imaging tool to assess inflammatory and autoimmune disease activity and thus it has been applied in the study of SS patients. Recent research has shown that increased FDG uptake may be observed in the salivary glands, lymph nodes, and lungs of SS patients. A new PET/CT activity score has been proposed, which correlates with the recently established the European League Against Rheumatism (EULAR) Sjögren's Syndrome Disease Activity Index (ESSDAI) and gammaglobulin levels in SS patients. This could lead to the future use of PET/CT in assessing disease activity[77] in patients with SS.

The advantages and disadvantages of each method of imaging, as well as their indications, are listed in Table 10-2.

Salivary Gland Biopsy

Definitive diagnosis of salivary pathology may require histologic examination. The labial minor salivary glands are most commonly biopsied since they provide the most accessible source of tissue, especially where SS is suspected. Biopsy of minor glands can also be used to diagnose amyloidosis and sarcoidosis and in diagnosing and monitoring chronic graft-versus-host disease (cGVHD).

The Minor Salivary Gland Biopsy

The MSGB is a minimally invasive procedure that can be performed with limited morbidity using appropriate techniques.[78] An incision is made on the inner aspect of the lower lip, near the midline, so that it is not externally visible. Six to ten minor gland lobules from just below the mucosal surface are removed and submitted for examination. The incision should be made through normal-appearing mucosa, avoiding areas of trauma or inflammation that could influence the appearance of the underlying minor glands. One pitfall in the MSGB for SS is failure to obtain sufficient minor salivary gland tissue for pathologic diagnosis. Recent use of corticosteroids, smoking, and exposure to radiation in the area of biopsy may also adversely affect the results.[79] Complications associated with MSGB include long-term lower lip numbness (reported at 0%–6%) and mucocele formation.[79]

The MSGB performed when SS is suspected is considered to be the most accurate sole criterion for diagnosis of the salivary component of this disorder.[80] Histologically, the presence of focal lymphocytic sialadenitis allows for diagnosis. The pathologic grading system used involves the generation of a "Focus Score" (FS), which relates to the number of aggregates of 50 or greater lymphocytes per 4 mm² of salivary gland tissue. A FS of greater than or equal to 1 is considered positive for SS.[79] A recent systematic review assessing the diagnostic value of the MSGB among patients presenting with sicca symptoms or other features suggesting SS showed that the MSGB had high specificity and a sensitivity ranging from 63.5% to 93.7% with respect to SS.[81]

Major Salivary Gland Biopsy

Biopsy of the parotid and submandibular glands usually requires an extraoral approach, although the sublingual glands are often approached intraorally. There is minimal morbidity associated with parotid biopsy, and it is done routinely as an outpatient procedure. With respect to SS, biopsy of the parotid gland has not been shown to offer diagnostic superiority to the minor gland procedure[82] but may offer unique value in assessing disease activity and progression.[83] The parotid gland biopsy has, however, been shown to be superior to the MSGB with respect to diagnosis of several conditions including sarcoidosis and lymphomas.[83] In cases of suspected lymphoma, histopathologic analysis combined with techniques such as flow cytometry, fluorescence in situ hybridization, and fluorescence-activated cell sorting analysis may be employed for definitive diagnosis and characterization of a lymphoma.

The parotid gland as a biopsy site offers several other advantages over the MSGB including allowing for repeat specimens to be obtained from the same gland in combination with saliva samples from the gland and the potential for early diagnosis of mucosa-associated lymphoid tissue (MALT) and non-Hodgkin lymphoma (NHL), often prior to clinical manifestation. This is especially important as these lymphomas are rarely observed in labial salivary glands.[84] Risks associated with the parotid biopsy include sialocele and salivary fistula formation, injury to the facial nerve and visible external incision. An intraoral approach of parotid biopsy requires deep dissection through the buccinator muscle and the buccal fat pad and does not offer a reduction in risk of damage to the facial nerve.[79]

Fine-Needle Aspiration Biopsy

FNAB is a simple and effective technique that aids the diagnosis of solid lesions.[85] Some studies have shown that preoperative fine-needle aspiration (FNA) cytology may prevent a significant minority of patients presenting with salivary gland lesions from undergoing a surgical procedure.[86] FNAB may also be useful for elderly patients who cannot tolerate an excisional biopsy because of medical considerations.

The reported diagnostic sensitivity and specificity for FNAB of salivary gland lesions has been reported as above 80% and 95%, respectively.[86] Limitations include inadequacy of specimen, difficulty in interpretation of tumor grade (i.e., discerning between high and low grade), and reduced accuracy with respect to nonneoplastic processes.[86] FNAB also does not provide any information on anatomic structure.

Core Needle Biopsy

Recent studies have suggested the use of core needle biopsy (CNB), employing a larger-bore needle than in the FNAB to remove cylinders of tissue, in the preoperative evaluation of salivary gland lesions. This technique has the advantages of having a low rate of complications (bruising being the most commonly reported problem) and reduced risk of tumor seeding.[86] CNB also provides increased material over FNAB, is able to preserve histologic architecture, and may allow for evaluation of extracapsular tumor invasion. Immunohisto-chemical stains are also more likely to be reliable with core biopsy specimens. The disadvantages to CNB include the requirement of local anesthesia and possibly increased pain and morbidity. A recent systematic review of 512 procedures from 5 studies shows a sensitivity of 96%, a specificity of 100%, and a complication rate of 1.6%.[86]

Ultrasound-Guided Core Needle Aspiration

Employing ultrasound guidance for aspiration biopsies significantly improves the diagnostic rate.[87] Ultrasound-guided core needle aspiration is indicated for biopsy of distinct salivary gland masses of the major salivary glands or for evaluation of pathology involving the submandibular space. It is a considered a safe and accurate technique with a low nondiagnostic rate[88] and can also be used to investigate associated cervical lymphadenopathy. Failure to obtain an adequate sample for diagnosis by this technique is indication for an open biopsy procedure.

To establish a diagnosis accurately, it is important to have a well-trained cytopathologist familiar with salivary cytology examine the specimen. The cytologist inspects the individual cells aspirated from the lesion and offers a diagnosis based upon the cellular characteristics observed. Even if a definitive diagnosis is not made, it may be possible to determine whether a lesion is benign or malignant. Awareness of the biologic aggressiveness of the tumor prior to definitive surgery is helpful in planning optimal treatment.

Analysis of frozen sections can be performed at the time of surgery. Frozen section analysis can serve to establish the nature of the tumor (benign versus malignant) and to assess margins for tumor involvement. In the case of parotid gland surgery, frozen sections increase the chances of sparing the facial nerve.[89] More than 80% of the time, the diagnosis based on the frozen section agrees with the final pathologic diagnosis from fixed and stained tissue. Most errors involve a failure to recognize malignant lesions. Malignant tumors are incorrectly diagnosed as benign 5%–24% of the time, but benign tumors are incorrectly diagnosed as malignant only 0%–2% of the time. If frozen sections reveal a malignant tumor, the surgical margins may require extension.[90,91]

Serologic Evaluation

Laboratory blood studies are helpful in the evaluation of dry mouth particularly in suspected cases of SS. Although there is no single definitive laboratory test for the diagnosis of SS, a combination of abnormal test results is frequently observed: elevated erythrocyte sedimentation rate (ESR), mild normochromic normocytic anemia, leukopenia, and polyclonal hypergammaglobulinemia. Autoantibodies are present in the majority of SS cases: rheumatoid factor (RF), antinuclear antibodies (ANAs), and anti-SSA/Ro and anti-SSB/La are strongly indicative of SS, although not exclusive.[92] The most recently proposed classification criteria for SS by the American College of Rheumatology (ACR) requires at least two of three criteria for case definition; one of which is a positive serum anti-SSA/Ro and/or anti-SSB/La or positive RF and ANA of greater than or equal to 1:320 (see Sjögren's Syndrome—Diagnosis).

Approximately 80% of patients with SS will display antinuclear antibodies (ANAs) and about 60% will have anti-SSA/Ro antibodies.[14] This latter autoantibody is considered the most specific marker for SS, although it may be found in a small percentage of patients with systemic lupus erythematous or other autoimmune connective tissue disorders.

Another serologic marker that may prove useful for the diagnosis of salivary gland disorders is serum amylase. The salivary glands and the pancreas are the two greatest contributors to an individual's serum amylase levels; thus increased levels may be seen in cases of salivary gland inflammation[93,94] and where there is pancreatic involvement in SS.[95] Determination of amylase isoenzymes (pancreatic and salivary) will allow the recognition of salivary contributions to the total serum amylase concentration. Further research is required to determine the utility of this marker.

SPECIFIC DISEASES AND DISORDERS OF THE SALIVARY GLANDS

Developmental Abnormalities

Overview

Complete absence (aplasia or agenesis) of salivary glands is rare but may occur together with other developmental defects, especially malformations of the first and second brachial arch seen as various craniofacial anomalies. Patients with salivary gland aplasia experience xerostomia and increased dental caries; in fact, rampant dental caries in children who had no other symptoms has led to the diagnosis of congenitally missing salivary glands. Enamel hypoplasia, congenital absence of teeth, and extensive occlusal wear are other oral manifestations of salivary agenesis.[96]

Parotid gland agenesis has been reported alone and in conjunction with several congenital conditions, including hemifacial microstomia, mandibulofacial dysostosis (Treacher Collins syndrome), cleft palate, lacrimo-auriculo-dento-digital syndrome, and anophthalmia.[97] It has also been observed in ectodermal dysplasia. Hypoplasia of the parotid gland has been associated with Melkersson–Rosenthal syndrome. Congenital fistula formation within the ductal system has been associated with brachial cleft abnormalities, accessory parotid ducts, and diverticuli.[96,98–103] Although heredity is a significant factor, some patients may have no familial history of salivary agenesis.

Aberrant salivary glands are salivary tissues that develop at unusual anatomic sites. Ectopic salivary glands have been reported in a variety of locations, including the middle-ear, external auditory canal, neck, posterior mandible, anterior mandible, pituitary gland, and cerebellopontine angle. These are usually incidental findings and do not require intervention.[70,104–107]

The Stafne bone defect (SBD; also known as Stafne bone cyst) is an asymptomatic depression of the lingual surface of the mandible often associated with ectopic salivary gland tissue. However, it is not a true cyst as there is no epithelial lining. The most common location of the SBD is in the region of the third molar inferior to the mandibular canal. The reported occurrence rate of these lesions is 0.1%–0.48%.[108] There are several reports of an anterior variant of the SBD occurring in the premolar region of the mandible, which is thought to be associated with ectopic sublingual salivary glands. These can often appear similar to a residual cyst and therefore may require further investigation including CT scanning.[108]

The definitive etiology of the SBD has not been established. One theory suggests SBDs result from pressure exerted by adjacent glandular tissue. The finding of salivary gland tissue upon surgical exploration and MRI imaging of these defects is evidence to support this theory; however, other case reports have described finding muscular, lymphatic, or vascular tissues related to the cavity.[108]

SBDs are usually diagnosed via conventional plain film radiography. The radiographic appearance of the Stafne defect is one of a round, unilocular, well-circumscribed radiolucency. The characteristic location and radiographic appearance make the SBD easily recognized. In some cases, sialography, CT, CBCT, and MRI may be required to reach a definitive diagnosis. On occasion, palpation of the salivary gland tissue can be achieved. Surgical intervention is reserved for atypical situations in which the diagnosis is unclear and a tumor is suspected. Where indicated, FNA biopsy is an accurate, cost-effective diagnostic tool for these and other lesions.[109–111]

Accessory Salivary Ducts

Accessory salivary ducts are common and do not require treatment. In a study of 450 parotid glands by Rauch and Gorlin, half of the patients had accessory parotid ducts. The most frequent location was superior and anterior to the normal location of Stensen's duct.[112]

Diverticula

By definition, a diverticulum is a pouch or sac protruding from the wall of a duct. Diverticula in the ducts of the major salivary glands often lead to pooling of saliva and recurrent sialadenitis. Diagnosis can be made by sialography. Patients with diverticula are encouraged to regularly milk the involved salivary gland and to promote salivary flow through the duct.[113]

Darier's Disease

Salivary duct abnormalities have been reported in Darier's disease (also known as dyskeratosis follicularis). Sialography of parotid glands in this condition revealed duct dilation, with periodic stricture affecting the main ducts. Symptoms of occasional obstructive sialadenitis have been reported. Progressive involvement of the salivary ducts in Darier's disease may be more common than reported previously.[114]

Sialolithiasis (Salivary Stones)
Description and Etiology

Sialoliths (also termed salivary calculi or salivary stones) are typically calcified organic masses that form within the secretory system of the major salivary glands. The true prevalence of sialolithiasis is difficult to determine since many cases are asymptomatic or may involve sialomicroliths detected only microscopically. Clinical and experimental research has shown that sialoliths form secondarily to chronic obstructive sialadenitis.[115] The etiologic factors favoring salivary stone formation may be classified into two groups: factors favoring saliva retention (i.e., irregularities in the duct system, local inflammation, dehydration, medications such as anticholinergics and diuretics) and saliva composition (i.e., calcium saturation and deficit of crystallization inhibitors such as phytate). Bacterial infection also promotes sialolith formation due to an associated increase in salivary pH favoring calcium phosphate supersaturation.[116] Although no causal relationship between tobacco smoking and an increased risk of sialolithiasis has been definitively shown, an association appears plausible given that smoking is known to adversely affect the cytotoxic activity of saliva and salivary amylase.[117]

Sialolithiasis can occur in a wide age range of patients and has been reported in children. It occurs more commonly in males. The average age of patients with sialolithiasis is 40.5 years for the submandibular gland, 47.8 years for the parotid gland, and 50 years for the minor salivary glands. Since the underlying cause is unknown and uncorrected in most patients, the recurrence rate is estimated at around 20%.[118,119]

Salivary stones occur most commonly in the submandibular glands (80%–90%), followed by the parotid (5%–15%) and sublingual (2%–5%) glands and only very rarely occur in the minor salivary glands. The higher rate of sialolith formation in the submandibular gland is due to (1) the torturous course of Wharton's duct, (2) the higher calcium and phosphate levels of the secretion contained within, (3) the dependent position of the submandibular glands that leaves them prone to stasis,[118,119] and (4) the increased mucoid nature of the secretion. In addition, since the submandibular and parotid glands' secretion is dependent on nervous stimulation, when there is an absence of stimulation, secretory inactivity increases the risk of stone development.

Spontaneous secretion in the minor and sublingual salivary glands provides some continuous salivary flow in these glands preventing stasis.[115] Fifty percent of parotid gland sialoliths and 20% of submandibular gland sialoliths are poorly calcified. This is clinically significant as these sialoliths will not be detected radiographically.[118–121]

Although the exact mechanism of sialolith formation has not been proven, it has been proposed that microcalculi are intermittently formed in salivary ducts due to secretory inactivity. Food debris and bacteria from the oral cavity may then migrate into the main ducts. In time, the result of the impacted sialomicrolith in a small intraglandular duct results in focal obstructive atrophy. Since this nidus is protected from flushing and the antimicrobial effects of saliva and systemic immunity, bacteria may proliferate resulting in local inflammation and further atrophy. The inflammatory process may then spread to involve adjacent lobules resulting in swelling and fibrosis of the large intraglandular ducts. The resulting partial obstruction leads to ductal dilatation and stagnation of calcium-rich secretory material resulting in further lamellar calcification.[115]

Salivary stones are composed of organic and inorganic substances including calcium carbonates and phosphates, cellular debris, glycoproteins, and mucopolysaccharides.[117] They contain cores that may vary from purely organic to heavily calcified material, surrounded by less-calcified or purely organic lamellae.[115] Hydroxyapatite is the most common mineral found in sialoliths but other minerals such as whitlockite and octacalcium phosphate are variably present depending on the mineral microenvironment.[115] Sialoliths also often contain trace amounts of magnesium, potassium chloride, and ammonium salts.

With the exception of gout, in which the calculi consist mainly of uric acid, there has been no proven link between sialolithiasis and development of stones in other areas of the body. There are some reports suggesting that patients with sialolithiasis are more likely to suffer from nephrolithiasis.[122] In addition, patients with hyperparathyroidism demonstrate an increased incidence of sialolithiasis and those with hyperparathyroidism and sialolithiasis show a greater incidence of nephrolithiasis than those without sialolithiasis indicating that hypercalcemia may be a contributing factor.[115]

Additional reports have also associated high dietary intake of calcium with the development of sialoliths.[123] The saliva of patients with calcified sialoliths has been found to contain more calcium and less phytate than that of a healthy group and of patients with purely organic sialoliths.[103] Dietary phytate is obtained from plant tissue, particularly bran and seeds and is a potent inhibitor of hydroxyapatite crystallization.[115]

Clinical Presentation

Patients with sialoliths most commonly present with a history of acute, colicky, periprandial pain and intermittent swelling of the affected major salivary gland. The degree of symptoms is dependent on the extent of salivary duct obstruction and the presence of secondary infection. Typically, salivary gland swelling will be evident upon eating since the stone completely or partially blocks the flow of saliva resulting in salivary pooling within the gland ductal system. Since the glands are encapsulated and there is little space for expansion, enlargement causes pain. If there is only partial obstruction of the duct by the sialolith, swelling will subside when salivary stimulation ceases and output decreases.[122,124]

Stasis of the saliva may lead to infection, fibrosis, and gland atrophy. If there is concurrent infection, there may be expressible suppurative or nonsuppurative drainage and erythema or warmth in the overlying skin. Sialolithiasis without infectious sialadenitis is predominately unilateral without drainage or overlying erythema and presents without systemic manifestations such as fever. Often, there is a history of sudden onset of swelling and pain.[125]

The involved gland is often enlarged and tender to palpation. The soft tissue adjacent to the salivary gland duct may be edematous and inflamed. Using bimanual palpation directed in a posterior to anterior fashion along the course of the involved duct, it may be possible to detect a stone.[125] Fistulae, a sinus tract, or ulceration may occur in the tissue covering the stone in chronic cases. Other complications from sialoliths include acute sialadenitis, ductal stricture, and ductal dilatation.[124]

Diagnosis

Plain film radiographs are helpful to visualize sialoliths; they are inexpensive, readily available, and result in minimal radiation exposure. Since small and poorly calcified stones may not be readily identifiable (see Figure 10-7), this modality is most useful in cases of suspected submandibular sialolithiasis where an occlusal radiograph taken at 90° from the floor of the mouth is recommended. However, other calcified entities such as phleboliths (stones that lie within a blood vessel), calcified cervical lymphadenopathy, and arterial atherosclerosis of the lingual artery can also appear on these films.[125]

Stones in the parotid gland can be more difficult to visualize for several reasons. Due to the superimposition of other anatomic structures, sialoliths may be obscured and therefore the choice of radiographic views is important. An AP view of the face or an occlusal film placed intraorally adjacent to the duct may be useful in these cases. In addition, since only 20%–30% of parotid stones are radiopaque, they may not be visualized even with proper positioning.

Conventional sialography using panoramic, occlusal, and periapical radiographs remains an appropriate first-line imaging modality in cases where there is a strong clinical suspicion of inflammation or salivary stone disease.[67] Contrast sialography using iodinated contrast media may be used to visualize the parotid and submandibular ductal systems. Sialography can also aid in differentiating calcified phleboliths from sialoliths since the former lie within a blood vessel, where as the latter occur within the ductal structure.

Sialography may be combined with therapeutic salivary interventional procedures such as stone retrieval.[126] Limitations of this modality include the use of ionizing radiation, dependence on successful ductal cannulation, pain during and after the procedure, and potential allergy to the contrast medium. The use of contrast sialography is also contraindicated in the presence of acute sialadenitis.[127]

Ultrasound (US) is widely used as a first-line imaging modality to assess the presence of salivary gland calculi.[127] Transoral sonography using an intraoral approach has been employed as an imaging modality in suspected sialolithiasis. US is noninvasive, less costly than other imaging, and may be able to visualize radiolucent calculi. However, US may not be able to allow for correct assessment of the precise number of calculi where multiple stones are present and calculi less than 2 mm may not produce an acoustic shadow.[6] It is because of this that the use of US alone may not be sufficient. There is much debate in the literature regarding the true sensitivity, specificity, and positive and negative predictive values of this modality.[127]

Noncontrast CT images using a slice thickness of 0.2–0.5 mm may be used for the detection of sialoliths and have a 10-fold greater sensitivity than plain film radiography for detecting calcifications. CT is the technique of choice for identification of small calculi within the salivary glands or ducts but at the expense of high radiation exposure. Since small opacified blood vessels may simulate small sialoliths in a contrast-enhanced CT, nonenhanced scans are indicated where sialolithiasis is suspected.[44]

CBCT provides the advantages of reduced superimpositions and distortions of anatomical structures and high sensitivities over two-dimensional radiography and reduced radiation exposure over medical CT.[128] CBCT also offers superior imaging of the ductal system over conventional sialography.[67] CBCT imaging in sialography has been proposed where plain film sialography has been found to be inadequate in imaging more complex cases of salivary duct obstruction.[129]

MRI sialography, although not widely available, is another alternate imaging modality and maintains some advantages over conventional sialography. Although contraindicated in individuals with pacemakers or claustrophobia, because it does not employ a contrast medium, it can be used in those with iodine or contrast media allergies or acute infection. It also does not employ ionizing radiation.[130]

Sialendoscopy has emerged as a diagnostic and therapeutic technique for many salivary gland disorders. Its advantages include allowing for access to deeper segments of a duct and potentially the inner areas of the gland and, where feasible, simultaneous visualization and removal of sialoliths. Sialendoscopy allows for the assessment of the intraductal and intraglandular anatomy using a small camera and can allow for visualization of strictures or secondary channels within the duct.[131] Introduction of customized surgical instruments into the duct can allow for removal of calcified material or soft tissue biopsy. Following the endoscopic procedure, a stent is placed allowing for healing of the duct and maintenance of salivary flow. Sialendoscopy may also be combined with sialography in the diagnosis and treatment of salivary gland obstructions.[131] Prior to sialendoscopy, ultrasound,[132] conventional sialography, contrast-enhanced CT, and MR sialography may be used to assess the salivary ductal system.[133]

Treatment

During the acute phase of sialolithiasis, therapy is primarily supportive. Standard treatment during this phase often involves the use of analgesics, hydration, antibiotics, and antipyretics, as necessary. Sialogogues, massage and heat applied to the affected area may also be beneficial. Stones at or near the orifice of the duct can often be removed transorally by milking the gland, but deeper stones require intervention with conventional surgery or sialendoscopy.

The conventional treatment of sialoliths has shifted from open surgical-based techniques such as open duct exploration or gland resection to endoscopic-based, gland preservation methods such as sialendoscopy. Interventional sialendoscopy has been shown to be effective in the treatment of sialolithiasis even in cases of multiple calculi. It has been proven to be effective in removal of stones up to 4–5 mm in diameter especially those that lie freely in the duct lumen. Larger sialoliths may be amenable to mechanical or laser fragmentation to facilitate their removal.[134] Dilation of the ductal opening or papillotomy to increase the ductal orifice size is performed prior to the introduction of surgical instruments such as the Dormia basket, graspers, or laser fibers to access the stones. Irrigation with saline or steroid instillation is then performed to flush out debris and treat ductal inflammation.[135] Following removal of the stone, the endoscope is used to explore the duct to ensure all calculi have been removed and a stent is placed to maintain patency of the duct.[132]

Extracorporeal shock wave lithotripsy (ESWL) also allows for fragmentation of large sialoliths of any size or location. A minimally invasive procedure, ESWL uses high-energy shock waves to pulverize stones so that they may be flushed out by physiologic saliva flow.[136] Successful treatment of sialoliths by ESWL may require multiple treatment sessions[134] and is contraindicated in cases of complete distal duct stenosis, pregnancy, patients with cardiac pacemakers, acute sialadenitis, or other acute inflammatory processes of the head and neck.[136] Currently, ESWL is not approved by the US FDA for management of salivary stones in the United States.[137]

Failing gland-sparing techniques and in the case of fixed intraparenchymal stones, sialoadenectomy remains a treatment option.[137] Very large stones and a long-standing history of recurrent sialadenitis may also be an indication for gland removal. Conventional management consists of superficial parotidectomy and transcervical submandibulectomy. Some postoperative complications associated with parotidectomy include transient (2%–76%) or permanent (1%–3%) facial nerve injury, sensory loss of the greater auricular nerve (2%–100%), or Frey's syndrome (8%–33%). Risks associated with submandibular gland removal include temporary (1%–2%) or permanent (1%–8%) injury to the marginal mandibular nerve, temporary (1%–2%) or permanent (3%) hypoglossal nerve palsy, or temporary (2%–6%) or permanent (2%) lingual nerve damage. Other complications include hematomas, salivary fistulas, sialoceles, wound infection, hypertrophic scars, and inflammation caused by residual stones.[136]

Extravasation and Retention Mucoceles and Ranulas

Mucocele

Description and Etiology

Mucocele is a clinical term that describes swelling caused by the accumulation of saliva at the site of a traumatized or obstructed minor salivary gland duct. Mucoceles can be classified histologically as extravasation types or retention types[138]; the extravasation type of mucocele being more common. Although often termed a "mucous retention cyst, " the extravasation mucocele does not have an epithelial lining or a distinct border. The formation of an extravasation mucocele is believed to be the result of trauma to a minor salivary gland excretory duct. Laceration of the duct results in pooling of saliva in the adjacent submucosal tissue and consequent swelling. The retention type mucocele is caused by obstruction of a minor salivary gland duct often by sialolith, periductal scaring, or tumor.[139] The blockage of salivary flow results in the accumulation of saliva and dilation of the duct.

Clinical Presentation

Mucoceles often present as discrete, painless, smooth-surfaced swellings that can range from a few millimeters to a few centimeters in diameter. Superficial lesions frequently have a characteristic blue hue. Deeper lesions can be more diffuse, covered by normal-appearing mucosa without the distinctive blue color. The lesions vary in size over time; superficial mucoceles are frequently traumatized, causing them to drain and deflate. Mucoceles that continue to be traumatized are most likely to recur and may develop surface ulceration (Figure 10-12). Although the development of a bluish lesion after trauma is highly suggestive of a mucocele, other lesions (including salivary gland neoplasms, soft tissue neoplasms, vascular malformations, and vesiculobullous diseases) should be considered in the differential diagnosis.

Extravasation mucoceles most frequently occur on the lower lip, where trauma is common. The buccal mucosa, tongue, floor of the mouth, and retromolar region are other commonly traumatized areas where mucous extravasation may be found. These types of mucoceles are most commonly seen in children and teenagers. The glands of Blandin and Nuhn located on the ventral surface of the tongue are also

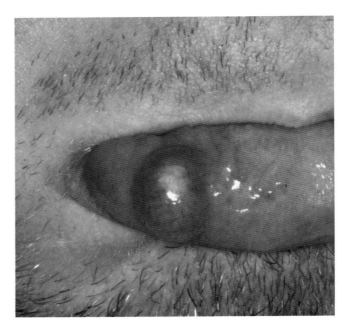

FIGURE 10-12 Mucocele of the lower right labial mucosa.

susceptible to mucocele formation. Mucoceles found in this area characteristically appear as a soft fluctuant polypoid mass.[140]

Mucous retention cysts are more commonly found on the upper lip, palate, buccal mucosa, floor of the mouth, and rarely the lower lip and usually afflict an older patient population than the extravasation mucoceles. Ductal narrowing associated with mucous retention cysts has also been associated with frequent use of hydrogen peroxide as a mouth rinse and tartar-control toothpastes.[139]

Treatment

Conventional definitive surgical treatment of mucoceles involves removal of the entire lesion along with the feeder salivary glands and duct. Incomplete removal of the mucocele may result in recurrence. Surgical management can be challenging since it can cause trauma to adjacent minor salivary glands and lead to the development of a new mucocele.

Alternative treatments that have been explored with varying degrees of success include electrosurgery, cryosurgery using liquid nitrogen, [141] laser surgery and micromarsupialization,[142] intralesional injections of corticosteroids, and sclerotherapy with pingyangmycin.[143]

Ranula

Description and Etiology

A form of mucocele located in the floor of the mouth is known as a *ranula* (Figure 10-13), named due to its resemblance to the underbelly of a frog (Latin rāna["frog"]). Ranulas are believed to arise from the sublingual gland usually following mechanical trauma to its ducts of Rivinus, resulting in extravasation of saliva. Other possible causes include an obstructed salivary duct or a ductal aneurysm.

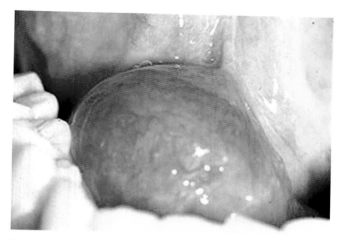

FIGURE 10-13 Sublingual salivary gland ranula. (Courtesy of Dr. Michael D. Turner, New York University.)

The predilection of ranulas in the sublingual glands has been thought to be due to the gland's continuous salivary secretion that precludes effective sealing of the mucous extravasation via fibrosis, in contrast to salivary secretion in the parotid and submandibular glands, which is dependent on gustatory stimulation.[144] Ranulas are most common in the second decade of life and in females.[145]

Ranulas are categorized as being "oral" ("simple", "superficial", "nonplunging"), "plunging" ("cervical", "diving"), or mixed, having both oral and plunging components.[145] The oral ranula remains confined to the sublingual space, while the plunging ranula dissects along facial planes beyond the sublingual space inferior to the mylohyoid muscle.[69] A congenital predisposition toward development of ranulas has been suggested, particularly in those of Asian descent.[146] In addition, particular anatomic variations of the ductal system of the sublingual gland may contribute to the formation of ranulas.[147]

Clinical Presentation

The most common presentation of the "oral" ranula is a painless, slow-growing, fluctuant, movable mass located in the floor of the mouth (see Figure 10-13). Usually, the lesion forms to one side of the lingual frenulum; however, if the lesion extends deep into the soft tissue, it can cross the midline. As observed with mucoceles, superficial ranulas can have a typical bluish hue, but when the lesion is deeply seated, the overlying mucosa may have a normal appearance. The size of the lesions can vary, and larger lesions can cause deviation of the tongue. In a "plunging" ranula, extravasated mucus from ruptured acini of the sublingual gland passes around the posterior border of the mylohyoid muscle or through a hiatus in the muscle. It will present as a swelling involving the submandibular triangle or other cervical space.

Diagnosis

Imaging to diagnose an oral ranula may not be necessary due to its characteristic clinical appearance, but to rule out other cystic lesions (e.g., thyroglossal duct cyst, epidermoid cyst, cystic hygroma), FNA, ultrasound, CT with contrast, and MRI have been used.[148] Ultrasound has been recommended for oral ranulas, while CT with contrast and MRI are the suggested modalities for evaluation of suspected plunging ranulas.[148]

Treatment

The most predictable method of eradicating both oral and plunging ranulas is to remove the associated sublingual gland because this will almost certainly eliminate recurrences.[139] Sublingual gland adenectomy combined with intraoral excision of the ranula is suggested for the simple ranula, while intraoral excision of the sublingual gland with cervical incision and drainage is the suggested treatment for the plunging ranula.[148] Other procedures used for the treatment of ranulas have included simple excision, marsupialization, injection of the sclerosing agent OK-432, silver nitrate, and botulinum toxin (BoNT)[149] all with varying rates of success. Large case studies indicate that marsupialization or excision of the ranula alone result in an unacceptably high recurrence rate.[145] Reports of spontaneous regression of ranulas exist and some would advocate deferring treatment for at least six months.[148]

Postsurgical complications include lesion recurrence, sensory deficits of the tongue, and damage to Wharton's duct.[150] Frequency of recurrence is related to the surgical technique selected and has been reported as 67% with marsupialization, 58% with excision alone, and 1% with sublingual gland excision.[145]

Inflammatory and Reactive Lesions
Necrotizing Sialometaplasia
Description and Etiology

Necrotizing sialometaplasia (NS) is a benign, self-limiting, reactive inflammatory disorder of salivary tissue. Clinically and histopathologically, NS can resemble a malignancy and its misdiagnosis has resulted in unnecessary radical surgery. The etiology is unknown, although it likely represents a local ischemic event, infectious process, or perhaps an immune response to an unknown allergen.[151] Development of NS has been associated with smoking, local injury, blunt force trauma, denture wear, and surgical procedures. It has been reported in pregnant patients and those with diabetes mellitus, sickle-cell disease, cocaine abuse, bulimia, and chronic vomiting.[152] The incidence of NS appears to be higher in male patients and especially in those older than 40 years.[152]

Clinical Presentation

NS has a spectrum of clinical presentations. Most commonly it presents as a painful, rapidly progressing swelling of the hard palate with central ulceration and peripheral erythema. The associated pain is often described as sharp in character and may precede mucosal changes. Numbness or anesthesia in the associated area may be an early finding.[153]

The lesions are typically of rapid onset and range in size from 1 to 3 cm.[153] Lesions occur predominantly on the palate; however, lesions can occur anywhere salivary gland tissue resides, including the lips, retromolar trigone, buccal mucosa, tonsils, tongue, nasal cavity, trachea, and maxillary sinus.[152] Although the lesions are usually unilateral, bilateral cases have been reported. Lesion affecting the hard palate clinically resemble salivary gland malignancies particularly mucoepidermoid carcinoma and adenoid cystic carcinoma although the rapid onset of NS may be a distinguishing feature.

Lesions often occur shortly after an inciting event to the area such as oral surgical procedures, restorative dentistry, or administration of local anesthesia, but lesions have also been reported to develop weeks after a dental procedure or trauma. It is also not uncommon for lesions to develop in an individual with no obvious history of trauma or oral habit.

Diagnosis

If histopathologic diagnosis is warranted to rule out a malignant process, biopsy specimens should be submitted to a pathologist with extensive training in oral and maxillofacial pathology. The specimen should include a margin of clinically uninvolved tissue adjacent to the lesion. Electrocautery or use of a laser should be avoided prior to removal of the biopsy specimen so as to avoid obfuscating thermal artifact. A complete clinical history, medical history, and ideally, clinical photos should be submitted with the specimen.

Histopathologically, NS also may present with an array of findings. Typically, there is necrosis of the salivary gland, with preservation of the lobular architecture of the gland, granulation tissue, and a mixed inflammatory cell infiltrate including lymphocytes, histiocytes, neutrophils, and eosinophils. There may also be pseudoepitheliomatous hyperplasia of the mucosal epithelium and squamous metaplasia of the salivary ducts. Critically, there are no malignant cells and the lobular architecture is preserved even though necrosis is present.[154,155] In later biopsies, necrosis may not be as evident and pseudoepitheliomatous hyperplasia and ductal metaplasia are more predominant.[153]

Treatment

NS is considered a self-limiting condition typically resolving within 3–12 weeks. During this time, supportive and symptomatic treatment is usually adequate. Appropriate analgesics combined with use of an antiseptic mouthwash such as 0.12% chlorhexidine gluconate have been recommended. Surgical intervention is typically not required in cases of NS; however, there are reports of resolution following débridement for particularly large lesions and those secondarily infected with bacterial species and *Candida*.[153]

Cheilitis Glandularis
Description and Etiology

Cheilitis glandularis (CG) is a chronic inflammatory disorder affecting the minor salivary glands and their ducts in which thick saliva is secreted from dilated ductal openings.

Although the etiology of CG is still undetermined, it has been suggested that it is an autosomal dominant hereditary disease. In addition, external factors (mainly UV rays) have been implicated as the condition occurs more frequently in fair-skinned adults and albino patients appear particularly prone to this condition. Additional proposed predisposing factors include poor oral hygiene, chronic exposure to sunlight and wind, smoking, and an immunocompromised state. Most reports of CG have been in middle-aged and elderly men with only a few cases reported in women and children.

Recently, there is evidence that the expression and possibly the function of some of the aquaporin proteins in the minor salivary glands may be altered in CG resulting in abnormalities in water flow mechanism and subsequent alteration in salivary composition leading to the characteristic thick saliva seen in CG.[156]

Clinical Presentation

CG presents with a secretion of thick saliva secreted from dilated ostia of swollen labial minor salivary glands. This saliva often adheres to the vermilion causing discomfort to the patient. Edema and focal ulceration may also be present. CG primarily affects the lower lip, but there are reports of upper lip and even palatal involvement. CG may present a diagnostic challenge to clinicians since its appearance is akin to orofacial granulomatosis and actinic cheilitis. The differential diagnosis of CG also includes multiple mucocele, chronic sialadenitis of the minor salivary glands, and factitious cheilitis.

Historically, CG has been subclassified into three clinical types: simple, superficial suppurative, and deep suppurative. In simple CG, there are multiple painless lesions, dilated ductal openings, and numerous small nodules that may be palpable. There is a lack of inflammation but mucinous material can be extruded on application of pressure to the lip. Infection of the simple type lesions may result in progression to the superficial or deep suppurative types. Superficial suppurative CG is characterized by superficial ulceration, painless crusting, swelling, and induration of the lip; a mucinous exudate is apparent at the ductal openings. In the deep suppurative type, infection of the deeper tissues is associated with abscess formation and fistulae.[157]

Diagnosis

The characteristic clinical presentation and biopsy are used to make the diagnosis of CG. The histopathologic features of CG are nonspecific and include variably dilated and tortuous minor salivary gland ducts, accumulation of mucus in the ductal lumina, and chronic sialadenitis. In addition, the histopathologic features may vary depending on the progression of the disease.

Treatment

Elimination of potential predisposing factors and the use of lip balms, emollients, and sunscreens for those with excessive exposure to the sun and wind are advised. Conservative treatment of CG may involve using topical, intralesional or systemic steroids, systemic anticholinergics, systemic antihistamines, and/or antibiotics. Refractory cases require surgical intervention such as cryosurgery, vermillionectomy, and/or labial mucosal stripping. Patients with CG, especially of the deep suppurative type, should be considered for surgical excision.

Several reports documented the development of squamous cell carcinoma in areas affected by CG, leading some to call CG a premalignant lesion. Currently, the association between CG and squamous cell carcinoma is not well defined, but it does appear that a co-occurrence of lower lip CG with actinic change represents an increased risk of development of squamous-cell carcinoma and therefore close clinical monitoring is advised.[158]

External Beam Radiation–Induced Pathology

Description and Etiology

External beam radiation therapy is standard treatment for head and neck cancers, and the salivary glands are often within the field of radiation.[159] Although therapeutic dosages for cancer are typically in excess of 65 Gy, permanent salivary gland damage and symptoms of oral dryness can develop after only 24–26 Gy.[160–162] The etiopathogenesis of radiation-induced salivary gland destruction is multifactorial, including programmed cell death (apoptosis) in conjunction with production of reactive oxygen species and other cytotoxic products. Radiation-associated impaired blood flow may also contribute to the destruction of glandular acinar and ductal cells.[163]

Clinical Presentation

Acute effects on salivary function can be recognized within a week of initiating radiotherapy, with symptoms of oral dryness and thick, viscous saliva developing by the end of the second week. Oral mucositis is a very common consequence of treatment and can become severe enough to alter the radiation therapy regimen.[163,164] Mucositis appears as a sloughing of the oral mucosa with erythema and ulceration. The pain associated with mucositis is described as a burning. Mucositis generally persists throughout radiotherapy, peaks at the end of the irradiation, and continues for one to three weeks after cessation of treatment.[165]

By the end of a typical six- to seven-week course of radiotherapy, salivary gland function is nearly absent. Hypofunction remains at a steady rate postradiation, with only small increases to two years post-radiotherapy (post-RT).[166] This can be permanent if the major salivary glands receive more than 24–26 Gy. With intensity-modulated radiation therapy (IMRT), a systematic review of published data demonstrated a lower prevalence of xerostomia with IMRT versus conventional therapy at two years post-RT (68% vs. 91%).[166] Permanent xerostomia and oral complications of salivary hypofunction impair a patient's quality of life

(Figure 10-14).[167,168] Signs and symptoms of radiation-associated xerostomia include a burning sensation of the tongue, fissuring of the tongue and lips, new and recurrent dental caries, difficulty in wearing oral prostheses, and increased thirst. Additional sequelae of radiation-induced salivary dysfunction include candidiasis, microbial infections, plaque retention, gingivitis, difficulty in speaking and tasting, dysphagia, and mucosal pain.[163,167,169,170] *Radiation caries* is the term commonly used to describe rapidly advancing caries, which characteristically occur at the incisal or cervical aspects of the teeth, starting with the incisors and canines[171] (Figure 10-14). Radiation caries may become evident as early as three months following the start of radiotherapy and can progress at an alarming rate. Interestingly, there is rarely any acute pain associated with these lesions. In spite of meticulous oral hygiene, the caries rate is often difficult to control and poses a diagnostic, preventive, and treatment challenge.

Patients are also at risk of developing osteoradionecrosis (ORN), a necrotic avascular condition, most commonly occurring in the mandible after more than 60 Gy exposure.[172,173] Hard tissues affected by radiation become hypovascular, hypocellular, and hypoxic. Risk increases with time after radiotherapy and persists for the remainder of a patient's life. The diagnosis of ORN is based on a history of radiation and clinical signs of severely painful, nonhealing exposed bone in the treatment area. Fistulae, sequestra, and pathologic fracture are other complications seen with ORN.[163] There is also an increased incidence of second primary tumors involving the radiated tissues and salivary gland neoplasms.[174,175]

Additional clinical consequences of radiation include taste loss or altered taste sensation, changes to the periodontium and trismus. Alteration in taste is an early response to radiation and often precedes mucositis. It is believed to be not only due to direct irradiation damage to the taste buds

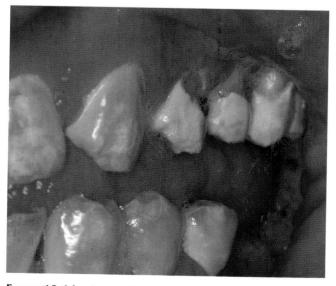

Figure 10-14 Severe salivary hypofunction in a patient who was treated with head and neck radiation therapy.

but also due to hyposalivation. Loss of taste is usually transient and may return to normal or near-normal levels within one year after radiation but may take as long as five years. As a consequence of these taste changes, patients often shift to a softer, stickier, carbohydrate-predominant diet, which further contributes to the higher caries rate reported in irradiated patients.[163]

Prevention and Treatment

Radiation planning is critically important for protecting salivary gland tissue from external beam radiotherapy. IMRT using three-dimensional conformal CT-assisted radiation delivery techniques has proven successful in delivering therapeutic radiation dosages to tumors and those head and neck regions at risk of tumor spread[176-180] while limiting exposure of the salivary glands considered to be at low risk. Recurrence rates with IMRT have not been significantly different compared with nonsalivary sparing techniques.[181,182]

In a recent systematic review of prevention and treatment strategies of salivary gland hypofunction and xerostomia in cancer patients treated with radiotherapy, the following were recommended based on the level of evidence and recommendation grade[183]:

- The use of parotid sparing IMRT for prevention of salivary gland hypofunction and xerostomia in head and neck cancer patients (level of evidence II, recommendation grade A).
- The use of oral pilocarpine following radiation therapy in head and neck cancer patients for improvement of xerostomia. The improvement of salivary gland hypofunction may be limited (level of evidence II, recommendation grade B).
- The use of oral mucosal lubricants/saliva substitutes for short-term improvement of xerostomia following radiation therapy in head and neck cancer patients (level of evidence II, recommendation grade B).
- The obtained level of sparing by submandibular salivary gland transfer might be of clinical significance (level of evidence IV, recommendation grade B).
- The use of acupuncture to stimulate salivary gland secretion and to alleviate xerostomia (level of evidence II, recommendation grade C).

No guideline or recommendation was possible for the following management strategies:

- Cannot recommend the use of oral pilocarpine during radiotherapy in head and neck cancer patients for improvement of xerostomia as the results of the various randomized clinical trials were equivocal (level of evidence II, recommendation grade C).
- No guideline possible for use of amifostine to prevent xerostomia during RT for head and neck cancer due to lack of consensus on the interpretation of existing evidence (level of evidence II, recommendation grade C).

- No guideline possible for use of gustatory and masticatory stimulation due to little evidence on which to base a guideline since this has been sparsely addressed specifically for patients suffering from xerostomia induced by cancer therapies (level of evidence III, recommendation grade D).
- No guideline possible for hyperbaric oxygen treatment of xerostomia due to no evidence on which to base a guideline (level of evidence IV, recommendation grade D).

All patients who have been referred for radiation therapy require a comprehensive dental examination several weeks prior to the initiation of radiation therapy and continued periodic examinations throughout active treatment and beyond. Patients experiencing the plethora of oral side effects from external beam radiotherapy require regular follow-up and aggressive treatment for salivary hypofunction (see section "Management of Xerostomia"), Candidal and other microbial infections, dental caries, and gingivitis. A prescribed daily oral hygiene regimen and use of prescription-strength topical fluorides are necessary to prevent dental caries. Prevention of dental disease is important to reduce the need for dentoalveolar surgery, which could induce ORN of irradiated bone.

Internal Radiation-Induced Pathology
Description and Etiology

Radioactive iodine (RAI) is the standard treatment in cases of papillary and follicular thyroid carcinomas following thyroidectomy or in cases of suspected or known metastases. A significant portion of the RAI taken up by thyroid tissue is concentrated and secreted through the salivary gland tissue resulting in radiation exposure of the salivary parenchyma and possible damage. Standard doses of RAI often cause obstructive duct symptoms, while hyposalivation from parenchymal damage is usually observed with larger or repeated doses of RAI. Acute risks associated with RAI include ageusia, salivary gland swelling, and pain, while long-term side effects include recurrent sialadenitis with xerostomia, stomatitis, and dental caries.[184] In some circumstances, RAI treatment may lead to glandular fibrosis and permanent salivary gland hypofunction.[185-188] In a systematic review of published data on salivary hypofunction and xerostomia in patients treated with RAI, the weighted prevalence of xerostomia was 33.6–37.8% at 1–2 years after treatment and the unstimulated and stimulated whole saliva flow rates were reduced by 27–41% and 27–36%, respectively 4 months to 20 years after treatment.[166]

Clinical Presentation

The glandular effect of RAI can be mild to severe. Patients may be asymptomatic or may complain of parotid gland swelling (usually bilaterally), pain, xerostomia, and decreased salivary gland function almost immediately after treatment.[189,190] In contrast to external beam radiotherapy, RAI effects within the oral cavity are limited to the salivary glands (as opposed to all hard and soft tissue), and it causes less destruction to the salivary glands.

Signs and symptoms of the effects of RAI on salivary flow may initially go unnoticed as the more radioresistant submandibular and sublingual salivary glands compensate for the decreased function of the parotid glands.[191] Symptoms of acute, early sialadenitis usually abate within a few days after RAI but persistent salivary gland swelling may occur. This may be accompanied by obstructive symptomatology with swelling and pain during salivary stimulation, not unlike symptoms associated with sialolithiasis. The patient may also complain of a salty taste.[189] Ageusia or dysgeusia immediately following RAI may be temporary or, at higher doses, permanent.

Diagnosis

A history of ^{131}I administration will help establish the diagnosis. Symptoms of chronic salivary gland dysfunction can be observed even after a single RAI dose.[192] SGS using IV technetium 99m pertechnetate may be used to determine the extent of parenchymal damage.[193] This procedure allows for assessment of acinar and ductal functions for both the parotid and the submandibular glands.[191] Parotid gland dysfunction tends to develop more frequently and with a greater severity than submandibular gland dysfunction after RAI treatment reflecting the greater radiosensitivity of the serous acinar cells of the parotid glands.[192]

Prevention and Treatment

RAI-induced salivary gland injury is irreversible; however, residual functioning salivary gland tissue is often present and responsive to therapy.[191] Following administration of ^{131}I, patients should undergo an aggressive salivary stimulation routine that includes sugar-free lozenges, sour candies, and gums to stimulate salivary flow.[189] This will aid in clearing the ^{131}I from the salivary glands and potentially decrease salivary gland damage. Stimulation of salivary flow by these means, however, should not be initiated within the first 24 hours after ^{131}I therapy as this has been shown to potentially increase the salivary gland side effects of the RAI.[185] Pilocarpine and cevimeline used before and after RAI treatment may decrease transit time through the salivary glands, thereby diminishing exposure. Avoidance of anticholinergic medications during RAI treatment is also helpful.[189]

In cases of RAI-associated sialadenitis, external massage of the gland or use of duct probing to encourage outflow of retained saliva and debris may be indicated. Antibiotics may be necessary if infection is suspected upon observation of suppuration or fever.[189] Other therapeutic protocols should be followed as with any other patient with hyposalivation to prevent development of further oral-pharyngeal complications.

Although amifostine has been used as a radioprotector in patients undergoing external radiation therapy for head and neck tumors to reduce damage to the salivary glands, clinical trials have not shown any significant effects of amifostine therapy on the incidence of xerostomia and hypogeusia[194] or any cytoprotective effects[195] in patients undergoing high-dose RAI therapy.

IgG4-Related Disease

In 2003, Kamisawa and Okamoto proposed the existence of a new clinicopathologic entity: IgG4-related disease. The basis of their proposal was the observation that there were several multiorgan, inflammatory, mass-forming lesions with increased IgG4-positive plasma cells and common histopathologic findings. These conditions have since been observed in multiple organ systems including the salivary glands, pancreas, kidneys, lung, lymph nodes, and thyroid. Chronic sclerosing sialadenitis (also known as the Küttner Tumor) and Mikulicz's disease are now considered to be manifestations of IgG4-related disease.[196] The features common to all IgG4-related disease are elevated serum and tissue levels of IgG4, a common histologic appearance and a response to immunosuppressive treatment.[196] The disease is found to affect mainly older men.[197]

Clinical Presentation

Chronic sclerosing sialadenitis (Küttner Tumor) is a chronic inflammatory disease primarily of the submandibular salivary gland, [198,199] although it has been reported in the parotid and minor salivary glands.[199,200] Histopathologically, chronic sclerosing sialadenitis is characterized by progressive periductal fibrosis, dilated ducts with a dense lymphocyte infiltration, and lymphoid follicle formation with acinar atrophy.[201] It has been reported that some patients with sclerosing sialadenitis showed a dense infiltration of IgG4-positive plasma cells and may have associated sclerosing manifestations in extra-salivary gland tissue such as autoimmune pancreatitis.

Mikulicz's disease is a bilateral, painless, symmetric swelling affecting the lacrimal, parotid, and submandibular glands and is considered by some to be a subtype of SS. Patients with Mikulicz's disease, however, lack anti-SSA and anti-SSB antibodies but often have elevated IgG4 serum levels. In addition, infiltration of the lacrimal and salivary glands by IgG4-positive cells has been observed in Mikulicz's disease.[197]

Diagnosis

In 2012, an international symposium proposed guidelines for the diagnosis of IgG4-related disease based on the presence of the characteristic histopathologic features and increased number of IgG4-positive plasma cells. Key histopathologic findings include a dense lymphoplasmacytic infiltrate, a storiform pattern of fibrosis, and obliterative phlebitis. However, exceptions are made for the minor salivary glands and lacrimal glands where storiform fibrosis or obliterative phlebitis may be inconspicuous or absent. Definitive diagnosis of IgG4-related disease, therefore, relies upon both the presence of the characteristic histopathologic appearance and elevated IgG4-positive plasma cells (or elevated IgG4:IgG ratio). The consensus established that in salivary gland lesions, greater than 100 IgG4-positive cells per high-powered field or an IgG4+:IgG+ cell ratio greater than 0.4 is indicative of disease.[196]

It has been recommended that patients with IgG4-related disease undergo a systemic workup at diagnosis to determine the extent of disease and to screen for NHL, since a history of IgG4-related disease may be a predisposing condition for lymphoma.[202,203]

Treatment

High-dose corticosteroid therapy is the current mainstay treatment for IgG4-related disease; the regimen indicated will be dependent on the organs involved and manifestations observed. The use of azathioprine in addition to steroid therapy[204] or as an alternative where steroids have failed[205] has been successful in a few cases. Other therapies that have been used are disease-modifying antirheumatic drugs and B-cell depletion therapy with rituximab.[205,206] A large retrospective study showed that 18F-FDG PET/CT imaging is useful in the staging and monitoring the treatment response in patients with IgG4-related disease.[207]

Acute and Chronic Allergic Sialadenitis

Description and Etiology

Acute allergic sialadenitis (AAS) is an uncommon form of sialadenitis due to allergic effects of allergens on the salivary glands. Enlargement of the salivary glands has been associated with exposure to various pharmaceutical agents and allergens (Table 10-3). It is unclear whether all of the reported cases are true allergic reactions or whether some represent secondary infections resulting from medications that reduced salivary output. Histopathologically, AAS presents with a mixed inflammatory infiltrate affecting the periductal and perivascular tissues composed of leukocytes, lymphocytes, histiocytes, and eosinophils and partial destruction of the acinar cells.[208] Chronic allergic sialadenitis (CAS) is seen in conjunction with sarcoidosis, Crohn's disease,

TABLE 10-3 Compounds Associated With Allergic Sialadenitis

Ethambutol
Heavy metals
Iodine compounds
Isoproterenol
Phenobarbital
Phenothiazine
Sulfisoxazole

cheilitis granulomatosa, and granulomatosis with polyangiitis (GPA; Wegener's granulomatosis).[208]

Clinical Description

The characteristic feature of allergic sialadenitis is acute salivary gland enlargement, often accompanied by itching over the gland. Cases have been reported of salivary gland enlargement without rash or other signs of allergy.

Diagnosis

The diagnosis of allergic reaction should be made judiciously, especially when salivary gland enlargement is not accompanied by other signs of an allergic reaction. The possibility of infection or autoimmune disease should also be considered.

Treatment

Allergic sialadenitis, when due to exposure to an allergen is self-limiting. Avoidance of the allergen, maintaining hydration, and monitoring for secondary infection are recommended.[209] Treatment for CAS is dependent on the underlying cause.

Eosinophilic Granulomatosis With Polyangiitis and Sialodochitis Fibrinosa

Two other allergy-associated forms of sialadenitis are worthy of mention especially since sialadenitis, when an allergic etiology is at play, is often accompanied by systemic eosinophilia and bronchial asthma.[208]

Eosinophilic granulomatosis with polyangiitis (EGPA; Churg–Strauss syndrome) is an unusual form of vasculitis affecting small- and medium-sized vessels, which can affect the major salivary glands. Histopathologically, it is characterized by eosinophilic and necrotizing granulomas in the vessel walls and perivascular tissue and is generally associated with a history of asthma, allergic rhinitis, and eosinophilia.[210] Because of this, vasculitis must be considered among the differential diagnoses in cases of salivary gland enlargement.[210] Treatment for EGPA involves glucocorticoid therapy or combinations of glucocorticoids and immunosuppressants. Newer therapeutic options investigated include the anti-IL5 antibody mepolizumab and the B-cell-depleting agent rituximab.[211]

Sialodochitis fibrinosa, a rare salivary disorder with a likely allergic etiology, was first reported by Kussmaul in 1879. Currently, however, the definitive etiology and pathophysiology have not been established. The presentation of sialodochitis fibrinosa is one of paroxysmal recurrent salivary gland swelling and a history of allergy-associated diseases such as asthma, allergic rhinitis, urticaria, and food allergy.

Other findings include increased serum eosinophils and/or increased serum IgE levels, secretion from the Stensen's duct(s) of eosinophil-laden mucous plugs, and abnormalities including ectasia on sialogram. Histopathologic findings of duct thickening and/or periductal lymphocytic and eosinophilic infiltration are seen.[212]

Management of sialodochitis fibrinosa is dependent on the severity of symptoms. Massage to encourage removal of obstructing mucous plugs has been successful in case reports. Other considerations for treatment include the use of systemic antihistamines and steroids, irrigation of the Stensen's ducts with a steroid solution, or parotidectomy in refractory cases.[212] A recent case reported successful use of the leukotriene receptor antagonist montelukast.[213]

Viral Diseases
Overview

Several viruses have been associated with acute nonsuppurative salivary gland enlargement. The viruses responsible for the majority of virally induced salivary gland enlargement are the mumps paramyxovirus, cytomegalovirus (CMV), HIV, and hepatitis C virus (HCV). Echoviruses, the Epstein–Barr virus (EBV), parainfluenza viruses, and choriomeningitis virus infections have also been linked to occasional reports of nonsuppurative salivary gland enlargement.

Mumps (Paramyxovirus or Epidemic Parotitis)
Description and Etiology

Mumps is an acute viral infection caused by an enveloped, RNA-containing paramyxovirus. The virus can be found in saliva and urine and is transmitted by inhalation of infectious droplets, by direct contact or by autoinoculation(i.e., interaction with virus-laden fomites followed by contact with the nose or mouth).[214] The Centers for Disease Control and Prevention (CDC) began recommending measles-mumps-rubella (MMR) vaccination for children in 1977. Current guidelines call for an initial vaccination at 12–18 months of age and a second dose at 4–6 years of age. Mumps virus vaccine is not recommended for severely immunocompromised children because the protective immune response often does not develop and risk of complications exists.[215,216] No epidemiologic studies have demonstrated a direct link between the MMR vaccine and autism or inflammatory bowel disease, yet some parents have refused vaccination for their children, raising the possibility of reemergence of the disease.[217] Therefore, this infection must be considered in cases of acute nonsuppurative salivary gland inflammation in unvaccinated patients who have not had mumps.

Despite widespread vaccination campaigns, mumps has made a comeback in many countries including those that had previously reported good control. In the past decade, outbreaks have been reported in the United States, the United Kingdom, Sweden, the Netherlands, Canada, Australia, Belgium, and a number of other countries.[214]

Clinical Presentation

Mumps typically occurs in children between the ages of 4 and 6 years. The incubation period is two to three weeks. Mumps usually presents with one to two days of malaise, anorexia, and low-grade pyrexia with headache followed by nonpurulent gland enlargement. Glandular swelling increases over the next few days, lasting about one week. Twenty-five percent of cases may involve unilateral salivary gland swelling, or swelling may develop in the contralateral gland after a time delay, which can complicate diagnosis unless there is a high index of suspicion.[218] Ninety-five percent of symptomatic cases involve the parotid gland only, while about 10% of cases involve the bilateral submandibular and sublingual glands concomitant with the parotid swelling.[218] A minority of cases may involve the submandibular glands alone (Figure 10-15).

The salivary gland enlargement is sudden and painful to palpation with edema affecting the overlying skin and the duct orifice. If partial duct obstruction occurs, the patient may experience pain while eating. Complications of mumps include mild meningitis and encephalitis; mumps encephalitis has an approximately 1.5% mortality rate.[218] Deafness, myocarditis, thyroiditis, pancreatitis, hepatitis, and oophoritis are additional complications. Males can experience epididymitis and orchitis, resulting in testicular atrophy and infertility if the disease occurs in adolescence or later.

Diagnosis

The clinical diagnosis of mumps relies upon the standard case definition of an acute onset unilateral or bilateral salivary gland swelling lasting two or more days without any other apparent cause.[219] This, of course, will miss cases where parotid gland swelling is absent or not prominent. Laboratory-confirmed mumps as defined by the CDC requires clinical symptoms compatible with mumps with positive mumps IgM antibody (without previous immunization in the last six weeks) or seroconversion as defined by a fourfold rise in IgG titer to mumps, or isolation of mumps virus, or detection of mumps RNA in saliva, urine, or cerebrospinal fluid.[214]

Diagnosis during an acute mumps infection can be done using a buccal swab. To perform this, the patient's parotid gland is massaged to express infected saliva and a swab is rubbed along the buccal mucosa near Stenson's duct.

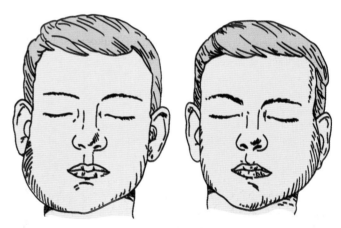

FIGURE 10-15 Left: Typical location and configuration of swelling associated with viral mumps. Right: Usual location and configuration of swelling associated with abscessed mandibular molars.

The swab is then placed in the appropriate viral transport medium and shipped to the laboratory at 4°C.[214] Nucleic acid–based tests including reverse transcriptase polymerase chain reaction(PCR) have been developed for detection of viral mumps in clinical samples. These methods are faster and more sensitive than tests relying on tissue culture.[214]

Treatment

The treatment of mumps is symptomatic and may involve the use of analgesics and antipyretics.

Prevention

Live-attenuated mumps vaccines have been available for more than 30 years and are usually given in combination with MMR and more recently with the varicella vaccine.[214] Currently, the CDC recommends mumps patients be isolated and standard and droplet precautions be followed for five days after parotitis onset.[220]

Anesthesia Mumps/Postoperative Sialadenitis

Anesthesia mumps, also known as "surgical mumps, " is a rare complication of general anesthesia, which presents as an acute transient swelling of the parotid glands. It typically presents unilaterally. The etiology of anesthesia mumps is currently unknown; some possible mechanisms involve trauma, straining during anesthesia, vascular congestion of the head and neck, anesthetic drugs, dehydration, and head and neck positioning during surgery. Some medical conditions that may predispose the salivary ducts to occlusion are associated with anesthesia mumps such as diabetes mellitus, hypothyroidism, SS, and malnutrition. In addition, xerogenic medications such as antihistamines, antihypertensives, tranquilizers, and muscle relaxants, which predispose patients to dehydration and salivary stasis, can place patients at an increased. Anesthesia mumps usually causes temporary esthetic local problems such as swelling of the face or neck. Massive facial, oral, and pharyngeal edema associated with anesthesia mumps can cause airway obstruction and can necessitate tracheostomy.

Anesthesia mumps is usually a self-limited condition that rapidly improves with symptomatic therapy including rehydration and anti-inflammatory medications such as nonsteroidal anti-inflammatory drugs.

CMV Infection

Description and Etiology

CMV (HHV-5) is a member of the Herpesviridae family. It commonly infects salivary glands in humans and is the major cause of non-EBV infectious mononucleosis in the general population. As is characteristic to other members of Herpesviridae, CMV can become latent after initial exposure and infection and may become reactivated when favorable conditions are present. The majority of CMV infections are asymptomatic, especially in healthy individuals; however, in immunocompromised patients and neonates, infection can be life threatening.[221,222]

CMV can be cultured from blood, saliva, feces, respiratory secretions, urine, and other body fluids. Horizontal transmission occurs through blood transfusion, allograft transplants, and sexual contact. High rates of seropositivity are found in homosexual males, intravenous drug users, prostitutes, and individuals who have undergone multiple transfusions.[223–226] Transmission from children to adults or between children occurs through fomites, urine, saliva, and respiratory secretions. Between 11% and 24% of children attending day-care centers have CMV in their saliva.[227,228] A large percentage of healthy adults have serum antibodies to the virus. Vertical transplacental transmission results in congenital infection and malformations. Perinatal infection occurs in 3% of all live births and is thought to be due to transmission from breast milk, saliva, fomites, or urine.

Clinical Presentation

In the young adult, acute CMV infection presents as a mild, self-limiting mononucleosis-like disease. Patients will commonly experience fever, malaise, and myalgia; pharyngitis and lymphadenopathy are seen less frequently than in EBV-associated mononucleosis. Acute sialadenitis, seen as a diffuse, painful swelling of the parotid and submandibular glands with associated xerostomia, [229] may also occur.

Transplacental transmission of CMV can result in congenital CMV infection, which may vary in presentation from being asymptomatic to a congenital syndrome involving prematurity, low birth weight, and various congenital malformations. The mortality rate has been recently estimated as less than 5% of cases in symptomatic neonates.[230] In clinically evident acute infection in neonates, the child will appear ill within a few days. A sepsis-like syndrome occurs most commonly and is associated with hepatosplenomegaly, abnormal blood counts with lymphopenia, neutropenia and thrombocytopenia, abnormal transaminases, and pneumonitis.[231] Long-term sequelae of early postnatal CMV infection may involve neurological problems such as sensorineural hearing loss. Developmental tooth detects may also be a consequence of neonatal CMV infection including diffuse enamel hypoplasia, attrition, enamel hypomaturation, and yellow coloration from the underlying dentin.[229] CMV can also cause parotitis in infants.[232]

In immunocompromised adults, the impaired immune system allows the virus to replicate and a disseminated infection to occur. Patients taking immunosuppressive medications and patients with hematologic abnormalities or HIV infection are susceptible to severe CMV infections. Infection may result from reactivation of endogenous virus, a transplanted organ, or blood product transfusion. Oral and maxillofacial manifestations of CMV in immunosuppressed patients typically present as persistent oral ulcerations and major salivary gland infections, with or without concomitant alterations in salivary flow.[232] In HIV-positive patients, the degree of CMV-induced sialadenitis and/or xerostomia was found to be proportional to the HIV load and inversely proportional to the CD4+ cell count.[232]

Diagnosis

Several diagnostic modalities for CMV are available including serology, qualitative and quantitative PCR, and histopathology. The choice of test is based on the status of the immune system of the patient. Diagnosis of primary CMV infection in immunocompetent hosts is usually made using serologic studies: either the detection of CMV-specific IgM or a fourfold increase in CMV-specific IgG. Diagnosis of CMV disease in immunocompromised patients relies on clinical history and presentation and quantitative PCR tests for detecting viral DNA.

Histopathologic examination of CMV-infected tissue may show large atypical cells with inclusion bodies, [233] resulting in a characteristic "owl eye" appearance. However, these cells may be scarce and undetectable, and therefore, CMV-specific immunohistochemistry staining is additionally recommended.[234]

Treatment

Most cases of primary CMV infection in immunocompetent adults present with minimal or no symptoms. In those with symptomatic, mononucleosis-like infection, the disease typically lasts for a few days to weeks and only supportive, symptomatic care (i.e., analgesics, rest, hydration) is required.

Immunocompromised patients require aggressive antiviral therapy that may be in the form of ganciclovir, valganciclovir, foscarnet, or cidofovir. Ganciclovir has also been recommended for prophylactic or preemptive treatment of CMV disease in transplant recipients.[235] The recommended length of treatment is dependent on CMV viral loads, which are monitored on a weekly basis and continues until one or two consecutive negative samples are obtained. A treatment course of at least two weeks minimizes the development of resistance and recurrence.[236]

HIV-Associated Salivary Gland Disease
Overview

Neoplastic and nonneoplastic salivary gland lesions occur with increased frequency in HIV-positive patients. The most common salivary gland presentation in these patients is one of salivary gland swelling usually attributed to either acute sialadenitis or HIV-associated salivary gland disease (HIV-SGD). AIDS-related neoplasms (e.g., Kaposi's sarcoma, lymphoma) and a SS–like phenomenon[237] can also manifest as salivary gland enlargements.[238] HIV-positive individuals have also been shown to have reduced salivary flow rates from the major salivary glands and changes in composition of saliva with respect to sodium, chloride, lysozyme, peroxidase, lactoferrin, and immunoglobulin A levels.[239–241] The antiviral drugs didanosine, lamivudine, indinavir, nelfinavir, ritonavir, and saquinavir are associated with xerostomia and hyposalivation.

Parotid gland enlargement in HIV-positive patients is reported to occur in 1%–10% of patients.[238] This enlargement may represent one of several pathologies including LELs, hyperplastic reactive lymphadenopathy, benign lymphoepithelial cysts (BLEC), lymphoma, benign or malignant neoplasms, bacterial, fungal, or viral infections, or diffuse infiltrative lymphocytosis syndrome (DILS).[242] Parotid gland swelling has also been observed in patients undergoing antiretroviral therapy.[243]

Description and Etiology

The term *HIV-associated salivary gland disease* was coined by Schiødt et al. in 1989 to describe major salivary gland enlargement and/or xerostomia in HIV patients in the absence of xerogenic agents, medications, and diseases known to cause xerostomia.[244] Typically, HIV-SGD presents as a unilateral or a bilateral diffuse swelling of the major salivary glands, resulting in facial disfigurement, which may or may not be painful. It may also be accompanied by generalized lymphadenopathy. When the labial minor salivary glands are affected, features of sialadenitis are present. HIV-SGD is considered a premalignant lesion since a reported 1%–2% of patients develop lymphoma associated with the glandular lesions.[233,245]

HIV-SGD is observed in both adults and children; however, it occurs more commonly in the pediatric population and may in fact represent a different disease process.[238] It has been proposed that HIV-SGD is due to a reactivation of a latent virus.[246] HIV-SGD presents similarly to the phenomenon known as immune reconstitution disease, which is thought to be a consequence of a pre-existing occult opportunistic or subclinical infection becoming "unmasked" as HIV viral load decreases and CD4 count increases upon the initiation of highly active antiretroviral therapy (HAART). Since the advent of HAART in the mid-1990s, the prevalence of many HIV-associated oral lesions has decreased; HIV-SGD is the exception.

A SS–like phenomenon has been described in HIV-positive patients, which involves salivary gland enlargement, xerostomia, and keratoconjunctivitis sicca. DILS is a broader term involving both sicca syndrome and extraglandular manifestations, which may involve the lung, gastrointestinal tract, kidney, liver, muscle, or nerves. DILS occurs in HIV-positive patients with low CD4 counts. Both the American-European Consensus Group (AECG) and the ACR list AIDS in the exclusion criteria for SS.

Diagnosis
Imaging and Biopsy

Persistent major salivary gland enlargement for no other discernible cause warrants further investigation by imaging and possibly biopsy. Imaging modalities employed for evaluation of salivary gland enlargement has been discussed in detail earlier in this chapter and in HIV-SGD may consist of the use of US, CT, and/ or MRI. US is particularly advantageous in the pediatric patient as there is no radiation exposure and sedation is rarely required. Ultrasound pathologic presentations of parotid glands affected by HIV may be one of four distinct patterns: lymphocytic aggregations, LECs, fatty infiltration, or lymphadenopathy only. Observation of multiple thin-walled cysts with diffuse cervical lymphadenopathy within the parotid gland in itself is an indication for HIV testing.[238] Scintiscan using technetium pertechnetate has been found to be of little value in delineating salivary lesions in HIV-positive patients.

Since HIV-SGD frequently resembles SS, appropriate salivary, ophthalmologic, and serologic evaluation must be performed.[237] Salivary flow rates may be reduced, and salivary immunoglobulin A (IgA) may be elevated in both patients with SS and patients with HIV-SGD. Peripheral blood changes can resemble those observed in patients with SS and include hypergammaglobulinemia, circulating immune complexes, and RFs. However, anti-SSA and anti-SSB autoantibodies are usually negative in HIV-SGD.

A MSGB may be indicated, and histologic findings resemble changes seen in cases of SS (including focal mononuclear cell infiltration). Using immunohistochemical stains to differentiate the infiltrating cells, there is a preponderance of CD8+ cells in HIV-SGD compared with the CD4+ infiltrates that predominate in SS. HIV-SGD may also feature hyperplastic, intraparotid lymph nodes, cystic cavities,[247] and/or a predominantly CD8+ T-cell lymphocytic infiltrate within the salivary gland tissue.[248] In DILS, CD8+ lymphocytic infiltrates are found in the salivary glands, lungs, gastrointestinal tract, and liver.[233,249]

BLECs tend to have a slow progression and therefore any acute change in size warrants further investigation. As patients with HIV-SGD are at an increased risk for the development of an EBV-associated B-cell lymphoma, tissue acquisition using FNAB is recommended.

Treatment

HIV-SGD-related xerostomia can be managed with increased hydration, the use of sugar-free lozenges, candies, and gums, dry mouth products and using saliva substitutes or other pharmacologic agents such as sialogogues (see section Management of Xerostomia). Patients with salivary hypofunction should be encouraged to follow a rigorous daily oral hygiene regimen incorporating the use of topical fluoride and to maintain a regular schedule of dental examinations and hygiene appointments.

Treatment with HAART can result in the resolution of the histologic changes associated with SLS[250] and DILS. Treatment for parotid gland BLEC is not definitively established. Options involve (1) close observation, (2) repeat aspiration, (3) antiretroviral medication, (4) sclerosing therapy, (5) radiation therapy, and (6) surgery.[238] Sclerosing agents such as bleomycin, sodium morrhuate, alcohol, tetracycline,

and doxycycline have been used.[251] The use of external beam radiation therapy (24 Gy in 1.5 Gy doses) has been reported to have some success but has the potential for radiation-induced malignancy and xerostomia.

Hepatitis C Virus Infection
Description and Etiology

The HCV is an enveloped, single-stranded RNA virus of the family Flaviviridae. The virus is hepatotropic, lymphotropic, and sialotropic. HCV has been associated with sialadenitis and sicca syndrome. The reported occurrence of HCV-related sicca syndrome ranges from 4% to 57% of chronic HCV patients; the large range may reflect differences in diagnostic criteria.[252] The mechanism by which HCV results in sicca syndrome has not been defined but studies show that HCV-related sicca syndrome is likely the product of a host immune-mediated mechanism rather than a direct viral effect since HCV has not been shown to directly infect salivary gland tissue.[252]

Xerostomia is common in patients with chronic hepatitis C, with prevalence ranging from 10% to 35%. Pegylated interferon/ribavirin (PegIFN/Rbv) therapy used to treat hepatitis C has been associated with the development of xerostomia and temporary salivary gland hypofunction.[253] The reported prevalence of hyposalivation in chronic hepatitis C patients ranges from 13% to 33%. A weak association between xerostomia and salivary gland hypofunction in HCV patients has been suggested.[254] In a study analyzing the prevalence of HCV RNA in saliva of patients with chronic hepatitis C and its possible association with xerostomia and hyposalivation, it was suggested there is a lack of association between the presence of HCV in saliva and the measures of salivary flow. These data indicate that the detection of HCV in saliva does not contribute to hyposalivation or xerostomia in patients with chronic hepatitis C.[254]

Since patients with HCV infection may exhibit sicca syndrome, and focal sialadenitis, HCV infection is an exclusion criterion for the ACR with respect to diagnosis of SS and the AECG for the Classification of SS with respect to diagnosis of secondary SS.[255]

The majority of HCV-associated lymphomas are extranodal and are located in the liver and salivary glands.[256, 257] MALT lymphoma is the most frequent histotype among the primary lymphomas of salivary glands and represents 1.7%–8.6% of all salivary gland tumors and about 1% of all NHL cases.[258260]

There is evidence for an oncogenic role of HCV in NHL. The association between HCV and NHL is strongest in geographic areas with highest prevalence of the viral infection. HCV RNA and HCV-related antigens have been detected in the epithelial cells of salivary glands of HCV-positive patients and in residual epithelial structures in a NHL of the parotid.[261,262] HCV is considered a classic example of an infectious agent causing NHL through persistent immune stimulation. Althoguh a direct oncogenic role of HCV through B-cell infection and deregulation has been proposed, since the virus is lymphotropic, this has never been proven.[263]

Clinical Manifestations

HCV infection has many extrahepatic manifestations, including sialadenitis and chronic major salivary gland enlargement and complaints of xerostomia and sicca syndrome are common.[264,265] Additional signs and symptoms of acute HCV infection (clinical signs or symptoms of hepatitis within six months of presumed HCV exposure) include jaundice, nausea, dark urine, and right upper quadrant pain. However, most patients who are acutely infected with HCV are asymptomatic. Chronic HCV infection is usually slowly progressive and may not result in clinically apparent liver disease in many patients. Most patients with chronic infection are asymptomatic or have only mild nonspecific symptoms. The most frequent complaint is fatigue; other less common manifestations include nausea, anorexia, myalgia, arthralgia, weakness, and weight loss.

Diagnosis

The diagnosis of HCV infection is established by the serologic detection of anti-HCV antibodies by ELISA and HCV DNA by PCR. HCV RNA is first detectable in serum by PCR within days to eight weeks following exposure, while development of antibodies may be delayed up to several years in patients who have subclinical infection. Distinguishing acute from chronic infection has important treatment implications since patients with acute HCV who do not spontaneously clear the virus should receive treatment with an interferon-based regimen.

Treatment

Patients with acute HCV infection receive weekly PegIFN-alpha or standard interferon. PegIFN/Rbv is the standard of care for chronic hepatitis C. Hepatitis-associated sialadenitis and xerostomia are treated symptomatically. Treatment for HCV-associated lymphoma of the salivary glands is dependent on the histotype. With respect to MALT lymphoma of the salivary glands, the treatment may involve surgery, radiotherapy, and chemotherapy.

Bacterial Sialadenitis
Acute and Chronic Bacterial Sialadenitis
Description and Etiology

Acute bacterial sialadenitis refers to a sudden onset of a swollen and painful infected salivary gland, whereas repeated bacterial glandular infection is termed *chronic bacterial sialadenitis.* Recurrent infections can occur in a gland where strictures develop following an episode of infectious sialadenitis.[125]

Bacterial infections of the salivary glands are most commonly seen in patients with salivary gland hypofunction[266] or with conditions that inhibit salivary flow. Risk factors include dehydration, the use of xerogenic drugs, salivary gland diseases, nerve damage, ductal obstruction, irradiation, and chronic diseases such as diabetes mellitus and SS.

Retrograde bacterial parotitis following surgery under general anesthesia is a well-recognized complication. It is due to the markedly decreased salivary flow during anesthesia, often as the result of anticholinergic drugs and relative dehydration. Although the incidence has decreased tremendously in the era of perioperative antibiotics, parotitis still complicates between 1 in 1000 and 1 in 2000 operative procedures. This condition usually occurs within two weeks of the surgery, with major surgeries comprising the greatest risk.[125]

Although bacterial sialadenitis occurs most frequently in the parotid glands, it can occur in any of the glands. It is thought that the antimicrobial activity of mucin, found in the saliva of the submandibular and sublingual glands, may competitively inhibit bacterial attachment to the epithelium of the salivary ducts.[125] The serous parotid gland saliva also contains less lysosomes, IgA antibodies, and sialic acid.[125] Anatomy may also play a protective role; tongue movements tend to clear the floor of the mouth and protect Wharton's duct. In contrast, the orifice of Stensen's duct is located adjacent to the molars, where heavy bacterial colonization occurs.[267]

Today, the majority of bacterial infections occur in patients with disease- or medication-induced salivary gland hypofunction. Commonly prescribed xerogenic drugs include antidepressants, anticholinergics, antispasmodics, antihistamines, antihypertensives, sedatives, diuretics, and bronchodilators.[9] Reduced salivary flow results in diminished mechanical flushing, which allows bacteria to colonize the oral cavity and then to invade the salivary duct in a retrograde fashion and cause an acute bacterial infection. Poor oral hygiene contributes to these infections, and older adults are particularly susceptible to bacterial sialadenitis due to the frequent combination of medication-induced salivary hypofunction and poor oral hygiene. Thus, although suppurative parotitis can affect persons of any age, it is predominately a disease of the middle aged and elderly; most patients are between the ages of 50 and 60 years.[125]

Clinical Presentation

Patients usually present with a sudden onset of unilateral or bilateral salivary gland enlargement. Approximately 20% of the cases present as bilateral infections. Complaints of fevers, chills, malaise, trismus, and dysphagia may accompany these findings. Observation of dry oral mucosa may indicate systemic dehydration.

The involved gland is enlarged, warm, painful, indurated, and tender to palpation.[268] If Stensen's duct is involved, it may appear erythematous and edematous. There may also be erythema of the overlying skin. Clinical examination of the involved glands involves bimanual palpation along the path of the excretory duct. In approximately 75% of cases, purulent discharge may be expressed from the orifice. Ductal obstruction or early stage disease, however, may preclude observation of drainage. Clinical examination may also reveal the presence of an obstructing sialolith.

Diagnosis

Bacterial parotitis is largely a clinical diagnosis. If purulent discharge can be expressed from the duct orifice, samples should be cultured for aerobes, anaerobes, fungi, and myco-bacteria (Figure 10-16)[269] taking care to avoid contamina-tion with intraoral flora. A second specimen should be sent for testing with a Gram stain. In addition, although not a requirement for diagnosis, laboratory studies may show leuk-ocytosis with neutrophilia.

Salivary gland hypofunction can result in decreased oro-pharyngeal salivary clearance and subsequent colonization of the oral cavity with *Staphylococcus aureus*. As a consequence, this species is by far the most common isolated pathogen seen in bacterial parotitis and is responsible for 50%–90% of cases of hospitalized patients.[270]

Infections are often polymicrobial. The predominant isolated aerobes in addition to *S. aureus* are *Haemophilus influenzae*, *Streptococcus viridans*, *Streptococcus pneumoniae*, and *Escherichia coli*. Common anaerobes are Gram-negative bacilli (including pigmented *Prevotella* and *Porphyromonas* species), *Fusobacterim* species, and *Peptostreptococcus* species.[269] Institutionalized individuals are particularly susceptible to infections caused by methicillin-resistant *S. aureus* (MRSA).

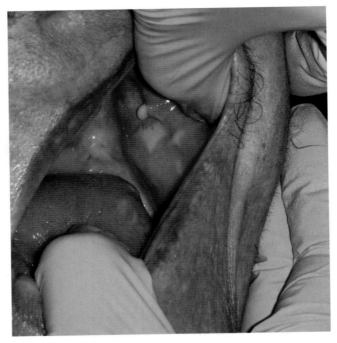

FIGURE 10-16 Acute bacterial sialadenitis and purulent discharge from Stensen's duct. Culture and sensitivity testing will indicate appropriate antibiotic therapy.

Actinomyces species, *Mycobacterium tuberculosis*, and atypical mycobacteria are rare causes of infection.[125]

Differentiating between viral and bacterial infectious parotitis can be challenging. In general, viral infections are bilateral, affect younger patients, have prodromal symptoms, do not involve purulent drainage, and patients appear to have less toxicity. Although systemic symptoms follow the devel-opment of a symptomatic gland in suppurative parotitis, the order is usually reversed in viral parotitis.

Due to the dense capsule surrounding the salivary glands, it is difficult to determine, based on physical examination alone, whether an abscess has been formed. A maxillofacial CT with intravenous contrast is the most sensitive and com-monly used tool for detecting an abscess. Sialoendoscopy, US, CT, MRI sialography, or percutaneous aspiration[125] may be helpful to rule out chronic salivary gland infections, cysts, obstructions,[268,271-273] or neoplasms.

Treatment

Treatment goals of bacterial sialadenitis include resolu-tion of signs and symptoms of infection, elimination of the causative bacteria, rehydration, and elimination of obstruc-tion where present. This may involve the use of antibiot-ics, analgesics, heat application, fluids, glandular massage, oral hygiene products, and sialogogues. Anti-inflammatory agents including steroids may help to rapidly reduce pain and swelling. Patients should also be instructed to massage the gland several times a day. Where possible, medications implicated in salivary gland hypofunction should be dis-continued. With these measures, significant improvement should be observed within 24–48 hours. If this does not occur, incision and drainage should be considered.[268] Where abscess formation is evident, surgical drainage is necessary.[125] Intraductal instillation of penicillin or saline is an alternat-ive for the treatment of chronic bacterial parotid or sub-mandibular sialadenitis.[274]

Appropriate empiric antibiotic regimens should include coverage for *S. aureus* as well as oral polymicrobial aerobic and anaerobic infections. It is estimated that up to 75% of infections are caused by β-lactamase–producing bacteria, and therefore, treatment with anti-Staphylococcal penicillin, a combination β-lactamase inhibitor, or a first-generation cephalosporin is appropriate. Macrolides such as azithromy-cin with metronidazole can be an alternative for those with a penicillin allergy. Antibiotics should not be started routinely unless bacterial infection is clinically obvious. Under all cir-cumstances, purulent discharge from the salivary gland should be cultured to confirm the diagnosis and determine antibiotic sensitivity.[266] Antibiotic therapy may need to be modified later based on culture results.

The mortality rate for bacterial sialadenitis has been reported to be as high as 20%–40%. Additional potential complications include facial nerve palsy, sepsis, mandibular osteomyelitis, internal jugular vein thrombophlebitis, and respiratory obstruction.[125]

Neonatal Suppurative Parotitis
Description and Etiology

Neonatal suppurative parotitis (NSP), also known as acute suppurative parotitis, is a rare condition in the neonate often attributable to infection by *S. aureus* or other Gram-positive cocci, and Gram-negative bacilli or anaerobic bacteria. Several recent reports have also implicated a MRSA in cases of NSP.[275]

Clinical Presentation

NSP may affect infants between the ages of 2–4 weeks. Presentation includes a swelling of the affected gland or glands with overlying erythema and may be accompanied by systemic symptoms and signs including fever, poor oral intake, and irritability.[275]

Diagnosis

Diagnosis of NSP is reliant on the presence of parotid swelling, which may be unilateral or bilateral, and expression of a purulent exudate from Stensen's duct in which pathogenic bacteria are identified on culture.[276] Diagnosis is aided by ultrasound examination, which may show an enlarged gland and hypoechoic areas characteristic of parotitis. Ultrasound may also help to determine whether there is an additional glandular mass or abscess.[276] The risk factors include dehydration, male gender, low birth weight, immune suppression, ductal obstruction, oral trauma, and structural abnormalities of the parotid gland.

Treatment

NSP is amenable to treatment by antibiotics with supportive therapy such as adequate hydration. However, in the event of intraglandular abscess, surgical drainage may be necessary.[276] Antimicrobial therapy is based on culture and sensitivity assays of the expressed suppurative fluid.[276] Complications reported with NSP have included facial palsy, recurrent infection, bacteremia, and sepsis and respiratory distress. Although potential morality has been associated with NSP, no deaths have been reported in the English-language literature since 1970 possibly due to improvement in antibiotic therapy.[275]

Systemic Conditions With Salivary Gland Involvement
Diabetes Mellitus

Diabetes mellitus is a common endocrine disease that produces multiple metabolic abnormalities and long-term complications, such as renal hypertension, neuropathies, and ophthalmic disease.

Many patients with uncontrolled diabetes report dry mouth and experience salivary hypofunction.[277–280] It appears that salivary disorders may be related to the efficacy of control of diabetes, with poorly controlled patients experiencing more salivary gland dysfunction than well-controlled patients or controls.[277,279] Children with diabetes are also affected by impaired salivary flow rates[281] and salivary compositional changes.[282]

The etiology of diabetic salivary gland dysfunction may be related to multiple problems, including polyuria, poor hydration, or underlying salivary gland pathology, including alterations in the basement membranes of salivary glands.[283] Poor glycemic control,[277,278,281] autonomic nervous system dysfunction,[279] and concomitant medications[284] may also account for salivary dysfunction. Complaints of xerostomia in those with diabetes could also be attributed to thirst, a common manifestation of diabetes.

Anorexia Nervosa/Bulimia

Salivary gland enlargement and dysfunction can occur in patients with anorexia nervosa and bulimia[285,286] possibly due to nutritional deficiencies and the habit of repeated induced vomiting. One case study reported histopathologic findings of acinar enlargement and reduced interstitial fat.[286] In bulimia, total and salivary specific amylase levels are increased. Salivary amylase tends to increase with the frequency of binge eating,[285,287] and salivary cortisol has been correlated with plasma cortisol, demonstrating the overdrive of the hypothalamic-pituitary-adrenal axis in these patients.[288] Salivary gland enlargement usually resolves when patients return to normal weight and discontinue unhealthy dietary habits. However, benign hypertrophy may persist and be of cosmetic concern. Although superficial parotidectomy will reduce salivary hypertrophy, surgical management is contraindicated for patients with an eating disorder due to the increased risk associated with the patient's metabolic imbalance and psychological profile.

Eating disorders are difficult to diagnose because of the secretive nature of the condition. To facilitate early diagnosis and treatment, dentists should be aware of the common associated oral findings (i.e., erosion, xerostomia, salivary gland enlargement, mucosal erythema, and cheilitis). Patients should be questioned directly when an eating disorder is suspected and an appropriate medical referral should be made. Eating disorders must be considered in the differential diagnosis of salivary gland hypofunction and hypertrophy.

Chronic Alcoholism

Chronic alcoholism is associated with salivary gland dysfunction and bilateral salivary gland enlargement, usually involving the parotid glands. The exact etiology is unclear, but the decreased salivary flow may be attributed to dehydration and poor nutrition.[289] Enlarged salivary glands in alcoholic patients demonstrate fatty tissue changes,[290] acinar hypertrophy and structural changes in the striated ducts,[291] and accumulation of secretory granules in the cytoplasm of acinar cells.[292] The enlargement of lumina within the ductal system could be the principal cause of glandular hypertrophy.[292]

Dehydration

Normal salivary output requires movement of water from the systemic circulation through acinar cells, into the salivary ductal system, and ultimately into the mouth. Dehydration has been demonstrated to result in diminished salivary output and increased symptoms of dry mouth.[293] Dehydration causes a greater and more prolonged period of salivary hypofunction in older adults compared with younger adults, probably due to an age-associated diminished secretory reserve capacity in older adults.[294] Patients should be questioned regarding their daily fluid intake, taking into account dehydrating liquids such as coffee and alcoholic beverages and the use of dehydrating medications such as diuretics. Requirements for daily water intake will vary based on an individual's body size, activity level, and additional factors. Reliance on thirst sensation alone to stimulate water intake may be inadequate. Patients can be counseled to take frequent sips of water throughout the day to prevent dehydration and concomitant xerostomia.

Medication-Induced Salivary Dysfunction

It is estimated that greater than 500 medications are associated with xerostomia.[295] Medication-induced salivary hypofunction is the most common cause of salivary disorders in the elderly.[296–299] In addition, the elderly are more likely to be engaged in polypharmacy, which further increases the likelihood of salivary hypofunction. When compared with younger adults, older healthy adults experience a more severe and longer duration of salivary hypofunction,[7] which may be due to a diminishment in secretory reserve capacity with aging.[300]

Due to insufficient clinical investigations, relatively few drugs have been shown definitively to reduce salivary function. Some drugs may not actually cause impaired salivary output but may produce alterations in saliva composition that lead to the perception of oral dryness. Table 10-4 summarizes the drug categories most commonly associated with salivary hypofunction. Medication-induced salivary hypofunction usually affects the unstimulated output, leaving stimulated function intact.

The pathogenesis of medication-induced salivary dysfunction differs with different classes of drugs. The anticholinergic drugs, the most common drug class associated with hyposalivation, inhibit acetylcholine binding to muscarinic receptors on salivary gland acinar cells preventing water movement through the ductal system and into the mouth. Other medications such as antihistamines and the alpha- and beta-blocker antihypertensives also inhibit neurotransmitter binding to the salivary gland acinar cells or perturb ion transport pathways resulting in changes in the quality and quantity of salivary secretion.[301]

TABLE 10-4	Common Drug Categories Associated With Salivary Hypofunction
Analgesics	
Anticholinergics	
Antidepressants	
Antihistamines	
Antihypertensives	
Antiparkinsonian	
Antipsychotics	
Antiseizure	
Cytotoxic agents	
Diuretics	
Muscle relaxants	
Sedatives and anxiolytics	

Ideally, prevention of medication-induced salivary dysfunction would be accomplished by discontinuation or substitution of the offending xerogenic drugs with a similar drug with little or no xerogenic potential. For example, serotonin-specific reuptake inhibitors have been reported to cause less dry mouth than tricyclic antidepressants.[302,303] Additional strategies to reduce xerostomia may require alteration in how the drug is administered. For example taking xerogenic drugs earlier during the day may diminish nocturnal xerostomia since salivary output is lowest at night.[295] Furthermore, if drug dosages can be divided, unwanted side effects from a large single dose can be minimized or avoided.

Polypharmacy is a common problem among the elderly. A critical review of a patient's medications is warranted not only to attempt to identify potential xerogenic drugs but also to determine whether the drug in question is still appropriate. Often, due to a lack of follow-up, the initial indication for the medication is no longer relevant but the patient may continue to take the medication. Where a patient has seen multiple health-care providers, there may be redundancy in their prescribed medications. Review of their current medications (both prescription and nonprescription) and medical history and coordination with a patient's primary care provider may help to eliminate drug-induced hyposalivation.

Drug-Induced Parotitis
Medication-Induced Salivary Dysfunction

Drug-induced parotitis, although rare, has been reported with numerous drugs but has only been definitively linked with a few. The most commonly associated medicines are iodine-containing drugs such as those used as imaging contrast media: hence the term "iodine mumps." Other drugs inducing parotitis are the antineoplastic drug L-asparaginase, clozapine, and phenylbutazone.[304] Most cases of drug-induced parotitis are bilateral due to the systemic distribution of the drug, but unilateral cases have been reported, which may be attributed to ductal obstruction.

With respect to the antipsychotic clozapine, there are two competing theories as to the pathogenesis of associated parotitis. One theory proposes that it is the immunomodulating properties of clozapine that sensitize mononuclear blood cells leading to a sialadenitis. The second hypothesis posits that clozapine-induced hypersialorrhea results in a chronic inflammatory state leading to parotid sialolithiasis and subsequent parotitis.[305] In the majority of cases, the condition resolves with discontinuation of the causative agent.

Parotid Lipomatosis

Parotid lipomatosis is the salivary gland manifestation of lipodystrophy syndrome associated with long-term HAART for HIV/AIDS. It has been associated with the antiviral medications indinavir, nelfinavir, amprenavir, ritonavir, and saquinavir. Parotid lipomatosis presents as painless, progressive enlargement of the parotid glands, which often becomes of cosmetic concern. MRI of a patient with parotid lipomatosis will show fatty replacement with no cystic change or masses. Histologically, it will be seen as an infiltration of the normal glandular parenchyma with benign-appearing adipocytes.[306] Case reports on treatment for parotid lipomatosis involve bilateral total superficial parotidectomy via a facelift approach, sparing the facial nerve.[306] Long-term follow-up is advised due to the likelihood of recurrence.

Immune Conditions
Sjögren's Syndrome (Primary and Secondary)

SS is a chronic autoimmune disease characterized by symptoms of oral and ocular dryness, exocrine dysfunction, lymphocytic infiltration, and destruction of exocrine glands.[14,307] The salivary and lacrimal glands are primarily affected, but SS can have wide-spread and diverse manifestations. Dryness may affect other mucosal areas such as the skin, nasopharynx, throat, trachea, and vagina. Signs of systemic autoimmune disease with musculoskeletal, pulmonary, gastric, hematologic, dermatologic, renal, and neurologic manifestations many also be evident in patients with SS.[308] SS patients frequently experience fatigue, arthralgias, myalgias, peripheral neuropathies, and rashes.

The definitive etiology of SS is unknown, and currently, there is no cure. Genetic studies have identified an association with HLA haplotypes and susceptibility genes in cytokine genes and genes involved in B-cell differentiation. Studies have suggested a hereditary link, and in fact, 35% of patients with SS have relatives with other autoimmune diseases.[308]

SS is classified as primary or secondary. Primary Sjögren's syndrome (pSS) occurs in the absence of another autoimmune disease, whereas secondary SS occurs in the setting of autoimmune diseases such as systemic lupus erythematosus, rheumatoid arthritis, and scleroderma. SS most commonly

affects perimenopausal and postmenopausal women; it is estimated that pSS affects 0.2%–3.0% of the population with a female-to-male ratio of 9:1. Younger individuals and children may also be affected. In addition, women with SS are at an increased risk of having offspring with congenital heart block, which is attributed to autoantibody-mediated damage of the atrioventricular node. Although the risk is slightly increased, estimated at approximately 2% in all infants born to women with anti-Ro/SSA antibodies and 3% in all infants born to women with anti-La/SSB, counseling for women with SS of childbearing age is necessary.[309]

Clinical Manifestations

Patients with SS experience the full spectrum of oral complications that result from decreased salivary function.[307] Virtually all patients complain of dry mouth and attendant difficulties in speaking, tasting, and swallowing and the need to sip liquids throughout the day. Xerostomia may first become evident with nocturnal awakening with thirst and the need to have chewing gum or lozenges to stimulate saliva production. Other subjective complaints include dysgeusia or hypogeusia, coughing episodes, and choking.

The mucosa may be painful and sensitive to spices and heat. Patients often have dry, cracked lips and angular cheilitis. Intraorally, the mucosa is pale and dry, friable, or furrowed; minimal salivary pooling is noted; and the saliva that is present tends to be thick and ropy. The tongue is often smooth (depapillated) and painful. Mucocutaneous candidal infections are common, particularly of the erythematous form. Due to the lack of lubricating saliva, traumatic or frictional injury is increased. Removable prostheses are less well tolerated due to a reduction in retention usually afforded by saliva.

Report of swollen salivary glands is common in the SS population. The American European Consensus Criteria for diagnosis of SS contains within its patient questionnaire a question as to whether the patient has had swollen salivary glands as an adult. A reported 20%–40% of patients with SS experienced enlarged salivary glands (Figure 10-17).[310] Bilateral parotid gland enlargement has been found in 25%–60% of all patients.[311] Parotid gland enlargement can be unilateral or bilateral, acute or chronic, and can be due to a retrograde salivary gland infection due to stasis or may be secondary to inflammation but may also represent a lymphoma as this population is at an increased risk.

An oral burning sensation, stomatitis, or glossodynia is a common complaint in SS patients and is most likely secondary to a fungal infection. However, it may be due to SS-associated neuropathies (see below). Alternate causes of oral burning sensation due to hematinic deficiencies, allergies, oral lesions, or burning mouth syndrome must be ruled out. The prevalence of peripheral nervous system involvement in SS has been estimated at 5%–20% and is most commonly reported as excruciating, burning pain of the extremities, or when the cranial nerves are involved, presents as a trigeminal neuropathy.

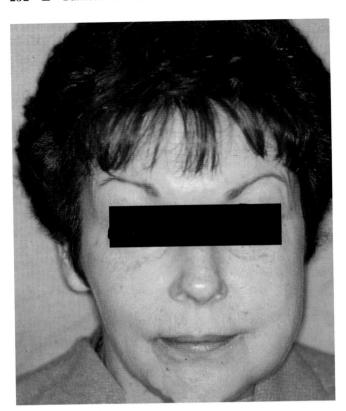

Figure 10-17 Chronic unilateral parotid salivary gland enlargement in a patient with Sjögren's syndrome.

Changes in volume and composition of saliva may lead to an increased caries index, which may alert a clinician to suspect SS. Patients with SS have a much lower pH and buffering capacity, which, coupled with the increased time for sugar clearance due to diminished salivary flow, leads to an increased rate of decay. Patients with SS also have higher levels of cariogenic and acidophilic bacteria such as *Lactobacillus acidophilus* and *Streptococcus mutans*. The decay pattern in patients with SS is distinctive: caries are usually seen to occur at tooth-restoration interfaces and locations that are usually more resistant to decay such as the root and facial surfaces and cusp tips.

Both primary and secondary SS patients usually have prominent serologic signs of autoimmunity, including hypergammaglobulinemia, autoantibodies, an elevated sedimentation rate, decreased white blood cells, hypocomplementemia, and monoclonal gammopathies.[14] Monoclonal gammopathy is predictive of a poor outcome in primary SS patients and should be routinely included in both the diagnostic and follow-up laboratory profiles. Monoclonal gammopathy was associated with a higher prevalence of parotid enlargement, extraglandular features, hypergammaglobulinemia, cryoglobulinemia and related markers (RF, hypocomplementemia), and with a poor prognosis (development of neoplasia and death).[312]

It has been established that primary SS patients are at an increased risk of developing a NHL, most commonly mucosa-associated B-cell lymphomas (MALT lymphomas) involving the salivary glands. However, the other NHL found in SS patients is the more aggressive diffuse large B-cell lymphoma (DLBCL) and some studies have found up to 10% of those with SS-MALT lymphomas transform into DLBCL. On average, 4.3% of patients develop NHL around 7.5 years after initial diagnosis. It has been estimated that primary SS patients have a 20- to 40-fold increased risk of lymphoma.[313,314]

Diagnosis

Currently, there is no single objective diagnostic gold standard for SS but rather classification criteria have been proposed. These criteria are dynamic and continue to evolve as understanding of the disease progresses. In 2002, the AECG criteria were published as a response to criticism regarding the European Study Group on Classification for SS, which were developed and validated between 1989 and 1996. The widespread acceptance of these AECG classification criteria in the research community has greatly aided standardization of diagnosis and definition of patients. The AECG classification criteria involve six criteria. Patients can meet classification criteria of pSS having met four of the six categories: ocular symptoms, oral symptoms, ocular signs, histopathology, salivary signs, and autoantibodies (anti-SSA [Ro] and anti-SSB [La]). Critically, either a positive labial MSGB or the presence of at least one of the auto antibodies is required to establish a definitive case. Alternatively, if three of the four objective criteria are satisfied (i.e., ocular signs, histopathology, salivary signs, and presence of autoantibodies), classification criteria are met. These criteria were found to have acceptably high sensitivity and specificity, are clinically practical, and greatly aid in evaluation of patients. Criticisms of the AECG criteria included the use of nonspecific, nonquantifiable subjective tests and led to the development of alternative classification criteria.

In 2012, the ACR proposed classification criteria, which employ three objective features. Patients with signs or symptoms suggestive of SS must have at least two of the following three objective features: (1) a positive anti-SSA or anti-SSB or a positive RF with ANA ≥1:320; (2) focal lymphocytic sialadenitis on a MSGB resulting in a Focus Score (FS) of ≥1 focus per 4 mm^2; and (3) keratoconjunctivitis sicca with ocular staining score of 3 or greater. These classification criteria also eliminated the distinction between primary and secondary SS. Exclusion criteria include a history of head and neck radiation therapy, hepatitis C infection, AIDS, sarcoidosis, amyloidosis, graft-versus-host-disease, and IgG4-related disease. These criteria are considered more stringent and may therefore have an effect on the reported prevalence of the disease.[315]

The labial MSGB is considered to be the best sole diagnostic criterion for the salivary component of SS (Figure 10-18A and Figure 10-18B).[80] A grading system exists for quantifying the salivary histologic changes seen in

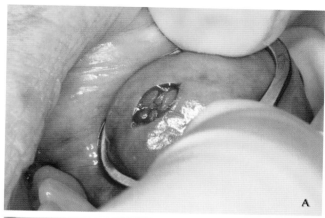

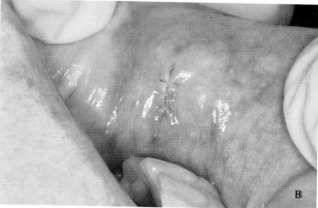

FIGURE 10-18 (A) Minor salivary gland biopsy of the lower labial mucosa. The minor salivary glands are readily accessible under the mucosal surface. (B) Primary closure after dissection and removal of the superficial minor salivary glands.

the minor glands,[316] as follows: (1) the numbers of infiltrating mononuclear cells are determined, with an aggregate of 50 or more cells being termed a focus; (2) the total number of foci and the surface area of the specimen are determined; and (3) the number of foci per 4 mm² is calculated. This constitutes the FS. The range is from 0 to 12, with 12 denoting confluent infiltrates. A FS of ≥1 is considered positive for salivary involvement consistent with SS. Acinar degeneration, with the relative preservation of ductal structures, is also noted (Figure 10-19).

Although parotid gland biopsy has been shown to be an alternative to the MSGB under the AECG's classification, currently it is not validated with respect to the ACR classification criteria. Histopathologically, in the affected parotid gland, epimyoepithelial islands with lymphoid stroma and LELs can be present, in addition to the characteristic lymphocytic infiltration. Histologic criteria for diagnosis of SS using a parotid gland biopsy requires one of the following two criteria: (1) a FS of greater than or equal to one per 4 mm² of glandular parotid tissue (including adipose tissue) regardless of the presence of benign LELs and/or (2) small lymphocytic infiltrates not fulfilling the criterion of a FS of greater than one, in combination with the presence of benign LELs. Sublingual salivary gland biopsy is also not validated with respect to classification criteria, and there are few reports of biopsy for diagnosis of SS. In addition, difficulty in access and postoperative complications, including damage to the Wharton's duct from suture placement, swelling, and bleeding at the floor of the mouth, make the sublingual gland biopsy for SS less desirable.[317]

Sialography remains the best performing diagnostic imaging technique with respect to SS with accuracy greater

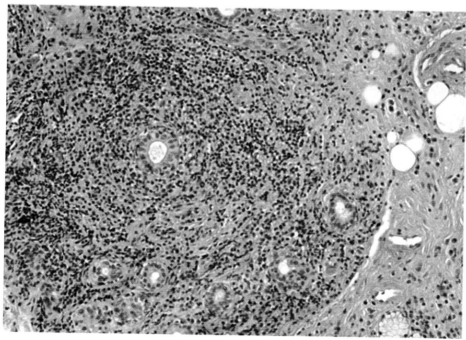

FIGURE 10-19 Histologic section of a biopsy of a labial minor salivary gland in a patient with Sjögren's syndrome. There is generalized chronic lymphocytic sialadenitis with fibrosis and atrophy of the gland parenchyma and cystic dilatation of ducts.

than that of MRI and US. Sialography shows characteristic changes (sialectasis) and may be useful in the evaluation of SS. MRI or CT can also be helpful, particularly in the assessment of enlarged glands and suspected lymphadenopathies. MRI is preferable to CT unless a stone is suspected or other calcified structure requires visualization, since MRI provides superior soft tissue resolution. Tc 99m radionuclide studies may also be used to determine salivary gland function. Scintigraphy, in spite of being an optional part of the American-European criteria, scored poorly when compared with sialography, MRI, and US.[318]

The presence of anti-SSA/Ro and anti-SSB/La antibodies is associated with a higher rate of extraglandular manifestations of SS and more active immunological status, when compared with seronegative SS cases. Anti-SSA/B-positive patients with SS can show severe hypergammaglobulinemia and cryoglobulinemia, and are at a higher risk of developing lymphoma. Circulating levels of anti-SSA/B do not correlate with disease activity but the IgA anti-SSA/Ro titer seems to be associated with the rate of lymphocyte glandular infiltration.[92]

Recent findings indicate that low vitamin D levels in patients with SS could be associated with severe complications such as lymphoma and peripheral neuropathy.[92] In addition, since patients with primary SS are at an increased risk of NHL and that there is some evidence that a low dietary intake of vitamin D is also associated with an increased risk of NHL, it has been proposed that evaluation of vitamin D levels and appropriate supplementation in SS patients be considered.[92]

The potential role of infectious agents in the development of autoimmune diseases has been the subject of much research. Several multicentre studies have found that in patients with SS, the prevalence and titres of antibodies against EBV early antigens were significantly higher than in a control group. In addition, a lower prevalence and titres of rubella and CMV antibodies (IgM) were detected in patients with SS compared to controls indicating that some infectious agents may provide a protective effect.[92] Further research is required to definitively elucidate the association between these infectious agents and autoimmune disease.

Lymphoma

Salivary gland lymphomas associated with SS are often indolent and progress very slowly necessitating close clinical monitoring of all patients. This involves periodic physical examination (including a thorough head and neck examination) and assessment of immunoglobulin levels. Suspicious clinical signs associated with NHL lymphoma in SS patients include unilateral or bilateral parotid gland enlargement, palpable purpura, splenomegaly, lymphadenopathy, leg ulcers secondary to vasculitis, mixed cryoglobulinemia, and low C4 level.[311] Chronic salivary gland enlargement or any lymphadenopathy in SS patients should be viewed with caution. Laboratory studies should determine whether a monoclonal gammopathy is present. Clinical suspicion

for lymphoma warrants a biopsy for further investigation. Incisional biopsy of extranodal tissue should be performed along with excisional lymph node biopsies if appropriate. Characterization of a lymphoma may be made using flow cytometry, fluorescence in situ hybridization and fluorescence-activated cell sorting analysis. Detection of lymphoma or monoclonal gammopathy requires prompt referral to an oncologist. Further characterization of the lymphoma may include evaluation of Waldeyer's ring, imaging of the neck, chest, abdomen and pelvis, and blood work including a complete blood count and chemistry panel.[311]

Treatment

Treatment for SS has advanced a great deal in the last decade.[319]

Currently, there is no single treatment that has proven to be effective in modifying the course of the disease. Therapeutic management of SS revolves around symptomatic treatment of glandular manifestations and on the use of disease-modifying drugs for systemic involvement.[92] Management of extraglandular manifestations must be tailored to the organ or system involved and may include the use of antimalarials, glucocorticoids, immunosuppressive drugs, and biologic agents. Comprehensive treatment of patients with SS requires a collaborative multidisciplinary approach involving referral to specialists to manage the glandular and extraglandular manifestations specific to the patient.

Here, we will focus primarily on the management of xerostomia and salivary gland hypofunction in SS patients. Management of salivary gland hypofunction in these patients is not dissimilar to those employed for other causes of secretory damage and revolves around the use of symptomatic therapies such as secretagogues, oral rinses and gels, mouthwashes, artificial saliva, and water sipping (see "Treatment of Xerostomia", pp. 41–44).[296,320] Symptomatic treatment not only has beneficial effects on oral dryness but can also prevent or lessen complications of sicca syndrome such as dental caries and oral candidiasis.

Secretagogues. Patients with remaining salivary function can stimulate salivary flow by the use of non pharmacologic secretagogues such as sugar-free gum or sugar-free candies. Parasympathomimetic secretagogues have shown the most success for xerostomia relief in SS patients with residual salivary gland function. There are two FDA-approved medications for the relief of dry mouth in SS: pilocarpine and cevimeline. Both medications are muscarinic agonists, which induce a transient increase in salivary output and statistically significant improvement in complaints of oral dryness.[321,323] Cevimeline has a reported increased specificity to M1 and M3 muscarinic receptors as compared with pilocarpine, which might result in a lowered potential for side effects,[324,325] but a lesser side-effect level has not been seen in clinical trials.

Common side effects of these medications include sweating, flushing, urinary urgency, nausea, and gastrointestinal discomfort. Although these side effects are frequent, they are rarely severe or serious, but they may be significant enough to be intolerable to patients. Parasympathomimetics are contraindicated in patients with uncontrolled asthma, narrow-angle glaucoma, or acute iritis and should be used with caution in patients with significant cardiovascular disease, Parkinson's disease, asthma, or chronic obstructive pulmonary disease. Currently, pilocarpine is recommended at a dosage of 5 mg up to four times daily, and cevimeline is commonly prescribed at 30 mg three times daily. Pilocarpine has also been approved for treatment of xerostomia related to head and neck radiotherapy.[326,327]

In two large RCTs, pilocarpine at 5 mg and 7.5 mg every six hours resulted in improved oral, ocular, nasal, vaginal and skin dryness, and salivary flow rates.[328] In a dose-adjustment-RCT, pilocarpine at the currently recommended dosage of 5 mg up to four times daily resulted in similar efficacy with more tolerable side effects.[328]

Salivary Substitutes. Saliva substitutes are thought to have a positive effect on nocturnal oral dryness without appreciable side effects. However, clinical trial data have not shown a significant difference in efficacy between some salivary substitutes and a placebo although some RCTs show improvement in several oral symptoms but not salivary flow rates. Although there is no reported superiority in preparations with mucin versus carboxymethylcellulose-containing substitutes, mucin-containing agents tend to be preferred by patients. Data from uncontrolled studies have shown considerable improvement in xerostomia and salivary flow with the use of a hydroxymethylcellulose-containing oral spray.[328] Agents incorporating salivary substitutes may be found in a range of products including lubricating gels, mouthwashes, lozenges, toothpastes, and oral sprays.[92]

Disease-Modifying Drugs

In SS, there have been substantial efforts to improve salivary function and oral symptoms with systemic therapies directed at the underlying disease process. Therapeutic strategies include hormone modulation, general and targeted anti-inflammatory approaches, blunting of the B-cell response, and treatment of potential viral etiologies.

Numerous clinical trials have been conducted evaluating systemic agents to treat the underlying exocrinopathy through manipulation of the immune system. However, these remain experimental, and most available treatment modalities are primarily symptomatic.

Corticosteroids. The frequent use of glucocorticoids for the treatment of primary SS is not supported by reliable scientific data. Although corticosteroids at high doses downregulate the immune inflammatory process within the salivary and lacrimal glands, data showing that they increase salivary and lacrimal flow rates are lacking. Corticosteroid use in patients

with SS is employed primarily in those with extraglandular manifestations or in those with parotid swelling.[92]

Antimalarial Agents. Antimalarial agents have been shown to reduce sicca and constitutional symptoms such as fatigue and arthromyalgia. In addition, hydroxychloroquine has been reported to increase salivary flow rate and reduce some inflammatory indices such as ESR and C-reactive protein, and result in an improved immunologic profile involving RF, anti-SSA, and anti-SSB. Owing to its antineoplastic properties, hydroxychloroquine also has the potential to reduce the risk of lymphoma development in those with SS.[92]

Immunosuppressant Agents. Immunosuppressant agents such as cyclosporine A, azathioprine, methotrexate, mycophenolic acid, and leflunomide are used for some extraglandular manifestations of SS; however, there is currently insufficient evidence to show efficacy. There are reports showing improvement in sicca symptoms with the use of cyclosporine A, methotrexate, and mycophenolic acid, but there were no improvements in objective tests. This class of drugs is also associated with a significant rate of adverse events (41%–100%).[328]

Biologic Agents. Although no biologic agents are currently approved for use in SS, there have been a number of clinical trials involving agents such as tumor necrosis factor (TNF) alpha antagonists (e.g., etanercept and infliximab) and interferon-α. In addition, recently, there has been much research related to direct B-cell-targeted therapies such anti-CD20 (e.g., rituximab) and anti-CD22 monoclonal antibodies (mAbs). Newer targets proposed involve major cytokines of B-cell homeostasis (e.g., B-cell-activating factor [BAFF], interleukin [IL]-6, and lymphotoxin-b).

Anti-TNF Alpha Antagonists. Despite several open-label studies in which anti-TNF alpha agents were shown to improve glandular and extraglandular manifestations, two RCTs failed to demonstrate the superiority of infliximab and etanercept over placebo.[329,330]

Since then, no further studies with the use of these agents have been carried out.

Interferon-α. Some controlled studies involving patients with SS evaluating the use of 150 IU of oral IFN-α three times per day reported an improvement in sicca symptoms, salivary flow, and lymphocytic infiltration, while others showed only an improvement in unstimulated salivary flow and an increase in adverse gastrointestinal events when compared with a placebo. A small uncontrolled comparative study showed increased tear and saliva production in those treated with 3.1 million units of oral IFN-α three times per week in comparison to those receiving 6 mg per kg of hydroxychloroquine daily.[328] Further trials will be necessary to determine the efficacy of this agent in SS.

Direct B-Cell-Targeted Therapy

Anti-CD20 Monoclonal Antibodies. Since the pathogenesis of SS is believed to be related to B-cell activity, recent focus has been on several B-cell-targeting therapies such as the anti-CD20 mAb rituximab. Several recent open-label studies suggest an efficacy of rituximab on improving sicca symptoms and extraglandular manifestations.[55] Rituximab was also associated with significant improvement in fatigue and joint pain and an overall improvement in quality of life. The recent "Tolerance and Efficacy of rituximab in primary Sjögren's syndrome" (TEARS) study, a multicenter, randomized, double-blind placebo-controlled trial, evaluating the efficacy of rituximab in 122 patients showed a moderate improvement in subjective and objective signs.[55] Additional smaller studies have shown treatment with rituximab to be relatively safe and effective. Adverse events reported with rituximab include severe infusion reaction, cardiac arrest, and infection. Controlled clinical trials are necessary to validate the use of rituximab in SS patients with systemic involvement.

Anti-CD22 Monoclonal Antibodies. Epratuzumab is a humanized anti-CD22 mAb that has been used recently in a small open-label study in which response was defined as improvement by at least 20% in at least two out of the following five items: Schirmer's test, unstimulated whole salivary flow, fatigue, ESR, and IgG level. The reported responder rate was 53% at 6 weeks and 67% at 32 weeks indicating that this mAb could be a future treatment for SS depending on results of randomized placebo-controlled trials.

Indirect B-Cell-Targeted Therapies

Abnormal cytokine production in pSS has also been the target of several investigations most notably the cytokines BAFF and a proliferation-inducing ligand (APRIL), both members of the TNF ligand family. Belimumab, a mAb targeting soluble BAFF, has been utilized in two phase II multicenter, open-label studies (Efficacy and Safety of Belimumab in Subjects with Primary Sjögren's syndrome [BELISS]) involving patients with pSS. Although there was no significant effect on salivary flow and Schirmer's test scores, systemic activity measured by the the EULAR ESSDAI was significantly decreased,[331] which may prompt further research into this treatment modality.

Chronic Graft-Versus-Host Disease

cGVHD is a complex clinical entity that occurs following bone marrow transplantation. Dysfunction of the major salivary glands with hyposalivation and xerostomia are some of the more common manifestations of cGVHD. This is due to the infiltration of autoreactive T lymphocytes into the salivary glands. Salivary gland involvement in cGVHD tends to develop rapidly and be very severe, while recovery often does not occur until at least one year following transplantation. Changes in both saliva composition and quantity have been observed.

The histopathologic changes seen in cGVHD resemble those seen in SS: lymphocytic infiltration of minor salivary glands, parenchymal destruction, and fibrosis. In general, cGVHD treatment consists of the use of immunosuppressive agents such as methylprednisolone and cyclosporine. Treatment of hyposalivation and xerostomia in patients with cGVHD with pilocarpine has been reported as successful.[332]

Granulomatous Conditions

Tuberculosis

Tuberculosis (TB) is a bacterial infection, caused by *M. tuberculosis*, leading to the formation of caseating granulomas in the infected tissues. The lungs are most commonly affected, but other tissues, including the salivary glands, may be involved.[333–335] TB is more commonly confined to the intraglandular and periglandular lymph nodes; involvement of the salivary gland parenchyma is rare and usually represents spread from the adjacent lymph nodes.[336]

TB of the major salivary glands may have a varied clinical appearance. Most commonly, it presents as a slow-growing, firm mass with a variable degree of fixation and is typically unilateral. Diffuse glandular enlargement and acute sialadenitis may also be seen if there is parenchymal involvement. It may alternatively present as a peri-auricular fistula or abscess.[337] Patients with TB of the salivary glands may experience xerostomia and/or salivary gland swelling, with granuloma or cyst formation within the affected glands.[336] Salivary gland enlargement usually presents as part of a characteristic symptom complex; however, salivary gland changes have been reported in the absence of systemic symptoms.

Salivary gland TB may present a diagnostic challenge in the absence of additional signs and symptoms of TB. In addition, the clinical appearance is indistinguishable from that of some salivary gland neoplasms. Imaging and FNAC are often inconclusive, and therefore, sialadenectomy may be required for definitive diagnosis. Where TB of the salivary gland is suspected, diagnosis is made by means of the patient's history, physical examination, radiographic images, microbiologic tests, molecular biologic assays, and histological evaluations such as FNAC or biopsy.[334] Definitive diagnosis of TB requires the isolation and identification of mycobacteria from a diagnostic specimen.[338]

PCR when applied to FNAC specimens can enhance specificity and sensitivity. Using PCR-based salivary assays, evidence of *M. tuberculosis* was found in 98% of infected patients, a detection rate significantly better than culture (17%), suggesting that in the future, salivary tests may be helpful for the diagnosis of TB.[339]

Treatment of salivary gland TB requires standard multidrug chemotherapy using a combination of antibiotics including isoniazid, rifampicin, pyrazinamide, and ethambutol. Additional chemotherapy and salivary gland surgery occasionally may be required to treat persistent salivary gland disease.[340,341]

Sarcoidosis

Sarcoidosis is a chronic condition of unknown etiology in which T lymphocytes, mononuclear phagocytes, and granulomas cause destruction of affected tissue. Of the major salivary glands, parotid gland involvement occurs most frequently and has been reported in approximately 6% of patients with sarcoidosis.[342] Involvement of the minor salivary glands in patients with sarcoidosis has been reported to range from 19% to 58% and may help differentiate sarcoidosis from SS.[343]

Salivary gland involvement with sarcoidosis may present with glandular swelling and xerostomia. The diagnosis of sarcoidosis is made by the presence of supporting clinical features with the presence of noncaseating granulomas in the biopsy specimen. Serum angiotensin 1–converting enzyme (ACE) levels may be increased in cases of active sarcoidosis.[343] Treatment of sarcoidosis may range from observation to the use of systemic corticosteroids and steroid-sparing agents. Infliximab, a mAb targeted against TNF alpha has been found to be helpful in refractory sarcoidosis. Salivary gland involvement of sarcoidosis is usually responsive to systemic treatment but surgical excision of granulomatous tissue may be required. Sarcoidosis-associated xerostomia may be treated symptomatically.[343]

Heerfordt's syndrome (uveoparotid fever) is a form of sarcoid that can occur in the presence or absence of systemic sarcoidosis. The syndrome is defined by the triad of parotid swelling, inflammation of the uveal tract of the eye, and facial nerve palsy.[247] Sarcoidosis can also occur in conjunction with SS or could mimic SS.[344] The typical clinical presentation is of bilateral, painless, and firm salivary gland enlargement with diminished salivary output from affected glands,[344] but unilateral salivary gland enlargement has been reported. Examination of a MSGB specimen and serum laboratory assays including calcium level, autoimmune serologies, and ACE concentration can confirm or refute the diagnosis of sarcoidosis.[345]

Crohn's Disease

Crohn's disease is an inflammatory condition of the gastrointestinal tract, which can present with oral signs that may precede any intestinal manifestations. Apart from the more commonly known serpiginous lesions of pyostomatitis vegetans, there are reports of Crohn's disease presenting as multiple submucosal nodules arising in minor salivary glands of the oral cavity.[208,346] Histopathologically, these nodules were composed of noncaseating granulomas within the walls of the minor salivary gland ducts. Additional findings in the minor salivary glands of patient's with Crohn's disease are foci of lymphocytes within the stromal connective tissue

and signs of acinar atrophy and ductal hyperplasia.[347] Often both the oral lesions and gastrointestinal symptoms of Crohn's disease resolve after appropriate therapy typically involving anti-inflammatory drugs such as steroids.

Granulomatosis With Polyangiitis

GPA, formerly known as Wegener's granulomatosis, is a systemic disease characterized by necrotizing granulomas involving the upper and/or lower respiratory tract, with small vessel vasculitis and focal glomerulonephritis. The head and neck are involved in nearly 90% of cases; most commonly affected areas are the nose, eyes, ears, and mouth. Although salivary gland involvement is a rare presenting clinical feature of GPA, involvement of the major salivary glands may be the initial manifestation allowing for prompt treatment, which may prevent irreversible organ damage.

Of the major salivary glands, GPA usually affects the parotid and submandibular glands. Glandular swelling is present, with or without pain, and there may be facial nerve weakness. A cutaneous fistula overlying the parotid gland has been reported in many cases. Depending on the extent of disease, the patient may additionally present with rhinitis, severe rhinorrhea, epistaxis, sinusitis, a saddle nose deformity, nonspecific oral ulcerations, and hyperplastic gingival lesions with petechial hemorrhages known as "strawberry gingivitis." Related constitutional symptoms include fever, migratory arthralgias, malaise, anorexia, and weight loss; where there is lung involvement, hoarseness, cough, and dyspnea may be present.

Diagnosis is made using a combination of clinical, laboratory, and histopathologic analyses. An open biopsy is indicated if FNAB is nondiagnostic. Cytoplasmic antineutrophil cytoplasmic antibodies (c-ANCA) levels are highly specific but have variable sensitivity dependent on the activity of the disease; the results may be negative in 15%–33% of patients, especially where there is renal involvement.[348]

Effective treatment of GPA can result in the resolution of the salivary gland manifestations of the disease without surgical intervention and healing of both the organ and the tissue manifestations. Treatment includes the use of cyclophosphamide and prednisone with or without the addition of cyclosporine.

Sialorrhea
Description and Etiology

Sialorrhea (hypersalivation or ptyalism) is defined as an excessive production of saliva[349] and is the result of either an increase in saliva production or decrease in salivary clearance.[350,351] Sialorrhea can lead to drooling, which is defined as excess saliva beyond the lip margin. Hypersalivation can be associated with certain medications (Table 10-5),[352] hyperhydration, infant teething, the secretory phase of menstruation, idiopathic paroxysmal hypersalivation, heavy metal poisoning, organophosphorus (acetylcholinesterase) poisoning, nausea, gastroesophageal reflux disease, obstructive

TABLE 10-5	Medications and Conditions That Cause Hypersalivation and Drooling
Medications	
Pilocarpine	
Cevimeline	
Lithium	
Bethanechol	
Physostigmine	
Clozapine	
Risperidone	
Nitrazepam	
Neurologic diseases	
Parkinson's disease	
Wilson's disease	
Amyotrophic lateral sclerosis	
Down syndrome	
Fragile X syndrome	
Autism	
Cerebral palsy	
Heavy metals	
Iron	
Lead	
Arsenic	
Mercury	
Thallium	

esophagitis, neurologic changes such as in a cerebral vascular accident (CVA), neuromuscular diseases, neurologic diseases, and central neurologic infections.[353] Minor hypersalivation may result from local irritations, such as aphthous ulcers or an ill-fitting oral prosthesis.

Clinical Presentation

Hypersalivation can cause drooling, which can produce social embarrassment and a severe impairment in the quality of a person's life.[354] In severe cases, a partial or total blockage of the airway can occur, producing aspiration of oral contents and possibly aspiration pneumonia. Hypersalivation can also lead to perioral irritations, malodor, and traumatic ulcerations that can become secondarily infected by fungal or bacterial organisms.

Diagnosis

Since there are a multitude of etiologic causes of hypersalivation, it is essential to obtain the exact history of the hypersalivation as well as a thorough and complete medical history. A systematic oral evaluation should be performed, focusing on salivary gland enlargements, oral ulcerations, head/neck/oral masses, neuromuscular function, and condition of removable intraoral prostheses. Since most cases of hypersalivation are related to secretion clearance, a swallowing study should be obtained from a clinician with expertise in speech and swallowing. If it becomes evident that secretion clearance is within normal limits, a salivary flow rate should be obtained. The normal rate of unstimulated salivary output from all glands is approximately 2.0–3.5 mL in five minutes.[21] Collection of unstimulated WS using a drooling technique into a pre weighed container that results in more than 5.0 mL in five minutes suggests greater than normal production of saliva and can help determine whether there is an overproduction of saliva rather than problem of salivary clearance. Blood samples should also be obtained and evaluated for heavy metals (see Table 10-5) and organophosphate pesticides. Premenopausal women should be evaluated for potential pregnancy, and in postmenopausal or male patients, androgen levels should be determined to rule out an androgen-excreting tumor. If the onset is acute, a CT scan of the brain should be obtained to rule out a CVA or a central nervous system mass.

Treatment

Treatment for hypersalivation should take into consideration the etiology of the hypersalivation, the risks and benefits of treatment, and, most importantly, the effect on patient quality of life.[355] Depending on the etiology, there are several categories of treatments for hypersalivation: physical therapy, medications, surgery, and rarely, radiation therapy. Additional strategies may involve changes in diet or medications, oral habits, or behavior modification. The management of drooling may require a multidisciplinary approach incorporating speech and language therapists, physiotherapists, or occupational therapists, for example.

Physical therapy can be used to improve neuromuscular control, but patient cooperation is essential. Speech and swallowing therapy should be attempted prior to medical or surgical interventions. Oral-motor exercises and intraoral devices such as palatal training devices have been used. Unfortunately, studies have shown a low success rate with these therapeutic modalities.

Drug-based treatments for hypersalivation are devised based on etiology. If the patient is experiencing hypersalivation secondary to a pharmaceutical treatment, alternate medications should be evaluated, and if the therapeutic regimen cannot be altered, compatible xerogenic agents (glycopyrrolate, scopolamine, benztropine, amitriptyline, atropine, tropicamide, and diphenhydramine hydrochloride) should be considered.[354] These anticholinergic agents downregulate acetylcholine resulting in decreased saliva secretion via the parasympathetic nervous system. However, they have side effects that may make them intolerable in elderly patients. A glycopyrrolate oral solution has been approved in the United States for drooling in children with neurologic conditions. Intraoral tropicamide films are also available, which provide short-term relief of sialorrhea.

One randomized, double-blind, placebo-controlled, crossover study reported that amisulpride (400 mg/d uptitrated from 100 mg/d over one week) produced significant improvements in a hypersalivation rating scale.[356]

Consultations should be made with the patient's physician to prevent deleterious drug–drug interactions or side effects. Hypersalivation that occurs secondary to chronic nausea (e.g., during chemotherapy) can be treated with antiemetic medications. Hypersalivation due to gastroesophageal reflux disorder (GERD) is a protective buffering response to acids encountered in the oral cavity. Under most circumstances, when GERD is appropriately addressed, hypersalivation resolves. Neurologic and neuromuscular conditions (e.g., CVA, Down syndrome, central neurologic infections) can result in neuromuscular incompetence in swallowing function, resulting in salivary pooling in the anterior floor of the mouth and salivary spillage from the oral cavity (drooling). A trial of xerogenic medications (see above) can be considered for these conditions.

Based on a number of open-label, retrospective studies, case studies, and controlled clinical trials, botulinum toxin (BoNT) has been reported to be effective in the treatment of sialorrhea.[357] Currently, three type A and one type B toxins are approved for use in the United States. There is strong evidence that both A and B types of BoNT are effective treatments of sialorrhea, produce similar effects, and have a low incidence of side effects.[357]

BoNT works by reversibly blocking the presynaptic release of acetylcholine and other neurotransmitters at the neuroglandular junction. Recently, BoNT-A injections have been used to treat sialorrhea in adults with Parkinson's disease, head and neck cancer, stroke, and neurodegenerative disease. BoNT-A has also been effective for sialorrhea in children with cerebral palsy or other neurologic disease.[192]

The therapeutic effects of BoNT-A when injected into the salivary glands have been reported to last for six to nine months.[192] Since they are the greatest contributors to saliva volume, the submandibular and parotid glands are the most commonly injected sites. Injection into these glands can be performed using either anatomical landmarks or under ultrasound guidance. Currently, there is no consensus as to the dosage or injection technique for the use of BoNT-A for sialorrhea. The most commonly reported side effect is a transient dysphagia, which typically resolves in two weeks. This side effect must be taken into consideration in patients with sialorrhea already experiencing dysphagia due to their condition (e.g., in ALS). Other reported side effects include increased saliva thickness, xerostomia, pain at the site of injection, facial nerve paralysis, and pneumonia. Some limitations to BoNT injection include cost, necessity for retreatment, and possible need for sedation in the pediatric population.

There are a multitude of surgical techniques that have been devised to treat hypersalivation, particularly in patients with poor or deficient neuromuscular function; however, there are no recent studies on surgical management in adults. In general, surgical intervention is reserved for the most severe cases of sialorrhea. Surgical interventions include salivary gland excision, denervation of the salivary gland, and transposition or ligation of the salivary ducts.[358] Historically, redirection of the submandibular ducts and parotid ducts posteriorly to the tonsillar pillars has been performed with good success, although patients with poor salivary clearance will not benefit from this technique.[359–361]

Bilateral tympanic neurectomy has also been performed, but this leaves a permanent anesthesia affecting the anterior portion of the tongue and is therefore not recommended. Other techniques involve redirection of submandibular glands and excision of sublingual glands[362] or ductal ligation of all major submandibular/sublingual ducts.[363] These techniques are successful in reduction of drooling approximately 80% of the time, with occasional postoperative complications such as ranula formation, pain, and numbness.[360] The advantage of the duct ligation technique is that it involves an intraoral surgical approach, thereby reducing the risk of damaging the facial nerve. A final strategy is excision of one or more major salivary glands. Although this does provide a permanent cure for hypersalivation, it subsequently produces salivary hypofunction and severe xerostomia. All surgical procedures involving the salivary glands involve risk factors such as xerostomia, ductal stenosis, postoperative cyst development, salivary fistulae, infection, and wound dehiscence.[364]

Radiation therapy is only very rarely used for this indication and is typically reserved for elderly patients who are not candidates for surgery or other medical therapies.[365] Side effects include xerostomia, pain, and increased salivary viscosity. Due to the risk of development of radiotherapy-associated neoplasia and other complications, radiation is not a routine treatment option.

MANAGEMENT OF XEROSTOMIA

Treatments available for the dry mouth patient may be divided into five main categories: (1) preventive therapy, (2) symptomatic (palliative) treatment, (3) local or topical salivary stimulation, (4) systemic salivary stimulation, and (5) therapy directed at an underlying systemic disorder. Based on the current literature and best clinical practice, the overall management strategy for xerostomia and salivary gland hypofunction should include a combination of supplemental fluoride, topical palliative agents, and a secretogogue.[16,296,319,366–369] Management approaches are summarized in Table 10-6.

Preventive Therapy

The use of topical fluorides in a patient with salivary gland hypofunction is critical to control dental caries. There are many different fluoride therapies available, from low-concentration over-the-counter fluoride rinses to more potent, highly concentrated prescription fluorides (e.g., 1.1% sodium fluoride) that are applied by brush or in a custom carrier. Oral health care practitioners may also apply fluoride varnishes. The dosage, method, and frequency of application (from daily to once per week) should be determined based on the severity of the salivary dysfunction, the patient's ability to perform oral care at home and the rate of caries development.[370]

It is essential that patients maintain meticulous oral hygiene. Patients with xerostomia require frequent dental

TABLE 10-6   Management of Xerostomia

Management Approach	Examples
Preventive therapies	Supplemental fluoride; remineralizing solutions; optimal oral hygiene; non cariogenic diet
Symptomatic (palliative) treatments	Water; oral rinses, gels, mouthwashes; increased humidification; minimize caffeine and alcohol
Local or topical salivary stimulation	Sugar-free gums and mints
Systemic salivary stimulation	Parasympathomimetic secretagogues: cevimeline and pilocarpine
Treatment of underlyingsystemic disorders	Anti-inflammatory therapies to treat the autoimmune exocrinopathy of Sjögren's syndrome

visits (usually every 3–4 months) and must work closely with their dentist to maintain optimal oral health.[371] Patients should be counseled as to diet, avoiding cariogenic, acidic and dehydrating foods, and beverages. Chronic use of alcohol and caffeine can increase oral dryness and should be minimized. In the absence of the remineralizing properties of saliva, tooth demineralization is unchecked, speeding the loss of tooth structure. Remineralizing solutions may be used to alleviate some of the effects of the loss of normal salivation.[372]

Patients with dry mouth may also experience an increase in oral infections, particularly mucosal candidiasis.[296,373] This often takes an erythematous form (without the easily recognized pseudomembranous plaques), and the patient may present with redness of the mucosa and complaints of a burning sensation of the tongue or other intraoral soft tissues. A high index of suspicion should be maintained, and appropriate antifungal therapies should be instituted as necessary (see Chapter 3, "Pharmacotherapy for Orofacial Infections"). Patients with salivary gland dysfunction may require prolonged treatment periods and periodic retreatment to eradicate oral fungal infections.[307]

Symptomatic Treatment

Several symptomatic treatments are available. Water is by far the most important. Patients should be encouraged to sip water throughout the day to help moisten the oral cavity, hydrate the mucosa, and clear debris from the mouth. The use of water with meals can make chewing and forming the food bolus easier, ease swallowing, and may improve taste perception. Use of sugar-free carbonated drinks is not recommended as the acidic content of many of these beverages is high and may promote tooth demineralization. As a function of normal diurnal variation, salivary flow drops almost to zero at rest, and in individuals with secretory hypofunction, desiccation of the mucosa is particularly troublesome. This may result in frequent awakening at night, which may prevent restorative sleep. The use of room humidifiers, particularly at night, may lessen discomfort markedly.

There are a number of oral rinses, mouthwashes, and gels available for dry mouth patients.[372] Patients should be cautioned to avoid products containing alcohol, sugar, or strong flavorings that may irritate sensitive, dry mucosa. Moisturizing and lubricating products may provide additional comfort and help prevent friction-associated lesions

and a burning sensation. The frequent use of products containing aloe vera or vitamin E should be encouraged. Manifestations of angular cheilitis, usually seen as persistent cracking and erythema at the corners of the mouth, should be investigated for a fungal and/or bacterial cause and treated accordingly.

There are many commercially available salivary substitutes, usually in the form of an aerosol or a liquid. These are typically composed of a mix of buffering agents, cellulose derivatives (to promote adherence to the mucosa and to provide moisture), and flavoring agents. However, in general, saliva replacements ("artificial salivas") are not well tolerated by most patients. Saliva substitutes are quickly swallowed, providing only temporary relief and therefore require frequent application. Although there is a role for the use of saliva replacements, particularly in individuals who have no residual salivary gland function, it must be recognized that this is not a highly effective symptomatic therapy.[374]

Salivary Stimulation
Local or Topical Stimulation

Several approaches are available for stimulating salivary flow. Chewing will stimulate salivary flow effectively, as will sour and sweet tastes. The combination of chewing and taste, as provided by gums or mints, can be very effective in relieving symptoms for patients who have remaining salivary gland function. However, patients with dry mouth must be told not to use products that contain sugar as a sweetener due to the increased risk of dental caries.

Neuroelectrostimulating devices have been developed recently as a means of stimulating residual functioning salivary gland tissue. Extraoral use of a transcutaneous electric nerve stimulation (TENS) unit over the parotid gland was reported to increase saliva production in healthy individuals and patients with radiation-induced xerostomia.[375] More recently, implantable devices in the form of an oral osteointegrated implant with an embedded wetness sensor have been developed. These devices are designed to monitor oral dryness and provide an automatic or patient-controlled stimulus to the adjacent tissue resulting in salivation.[376] Although these devices hold some promise for treatment of hyposalivation, further research, development, and clinical trials are necessary.

Acupuncture, with application of needles in the perioral and other regions, has been proposed as a therapy for salivary gland hypofunction and xerostomia. A recent Cochrane review reported that there is some low-quality evidence that acupuncture results in a small increase in saliva production in patients with dry mouth following radiotherapy. Reported adverse effects of acupuncture are mild and of short duration, and there were no reported adverse effects from electrostimulation.[377]

Systemic Stimulation

The use of systemic secretagogues for salivary stimulation has long been examined, with the earliest reports dating from the late 1800s. More than 24 agents have been proposed as means of stimulating salivary output systemically. Of these, four have been examined extensively in controlled clinical trials; these are bromhexine, anetholetrithione, pilocarpine HCl, and cevimeline HCl. Only pilocarpine and cevimeline are currently in wide-spread use.

Bromhexine is a mucolytic agent used in Europe and the Middle East but not available in the United States. The proposed mechanism of action for salivary stimulation is unknown. No proven benefit to salivary function has been shown in controlled clinical trials. Bromhexine may stimulate lacrimal function in patients with SS, although this is controversial.[378,379]

Anetholetrithione is a mucolytic agent that has been shown in clinical trials to increase salivary output with mild adverse effects. The mechanism of action is not known definitively, but it has been suggested that anetholetrithione may upregulate muscarinic receptors. In patients with mild salivary gland hypofunction, anetholetrithione significantly increased saliva flow.[380] However, it was ineffective in patients with marked salivary gland hypofunction.[381] One study suggested a possible synergistic effect of anetholetrithione in combination with pilocarpine.[382] This agent is unavailable in the United States.

Pilocarpine HCl is an FDA-approved drug specifically for the relief of xerostomia following radiotherapy for head and neck cancers and for those with SS.[323,326,327] It is a parasympathomimetic drug, functioning as a muscarinic cholinergic agonist, which increases salivary output and stimulates remaining gland function. Adverse effects of pilocarpine in human studies are commonly reported, are generally mild, and are consistent with the known mechanism of action of the drug. Sweating is the most common side effect. Other frequently reported side effects include hot flashes, urinary frequency, diarrhea, and blurred vision.

Following administration of pilocarpine, salivary output increases fairly rapidly, usually reaching a maximum within one hour. The best-tolerated doses are those of 5.0–7.5 mg, given three or four times daily.[383] The duration of action is approximately two to three hours. Pilocarpine is contraindicated for patients with pulmonary disease, uncontrolled asthma, cardiovascular disease, and narrow angle glaucoma. Tolerance to pilocarpine does not appear to occur even with prolonged use. Pilocarpine has been shown to be a safe and effective therapy for patients with diminished salivation but with some remaining secretory function.

Cevimeline HCl is another FDA-approved parasympathomimetic agonist indicated for the treatment of symptoms of oral dryness in SS patients.[321,322] Cevimeline is prescribed at 30 mg three times daily. This medication reportedly selectively targets the M1 and M3 muscarinic receptors of the salivary and lacrimal glands.[324,325] Despite this reported increased selectivity, its side effect profile is similar to that of pilocarpine. It is contraindicated in patients with asthma and glaucoma and must be used with caution in patients with a history of cardiovascular, respiratory, or gallbladder disease and in patients who use certain medications. The duration of secretagogue activity is longer than pilocarpine (3–4 hours), but the onset is somewhat slower. Clinical trials have indicated that cevimeline is well tolerated in patients with xerostomia following radiation therapy for head and neck cancer.[384]

Pilocarpine HCl and cevimeline HCl are the only systemic sialagogues that are available in the United States. Both are effective at transiently relieving symptoms of oral dryness and increasing salivary output. Consultation with the patient's physician prior to prescribing these drugs for patients with significant medical conditions may be indicated, although they have a good safety record in many years of use. Increased understanding of the causes of xerostomia and salivary gland dysfunction undoubtedly will lead to improvement in the available treatments through the design and testing of more specific therapies with alternate mechanisms of action.

Stem Cell Therapy

The majority of therapies for salivary gland hypofunction provide transient relief of symptoms and often do not address the underlying lack of functioning salivary gland tissue. Recent research has focused on the use of stem cell replacement therapy for the treatment of radiation-induced hyposalivation. It has been determined that within the ducts of salivary glands reside cells capable of proliferation and differentiation known as a stem/progenitor cell population. Application of specific growth factors to these cells induces differentiation into functional units. Theoretically, prior to radiation therapy, these progenitor cells could be harvested and cultured in vitro and transplanted following radiation therapy to provide additional functional salivary gland tissue. Although many hurdles are faced in the development of therapies such as these, researchers are optimistic given the current use of adult stem cells in bone marrow transplantation.[385]

Treatment of Underlying Systemic Disorders

Most clinical work has been done in SS, and therapeutic trials are discussed in detail in the section on treatment of SS. Also, therapies used during head and neck radiotherapy to minimize salivary gland dysfunction are detailed in the section on management of radiation-induced salivary disease.

SALIVARY GLAND TUMORS

There are nearly 40 different entities of major and minor salivary gland tumors, ranging from benign to aggressively malignant.[386–389] The majority of salivary gland tumors (about 80%) arise in the parotid glands.[390,392] The submandibular glands account for 10%–15% of tumors, and the remaining tumors develop in the sublingual or minor salivary glands. Approximately 80% of parotid gland tumors and approximately half of submandibular gland and minor salivary gland tumors are benign. In contrast, more than 60% of tumors in the sublingual gland are malignant. For minor salivary glands, pleomorphic adenoma is the most common benign tumor, and mucoepidermoid carcinoma is the most common malignant tumor.[393]

The risk of malignancy for all salivary tumors increases as the size of the tumor increases, which supports the importance of early detection.[389,394] Over 85% of salivary gland tumors occur in adults. Salivary tumors in children are most often located in the parotid glands, with more than half being benign.[395] The most common malignant lesions in children are mucoepidermoid carcinoma and acinic cell carcinoma.[396] Treatments for patients of any age involve surgical removal and adjuvant radiotherapy for more advanced cancers.[397–399] Brachytherapy is an effective technique for delivering postoperative radiotherapy to small malignant minor salivary gland tumors.[400] Efficacy of treatment of malignant tumors is dependent upon stage, location, presence of perineural invasion, treatment modality, histologic type, and presence of regional invasion.[401] Clinicians should be cognizant of the possibility of development of salivary gland tumors as second cancers in patients who have previously received radiotherapy.[402]

Table 10-7 demonstrates the diverse types of tumors affecting the salivary glands. Clinicians are advised to consult an oral pathology text for more details of these and to examine recent literature for the most current treatment modalities.

TABLE 10-7 Benign Tumors of the Salivary Glands
Pleomorphic adenoma
Monomorphic adenoma
Papillary cystadenoma lymphomatosum
(Warthin's Tumor)
Oncocytoma
Basal cell adenomas
Canalicular adenoma
Myoepithelioma
Sebaceous adenoma
Ductal papilloma

Selected Readings

Abdullah A, Rivas FF, Srinivasan A. Imaging of the salivary glands. *Semin Roentgenol.* 2013;48(1):65-74.

Armstrong MA, Turturro MA. Salivary gland emergencies. *Emerg Med Clin North Am.* 2013;31(2):481-499.

Brennan MT. Sjögren's syndrome. *Oral Maxillofac Surg Clin North Am.* 2014;26(1):ix.

Burke CJ, Thomas RH, Howlett D. Imaging the major salivary glands. *Br J Oral Maxillofac Surg.* 2011;49(4):261-269.

Colella G, Cannavale R, Vicidomini A, et al. Salivary gland biopsy: a comprehensive review of techniques and related complications. *Rheumatology (Oxford).* 2010;49(11):2117-2121.

Deshpande V, Zen Y, Chan JK, et al. Consensus statement on the pathology of IgG4-related disease. *Mod Pathol.* 2012;25:1181-1192.

Doumas S, Vladikas A, Papagianni M, et al. Human cytomegalovirus-associated oral and maxillo-facial disease. *Clin Microbiol Infect.* 2007;13(6):557-559.

Harrison JD. Modern management and pathophysiology of ranula: literature review. *Head Neck.* 2010;32(10):1310-1320.

Jeffers L, Webster-Cyriaque JY. Viruses and salivary gland disease (SGD): lessons from HIV SGD. *Adv Dent Res.* 2011;23(1):79-83.

Jensen SB, Pedersen AM, Vissink A, et al. A systematic review of salivary gland hypofunction and xerostomia induced by cancer therapies: management strategies and economic impact. *Support Care Cancer.* 2010;18(8):1061-1079.

Kamisawa T, Okamoto A. IgG4-related sclerosing disease. *World J Gastroenterol.* 2008;14(25):3948-3955.

Kaplan I, Alterman M, Kleinman S, et al. The clinical, histologic, and treatment spectrum in necrotizing sialometaplasia. *Oral Surg Oral Med Oral Pathol Oral Radiol.* 2012;114(5):577-585.

Liu B, Dion MR, Jurasic MM, et al. Xerostomia and salivary hypofunction in vulnerable elders: prevalence and etiology. *Oral Surg Oral Med Oral Pathol Oral Radiol.* 2012;114(1):52-60.

Mandel SJ, Mandel L. Radioactive iodine and the salivary glands. *Thyroid.* 2003;13(3):265-271.

Neville BW, Damm DD, Allen CM, Bouquot JE, eds. *Oral and Maxillofacial Pathology.* 2009:3rd ed. Philadelphia, PA: WB Saunders.

Ramos-Casals M, Brito-Zerón P, Sisó-Almirall A, et al. Topical and systemic medications for the treatment of primary Sjögren's syndrome. *Nat Rev Rheumatol.* 2012;8(7):399-411.

Shanti RM, Aziz SR. HIV-associated salivary gland disease. *Oral Maxillofac Surg Clin North Am.* 2009;21(3):339-343.

Ship JA. Xerostomia: aetiology, diagnosis, management and clinical implications. In: Edgar M, Dawes C, O'Mullane D, eds. *Saliva and Oral Health.* 3rd ed. London, UK: British Dental Association; 2004:50-70.

Theander E, Henriksson G, Ljungberg O, et al. Lymphoma and other malignancies in primary Sjogren's syndrome: a cohort study on cancer incidence and lymphoma predictors. *Ann Rheum Dis.* 2006;65:796-803.

Vinagre F, Santos MJ, Prata A, et al. Assessment of salivary gland function in Sjögren's syndrome: the role of salivary gland scintigraphy. *Autoimmun Rev.* 2009;8(8):672-676.

Vissink A, Jansma J, Spijkervet FK, et al. Oral sequelae of head and neck radiotherapy. *Crit Rev Oral Biol Med.* 2003;14:199-212.

Wong DT. Salivaomics. *J Am Dent Assoc.* 2012;143(10 suppl):19S-24S.

For the full reference lists, please go to http://www.pmph-usa.com/Burkets_Oral_Medicine.

CHAPTER 11

Temporomandibular Disorders

Richard Ohrbach DDS, PhD
Bruce Blasberg DMD, FRCD(C), FDS RCSEd
Martin S. Greenberg DDS, FDS RCSEd

This chapter focuses on the assessment and management of disorders of the masticatory system. The masticatory apparatus is a specialized unit that performs multiple functions, including those of suckling, cutting and grinding food, swallowing, and communication. The loss of these functions in association with pain is characteristic of masticatory system disorders and causes significant distress that can be severely disabling.

In the past, disorders of the masticatory system were generally treated as one condition or syndrome, with no attempt to differentiate subtypes of muscle and joint disorders. With increased understanding, the ability to identify different muscle or joint disorders has become possible; this should lead to a better understanding of the natural course, more accurate predictions of prognosis, and more effective treatments. The term *temporomandibular disorder(s)* (TMD) used in this chapter is a collective term embracing a number of clinical problems that involve the masticatory muscles, the temporomandibular joints (TMJs) and associated structures, or both.[1] These disorders are characterized by (1) facial pain in the region of the TMJs and/or muscles of mastication, (2) limitation or deviation in mandibular movements, (3) hyperalgesia of the musculoskeletal structures, and (4) TMJ sounds during jaw movement and function.[2,3]

The cause of most TMD remains unknown, although numerous hypotheses have been proposed. The relationship of occlusal disharmony and TMD became a focus after Costen reported that a group of patients with multiple complaints associated with the jaws and ears improved after their occlusal-vertical dimension was altered.[4] Despite the lack of anatomic support for occlusal-vertical dimension as a mechanism,[5] the occlusal hypothesis was nevertheless expanded to include other occlusal parameters, each believed to be responsible for causing TMD, in addition to loss of vertical dimension.[6,7] During the 1950s and 1960s, a muscular cause not directly related to occlusion was proposed; the proposed mechanisms were generic for similar pains elsewhere in the body, thereby highlighting the high plausibility of the model.[8-10] In contrast, because this particular model ignored occlusion as a cause of TMD, the model proved to be very controversial within dentistry, setting the stage for ongoing controversy for any model that did not include occlusion as a cause. In the late 1970s, advances in diagnostic imaging resulted in a better understanding of intracapsular dynamics of the TMJ, and the focus was renewed upon so-called abnormalities of structure as the cause of TMD.[11,12] The lack of a clear understanding with regard to cause, the existence of multiple hypotheses, and strongly held beliefs by some clinicians have resulted in a wide spectrum of views about what TMD constitutes. The absence of standardized methods for assessment, classification, and treatment within much of the clinical TMD literature has diminished its value, particularly in light of the knowledge that has emerged over the past 20–25 years based on using standardized methods for assessment and classification as well as randomized clinical trials for evaluating treatments. This chapter presents a general but evidence-based approach to the diagnostic assessment and nonsurgical management of the most common TMD.

FUNCTIONAL ANATOMY

Temporomandibular Joint

The TMJ articulation is a joint that is capable of hinge-type and gliding movements. The bony components are enclosed and connected by a fibrous capsule. The mandibular condyle forms the lower part of the bony joint and is generally elliptical, although variations in shape are common.[13] To date, there is no evidence of any clinical significance of these variations in shape, in the absence of other markers of a disease process within the joint. The articulation is formed by the mandibular condyle occupying a hollow in the temporal bone

(the mandibular or glenoid fossa) (Figures 11-1 and 11-2). The S-shaped form of the fossa and eminence develops at about 6 years of age and continues into the second decade.[14] During wide mouth opening, the condyle rotates around a hinge axis and glides, causing it to move beyond the anterior border of the fossa, which is identified as the articular eminence.[15] Rotation of the condyle contributes more to normal mouth opening than translation.[16] Rotational movement of the condyle during closing has a rigid end point determined by tooth contact.

The capsule is lined with synovium, and the joint cavity is filled with synovial fluid. The synovium is a vascular connective tissue lining the fibrous joint capsule and extending to the boundaries of the articulating surfaces. Both upper and lower joint cavities are lined with synovium. The synovial membrane consists of macrophage-like type A cells and

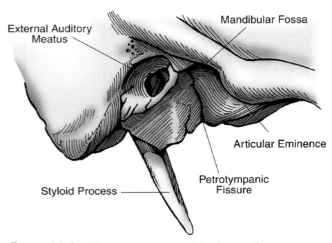

FIGURE 11-1 The S-shaped form of the fossa and eminence develops at about 6 years and continues into the second decade. The mandibular condyle occupies the space of the fossa, with enough room to both rotate and translate during mandibular movements.

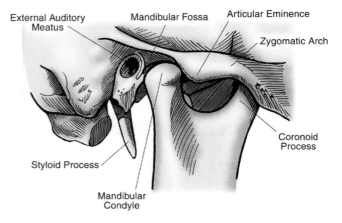

FIGURE 11-2 The articulation is formed by the mandibular condyle occupying a hollow in the temporal bone (the mandibular or glenoid fossa) during wide mouth opening; the condyle rotates around an axis and glides, causing it to move beyond the anterior border of the fossa, the articular eminence.

fibroblast-like type B cells identical to those in other joints. The macrophage-like type A cells react with antimacrophage and macrophage-derived substances, including the major histocompatibility class II molecule, and show a drastic increase in their number in the inflamed synovial membrane.[17] Synovial fluid is a filtrate of plasma with added mucins and proteins. Its main constituent is hyaluronic acid. Fluid forms on the articulating surfaces and decreases friction during joint compression and motion.[18] Joint lubrication is achieved by mechanisms described as weeping lubrication and boundary lubrication. Weeping lubrication occurs as fluid is forced laterally during compression and expressed through the unloaded fibrocartilage.[19] As the adjacent areas become loaded, the weeping lubrication aids in reducing friction. Boundary lubrication is a function of water that is physically bound to the cartilaginous surface by a glycoprotein.[20] Collectively, the fluid dynamics depend on appropriate loading and unloading of the joint through normal function to maintain continuous lubrication as well as maintenance of the tissue health.

Distinguishing features include a covering of fibrocartilage rather than hyaline cartilage on the articulating surfaces; these surfaces in each of the right and left joints are held in a rigid relationship to each other via the connecting mandible. It is likely that the yoked functioning of the two joints has clinical implications, but these are as yet poorly understood. Fibrocartilage is less distensible than hyaline cartilage due to a greater number of collagen fibers. The matrix and chondrocytes are decreased because of the larger irregular bundles of collagen fibers. Fibrocartilage derives its nutrition from the diffusion of nutrients into the synovial fluid that then diffuse through the dense matrix to the chondrocytes.

Articular Disc

A fibrocartilage is made up primarily of dense collagen of variable thickness and referred to as a disc occupies the space between the fibrocartilage coverings of each of condyle and mandibular fossa (Figures 11-3 and 11-4). The disc consists of collagen fibers, cartilage-like proteoglycans,[21] and elastic fibers.[22] The disc contains a variable number of cells that resemble fibrocytes and fibrochondrocytes.[23] Collagen fibers in the center of the disc (often referred to as the intermediate zone) are oriented perpendicular to its transverse axis and thereby in-line with loading on that zone. The collagen fibers become interlaced as they approach the anterior and posterior bands, and many fibers are oriented parallel to the mediolateral aspect of the disc. Cartilage-like proteoglycans contribute to the compressive stiffness of articular cartilage.[24] The disc is primarily avascular and has little sensory nerve penetration. The disc is attached by ligaments to the lateral and medial poles of the condyle. The ligaments consist of both collagen and elastic fibers.[25] These ligaments permit rotational movement of the disc on the condyle during mouth opening and closing. The normal disc is thinnest in the intermediate zone and thickens to form anterior and posterior bands. This arrangement is considered to help stabilize the condyle in the glenoid fossa. Over time, discs may

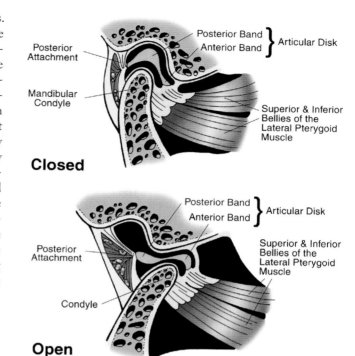

FIGURE 11-3 The temporomandibular joint is capable of hinge-type movements and gliding movements. The articular disc has ligamentous attachments to the mandibular fossa and condyle. The disc's attachments create separate superior and inferior joint compartments.

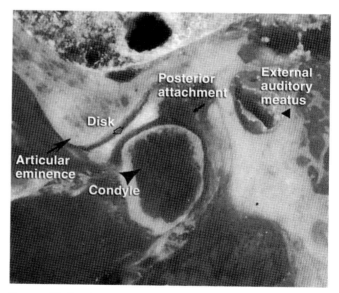

FIGURE 11-4 A cadaver section through the temporomandibular joint shows the relationship of the condyle, fossa, and articular disc.

exhibit changes in this conformation; the central intermediate zone may become elongated or nonexistent, the anterior band may become thinner, or the posterior band may become either thinner or thicker. These conformation changes, while presumably affecting the ideal function of the disc in stabilizing the condyle during loading, are currently regarded as a variation on normal in the absence of any clinical manifestation of disordered function.

The disc provides an interface for the condyle as it glides across the temporal bone. The disc and its attachments divide the joint into upper and lower compartments that normally do not communicate. The passive volume of the upper compartment is estimated to be 1.2 mL and that of the lower compartment is estimated to be 0.9 mL.[25] The roof of the superior compartment is the mandibular fossa, whereas the floor is the superior surface of the disc. The roof of the inferior compartment is the inferior surface of the disc and the floor is the articulating surface of the mandibular condyle.[25] At its margins, the disc blends with the fibrous capsule. Muscle attachments inserting into the anterior aspect of the disc have been observed in a relatively small number of individuals.[26] Fibers of the posterior one-third of the temporalis muscle and of the deep masseter muscle may attach on the anterolateral aspect, and fibers of the superior head of the lateral pterygoid have been observed to insert into the anteromedial two-thirds of the disc.[26] Clinical significance of these anatomic variations in muscle attachment to the disc has received much speculation but little data.

Retrodiscal Tissue

A mass of soft tissue occupies the space behind the disc and condyle. It is often referred to as the posterior attachment. The posterior attachment is a loosely organized system of collagen fibers, branching elastic fibers, fat, blood and lymph vessels, and nerves. Synovium covers the superior and inferior surfaces. The attachment has been described as being arranged in two lamina of dense connective tissue,[27] but this has been challenged.[28] Between the lamina, a loose areolar, highly vascular, and well-innervated tissue has been described. The superior lamina arises from the posterior band of the disc and attaches to the squamotympanic fissure and tympanic part of the temporal bone. The superior lamina consists primarily of elastin.[27,29] The inferior lamina arises from the posterior band of the disc and inserts into the inferior margin of the posterior articular slope of the condyle and is composed mostly of collagen fibers.[27]

Temporomandibular Ligaments
Capsular Ligament

The capsular ligament is a thin inelastic fibrous connective tissue envelope that attaches to the margins of the articular surfaces (Figure 11-5). The fibers are oriented vertically and do not restrain joint movements. The medial capsule is composed of loose areolar connective tissue.[28] The capsule and the lateral discal ligament join and attach to the lateral aspect of the neck of the condyle.[30]

Lateral Temporomandibular Ligament

The lateral temporomandibular ligament is the main ligament of the joint, lateral to the capsule but not easily separated from it by dissection. Its fibers pass obliquely from bone lateral to

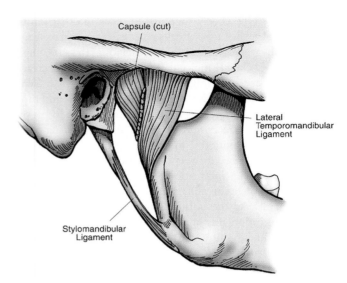

FIGURE 11-5 The capsular ligament is a thin, inelastic, fibrous connective tissue envelope, oriented vertically, that attaches to the margins of the articular surfaces. The capsular ligament does not restrain condylar movements. The temporomandibular ligament is lateral to the capsule but is not easily separated from it by dissection. Its fibers pass obliquely from bone lateral to the articular tubercle in a posterior and inferior direction to insert in a narrower area below and behind the lateral pole of the condyle.

the articular tubercle in a posterior and inferior direction and insert in a narrower area below and behind the lateral pole of the condyle (see Figure 11-5). In earlier literature, this ligament was identified as an oblique band from the condylar neck to the anterosuperior region on the eminence and as a horizontal band from the lateral condylar pole to an anterior attachment of the eminence.[25] A recent study was unable to confirm a distinct structure separate from the capsule.[30]

Accessory Ligaments

The sphenomandibular ligament arises from the sphenoid bone and inserts on the medial aspect of the mandible at the lingula. It is not considered to limit or affect mandibular movement. The stylomandibular ligament extends from the styloid process to the deep fascia of the medial pterygoid muscle. It is thought to become tense during protrusive movement of the mandible and may contribute to limiting protrusive movement.

Muscles of Mastication

The muscles of mastication are the paired masseter, medial and lateral pterygoids, and temporalis (Figures 11-6–11-8). Mandibular movements toward the tooth contact position are performed by contraction of the masseter, temporalis, and medial pterygoid muscles. Masseter contraction contributes to moving the condylar head toward the anterior slope of the mandibular fossa. The posterior part of the temporalis contributes to mandibular retrusion. Unilateral contraction of the medial pterygoid contributes to a contralateral movement of

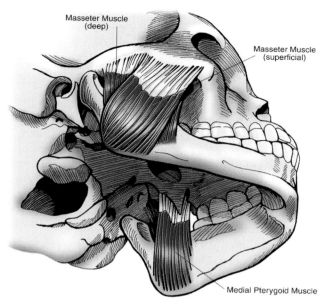

FIGURE 11-6 The masseter and medial pterygoid muscles have their insertions at the inferior border of the mandibular angle. They join together to form a sling that cradles the ramus of the mandible and produces the powerful forces required for chewing. The masseter muscle has been divided into a deep portion and a superficial portion.

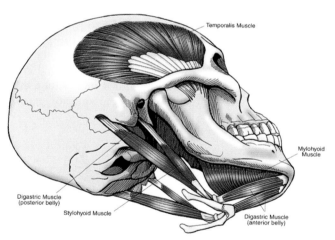

FIGURE 11-7 The digastric muscle is a paired muscle with two bellies. The anterior belly attaches to the lingual aspect of the mandible at the parasymphysis and courses backward to insert into a round tendon attached to the hyoid bone. Contraction produces a depression and retropositioning of the mandible. The mylohyoid and geniohyoid muscles contribute to depressing the mandible when the infrahyoid muscles stabilize the hyoid bone during mandibular movement. These muscles may also contribute to retrusion of the mandible. The temporalis muscle is broadly attached to the lateral skull. The muscle fibers converge to insert on the coronoid process and anterior aspect of the mandibular ramus. The posterior part traverses anteriorly and then curves around the anterior root of the zygomatic process before insertion. The posterior part of the temporalis contributes to mandibular retrusion.

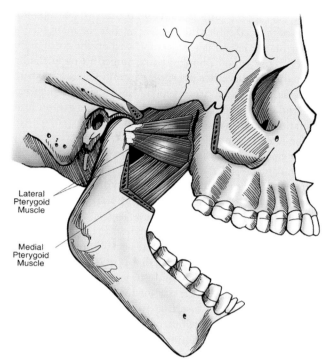

FIGURE 11-8 The lateral pterygoid muscle is the main protrusive and opening muscle of the mandible. It is arranged in parallel-fiber units that allow for greater displacement and velocity compared to that of the multipennate-based closing muscles. The lateral pterygoid muscle is divided into two parts. The inferior part originates from the outer surface of the lateral pterygoid plate of the sphenoid and the pyramidal process of the palatine bone. The superior part originates from the greater wing of the sphenoid and the pterygoid ridge. The fibers of the upper and lower heads course posteriorly and laterally, fusing in front of the temporomandibular joint. They insert into the anteromedial aspect of the condylar neck. Some of the fibers insert into the most anterior medial portion of the disc, but most of the lateral pterygoid fibers insert into the condyle. Translation of the condylar head onto the articular eminence is produced by contraction of the lateral pterygoid.

the mandible. The masseter and medial pterygoid muscles have their insertions at the inferior border of the mandibular angle. They join together to form a sling that cradles the mandible and produces the powerful forces required for chewing. The masseter is divided into deep and superficial parts. The deep masseter in some individuals overlaps the anterior aspect of the TMJ, such that pain localized to the pre-auricular region may be associated with masseter, TMJ, or both structures.

The temporalis muscle is broadly attached to the lateral skull and has been divided into anterior, middle, and posterior parts. The muscle fibers converge into a tendon that inserts on the coronoid process and anterior aspect of the mandibular ramus. The anterior and middle fibers are generally oriented in a straight line from their origin on the skull to their insertion on the mandible. The posterior part traverses anteriorly and then curves around the anterior root of the zygomatic process before insertion.

The lateral pterygoid is the main protrusive and opening muscle of the mandible. The inferior head is the main section responsible for lateral jaw movements when the teeth are in contact.[31] The lateral pterygoid is arranged in parallel-fiber units, whereas the other muscles are multipennate in structure. This differential arrangement allows greater displacement and velocity in the lateral pterygoid versus greater force generation in the elevator muscles.[32]

The lateral pterygoid muscle arises from two heads. The inferior head originates from the outer surface of the lateral pterygoid plate of the sphenoid and the pyramidal process of the palatine bones. The superior head originates from the greater wing of the sphenoid and the pterygoid ridge. The fibers of the upper and lower heads course posteriorly and laterally, fusing in front of the condyle.[33] They insert into the anteromedial aspect of the condylar neck. Some of the fibers insert into the most anterior medial portion of the disk (or capsule), but most of the lateral pterygoid fibers insert into the condyle.[33] The superior part of the insertion consists of an identifiable tendon inserting through fibrocartilage. The inferior part of the insertion consists of muscle attached to periosteum.[34] Debate continues about the functional anatomy of the lateral pterygoid. The superior head is thought to be active during closing movements, and the inferior head is thought to be active during opening and protrusive movements.[35–37] Translation of the condylar head onto the articular eminence is produced by contraction of the lateral pterygoid.

The digastric muscle is a paired muscle with two bellies. The anterior belly attaches to the lingual aspect of the mandible at the parasymphysis and courses backward to insert into the hyoid bone. Contraction produces a depression and retropositioning of the mandible. The mylohyoid and geniohyoid muscles contribute to depressing the mandible when the infrahyoid muscles stabilize the hyoid bone. These muscles may also contribute to retrusion of the mandible. The buccinator attaches inferiorly along the facial surface of the mandible behind the mental foramen and superiorly on the alveolar surface behind the zygomatic process. The buccinator fibers are arranged horizontally; anteriorly, fibers insert into mucosa, skin, and lip. The buccinator helps position the cheek during chewing movements of the mandible. The functional activity of these accessory muscles depends on simultaneous activation of the primary masticatory muscles for stabilizing the position of the mandible, which, given the basal functions of the masticatory system, has implications with respect to the functional limitation and disability often associated with a TMD.

Vascular Supply of Masticatory System Structures

The external carotid artery is the main blood supply for the masticatory system structures. The artery leaves the neck and courses superiorly and posteriorly embedded in the substance of the parotid gland. The artery sends two important branches, the lingual and facial arteries, to the region. At the level of the condylar neck, the external carotid bifurcates into the superficial temporal artery and the internal maxillary artery. These two arteries supply the muscles of mastication and the TMJ. Arteries within the temporal bone and mandible also send branches to the capsule.

Nerve Supply of Masticatory System Structures

The masticatory structures are innervated primarily by the trigeminal nerve, but cranial nerves VII, IX, X, and XI and cervical nerves 2 and 3 also contribute. The peripheral nerves synapse with nuclei in the brainstem that are associated with touch, proprioception, and motor function. The large spinal trigeminal nucleus occupies a major part of the brainstem and extends to the spinal cord. The spinal trigeminal nucleus is thought to be the main site for the reception of impulses from the periphery involved in pain sensation. The mandibular division of the trigeminal nerve supplies motor innervation to the muscles of mastication and the anterior belly of the digastric muscle. Branches of the auriculotemporal nerve supply the sensory innervation of the TMJ; this nerve arises from the mandibular division in the infratemporal fossa and sends branches to the capsule of the joint (Figure 11-9). The deep temporal and masseteric nerves supply the anterior portion of the joint. The auriculotemporal nerve, a branch of the mandibular portion (V3) of the trigeminal nerve, provides innervation of the TMJ. About 75% of the time, the masseteric nerve, a branch of the maxillary division of the trigeminal nerve (V2), innervates the anteromedial capsule of the TMJ. In about 33%, a separate branch from V2 comes through the mandibular notch and innervates the anteromedial capsule.[38] These nerves are primarily motor nerves, but they contain sensory fibers distributed to the anterior part of

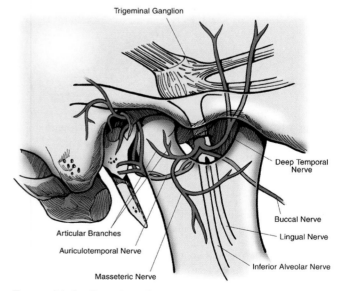

Figure 11-9 Branches of the auriculotemporal nerve supply sensory innervation of the TMJ. This nerve arises from the mandibular division in the infratemporal fossa and sends branches to the capsule of the joint.

the TMJ capsule. The autonomic nerve supply is carried to the joint by the auriculotemporal nerve and by nerves traveling along the superficial temporal artery.

ANATOMY OF CLINICAL INTEREST

Jaw Jerk Reflex

The jaw jerk reflex, analogous to the knee jerk reflex, is a stretch reflex that occurs by applying a downward tap on the chin. The tap produces a monosynaptic reflex contraction of the jaw closing muscles. It demonstrates the existence of a feedback loop from the jaw-closing muscles to their own motor neurons in the central nervous system (CNS). This reflex is thought to relate to the fine control of jaw movements required to masticate different consistencies of food.[39] Neurosensory testing for examination, diagnosis, and classification of orofacial pain disorders has received attention in the research community, but measuring and interpreting the jaw jerk reflex has not yet become a valuable clinical test.[40]

Jaw-Opening Reflex

Stimulating mechanoreceptors or nociceptors in the mouth triggers the jaw-opening reflex. The pathway is polysynaptic; the first synapse is in either the trigeminal sensory nuclei or the adjacent reticular formation and the final synapse is in the trigeminal motor nucleus. The reflex results in an inhibition of the activity of the jaw-closing muscles. This reflex is thought to help prevent injury when biting or chewing objects that may cause damage.[39]

The jaw-opening reflex has been used to study lingual nerve injuries. Differences in the reflex were found when stimulating tongue mucosa on the injured side, but the difference was not helpful in predicting recovery.[41]

Rest Position

When the mandible is not functionally active, it adopts a so-called rest position in which the condyle occupies a relatively neutral position in the glenoid fossa with the teeth separated. The rest position is considered to be associated with minimum muscular activity and with the articulating surfaces of the mandibular teeth a few millimeters from the occlusal contact position with the opposing teeth.[42] "Rest position" is, however, somewhat of a misnomer since a wide range of activity in the masticatory muscles is observed, under the presumed condition of "rest," across individuals and within individuals across time; the masticatory muscles seldom exhibit a reliable level of lowest activity. Consequently, the muscle activity and mandibular position vary for a number of reasons (e.g., head posture, emotion, cognition, pain) and "rest position" is not an exact position.[43] Clinical diagnoses that require an interpretation of rest position must be considered very cautiously.

Centric Relation

Centric relation is a position that has traditionally relied on guiding the condyles into a position to rotate around a stationary axis in the mandibular fossa. The definition from the "The Glossary of Prosthodontic Terms" is "the maxillomandibular relationship in which each condyle articulates with the thinnest avascular portion of the disc in an anterosuperior position against the posterior slope of the articular eminence."[44] This position of condylar rotation about a stationary axis can be reproduced and transferred to an articulator, and although that is useful clinically for restorative dentistry, a biological basis for the manipulated position has not been defined. That is, a mandibular position usefully defined in operational terms for purposes of restorative dentistry should not be confused with necessarily having diagnostic value beyond the operational definition. Adjusting the maximum intercuspal position to be coincident with centric relation has been recommended by some clinicians to treat TMDs, but the evidence for this as a standard treatment is lacking.[45] In contrast, the available evidence indicates that the "stationary axis" is itself dynamic: for example, restoring a dentition for centric relation coincidence with maximum intercuspal position results in the development of a new centric relation position over time,[46] implying that centric relation is a boundary of a zone used for regular movement.

Mandibular Range of Motion

Mandibular motion during normal function is composed of rotation and translation of the condyles. Gallo et al. calculated the average rotation of the condyle to be 24° and the condylar translation to extend 13–15 mm before achieving maximum opening.[47] During translation, the disc and condyle move downward and forward along the posterior slope of the articular eminence. The articular disc translates with the condyle, and simultaneously it rotates posteriorly as the condyle moves anteriorly; consequently, the movement of the disc across the fossa is limited to a range of 5–9 mm.[48] At maximum mouth opening, the condyle moves to the crest of the articular eminence or beyond. The temporomandibular, sphenomandibular, and stylomandibular ligaments, together with the articular eminence, have been suggested as the main constraints of jaw opening.[49] In addition, a muscular constraint of jaw opening has also been proposed.[50] Measuring the gap between the maxillary and the mandibular incisors during opening remains the most common assessment method.[51,52] A wide variation in maximal vertical mandibular movement exists; males open a few millimeter greater than females, and 40–45 mm represents the mean extent (with standard deviation around 10) across studies of pain-free opening among asymptomatic individuals. Individuals with TMD exhibit a notable decrease in pain-free opening,[53,54] and pain, not structural problems, is the most common cause of the restricted opening.

Articular Covering

The fibrocartilage found on the articulating surfaces of the TMJ is believed to provide more surface strength against forces in many directions while allowing more freedom of movement that would be possible with hyaline cartilage. Fibrocartilage also forms the articular disc. This covering is thickest on the posterior slope of the articular eminence and on the anterior slope of the condylar head; these are the areas thought to receive the greatest functional load. The thinnest part of the fibrocartilage covering is on the roof of the mandibular fossa. Fibrocartilage has a greater repair capacity than hyaline cartilage. This may affect how the TMJ responds to degenerative changes.[55]

Disc Displacements

Demonstration of the lateral pterygoid's attachment to the anterior articular disc has led to the theory that some anterior disc displacements may be related to lateral pterygoid muscle dysfunction. The theory suggests that hyperactivity of the superior head of the lateral pterygoid is capable of pulling the disc forward from its normal position over the mandibular condyle.[56] Research on cadaver specimens has indicated that muscle fibers inserting into the disc or the condyle are not differentiated into inferior and superior heads.[33,57] The muscle fibers that do insert into the disc are located primarily at the medial portion. Carpentier et al. postulated that the two heads did not have distinct independent actions and that the lateral pterygoid was not a significant cause of disc displacement.[33] The inferior lamina of the posterior attachment is considered to be the primary restraint preventing the disc from moving forward. Injury to this ligament has been proposed as the cause of disc displacements.[58]

Clicking has been reported as the most common TMJ irregularity detected during clinical examination and may occur as an isolated finding.[59] An estimated one-third of asymptomatic and normally functioning volunteers on magnetic resonance imaging (MRI) examination of the TMJs had disc displacements.[60] Although the sounds of TMJ clicking can be produced by disc reduction and displacement during, respectively, the opening and closing mandibular movements, clicking is not specific to disc displacements. Rather, clicking noises can be produced by several phenomena (described below), and disc displacements can be completely silent. Therefore, the phenomenon of clicking, based on reported patient history or clinical examination, must be distinguished from disc displacements as observed on imaging such as magnetic resonance (MR).

The angle or steepness of the mandibular fossa has been considered a contributing factor in the development or aggravation of intra-articular disorders. However, the steep, vertical form of the fossa has been inconsistently associated with articular disc displacements (ADDs) across studies. Differing levels of muscle activity, for example, as one possible contributing variable, may explain disparate findings, but such research is only now being conducted.[61] The form and steepness of the fossa has also been considered a contributing factor in chronic subluxation or dislocation of the condyle, but the co-existence of a disc displacement often accompanies problematic subluxation (or dislocation). Osseous changes in response to the disc displacement have been found suggesting that the steepness of the eminence may be a consequence of disc displacement rather than a cause.[62] In

contrast, Bell[63] suggested that subluxation (or dislocation) occurs due to a combination of fossa steepness and increased activity of the masticatory elevator muscles preventing the condyle from translating posteriorly around the eminence during the closing phase of mandibular movement. Surgical treatments that modify the steepness or flatten the eminence have been recommended but controlled outcomes do not yet exist for any treatment approach.

In addition to sudden locking associated with disc displacement with reduction, Nitzan and Etsion proposed that adhesion of the disc in the fossa might cause acute closed lock,[64] which can occur with both normal discs and displaced discs. Adhesion occurs when hyaluronic acid and associated phospholipids are degraded. Support for this hypothesis is the immediate and generally stable improvement of mouth opening after arthrocentesis.[64] In fact, this procedure can be effective treatment for a significant number of patients, but the specific clinical characteristics of those for whom it is effective remain poorly defined.

Joint Noises

ADDs are thought to be the most common cause of joint noises, specifically clicking. Clicking can occur in individuals who have a normal disc position on MRI.[65] Other explanations for TMJ clicking include condylar hypermobility, enlargement of the lateral pole of the condyle, structural irregularity of the articular eminence, loose intra-articular bodies other than the disc, and dysfunctional movement patterns or incoordination.[66,67] A report of clicking that interferes with function or is accompanied by pain warrants clinical attention, regardless of whether the MRI demonstrates disc displacement,[68] highlighting the need to consider multiple levels of complexity and function in addition to the relevant anatomy.

Nerve Entrapment

Compression of nerves due to decreased occlusal vertical dimension and variations in their course close to the mandibular condyle was an early hypothesis proposed by Costen to explain TMD pain.[4] Close proximity of the auriculotemporal nerve to the medial aspect of the condyle has been described. Medial displacement of the articular disc exposing the auriculotemporal nerve to mechanical irritation has been described as a possible cause.[69] However, anatomic study of the condyle and its relationship to the auriculotemporal nerve make this an unlikely cause of TMDs.[70]

Occlusion

The intercuspal position is achieved when maximum intercuspation of opposing teeth occurs.[48] Occlusal stability has been defined as "the equalization of contacts that prevents tooth movement after closure."[71] A physiologic occlusion has been defined as "an occlusion in which a functional equilibrium or state of homeostasis exists between all tissues of the masticatory system."[72] This definition has been interpreted both narrowly and broadly. The narrow interpretation, one with general agreement, is that occlusal forces at the inter-cuspal position are best directed toward the long axes of teeth[73,74] and that all teeth should contact at the same time with approximately equal force. The broad interpretation, one with little agreement, has encompassed all possible attributes of occlusion to define a normal occlusion; a very large volume of research has as yet failed to find associations between occlusal attributes and TMD. For example, a reduced num-ber of contacting teeth in the intercuspal position and loss of posterior teeth have been hypothesized to be risk factors for the subsequent development of TMD,[75] but at present no lon-gitudinal evidence exists for this hypothesized relationship.

To date, as summarized elsewhere,[73] TMD has a reliable association with only a very few attributes of a static occlusion, and the magnitude of the association is relatively small. These associations are based on cross-sectional study designs, not longitudinal designs, and collectively suggest that the specific occlusal features have a complex relationship to TMD pain. The available evidence indicates that that complex relation-ship, pointedly, does not include a direct causal role. Just as the evidence has not supported occlusal attributes as cause of TMD, the research literature has not supported any efficacy of occlusal treatment for TMD.[76] Overall, studies examining occlusal characteristics and TMD symptoms have failed to identify a strong association.[77] Returning to the early work of Costen, the loss of occlusal vertical dimension has been (and perhaps continues to be) considered a cause of TMD, but contemporary evidence for this remains lacking.[78]

Ear Symptoms Associated With TMDs

Earache, tinnitus, and fullness or a feeling of stuffiness are complaints that are often reported by patients with TMD.[79,80] One purported mechanism for the association is a ligament connecting the disc and the malleus, which has been observed in anatomic specimens.[81] The superior retrodiscal lamina has been considered to be a remnant of the ligament connecting the lateral pterygoid tendon to the mal-leus through the squamotympanic fissure in the fetus.[82] This anatomic finding has been used to explain the prevalence of auditory symptoms in TMDs, but research has not estab-lished that this is a functioning ligament between the TMJ and the middle ear.[83,84] Pressure on the anterior tympanic artery that enters the petrotympanic fissure in the mandibu-lar fossa is an alternative hypothesis. The most common dis-orders associated with ear pain unrelated to ear disease are cervical spine disorders, TMDs, or both,[85] suggesting that multiple mechanisms might exist or that both TMD and cervical problems have shared mechanisms responsible for ear symptoms; such shared mechanisms point away from the isolated anatomical findings described here that are specific for a TMD cause of ear symptoms.

Injection Sites

Injections to anesthetize sensory innervation of the joint may be a part of the diagnostic assessment or injecting medica-tion such as corticosteroids may be part of therapy. The site

of injection should be anterior to the tragus to minimize the risk of intravascular injection of the external carotid artery or the accompanying vein. Because the auriculotemporal nerve enters the capsule from the medial aspect, injections (normally given from the lateral aspect) may not completely anesthetize the joint.[86] Fernandes et al. found the auricu-lotemporal nerve to be 10–13 mm inferior to the superior surface of the condyle and 1–2 mm posterior to the neck of the condyle.[70]

Muscle Palpation

The most widely used clinical test for the assessment of TMD is applying pressure to muscles and joints to determine whether pain is elicited by the stimulus, known as palpation for pain. Although this procedure is deemed fully valid and appropriate for the extraoral muscles, intraoral palpation of the lateral pterygoid muscle has been challenged because of its location and inaccessibility (Figure 11-10).[87] In addition to poor reliability associated with its examination, the exam-ination procedure is likely to cause discomfort in individuals without a TMD, diminishing the value of lateral pterygoid palpation as a diagnostic test.[88] The fibers of the deep mas-seter muscle are intimately related to the lateral wall of the joint capsule, which may explain the frequent localization by patients of the pain complaint to the preauricular area broadly. This anatomic characteristic makes differentiating muscle and joint pain in this area difficult.[89,90]

Jaw Jerk Reflex and the Silent Period

Masseter and temporalis muscles exhibit suppressed peri-ods of electromyographic (EMG) activity when subjected to mechanical stimuli or electric shocks.[91] A prolonged period of electrical inactivity on EMG recordings has been observed in TMD patients,[92] but because this "silent period" is a func-tion of decreased bite force secondary to pain inhibition, the "silent period" has not been established as a valuable test for the diagnosis of TMDs.

ETIOLOGY, EPIDEMIOLOGY, AND CLASSIFICATION

Etiology

The etiology of the most common TMDs is unknown. The literature has been dominated by several hypothesized causes: occlusal disharmony, muscle hyperactivity, central pain mechanisms, psychological distress, and trauma. Clear and convincing evidence for so-called occlusal disharmony as a primary etiology does not exist,[73] as discussed earlier. Research studying discrepancies between centric relation and centric occlusion, nonworking side occlusal interfer-ences, and Angle's occlusal classification has not established a strong association in patients with myofascial pain compared with controls.[93–96] Significant differences in occlusal char-acteristics are not found between patients with myofascial pain compared with control subjects.[97] Premature occlusal

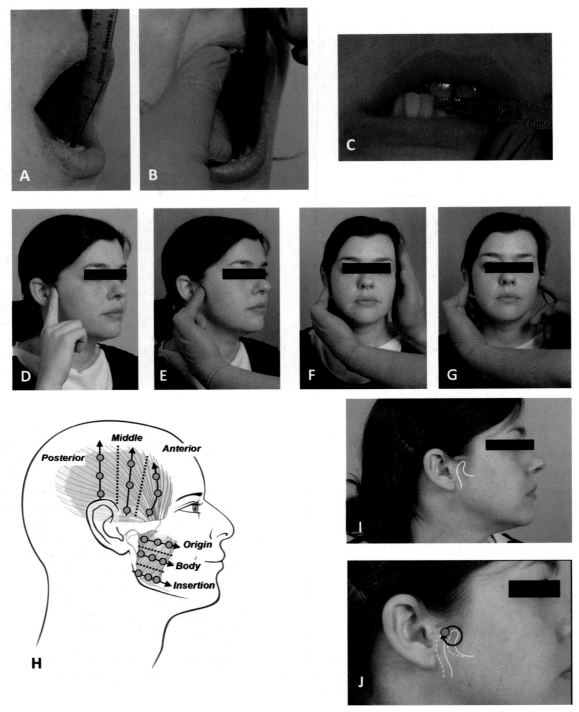

FIGURE 11-10 The core components of the clinical examination. A, Measuring pain-free opening and maximal unassisted opening. B, Measuring maximal assisted opening. C, Measuring right lateral movement of the mandible; this is repeated for movement of the mandible to the left, and then in protrusive. D, Patient points to location of pain, which is asked after each of maximal unassisted and maximal assisted opening, right and left lateral movement, and protrusive. E, Examiner confirms structure that the patient had pointed to as painful from the range of motion procedure. F, Position of hands for palpation of single TMJ during range of motion. G, Position of hands for simultaneous bilateral palpation of the TMJ during range of motion. H, Location of palpation sites for palpation for pain of the temporalis and masseter muscles. I, Visualization of lateral pole for palpation for pain of the lateral pole; finger is placed directly on the pole. J, Visualization of starting finger position (*green dot*) for circumpolar palpation for pain of the TMJ; the finger rotates around the condyle, as shown by the black arrow. Illustrations and photos are adapted from Ohrbach et al.[52] See Protocol for full set of illustrations and instructions for the clinical examination.

contacts such as faulty restorative dentistry are traditionally believed to initiate sleep bruxism. This actually triggers the opposite in healthy subjects: a decrease in the activity of masticatory elevator muscles during sleep in healthy individuals.[98] In contrast, the same trigger in individuals with TMD or a prior history of TMD will cause an increase during sleep of the activity of the masticatory elevator muscles.[99] Overjet and overbite do not have a strong relationship with joint clicking, crepitus, pain, or limited opening.[100,101] It may be premature to completely dismiss occlusal attributes for possible causal roles in TMD; a major limitation in a majority of studies of occlusion as a putative cause of TMD are that terms such as "disharmony" are used without an adequate definition, leading to research that is not reproducible.

A relationship between tooth loss and osteoarthrosis has been observed in patients with TMD[102] but not in nonpatient populations.[103] In contrast, incisal relationships, condylar position, and joint sounds do not differentiate symptomatic individuals and nonpatient populations.[104] An observed relationship between severe overbite and TMD symptoms has not been consistently observed.[105,106]

Much research on occlusal characteristics as a cause of TMD has focused on the quality of the occlusion (e.g., the so-called occlusal prematurity) within cross-sectional study designs, and in such studies, it is equally logical to assume a reversed causal pattern: that some aspect of the TMD caused the observed occlusal attribute. The most obvious example of malocclusion being the result of another process is that of anterior open bite, which may be the result of anatomic changes in the TMJs due to inflammation and degenerative changes associated with rheumatoid arthritis (RA).[107] Patients sometimes present with acute unilateral posterior open bite and premature contact on the contralateral side due to lateral pterygoid splinting or spasm on the side of the open bite. Some patients with unilateral nonreducing ADD will report, on questioning, hyperocclusion of the molars on the ipsilateral side. As another example, premature contacts in one dental segment coupled with balancing interferences on that same side could be due to unilateral guarding behavior in response to the TMD pain. Masseter pain induced by saline injections caused a shift in the apex point of the gothic arch, suggesting that pain might be a factor in producing the occlusal changes that are sometimes reported by patients with TMD.[108] A number of studies have been performed to investigate a possible relationship between orthodontic treatment and the development of TMD, but the results do not support a causal relationship.[109–111]

Masticatory muscle hyperactivity—muscle activity without functional purpose—has been proposed for more than 50 years as a cause of myofascial pain. The diagnostic terms *myospasm*, *muscle spasm*, and *reflex splinting* have also been used to describe this condition which is characterized by a "vicious cycle" of pain and hyperactivity mutually reinforcing each other.[112] Muscle hyperactivity is usefully separated into sleep bruxism and waking parafunction,

corresponding, respectively, to sleep versus waking states. The favored hypothesis for many years was that sleep bruxism is caused by abnormalities of occlusion, but this was based on flawed research.[113,114] Currently, evidence strongly supports sleep bruxism as a parasomnia type of sleep disorder; specifically, sleep bruxism events are related to microarousals during sleep.[115,116] Although microarousals are a normal part of sleep architecture in everyone, microarousals selectively trigger bruxism events in those individuals with the disorder, and do not do so in individuals without the disorder for reasons as yet unknown. The evidence to date is circular, and it does not support microarousals as the cause of sleep bruxism; rather, individuals at risk for sleep bruxism may be differentially primed to respond to microarousals with bruxism events.

A variety of studies have linked sleep bruxism to pain.[117–122] The common explanation is that the pain is simply due to overuse of the muscle during sleep, as in postexercise pain. Clinical observations have indicated, however, that severe sleep bruxism, as measured by extensive tooth wear, can occur without symptoms. Moreover, empirical data demonstrate that not only pain but also TMJ clicking and masticatory muscle tenderness are unrelated to severe tooth wear from sleep bruxism.[123] These contradictory findings lead to an important paradox: how could the most severe form of a disorder not produce pain while the less severe form presumably does? Polysomnography-based measurement of jaw muscle activity during sleep demonstrates that sleep bruxism has, at best, a weak relationship to pain on waking the following morning.[124] In other words, individuals with TMD pain may simultaneously have evidence of sleep bruxism and report jaw pain on awakening, but the bruxism does not appear to directly cause the pain.

Parafunction while awake has for more than 50 years been regarded as a cause of TMD pain, but only recently has any substantial evidence emerged. Waking parafunction has classically been depicted as excessive tooth clenching, but waking parafunction appears to be a much more complex process in terms of a wide range of behaviors (e.g., bracing, pushing, guarding, pressing), a high frequency of occurrence, and lower forces than previously assumed. The duration of such behaviors necessary to cause pain appears to vary across individuals. As described previously, muscle activity at so-called rest does not differ between painful and non-painful jaw-closing muscles,[125] suggesting that jaw behavior is very dynamic across the span of a day. Waking behaviors such as tooth clenching or muscle guarding are remarkably concrete and reliable in how they manifest across persons with or without TMD.[126,127] Experimental evidence suggests that tooth clenching at a relatively low but sustained level might be a source of pain in some individuals.[128] As primary evidence that parafunctional behaviors can cause pain, positive findings on muscle examination are more frequent in individuals who perform tooth-clenching activities.[129] In addition, among individuals who have developed a first lifetime episode of TMD pain, parafunctional behaviors are reported at a much higher rate prior to the development of the TMD compared to those who do not develop TMD, demonstrating the potential of these behaviors to contribute to the development of TMD.[130] Oral parafunctional behaviors exhibit a substantial association with chronic TMD pain, suggesting that the parafunctional behaviors have both contributed to the persistence of the TMD and become a result of the TMD pain.[53]

The Pain-Adaptation Model has been proposed as an alternative to the "vicious cycle" hypothesis regarding pain and muscle hyperactivity. The Pan-Adaptation Model is based on observations that EMG activity and force output of the muscle are lower in patients with musculoskeletal pain.[130] The reduction in muscle activity is thought to be protective to prevent further injury, and for acute pain, this model is both sensible and clinically useful. The Pain-Adaptation Model and the vicious cycle hypothesis are not incompatible, however; in that experimental evidence indicates that persistent parafunctional behaviors occurring at low levels of contractile activity are sufficient to cause pain. Moreover, in chronic pain, the Pain-Adaptation Model fails to have the same relevance in that goal-oriented behavior can override the model-specified inhibition in behavior, as one aspect of adaptation to the disorder: for example, a person will chew desired foods regardless of the pain. In recognition of this clearly observed discrepancy between clinical presentations and the Pain-Adaptation Model, Minami and colleagues recently provided experimental evidence demonstrating the limits of the Pain-Adaptation Model in understanding pain and behavior.[131] Overall, the available evidence provides strong support for parafunctional behaviors having a strong role in the etiology of TMD and a strong role as a contributing factor for persistence of TMD.

In addition to local factors affecting muscle function, the results of a number of experimental studies of myofascial pain support the hypothesis that the pain is caused by altered CNS processing.[132–136] However, these studies have not been able to distinguish whether the findings are a consequence of the pain rather than the cause of the pain. More recent evidence, however, suggests that altered CNS processing related to pain amplification occurs in response to having a pain disorder rather than contributing to the etiology of the disorder.[137]

The psychological distress hypothesis proposes that TMD evolves as a consequence of pre-existing problems in overall functioning, usually due to the individual's stressful environment coupled with poor coping skills and which leads to distress in the form of depression, anxiety, or both. Two pathways by which the psychological distress leads to TMD have been proposed. The most common pathway in the TMD literature specifies that distress leads to oral parafunctional behaviors (as described earlier) that then result in muscle pain.[138–140] The second pathway, which is common in the general pain literature, specifies that psychological distress results in an overall increased risk for an individual to experience pain in response to some event (e.g., a traumatic yawn). A challenge that is continually faced in the clinic when evaluating patients with chronic pain disorders is determining how much of the psychological distress is a cause or a consequence of chronic pain.[141] The weight of the evidence has suggested that the emotional distress is more likely a consequence than a cause of pain.[142] That evidence has been, however, largely cross-sectional at the time of entry into the clinic, and prior functioning was assessed retrospectively. In contrast, recent evidence from a large-scale prospective longitudinal study indicates that psychological distress, in the form of depression, anxiety, and problems with stress and coping, exerts a long-term effect on the individual with respect to increased risk for subsequent development of TMD and, consistent with the prior cross-sectional evidence, chronic TMD is associated with greater extent of distress.[143,144]

The role of trauma as a primary etiology for TMD varies from self-evident (pain or mechanical TMJ problem following direct blow to the jaw) to purely inferential (jaw pain six months after a motor vehicle collision). Although the literature points to some trauma events as having greater likelihood of being a sufficient cause of TMD and other trauma events as not sufficient on their own to cause TMD, conflicting conclusions emerge from other studies. The best evidence to date may come from two studies using the same methods and conducted in parallel. In a case-control study, individuals with chronic TMD reported trauma at a high rate, compared to individuals with no lifetime history of TMD,[53] whereas in the parallel study of individuals with no lifetime history of TMD, trauma history taken at the time of study entry was not predictive of who subsequently developed TMD.[145] Regardless of actual causation, trauma associated with the onset of TMD has always been considered to be a factor likely to increase severity and extend the course of the disorder—that is, trauma as a perpetuating factor. However, the literature regarding this role of trauma is also complex. In a comparison of treatment response between TMD associated with trauma and TMD without trauma, findings have varied from no difference in the treatment outcome, to posttraumatic TMD patients with a decreased response to treatment and requiring more treatment than a nontrauma patient group.[146,147] Collectively, the research suggests that unless a traumatic event has a self-evident relationship to symptom onset, a simple cause–effect relationship may not adequately describe the potential relationship between such events and TMD symptoms. Clearly, more research is needed for this complex relationship.

Although one major factor may be the direct and self-evident cause of acute TMD—for example, a direct blow to the jaw, this is relatively uncommon. More commonly, the initial patient history will either reveal the absence of an identified cause or point to an event as a possible cause that has some ambiguity surrounding it. For example, a commonly stated event prior to symptom onset is third molar extraction; if the event is not described as having traumatic features or if the event occurred sometime before symptom onset, should it be considered a cause of the symptoms? Similarly, another commonly stated event prior to symptom onset is increased stress due to a particular situation; this type of event will often exhibit a long time period before symptoms really manifest, and if so, should it be considered a cause of the symptoms? These are challenging questions to answer in the context of an individual patient. Consequently, the lack of a clear single cause of TMD is notable in the majority of individuals, and in such individuals, TMD is increasingly thought to emerge in response to multiple risk determinants: no one factor by itself is sufficient to cause the disorder, whereas multiple factors increase the risk. A final initiating event may even be relatively minor, but if it occurs in conjunction with other already active determinants, then critical thresholds can be exceeded and symptoms emerge. In other words, multiple factors often come together contributing to the initiation, aggravation, and/or perpetuation of the disorder. Given the available evidence, the factors that have supporting evidence and at least some biological plausibility are, from local to systemic, summarized as follows:

1. Instability of maxillomandibular relationships[148]
2. TMJ hypermobility[149–151]
3. Trauma (e.g., dental procedures, oral intubations for general anesthesia, yawning, hyperextension associated with cervical trauma)[152–158]
4. Parafunctional behaviors (e.g., sleep bruxism, tooth clenching, jaw guarding, lip or cheek biting)[53,145,159–162]
5. Sleep disturbance[163,164]
6. Comorbidity in the form of other rheumatic, musculoskeletal, or pain disorders[165,166]
7. Emotional distress[143,144,167,168]
8. Poor general health and an unhealthy lifestyle[169,170]

The aforementioned factors vary in the strength of both evidence and association with TMD. Each factor can occur, for the most part, along continua defined by magnitude (i.e., weak to strong), frequency (seldom to continuous), and duration (short term to enduring). The actual threshold by which each factor exerts an influence on a given individual is unknown. In a reflexive manner, it would seem that individuals vary in their susceptibility to each factor for its potential to cause problems for the organism. And, each TMD would appear to have its own profile of risk factors. For example, myofascial pain with arthralgia and myofascial pain alone were associated with trauma, clenching, third molar removal, somatization, and female gender.[170] Emerging research will likely provide much better estimates regarding the relative significance of these and other factors.

Epidemiology

Between 65% and 85% of people in the United States experience one or more symptoms of TMD during their lives,

but the symptoms are self-limiting for most individuals and resolve without professional intervention.[171] Incidence of first lifetime onset of TMD appears to be between 2% and 4% per annum.[54,172,173] Although the prevalence of one or more signs of mandibular pain and dysfunction is high in the population, only about 5% to 7% have symptoms severe enough to require treatment.[94,171,174] Among those who develop TMD, approximately 12% experience prolonged pain that results in disability,[171] and more recent estimates indicate that approximately 25% of individuals with acute TMD develop chronic pain in the absence of appropriate intervention.[175] In terms of symptom profile, individuals with TMD are similar to those with headache and back pain with respect to pain intensity, frequency, chronicity, disability, psychosocial distress, and disability.[176,177] These profiles appear to be similar in individuals with TMD across cultures; for example, Asian, Swedish, and American populations with TMD share similar characteristics.[178]

Available evidence indicates that TMDs are most prevalent between the ages of 20 and 40 years and that prevalence then decreases by age 60, after which it decreases substantially. The lower prevalence of TMD in older age groups suggests that the disease course in a significant proportion of individuals with TMD is strongly influenced by situational factors that resolve with aging. TMD in the community occurs at about twice the rate in women as in men, yet women are eight times more common in the clinic population, compared to men. The reason why women make up the majority of patients presenting for treatment is still unclear. Although the natural course of TMD is poorly understood, gender apparently affects the disease course as well.[179] For example, oral contraceptives and estrogen replacement in women older than 40 years substantially increases the risk of developing TMD.[180]

Signs and symptoms of masticatory muscle and TMJ dysfunction are also commonly observed in children and adolescents.[181–183] Among adolescents in Sweden between the ages of 12 and 19 years, 4.2% reported TMD pain, and girls reported TMD pain approximately twice more frequently than boys, 6% compared with 2.7%.[184] Surprisingly, a wide variety of TMD characteristics observed in adults also occur to largely the same extent in children and adolescents. For example, among a group of 40 children aged 10–16 years and presenting with signs and symptoms of TMD, 14 (35%) were diagnosed as having acute reactive depression.[185] Arthrography and computed tomography (CT) were performed on 31 children complaining of TMJ pain and dysfunction; 12 (39%) exhibited disc displacement with reduction, and 17 (55%) exhibited disc displacement without reduction.[186] Among the 29 individuals with internal derangement, causation was attributed to previous injury in 12 individuals. Yet, in a survey of 1000 twelve-year-old children, only 1% had a maximum mouth opening of less than 40 mm, indicating that the norm for expected opening range is established prior to the final growth phase in adolescents. Despite this extent of abnormal findings, only a small proportion of children presented with clinical findings severe enough to warrant treatment.[187]

Classification

Due to the uncertainty about etiology, the present diagnostic classifications of TMD have been based only on signs and symptoms. Substantial evidence is now emerging regarding the myriad factors that predict the first lifetime episode of TMD,[188] and collectively, the evidence indicates that TMD is a complex disease. A complex disease is one that does not follow simple classical etiologic pathways, whereby a single necessary and sufficient etiologic factor exists; instead, epigenetic factors, phenotypic factors, and environmental factors are dynamic and interact over time. Part of this interaction may also include feedback loops, whereby the activity of a particular factor will facilitate its emergence again; for example, stress experience due to poor coping tends to progress in a downward spiral. This type of complexity requires multidimensional assessment and, correspondingly, multiaxial classification. Current perspectives on taxonomy development point to the inadequacy, both scientific and clinical, of classification systems for complex disease developed according to traditional methods. For the future, we envision the merger of genetics, pain medicine, neuroscience, psychology, and bioinformatics as underlying the next major diagnostic system for TMD.[189–193] In addition, we envision that diagnostic systems designed for each domain (jaw, head, back, etc.) will be integrated into one system based on a standard set of rules.[194] Currently, the traditional taxonomic approach based on signs and symptoms will continue to be used and, despite the limitations inherent in that approach, it does have clinical utility. For example, the present validated system[195] minimizes false-positive diagnoses and thereby unnecessary treatment.

In the late 1980s and early 1990s, TMD classification was influenced by several independent developments. The first development emphasized a concise symptom- and sign-based classification system that was developed for use by the practicing clinician.[196,197] The American Academy of Orofacial Pain (AAOP) published a more far-reaching general classification of disorders that affect the cranial bones, TMJs, and masticatory muscles.[198] This classification system was developed by a broad group of experts who applied available knowledge to the development of an acceptable and useful system for clinical practice. The system was considered useful because it included for a given diagnosis all of the clinical characteristics associated with a given disorder and it was inclusive of all disorders a clinician might encounter. By virtue of being inclusive, one intent was to assist clinical decision making. However, this classification system was not assessed for validity, no doubt a function of its very structure. For example, supporting signs in disc disorders that may have additional clinical value were included as "clinical findings that may support the diagnosis." Such ambiguity leads, over time, to unreliable diagnoses. Both the AAOP system and other contemporary classification systems recognized the need for allowing multiple diagnoses to better reflect the zThe above developments, while helpful to clinicians and a clear improvement over prior systems, unfortunately did not

facilitate research. Dworkin and LeResche developed an evaluation and classification system for the most common TMD to enhance clinical research. The Research Diagnostic Criteria for TMD (RDC/TMD) was published as a system "offered to allow standardization and replication of research into the most common forms of muscle and joint-related TMD."[51] The assessment of physical status (Axis I) was described in detail, which provided a means for standardizing data collection and allowing reliable diagnoses as well as comparison of findings across clinical investigators. Because pain transcends a given organ system, a classification system that reflects psychological, behavioral, and social issues is as important as an accurate description of the physical pathology. Consequently, the RDC/TMD classification contained a separate Axis II to assess psychosocial status and pain-related disability. Although the RDC/TMD was designed for research, and thereby less comprehensive than either of the other two systems designed for clinical use (i.e., Clark and coworkers, AAOP), the RDC/TMD permitted far more reliable diagnoses of the disorders the clinician encounters most often. Tension, however, existed between clinical and research settings regarding which system was "best."

The RDC/TMD classification was subsequently assessed in a multicenter study for validation, and initial findings demonstrated areas where the RDC/TMD was good and areas where it could be improved. Extensive efforts to improve the RDC/TMD while retaining the core features described earlier ensued,[201] leading to three parallel publications: a diagnostic criteria for TMD (DC/TMD),[195] an overall taxonomy and draft criteria for the less common TMD,[202] and incorporation of both into the current version of the AAOP guidebook.[203] In summary, a reliable and valid TMD classification system based on signs and symptoms was developed for both clinical and research use. The overall TMD classification is listed in Table 11-1.

Like the RDC/TMD, the new DC/TMD allows, for each individual, multiple TMD diagnoses: several pain diagnoses and, for each joint, pain, disc displacement, degenerative joint disease (DJD), and subluxation diagnoses. See Tables 11-2 and 11-3. The terms used are clearly defined, the clinical examination procedures are completely specified, and the criteria required to meet the diagnosis are specific. The pain diagnoses exhibit excellent sensitivity and specificity. In contrast, the joint disorders, with one exception, exhibit unacceptable sensitivity and specificity based only on clinical assessment. The one exception among the joint disorders is disc displacement without reduction, with limited opening, which does have acceptable sensitivity and specificity from clinical examination procedures.

In clinical practice, it has been generally believed that rigidly adhering to the criteria of a system such as the RDC/TMD may not be possible due to the assumption that the common TMD, for example, exhibit a wide spectrum of signs and symptoms. However, recent evidence indicates that each of the common TMD has reliable characteristics; for the very large majority of patients, the stated criteria clearly define the disorder. The consequence is that the clinician, using the described clinical assessment methods, can reliably and

TABLE 11-1　Taxonomic Classification for Temporomandibular Disorders

I. *Temporomandibular joint disorders*
  1. Joint pain
    A. Arthralgia
    B. Arthritis
  2. Joint disorders
    A. Disc disorders
      1. Disc displacement with reduction
      2. Disc displacement with reduction with intermittent locking
      3. Disc displacement without reduction with limited opening
      4. Disc displacement without reduction without limited opening
    B. Hypomobility disorders other than disc disorders
      1. Adhesions/adherence
      2. Ankylosisa
        a. Fibrousb
        b. Osseous
    C. Hypermobility disorder
      1. Dislocationsa
        a. Subluxationb
        b. Luxation
  3. Joint diseases
    A. Degenerative joint disease
      1. Osteoarthrosis
      2. Osteoarthritis
    B. Systemic arthritides
    C. Condylysis/idiopathic condylar resorption
    D. Osteochondritis dissecans
    E. Ostronecrosis
    F. Neoplasm
    G. Synovial chondromatosis
  4. Fractures
  5. Congenital/developmental disorders
    A. Aplasia
    B. Hypoplasia
    C. Hyperplasia
II. *Masticatory muscle disorders*
  1. Muscle pain
    A. Myalgia
      1. Local myalgia
      2. Myofascial pain
      3. Myofascial pain with referral
    B. Tendonitis
    C. Myositis
    D. Spasm
  2. Contracture
  3. Hypertrophy
  4. Neoplasm
  5. Movement disorders
    A. Orofacial dyskinesia
    B. Oromandibular dystonia
  6. Masticatory muscle pain attributed to systemic/central pain disorders
    A. Fibromyalgia or widespread pain
III. *Headache*
  1. Headache attributed to TMD
IV. *Associated structures*
  1. Coronoid hyperplasia

Abbreviation: TMD, temporomandibular disorder.
Source: Reprinted with permission from *Journal of Oral & Facial Pain and Headache* and *Journal of Oral Rehabilitation.*

validly provide diagnoses for most individuals with TMD pain. Imaging will be required to establish a disc disorder diagnosis such as "disc displacement without reduction." See Table 11-4 for validated imaging criteria. The clinician should recommend diagnostic imaging as part of the assessment when the prognosis or choice of treatment might benefit. The reader is referred to the publication by Schiffman et al. for a full description of the DC/TMD, by Peck et al. for DC for the less common TMD, by DeLeeuw and Klasser for a comprehensive guidebook to evaluation, diagnosis, and treatment, and the website of the International RDC-TMD Consortium Network (http://rdc-tmdinternational.org/) for clinical examination specifications, training video, and all patient assessment instruments.

ASSESSMENT

Although examination methods have been traditionally considered to lack the ability to accurately differentiate individuals with a TMD from those without TMD,[204] recent developments have dramatically changed the diagnostic terrain of TMD. The most valuable aspect of the diagnostic assessment is a thorough history[205]; pain disorder diagnoses rely predominantly on the history, and the diagnosis of some pain disorders, for example, headache, relies exclusively on the history.[206] For some disorders (e.g., headache), the history serves to rule out other forms of pathology; for TMD, the examination is now confirmatory for a pain diagnosis but remains only suggestive for most of the joint disorders. An examination for a particular disorder (e.g., the comprehensive examination of TMD, as described[201]) must be supplemented by examination procedures as needed for a differential diagnosis, for example, ruling out odontogenic causes of regional masticatory system pain. In contrast to the situation 20 years ago when TMD diagnostic tests were not validated or standardized,[197] the clinical tests most needed for the assessment of a person with TMD are now standardized, reliable, and valid.[195,207] In contrast, diagnostic tests such as ultrasonography of joint sounds, thermography, jaw tracking, and EMG, all of which exhibit high measurement reliability and precision, do not offer the assurance of a more accurate diagnosis or better treatment outcomes.[208] These devices were reviewed for their diagnostic value in assessing patients with temporomandibular complaints and were judged 20 years ago to not have the necessary sensitivity and specificity for a valid diagnosis.[205] No additional supporting evidence has emerged over the past several decades. However, claims that they are adjunctive tests must be accompanied by the same evidence as required for any diagnostic test; if an adjunctive test is to be useful, incremental validity must be demonstrated. Incremental validity refers to the ability of an additional test to provide unique information that improves the sensitivity or specificity of the information obtained prior to the additional test. For example, analysis of TMJ synovial fluid is an active area of research but has not yet become a standard procedure in diagnosis or the selection

TABLE 11-2   Diagnostic Criteria for the Most Common Pain-Related Temporomandibular Disorders

Myalgia (ICD-9 729.1)

Description		Pain of muscle origin that is affected by jaw movement, function, or parafunction, and replication of this pain occurs with provocation testing of the masticatory muscles.
Criteria	History	1. Pain[a] in the jaw, temple, in the ear, or in front of ear; and 2. Pain modified with jaw movement, function or parafunction.

	and
	
	Exam
		1. Confirmation[b] of pain location(s) in the temporalis or masseter muscle(s); and
		2. Report of familiar pain[c] in the temporalis or masseter with at least one of the following provocation tests:
		   a. Palpation of the temporalis or masseter muscle(s); or
		   b. Maximum unassisted or assisted opening.

Validity		Sensitivity 0.90; specificity 0.99
Comments		The pain is not better accounted for by another pain diagnosis. Other masticatory muscles may be examined as dictated by clinical circumstances but the sensitivity and specificity for this diagnosis based on these findings has not been established.

Myofascial Pain with Referral (ICD-9 729.1)

Description		Pain of muscle origin as described for myalgia with referral of pain beyond the boundary of the masticatory muscle(s) being examined when using the myofascial examination protocol. Myofascial pain with referral is a subtype of myalgia.
Criteria	History	1. Pain[a] in the jaw, temple, in the ear, or in front of ear; and 2. Pain modified with jaw movement, function, or parafunction.
	and Exam	1. Confirmation[b] of pain location(s) in the temporalis or masseter muscle(s); and 2. Report of familiar pain[c] with palpation of the temporalis or masseter muscle(s); and 3. Report of pain at a site beyond the boundary of the muscle(s) being palpated.
Validity		Sensitivity 0.86; specificity 0.98
Comments		The pain is not better accounted for by another pain diagnosis. Other masticatory muscles may be examined as dictated by clinical circumstances, but the sensitivity and specificity for this diagnosis based on these findings has not been established.

Arthralgia (ICD-9 524.62)

Description		Pain of joint origin that is affected by jaw movement, function, or parafunction, and replication of this pain occurs with provocation testing of the TMJ.
Criteria	History	1. Pain[a] in the jaw, temple, in the ear, or in front of ear; and 2. Pain modified with jaw movement, function, or parafunction.

	and
	
	Exam
		1. Confirmation[b] of pain location in the area of the TMJ(s); and
		2. Report of familiar pain[c] in the TMJ with at least one of the following provocation tests:
		   a. Palpation of the lateral pole or around the lateral pole; or
		   b. Maximum unassisted or assisted opening, right or left lateral movements, or protrusive movements.

Validity		Sensitivity 0.89; specificity 0.98
Comments		The pain is not better accounted for by another pain diagnosis.

Headache attributed to TMD (ICD-9 339[d])

Description		Headache in the temple area secondary to pain-related TMD[e] that is affected by jaw movement, function, or parafunction, and replication of this headache occurs with provocation testing of the masticatory system.
Criteria	History	1. Headache1 of any type in the temple; and 2. Headache modified with jaw movement, function, or parafunction.

	and
	
	Exam
		1. Confirmation[b] of headache location in the area of the temporalis muscle(s); and
		2. Report of familiar headache[c] in the temple area with at least one of the following provocation tests:
		   a. Palpation of the temporalis muscle(s); or
		   b. Maximum unassisted or assisted opening, right or left lateral movements, or protrusive movements.

Validity		Sensitivity 0.89; specificity 0.87
Comments		The headache is not better accounted for by another headache diagnosis.

Abbreviations: ICD, *International Classification of Diseases*; TMD, temporomandibular disorder. TMJ, temporomandibular joint.

[a]The time frame for assessing pain including headache is in "the last 30 days" since the stated sensitivity and specificity of these criteria were established using this time frame. Although the specific time frame can be dependent on the context in which the pain complaint is being assessed, the validity of this diagnosis based on different time frames has not been established.

[b]The examiner must identify with the patient all anatomical locations that they have experienced pain in the last 30 days. For a given diagnosis, the location of pain induced by the specified provocation test(s) must be in an anatomical structure consistent with that diagnosis.

[c]"Familiar pain" or "familiar headache" is based on patient report that the pain induced by the specified provocation test(s) has replicated the pain that the patient has experienced in the time frame of interest, which is usually the last 30 days. "Familiar pain" is pain that is similar or like the patient's pain complaint.

[d]The ICD-9 has not established a specific code for *Headache attributed to TMD;* ICD-9 339 is for *"other headache syndromes."* If a primary headache is present (*e.g., tension type headache*), then the headache can be classified according to the primary headache type.

[e]A diagnosis of painful TMD (e.g., myalgia, myofascial pain with referral, or TMJ arthralgia) is derived using valid diagnostic criteria.

Source: Reprinted by permission of J Oral & Facial Pain and Headache

TABLE 11-3 Diagnostic Criteria for the Most Common Intra-articular Temporomandibular Disorders

Disc Displacement With Reduction (ICD-9 524.63)

Description		An intra-capsular biomechanical disorder involving the condyle–disc complex. In the closed mouth position, the disc is in an anterior position relative to the condylar head, and the disc reduces upon opening of the mouth. Medial and lateral displacement of the disc may also be present. Clicking, popping, or snapping noises may occur with disc reduction. A history of prior locking in the closed position coupled with interference in mastication precludes this diagnosis.
Criteria	History	1. In the last 30 days,[a] any TMJ noise(s) present with jaw movement or function, or 2. Patient report of any noise present during the exam.
	and	
	Exam	1. Clicking, popping and/or snapping noise detected during both opening and closing, with palpation during at least one of three repetitions of jaw opening and closing; or 2. Clicking, popping, and/or snapping noise detected with palpation during at least one of three repetitions of opening or closing; and 3. Clicking, popping, and/or snapping noise detected with palpation during at least one of three repetitions of right or left lateral movements, or protrusive movements.
Validity		Without imaging: sensitivity 0.34; specificity 0.92. Imaging is the reference standard for this diagnosis.
Imaging		When this diagnosis needs to be confirmed, then TMJ MRI criteria[252] are positive for both of the following: 1. In the maximum intercuspal position, the posterior band of the disc is located anterior to the 11:30 position and the intermediate zone of the disc is anterior to the condylar head; and 2. On full opening, the intermediate zone of the disc is located between the condylar head and the articular eminence.

Disc Displacement With Reduction With Intermittent Locking (ICD-9 524.63)

Description		An intracapsular biomechanical disorder involving the condyle–disc complex. In the closed mouth position, the disc is in an anterior position relative to the condylar head, and the disc intermittently reduces with opening of the mouth. When the disc does not reduce with opening of the mouth, intermittent limited mandibular opening occurs. When limited opening occurs, a maneuver may be needed to unlock the TMJ. Medial and lateral displacement of the disc may also be present. Clicking, popping, or snapping noises may occur with disc reduction.
Criteria	History	In the last 30 days,[a] any TMJ noise(s) present with jaw movement or function; or Patient report of any noise present during the exam.
	and	and In the last 30 days,[a] jaw locks with limited mouth opening, even for a moment, and then unlocks.
	Exam	Same as specified for Disc Displacement with Reduction. Although not required, when this disorder is present clinically, examination is positive for inability to open to a normal amount, even momentarily, without the clinician or patient performing a specific manipulative maneuver.
Validity		Without imaging: sensitivity 0.38; specificity 0.98. Imaging is the reference standard for this diagnosis.
Imaging		When this diagnosis needs to be confirmed, then the imaging criteria[252] are the same as for disc displacement with reduction if intermittent locking is not present at the time of imaging. If locking occurs during imaging, then an imaging-based diagnosis of disc displacement without reduction will be rendered and clinical confirmation of reversion to intermittent locking is needed.

Disc Displacement Without Reduction With Limited Opening (ICD-9 524.63)

Description		An intracapsular biomechanical disorder involving the condyle–disc complex. In the closed mouth position, the disc is in an anterior position relative to the condylar head, and the disc does not reduce with opening of the mouth. Medial and lateral displacement of the disc may also be present. This disorder is associated with persistent limited mandibular opening that does not resolve with the clinician or patient performing a specific manipulative maneuver. This is also referred to as "closed lock."
Criteria	History and Exam	1. Jaw lock or catch so that the mouth would not open all the way; and 2. Limitation in jaw opening severe enough to limit jaw opening and interfere with ability to eat. Maximum assisted opening (passive stretch) <40 mm including vertical incisal overlap.
Validity		Without imaging: sensitivity 0.80; specificity 0.97. Imaging is the reference standard for this diagnosis.
Imaging		When this diagnosis needs to be confirmed, then TMJ MRI criteria[252] are positive for both of the following: 1. In the maximum intercuspal position, the posterior band of the disc is located anterior to the 11:30 position and the intermediate zone of the disc is anterior to the condylar head, and 2. On full opening, the intermediate zone of the disc is located anterior to the condylar head. Note: Maximum assisted opening of <40 mm is determined clinically.
Footnote		Presence of TMJ noise (e.g., click with full opening) does not exclude this diagnosis.

TABLE 11-3 Diagnostic Criteria for the Most Common Intra-articular Temporomandibular Disorders (*Continued*)

Disc Displacement Without Reduction Without Limited Opening (ICD-9 524.63)

	Description	An intracapsular biomechanical disorder involving the condyle–disc complex. In the closed mouth position, the disc is in an anterior relative the condylar head and the disc does not reduce with opening of the mouth. Medial and lateral displacement of the disc may also be present. This disorder is not associated with limited mandibular opening.
Criteria	History and Exam	Same as specified for Disc Displacement Without Reduction With Limited Opening.
		Maximum assisted opening (passive stretch) >40 mm including vertical incisal overlap.
	Validity	Without imaging: sensitivity 0.54; specificity 0.79. Imaging is the reference standard for this diagnosis.
	Imaging	When this diagnosis needs to be confirmed, then TMJ MRI criteria[252] are the same as for disc displacement without reduction with limited opening. Note: Maximum assisted opening of ≥40 mm is determined clinically.
	Footnote	Presence of TMJ noise (e.g., click with full opening) does not exclude this diagnosis.

Degenerative Joint Disease (ICD-9 715.18)

	Description	A degenerative disorder involving the joint characterized by deterioration of articular tissue with concomitant osseous changes in the condyle and/or articular eminence.
Criteria	History and Exam	1. In the last 30 days[a] any TMJ noise(s) present with jaw movement or function; or 2. Patient report of any noise present during the exam. At least one of the following must be present: 1. Crepitus detected with palpation during opening, closing, lateral, or protrusive movements.
	Validity	Without imaging: sensitivity 0.55; specificity 0.61. Imaging is the reference standard for this diagnosis.
	Imaging	When this disorder is present, then TMJ CT criteria[252] are positive for at least one of the following: Subchondral cyst(s), erosion(s), generalized sclerosis, or osteophyte(s). Note: Flattening and/or cortical sclerosis are considered indeterminant findings for DJD and may represent normal variation, aging, remodeling, or a precursor to frank DJD.

Subluxation (ICD-9 830.1)

	Description	A hypermobility disorder involving the disc-condyle complex and the articular eminence: In the open mouth position, the disc-condyle complex is positioned anterior to the articular eminence and is unable to return to a normal closed mouth position without a specific manipulative maneuver. The duration of dislocation may be momentary or prolonged. When prolonged the patient may need the assistance of the clinician to reduce the dislocation and normalize jaw movement; this is referred to as luxation. This disorder is also referred to as "open lock".
12	History and Exam	1. In last 30 days,[a] jaw locking or catching in a wide open mouth position, even for a moment, so could not close from the wide open position; and 2. Inability to close the mouth without a specific manipulative maneuver. Although no exam findings are required, when this disorder is present clinically, examination is positive for inability to return to a normal closed mouth position without the patient performing a specific manipulative maneuver.
	Validity	Without imaging and based only on history: sensitivity 0.98; specificity 1.00.
	Imaging	When this disorder is present, then imaging criteria are positive for the condyle positioned beyond the height of the articular eminence.

Abbreviations: CT, computed tomography; DJD, degenerative joint disease; ICD, *International Classification of Diseases*; MRI, magnetic resonance imaging; TMD, temporomandibular disorder; TMJ, temporomandibular joint.

[a]The time frame for assessing selected biomechanical intra-articular disorders is in "the last 30 days" since the stated sensitivity and specificity of these criteria was established using this time frame. Although the specific time frame can be dependent on the context in which the pain complaint is being assessed, the validity of this diagnosis based on different time frames has not been established.

Source: Reprinted with permission from *Journal of Oral & Facial Pain and Headache.*

of treatment. These tests require sophisticated instrumentation that would increase health care costs to the patient that, for the present, are not justified.

Consequently, history, clinical examination, and imaging when indicated remain the recommended diagnostic approach for most patients.[109,210] Diagnostic imaging is of value in selected conditions but not as a routine part of a standard assessment. Diagnostic imaging can increase accuracy in the detection of internal derangements[211] and abnormalities of articular bone.[212] The clinical meaningfulness of such tests, however, must be determined prior to ordering the test; a special test should be preceded by a clinical hypothesis (differential diagnosis) that the test will be able to answer, and the clinical hypothesis should be related to a particular course of action. For example, if treatment for what appears to be a painful recurrent mechanical joint problem will proceed in one

TABLE 11-4 Imaging-Based Diagnosis of Soft- and Hard-Tissue TMJ Disorders

Disorder	Criteria
Disc diagnosis for the TMJ, based on MRI[a]	
Normal	Disc location is normal on closed and open mouth images.
Disc displacement with reduction	Disc location is displaced on closed mouth images but normal on open mouth images
Disc displacement without reduction	Disc location is displaced on both closed mouth and open mouth images.
Indeterminate	Disc location is not clearly normal or displaced in the closed mouth view
Disc not visible	Neither signal intensity nor outlines make it possible to define a structure as the disc in the closed mouth and open mouth views. If the images are of adequate quality in visualizing other structures in the TMJ, then this finding is interpreted to indicate a deterioration of the disc, which is associated with advanced disc pathology.
Osseous diagnoses for the TMJ, based on CT[b]	
Normal	a. Normal relative size of the condylar head; and b. No subcortical sclerosis or articular surface flattening; and c. No deformation due to subcortical cyst, surface erosion, osteophyte, or generalized sclerosis.

Indeterminate for osteoarthritis	a. Normal relative size of the condylar head; and
	b. No deformation due to subcortical cyst, surface erosion, osteophyte, or generalized sclerosis; and
	c. Either of:
	  i. Subcortical sclerosis; or
	  ii. Articular surface flattening

Osteoarthritis	a. Deformation due to subcortical cyst, surface erosion, osteophyte, or generalized sclerosis

Abbreviations: CT, computed tomography; MRI, magnetic resonance imaging; TMJ, temporomandibular joint.
[a]Adapted from Table IV, Ahmad et al.[252]
[b]Adapted from Table II, Ahmad et al.[252]

direction if the problem is a disc displacement but in another direction if the disc is normal, then imaging would be well justified. If, on the other hand, both treatments for this stated example would be pursued, each for four to six weeks and with no or minimal risk of adverse effects, then the treatment trial without imaging may be more prudent, thereby not unnecessarily expending health-care resources. A painful clicking joint should be treated, regardless of whether the problem is due to an internal derangement.[68] If the choice of treatment depends on a more accurate diagnosis, then imaging would be indicated.

Similarly, other tests should be ordered when the differential diagnosis warrants further diagnostic exploration. Examples follow. Facial pain similar to the pain of a TMD may be associated with serious undetected disease. Muscle or joint pain may be a secondary feature of another disease or may mimic a TMD. A diagnosis of a more serious condition may be missed or delayed.[213,214] Severe throbbing temporal pain associated with a palpable nodular temporal artery, increasingly severe headache associated with nausea and vomiting, and documented altered sensation or hearing loss are all indications of serious disease requiring timely diagnosis and management. Table 11-5 lists, for many TMDs, characteristics which, if present and clinically significant, may require focused assessment in conjunction with the standard evaluation. In short, TMD diagnosis (and management) requires ongoing use of clinical decision-making skills.

History

The most common symptom related to TMD is pain, and it is the overwhelming reason why people seek care. Pain may be present at rest, may be continuous or intermittent, and characteristically increases with jaw functions such as chewing or opening wide. Reported pain among community cases is somewhat lower in intensity compared to clinic cases,[163] suggesting that processes that affect pain amplification or pain modulation differ across time, and eventually a community case will decide to seek care. Other chief complaints in relation to seeking care for a TMD include restricted jaw movement (independent of pain), painful or loud TMJ clicking or crepitus, and jaw locking.

Pain severity or intensity is a subjective measure provided by the patient and can be rated in several ways.[215] A rating scale can be either numeric or verbal. A numeric scale asks the patient to rate pain by identifying a number, typically between 0 and 10, that best reflects pain intensity. Verbal descriptors such as no pain, mild pain, moderate pain, and severe pain can also provide an equally valid assessment. If an estimate with greater precision is needed, a visual analogue scale (VAS) can provide an estimate that has high sensitivity to change and better independence when using repeated measures. A VAS uses a 10-cm line anchored on the left side with the descriptor of "no pain" and on the right an extreme descriptor such as "the worst pain ever experienced." The patient is asked to mark his or her pain intensity by placing a mark on the line, and the score is obtained by measuring

TABLE 11-5 Selected TM Disorders and Supplemental Characteristics

Disorder	Characteristics
Deviation in form Note: Painless mechanical dysfunction or altered function due to irregularities or aberrations in the form of intracapsular soft and hard articular tissues. Does not require intervention.	• Complaint of faulty or compromised joint mechanics • Reproducible joint noise, usually at the same position during opening and closing • Radiographic evidence of structural bony abnormality or loss of normal shape
Disc displacement with reduction Note: Clinical significance is related to pain associated with the noise, to mechanical locking, or interference in mastication or other functional activities.	• Pain (when present) is directly associated with joint noise during movement • Clinical assessment is often unreliable due to poor stability of the noise • Mandibular deviation during opening or closing coinciding with a click
Disc displacement without reduction	• History of clicking that stopped when the locking began • Pain clearly localized to the TMJ precipitated by function, when acute • Marked limited mandibular opening when acute • Uncorrected deviation to the affected side on opening and marked limited laterotrusion to the contralateral side when acute • Localized pain precipitated by forced mouth opening • Ipsilateral hyperocclusion, when acute
Synovitis or capsulitis Note: Inflammation of the synovial lining or loading of capsular lining. Difficult to clearly differentiate from arthralgia.	• Localized pain at rest exacerbated by function, especially with superior and posterior joint loading • Limited range of motion secondary to pain • T2-weighted MRI may show joint fluid
Osteoarthrosis Note: Degenerative noninflammatory condition of the joint, characterized by structural changes of joint surfaces secondary to excessive strain on the remodeling mechanism. Distinguish from osteoarthritis, which is a secondary inflammatory condition. Both osteoarthrosis and osteoarthritis are subsumed within degenerative joint disease in the DC/TMD.	• Crepitus on examination • Absence of joint pain
Myofascial pain Note: Is a regional disorder, distinguishing it from fibromyalgia. When the pain is local to the area of stimulation, this disorder is termed myalgia in the DC/TMD to note the presence of hyperalgesia without spreading, referral, or autonomic reactions. The clinical significance of these additional characteristics is with differential diagnosis; the requirement for specific treatments when referral is present remains untested but anecdotally rich.	• Taut bands and trigger points are hallmark characteristics but exhibit only fair examiner reliability • Reduction in pain with local muscle anesthetic injection or vapocoolant spray, coupled with stretch of the muscle
Protective muscle splinting Note: Restricted or guarded mandibular movement due to co-contraction of muscles as a means of avoiding pain caused by movement of the parts. Should be distinguished from fear-avoidance behavior by ruling out local nociceptive source, by either history or examination.	• Severe pain with function but not at rest • Marked limited range of motion (generally, pain-free opening and maximal unassisted opening will be similar), and opening is only minimally responsive to attempted passive stretch (maximal assisted opening) initially, and active resistance to further attempts at stretch can be noted
Contracture Note: Chronic resistance of a muscle to passive stretch as a result of fibrosis of the supporting tendon, ligaments, or muscle fibers themselves.	• Limited range of motion • Unyielding firmness on passive stretch • History of trauma or infection

Abbreviations: DC/TMD, diagnostic criteria for temporomandibular disorder; MRI, magnetic resonance imaging; TMJ, temporomandibular joint.
Source: Adapted from McNeill.[198]

from the left end to the mark. Any of these rating scales can be used to assess current, minimum and maximum in the past, or average pain ratings. For rating prior periods (past minimum and maximum, average), a time span is required; common ones are last 30 days, last 3 months, and last 6 months. The DC/TMD explicitly uses the "last 30 days" for two reasons: memory for prior pain is better with shorter time periods, and in general, the last 30 days is sufficient for an active chief complaint of pain to reference concurrent symptom states. In addition, an empirical limitation is that the Validation Project dataset (from which the DC/TMD validity statistics were derived) was based, for these 2 reasons, on a 30-day period as well. However, that time period should be modified for a given patient as circumstances dictate; the most common is the patient presenting with a chief complaint of a prior pain bout that has resolved but now wants a diagnosis and recommendations for prevention or management in the future. The time period of interest is accordingly modified for the particular history questions, for assessing pain intensity, and, later in the examination, for assessing familiar pain from any positive provocation findings.

As defined by the DC/TMD, regional masticatory system pain should be influenced by mandibular function, or an alternative diagnosis should be suspected. Table 11-2 indicates that pain aggravated by function is a criterion for a diagnosis of either myalgia or arthralgia. Mandibular functions shown to reliably affect myofascial pain include chewing hard or tough food, opening the mouth or moving the jaw, jaw behaviors such as clenching, and other jaw activities such as talking or yawning. Table 11-6 lists questions that are useful (as part of the history) for assessing mandibular function.

A pain drawing that contains the full body is helpful in defining the extent of pain; the recording of other body regions helps identify patients who have multiple sites of pain, which suggests a more systemic or generalized disorder. A pain drawing completed at initial evaluation may also be used to assess treatment progress of the TMD. Following the initial evaluation, a pain diary can be a useful tool for identifying events or times of increased and decreased pain;

it may also serve to identify behaviors or situations that are contributing to the persistence of symptoms.[216]

A range of other symptoms is sometimes reported in association with a TMD and include dizziness; nausea; ear symptoms of fullness, ringing, diminished hearing, or, especially common, earache; facial swelling; redness of the eyes; nasal congestion; altered sensation such as numbness, tingling, or burning; altered vision; muscle twitching; altered occlusion; and jaw misalignment. The presence of these symptoms is sometimes used to substantiate the diagnosis of a TMD; the risk of circular reasoning should be considered, however. None of these symptoms define a TMD, as currently conceptualized, and most of the aforementioned symptoms not only are observed in relation to other disorders but also are considered functional in nature—a reported change in the body without observable characteristics. An example of a functional symptom is facial swelling: reported by TMD patients but seldom observed clinically. If the patient history is consistent with criteria for, say, masticatory myalgia and the only clinical examination finding is palpation pain but without replication, should the presence of any of these associated symptoms be used to therefore substantiate a TMD diagnosis, given their oft association with TMD? Consider the following example: A particular patient meets criteria for myalgia of the masticatory muscles and that patient also complains of earache accompanied by negative ear examination for local nociceptive source. Given the negative ear examination, is the earache necessarily then related to the myalgia? If adequate testing is performed to determine the presence of the myalgia subtype of myofascial pain with referral and the earache is thereby replicated, then the earache is likely secondary to TMD (at least based on available clinical data).

TABLE 11-6   Assessment of TMD History[a]
Where is the pain located? Is there pain in any other areas of the body?
When did the pain first begin? What has been the pattern over time; have there been notable periods of remission, or notable periods of exacerbation, and what were the circumstances?
How often do episodes (or, if pain is continuous: flare-ups) occur, duration, temporal pattern to the bouts (time of day, day of week), and how managed?
When is pain at its worst (morning [on awakening] or as day progresses [toward evening])?
What aggravates the pain (e.g., when using the jaw such as opening wide, yawning, chewing, speaking, or swallowing; stress or deadlines; postural positions)?
What alleviates the pain (e.g., rest, analgesic, holding the jaw rigid in specific positions)?
(If other pains such as headaches, earaches, neckache, or cheek pain are present] When did the other pain(s) begin, did they worsen when the jaw pain worsened, did they respond to treatment for the jaw pain?
Is there pain or thermal sensitivity in the teeth? Does biting on any teeth cause pain?
Do jaw joint noises (clicking, popping, grinding, or crepitus) occur when moving the jaw or when chewing?
Does the jaw ever hesitate, get stuck, or lock when trying to open or when trying to close from a wide-open position?
Does jaw motion feel restricted?
Has the jaw ever been injured?
Has there been an abrupt change in the way the teeth meet or fit together? Does the bite feel "off" or uncomfortable?
What treatments have been provided? What was the outcome? What was the compliance with treatment requirements?

[a]Miscellaneous symptoms sometimes reported in association with TMD related include: dizziness; nausea; fullness or ringing in the ears; diminished hearing; facial swelling; redness of the eyes; nasal congestion; altered sensation such as numbness, tingling, or burning; altered vision; and muscle twitching.

If adequate testing for referral mechanisms fails to replicate the earache, the appropriate interpretation of findings would be, given available clinical data, that the earache is likely a result of some other nociceptive source. Similarly, a positive history of myalgia but without sufficient clinical findings to meet criteria should not then incorporate the earache as an additional finding to substantiate the diagnosis. The problem list was designed for exactly this situation: elevate the findings to as high a level of clinical conceptualization as warranted by the data, but no higher; a problem list entry could be a diagnosis, or it could be a symptom description, based on available data. The patient can be informed that the additional symptoms (or complaints) may be secondary to the TMD, but verification through other diagnostic testing or parallel treatment response is needed.

Behavioral Assessment

Assessment should result in a diagnosis of a TMD and an evaluation of the person; the latter should be composed, at least, of assessment for psychological distress and pain-related disability. Some TMDs evolve into a chronic pain disorder, resulting in psychological distress and disruption of interpersonal relationships and an inability to perform daily activities, including work. Psychosocial factors are considered more important in predicting treatment outcome than physical factors.[130,217] The lack of a direct relationship between physical pathology and intensity of pain and subsequent disability emphasizes the need to assess the psychological and behavioral effects of the disorder to better understand (1) the reported pain and not assume that as-yet undetected physical pathology is responsible, (2) anticipated barriers to successful treatment, and (3) the potential for relapse.

Complex disease is characterized by multiple manifestations, and although the physical disorder is conveniently captured with a diagnosis, often more than one diagnosis co-exists. In addition, contributing factors—a rubric of things that may not have the status of "diagnosis" but nevertheless impact on the disorder or the person—should be identified and noted. Consequently, a problem list of diagnoses and all contributing factors associated with the TMD should be developed.[218] Contributing factors may affect the symptom control and the long-term success of treatment. Table 11-7 lists multiple potential contributing factors, organized by domain, often reported in the pain research literature.[218] No one health-care professional can be expected to manage the physical pathology of the temporomandibular structures and all of the various lifestyle, emotional, cognitive, and social issues that may affect the individual with chronic pain. Chronic TMDs are best managed in a multidisciplinary or interdisciplinary setting.

The number of lifestyle, emotional, cognitive, and social issues can seem daunting in terms of the complexity that could occur. However, that complexity can be somewhat simplified. Rudy et al. classified TMD patients based on psychosocial and behavioral parameters into three unique subgroups: dysfunctional, interpersonally distressed, and adaptive copers.[219] TMD patients have been found to have psychosocial and behavioral profiles similar to those of back pain patients and headache patients, the two comparison groups used in that research.[176,220] These findings not only highlight the substantial overlap in important phenotypic characteristics exhibited by people with TMD, compared to other disorders, but also point to a relatively straightforward conceptualization of person functioning. Interventions targeting pain and psychological distress are of equal importance to the pathophysiology of temporomandibular structures in managing a chronic TMD. Turner et al. showed that TMD patients who catastrophized had higher scores on clinical examination, more activity interference, and greater health-care use regarding the TMD than TMD patients who did not.[221] Clinical evaluations that focus only on physical findings have a high risk for tagging the individual with a more serious physical diagnosis to explain the pain, on the wrong assumption that the extent of physical findings is directly indicated by the extent of reported pain, and this leads, in turn, to more aggressive treatment.

Psychosocial assessment should provide the clinician with an appreciation of the extent to which pain and dysfunction interfere with or diminish the patient's quality of life. A measure of the severity of limitation in activity will provide a reflection of the magnitude of the condition.[222,223] For example, Von Korff et al. reported that approximately 16% of TMD patients experienced significant activity limitation compared with approximately 3% of healthy individuals.[224]

A systematic method of evaluating for relevant psychosocial factors is necessary to efficiently and reliably assess these constructs. A construct is an attribute that is not objectively measureable, such as pain. And dentists, like all health

TABLE 11-7 Problem List of Domains and Specific Factors Contributing to Persistence and Symptom Amplification in Temporomandibular Disorders

Lifestyle	Emotional Factors	Cognitive Factors	Biologic Factors	Social Factors
Diet	Prolonged anger	Negative self-image	Other illnesses	Work stresses
Sleep	Anxiety	Unrealistic expectations	Past trauma	Unemployment
Alcohol	Excessive worry	Inadequate coping	Past jaw surgery	Family stresses
Smoking	Depression			Litigation
Overwork				Financial difficulty

Source: Adapted from Fricton.[218]

professionals, do not accurately assess constructs such as pain-related psychosocial factors in TMD patients when relying solely on interview skills.[225] Therefore, the DC/TMD recommends either a short set of instruments for screening for the most critical constructs, or a comprehensive set of instruments that provides better reliability of two critical constructs (depression, anxiety) as well as assessment of other domains. The reader is referred to the study by Schiffman et al.[195] for further discussion of the screening versus comprehensive approach and to the Consortium website for the assessment instruments (http://rdc-tmdinternational.org/).

It is difficult to determine the presence of active oral parafunctional behaviors. Direct interview will produce a high rate of false negatives due to the unconscious character of the target behavior. Patients are often unaware of tooth clenching or other behaviors associated with jaw hyperactivity during the waking hours. There are several methods that can improve this assessment. Use of a checklist that describes the common types of parafunctional behaviors appears to trigger intentional access to memory via the patient deciding to "test" each listed behavior to determine whether the behavior feels familiar (i.e., I must do this one) or not familiar (i.e., I probably don't do that one). Field monitoring of daytime jaw activity, reports by friends and coworkers of observed behaviors (e.g., clenching with associated observable masseter contraction), and reports by a bedroom partner of tooth-grinding noises during sleep are helpful. Finally, teaching the therapeutic jaw relaxation posture will often uncover the otherwise denied behaviors via recognition, typically by both patient and clinician, that the target therapeutic behavior is very challenging.

Clinical characteristics that are indicators of the need for expert psychological evaluation of a person with TMD include the following[226]:

1. The persistence of pain beyond the expected healing time and no clear physical explanation is identified
2. Inconsistent or poor response to usual treatments
3. Significant psychological distress, as revealed via self-report instruments and confirmed through clinical interview
4. Disability greatly exceeds what is expected on the basis of the clinical findings
5. Excessive or inappropriate use of health-care services, including tests and treatments
6. Prolonged use or excessive reliance on opioids, sedatives, minor tranquilizers antianxiety medications, or alcohol for pain control.

Physical Examination

There is no single pathognomonic physical finding that can be relied on to establish a TMD diagnosis. Historically, and as described previously for the AAOP Guidelines approach, a set of possible physical findings was listed for each type of TMD, but in the absence of clear data regarding what constituted a given problem, the diagnostic rubric was based on the presence of any of the findings. By extension, the more

such findings occur, either the more severe the disorder or the more certain the diagnosis? For the common TMDs, as initiated by the RDC/TMD and now validly described in the DC/TMD,[195] each disorder is defined by, or constituted of, specific characteristics, and all of them must be present for the putative diagnosis to correctly identify the problem. For the uncommon TMD,[202] each disorder is less strongly defined by the stated characteristics, simply because there are, at present, little data to empirically characterize each of those disorders. Distinguishing clinical decision making when we have sufficient data versus when we do not is a critical function of being an expert: knowing when and when not to use the rules.[227] In recognizing that the DC/TMD is not 100% accurate, the clinician must consequently know when exceptions to the rules are optimally invoked. Taking a history prior to the examination has a seminal role: serve as sufficient information by which the clinician has developed clinical hypotheses (i.e., differential diagnoses) and then knows what to look for in the examination. Unexpected findings should be appropriately followed up. A standardized examination procedure (as defined by the DC/TMD and available as a full set of specifications[52] from the Consortium Network and as a video for examiner training[228]) simplifies the task of the examiner: a reference frame emerging from consistent examinations better identifies unexpected findings. In general, the clinical features that distinguish patients from controls are decreased passive mouth opening,[229] and masticatory muscle pain provoked by maximal mouth opening and especially palpation.[230] In contrast, the literature has described an uncorrected deviation on maximum mouth opening as characteristic of acute disc displacements without reduction[171]; although common in the individual with an acute joint, such deviation is less reliable than assumed, and in chronic conditions, deviations are far more variable as both a finding and, when present, due to a disc displacement versus unilateral contractures or especially guarding behavior. Among all individuals with a TMD, masticatory muscle tenderness on palpation (see Figure 11-10) is the most consistent examination feature present in TMDs.[199] Components of the physical examination that are discussed in this section are summarized in Table 11-8.

Mandibular Range of Motion

Mandibular range of motion (ROM) comprises three procedures in the vertical plane and three procedures in the horizontal plane. Measurements of vertical ROM are generally far more useful clinically, compared to those of the horizontal ROM. The three vertical ROM procedures include maximal opening without pain, as wide as possible with pain, and after opening with clinician assistance; each of these is operationalized accordingly. These measures are termed in the DC/TMD pain-free opening, maximal unassisted opening, and maximal assisted opening, respectively. Vertical measurements are made with a ruler between opposing maxillary and mandibular incisal edges; the measurement can

TABLE 11-8 Physical Examination of the Masticatory System for TMD

Examination Component	Observations
Inspection	Facial asymmetry, swelling, and masseter and temporal muscle hypertrophy Opening pattern (corrected and uncorrected deviations, uncoordinated movements, limitations)
General palpation	Parotid and submandibular areas Lymph nodes
Mandibular ROM	Vertical jaw movements: pain-free opening, maximal opening with pain, and maximal assisted opening Horizontal jaw movements: lateral and protrusive movements Pain provocation, location, and replication are assessed with each movement
TMJ noises	Any noise produced by vertical or horizontal movements, as reported by the patient and as identified as to type by the examiner (e.g., click vs. crepitus), any pain and replication with noise, and any locking
Palpation for pain	Masticatory muscles Temporomandibular joints
Additional provocation tests as indicated	Static pain test (no mandibular movement to pressure) Dynamic pain test (active mandibular movement against resistance) Pain in the joints or muscles with tooth clenching or unilateral biting Reproduction of symptoms with chewing (wax, sugarless gum)
Other systems	Cervical ROM Palpation for pain of neck muscles and accessory muscles of mastication Neurologic screening, sensory testing
Intraoral examination	Signs of parafunction: cheek or lip biting, accentuated linea alba, occlusal wear Dental pathology: tooth mobility, percussion, thermal testing, fractures of enamel and restorations General soft tissue: scalloped tongue borders, parotid gland patency

Abbreviations: TMD, temporomandibular disorder; TMJ, temporomandibular joint; ROM, range of motion.

be corrected by the extent of vertical overlap of the teeth, if a measure of full mobility is desired. Mouth opening with assistance is accomplished by applying mild to moderate pressure against the upper and lower incisors with the thumb and index finger. All three of these measures exhibit excellent reliability (Intra-class correlation coefficient (ICC) > 0.90) among trained examiners and thereby are excellent measures for monitoring status of the disorder over time.

The three horizontal ROM procedures include right and left lateral, and protrusive movements of the mandible, and all are executed with the teeth slightly separated and "as far as possible, even if painful." Lateral movement measurements are made with the ruler measuring the displacement of the lower midline from the maxillary midline and adding or subtracting the lower-midline displacement at the start of movement. Protrusive movement measurement is made by adding the horizontal distance between the upper and the lower central incisors during full closure and adding the distance the lower incisors travel beyond the upper incisors. All three of these measures exhibit acceptable reliability (ICC > 0.80) among trained examiners; because the range is relatively constricted, compared to vertical range, these measures are less useful clinically.

Normal maximum mouth opening is ≥40 mm. In a study of 1160 adults, the mean maximum mouth opening was 52.8 mm (with a range of 38.7–67.2 mm) for men and 48.3 mm (with a range of 36.7–60.4 mm) for women.[231] Normal lateral and protrusive movements are ≥7 mm.[232-234] Measures of the mandibular range of movement are similarly performed in children. The mean maximum mouth opening

recorded in 75 boys and 75 girls aged 6 years was 44.8 mm.[235] Similar values (a mean maximum opening of 43.9 mm, with a range of 32–64 mm) were observed in 189 individuals with a mean age of 10 years.[236] The means of left, right, and protrusive maximal movements were each approximately 8 mm.

ROM assessments have two types of diagnostic significance. The first is that following each of the tests (with the exclusion of pain-free opening), the patient is asked whether the movement caused pain, and if so, to point to the area of pain and to indicate whether that pain replicated pain of complaint (see "Palpation for Pain" for further explanation). The second is by using maximal assisted opening for distinguishing the subtype of with versus without limitation, for the disorder of disc displacement without reduction. More generally, observed findings from the three vertical measures, and sometimes the three horizontal measures, are evaluated in relation to the history and other clinical findings: These are the ROM measures expected or unexpected?

There are several noncriterion-based uses of the ROM measures, particularly when comparing findings across all three procedures. Passive stretching (mouth opening with assistance) is a technique that may assist in differentiating limitation due to a muscle or joint problem, but clinical judgment is needed to interpret. In performing maximal assisted opening, the examiner can evaluate the quality of resistance at the end of the movement. Muscle restrictions are associated with a soft end feel and should result in an increase of >5 mm beyond the maximal unassisted opening. Joint disorders such as acute nonreducing disc displacements are described as having a hard end feel and characteristically limit assisted opening to <5 mm. However, limited movement in response to attempted assisted opening can be due to two other causes: muscle contracture and guarding behavior by the patient. The latter can be especially meaningful when considering other biobehavioral factors, such as fear avoidance or kinesophobia,[237,238] for the direction of treatment. The difficulty in operationalizing guarding behavior for reliable assessment, however, is noteworthy.

TMJ Noises

Palpation of the TMJs is first performed to detect irregularities during condylar movement, described as clicking or crepitus. The lateral pole of the condyle is most accessible for palpation during mandibular movements. In addition to joint noise, there may be palpable differences in the form of the condyle comparing right with left. A condyle that does not translate may not be palpable during mouth opening and closing. This may be a finding associated with an ADD without reduction. A click that occurs on opening and closing and is eliminated by bringing the mandible into a protrusive position before opening is most often associated with ADD with reduction, but this maneuver for eliminating reciprocal clicks does not assure a diagnosis of ADD with reduction.[207]

Palpation for Pain

Although pain is reported in response to ROM procedures among individuals with TMD, pain is elicited at a much higher rate from palpation of the masticatory muscles and TMJs. Because palpation is a discrete stimulus, the response can be separated into reported pain local to the area of stimulation, pain spreading beyond the area of stimulation, and pain perceived in a different area (i.e., referred pain to another structure). These categories of pain response are particularly relevant for muscle tissue, but spreading and referral also occur, albeit at a much lower rate, in response to palpation of the TMJs. A critical aspect of the DC/TMD examination is to inquire whether provoked pain (whether from ROM or palpation procedures) is "familiar" to the person's usual pain (i.e., the examination procedure has provoked replication of the pain of complaint); this specific finding is part of the criteria for the pain-related diagnoses. Another level of pain replication from palpation (but not ROM) is whether spreading or referral response is also familiar, and although familiar spreading or referral are not, at this time, part of the criterion for the respective subtypes of myalgia, inquiring of the patient during the palpation examination is recommended. Differential diagnosis (e.g., TMD vs. odontogenic pain) sometimes depends critically on elicitation of referral response, its replication of pain of complaint, and the specificity in identifying the target tissue of the referral.

Many methods for palpation are advocated, and parameters that affect palpation, as a procedure, include amount of loading to the tissue, surface area of the loading, duration of loading, and where the loading is applied. The RDC/TMD guidelines recommended 2 lbs of loading for the muscles and 1 lb of loading for the joint, as based on population and clinical samples,[51] and an extensive range of research has generally supported this parameter. The RDC/TMD Validation Project assessed the extent of loading and determined that the loading to muscle should be at least 2 lbs (which was simplified to at least 1.0 kg for international purposes), but that 1 lb to the joint needed to be supplemented by an additional dynamic palpation around the condyle, which should be at least 2 lbs (i.e., 1.0 kg) for valid diagnosis of arthralgia. Palpation is usually specified in terms of pressure (e.g., 2 lbs pressure) but calibration is usually in terms of loading (e.g., 2 lbs, as measured by some type of scale) when a fingertip is used to palpate. In recognition that fingertips used for palpation vary considerably in surface area, the indicated loadings will ultimately vary in terms of pressure to the peripheral receptors in the patient's tissue, and thereby introduce error in the palpation procedures. Hence, the DC/TMD specified that loading should be "at least" to the stated criterion. The alternative, for better standardization, is to use a simple algometer that will provide consistent pressure (loading/square area); one example is the Palpeter, which is easy to use and has excellent reliability.[239] Population and clinical samples, as well as the reference standard procedures used in the Validation Project, appear to provide sufficient empirical support for the stated magnitudes of palpation in terms of maximizing true positives and negatives and minimizing false positives and negatives. Although the use of fingertips introduces a source of error into palpation, classification does not appear to be compromised by this problem. During loading, the muscles should be in a noncontracted state. As further explained below, muscles may be placed on a stretch prior to palpation.

As an alternative to standardized loading, some clinicians have recommended that palpation loading be normalized to the individual's pain threshold: establish a baseline (to serve as a general guide or reference) by squeezing a muscle between the index finger and thumb or by loading the center of the forehead or thumbnail to gauge the minimum extent that becomes painful. Although perhaps intuitively sensible, this approach has two problems: circularity through the assumption that the individually tailored threshold for painful loading is "normal" for that person and thereby sidestepping the considerable problem of widespread body tenderness as either a comorbid condition or simply as a reflection of central sensitization,[240] and likely poor reliability in applying the individually tailored loading (which will vary from patient to patient) during the next phase of the examination.

In contrast to palpation loading, duration of palpation is more nebulous in terms of empirical support. Patients report that fast palpation (e.g., loading of the tissue for less than one second) is too quick to feel confident about the response (e.g., painful yes or no?), whereas a stimulus that is at least two seconds in duration (including ramp up and down) appears to be sufficient to respond to. Referred pain phenomena, in contrast, seldom occur in relation to a stimulus as short as two seconds; the minimum duration to elicit referral is unknown, and a stimulus at least 10 seconds in duration has been recommended.[241] The DC/TMD attempts to provide a starting point for further research by requiring the stimulus to be at least five seconds in duration if referral is of interest; this stimulus duration is sufficient for at least a reliable diagnosis of referred pain. Clinically, if referral phenomena are suspected and are important for, say, differential diagnosis, then extending the palpation duration to 10 (or more) seconds would be justified, as based on reported observations; in addition, as Travell and Simons indicate, placing the muscle on a stretch prior to the palpation can reportedly facilitate elicitation of referral.[241] Whether increasing the magnitude of the loading is as important as the duration of the loading (to trigger temporal summation) is unknown. The necessary stimulus duration for elicitation of spreading phenomena is unknown, but because the mechanism is likely similar to that underlying referral, the same five seconds duration is recommended at this time.

Where to palpate is another parameter with much clinical lore. For simple myalgia, it seems that a sampling approach (e.g., divide the temporalis and masseter muscles into three zones each, and distribute three palpation sites across each zone) to the underlying tissue is sufficient. Critically, this method is reliable.[242] For eliciting referral phenomena, in contrast, the finding of "bands" and "trigger point nodules" is advocated, yet this method is only marginally reliable and then only with extensive training.[243] One problem affecting reliability in the examination of trigger points is that their location is not stable across relatively short periods of time.[244] Abnormalities such as trigger points and taut bands in muscle have not been sufficiently characterized in the masticatory muscles to enable the clinician to reliably distinguish these sites anatomically from normal muscle. If there is a particular clinical question (e.g., differential diagnosis) that needs to be answered with regard to presence of referred pain, then the most reliable method of detection is probably to sample the muscle in a systematic manner: divide the muscle into enough zones and each zone into enough palpation sites, such that the areas of stimulation via the fingertip are contiguous. Only this will be sufficiently reliable. If subtyping myalgia into local myalgia, spreading, or referral is important primarily for adequate capture of the stated symptom descriptions, then the standard sampling method of the DC/TMD will likely be sufficient: palpate temporalis and masseter muscles at 1 kg loading, for five seconds at each of nine palpation sites within each muscle.

Related to where to palpate each muscle is which muscle to palpate. The muscles of mastication include not only the temporalis and masseter, as the muscles most commonly associated with location of pain complaints, but also additional muscles of the two pterygoids, the hyoids, and the digastrics on each side. Yet, in terms of incremental validity, little is often gained by palpating these additional muscles versus the information gained from initially examining the

temporalis and masseter muscles. The lateral pterygoid is in a position that does not allow access for adequate palpation examination even though there are examination protocols and descriptions for palpating this muscle.[245] Hence, the DC/TMD requires palpation of temporalis and masseter, and palpation of the other muscles is optional and should be determined by the nature of the chief complaint.

Where to palpate the TMJ for pain, and its interpretation, has a range of perspectives. Traditionally, palpating the lateral pole and through the ear canal was believed to be sufficient to provoke pain associated with the capsular ligament. However, the Validation Project determined that lateral pole palpation alone was insufficient and that the false-negative rate of arthralgia diagnosis was too high. Consequently, a circumpolar dynamic palpation, with loading at a minimum of 1.0 kg, was recommended; the full circle around the lateral pole should take approximately five seconds. The clinical literature states that pain elicited in one part of the joint is indicative of a posterior capsulitis, while pain from another part of the joint is indicative of a synovitis, and so on; although such differentiations may be possible in principle, the available empirical data only identify arthralgia as a reliable diagnosis.

The severity of the pain provoked from palpation can be assessed (e.g., using a 4-point verbal scale of none, mild, moderate, or severe or by using a 0–10 numeric rating scale), but this type of finely granular response has not, in the research literature, been shown to be more useful than the simple binary report of pain yes versus no with respect to disorder classification or overall severity of the condition. For monitoring pain sensitivity of a single muscle, the severity ratings could help. The report of pain is followed by the question of whether the provoked pain is familiar—whether it replicates the pain of complaint. Because pain sensitivity varies across individuals, some patients even after treatment may well report that palpation still induces pain, but if the patient no longer has pain, then the pain replication question will be negative, which would be essential for assessing treatment progress.

Provocation Tests

Provocation tests are designed to elicit the pain of complaint. Assessing jaw ROM and palpation for pain are types of provocation tests. Since pain is often aggravated by jaw use according to the patient's history, an appropriate clinical test would assess function; a positive response adds support for a diagnosis of TMD even though functional tests such as clenching the teeth (i.e., involving sustained muscle contraction) did not provide additional information that improved sensitivity and specificity for a TMD compared to a nonpain control.[207] In contrast, functional tests improved diagnostic validity of TMD versus a comparison pain condition of odontogenic pain.[246] Consequently, including functional testing when the history or findings from the standardized clinical examination yield an ambiguous diagnostic outcome is very sensible and represents good practice. Four types of functional tests have been recommended and which continue to be sensible at least in terms of face validity. These tests include static muscle contraction test, dynamic muscle contraction test, bilateral loading via clench, and unilateral loading via clench.

The static pain test involves having the mandible slightly open and remaining in one position while the patient resists the slowly increasing manual force applied by the examiner in each of right lateral, left lateral, upward, and downward directions. If the mandible remains in a static position during the test, the muscles will be subjected to activation, and any pain should be specific to muscle. However, the ability of this test to discriminate between muscle and joint pain is not known. In the dynamic test, the mandible slowly moves against resistance, in each of the same directions as for the static test; any provoked pain should be specific to the joint. As for the static test, however, the specificity of response in muscle versus joint does not seem to accord with the putative principle. Nevertheless, dynamic and static tests exhibited excellent specificity: 84% of dental pain cases were negative for these tests.[245] Neither of the static or dynamic tests added incremental validity to the provocation tests of ROM and palpation procedures for a myalgia diagnosis.[207]

Clenching the teeth or chewing wax or gum is expected to load the joints and muscles. According to one study, approximately 50% of TMD patients who chewed half of a leaf of 28-gauge casting wax for three minutes reported increased pain, but 30% reported decreased pain, and 20% reported no change.[247] This is not surprising, given the report by many patients who participate in examiner reliability studies: it is not unusual that despite the considerable provocation of painful muscles by palpation across four examiners, the repeated maximal opening and other jaw movements become therapeutic for some of the subjects. In the clinic, some patients will clearly report that chewing gum improves their pain (and they are seeking consultation primarily to rule out a more complex disorder; they will henceforth use gum more frequently). Biting on unilateral cotton roll or tongue blade has been recommended for many years as an important diagnostic test; however, fewer experts seem to utilize these tests currently, no doubt due to the lack of any published sensitivity and specificity as well as the difficulty in simple interpretation of the findings. Nevertheless, it is a simple test to perform and likely especially useful (despite the interpretation ambiguity) when the patient complaint points to unilateral chewing as the proximal trigger for a pain bout.

Assessment of Consequences or Correlates of Parafunctional Behaviors

Each of tooth wear, soft tissue changes (evidence of lip or cheek chewing, an accentuated occlusal line, and scalloped tongue borders), and hypertrophic jaw-closing muscles has been suggested as an objective means of assessing for parafunctional behaviors (or muscle hyperactivity). The face validity, with regard to pathophysiology or cause-and-effect with parafunction, varies across these different types of findings, with tooth wear and muscle hypertrophy seemingly

high and scalloped tongue borders seemingly lower. However, the interexaminer reliability of assessing tooth wear is fair at best,[248] and the other assessments also exhibit poor reliability, thereby decreasing the clinical utility of these procedures.

Cervical Region: ROM and Palpation of Muscles

Patients with TMDs often have musculoskeletal problems in other regions, particularly the neck.[249,250] The upper cervical somatosensory nerves send branches that synapse in the spinal trigeminal nucleus, which is one proposed mechanism to explain referral of pain from the neck to the orofacial region. The sternocleidomastoid and trapezius muscles are often part of cervical muscle disorders and may refer pain to the face and head. The cervical area and the masticatory area, therefore, share several linkages: mechanical, motor control, and afferent.

Consequently, the cervical region warrants at least a screening examination. Mobility is assessed during flexion, extension, rotation, and side-bend of the neck. Using an observational method, the head should, in general, flex to the extent that the chin can touch the sternum, extend until the face is parallel to the ceiling, rotate 90° to either direction, and side-bend 45° to either direction. Methods, including ruler or goniometry, can be used for quantitative assessment, but utility of higher precision should be considered if the goal is screening. For palpation, the trapezius, levator scapula, and suboccipital muscle groups seem adequate for screening; other cervical muscle groups of sternocleidomastoid (SCM), splenius capitis, and semispinalis capitis can be included. The inclusion of examination and treatment of the cervical area, in relation to a TMD, is strongly advocated in the clinical literature, but there are little data at this time to draw on. One substantially limiting factor is that research has been largely nonreplicable due to no universally held evaluation and diagnostic standard (e.g., a hypothetical RDC/cervical). One cervical parameter that seems to have sufficient agreement regarding assessment method is forward head posture; however, there is no reliable relationship between static head posture and TMD.[251] Some type of RDC for cervical musculoskeletal pain problems is urgently needed to have a better basic classification, from which science can move forward.

Diagnostic Imaging

TMJs can be examined by using plain-film radiography, plain-film tomography, arthrography, CT, MR, single-photon emission CT, and radioisotope scanning (Figures 11-11 and 11-12). Imaging should be part of the assessment whenever any of the following are present: history or clinical findings suggest a progressive pathologic condition of the TMJs, recent injury, sensory or motor abnormality, severe restriction in mandibular motion, nonresponse to usual treatment for a joint condition, differential diagnosis dictating change in treatment direction, or acute alterations of the occlusion. The most frequent abnormalities that are imaged in TMD patients are disc displacements and degenerative changes of the articular bones. Acceptable and valid parameters and interpretation

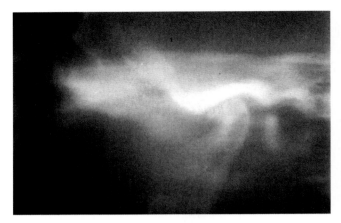

FIGURE 11.11 Temporomandibular joint tomogram displaying flattening of the condylar head in degenerative joint disease.

for using MR and CT have been established and were recently updated.[252] For the majority of TMDs, however, the information from diagnostic imaging has not proven to be important for directing treatment, predicting treatment outcome, and determining long-term prognosis. Consequently, imaging should be ordered only when a clinical hypothesis can be answered by incorporating such information.

A large variation exists in condylar position as observed in plain-film radiographic and tomographic studies, making the condyle–fossa relationship of little value in the diagnosis or treatment of TMD.[253] No differences were found in joint-space narrowing in the centric occlusion position in symptomatic and asymptomatic patients by transcranial plain-film radiography and tomography.[254,255] Using plain films (such as transcranial radiography) to determine condylar position or using the condylar position on these films to infer disc position is not recommended.[254–256]

CT is the imaging of choice to document osteodegenerative joint disease. CT comprises multiple detector computed tomography (MDCT) and cone-beam computed tomography and both are considered equally valid although MDCT appears to have greater resolving power for distinguishing type of tissue at the pixel level.[257,258] CT provides detail for bony abnormalities and is an appropriate study when considering ankylosis, fractures, tumors of bone, and DJD.

An MR is the method of choice for establishing alterations in articular disc form and position in closed and open mouth positions (Figure 11-13). MR studies in asymptomatic volunteers have shown disc position abnormalities in approximately one-third of subjects.[259] With the use of T2-weighted MR, a correlation between joint pain and joint effusion has been suggested, but the results are conflicting.[260–262] TMJ effusion is associated with an elevated concentration of synovial fluid proteins, including proinflammatory cytokines, but the ability to confirm the presence or absence of synovitis in the joint has not been established.[263] It is still not possible to predict the presence of pain based on MR findings. Individual features on MR of internal derangement, osteoarthrosis, effusion, and bone marrow

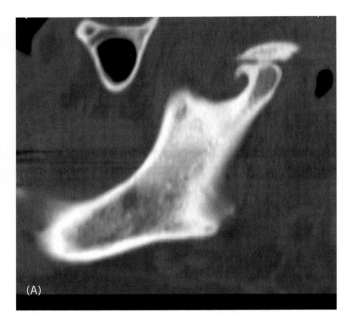

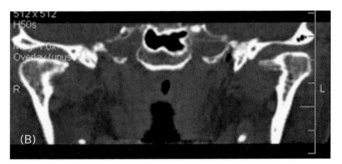

FIGURE 11-12 Sagittal (A) and coronal (B) CT images demonstrating flattening and beaking of the mandibular condyles in a patient with degenerative joint disease.

edema are not predictive of TMJ pain, but when these features occur together, an increased risk of TMJ pain has been observed.[264]

Radioisotope scanning for detecting increases in metabolic activity has been used to detect condylar hyperplasia. Bone scanning is a sensitive indicator of metabolic bone activity and will show similar activity in a joint that is undergoing physiologic remodeling as well. Scintigraphy is a sensitive test but is not specific for TMJ disease. Bone scintigraphy in combination with other imaging and clinical findings (including findings on periodic examinations) is usually effective in diagnosing continued condylar change due to hyperplasia.

Diagnostic Local Anesthetic Nerve Blocks

Injections of anesthetics into the TMJ or selected masticatory muscles may help confirm a differential diagnosis. Immediate elimination of or a significant decrease in pain and improved jaw motion should be considered a positive test result. In situations in which a joint procedure (such as surgical intervention) is being considered, local anesthetic injection of the joint may confirm the joint as the source of pain.

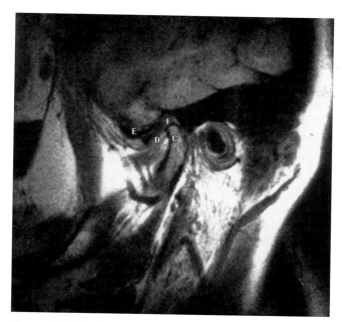

Figure 11-13 An MR image of an anterior disc displacement in the closed mouth position. The disc and critical bone image darker than surrounding tissue. C, condyle; D, disc; E, eminence; F, fossa; MRI, magnetic resonance imaging.

Kopp has described a technique for TMJ injection.[265] Injecting trigger points or tender areas of muscle should eliminate pain from the site and should also eliminate referred pain associated with the injected trigger point.[241] These tests, like all others, require interpretation in the context of all the diagnostic information since a positive result does not ensure a specific diagnosis.

PREDICTION OF CHRONICITY

Although most TMD patients respond, at least in part, to nonsurgical management that can be provided or coordinated by a dentist, a substantial number of individuals with TMD evolve into a chronic musculoskeletal pain disorder that results in significant disability. With chronic TMD comes great psychological distress, disruption of normal daily activities, and ongoing access to healthcare resources. Predicting which individual who is likely to become chronic is important to provide alternative or additional interventions, earlier in the scope of treatment. Early treatment that addresses biobehavioral factors appears to decrease the likelihood of acute pain becoming chronic,[266] but the overall risk factors for the transition from acute to chronic are as yet not known for TMD. Patient histories suggest that most individuals with acute TMD do not immediately seek care; instead, they wait for weeks or perhaps months for it to resolve on its own, much as one might with a flu, the common cold, or a joint sprain. Consequently, in clinical settings, most patients with TMD have already either begun the transition to having chronic pain or already have chronic pain, increasing the

importance of utilizing comprehensive treatment models routinely for all patients with TMD.

Chronic pain has been traditionally defined in three different ways: pain that extends beyond a certain period; pain that persists beyond the time of usual healing; or pain that does not respond to usual treatment. When using the time period criterion, typically six months is selected,[267] and one rationale for using a time period is that the commonly recognized behavioral or social changes that accompany persisting pain have their own latency period. Some changes, such as worry, appear early, while financial and work-related problems tend to occur later. Whether depression is a cause of chronic pain or a consequence has been rigorously debated for many years; current evidence from the OPPERA project indicate that it is probably both: depression appears to be a significant risk factor for developing chronicity, and once pain becomes chronic, the CNS burden of ongoing pain leads to alterations at multiple levels in the CNS, and the state of depression is one manifestation, in terms of behavior and mood, of the CNS changes. Persisting depression only further exacerbates persistent pain; two obvious direct mechanisms for how depression worsens pain include dampening of descending modulatory systems and the impact on motivation and intentional behavior, necessary for adherence to any treatment that involves the development and use of self-regulatory skills. This type of recursive involvement of a factor, such as depression, readily illustrates the complex disease character of TMD. In recognition of the range of morbidity that can accompany chronic pain, shorter time periods for defining chronic pain have been suggested, for example, three months. The neurophysiological evidence indicates that three months, however, is probably still too long, in that sustained bouts of nociception over the period of a minute can be sufficient to initiate sensitization that persists for hours.[268] The other two definitions of chronic pain—pain persisting beyond healing period or pain nonresponsive to usual treatments—are very sensible and useful for patient discussions regarding treatment recommendations.

The available evidence has consistently indicated that across pain conditions, psychosocial factors have been better predictors of treatment outcome compared to physical findings, diagnosis, or how much treatment was pursued.[269] In addition, psychological factors seem to be more important than peripheral injury or physical disease of the masticatory system in predicting chronicity.[175,270–272] Epker et al. found that the combination of high pain intensity (as measured by the Graded Chronic Pain Scale) and a myofascial pain diagnosis was predictive of persisting TMD symptoms in their study sample.[266]

From a clinical perspective, any patient who comes for a consultation should be considered for chronicity. Although the traditional definitions remain useful for initial clinical assessment, a dynamic conception of chronic pain is emerging, one far more relevant for the here-and-now reality of a new clinical consultation: what is the likelihood that this patient, today, will still have pain six months from now? And, a small constellation of variables can provide that prediction: pain intensity, pain-related disability, depressive symptoms, number of pain sites, and pain days.

Comorbidity with widespread musculoskeletal pain is likely to contribute toward the development of a chronic TMD. Individuals with fibromyalgia, a chronic widespread musculoskeletal pain disorder, have a significantly higher frequency of masticatory myofascial pain than the general population.[273,274] The presence of pain in other body sites in individuals with a TMD pain diagnosis is high[53] and may indicate that a musculoskeletal problem affecting the jaws is part of a more generalized pain disorder. In a follow-up study on TMD patients, the group that self-reported the coexistence of fibromyalgia had a higher frequency of chronic TMD symptoms.[275]

Overall, chronicity is a function of multiple factors, and focusing primarily on seemingly obvious ones such as trauma (with a presumed biological impact) to the exclusion of other, more abstract ones such as depression, anxiety, or pain-related disability is to contribute to the patient's pain chronicity.

GENERAL PRINCIPLES OF TREATING TEMPOROMANDIBULAR DISORDERS

The most important feature of TMD is, in general, pain, and consequently, pain is the most important patient-reported outcome (PRO) with regard to whether a treatment was helpful. Other common and important features that can serve as a target for a PRO include inability to eat hard-to-chew foods, restricted range of mandibular movement, and mechanical joint problems that interfere with function. Chronic TMD pain (like all chronic pain) results in psychological, behavioral, and social disturbances, and although these characteristics may be a dominant part of the overall symptom presentation, they seem to be less often regarded as important by the patient with TMD. However, patient education into how biobehavioral factors are linked to their pain can make such variables more relevant as indicators for specific treatment types as well as important PRO measures.

Treatment goals for TMDs can be divided into two levels, both of which are equally relevant. The first level includes control pain, improve mandibular motion, and restore function as close to normal as possible. The second level concerns impact to the person by the pain, methods to restore general functioning, and strategies for relapse prevention. The relative importance and timing of implementing each level is determined by many patient-specific factors and available health-care expertise. Explanatory models[276,277] held by each of patient and clinician will affect how treatments oriented to each of the two levels will proceed; when pain is the dominant symptom (as it typically is at the first consultation), addressing the pain directly is generally the first priority, and success in reducing or better controlling the pain helps patients incorporate other treatment recommendations that may exist outside their explanatory model

of illness. Unless an obvious and clearly causal source of nociception is identified for the TMD pain and which warrants invasive therapy (e.g., chronic pulpitis presenting as a TMD), initial treatment should focus on noninvasive therapies that also have desirable nonspecific effects and that readily permit the integration of therapies across the two levels described here.

Clinical case studies and a variety of randomized controlled trials suggest that the majority of individuals with TMD respond to conservative noninvasive therapy, making the use of invasive procedures unwarranted as initial therapy. No one treatment has emerged as superior, although many of the treatments studied have shown beneficial effect.[278] The symptoms of TMD tend to be intermittent, fluctuate over time, and are often self-limiting.[279–281] A five-year follow-up indicated that TMD patients could be allocated roughly into thirds: remission, recurring symptoms, or persisting symptoms.[282] The process of deciding whether to treat and how aggressively to treat should take into account the course of symptoms. Patients who are improving at the time of assessment may require a minimum of care and follow-up compared with the individual whose symptoms are becoming progressively more severe and disabling.

The variations in types of treatment recommended by dentists have been explained by the gap between published information in the medical and dental literature and individual dentist's beliefs and attitudes.[276,283] Yet, because the different types of TMD treatment appear to have more or less equivalent efficacy, the treatment effect may be nonspecific and related more to the therapeutic relationship established between therapist and patient than to the specific attributes of the treatment.[284] These factors further support the use of noninvasive reversible therapies for managing TMD.

Management, not cure, is the guiding principle for selecting and deciding when, if at all, to escalate treatment of TMD. Widely known and generally accepted clinical observations are highly informative. Patients with irreversible anatomic abnormalities such as disc disorders are nevertheless able to regain pain-free jaw function.[285,286] Decreased pain and improved physical findings are not directly related.[217,287] The presence of joint noises and deviations from the ideal in occlusion, in maxillomandibular relationships, and in the morphology of bony structures such as the condyle are relatively common in the general population. Evidence indicating prophylactic treatment of these anatomic abnormalities when no pain, impairment of function, or disability exists is lacking. Rather, treatment should be based on the severity of pain and disability and should be directed toward those factors that are considered important in initiating, aggravating, or perpetuating the disorder.

Episodes of pain and dysfunction may recur even after successful symptom control. Reinjury or factors that contributed to earlier episodes of symptoms may be responsible. Recurrence should not be considered a treatment failure and therefore indicate the need to escalate treatment; rather it is more prudent to first consider the initiation of previous treatment that was successful. Myogenous disorders appear to relapse more often and therefore require retreatment more frequently than do articular disorders.[288]

For the smaller group of patients in whom TMD progresses to a chronic pain disorder, treatment becomes more complex. These patients may still benefit from local therapies; however, it is essential for the provider to more carefully consider the need for more comprehensive management to address the emotional and behavioral disabilities that result from chronic pain. Drug therapy of chronic pain is becoming increasingly complex, requiring knowledge and experience that are not common in general dental practice. These patients are often at risk for unnecessary investigations or treatments that may be harmful and that may further complicate their problems.[289,290] Persistence of pain does not necessarily indicate progressive disease; one task for the clinician is to monitor for possible disease progression (and thereby reassure the patient), while simultaneously holding the reins on a management treatment model.

A National Institutes of Health conference on TMD therapy, while now somewhat dated, produced the following conclusions, which remain worth considering[291]:

1. Significant problems exist with present diagnostic classifications because these classifications are based on signs and symptoms rather than etiology.
2. No consensus has been developed regarding which TMD problems should be treated and when and how they should be treated.
3. The preponderance of the data does not support the superiority of any method for initial management, and the superiority of such methods to placebo controls or to no treatment controls remains undetermined.
4. Because most individuals will experience the improvement or relief of symptoms with conservative treatment, the majority of TMD patients should be initially managed with noninvasive and reversible therapies.
5. The efficacy of most treatment approaches for TMD is unknown because most have not been adequately evaluated in long-term studies and because virtually none have been studied in randomized controlled group trials.
6. Therapies that permanently alter the patient's occlusion cannot be recommended on the basis of current data.
7. Surgical intervention should be considered for the small percentage of patients with persistent and significant pain and dysfunction who show evidence of pathology or evidence that an internal derangement of the TMJ is the source of their pain and dysfunction and for whom more conservative treatment has failed.
8. Relaxation and cognitive-behavioral therapies (CBTs) are effective approaches to managing chronic pain.

Referral to a Pain Specialist

Many patients with TMD respond to usual treatments oriented toward symptom reduction, improvement of jaw mobility, and restoration of normal physical jaw function. Such treatment is appropriately managed by dental professionals. More severe myofascial pain or presence of comorbid cervical problems warrants the inclusion of physiotherapists. For patients who have depression, anxiety, comorbid pain disorders, multiple nonspecific physical symptoms, or pain-related disability, psychologists are helpful. Other health-care professionals become important for conditions such as neuropathic pain or simultaneous migraine headache (neurologist), or for multiple joints with osteoarthritis (rheumatologist). Some patients may be more appropriately managed by a pain specialist within a setting of a multidisciplinary pain clinic. This may be indicated when (1) the disability greatly exceeds what is expected on the basis of physical findings, (2) the patient makes excessive demands for tests and treatments that are not indicated, (3) the patient displays significant psychological distress (e.g., depression), (4) the patient displays aberrant behavior, such as continual nonadherence to treatment, or (5) the patient is unable to sufficiently control significant contributing environmental factors such as family reaction to the patient's illness or persistent problems in illness behavior.

SPECIFIC DISORDERS AND THEIR MANAGEMENT

The majority of patients likely to present in a dental practice with a complaint of temporomandibular pain and dysfunction can be broadly categorized into muscle disorders, articular disc disorders, and disorders affecting the articular bones. The most common muscle disorder is myalgia (as per the DC/TMD; also commonly referred to as myofascial pain that remains localized to the hyperalgesic tissue upon provocation). This pain is not associated with an identifiable anatomic muscle abnormality.

Intracapsular disorders affecting the TMJ are divided into two broad categories: articular disc disorders and DJD. Either may be present without causing symptoms or impairment. It is important for the clinician treating patients with TMD to distinguish clinically significant disorders that require therapy from incidental findings in a patient with facial pain from other causes. TMJ abnormalities are often discovered on routine examination and may not require treatment. The need for treatment is largely based on the level of pain and dysfunction and the progression of symptoms. The discovery of an anatomic abnormality such as a longstanding joint noise that is otherwise asymptomatic and consistent with a disc displacement is usually not treated given what is currently known about the longitudinal course of such disorders and the currently available treatments. Diagnostic imaging using MR has identified disc displacements in about 30% of individuals who do not have temporomandibular symptoms or a TMD requiring treatment.[292]

Myalgia and Myofascial Pain of the Masticatory Muscles

The terms most commonly used for muscle pain produced on palpation are myalgia or *myofascial pain*. The DC/TMD considers myalgia as the general disorder for muscle pain, and local myalgia and myofascial pain are subtypes of myalgia. Local myalgia refers to pain that remains local to the provoked muscle, and it contrasts with *myofascial pain* that can be associated with either spreading or radiating of the pain within the muscle or referral to a different structure when the muscle is stimulated during palpation.[195,202] Understanding the pathophysiology associated with muscle pain is still a challenge for further research. Since treatment cannot yet be designed to address a particular cause, multiple therapies for controlling symptoms and restoring range of movement and jaw function are usually combined in a management plan.[203] These therapies are more effective when used together than when used alone.[200,293–296] Given the complex disease character of TMD, it may be that even when etiology is better understood, the multimodal approaches to treatment currently used for any pain condition may still be the primary form of treatment for TMD.

Most of the research on the natural course of this disorder suggests that for most individuals, symptoms are intermittent and usually do not progress to chronic pain and disability. The dentist is the appropriate clinician to first conduct a comprehensive history and examination and thereby provide a differential diagnosis; management of these patients then logically follows. The principles of treatment provided here are based on a generally favorable prognosis and an appreciation that only a small number of clinically controlled trials exist indicating the superiority, predictability, and safety of the respective treatments. The literature suggests that many treatments have some beneficial effect; moreover, the literature suggests that the treatment effect may be nonspecific and not directly related to the particular treatment. Surgery for a chronic muscle pain disorder has no value.

Priority should be given to treatments that have the following characteristics: relatively accessible, not prohibitive due to expense, safe, and reversible. Treatments with these characteristics include education, self-care, physical therapy, intraoral appliance therapy, short-term pharmacotherapy, behavioral therapy, and relaxation techniques (Table 11-9). Evidence suggests that combining treatments produces a better outcome.[297] Despite evidence clearly to the contrary, occlusal therapy continues to be recommended by some clinicians as an initial treatment or as a requirement to prevent recurrent symptoms. Research does not support occlusal abnormalities as a significant etiologic factor,[298] and also it does not support the use of occlusal treatment (e.g., occlusal adjustment) for TMD.[299,300] The evaluation of occlusion and correction of occlusal abnormalities are an important part of dental practice but should not be a standard treatment for TMDs.

Education and Information

A source of great anxiety for patients is the possibility that their condition is progressive and degenerative and will lead to greater pain and disability in the future. Patients may have sought prior consultations from other physicians and dentists who were not able to establish a diagnosis or explain the nature of the problem. This often leads to fears of a more catastrophic problem, such as a brain tumor or other

TABLE 11-9 Initial Treatment of Myofascial Pain	
Treatment Component	**Description**
Education	Explanation of the diagnosis and treatment Reassurance about the generally good prognosis for recovery and natural course Explanation of patient's and doctor's roles in therapy Information to enable patient to perform self-care
Self-care	Control parafunctional oral behaviors (e.g., tooth clenching, chewing gum, bracing the jaw) Provide information on jaw care associated with daily activities
Physical therapy	Education regarding biomechanics of jaw, neck, and head posture and integrated movement patterns Passive modalities (heat and cold therapy, ultrasound, laser, and TENS) for pain Passive stretching and range of motion exercises Posture therapy sufficient to regain a neutral zone General exercise and conditioning program
Intraoral appliance therapy	Cover all the teeth on the arch the appliance is seated on Adjust to achieve simultaneous contact against opposing teeth Adjust to a stable comfortable mandibular posture Does not alter mandibular position Use during sleep and rely on behavioral methods for waking hours
Pharmacotherapy	NSAIDs, acetaminophen, muscle relaxants, antianxiety agents, tricyclic antidepressants
Behavioral/relaxation techniques	Relaxation therapy Hypnosis Biofeedback Cognitive-behavioral therapy

Abbreviations: NSAIDs, nonsteroidal anti-inflammatory drugs; TENS, transcutaneous electrical nerve stimulation.

life-threatening disease. Explaining the nature of the pain, its source, and the varied nature of the symptoms that may occur is an important part of treatment to reduce anxiety that results in an amplification of pain and increased disability. Education is the basis for self-care activities that patients must perform for symptom control as well as longer term rehabilitation. Successful patient education requires enough time in an unhurried environment for the dentist to provide information and to allow the patient to express his or her concerns and to ask questions. This interaction is the basis for the therapeutic relationship. Education and information provide the patient with an understanding of the condition and the ability to perform activities and make choices that have a direct effect on the symptoms. The patient has to participate in developing strategies to avoid stresses that aggravate symptoms or interfere with the ability to manage therapy.

Self-Management

Self-management consists of a range of activities that are synergistic in their effectiveness. The core activities include muscle stretching, use of thermal agents, avoidance of strain or overuse while chewing, and parafunctional behavior control (see "Parafunctional Behavior Control"). Muscle stretching, for most patients, should be performed 2–3 times each day; about 10 repetitions seem sufficient. Stretching should be performed within the limits of pain threshold—that is, in a comfort zone; excessive stretching elicits a stretch-reflex, which causes simultaneous activation of alpha-motor neurons, undermining the efficacy of the stretching. The mouth-opening and mouth-closing phases of stretching should be monitored to insure that the jaw moves in a straight line at a steady rate. Monitoring is best achieved by the patient using a mirror (as an inexpensive form of biofeedback) and watching the movement of the jaw. An alternative form of this variant on stretching is to maintain the tongue in contact with the palate to control mouth-opening in terms of both encouraging primarily rotational movement of the TMJ as well as limiting the overall opening extent; both aspects are sometimes strategically implemented when painful popping is interfering with full stretching. A three-month study of treatment consisting of education only or education plus a home physical therapy program found that education plus home physical therapy was more effective.[301]

Thermal agents consist of the application of moist heat to the affected areas for 15–20 minutes twice daily, as well as ice packs for about 10 minutes.[301,302] Ice has traditionally been considered to be primarily for acute problems, especially joint injury, but clinical experience has shown that ice seems to be more effective than heat for not all but certainly a larger number of patients with chronic problems than previously thought. Ice is particularly effective prior to stretching and especially when very tender or irritable areas of muscle or joint are present.

A common treatment recommendation is to eat only softer foods; the rationale is that avoidance of tougher or harder foods will facilitate recovery. Resting a painful body part is a traditional and intuitively understood action. However, too much "rest" leads to atrophy and thereby, via a negative feedback loop, to further restrictions in activities. In contrast, emphasizing resumption of normal textured foods facilitates recovery rather than blocks it.[303] As part of avoidance behavior, many patients with TMD will start to chew on only one side, and unilateral chewing is one of the very few "dental" factors associated with TMD.[129] Before resuming a normally textured diet, the patient who chews unilaterally should retrain to chew bilaterally; this is best facilitated by judicious use of a mechanical soft diet for perhaps two weeks at most, and then gradually resuming more normally textured foods. Hard or brittle food should still be avoided until symptoms improve. Chewing restores strength, which aids relaxation.

Parafunctional Behavior Control

Attention to jaw activities that are unrelated to function (such as tooth clenching, jaw-posturing habits, jaw-muscle tensing, and leaning on the jaw) is a critical beginning. Those parafunctional behaviors associated with clinically relevant hyperactivity need to be replaced with restful jaw postures, and this should be part of any initial therapy. Parafunctional behavior control is simultaneously the same thing as fully resting or relaxing the jaw. Parafunction control is helpful in reducing pain in myofascial pain patients.[304] Patients need education, training, support, and reinforcement to have the skills to appropriately monitor and control their parafunctional behaviors and to simultaneously critically evaluate the relative contribution such behaviors contribute to the aggravation or persistence of symptoms (Table 11-10).

Physiotherapy

Although clinical trials necessary to confirm the effectiveness of physiotherapy are generally lacking, the clinical literature suggests that physiotherapy is a reasonable part of initial therapy.[305] Physiotherapy has been shown to be better than placebo, but no differences between various physical therapies have been demonstrated.[306] Both passive and active treatments are commonly included as part of therapy. Posture therapy has been recommended to avoid forward head positions that are thought to adversely affect mandibular posture and masticatory muscle activity; research evidence, however, suggests that forward head posture, by itself, is not strongly associated with having TMD.[307] This leads to a conundrum in how to best use evidence to guide treatment: clinical practice of physical therapy, when done in a manner that reliably helps symptoms, typically includes many elements, most of which either have not been adequately researched or, as in the case of forward head posture, have disconfirming data. Explanatory models for how physical therapy works are plentiful but critical data are absent. Appropriate goals of physical therapy (PT) are to restore normal muscle tone and resilience, improve joint movement, reduce pain, and improve function.

Passive modalities such as ultrasound, cold laser, and transcutaneous electrical nerve stimulation (TENS) are

TABLE 11-10 Instructions to Patients for Self-Care as Part of Initial Therapy
Be aware of and control oral parafunctional behaviors.
Teeth should only contact during chewing and swallowing.
Monitor jaw at regular intervals through the day for any clenching, grinding, touching, or tapping of teeth or any tensing or rigid holding of the jaw muscles.
Monitor jaw for parafunctional behaviors during specific situations such as while driving, studying, using computer, reading, engaging in athletic activities, when at work, or in social situations, and when experiencing overwork, fatigue, or stress.
Practice neutral jaw posture: Place the tip of the tongue behind the top teeth or in the floor of the mouth, separate the teeth slightly, and allow the jaw to "hang" in this position; maintain this position when the jaw is not being used for functions such as speaking and chewing.
Modify the food texture in your diet.
Choose softer foods and only those foods that can be chewed without pain.
Cut foods into smaller pieces; avoid foods that require wide mouth opening and biting off with the front teeth or foods that are chewy and sticky and that require excessive mouth movements.
Do not chew gum.
Avoid certain postures or movements.
Do not lean on or cup the chin when performing desk work or at the dining table.
Do not test the jaw by opening wide or moving the jaw around excessively to assess pain or motion.
Avoid habitually maneuvering the jaw into positions to assess its comfort or range.
Avoid habitually clicking the jaw if a click is present.
Do not sleep on the stomach or in postures that place stress on the jaw.
Avoid elective dental treatment while symptoms of pain and limited opening are present.
During yawning, support the jaw by providing mild counter-pressure underneath the chin with the thumb and index finger or with the back of the hand.
Use thermal agents to control pain.
Apply moist hot compresses to the sides of the face and to the temple areas for 10–20 min twice daily.
Apply ice packs to targeted areas for 10 min; can alternate with heat.

typically used initially to reduce pain. Passive modalities are often used as a prelude to active treatments of joint mobilization and muscle stretching to reduce discomfort associated with the active treatments. Ultrasound relies on high-frequency oscillations that are produced and converted to heat as they are transmitted through tissue; it is a method of producing deep heat more effectively than the patient could achieve by using surface warming. Ultrasound is generally regarded as effective; however, whether it is effective alone is questionable.[308] Cold laser is heavily promoted for its role in effecting cellular metabolism,[309] and it appears to be effective for at least some types of pain[310,311]; its use in chronic pain has, so far, not been supported by strong evidence.[312] TENS uses a low-voltage biphasic current of varied frequency and is designed for sensory counterstimulation for the control of pain. It is thought to increase the action of the modulation that occurs in pain processing at the dorsal horn of the spinal cord and (in the case of the face) the trigeminal nucleus of the brainstem. The general principle in the use of TENS is to consider it for therapeutic trial, recognizing that long-term efficacy is highly idiosyncratic. Physical therapists will commonly add more jaw exercises such as active stretching to increase the range of jaw motion, and isotonic and isometric exercises to facilitate strength and coordinated movement. Providing too many exercises too quickly can lead to poor compliance; the addition of exercises to the

home program should be titrated based on the performance and adherence.

Some physiotherapists apply mobilization techniques to increase mandibular motion. These are done passively under the control of the physiotherapist and will usually include distraction and some combination of lateral and protrusive gliding movements. The choice and timing of treatment are individual considerations since the literature is not developed enough to provide specific guidelines.

In addition to the benefits of the therapeutic relationship between the dentist and patient, a physiotherapist trained in managing TMDs is likely to interact with the patient periodically for review and coaching regarding physical self-management, education regarding the disorder, and further provision of physical therapy. A physiotherapist can reinforce management from a biopsychosocial approach contributing to a successful treatment outcome.

Intraoral Appliances

Intraoral appliances (variously termed splints, orthotics, orthopedic appliances, bite guards, nightguards, or bruxing guards) are used in TMD treatment. When carefully used, an intraoral appliance is considered to be a reversible form of therapy; however, appliances also have adverse effects as well. A number of studies on splint therapy have demonstrated a treatment effect, although researchers disagree as to the reason for the effect.[281,296,313,314] In an early review of the literature on splint therapy, Clark found that patients reported a 70% to 90% improvement with splint therapy.[315] A number of qualitative and systematic reviews have carefully considered the question of appliance treatment, concluding in general that the use of appliances in TMD treatment is beneficial, but available high-quality evidence and a plausible mechanism of action are still lacking.[76,316–321]

A decrease in masticatory muscle activity has been associated with splint therapy and might be the reason for the effects of splint therapy.[322] Alternatively, a nonspecific treatment effect has been proposed.[323] Other explanations for the effects of splint therapy include occlusal disengagement, altered vertical dimension, realigned maxillomandibular relationship, mandibular condyle repositioning, and cognitive awareness of mandibular posturing and habits.[324] The nature of treatment effects of appliance therapy will require further research. For the present, however, intraoral appliance therapy is considered to be a reversible treatment. When to include an intraoral appliance differs considerably across practice settings; some practices start treatment with an appliance, whereas more behaviorally oriented practices will include an appliance only after specific goals have been met with regard to self-care and behavioral treatments. Early use of an appliance can facilitate treatment response,[325] but early use can also diminish the value and adherence to the other self-care treatments. Excessive reliance on appliances typically leads to poor treatment outcomes of TMD.

The choice of material for the construction of an appliance remains one of individual preference. In comparing hard versus soft material appliances, a 3-month trial found no difference in outcome when either the hard or the soft appliance was used,[326] and a 12-month trial had the same findings.[327] In contrast to the equivocal study results, a survey of dentists and dental specialists reported that a flat-plane splint made of hard acrylic was used more frequently than any other design or material.[328] Reasons for this preference of hard appliance include adherence to occlusion models and the belief that appliances should replicate an occlusal scheme, belief that dental proprioception facilitated by the hard appliance is beneficial to muscle retraining, greater longevity, and reports by patients that soft appliances often feel bulky or provoke clenching that was not previously present.

The most common purposes advocated for appliance therapy are to provide joint stabilization, protect the teeth, redistribute forces, relax elevator muscles, and decrease or control the effects of bruxism.[324] The appliance most commonly used for these purposes is described as a stabilization appliance or muscle relaxation splint (Figure 11-14). Such appliances are designed to cover a full arch and are adjusted to avoid altering jaw position or placing orthodontic forces on the teeth. Long-term continuous wearing of an occlusal appliance is a risk for a permanent change in the occlusion.[329] This is a greater concern with appliances that provide only partial coverage or that occlude only on selected opposing teeth.[330] Not because of occlusal theory related to TMD

but rather because appliance treatment should not cause teeth to move, the appliance should be adjusted to provide bilateral, even contact with the opposing teeth on closure in a comfortable mandibular posture. Anterior guidance during excursive movements is often preferred and can be achieved with an appropriate acrylic contour; however, anterior guidance patterns do not improve appliance efficacy.[331]

During the period of treatment as symptoms improve, the appliance should be reexamined periodically and readjusted as necessary to accommodate changes in mandibular posture or muscle function that may affect the opposing tooth contacts on the appliance. At the beginning of appliance therapy, a combination of appliance use during sleep and for periods during the waking hours is used by some providers; however, better behavioral management during the waking hours should preclude the need to rely on an appliance except during sleep. Each patient has his or her own needs and characteristics, and these should be monitored to determine the most effective schedule for appliance use. Factors such as tooth clenching when driving or exercising may be managed by increasing splint use during these times,

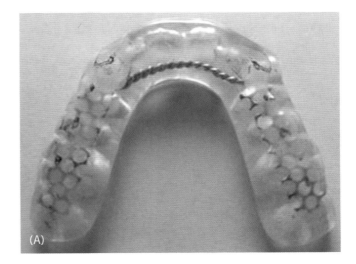

(A)

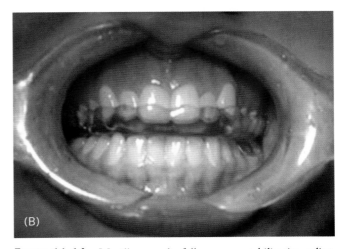

(B)

FIGURE 11-14 Maxillary acrylic full-coverage stabilization splint.

or perhaps such symptom-related events serve as a gateway for referral for stress management. Pain symptoms that tend to increase as the day progresses generally indicate pervasive parafunctional behaviors; the appliance can be used at various times during the day in response to such pain patterns, or behavioral management can be emphasized. Overall, to avoid the possibility of occlusal change, the appliance should certainly not be worn continuously (i.e., 24 hours per day) over prolonged periods, which suggests that behavioral management must remain the primary method for waking parafunction. Full-coverage appliance therapy during sleep is a common practice to reduce the effects of bruxing and is not usually associated with occlusal change. In addition, appliances seem to retain more efficacy if used for shorter periods (e.g., only during sleep); however, as discussed elsewhere in this chapter, alternative views exist regarding how to capitalize upon the apparent benefits of using appliances.

The choice of inserting a stabilizing appliance on the upper or lower arch is a clinical judgment related to how the appliance is to be used and the clinical findings. Placing the appliance on the arch with missing teeth allows for an increase in occlusal contact position. For patients who are likely to benefit from daytime wear, a lower appliance is usually less visible and does not interfere with speech as much as an upper appliance. When an appliance is to be used only at night, most clinicians choose the upper arch, but this choice seems to be more a function of tradition. There is no evidence that indicates one arch is the better home for an appliance in the treatment of TMD.

Splints that reposition the mandible anteriorly have been used effectively in treating disc displacements,[332] but they increase the risk of permanently altering the occlusion and should be used with caution. These splints have been made for the upper or lower arch, although the maxillary appliance is better able to maintain a forward mandibular posture by using a ramp extending from the anterior segment that guides the mandible forward during closure. These appliances were used with greater frequency in the past to correct disc position as a step toward more permanently altering mandibular position through permanent changes in the occlusion. This approach was associated with great technical difficulties, and the treatment failed to correct disc displacement in a significant percentage of patients. Repositioning appliances used for short periods intermittently can be useful in controlling symptoms arising from the mechanical instability of the disc–condyle relationship. Short-term intermittent repositioning therapy may be helpful when transient episodes of jaw locking occur due to disc displacement and are accompanied by pain and dysfunction.

In summary, a stabilizing oral appliance that fully covers one arch and does not reposition the mandible or alter the occlusion is considered a standard part of therapy of TMD. Continuous appliance wear, appliances that only provide partial coverage, and appliances that reposition the mandible and alter the occlusion have a greater chance of adverse effects.

Pharmacotherapy

Mild analgesics, nonsteroidal anti-inflammatory analgesic drugs (NSAIDs), antianxiety agents, tricyclic antidepressants, and muscle relaxants are medications used as part of initial treatment. All of these drugs may be of use in therapy, especially at the beginning of treatment, to enhance pain control. Because of the adverse effects of all of these drugs, short-term or intermittent use is preferred, but a smaller percentage of patients who evolve into a chronic musculoskeletal pain disorder are usually taking combinations of medications long term. Opioids are usually reserved for complex chronic pain disorders or briefly for acute injuries to the TMJs or muscles where moderate to severe pain is present. The use of opioid medication for nonmalignant pain remains an increasingly controversial issue, driven by differing views of pain and suffering as well as by the unfortunate practice by some patients of medication diversion. A related issue is pseudo-addiction, which is the reliance on adequate dosages of medication (often opioid, but it could be any type) to control a symptom but which is then viewed as "addiction." Knowing one's patient is essential, but careful prescribing is also essential.

Drug therapy as part of TMD management should follow the general principles of analgesic therapy and be used on a fixed-dose schedule according to time rather than as needed for pain. Drug therapy requires a thoughtful assessment of the potential risks relative to the benefits, including the clinician's own professional ability and confidence in using the particular drug or drugs.

NSAIDs are probably the most commonly prescribed medication for pain control in TMD therapy. The promise of the COX-2 inhibitors (e.g., rofecoxib) as safer alternatives to other NSAIDs has proven unfulfilled due to the association of cardiovascular incidents. There is modest evidence for efficacy of NSAIDs in TMD therapy.[333] In one study, ibuprofen 2400 mg daily for four weeks did not demonstrate a clear analgesic effect due to the drug.[334] Naproxen 500 mg twice daily in a six-week trial was more effective than placebo or celecoxib.[335] A trial of systemic NSAIDs is a reasonable part of initial therapy. NSAIDs for most TMDs should be used short term to supplement the other nondrug therapies that should reduce the need for long-term NSAID therapy. A mild analgesic such as acetaminophen might be a first choice for analgesic drug treatment since it is much less likely to cause adverse side effects when taken in the appropriate dose for short periods. A combination of ibuprofen and acetaminophen is commonly regarded as more effective than either medication alone for certain pains, but the data are inconclusive.[336,337]

Topical NSAIDs have demonstrated significant pain-reducing effects in acute and chronic musculoskeletal injuries. NSAIDs can be incorporated in transdermal creams for application on the skin over the painful joint or muscle. Ketoprofen, felbinac, ibuprofen, diclofenac, and piroxicam have significant efficacy. This efficacy holds true for chronic conditions such as arthritis. The incidence of local and systemic adverse events is low and no different from placebo.[338] Capsaicin cream (0.025% and 0.075%) has not been studied for TMD therapy, but it has been recommended as a topical analgesic when applied to the skin over a sore joint or muscle four times daily for at least two weeks. Capsaicin is a substance P depleter, a neurotransmitter responsible for increased nerve sensitization. Capsaicin was originally found to be of value in treating postherpetic neuralgia. Capsaicin therapy is limited due to its burning quality on application, which frequently causes the patient to abandon treatment.

The long-acting benzodiazepine clonazepam was effective in a pilot study of TMD treatment,[339] but more recently, 10 mg cyclobenzaprine, a muscle relaxant, taken at bedtime was found to be superior to clonazepam at managing jaw pain on awakening.[340] Muscle relaxants are a class of drugs that act in the CNS, inhibiting interneurons and depressing motor activity. These medications are used before sleep because of their sedative effects. Some patients taking 10 mg of cyclobenzaprine at bedtime experience continued sedation into the day, but they are able to tolerate a lower dose by splitting the tablet into two or four sections and taking one section. The sedative effects of cyclobenzaprine may contribute to their efficacy and, in addition, be of value in promoting sleep, which is often also compromised in individuals with pain. Sleep disorders may also require the use of hypnotics or other drug combinations to increase restorative sleep, but behavioral approaches should also be considered.

Tricyclic antidepressants, particularly amitriptyline, have proven to be effective in managing chronic orofacial pain. Amitriptyline is analgesic at low doses, has sedative effects, and promotes restful sleep; all of these effects can be helpful in treatment. It is the anticholinergic effects of the drug (dry mouth, weight gain, sedation, and dysphoria) that often make it intolerable. An effective dose can be as low as 10 mg at night but can be increased gradually to 75–100 mg, depending on the patient's tolerance of the side effects. Two clinical studies demonstrated a positive treatment effect using low-dose amitriptyline for TMD treatment.[341,342] Depression commonly accompanies chronic pain; referral for depression-relevant dosages of antidepressant medications should be considered.

Drug therapy with an NSAID, acetaminophen, amitriptyline, or cyclobenzaprine, along with the other components of initial therapy, may contribute to symptom control.[343] The choice of drugs and their management as a part of a complex chronic pain disorder is different and is not covered in this chapter.

Behavioral Therapy and Relaxation Techniques

Integrating behavioral therapy and relaxation techniques in chronic pain management is effective.[344] In some cases, self-care and awareness of parafunctional behaviors may not be sufficient to change behavioral patterns that are contributing to symptoms. A more structured program supervised by a clinician who is competent in behavioral therapy offers a greater chance of addressing issues that are contributing factors. There is general agreement in the literature that behavioral and educational therapies are effective in the management of chronic pain disorders, although the existing research is not sufficient to conclude that any one technique is superior. Relaxation techniques, biofeedback, hypnosis, and CBT have all been used to reduce symptoms in patients with TMD.[345] The mechanism of action of these techniques is likely complex.

Relaxation techniques generally decrease sympathetic activity and (possibly) arousal. Deep methods include autogenic training, meditation, and progressive muscle relaxation.[344] These techniques are aimed at producing comforting body sensations, calming the mind, and reducing muscle tone. Brief methods for relaxation use self-controlled relaxation, paced breathing, and deep breathing. Hypnosis produces a state of selective or diffuse focus to induce relaxation. The technique includes pre- and postsuggestion and is used to introduce specific goals. Individuals vary greatly in their susceptibility to hypnosis and suggestion. Hypnosis does not affect endorphin production, and its effect on catecholamine production is not known.

CBT, which often includes relaxation techniques, is primarily focused on changing patterns of negative thoughts. Hypnosis and CBT have been hypothesized to block pain from entering consciousness by activating the frontal limbic attention system to inhibit pain impulse transmission from the thalamic to the cortical structures.[344] Functional imaging data clearly demonstrate that CNS activity quickly changes in response to changes in thought patterns. A six-session CBT intervention enhanced the treatment effect of usual TMD treatment.[346]

Biofeedback is a treatment method that provides continuous feedback, usually by monitoring the electrical activity of muscle with surface electrodes or by monitoring peripheral temperature. The monitoring instruments provide patients with physiologic information that allows them to reliably change physiologic functions to produce a targeted system response similar to that produced by relaxation therapies. The patient develops strategies that are aimed at either lowering the electrical activity of the muscle or raising peripheral temperature. Repetitive practice using the biofeedback instrumentation provides the training for the patient to develop better motor control and more accurate proprioception, with the goal of ultimately achieving a more relaxed state; central to the success of biofeedback, in terms of generalizing treatment effects from the clinic to the environment, is developing a greater sensitivity to the environmental stimuli that have adverse effects on the individual.

Barriers to integrating behavioral and relaxation therapy exist in standard medical and dental care. The biomedical model of disease is emphasized in medical and dental education. The biomedical model emphasizes the anatomic and pathophysiologic aspects of disease and does not emphasize psychosocial issues, the importance of the patient's experience of disease, or the fundamental importance of self-regulation. In addition, behavioral therapies can be time intensive and may also not be supported by insurance companies.

For the patient who does not respond to initial treatment and who continues to have significant pain and disability, additional therapies beyond those described earlier are usually required. These patients are characterized more as having a chronic pain disorder than as having an anatomic abnormality that is unique to the masticatory system. Treatments used in the management of chronic pain are indicated for this group. A greater focus on behavioral therapies and coping strategies may provide additional benefits. Multidisciplinary pain clinic management may be required. The use of chronic pain medications, including opioids and the drugs described as adjuvant analgesics (tricyclic antidepressants, anticonvulsants, membrane stabilizers, and sympatholytics), may be part of a long-term management plan. Chronic pain disorders cause psychosocial changes that require management to reduce the associated disability.

Trigger Point Therapy

Trigger point therapy has used two modalities: cooling of skin over the involved muscle followed by stretching and direct injection of local anesthetic into the muscle.

"Spray and stretch" therapy is performed by cooling the skin with a refrigerant spray (e.g., fluoromethane) and stretching the involved muscle. Cooling allows for stretching without pain that causes a reactive contraction or strain. Travell and Simons described this technique in detail, introducing the method for the treatment of myofascial pain.[241] Patients who respond to this therapy can use a variation at home by first warming the muscle, then briefly icing it, and then gently stretching the jaw passively.

Intramuscular trigger point injections have been performed by injecting local anesthetic, saline, or sterile water or by dry needling without depositing a drug or solution. The choice of solution for injection exists because of the lack of established benefits of any one method.[347] Injection of sterile water was associated with greater injection pain than was injection of saline.[348] In a study in which myofascial pain patients were treated with injection of lidocaine or with dry needling, both groups reported decreased pain immediately after injection, but the group that received dry needling experienced greater soreness 48 hours after the procedure.[349] Procaine diluted to 0.5% with saline has been recommended because of its low toxicity to the muscle,[350] but 1% lidocaine is an alternative.

There are no tested protocols for trigger point injection therapy. Three- to five-weekly sessions has been recommended, and this may be continued with modification of the intervals between injections, depending on the response.[351] Injections can be given to a muscle group in a series of five weekly or biweekly treatments. If there is no response to the initial series of injections, treatment should be abandoned. Hopwood and Abram analyzed treatment outcomes for 193 patients who received trigger point injection therapy for myofascial pain.[352] They found that (1) unemployment due to pain increased the odds of treatment failure threefold, (2) a longer duration of pain and greater change in social activity increased the risk of failure twofold, and (3) constant pain (vs. intermittent pain) increased the likelihood of treatment failure by 80%. These results emphasize that chronic pain is a multidimensional and complex problem and that a variety of factors will influence treatment outcome.

Other TMD Treatments

The above sections highlight only the most common treatment methods and have not addressed many treatments that have been recommended for the management of TMDs. Acupuncture has been shown to be an effective part of the management of chronic pain. Botulinum toxin has been advocated for the treatment of TMDs,[353] but randomized clinical trials question the true efficacy of this treatment for pain beyond that of decreasing muscle tone.[354–356]

Acupressure, different forms of injection therapy using natural substances, massage therapy, naturopathic and homeopathic remedies, and herbal remedies are just a few of the treatments patients may pursue.[357] The Internet has produced treatment programs that even allow patents to evaluate their problem to determine whether the advertised treatment will be of benefit. There is a critical need (which will increase in the future) for dentists to help patients evaluate the treatments and products that are promoted for TMD therapy. Many of these treatments lack publication in the scientific literature that is even descriptive. The large variety of treatments promoted, coupled with the lack of clarity in the scientific research about cause, makes the need to establish a trusting doctor–patient relationship critical.

Restorative Dental Procedures in TMD Patients

Patients who require elective dental treatment should defer such procedures until the TMD symptoms have resolved or are under reasonable control. Patients who develop active dental disease requiring treatment while they are suffering from TMD pain are likely to have increased pain and dysfunction after dental procedures. The dentist should attempt to minimize the effect of a procedure on myalgia or joint strain by using a variety of procedures, as outlined in Table 11-11. One clinically proven method of minimizing symptom aggravation from dental treatment visits is the use of a mechanical support device for the mandible; both pain and fatigue are reduced, and focus groups report that its use by the dentist also minimizes jaw overextension during dental procedures.[358]

TABLE 11-11 Managing TMD Patients Requiring Dental Procedures

Prior to the procedure

Use hot compresses to masseter and temporalis areas 10–20 min two to three times daily for 2 d.

Use a minor tranquilizer or skeletal muscle relaxant (e.g., lorazepam, 1 mg; cyclobenzaprine, 10 mg) on the night and day of the procedure (patient must be accompanied by an adult).

Start a nonsteroidal anti-inflammatory analgesic the day of the procedure.

During the procedure

Use a child-sized surgical rubber mouth prop to support the patient's comfortable opening; remove periodically to reduce joint stiffness. Alternatively, an extraoral device that supports the jaw can be used.

Consider intravenous sedation and/or inhalation analgesia.

Provide frequent rest periods to avoid prolonged opening.

Apply moist heat to masticatory muscles during rest breaks.

Gently massage masticatory muscles during rest breaks.

Perform the procedure in the morning, when reserve is likely to be greatest.

After the procedure

Extend the use of muscle relaxant and NSAID medication as necessary.

Apply cold compresses to the TMJ and muscle areas during the 24 h after the procedure.

Abbreviations: NSAID, nonsteroidal anti-inflammatory drug; TMJ, temporomandibular joint.

Articular Disc Disorders of the TMJ

An ADD is an abnormal relationship between the disc, the mandibular condyle, and the articular eminence, resulting from the elongation or tearing of the attachment of the disc to the condyle and glenoid fossa. ADD may result in abnormal joint sounds, limitation and deviation of mandibular motion, and pain. The majority of individuals with an ADD, with or without reduction, in one or both TMJs have no pain or limitation in functioning; MR studies have demonstrated that ADD is present in 25% to 35% of the normal asymptomatic adult population.[359,360] This is comparable to the finding of asymptomatic clinically insignificant disc displacement that is well documented in the knee and spine.[361,362] ADD of the TMJ does not appear to affect children younger than 5 years.[363]

The most common disc displacement is anterior and medial to the condyle.[364] It is theorized that ADD occurs more frequently when the superior head of the lateral pterygoid muscle attaches to the disc. This attachment would pull a loosened disc anterior and medial to the condyle. Posterior disc displacement (when a portion of the disc is found posterior to the top of the condyle) is rare but has been reported in the literature.[365]

A specific etiology in the majority of cases of disc displacement is poorly understood. Some cases result from direct trauma to the joint from a blow to the mandible. It is also generally believed that chronic low-grade micro-trauma resulting from long-term bruxism or clenching of the teeth is a major cause of ADD. Studies using arthroscopic examination of the TMJ have demonstrated a relationship between intracapsular disorders and bruxism.[366] There is evidence that ADD may be associated with a generalized laxity of joints.[367] Craniofacial morphology may also play a role in ADD.[368]

Clinicians have also theorized that indirect trauma from cervical flexion extension injuries (whiplash-associated disorders [WAD]) or certain types of malocclusion may also predispose an individual to disc displacement. There is some support that WAD can affect the jaw in adverse ways,[369] but the evidence is weak because it is based on insufficient study designs for assessing causation. With respect to trauma, the particular events and presumed pathophysiology that may result in ADD are unknown. Based on available evidence it is less likely that any particular event causes an internal derangement, and, consistent with TMD as a complex disease, it is more likely that a combination of mechanisms related to the anatomy of the joint and the facial skeleton, connective tissue chemistry, and chronic loading of the joint increases the susceptibility of certain individuals to a disturbance of the restraining ligaments and displacement of the disc. ADD results in significant pain or dysfunction when accompanied by capsulitis and synovitis, but why specific joints with ADD may be accompanied by symptoms versus the much larger number of joints that remain asymptomatic across the lifespan is as yet unknown.

Clinical Manifestations

Disc displacement is divided into stages based on signs and symptoms combined with the results of diagnostic imaging. A simple classification system divides ADD into (1) anterior disc displacement with reduction (clicking joint), (2) anterior disc displacement with intermittent locking, and (3) anterior disc displacement without reduction (closed lock).

Anterior Disc Displacement With Reduction

This condition is caused by an articular disc that has been displaced from its position on top of the condyle due to elongation or tearing of the restraining ligaments. An alteration in the form or shape of the disc has also been proposed as a possible factor, with thinning of the posterior band presumably allowing the disc to migrate anteriorly over time. A reducing disc displacement is common in the general population, and a clicking or popping joint is of little clinical significance unless it is accompanied by pain, loss of function, and/or intermittent locking. An individual may seek professional advice regarding treatment of an audible click that is not accompanied by pain but that may be socially embarrassing. In such an instance, the "click" may be the appropriate treatment target, regardless of whether there is an associated internal derangement.[68]

The clinician must distinguish the patient with myofascial pain and coincidental TMJ clicking from the patient whose pain is directly related to disc displacement. In making this distinction with regard to treatment selection, the clinician should also be aware that symptoms of pain and dysfunction associated with anterior disc displacement with reduction usually resolve over time with minimal noninvasive therapy.[370]

Palpation and auscultation of the TMJ will reveal a clicking or popping sound during both opening and closing mandibular movements (reciprocal click). The clicking or popping sound due to anterior disc displacement with reduction is characterized by a click that may occur during opening, closing, lateral movements, protrusive movement, or any combination of these movements. The clicking sound of an ADD occurs due to relative movement of the disc while the condyle translates. Clinicians examining patients with ADD may observe a deflection of the mandible early in the opening cycle prior to the click with correction to the midline after the click, but this is a variable finding and deflection due to muscle guarding must be distinguished. Diagnostic sensitivity and specificity for ADD is fair to poor based on clinical findings, because joints without ADD may click and joints with ADD may not click. Palpation pain will be present when ADD is accompanied by capsulitis or synovitis, but a joint with an ADD may also exhibit palpation pain due to hyperalgesia without inflammation.

Anterior Disc Displacement Without Reduction (Closed Lock)

ADD without reduction is often referred to as a closed lock and occurs in three forms: intermittent lock lasting seconds to minutes, acute lock that is persistent (in the absence of treatment), and chronic closed lock as the resolution to the acute lock. These three forms appear to occur in stages, self-evident in the order as described, but apparently a tipping point must exist in that the majority of individuals with a clicking joint due to ADD do not progress to any locking phase. Closed lock may be the first sign of TMD occurring after trauma or severe long-term nocturnal bruxism. A patient with an acute closed lock will often have a history of a long-standing TMJ click that abruptly disappears followed by a sudden restriction in mandibular opening. This limited mandibular opening occurs due to disc interference with the normal translation of the condyle. Other findings of acute closed lock include pain directly over the joint during mandibular opening (especially at maximum opening), limited lateral movement to the side away from the affected joint, and deviation of the mandible to the affected side during maximum mouth opening. That is, the condyle on the affected side will not translate normally. In addition, the affected condyle will not be as palpable on examination. In chronic closed lock, the disc will deform and maximum mouth opening will gradually improve. The displacement of the disc exposes the posterior attachment to compression by the condyle. The posterior attachment has been shown to react to the change by depositing hyaline in the connective tissue[371] and has been called a "pseudomeniscus."[372] Symptoms typically remit as the joint progresses from the acute lock to the chronic lock.

Posterior Disc Displacement

Posterior disc displacement has been described as the condyle slipping over the anterior rim of the disc during opening, with the disc being caught and brought backward in an abnormal relationship to the condyle when the mouth is closed. The disc is folded in the dorsal part of the joint space, preventing full mouth closure.[373] The clinical features are (1) a sudden inability to bring the upper and lower teeth together in maximal occlusion, (2) pain in the affected joint when trying to bring the teeth firmly together, (3) displacement forward of the mandible on the affected side, (4) restricted lateral movement to the affected side, and (5) no restriction of mouth opening.[373]

Management

Longitudinal studies demonstrate that most symptoms associated with ADD resolve over time either with no treatment or with minimal conservative therapy.[374] One study of patients with symptomatic anterior disc displacement without reduction experienced resolution without treatment in 75% of cases after 2.5 years.[375] Since symptoms associated with anterior disc displacement with and without reduction tend to decrease with time, the clinician should not treat patients on the assumption that asymptomatic clicking will inevitably progress to painful clicking or locking. Painful clicking or locking should initially be treated with conservative therapy.

Recommended treatments for symptomatic ADD include splint therapy, physical therapy including manual manipulation, anti-inflammatory drugs, arthrocentesis, arthroscopic lysis and lavage, arthroplasty, and vertical ramus osteotomy. Many of these nonsurgical and surgical techniques are effective in decreasing pain and in increasing the range of mandibular motion, although the abnormal position of the disc is not usually corrected.[376]

Anterior Disc Displacement With Reduction

Patients with TMJ clicking or popping that is not accompanied by pain do not require therapy. Both flat-plane stabilization splints that do not change mandibular position and anterior repositioning splints have been used to treat painful clicking. Anterior repositioning splints maintain the mandible in an anterior position, preventing the condyle from closing posterior to the disc. One meta-analysis that summarized the results of previous studies concluded that repositioning splints were more effective than stabilization splints in eliminating both clicking and pain in patients with ADD.[377] Clinicians must weigh the potential benefits of using repositioning splints against the potential adverse effects that include tooth movement and open bite. Clinicians have advocated techniques that are designed to "recapture" the disc to its normal position, but splint therapy, arthrocentesis, or arthroscopy rarely corrects disc position and function. Painful symptoms resolve, although the disc remains displaced.

Anterior Disc Displacement Without Reduction

Some patients with closed lock may present with little or no pain, whereas others have severe pain during mandibular movement. Treatment options should depend on the degree of pain and limitation associated with the ADD. Management of a locked TMJ may be nonsurgical or surgical. The goals of successful therapy are to eliminate pain, restore function, and increase the range of mandibular motion. Correcting the disc position is not necessary to achieve these goals.

Patients who present with restricted movement but minimal pain frequently benefit from manual manipulation and an exercise program designed to increase mandibular motion. A flat-plane occlusal stabilization appliance to decrease the adverse effects of sleep bruxism on the affected joint is appropriate. There is no evidence to suggest that repositioning the mandible using oral appliance therapy is indicated as a treatment for ADD without reduction. Sato et al. reported that a combination of a flat-plane stabilization splint and anti-inflammatory drugs was successful in reducing pain and increasing the ROM in over 75% of patients.[374] The success of this therapy was attributed to decreased inflammation and to the gradual elongation of the posterior attachment, permitting increased translation of the condyle. In a multigroup randomized controlled trial, Schiffman et al. randomized individuals with severe closed lock to medical management, rehabilitation, arthroscopic surgery, or arthroplasty[378]; each of the surgical treatments included postoperative rehabilitation. At five years, all treatments resulted in equal improvement as based on symptoms and examination findings, and no treatment was superior, indicating that medical management or rehabilitation should be sufficient treatments.

Patients with severe pain on mandibular movement may benefit from either arthrocentesis or arthroscopy. Flushing the joint and deposition of intraarticular corticosteroids to decrease inflammation or sodium hyaluronate to increase joint lubrication and decrease adhesions have been reported to decrease pain associated with nonreducing disc displacements.[379,380] A significant reduction in the range of movement was associated with a less favorable treatment outcome.[381]

Kurita et al. reported on a 2½-year follow-up on patients with ADD without reduction. Approximately 40% of patients became asymptomatic, 33% continued to have symptoms at a decreased level, and 25% had no improvement. An association was noted between continued TMD symptoms and radiographically detectable degenerative changes.[370] Permanent disc displacement promotes the development of fibrous adhesions in the superior joint compartment.[382] In most cases, discs do not reduce but show increased mobility.[383]

Temporomandibular Joint Arthritis
Osteoarthritis (Degenerative Joint Disease)

DJD, also referred to as osteoarthrosis, osteoarthritis, and degenerative arthritis, is primarily a disorder of articular cartilage and subchondral bone, with secondary inflammation of the synovial membrane. It is a localized joint disease without systemic manifestations. The process begins in loaded articular cartilage that thins, clefts (fibrillation), and then fragments. This leads to sclerosis of underlying bone, subchondral cysts, and osteophyte formation.[384] The articular changes are essentially a response of the joint to chronic microtrauma or pressure. Microtrauma may be in the form of continuous abrasion of the articular surfaces as in natural wear associated with age or due to increased loading possibly related to chronic parafunctional activity. The fibrous tissue covering in patients with degenerative disease is preserved.[385] This may be a factor in remodeling and the recovery that is usually expected in osteoarthrosis and osteoarthritis of the TMJs. The relationship between internal derangements and DJD is unclear, but a higher frequency of radiographic signs of DJD was observed in subjects with disc displacement without reduction.[386] Whether intracapsular soft tissue changes precede bony changes, or the reverse, is unknown.[387]

DJD may be categorized as primary or secondary, although both are similar on histopathologic examination. Primary DJD is of unknown origin, but genetic factors play an important role. It is often asymptomatic and is most commonly seen in patients older than 50 years, although early arthritic changes can be observed in younger individuals. Secondary DJD results from a known underlying cause, such as trauma, congenital dysplasia, or metabolic disease.

Proposed risk factors include gender, diet, genetics, and psychological stress. Epidemiologic studies suggest a female predisposition to TMDs, including osteoarthritis.[180] How estrogen might contribute to osteoarthritis is unknown, but estrogen receptors have been identified on TMJ articular tissues.[388] The possibility that a diet of excessively hard or chewy foods might cause increased loads on the joints and lead to degenerative changes has been proposed but is speculative. Psychological stress leading to parafunctional activities such as tooth clenching or bruxing has been proposed as a factor. In addition to loading the joint, psychological stress might lead to biologic, biochemical, and hormonal changes that might contribute to changes in the joints, leading to osteoarthritis. A significant association has been observed between ADD and osteoarthritis.[389] The mechanisms and pathogenesis remain unknown.

The present model suggests that excessive mechanical loading on the joints produces a cascade of events leading to the failure of the lubrication system and destruction of the articular surfaces. These events include the generation of free radicals, the release of proinflammatory neuropeptides, signaling by cytokines, and the activation of enzymes capable of matrix degradation.[390]

Clinical Manifestations

DJD of the TMJ begins early and has been observed in over 20% of joints in individuals older than 20 years.[391] A study of patients younger than 30 years presenting to a TMD clinic demonstrated that two-thirds of the patients had degenerative changes detected on tomograms.[392] The incidence of degenerative changes increases with age. Degenerative changes are found in over 40% of patients older than 40 years. A direct relationship irrespective of age was observed between the rate and extent of dental attrition and degenerative disease of the TMJs in cadavers of aboriginal humans.[393] Many patients with mild to moderate DJD of the TMJ have no symptoms, although arthritic changes are observed on radiographs.

Degenerative changes of the TMJ detected on radiographic examination may be incidental and may not be responsible for facial pain symptoms or TMJ dysfunction; however, some degenerative changes may be underdiagnosed by conventional radiography because the defects are confined to the articular soft tissue. These soft tissues changes are better visualized with MR.[394]

Patients with symptomatic DJD of the TMJ experience pain directly over the affected condyle, limitation of mandibular opening, crepitus, and a feeling of stiffness after a period of inactivity. Examination reveals tenderness and crepitus on intra-auricular and pre-auricular palpation. Deviation of the mandible to the painful side may be present. Radiographic findings in DJD may include narrowing of the joint space, irregular joint space, flattening of the articular surfaces, osteophyte formation, anterior lipping of the condyle, and the presence of subchondral cysts. These changes may be seen best on tomograms or CT scans (see Figure 11-11). The presence of joint effusion is most accurately detected in T2-weighted MRs. Whether MR-depicted effusion in the TMJ is important clinically has not yet been determined[261]; because TMJ effusions are small relative to effusions observed in other joints (e.g., knee), their detection reliability is less, which may underestimate the potential association with clinical parameters.

Rheumatoid Arthritis

RA is an inflammatory disease primarily affecting periarticular tissue and secondarily bone. The percentage of RA patients with TMJ involvement ranges from 40% to 80%, depending on the group studied and the imaging technique used.[394–398] Studies using conventional radiography and tomography find fewer abnormalities than detectable on CT.[394] TMJ changes on CT were found in 88% of RA patients, but changes were also detected in more than 50% of controls.[397] CT changes did not correlate with clinical complaints. Avrahami et al. detected condylar changes in approximately 80% of RA patients using high-resolution CT.[394] Ackerman et al., using tomography, detected erosive condylar changes in two-thirds of RA patients and stated that symptoms were related to the severity of radiographic changes.[398] The disease process starts as a vasculitis of the synovial membrane. It progresses to chronic inflammation marked by an intense round cell infiltrate and subsequent formation of granulation tissue. The cellular infiltrate spreads from the articular surfaces eventually to cause an erosion of the underlying bone.

Clinical Manifestations

The TMJs in RA are usually involved bilaterally. Pain is usually associated with the early acute phase of the disease but is not a common complaint in later stages. Other symptoms often noted include morning stiffness, joint sounds, and tenderness and swelling over the joint area.[399] The symptoms are usually transient in nature, and only a small percentage of patients with RA of the TMJs experience permanent clinically significant disability.

The most consistent clinical findings include pain on joint palpation, limited mouth opening, and crepitus. Micrognathia and an anterior open bite are commonly seen in patients with juvenile idiopathic arthritis. Larheim attributes the micrognathia to a combination of direct injury to the condylar head and altered orofacial muscular activity.[400] Ankylosis of the TMJ related to RA is rare. Radiographic changes in the TMJ associated with RA may include a narrow joint space, destructive lesions of the condyle, and limited condylar movement. There is little evidence of marginal proliferation or other reparative activity in RA in contrast to the radiographic changes often observed in DJD. High-resolution CT of the TMJs in RA patients shows erosions of the condyle and glenoid fossa that are not detected on conventional radiography.[394]

Seronegative Spondyloarthropathies

Several arthropathies that are distinct from RA are not associated with positive serology (rheumatoid factor). These disorders, characterized by arthritis, are known as the seronegative spondyloarthropathies and include ankylosing spondylitis (AS), psoriatic arthritis (PA), and Reiter's syndrome. The TMJs can be involved in these arthropathies. The clinical manifestations are joint pain with function, limited mouth opening, and erosion of the superior surface of the condyle on radiography. There are no specific findings that are pathognomonic of involvement of the TMJs.

AS primarily involves the spine, although other joints are often involved. It causes inflammation that can lead to new bone formation, causing the spine to fuse, reducing mobility, and producing a forward, stooped posture. The disease usually involves the sacroiliac joints where the spine joins the pelvis. TMJ involvement has been reported in AS, but the prevalence has not been established. Wenneberg estimated that the TMJ was involved in about 15% to 20% of patients with AS.[401] Significantly decreased mouth opening, TMJ pain, crepitus, and muscle pain are frequent clinical findings.[402]

PA is a chronic disease characterized by psoriasis and inflammation of the joints. Approximately 10% of patients who have psoriasis develop joint inflammation. The skin lesions may precede the joint involvement by several years. PA commonly involves the fingers and spine, and pitting of the nails is common. The cause is unknown, and the disease presents in a variety of forms.[403]

The masticatory system is affected in about 50% of patients with PA.[404,405] The symptoms of PA of the TMJ are similar to those noted in RA, except that the signs and symptoms are likely to be unilateral.[406] TMJ pain with chewing is a common finding.[405] Limitation of mouth opening may occur.[407] The most common radiographic finding is erosion of cortical outline of the mandibular condyle.[408] Coronal CT is particularly useful in showing TMJ changes of PA.[410]

Reiter's syndrome includes polyarthritis, urethritis, and conjunctivitis. It is thought to be triggered by infection, but the arthritis is not septic. Reiter's syndrome occurs more frequently in males in the third decade. The syndrome usually follows venereal infection most often involving *Chlamydia*, *Mycoplasma*, or *Yersinia*. Approximately 25% of male patients with Reiter's syndrome reported recurrent pain, swelling, and/or stiffness of the TMJ.

Connective Tissue Disease

Connective tissue diseases that affect the TMJ include systemic lupus, systemic sclerosis (scleroderma), undifferentiated connective tissue disease, and mixed connective tissue disease. When the TMJ is involved, the clinical presentation is similar to other disorders causing inflammation and subsequent degenerative changes. A clinical examination supplemented with diagnostic imaging is usually adequate to confirm involvement of the TMJ.

Diseases Associated With Crystal Deposits in Joints

Gout is a disease that includes hyperuricemia, recurrent arthritides, renal disease, and urolithiaisis. The disease primarily affects men. Acute pain in a single joint is the characteristic clinical presentation. The TMJ is not commonly involved. Calcium pyrophosphate deposition is also known as pseudogout. Deposits of microcrystals in affected joints are responsible for the clinical manifestations. Examination of aspirated synovial fluid from the involved joint by polarized light and detection of monosodium urate crystals confirms the diagnosis. Treatment includes colchicine, NSAIDs, and intra-articular steroid injection. Pseudogout affecting the TMJ has been treated with colchicine and arthrocentesis.

Treatment

Osteoarthritis, the spondyloarthropathies, RA, and other connective tissue diseases that affect the TMJs result in TMJ inflammation. The process eventually leads to the degenerative changes that manifests as joint pain and crepitus, loss of function and range of movement, and, in severe cases, facial deformity. Treatment is directed toward the systemic disease with supportive local therapy consisting of jaw self-care, physiotherapy, oral appliance therapy, topical NSAID, and intra-articular corticosteroid injection.

DJD of the TMJ can usually be managed by conservative treatment with an emphasis on physical therapy and NSAIDS that control both pain and inflammation. In osteoarthritis, significant improvement is noted in many patients after nine months, and a "burning out" of many cases occurs after one year.[410] Nonsurgical management may consist of jaw self-management, including behavior modification, heat application, soft diet, physical therapy including jaw exercises, NSAID, and oral appliance therapy. When nonsurgical management is not effective, then direct joint therapy, such as intra-articular corticosteroid injection, is indicated.[411] Arthrocentesis is a relatively conservative joint procedure if intra-articular steroid injection is ineffective.[412] Arthroscopy, arthroplasty, and arthrotomy are surgical procedures that may be indicated depending on the response to more conservative treatment and the severity of pain and disablility.[413] It seems prudent to manage a patient with conservative treatment for six months to one year before considering surgery unless severe pain or dysfunction persists after an adequate trial of nonsurgical therapy. Only when there is intractable TMJ pain or disabling limitation of mandibular movement, surgery is indicated. Arthroplasty or condylectomy with placement of costochondral grafts has been performed successfully.[414]

Involvement of the TMJ in RA is usually treated with anti-inflammatory drugs in conjunction with the therapy for the systemic disease.[415] The patient should be placed on a soft diet during the acute exacerbation. Use of a flat-plane occlusal appliance may be helpful, particularly if parafunctional behaviors are present. An exercise program to increase mandibular movement should be instituted as soon as possible after the acute symptoms subside. Intra-articular steroids should be considered.[416] Prostheses appear to decrease symptoms in fully or partially edentulous patients.[417]

Surgical treatment of the joints, including placement of prosthetic joints, is indicated in patients who have severe functional impairment or intractable pain not successfully managed by other means. Orthognathic surgery and orthodontics are required for correction of facial deformity resulting from arthritis during growth.

Synovial Chondromatosis

Synovial chondromatosis (SC) is an uncommon benign disorder characterized by the presence of multiple cartilaginous nodules of the synovial membrane that break off resulting in clusters of free-floating loose calcified bodies in the joint. It is theorized that SC originates from embryonic mesenchymal remnants of the subintimal layer of the synovium that become metaplastic, calcify, and break off into the joint space.[418,419] SC most commonly involves one joint, but cases of multi-articular SC have been reported.[420] Some cases appear to be triggered by trauma, whereas others are of unknown etiology. The knee and elbow are most commonly involved, and fewer than 100 cases of SC of the TMJ have been reported in the world medical literature.

More sophisticated imaging techniques, such as CT and arthroscopy, have revealed cases of SC that previously would have received other diagnoses, causing authors of recent publications to suspect that SC is more common than previously believed.[421–424] Extension of SC from the TMJ to surrounding tissues (including the parotid gland, middle ear, or middle cranial fossa) may occur.[424]

Slow progressive swelling in the preauricular region, pain, and limitation of mandibular movement are the most common presenting features. TMJ clicking, locking, crepitus, and occlusal changes may also be present.[419] The extension of the lesion from the joint capsule and involvement of surrounding tissues may make diagnosis difficult, causing SC to be confused with parotid, middle ear, or intracranial tumors. Cases of SC that were mistaken for a chondrosarcoma have been reported. Intracranial extension may lead to neurologic deficits such as facial nerve paralysis. Conventional radiography may not lead to the diagnosis due to superimposition of cranial bones that may obscure the calcified loose bodies.[425] A CT scan should be obtained if SC is suspected after clinical evaluation. The lesion may appear as a single mass or as many small loose bodies.[421] Arthroscopy may be necessary for accurate diagnosis, particularly when the loose bodies are not calcified and cannot be visualized by conventional radiology or CT.[426]

Treatment should be conservative and consist of removal of the mass of loose bodies. This may be done arthroscopically when only a small lesion is present, but arthrotomy is required for larger lesions. The synovium and articular disc should be removed when they are involved. Lesions that extend beyond the joint space may require extensive resection.

Septic Arthritis

Septic arthritis of the TMJ most commonly occurs in patients with previously existing joint disease such as RA or underlying medical disorders (particularly diabetes). Patients receiving immunosuppressive drugs or long-term corticosteroids also have an increased incidence of septic arthritis. The infection of the TMJ may result from blood-borne bacterial infection or by extension of infection from adjacent sites, such as the middle ear, maxillary molars, and parotid gland.[427] Gonococci are the primary blood-borne agents causing septic arthritis in a previously normal TMJ, whereas *Staphylococcus aureus* is the most common organism involved in previously arthritic joints.[428]

Symptoms of septic arthritis of the TMJ include trismus, deviation of the mandible to the affected side, severe pain on movement, and an inability to occlude the teeth, owing to the presence of inflammation in the joint space. Examination reveals redness and swelling over the involved joint. In some cases, the swelling may be fluctuant and extend beyond the region of the joint.[428] Large tender cervical lymph nodes are frequently observed on the side of the infection. Diagnosis is made by detection of bacteria on Gram's stain and culture of aspirated joint fluid.

Serious sequelae of septic arthritis include osteomyelitis of the temporal bone, brain abscess, and ankylosis. Facial asymmetry may accompany septic arthritis of the TMJ,

especially in children. Of the 44 cases of ankylosis of the TMJ reviewed by Topazian, 17 resulted from infection.[429] The primary sources of these infections were the middle ear, teeth, and the hematologic spread of gonorrhea.

Evaluation of patients with suspected septic arthritis must include a review of signs and symptoms of gonorrhea, such as purulent urethral discharge or dysuria. The affected TMJ should be aspirated and the fluid obtained tested by Gram's stain and cultured for *Neisseria gonorrhoeae*.

Treatment of septic arthritis of the TMJ consists of surgical drainage, joint irrigation, and four to six weeks of antibiotics.

OTHER DISORDERS

Developmental Disturbances

Developmental disturbances involving the TMJ may result in anomalies in the size and shape of the condyle. Hyperplasia, hypoplasia, agenesis, and the formation of a bifid condyle may be evident on radiographic examination of the joint. Local factors, such as trauma or infection, can initiate condylar growth disturbances.

True condylar hyperplasia usually occurs after puberty and is completed by 18–25 years of age. Limitation and deviation of mouth opening and facial asymmetry may be observed.

Facial asymmetry often results from disturbances in condylar growth because the condyle is a site for compensatory growth and adaptive remodeling. The facial deformities associated with condylar hyperplasia involve the formation of a convex ramus on the affected side and a concave shape on the normal side. If the condylar hyperplasia is detected and surgically corrected at an early stage, the facial deformities may be prevented. Bone scintigraphy is recommended as part of a presurgical evaluation to identify activity in the joint.[430]

Deviation of the mandible to the affected side and facial deformities also are associated with unilateral agenesis and hypoplasia of the condyle. Rib grafts have been used to replace the missing condyle to minimize the facial asymmetry in agenesis. In cases of hypoplasia, there is a short wide ramus, shortening of the body of the mandible, and antegonial notching on the affected side, with elongation of the mandibular body and flatness of the face on the opposite side. Early surgical intervention is again emphasized to limit facial deformity.

Hyperplasia of the coronoid process is an uncommon cause of restricted mouth opening but may be missed in the differential diagnosis of restricted mouth opening. One study estimated that 5% of 163 patients had restricted mouth opening due to elongation of the coronoid process.[431]

Fractures

Fractures of the condylar head and neck often result from a blow to the chin (see Figure 11-15). The patient with a condylar fracture usually presents with pain and edema over

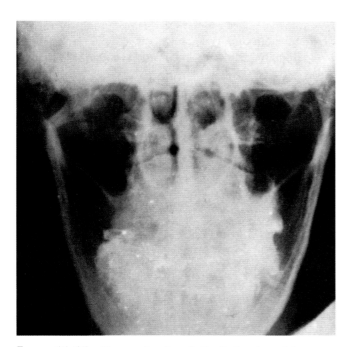

FIGURE 11-15 Fractured and medially displaced condyle.

the joint area and limitation and deviation of the mandible to the injured side on opening. Bilateral condylar fractures may result in an anterior open bite. The diagnosis of a condylar fracture is confirmed by diagnostic imaging. Intracapsular nondisplaced fractures of the condylar head are usually not treated surgically. Early mobilization of the mandible is emphasized to prevent bony or fibrous ankylosis.

Dislocation

In dislocation of the mandible, the condyle is positioned anterior to the articular eminence and cannot return to its normal position without assistance. This disorder contrasts with subluxation, in which the condyle moves anterior to the eminence during wide opening but is able to return to the resting position without manipulation. It has been demonstrated that subluxation is a variation of normal function and that the normal ROM of the condyle is not limited to the fossa.

Dislocations of the mandible usually result from muscular incoordination in wide opening during eating or yawning and less commonly from trauma; they may be unilateral or bilateral. The typical complaints of the patient with dislocation are an inability to close the jaws and pain related to muscle spasm. On clinical examination, a deep depression may be observed in the preauricular region corresponding to the condyle being positioned anterior to the eminence.

The condyle can usually be repositioned without the use of muscle relaxants or general anesthetics. If muscle spasms are severe and reduction is difficult, the use of intravenous diazepam (approximately 10 mg) can be beneficial. The

practitioner who is repositioning the mandible should stand in front of the seated patient and place his or her thumbs lateral to the mandibular molars on the buccal shelf of bone; the remaining fingers of each hand should be placed under the chin. The condyle is repositioned by a downward and backward movement. This is achieved by simultaneously pressing down on the posterior part of the mandible while raising the chin. As the condyle reaches the height of the eminence, it can usually be guided posteriorly to its normal position.

Postreduction recommendations consist of limiting mandibular movement and the use of NSAIDs to lessen inflammation. The patient should be cautioned not to open wide when eating or yawning because recurrence is common, especially during the period initially after repositioning. Long periods of immobilization are not advised due to the risk of fibrous ankylosis.

Chronic recurring dislocations have been treated with surgical and nonsurgical approaches. Injections of sclerosing solutions have been used but are not used as often now because of difficulty in controlling the extent of fibrosis and condylar limitation. Various surgical procedures have been advocated for treating recurrent dislocations of the mandible; these include bone grafting to the eminence, lateral pterygoid myotomy, eminence reduction, eminence augmentation with implants, shortening the temporalis tendon by intraoral scarification, plication of the joint capsule, and repositioning of the zygomatic arch.

Ankylosis

True bony ankylosis of the TMJ involves fusion of the head of the condyle to the temporal bone. Trauma to the chin is the most common cause of TMJ ankylosis, although infections also may be involved.[429] Children are more prone to ankylosis because of greater osteogenic potential and an incompletely formed disc. Ankylosis frequently results from prolonged immobilization following condylar fracture. Limited mandibular movement, deviation of the mandible to the affected side on opening, and facial asymmetry may be observed in TMJ ankylosis. Osseous deposition may be seen on radiographs. Ankylosis has been treated by several surgical procedures. Gap arthroplasty using interpositional materials between the cut segments is the technique most commonly performed.

Sleep Bruxism

Sleep bruxism is thought to aggravate or contribute to the persistence of pain symptoms associated with TMD. The etiology is not understood, but the evidence suggests that occlusal abnormalities are not the cause.[432,433] Occlusal appliances may protect the teeth from the effects of bruxism but cannot be expected to prevent or decrease the bruxism activity.[434] When bruxism is considered to be the cause or a factor of TMD symptoms, oral appliance therapy is effective, but symptoms are likely to return when appliance therapy is withdrawn.[435] In one report, nocturnal aversive biofeedback and splint therapy caused a decrease in the frequency and duration of bruxism, but bruxism activity returned after treatment was withdrawn.[436] Occlusal splints worn during sleep have not been found to stop bruxism but do reduce the signs of bruxing.[437]

Recently, reports of bruxism and symptoms of facial pain, earache, and headache associated with the use of selective serotonin reuptake inhibitors (SSRIs) have been published.[438] Symptoms of bruxing resolved when the dosage was decreased or when buspirone was added.[439] Buspirone has a postsynaptic dopaminergic effect and may act to partially restore suppressed dopamine levels associated with the use of SSRIs.

Tang and Jankovic injected severe bruxers in the masseter muscles with botulinum toxin in an open-label prospective trial and reported significant improvement in symptoms and minimal adverse effects.[440] The treatment effect lasted approximately five months and had to be repeated. Botulinum toxin exerts a paralytic effect on the muscle by inhibiting the release of acetylcholine at the neuromuscular junction.

Oral Dyskinesia and Dystonia

Oral dyskinesias are abnormal, involuntary movements of the tongue, lips, and jaw. The term *tardive dyskinesia* was introduced in 1964 to describe a dyskinesia associated with antipsychotic medication.[441] The prevalence of tardive dyskinesia in patients treated chronically with conventional antipsychotic medication is estimated to be approximately 20%.[442] Oral dyskinesias may be a factor contributing to muscle stiffness, TMJ degenerative changes, mucosal lesions, damage to teeth, and dental prostheses. Tardive dyskinesia has been reported to cause facial pain.[443] Complete loss of teeth is considered to be one cause of oral dyskinesia. Ill-fitting dentures or the lack of replacements may initiate dyskinesia.[444]

Dyskinesias are characterized clinically by the observation of involuntary mouth movements and the effects of these movements on the jaw muscles, TMJs, oral mucosa, and teeth. Emphasis on management is prevention because no one treatment is predictably effective and safe. A dentist observing dyskinesia in a patient taking conventional antipsychotics should inform the physician managing the medication. Tardive dyskinesia may be persistent even after drug therapy is stopped. Palliative treatment using tetrabenazine, a central monoamine depleter, clonazepam, and baclofen has been tried.[444]

Oromandibular dystonia produces involuntary and excessive contractions of tongue, lip, and jaw muscles. The etiology and pathophysiology are unknown. The proposed mechanism is related to defective inhibitory control of the basal ganglia of the forebrain, thalamus, and brainstem. Injection of botulinum toxin has been used in cases of oromandibular dystonia.[445] Severely disabling and refractory conditions have been treated with neurosurgical intervention.[446]

Selected Readings

Clark GT, Minakuchi H. Oral appliances. In: Laskin DM, Greene CS, Hylander WL, eds. *TMDs, an Evidence-Based Approach to Diagnosis and Treatment.* Chicago: Quintessence; 2006:377–390.

de Leeuw R, Klasser GD. *Orofacial Pain: Guidelines for Assessment, Diagnosis, and Management.* Hanover Park, IL: Quintessence Publishing; 2013.

Dworkin SF. Psychological and psychosocial assessment. In: Laskin DM, Greene CS, Hylander WL, eds. *TMDs, an Evidence-Based Approach to Diagnosis and Treatment.* Chicago: Quintessence; 2006:203–217.

Fricton J, Kroening R, Hathaway K. *TMJ and Craniofacial Pain: Diagnosis and Management.* St. Louis: Ishiyaku Euroamerica; 1988.

Kurita K, Westesson PL, Yuasa H, et al. Natural course of untreated symptomatic temporomandibular joint disc displacement without reduction. *J Dent Res.* 1998;77:361–365.

Lund JP. Muscular pain and dysfunction. In: Laskin DM, Greene CS, Hylander WL, eds. *Temporomandibular Disorders, an Evidence-Based Approach to Diagnosis and Treatment.* Chicago: Quintessence; 2006: 99.

Milam SB. TMJ osteoarthritis. In: Laskin DM, Greene CS, Hylander WL, eds. *TMDs, an Evidence-Based Approach to Diagnosis and Treatment.* Chicago: Quintessence; 2006:105–123.

National Institutes of Health. Management of temporomandibular disorders: NIH technology assessment statement. 1996.

National Institutes of Health Technology Assessment Conference on Management of Temporomandibular Disorders. Oral Surg Oral Med Oral Pathol Oral Radiol Endod 1997;83:49–183.

Ohrbach R, Gonzalez Y, List T, Michelotti A, Schiffman E. *Diagnostic Criteria for Temporomandibular Disorders (DC/TMD) Clinical Examination Protocol.* 2014; Available from: http://www.rdc-tmdinternational.org/Portals/18/protocol_DC-TMD/DC-TMD Protocol - 2013_06_02.pdf.

Sato S, Takahashi K, Kawamura H, Motegi K. The natural course of nonreducing disc displacement of the temporomandibular joint. *Int J Oral Maxillofac Surg.* 1998;27:173–178.

Schiffman E, Ohrbach R, Truelove E, Look J, et al. Diagnostic Criteria for Temporomandibular Disorders (DC/TMD) for Clinical and Research Applications: recommendations of the International RDC/TMD Consortium Network and Orofacial Pain Special Interest Group. *J Oral Facial Pain Headache.* 2014;28:6–27.

Scrivani SJ, Keith DA, Kaban LB. Temporomandibular disorders. *N Engl J Med.* 2008;359:2693–2705.

Wanman A. Longitudinal course of symptoms of craniomandibular disorders in men and women. A 10-year follow-up study of an epidemiologic sample. *Acta Odontol Scand.* 1996;54:337–342.

For the full reference lists, please go to http://www.pmph-usa.com/Burkets_Oral_Medicine.

CHAPTER 12

Orofacial Pain

Rafael Benoliel, BDS, LDS RCS Eng
Sowmya Ananthan, BDS, DMD, MSD
Julyana Gomes Zagury, DMD, MSD
Junad Khan, BDS, MPH, PhD.
Eli Eliav, DMD, MSc, PhD.

INTRODUCTION

Pain is a multifaceted experience involving physical, cognitive, and emotional aspects. Reflecting this complexity, pain has been defined as "an unpleasant sensory and emotional experience associated with actual or potential tissue damage, or described in terms of such damage."[1]

Acute pain resulting from injury will generally initiate a reflex withdrawal thus ensuring minimal or no tissue damage (nociceptive pain). If tissue has been damaged, a local inflammatory response ensues causing increased sensitivity in peripheral nociceptors (peripheral sensitization) and in dorsal horn neurons associated with pain transmission (central sensitization). Due to these effects, the injured region becomes sensitive to even light touch (allodynia) and over reactive to painful stimuli (hyperalgesia). As a result, the individual protects the injured area encouraging healing. Injury is, in most cases, followed by a healing period associated with variable levels of pain, but in most cases, resolves with no residual disability.

In contrast, chronic pain not associated with ongoing tissue damage or that continues beyond healing offers no tangible survival value. Instead chronic pain inflicts severe physical and emotional suffering on the individual. In many patients who develop chronic pain, this may be the result of primary or reactive changes in the nervous system. These changes include faulty pain modulation with deficient pain inhibition and often increased facilitation. These changes perpetuate the sensation of pain in the absence of an active injury; the system has malfunctioned and maladaptive pain remains.

Chronic pain is therefore often not a symptom but a disease in its own right. It is often hard to distinguish between pain as a *disease* from pain as a *symptom*. The latter signifies an expression of a pathological process that if treated will eradicate pain. The inability to perceive pain as a disease may result in repeated and unsuccessful interventions, all in an attempt to "to eliminate the cause of pain."

OROFACIAL PAIN

Orofacial pain (OFP) is prevalent in the general population; around 23%, of which 7%–11% is chronic.[2,3] Acute OFP is primarily associated with the teeth and their supporting structures. Most frequently, dental pain is due to dental caries, although a broken filling or tooth-abrasion may also cause dental sensitivity. Other oral pains are usually periodontal or gingival in origin.

Chronic orofacial pain (COFP) is a term used to describe painful regional syndromes with a chronic, unremitting pattern. Clinically COFP may be subdivided into three main symptomatic classes: musculoskeletal, neurovascular, and neuropathic.[4] Musculoskeletal entities are dealt with in Chapter 11, "Temporomandibular Disorders."

The best resources for diagnostic descriptions of OFP and headache entities are the classifications published by the International Headache Society (http://www.ihs-headache.org/frame_non_members.asp),[5] and by the american academy of orofacial pain.[6]

CHRONIC OROFACIAL PAIN

Neurovascular Pain

Neurovascular pains include the trigeminal autonomic cephalgias (TACs) and migraines (Table 12-1). In this section, we describe TACs and facial migraines; for a description of migraines and other primary headaches, see Chapter 13, "Headaches."

Trigeminal Autonomic Cephalgias

TACs are primary headaches with a common clinical phenotype consisting of trigeminal pain and autonomic signs (AS) and include cluster headache (CH), paroxysmal hemicrania (PH), short-lasting unilateral, neuralgiform headache attacks with conjunctival injection and tearing (SUNCT), short-lasting, unilateral, neuralgiform headache attacks with cranial autonomic features (SUNA), and hemicrania continua (HC).[5]

Pathophysiology of Trigeminal Autonomic Cephalgias

The current pathophysiologic model attempts to explain the three major features of the TACs; trigeminal pain, rhythmicity (particularly in CH), and AS. Taken together, current data suggest that CH and other TACs are conditions whose pathophysiological basis is in the central nervous system, including the hypothalamus, that drives the initiation of the clinical phenotype. Detailed pathophysiology may be obtained in reviews; see Leone et al.[7] and Holle et al.[8]

TABLE 12-1 Diagnosis of Neurovascular Pain

Diagnosis	Pain Intensity	Primary Location	Referral	Autonomic Signs	Clinical Symptoms	Examination Findings	Imaging
Migraine	Moderate to severe	Frontal, temporal, occipital	Maxillary sinus, intraorally	+	Throbbing, periodic, nausea and/or vomiting, photo- and phonophobia, unilateral>bilateral. Last 4–72 h. May wake from sleep—usually early morning.	Allodynia	Usually not needed. Note: Onset is in in childhood.
Facial migraine/ NVOP	Moderate to severe	Intraorally. Middle and lower third of the face	Infraorbitally, periauricular	+/-	Also pressing pain that may wake from sleep.	Thorough examination to exclude dental pathology. Often mild pericranial/ masticatory muscle tenderness is present. Cranial nerve examination and brain imaging should be performed to identify symptomatic cases.	Important to exclude dental pathology or sinusitis. In selected cases brain imaging to exclude pathology
CH	Severe	These entities are usually associated with a primarily periorbital location. SUNCT occurs throughout the face/head	Commonly to temporal, frontal and cervical regions. Very commonly to intraoral regions	+++	Also neuralgic. Occurs in cluster or chronic. Last 15–180 min and may occur up to 8/d. Restlessness.		Up to 4% of patients with pituitary tumors have CH.

TABLE 12-1 *(Continued)*

Diagnosis	Pain Intensity	Primary Location	Referral	Autonomic Signs	Clinical Symptoms	Examination Findings	Imaging
PH	Severe			++	More frequent (8–30/d) than cluster headache but shorter lasting (2–30 min).		Chronic PH is often associated with systemic disease.
SUNCT	Severe			++	Sharp, stabbing lasts 2–240 s. Extremely high frequency (2–200/d). May have trigger areas similar to trigeminal neuralgia.		Most common mimics of SUNCT are lesions in the posterior fossa or involving the pituitary gland.
Hemicrania continua	Moderate	Temporal, frontal, periorbital	Upper 2/3 of the face and intraorally	+	Continuous unremitting. Exacerbations resemble migraine.		

Abbreviations: CH, cluster headache; NVOP, neurovascular orofacial pain; PH, paroxysmal hemicrania; SUNCT, short-lasting, unilateral, neuralgiform, headache attacks with conjunctival injection and tearing.

Cluster Headache

CH is the archetypal TAC with severe pain and major autonomic activation.[5] The precise genetics of CH are unclear but is likely to involve an autosomal dominant gene with low penetrance.[9] First-degree relatives of CH patients are up to 14–48 times and second-degree relatives 2–8 times more likely to have CH than the general population.[9] CH typically appears between the ages of 20–29 years, is more common than previously thought, and seems to affect men more than women.[10]

A unique feature of episodic CH is the distinctive circadian and circannaual periodicity. Episodic CH commonly occurs at least once daily for a period of weeks, at the same time of day or night. Active periods (or "clusters" of 6–12 weeks) are followed by a temporary remission that may last from weeks to years (12 months). Attacks tend to be shorter and less severe at the beginning and toward the end of each cluster period. At its initial onset, CH active periods are seasonal, occurring around spring or autumn.

There are two distinct temporal presentations of CH; most (80%–85%) suffer from the episodic type characterized by at least two cluster periods lasting 7–365 days separated by pain-free periods of ≥ 1 month.[5,11] In chronic CH, repeated attacks recur over more than a year without remission or with remission periods lasting less than one month. Interictal pain may also be present between attacks or between clusters.[12] Of the 15% of patients with chronic CH, in two-thirds it usually begins as such and in the remaining evolves from the episodic form. Up to half of chronic CH patients report transition to an episodic pattern. Over the course of the disease, attack duration tends to lengthen in both episodic and chronic CH.

Interval till final diagnosis is reported atthree to six years: 34%–45% had consulted a dentist and 27%–33% an otolaryngologist before accurate diagnosis.[12,13] Atypical referral patterns, migrainous features, episodic attack patterns, and a young onset age tended to delay diagnosis.

Features

Pain in CH is usually periorbital or ocular, but varies. In "upper CH" the forehead, temporal, and parietal regions are involved,[14] whereas in "lower CH" the temporal and suboccipital regions are affected with radiation to the teeth, jaws, neck,[14] and cheeks.[12,15] Pain is unilateral and in 20% of cases may change sides. Attacks alternate sides more commonly between clusters than between attacks in the same cluster.

Severity is excruciating and rated as 8–10 on a visual analog scale. Quality is nonspecific and is variably described as throbbing or boring, burning, stabbing.[16] Patients may describe pain as a "hot poker" or a "stabbing" feeling in the eye.[15] CH attacks last 15–180 minutes reaching peak intensity very rapidly—within 3 minutes (up to 9–10 minutes).[16] Longer attacks lasting from 3 to 48 hours are rare[12] and frequency is one every other day to 8/d. Pain is most usually accompanied by at least one ipsilateral autonomic sign; conjunctival injection/lacrimation, nasal congestion/rhinorrhea, eyelid edema, forehead/facial sweating, miosis, and ptosis.

The vast majority (>80%) of patients are markedly restless during an attack. Patients appear agitated, continually move around, particularly during more severe attacks; in sharp contrast to the quiet-seeking behavior observed in migraine.

Additional Features

A considerable number of CH patients report nocturnal attacks that wake them. Pain typically awakens patients within 90 minutes coinciding with the onset of rapid eye movement sleep.[15] Additionally, CH patients significantly suffer from obstructive sleep apnea.[17] Alcohol is a common precipitant of CH attacks during active cluster periods.[18]

Premonitory symptoms may predict CH days before onset. CH prodromes include AS, blurred vision, sensitivity to smells, nausea, dyspepsia, hunger, irritability, tiredness, tenseness, and mild pain or non-painful sensations in the area that subsequently becomes painful. Migrainous features are common in CH and may confuse diagnosis.[19] Photophobia, phonophobia, nausea, and vomiting are reported in up to half of cases. It is important to note that phono- and photophobia are unilateral while in migraine these are bilateral.[20]

Differential Diagnosis and Secondary CH

CH is often misdiagnosed as dental or maxillary sinus pathology possibly due to referral patterns[12,13,21] and occurrence of "lower CH."[14] Secondary TACs, due to pathology, have no "typical" presentation and mimic 1ry TAC.[22,23] Neuroimaging must be performed for all TACs or atypical TAC-like syndromes.[24]

CH Treatment

Based on attack patterns, patients should avoid daytime naps, alcoholic beverages, and other triggers. Pharmacologic treatment may be abortive, transitional, or preventative. Abortive symptomatic relief may be rapidly attained with oxygen inhalation.[25] Subcutaneous sumatriptan is a very efficacious abortive therapy, but patients must be medically fit. Rapid transitional prophylaxis may be attained with corticosteroids that may be continued only for a limited period in selected patients.[26] In both episodic and chronic CH, prophylaxis is usually with verapamil, and topiramate as second-line therapy. Remission periods may increase with time, and beyond the age of 65–75 active CH is rare.

Paroxysmal Hemicrania

PH is rare with an estimated prevalence of 2–20 per 100,000.[27,28] Mean age of onset is usually 34–41 years, but children aged 6 and adults aged 81 years have been reported. The episodic form is considered to have an earlier mean age of onset (27 years) than the chronic form (37 years). Only 20% of PHs behave episodically, and many of these eventually developed into a chronic form.[29]

Features

PH is a unilateral, severe orbital, or periorbital pain. The vast majority of attacks do not change sides, but strong pain may cross the midline and very rarely becomes bilateral.[30] It may occur in temporal, periauricular, maxillary, and rarely occipital areas.[31] Referral to the shoulder, neck, and arm is quite common.[31]

Patients usually report 8–30 attacks/24 h that last 2–30 minutes, but may last nearly an hour. Pain onset is rapid and mostly peaks in less than 5 minutes.[29] A seasonal pattern of attacks has been described in PH patients and has led to the term "modified cluster pattern."[31] About one-third of PH patients report nocturnal attacks that wake.

Quality is mostly sharp but may also be throbbing, stabbing, or boring and its severity excruciating.[29] Accompanying ipsilateral AS include conjunctival injection/lacrimation, nasal congestion/rhinorrhea, eyelid edema, forehead/facial sweating, miosis, and ptosis. AS may occur bilaterally but are more pronounced on the symptomatic side. The most common are ipsilateral lacrimation, nasal congestion, conjunctival injection, and rhinorrhea. In patient series one "migrainous feature" was reported by nearly 90% of PH cases.[29,32]

Secondary Paroxysmal Hemicrania

Systemic diseases, malignancy, CNS disease, and benign tumors[33] have mimicked PH and therefore all cases require imaging.

Treatment

Most cases respond to indomethacin within 24 hours and this response to indomethacin is part of its classification criteria. Indomethacin should be initiated for 3 days at 75mg followed, if needed, by 150 mg for a further 3 days is recommended as trial therapy. High and persistent dosage requirements may indicate the underlying pathology. Prognosis in PH is good and long-term remission has been reported. A summary of therapies for PH, SUNCT, and HC is shown in Table 12-2.

SUNCT

SUNCT syndrome is a unilateral headache/facial pain characterized by brief paroxysmal attacks accompanied by ipsilateral local AS, usually conjunctival injection and lacrimation. The similarities of this syndrome to trigeminal neuralgia (TN) are marked, particularly the triggering mechanism, and some believe that SUNCT may be a TN variant.

Estimates suggest SUNCT/SUNA to be as common as PH.[10] SUNCT is presently considered only slightly more common in males[34,35] with a mean onset age of about 50 years.[34,36] SUNCT occurs in siblings and has been presented as "familial SUNCT."[37]

Features

SUNCT is a unilateral pain, usually ocular/periocular,[5] but may involve most head areas.[38] Pain spreading across the midline or changing sides is rare.[34] Quality is usually stabbing or pulsating but sometimes electric or burning.[34] Pain is moderate to severe[34] and accompanied by ipsilateral conjunctival injection and lacrimation.

Attacks last from 5 to 600 seconds, and three patterns of attack frequency are described.[24,38] These may be single attacks, groups of a number of stabs/attacks, or a "saw-tooth" pattern with numerous stabs/attacks lasting minutes. Frequency is from 3 to 200 daily, but this is inconsistent and irregular with an average of 28/d.[39]

TABLE 12-2 Treatment of Neurovascular Pain

Diagnosis	Treatment
Facial migraine/NVOP	Abortive: naproxen sodium (825 mg stat), other NSAIDs, analgesics, triptans (e.g., rizatriptan 10mg, zolmitriptan 2.5 mg, eletriptan 40 mg, frovatriptan 2.5 mg. No specific evidence for triptans in facial migraine/NVOP but works in selected cases) Prophylactic: β-blockers (propranolol SR 80–160 mg daily), AEDs (divalproex SR 500 mg daily, topiramate 25–200 mg/d), TCAs (amitriptyline 10–50 mg/d)
Cluster headache	Abortive: sumatriptan (IN 20 mg stat, SC 6–12 mg stat), dihydroergotamine (IN 0.5–1 mg stat), oxygen (5–10L/min for 15 min) Prophylactic: verapamil (160–480 mg/d), AEDs (topiramate 25–200 mg/d or gabapentin 900 mg/d), prednisone (initial control), lithium (for chronic, 300–900 mg/d)
Paroxysmal hemicrania	Indomethacin (75–225 mg/d), other NSAIDs
SUNCT	Lamotrigine (currently considered drug of choice: 100–300 mg/d), gabapentin (900–2700 mg/d), topiramate (50–200 mg/d)
Hemicrania continua	Indomethacin (25–300 mg/d), other NSAIDs

Abbreviations: AED, antiepileptic drug; NSAID, nonsteroidal anti-inflammatory drug; NVOP, neurovascular orofacial pain; SUNCT, short-lasting, unilateral, neuralgiform, headache attacks with conjunctival injection and tearing; TCA, tricyclic antidepressant.

Pain in SUNCT may be triggered by light mechanical stimuli in the areas innervated by the trigeminal nerve, with a short latency till onset but with no refractory period.[34] Extratrigeminal triggers including neck movements precipitate attacks.

SUNA

Essentially the accompanying AS differentiate it from SUNCT; SUNA may be accompanied by either autonomic sign, ipsilateral conjunctival injection or lacrimation but not both.

SUNCT/SUNA Treatment

Lamotrigine is the drug of choice and should be initiated at 25mg/d then increased very slowly and reach target dose in ≥7 weeks.[24,40] Other anticonvulsant drugs such as carbamazepine, topiramate, and gabapentin may induce some improvement. SUNCT may also respond to steroids. There are case reports of successful surgical microvascular decompression (MVD) and percutaneous trigeminal ganglion compression for SUNCT.[41] Spontaneous remissions have been observed and may last for several months.

Hemicrania Continua

HC is now considered a part of the TAC family.[5] As in other TACs, HC seems to be often misdiagnosed and mistreated; time to correct diagnosis may reach five years.[42]

Features

HC is a unilateral headache that has been present for >3 months and is daily and continuous. Pain is diffuse around half the head and face primarily in the frontal, temporal, and periorbital regions.[5] Two forms of HC have been described. The remitting form is characterized by headache that can last for some days followed by a pain free period lasting from 2 to 15 days.[43] Following a mean duration of 7.8 years one-third of remitting cases transform to the second form which is continuous.[43] Nocturnal attacks are reported in up to half of patients.[43]

Severity is moderate (VAS 4.7) and characterized by fluctuations.[43] Exacerbations result in severe pain (VAS 9.3) lasting 30 minutes to 10 hours and even up to 2–5 days.[43] These exacerbations are almost indistinguishable from migraine and about 40% of patients report they are temporarily disabled.[43] Pain quality may be throbbing.

There is usually a paucity of AS in HC. However, during exacerbation AS commonly appear singly or in various combinations but are still relatively mild. This strengthens the hypothesis that activation of AS is dependent on pain severity. The most common signs present in 30%–40% of patients are photophobia, nausea, conjunctival injection, phonophobia, and tearing. A sandy sensation in the eye has been reported.[44] During exacerbations up to 60% of patients display features such as photophobia, phonophobia, nausea, and more rarely vomiting.[43] HC with aura has also been described further linking HC to migraine pathophysiology.[45] More rarely (15%–18%) nasal stuffiness or rhinorrhea, vomiting, or ptosis may also be reported.[46] These features establish the HC phenotype as straddling both TACs and migraine.

Secondary Hemicrania Continua

HC is not usually accompanied by notable pathology or other abnormalities. Most published cases of HC with computerized scanning of the head, neurological examination, hematology, and serum biochemistry were all normal. However, cases of HC secondary to pathology or systemic disease have been reported.[33] HC like presentations secondary to medication abuse, head trauma, and surgery have also been reported.[43]

Treatment

Indomethacin is totally effective and relieves pain within hours or 1–2 days[5]; other NSAIDs are less effective.[47] Piroxicam-beta-cyclodextrin is a good alternative for selected cases.

Lower Facial Pain With Neurovascular Features

OFP with neurovascular features may occur as a result of referral in migraine or one of the TACs.[12,48] Some patients, however, present with primary lower facial pain accompanied by AS, nausea, and photo- or phonophobia.[49,50] These cases are often classifiable as lower CH or an atypically located but otherwise classical migraine (lower half migraine)

Alternatively, patients may present with neurovascular OFP that is not diagnosable as lower CH or lower half migraine, an entity we refer to as neurovascular orofacial pain (NVOP). The rational for introducing NVOP is based on features that segregate it from other primary neurovascular headaches, such as its intraoral and perioral locations (i.e., second and third divisions of the trigeminal nerve). Additionally, NVOP is a term that allows us to keep an open mind as data accumulate and point toward a possible pathophysiology.

Clinical Features

Pain location is most commonly reported in the oral and perioral areas (60%–70%).[51] Pain may refer to the infraorbital or to the periauricular regions.[51] Moderate-to-strong, episodic, unilateral (80%) pain is characteristic of NVOP. In 48%–65% of cases, pain throbs, and in 35%–48% wakes the patient from sleep,[51] particularly when the pain is more severe.[51] Pain may last from minutes to hours (45%–72% of cases) or continues for >24 hours (28%–55% of cases). Many NVOP patients present with daily chronic pain with a mean duration of 17 hours but may be as short as 1.7 hours.[51]

Pain can be accompanied by AS in 35% of cases.[51] Specifically tearing (10%–17%), nasal congestion (7%–9%), a feeling of swelling or fullness (7%) particularly in the cheek, and a complaint of excessive sweating (7%) were reported.[51] Other phenomena such as photo- or phonophobia and nausea (24%–30%) are observed.[51] Often patients report dental hypersensitivity to cold food or drink. Patients with NVOP are therefore commonly misdiagnosed and undergo unwarranted dental treatment.

The onset of NVOP is around 35–50 years of age, and it affects women more often than men.[51] Some patients have a positive history of migraine,[52] and in 30% of cases the onset of NVOP is associated with trauma,[51] often with previous migraine in cases. These cases exemplify the possible phenomenon of "relocation" of the original migraine to the orofacial region.[51,52]

In an attempt to establish diagnostic criteria we recently found that the combination of facial pain, throbbing quality, autonomic and/or systemic features (in particular nausea), and attack duration of >60 minutes gave a positive predictive value of 0.71 and a negative predictive value of 0.95 in the diagnosis of NVOP.[51]

Neuropathic Orofacial Pain

Neuropathic OFP (Table 12-3) includes a number of clinical entities; the most common are TN, painful posttraumatic neuropathies, and burning mouth syndrome (BMS). More rarely facial postherpetic neuropathy, central poststroke pain, and glossopharyngeal neuralgia (GN) are encountered.

Trigeminal Neuralgia
Introduction and Definition

TN is an excruciating, short-lasting, unilateral facial pain. The most common is the classical unrelated to pathology and most probably caused by neurovascular compression of the trigeminal nerve root. In the new classification, secondary forms have been classified separately, and these are related to a variety of clear pathologies including tumors, cysts, viral infection, trauma, and systemic diseases such as multiple sclerosis.[5] The vast majority (>85%) of TN patients are diagnosed with classical TN (CTN). Recent evidence suggests that most cases of CTN result from the compression of the trigeminal nerve root by a vascular malformation. Recognized by the current classification are TN cases that present with a continuous background pain in addition to the typical pain paroxysms. Up to one-third of patients (4%–35%) describe typical paroxysmal attacks on a background of dull persistent pain of varying duration.

TN and GN patients should undergo imaging (computerized tomography [CT] or magnetic resonance imaging [MRI]) at least once during diagnosis and therapy.[53] Imaging techniques such as magnetic resonance tomographic angiography (MRTA) may more accurately identify neurovascular compression.

Clinical Features and Diagnostic Criteria of CTN

Characterized by paroxysmal, excruciating pain in trigeminal dermatomes, most commonly in both the maxillary and mandibular branches of the trigeminal nerve (35%). In 36%–42% of cases CTN affects one branch: 16%–18% each in the maxillary or the mandibular branch, 2% in the ophthalmic branch, and all three branches in 14% of patients. CTN is strictly unilateral and pain radiation is generally within the dermatome of the origin.[5] Bilateral cases are extremely rare and begin unilaterally preceding the onset of contralateral pain by years.[54]

Pain is paroxysmal, shooting, sharp, piercing, stabbing, or electrical. Pain episodes are identical in location, duration, and intensity within individual TN patients, that is, stereotyped[5] but may vary considerably between patients. TN is characterized by spontaneous remissions lasting weeks to years but approximately 20% of TN patients suffer daily attacks with no respite. In fact, the majority of TN patients (90%) report increased attack frequency and severity.[55,56]

Attacks begin and end abruptly, lasting from a fraction of a second up to 2 minutes. Longer attacks, increasing with disease duration, have been reported.[57] Most paroxysms occur during waking hours, but may awaken the patient.[58] Pain paroxysms are usually accompanied by spasm of the ipsilateral facial muscles (hence the name *tic douloureux*).

TABLE 12-3 Diagnosis of Neurovascular Pain

Diagnosis	Pain Intensity	Primary Location	Referral	Clinical Symptoms	Examination Findings	Imaging
Posttraumatic neuropathy	Mild to severe	Initially localized, dermatomal	Adjacent structures, may cross midline	Onset associated with traumatic event. Burning or lancinating, electrical pain.	May be associated with areas of scar tissue. Affected areas demonstrate allodynia, dysesthesia, analgesia, redness. Temporal summation may occur.	May be associated with skeletal fractures or other pathology that induces nerve damage.
Burning mouth syndrome	Moderate (severe in some)	Tongue, lips	Localized	Idiopathic onset. Very frequently observed in postmenopausal women. Continuous burning sensation. May be associated with taste and salivary secretion disturbances.	Primary or idiopathic BMS must not be due to any local or systemic factor. Secondary BMS may occur in local mucosal disease, and a number of metabolic and endocrine disorders.	Irrelevant
TN	Severe	Second and third dermatomes of fifth CN	Usually dermatomal Referral to teeth very common	Short (seconds to 2–3 min), paroxysmal pain. May be triggered by innocuous stimuli or spontaneous. May have background pain (atypical TN) or begin in an uncharacteristic fashion pre-TN.	Usually none. Quantitative sensory testing may reveal mild sensory deficits. Focal neurological findings may indicate pathology. Trigger area may be identified that induces pain and subsequently becomes refractory.	Advanced techniques may show neurovascular contact at the CN5 nerve root. TN may also occur secondary to tumors and multiple sclerosis.
Postherpetic trigeminal neuropathy	Moderate to severe	Usually first dermatome of CN5	Usually localized but may spread if severe	Burning, constant pain. Superimposed flashes of pain.	Scars, hypopigmented regions. Scars may be hyposensitive or allodynic.	Irrelevant

Abbreviations: CN, cranial nerve; TN, trigeminal neuralgia.

Typically pain is precipitated by light, innocuous touch at sites called "trigger areas."[5] Many attacks are spontaneous, and trigger areas are not always clinically identifiable. Trigger areas are usually in the distribution of the affected trigeminal branch, usually the lips but may be extratrigeminal,[55] may be multiple, and may change location. Trigger *factors* such as noise, lights, and stress may also induce pain.

There are two attack-related phenomena that are particular to TN. *Latency* refers to the short period of time between stimulation of a trigger area and pain onset. A *refractory period* occurs following an attack and during this time pain may not be initiated.[5] Patients with CTN rarely complain of sensory loss[59] but sophisticated techniques may reveal these.

In patients with concomitant background pain, this is usually throbbing or burning. Patients with background pain demonstrate sensory loss and carry a poorer surgical prognosis.[60,61]

Pretrigeminal Neuralgia

An early form of TN termed "pretrigeminal neuralgia" (PTN) has been reported in 18% of TN patients and is characterized by a dull continuous pain (days to years) in one of the jaws. As PTN progresses it becomes more typical with characteristic flashes of pain. Thermal stimuli may cause triggering at a relatively higher rate, and a throbbing quality to PTN pain is sometimes present mimicking dental pathology. Indeed, these qualities combined with the success of regional anesthesia have led to misdiagnosis of PTN as pain of dental origin. PTN is however highly responsive to carbamazepine, and careful dental assessment should help differentiate it. Unfortunately, the lack of clear and consistent diagnostic criteria makes this a problematic entity to recognize; it is usually diagnosed when all other possibilities are exhausted or in retrospect once CTN develops.

Treatment (Table 12-4)
Pharmacological

Carbamazepine remains the drug of choice for TN. Initial low-dose therapy (100 mg with food) and a slow increase (by 100–200 mg) on alternate days will minimize side effects. In responsive cases, therapeutic effects are observed rapidly or within three days. Titration to final dose (1200 mg/d or more) should continue slowly based on response and side effects. Light-headedness, confusion,

dizziness, vertigo, blurred vision or diplopia, sedation, vomiting, nystagmus, and nausea are very common and cause 5%–20% of patients to request drug cessation. Transient elevation in liver enzymes may occur in 5%–10% and transient leucopenia in 5% of patients (persistent in 2%). Aplastic anemia is a serious effect that may occur in 1 of 15–200,000 cases. Hyponatremia is observed in 4%–22% of carbamazepine-treated cases and requires drug withdrawal. Skin rashes occur in up to 10% of patients and may signal the onset of antiepileptic drug hypersensitivity syndrome. This is a life-threatening syndrome (fever, rash, and lymphadenopathy) associated with some antiepileptic drugs (AEDs) and requires immediate drug cessation.

Clinically, about 300 mg of oxcarbazepine is approximately equivalent to 200 mg of carbamazepine and response occurs in 24–48 hours.[62] Baclofen has a strong synergistic effect with carbamazepine, making it suitable for combined therapy. Newer anticonvulsants have fewer side effects and have been shown to be effective for some cases either as monotherapy or add-on therapy. Lamotrigine is effective particularly as add-on therapy, and gabapentin may be useful in selected TN cases.

Initial response to carbamazepine is good (70%) but drops dramatically (20%) by 5–16 years. Similarly, oxcarbazepine-treated TN patients demonstrate a high failure rate leading to surgery.[56] The progressive nature of TN is also reflected by the fact that MVD has a significantly reduced prognosis in long-standing TN.[63]

TABLE 12-4 Treatment of Trigeminal Neuropathic Pain	
Diagnosis	Treatment Options
Posttraumatic neuropathy	Gabapentin (300 mg/d initial for 3 d; increase by 300 mg every 3 d till 300 mg × 3/d. If response is positive titrate up to 2700 mg/d) TCAs (amitriptyline 10 mg/d initially up to 50 mg daily; nortriptyline 10–25 mg/d titrate slowly) SNRIs (venlafaxine SR 37.5 mg/d initially up to 150 mg/d) Pregabalin Opioids Combination therapies (gabapentin/venlafaxine; gabapentin/opioids) Topical medications: 5% lidocaine patches, topical AEDs, or TCAs in stents
Burning mouth syndrome	Topical clonazepam (1 mg; "suck and spit" 3 times daily) Cognitive behavioral therapy Alpha-lipoic acid (600 mg daily) TCAs
TN	Carbamazepine (100–200 mg twicedaily of the slow release formulation. Increase as needed) Oxcarbazepine (300 mg × 3/d, titrate as needed) Baclofen (5–10 mg × 3/d, needs titrating down slowly. Usually used as add on therapy) Gabapentin (200–300 mg × 2/d) Lamotrigine (25 mg × 1–2/d. Needs very slow titration, use only if experienced) Surgical (best prognosis in typical TN early after onset): • Peripheral level • Ganglion level • Trigeminal root level
Postherpetic trigeminal neuropathy	Topical lidocaine TCAs Gabapentin Opioids

Abbreviations: AEDs, antiepileptic drugs; TCAs, tricyclic antidepressants; TN, trigeminal neuralgia.

Surgical

Surgery for TN is directed peripherally or centrally at the trigeminal ganglion or nerve root. Surgical procedures have a better prognosis when carried out on patients with typical CTN; MVD has the best prognosis when performed within seven years of TN onset.[63]

Peripheral Procedures

Success rates for neurectomy are conflicting and involve relatively small series with short-term follow-up.[64] Peripheral neurectomy carries the danger of inducing traumatic neuropathic pain and is not recommended. Cryotherapy of peripheral branches may give pain relief for six months.[65] Pain recurrence is at the original site, and repeated cryotherapy often produces better results. Up to one-third may develop persistent pain after cryotherapy. Historically, alcohol injections have been used but are painful and cause fibrosis. Alcohol may induce herpes zoster (HZ) reactivation and bony necrosis.[64] Pain control after alcohol block lasts just over one year, and there have been reports of postinjection neuropathic pain. Peripheral glycerol injection has been employed, but success seems short term. Reinjection is however possible with reportedly good results.[66]

Due to the risk of developing neuropathic pain, peripheral procedures should be reserved for patients with significant medical problems that make other procedures unsafe.[64]

Central Procedures

Percutaneous Trigeminal Rhizotomy

Three techniques are in use at the ganglion level: radiofrequency rhizolysis, glycerol injection, and balloon compression. These modalities result in excellent initial pain relief (around 90%) but are associated with high rates of recurrence and complications. Overall radiofrequency rhizolysis consistently provides the highest rates of pain relief but is associated with high frequencies of facial and corneal numbness.[67]

Microvascular Decompression

MVD surgically separates intracerebral arteries from the trigeminal nerve root. Complications may include hearing loss, meningitis, cerebral fluid leak, wound infection, and sensory changes (5%–10% of patients).[68,69] However, complication rates are lowest in hospitals with extensive experience.[70] After 10 years, 30%–40% of MVD patients will experience a relapse, but MVD remains the most cost-effective surgical approach to CTN.[71,72]

Gamma Knife

Gamma knife stereotactic radiosurgery (GKS) is a minimally invasive technique that precisely delivers radiosurgical doses (70–90 Gy) to the trigeminal nerve root at the point of vascular compression and provides good to excellent initial pain relief.[73,74] GKS has better long-term pain relief with less treatment-related morbidity than glycerol rhizotomy and may be indicated in patients who are poor candidates for MVD.[73,75] However GKS been extensively used as a second (salvage) procedure. Success rates of GKS as a first procedure are therefore higher.[76,77]

In summary, TN has a good initial treatment response to almost all modalities but a predictable relapse of up to 40%–50% over 15 years. Periods of pain relief are shortest for peripheral procedures, intermediate for drug therapy or rhizotomies, and longest for MVD.

Glossopharyngeal Neuralgia

Although similarities with TN are prominent, GN is characterized by a milder natural history with the majority of patients going into remission. Due to its location and features, GN is a difficult diagnosis and adequate treatment is often delayed for years.[78]

Features

The glossopharyngeal (IX) nerve has two main sensory branches: the auricular (tympanic) and the pharyngeal. In pharyngeal-GN, the pharynx or posterior tongue-base are involved. Pain radiates to the inner ear or the angle of the mandible, and may include the eye, nose, maxilla, or shoulder and even the tip of the tongue. In tympanic-GN, pain predominates in the ear but may radiate to the pharynx. Bilateral pain occurs in up to a quarter of patients.

GN is a paroxysmal, unilateral, severe painthat is sharp, stabbing, shooting, or lancinating.[5] Patients often feel a scratching or foreign body sensation in the throat. Pain intensity is usually milder than TN but may vary[79] and attacks last from a fraction of a second up to 2 minutes. GN attacks are stereotyped within patients. Trigger areas are located in the tonsillar region and posterior pharynx, and these display a refractory period.[5] Swallowing, chewing, talking, coughing and/or yawning, sneezing, clearing the throat, and rubbing the ear activate these areas.[80]

Frequency is around 5–12 every hour, and attacks may occur in clusters lasting weeks to months, then relapse for up to a number of years.[5] Spontaneous remissions occur in the majority of patients, but some have no periods of pain relief. GN may induce uncontrollable coughing, seizures, and cardiac arrhythmias, particularly bradycardia, and syncope.

Imaging of the head and neck to rule out pathology is indicated. An electrocardiogram should be performed prior to and after treatment. Preoperative MRTA is recommended to locate possible neurovascular contacts. The most common differential is TN particularly since co-occurrence of TN and GN is common.

Pathologies Mimicking GN

A significant association between symptomatic GN and multiple sclerosis has been reported.[80] Regional diseases such as infectious or inflammatory processes, tonsillar carcinoma, and other regional tumors (tongue, oropharyngeal) may cause GN. Cerebello pontine angle or pontine lesions may cause GN-like symptoms.[81] These entities are however rare. Persistent pain interictally and clinically detectable neurological deficits are characteristics of symptomatic GN.

Pathophysiology of GN

The pathophysiology is uncertain but is considered to probably be secondary to compression of the nerve root by a blood vessel. GN cases demonstrate nerve compression on MRI and on surgical exposure,[82] and nerve biopsy shows variable myelin damage and patches of demyelinated axons in close membrane-to-membrane apposition to one another.[83] These morphological changes are similar to those observed in patients with TN suggesting shared pathophysiology.

Treatment

Carbamazepine is usually successful and is the favored medication. Alternatives include baclofen, oxcarbazepine, gabapentin, lamotrigine, and phenytoin.[84] Patients with GN successfully treated with anticonvulsants may become resistant in which case there is a clear indication for surgery. Life-threatening arrhythmias may require cardiac pacing. MVD and GKS have been successful in patients with GN.[85] MVD induced immediate and complete relief of pain in 80%–95% of GN patients with stable long-term-results.[78,86] Permanent neurological deficits are rare and may include mild hoarseness and/or dysphagia, or facial nerve paresis.

Facial Pain Associated With Herpes Zoster
Acute Herpes Zoster

Acute HZ (shingles) is a reactivation of latent varicella virus infection that may occur decades after the primary infection. HZ is a disease of the dorsal root ganglion and therefore induces a dermatomal vesicular eruption. Definitive diagnosis may be obtained by identification of viral DNA from vesicular fluid employing the polymerase chain reaction.

Trigeminal and cervical nerves are involved in up to a quarter of cases each.[5] The ophthalmic branch is affected in more than 80% of the trigeminal cases, particularly in elderly males, and may cause sight-threatening keratitis. The vesicles and pain are dermatomal and unilateral and may appear intraorally when the maxillary or mandibular branches of the trigeminal nerve are affected.

Clinical Features

Usually begins with a prodrome of regional pain, itching and malaise.[5] Pain precedes typical vesicular eruption by <7 days, usually 2–3 days. The dermatomal vesicular or herpetic eruption will rupture and "dry out" over 7–10 days, but complete healing may last up to one month. Accompanying pain is moderate to severe (VAS 6) and may persist for three to six months.[87] Very rarely dermatomal pain occurs with no rash (zoster sine herpete).

Treatment

Therapy[88] is directed at controlling pain, accelerating healing, and reducing the risk of complications such as meningitis, postherpetic trigeminal neuropathy (PHN), and local secondary infection.[87] Antivirals should be initiated within 72 hours from onset of rash, and will significantly decrease rash duration, pain severity, and the incidence of PHN.[89,90] This is particularly effective in patients >50 years old. Fever and pain should be controlled initially by mild analgesics, but opioids may be used for stronger pain. Alternatively central analgesics may be used (amitriptyline or gabapentin). Use of glucocorticoids is controversial, but may help reduce acute pain[91]; they should always be used together with antivirals. Amitriptyline may reduce the incidence of PHN. Vaccinating at risk individuals markedly reduces the incidence of PHN among older adults.[92]

PHN

Up to one-fifth of acute HZ patients will suffer persistent pain three to six months after acute HZ. By one year however only 5%–10% suffer pain. Advanced age (>50), severe prodromal pain (VAS>5), severe acute pain, and severe rash are risk factors for persistent pain.[93,94] In patients older than 60 years, 50% or more will continue to suffer pain for more than one year.

Features of PHN

PHN is a dermatomal disease persisting or recurring ≥3 months after the acute HZ stage.[5] PHN rarely affects the trigeminal nerve and when it does it is mostly in the ophthalmic branch which accounts for 22% of PHN patients. Patients relate a previous herpetic (dermatomal) eruption that waspreceded by pain usually two to three days but up to six days prior.[5]

PHN is characterized by fluctuations from moderate background pain to excruciating, superimposed lancinating pains. Pain quality is burning, throbbing, stabbing, shooting, or sharp. Burning pain is significantly higher in patients not treated with antivirals for acute HZ. Itching is very common and prominent in trigeminal dermatomes[95] and may be subjectively graded as worse than pain. Pale, sometimes red/purple, scars that are usually hypoesthetic or anesthetic (but with allodynia and hyperalgesia) may remain in the affected area.

Treatment

Early treatment of established PHN improves prognosis.[96] Ophthalmic PHN per se seems to have the worst prognosis. Evidence-based treatment options for PHN include tricyclic antidepressant (TCA) drugs, gabapentin and pregabalin, opioids, tramadol, and topical lidocaine patches.[97]

Invasive therapies include epidural and intrathecal steroids and a variety of neurosurgical techniques.[98] The most promising surgical intervention seems to be dorsal root entry zone lesion that provides relief in 59% of treated cases. Central nervous system stimulation may also provide some relief.

Prevention with a vaccine has been advocated for the older population, particularly those at risk.

Burning Mouth Syndrome

BMS is a poorly understood pain condition that is most probably neuropathic. The condition is also known as stomatodynia and is characterized by a burning mucosal pain with no significant physical signs and is common in postmenopausal women.

BMS may be subclassified into "primary" or idiopathic BMS for which a neuropathological cause is likely and cannot be attributed to any systemic or local cause and "secondary BMS" (SBMS) resulting from local or systemic pathological conditions.[99] BMS is unfortunately characterized by resistance to a wide range of treatments and is one of the most challenging management problems in the field of OFP.[100]

Clinical Features

The primary location of the burning complaint is the tongue, usually the anterior 2/3. However, usually more than one site is involved and in addition to the tongue, hard palate, lips, and gingivae are frequently involved.

Pain is most commonly described as burning or hot[100] and intensity varies from mild to severe.[100] BMS is typically of spontaneous onset and lasts from months to several years.[101] The pain pattern may be irregular, but some patients may complain that pain increases toward the end of the day. Although a chronic unremitting pattern is usual, partial remission has been reported in about one half to two-thirds of patients, six to seven years after onset. Spontaneous remission is very rare.

Common aggravating factors include personal stressors, fatigue, and specific foods (acidic, hot, or spicy). More than two-thirds of the patients complain of altered taste sensation (dysgeusia) accompanying the burning sensation, in many cases described as a spontaneous metallic taste. Abnormal sensations, such as feeling of dry mouth, are common but true hyposalivation is less common and should be considered under secondary or symptomatic BMS.

As a group, BMS patients have shown no evidence for significant clinical depression, anxiety, and somatization but report fewer disruptions in normal activities relative to other chronic pain patients.[102] This suggests that although some BMS patients suffer significant distress the vast majority cope better than most chronic pain patients.[102]

Oral and perioral burning sensation as a result of local or systemic factors or diseases is classified as SBMS.[99] Local factors and diseases known to induce SBMS include oral candidiasis, lichen planus, and allergies. Systemic disorders that induce SBMS include hormonal changes, deficiencies of vitamin B_{12}, folic acid or iron, diabetes mellitus, side effects of medications, and autoimmune diseases.[99] Successful treatment of the primary disease will usually (but not invariably) alleviate the burning sensation in SBMS patients.

Treatment

BMS is frustratingly resistant to therapy and there are few evidence-based treatments.[100] Topical therapies may be effective and are useful in elderly, medically compromised patients. The most established is clonazepam (1 mg) which should be sucked and subsequently spat out three times daily.[103] Topical anesthetics may decrease or increase pain and are thereforeunpredictable.

Systemic therapies include paroxetine (20 mg/d) and sertraline (50 mg/d) or other selective serotonin reuptake inhibitors (SSRIs).[104] These may reduce pain and improve anxiety and depression. A two-month course of 600 mg daily of alpha-lipoic acid[105] may be beneficial, although these findings are not consistent.[106] A combination of alpha-lipoic acid (600 mg/d) and gabapentin (300 mg/d) results in greaterimprovement of the burning symptoms compared to these medications taken alone.[107] Clonazepam (0.5 mg/d) has been suggested as an option for short-term management.[108]

Pharmacotherapy-resistant BMS has been associated with underlying psychological distress, and these patients may particularly benefit from cognitive behavioral therapy.

Painful Posttraumatic Trigeminal Neuropathy

The term painful posttraumatic trigeminal neuropathy (PTTN) is novel and has recently been adopted by the International Headache Society (IHS).[5] Some patients develop chronic pain following negligible nerve trauma such as root canal therapy or following considerable injury to nerve bundles, such as in fractures of the facial skeleton.[109,110]

Following dental implant surgery 1%–8% and following orthognathic jaw surgery 5%–30% of patients may remain with permanent sensory dysfunction but the incidence of chronic pain is unclear.[111–113] Third molar extractions may lead to disturbed sensation in the lingual or inferior alveolar nerve for varying periods in 0.3%–1% of cases, but follow-up failed to identify any neuropathic pain cases.[114,115] Patient complaints of tongue dysesthesia after injury may remain in a small group of patients (0.5%). Persistent pain after successful root canal therapy was found in 3%–13% of cases,[110] whereas surgical root therapy resulted in chronic neuropathic pain in 5% of cases.

Features

Following identical injuries, onset of neuropathic pain and its characteristics vary from patient to patient. Such variability is probably due to a combination of environmental, psychosocial, and genetic factors. The presence and duration of pain in the tooth, tenderness to percussion, female gender, previous painful treatment in the orofacial region, and concomitant chronic pain issues are possible risk factors for the development of chronic pain following successful root canal therapy.[110]

The considerable complexity of the sensory processing in the scenario of nerve damage or neuritis (nerve inflammation) results in altered activity by different nerve fibers and hence clinical presentation. Painful neuropathies may present with a clinical phenotype involving combinations of spontaneous and evoked pain and of positive (e.g., dysesthesia) and negative symptomatology (e.g., numbness).

Pain is overwhelmingly unilateral and occurs in the area of injury, or at the distal dermatome of an injured nerve. Initially pain may be precisely located to the dermatome of the affected nerve, but it may become diffuse and spread across dermatomes. Pain is of moderate-to-severe intensity (VAS 5–9), usually burning in quality but also stabbing during exacerbations.[57] Positive or negative local neurological signs include clinically demonstrable sensory dysfunction, usually allodynia, hyperalgesia, or parasthesia.[57]

Most cases are continuous, but some report superimposed paroxysmal pain attacks.[57] Less frequently there may be short-lasting pain with associated mechanical trigger areas, mimicking TN.[57] Rarely, a subjective feeling of swelling, foreign body, hot or cold, local redness or flushing may be reported but these may not always be clinically verifiable.[57]

Treatment
Topical

Topical anesthetics may be successfully employed in the management of painful neuropathies.[116] Some benefits have been observed using topical capsaicin in a heterogeneous group of patients with oral neuropathic pain. A combination of topical drugs has been successfully applied to the treatment of oral neuropathies.[116] The authors conclude that topical medication as single treatment or in combination with systemic medications can reduce the severity of orofacial neuropathic pain.[116]

Systemic Pharmacotherapy

Available data confirm that AEDs and TCAs are most effective.[117–120] For many of the drugs used in the therapy of traumatic neuropathies, response is dose dependent and subsequently accompanied by significant side effects. Therapy of neuropathic pain with any one of the established drug groups (antidepressants, anticonvulsants, opioids) leads to improved quality of life, sleep, and mood. However, pain intensity is reduced by 20%–40% in only a subset of responders and is usually accompanied by significant side effects, particularly at the higher doses often required in neuropathic pain.[121–123] We have recently tested this stepped care protocol on a group of PTTN patients with only 10% achieving a significant improvement.[124] Although we strive to attain a 50% reduction in pain intensity or frequency, research has shown that a 30% reduction may represent meaningful pain relief for neuropathic pain patients.[125]

Antidepressants with mixed serotonin/noradrenaline (e.g., imipramine and amitriptyline) or specific noradrenaline reuptake inhibition (e.g., nortriptyline) are superior to the SSRIs, such as fluoxetine or paroxetine.[126] Newer AEDs such as gabapentin and pregabalin have an improved side-effect profile but for neuropathic, pain still seems inferior to antidepressants.

Patients should be initiated on a TCA such as amitriptyline. Amitriptyline commonly induces side effects and if these are severe nortriptyline, imipramine, desipramine, or venlafaxine (serotonin noradrenaline reuptake inhibitors) may be tried. If there is a medical contraindication to amitriptyline or if TCAs fail, the anticonvulsants gabapentin or pregabalin would be the first alternative drugs indicated.[118–120]

If initial TCAs or gabapentinoids are unsuccessful, patients should be transferred to their counterparts, that is, TCAs to gabapentinoids and vice versa. If individual drugs (TCAs, gabapentinoids) are partly successful, combination approaches may be employed.

Surgery

In the management of *nonpainful* neuropathies, microsurgery is well established and improves sensation in affected patients.[127] Response is marginally better in inferior alveolar than in lingual nerve surgeries, and the presence of a neuroma is a negative prognostic factor.[128,129] The efficacy of surgery for *painful* trigeminal neuropathies is unclear. This would also depend on the type of surgery performed, that is, nerve repair or interventional surgery to further remove pathology. Most cases that have undergone peripheral surgical procedures for traumatic trigeminal neuropathy end up with *more* pain. Some cases treated with peripheral glycerol injections enjoy some relief but we have found no controlled trials. There are no prospective trials in the literature on central procedures aimed at the trigeminal ganglion or the dorsal root entry zone for the treatment of such cases. Anecdotal evidence suggests that central procedures may be useful for recalcitrant cases. In a mixed group of patients, some with posttraumatic neuropathic pain, DREZ lesions was reported to significantly alleviate symptoms.

Selected Readings

Ashkenazi A, Schwedt T. Cluster headache–acute and prophylactic therapy. *Headache*. 2011;51(2):272–286.

Barry P, Cole T, Crawford P, et al. *Neuropathic Pain: The Pharmacological Management of Neuropathic Pain in Adults in Non-Specialist Settings*. http://www.nice.org.uk/cg96. Accessed January 18, 2010.

Benoliel R, Zadik Y, Eliav E, Sharav Y. Peripheral painful traumatic trigeminal neuropathy: clinical features in 91 cases and proposal of novel diagnostic criteria. *J Orofac Pain*. 2012;26(1):49–58.

Cohen JI. Clinical practice: herpes zoster. *N Engl J Med*. 2013;369(3): 255–263.

de Leeuw R, Klasser GD, editors. *Orofacial Pain: Guidelines for Assessment, Classification, and Management. The American Academy of Orofacial Pain*. 5th ed. Chicago, IL: Quintessence Publishing Co., Inc.; 2013.

Gan EY, Tian EA, Tey HL. Management of herpes zoster and post-herpetic neuralgia. *Am J Clin Dermatol*. 2013;14(2):77–85.

Goldman GS, King PG. Review of the United States universal varicella vaccination program: Herpes zoster incidence rates, cost-effectiveness, and vaccine efficacy based primarily on the Antelope Valley Varicella Active Surveillance Project data. *Vaccine*. 2013;31(13):1680–1694.

Haviv Y, Zadik Y, Sharav Y, Benoliel R. Painful traumatic trigeminal neuropathy: An open study on the pharmacotherapeutic response to stepped treatment. J Orofac Pain 2014. 28(1);52-60.

Heckmann SM, Kirchner E, Grushka M, et al. A double-blind study on clonazepam in patients with burning mouth syndrome. *Laryngoscope*. 2012;122(4):813–816.

Leone M, Proietti Cecchini A, Franzini A, et al. From neuroimaging to patients' bench: what we have learnt from trigemino-autonomic pain syndromes. *Neurol Sci*. 2012;33 Suppl 1:S99-S102.

Lim JNW, Ayiku L. *The Clinical Efficacy and Safety of Stereotactic Radiosurgery (Gamma Knife) in the Treatment of Trigeminal Neuralgia*. National Institute for Clinical Excellence (NICE). http://www.nice.org.uk/page.aspx?o=ip173systematicreview. Updated 2004. Accessed January 18, 2014.

Olesen J, Bendtsen L, Dodick D, et al. Headache classification committee of the International Headache Society (IHS). The International Classification of Headache Disorders, 3rd edition (beta version). *Cephalalgia*. 2013;33(9):629–808.

Olesen J, Bousser M-G, Diener HC, et al. *The International Classification of Headache Disorders*. 2nd ed; 2004. http://ihs-classification.org/en/. Accessed T*he international headache society* January 18, 2014.

Zakrzewska JM, Coakham HB. Microvascular decompression for trigeminal neuralgia: update. *Curr Opin Neurol*. 2012;25(3):296–301.

For the full reference lists, please go to http://www.pmph-usa.com/Burkets_Oral_Medicine.

CHAPTER 13

Common Headache Disorders

Scott S. De Rossi, DMD
J. Ned Pruitt II, MD

- ❐ PAIN-SENSITIVE STRUCTURES OF THE HEAD
- ❐ CLASSIFICATION OF HEADACHE
- ❐ GENERAL CLINICAL CONSIDERATIONS
- ❐ MIGRAINE
  Epidemiology
  Pathophysiology
  Vascular Theory
  Neuronal Theory and the Trigeminovascular System
  Role of Serotonin and Dopamine
  Clinical Findings
  Management
- ❐ TTH
  Epidemiology
  Pathophysiology
  Clinical Findings
  Management
- ❐ CLUSTER HEADACHE
  Epidemiology
  Pathophysiology

Clinical Features
Management
- ❐ TEMPORAL ARTERITIS
  Epidemiology
  Pathophysiology
  Clinical Features
  Management
- ❐ CHRONIC PAROXYSMAL HEMICRANIA
  Epidemiology
  Clinical Features
- ❐ OTHER CAUSES OF HEADACHES
  Brain Tumor
  Intracranial Hemorrhage
  Lumbar Puncture
  Idiopathic Intracranial Hypertension
  Headaches after Head Injury

Globally, it has been estimated that prevalence among adults of current headache disorder (symptomatic at least once within the last year) is 47%. Half to three quarters of the adults aged 18–65 years in the world have had headache in the last year and among those individuals, more than 10% have reported migraine. Headache on 15 or more days every month affects 1.7%–4% of the world's adult population. Despite regional variations, headache disorders are a worldwide problem, affecting people of all ages, races, income levels and geographical areas.[1–3] Headaches are relatively rare in children but increase with age. Headache in general and migraine specifically increase in frequency during adolescence, particularly in women of childbearing age.[3] As headache disorders are most troublesome in the productive years (late teens to 50s), estimates of their financial cost to society—principally from lost working hours and reduced productivity—are massive.[4] Appropriate treatment of headache disorders requires professional training of health professionals, accurate diagnosis and recognition of the condition, appropriate treatment with cost-effective medications, simple lifestyle modifications, and patient education. Since there is significant anatomic proximity of structures of the head and face and because dentists are often consulted to evaluate orofacial pain, it is imperative that dentists be familiar with the clinical manifestations of common headache disorders. This chapter reviews the pain-sensitive structures of the head and discusses the etiology and pathophysiology, diagnostic considerations, and treatment recommendations of headache appropriate for oral health professionals.

PAIN-SENSITIVE STRUCTURES OF THE HEAD

All somatic pain occurs when peripheral nociceptors are stimulated in response to tissue injury or inflammation. Visceral pain often arises from distention and may be referred to external locations. In such cases, pain is a normal physiologic response mediated by a healthy nervous system. However, pain can also be as a result of damaged or inappropriately activated pain-sensitive pathways of the central or peripheral nervous system. Headache pain may result from both mechanisms. Very few of the cranial structures are pain sensitive, with intracranial pain arising primarily from innervation blood vessels and meninges. (Table 13-1). Sensory stimuli from these intracranial tissues are conveyed to the central nervous system via the trigeminal nerve for areas above the tentorium in the anterior and middle cranial fossa and pain can often be referred to trigeminal distributions in the face and head. Causes of headache are multifactorial but can occur as the result of distention or dilation of intracranial or extracranial vessels; displacement of large intracranial vessels or their dural envelope; compression or inflammation of the cranial or spinal nerves; inflammation; trauma to cranial, facial, and cervical muscles; meningeal irritation; or increased intracranial pressure.[5]

CLASSIFICATION OF HEADACHE

A useful classification of the numerous types of headache has been established by the International Headache Society (IHS) based on specific inclusion and exclusion criteria (Table 13-2).[6] The International Classification of Headache Disorders is intended equally for research and for clinical practice. A classification and its diagnostic criteria should be reliable, valid and exhaustive. The International Classification of Headache Disorders has been shown to have fairly high degrees of reliability and validity. It has also proven to be exhaustive in several studies spanning from population-based studies to studies in headache clinics. Since there are no specific diagnostic tests to allow a guaranteed diagnosis, the clinical diagnosis of headache relies heavily on the ability of the examiner to elicit the relevant history, the reliability of patients to report accurately their symptoms, and the absence of other etiologic factors.

GENERAL CLINICAL CONSIDERATIONS

The first and most important consideration in evaluating patients with complaints of orofacial pain or headache is to rule out an underlying structural lesion or systemic disease, such as intracranial tumor, severe infection, aneurysm, uncontrolled hypertension, or stroke. Headache is generally a benign symptom, but it is estimated that 5% of patients with headache in emergency settings are found to have a serious

TABLE 13-1 Pain Sensitive Structures in the Head

	Sensitive	Insensitive
Extracranial	Skin, muscles, fascia Blood vessels Mucosa of sinuses Dental structures	Skull (except periosteum)
Intracranial	Large arteries near circle of Willis Large venous sinuses Dural arteries and parts of dura	Parenchyma of brain Pia mater, arachnoid mater, parts of dura mater Ependyma, choroid plexus

TABLE 13-2 International Headache Society Classification

Part 1 - Primary Headache

1. Migraine
2. Tension-type headache
3. Cluster headache and trigeminal autonomic cephalgias
4. Other primary headaches

Part 2 - Secondary Headache

5. Headache associated with head and/or neck trauma
6. Headache attributed to cranial or cervical vascular disorders
7. Headache associated with nonvascular intracranial disorders
8. Headache associated with substances or their withdrawal
9. Headache attributed to infection
10. Headache attributed to disorders of hemostasis
11. Headache or facial pain attributed to disorders of the cranium, neck, eyes, ears, nose, sinuses, teeth, mouth, or other facial or cranial structures
12. Headache attributed to psychiatric disorders

Part 3 - Cranial neuralgias, central and primary facial pain and other headaches

13. Cranial neuralgias and central causes of face pain
14. Other headache, cranial neuralgia, central or primary facial pain

underlying disorder, emphasizing the need for rapid and accurate diagnosis of headache.[6–8]

A good headache history allows the clinician to recognize a pattern that in turn leads to the correct diagnosis.[9] A comprehensive history needs time, interest, focus, and establishment of rapport with the patient. When to ask what question to elicit which information is an art that is acquired by practice and improves with experience—questions related to the time, severity, location, and frequency of the headache syndrome in general and the episode in particular are of vital importance.[9] The history of present illness, including the quality, location, duration, and timing of headache, along with the modifying factors that produce, worsen, or relieve headache, needs to be carefully reviewed in each patient. The clinician may find it helpful for the patient to complete a daily, weekly, or monthly headache diary to monitor the headache complaints or the response to treatment. (Box 13-1).

Box 13-1 Weekly Headache Diary

Day	Sunday	Monday	Tuesday	Wednesday	Thursday	Friday	Saturday
Dates							
Prodrome							
Aura							
Time of pain onset							
Severity of pain							
Treatment 1 (dose)							
Symptoms(nausea, throbbing, disability)							
Treatment 2 (dose)							
Treatment 3 (dose)							
Time to pain relief							
Noted Triggers (caffeine, menses, etc.)							
Type of headache (migraine, tension)							
Other comments or questions							

Ascertaining characteristic pain qualities are often helpful for diagnosis. For instance, most tension-type headaches (TTHs) are described as tight "band-like" pain or a deep, aching pain. The location of pain might be important in diagnosing a temporal arteritis since pain is localized to the side of the inflamed vessel. Pain duration and the time for pain to reach a maximal intensity are often diagnostically useful since ruptured aneurysm, migraine, and cluster headache all have unique pain peaks and duration. In general, progressive headaches that are associated with neurologic deficits are the most concerning and are often secondary to a serious underlying disorder.[10]

Patients who present with their first severe headache raise different diagnostic possibilities compared with those who have recurring headaches. Features or "diagnostic alarms" of acute, new-onset headache caused by underlying disorders are reviewed in Table 13-3. A complete neurologic examination is a vital first step in patient evaluation. Diagnostic imaging, such as computed tomography (CT) or magnetic resonance imaging (MRI), is useful in screening for intracranial pathology. Whereas CT is typically more readily available than MRI, MRI provides much greater sensitivity, particularly for vascular lesions and lesions in the posterior fossa. An MRI and magnetic resonance angiography of the brain with contrast is the most sensitive noninvasive diagnostic study for headache and should be the diagnostic modality of choice in nonemergent cases.[11] In addition, the psychological state of the patient needs to be assessed given the well-demonstrated relationship between head pain and depression. Finally, it is important to ask for disability or limitation of activities during headache, which usually happens with migraine. The extent of disability can be gauged using instruments such as a Migraine Disability Assessment (MIDAS) questionnaire.[12]

TABLE 13-3 Headache Symptoms Suggesting a Serious Underlying Disorder

First severe headache

"Worst" headache ever

Continuous headache worsening over days or weeks

Abnormal neurologic examination

Fever or other unexplained systemic signs/symptoms

Vomiting precedes headaches

Headache induced by bending, lifting, or coughing

Onset after age 55

Clinicians can reasonably sure of excluding "dangerous" headaches by the following:

- There should be no history of serious head or neck injury, of seizures or focal neurologic symptoms, or of infections that may predispose to meningitis or brain abscess.
- The patient should be afebrile.
- The diastolic blood pressure should not be greater than 120.
- The fundi should be normal.
- The neck should be supple.
- There should be no cranial bruits.
- The neurologic examination should be normal; the patient should not be lethargic or confused.
- In appropriate cases, complete blood cell count, ESR, cranial imaging, or neck x-rays should be obtained and be normal.

MIGRAINE HEADACHES

Epidemiology

The core features of migraine are headache, which is usually throbbing and often unilateral, and associated features of nausea, sensitivity to light, sound, and exacerbation with head movement. Migraine has long been regarded as a vascular disorder because of the throbbing nature of the pain. However, as we shall explore here, vascular changes do not provide sufficient explanation of the pathophysiology of migraine. Up to one-third of patients do not have throbbing pain. Modern imaging has demonstrated that vascular changes are not linked to pain and diameter changes are not linked with treatment.[13,14]

Migraine typically presents as an episodic "sick" headache that interferes with normal daily activities. The migraine headache is frequently accompanied by nausea, vomiting, photophobia (aversion to light), phonophobia (aversion to sound), and osmophobia (aversion to odors). It may be preceded by an aura of neurologic dysfunction, such as visual disturbances, vertigo, numbness, or weakness. The pain may be moderate or incapacitating. Migraine frequency varies considerably. In many patients, migraine is triggered by specific factors, such as menses, weather changes, irregular sleep, alcohol, or certain foods. Migraine is also often relieved by sleep. The lifetime prevalence of migraine is estimated to be near 35%, and it affects greater than 17% of women and 6% of men.[15] Migraine headache has a staggering economic impact, including absenteeism and loss productivity totaling $13 billion dollars in the United States.[4,12] The direct medical cost of caring for migraineurs is estimated at $1 billion yearly.[16,17]

Pathophysiology

There appears to be a genetic and familial risk as more than half of all migraineurs report having other family members who suffer from migraine. In addition, specific mutations leading to rare causes of vascular headache have been identified.[18] A strong familial influence in migraine has long been apparent and this has been demonstrated in twin studies.[19] The concordance for migraine in monozygotic twins is greater than that for dizygotic twins. However, it is also clear that the genetic background is complex. Additionally, research suggests that variations within the dopamine D2 receptor gene also may have some effect on susceptibility to migraine.[20] The pathogenesis of migraine is only now becoming more clearly understood but involves the role of serotonin and dopamine in both vascular and neuronal dysfunction. Neuronal calcium channels mediate serotonin (5-HT) release within the midbrain and dysfunction of these channels might impair serotonin release and predispose patients to migraine or impair their self-aborting mechanism.[21] In addition, acute migraine attacks occur in the context of an individual's inherent level of vulnerability. The greater the vulnerability or lower the threshold, the more frequent attacks occur.[22] Attacks are initiated when internal or environmental triggers are of sufficient intensity to activate a series of events which culminate in the generation of a migraine headache.

Vascular Theory

The aura of migraine was once thought to be caused by cerebral vasoconstriction and the headache by reactive vasodilation, which explained the throbbing quality of migraine and

the relief of pain by ergots. It is now believed that the aura is caused by neuronal dysfunction rather than ischemia.[23] Migrainous fortification spectra (an aura consisting of scintillating zigzag figures of bright luminous geometric lines and shapes) experienced by many patients corresponds to cortical changes in metabolism that begin in the visual cortex and spreads across the cortex at 2–3 mm/min and continues as the headache phase begins.[24] It is unlikely that these changes fully explain the symptoms of migraine. Specifically, the decreased vascular perfusion seen is not significant enough to cause focal neurologic symptoms.[25] Some cerebral blood flow changes do occur in aura, however, migraine without aura demonstrates no flow abnormalities; thus, it is unlikely that simple vasoconstriction and vasodilation are the fundamental pathophysiologic feature.

Clinically, the aura phase consists of focal neurological symptoms that persist up to one hour. Symptoms may include visual, sensory, or language disturbance as well as symptoms localizing to the brainstem. Within an hour of resolution of the aura symptoms, the typical migraine headache usually appears with its unilateral throbbing pain and associated nausea, vomiting, photophobia, or phonophobia. Without treatment, the headache may persist for up to 72 hours before ending in a resolution phase often characterized by deep sleep.

Neuronal Theory and the Trigeminovascular System

Migraine aura is believed to result from a slow-moving, spreading depression of cortical activity that liberates potassium and is preceded by a wavefront of increased metabolic activity, suggesting that dysregulation of normal neuronal function is a cause of migrainous attacks. Migraine probably results from pathologic activation of meningeal vessel nociceptors combined with a change in central pain modulation.[26] The trigeminal nerve, which innervates the meninges, is intricately involved in migraine. How the migraine is triggered and the cascade of events following the activation of migraine are not completely understood. However, there is increasing evidence that events intrinsic to the cerebral cortex are capable of affecting the pain sensitive dural vascular structures.[27] If this is the case, then this might explain on way in which the headache is activated in individuals experiencing the aura. Both headache and the associated neurovascular changes are served by the trigeminal system. Activation of the trigeminovascular system results in vasoactive polypeptide release, including substance P and calcitonin gene–related peptide (CGRP).[28] These neuropeptides and other cytokines interact with the blood vessel wall to produce dilation, plasma protein extravasation, and platelet activation producing a sterile inflammation that activates trigeminal nerve nociceptive afferents leading to further pain production.[29] Inhibiting this trigeminovascular activation is at the core of attempts to link headache with temporomandibular disorders (TMDs) and to treat headache with splint therapy and traditional treatments for TMDs.[30] The pathophysiology of migraine and the potential role of TMD as a mechanical trigger is summarized in Figure 13-1.

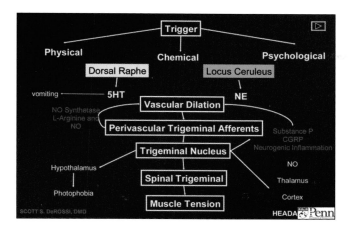

FIGURE 13-1 Pathogenesis of migraine. 5HT, 5-hydroxytryptamine; CGRP, calcitonin gene–related peptide; NE, Norepinephrine; NO, nitric oxide.

Role of Serotonin and Dopamine

Pharmacologic data point to a strong role of the neurotransmitter serotonin in migraine dating back to 40 years ago, when methysergide was found to antagonize certain peripheral actions of serotonin and was introduced as the first drug capable of preventing migraines.[31] More recently, the "triptan" class of drugs has renewed interest in the role of 5-hydroxytryptamine (5-HT) in migraine because of their ability to stimulate selectively a crucial subtypes of 5-HT receptors (i.e., $5\text{-HT}_{1B\&1D}$).[32] A growing body of data supports a role of dopamine in the pathophysiology of certain types of migraine. Biologic, genetic, and pharmacologic evidence includes the following: (1) most migraine symptoms can be induced by dopamine, (2) there is dopamine receptor hypersensitivity in migraineurs, and (3) dopamine receptor antagonists are effective agents in treating migraine.[33]

Clinical Findings

The clinical features of migraine are separated into two types of headache: migraine without aura (common migraine) and migraine with aura (classic migraine). In migraine without aura, there is an absence of focal neurologic symptoms preceding headache. Clinically, patients have moderate to severe pulsating, unilateral head pain aggravated by routine activity. In addition, nausea and vomiting, photophobia, and phonophobia are usually associated with the headache and the pain typically lasts 4–72 hours.

In migraine with aura, the headache is preceded by stereotyped sensory, motor, or visual symptoms. The most common premonitory symptoms in migraine include visual scotomas and fortification spectra, and approximately one-third of all migraineurs are affected.[34] Paresthesias follow a cortical somatotopic pattern and may involve the face, lips, and tongue; rarely focal motor weakness may occur. The median frequency of migraine attacks is 1.5 per month, and the typical headache begins unilaterally, has gradual-onset reaching a peak of pain in 2–4 hours, has a throbbing or pounding quality, and causes moderate to severe pain that is aggravated by movement. After the headache, there may be a resolution phase or "postdrome" in which the patient feels tired, irritable, and listless.

Management

Treatment of migraine begins with making an accurate diagnosis, appropriate patient education, and a treatment plan including nonpharmacologic and pharmacologic strategies. Generally, migraine management is divided into three specific components: (1) prophylactic or preventative therapy, (2) abortive therapy, and (3) palliative or rescue therapy. The mainstay of preventative pharmacologic therapy is the judicious use of one or more migraine-effective drugs. The selection of the most optimal drug regimen is dependent on several factors, including individual patient medical history, but primarily on the frequency and severity of the attacks. Patients experiencing more than three migraines per month are candidates for prophylactic therapy. Less frequent headaches can be managed with abortive therapy alone. Patients with migraines refractory to first line abortives may require rescue therapy to avoid frequent visits to the emergency room. A staged

TABLE 13-4 Symptoms Associated With Migraine			
Neurologic Symptoms	**Prodrome**	**Aura**	**Postdrome**
• Hemiparesis (this symptom defines hemiplegic migraine)	• Heightened sensitivity to light, sound, and odors	• Homonymous hemianopic or quadrantic field defects	• Tired, "washed out," or irritable feeling
• Aphasia	• Lethargy or uncontrollable yawning	• Central scotomas	• Unusually refreshed or euphoric feeling
• Confusion	• Food cravings	• Tunnel vision	• Muscle weakness or myalgias
• Paresthesias or numbness	• Mental and mood changes (e.g., depression, anger, euphoria)	• Altitudinal visual defects	• Anorexia or food cravings
	• Excessive thirst and polyuria	• Complete blindness	
	• Fluid retention		
	• Anorexia		
	• Constipation or diarrhea		

approach to the medical management of migraine is summarized in Table 13-5.

Mild migraine can often be successfully managed by oral agents, whereas fulminant attacks with accompanying nausea may require parenteral drugs. Most abortive agents for migraine fall into one of three classes: (1) non-steroidal anti-inflammatory agents, (2) 5-HT$_1$ agonists, and (3) dopamine antagonists. The response to migraine treatment is highly variable and must be individualized for each patient. Preventive protocols for migraine include a substantial number of drugs now available that have been shown to stabilize migraine. β-Adrenergic receptor blockers, anticonvulsants, tricyclic antidepressants, monoamine oxidase inhibitors, serotoninergic drugs, and calcium channel antagonists have all been used with varied success, although not all of them have received a specific indication for migraine by the Food and Drug Administration (FDA). These drugs must be taken daily and usually have a 2–6-week period before an effect is observed. A thorough medical and social history helps provide guidance in selecting the best preventive medication. Preventive agents are ultimately effective in at least 50%–75% of cases. A reasonable goal for preventive therapy is at least a 50% reduction in headache frequency and/or severity. To assess this, some idea of the baseline headache frequency and severity is essential prior to initiating therapy. Once effective stabilization is achieved, the drug should be continued for at least six months and then tapered to assess continued need.[35]

The mainstay of abortive therapy for migraine centers on the use of ergotamine derivatives and the "triptan" drugs, although both the severity and duration of migraine can be reduced by anti-inflammatory agents, especially when taken early in a migraine attack.[36] Specifically, the combination of acetaminophen, aspirin, and caffeine has been approved by the FDA for the treatment of mild to moderate migraine. Stimulation of 5-HT$_{1B}$ receptors can stop a migraine attack. Ergotamine derivatives are nonselective receptor agonists,

whereas the "triptan" drugs are selective 5-HT$_{1B}$ receptor agonists. Each of the "triptans" has similar pharmacologic properties, but they vary in clinical effectiveness. Available in oral, nasal, and parenteral formulations, "triptan" drugs unfortunately do not result in consistent, and complete relief in all migraine patients. Dopamine antagonists may be used as an adjunctive therapy in the treatment of migraine. Gastrointestinal drug absorption can be impaired during attacks because of decreased motility limiting the effectiveness of nonsteroidal anti-inflammatory drugs (NSAIDs) or oral "triptans". Dopamine antagonists can decrease nausea/vomiting and restore gastric motility. The drugs often used for treatment of acute migraine are reviewed in Tables 13-6 and 13-7.

TENSION-TYPE HEADACHES

Epidemiology

The most common cause of headache is tension-type headache (TTH). Over 80% of adults experience TTH, characterized by bilateral, tight, band-like discomfort periodically, and it is common in both adolescents and children. However, TTH is rarely disabling in its severity. Women tend to be affected more than men, and in some patients, anxiety and depression are coexisting diagnoses. TTH may be episodic or chronic (i.e., present for > 15 days per month). Indeed, musculoskeletal or tension-type headache is the most common cause of chronic daily headache.[37] Patients often describe a slow-building pain that fluctuates in severity. Most patients who experience TTH

Table 13-5 Staged Approach to Treating Migraine

Stage	Diagnosis	Therapy
Mild migraine	Occasional throbbing HA	NSAIDs
	No major impairment of daily function	Combination analgesics
		Oral serotonin agonists
Moderate migraine	Moderate to severe headache	Oral, nasal, or subcutaneous serotonin agonists
	Nausea	
	Some impairment of functioning	Oral dopamine antagonists
Severe migraine	Severe headaches (>3 times/mo)	Intramuscular or intravenous dopamine antagonists

HA, headache; NSAIDs, nonsteroidal anti-inflammatory drugs.

Table 13-6 Medications/Treatments Effective for Acute Migraine

Trade Name	Drug	Dose
Amerge	Naratriptan	2.5 mg tablet at onset; repeat once after 4h
Axert	Almotriptan	12.5 mg tablet at onset; repeat once after 2h
Ergomar	Ergotamine	One 2 mg sublingual tablet at onset and q30min
Excedrine Migraine	Acetaminophen, aspirin, caffeine	Two tablets q6h
Frova	Frovatriptan	2.5 mg tablet at onset; repeat once after 2h
Imitrex	Sumatriptan	50–100 mg tablet at onset; repeat once after 2h
		5–20 mg intranasal spray (2 sprays)
Maxalt	Rizatriptan	5–10 mg tablet at onset; repeat once after 2h
Migranal Nasal Spray	Dihydroergotamine	One spray (0.5 mg); repeat in 15 min
Zomig	Zolmitriptan	2.5 mg tablet at onset; repeat once after 2h
Relpax	Eletriptan	20–40 mg tablet at onset; repeat once after 2h

rely on over-the-counter remedies rather than seek medical attention for their symptoms.[38] A well-recognized "analgesic rebound syndrome" or "medication over-use headache" due to analgesic overuse is a major contributing factor to the transformation from episodic TTH to chronic daily headache.[39] Most patients are not aware that they can develop a tolerance and even a dependence on over-the-counter analgesics and that more than an occasional use of these drugs can be counterproductive. Determining the frequency and dosing of over-the-counter analgesics is an important part of the headache history. In many cases, dramatic improvements can be achieved simply by stopping or limiting daily analgesics, albeit with increased discomfort for the first few days.

Pathophysiology

Although tension-type headaches are common, the pathophysiology and likely mechanism remain unclear. Many investigators believe that periodic TTH is biologically indistinguishable from migraine, whereas others believe that TTH and migraine are, in fact, two distinct clinical entities.[40] It is generally agreed that TTH is often triggered by psychophysiologic changes related to stress, anxiety, and depression.[41] Controversy arises because an electromyogram (EMG) often cannot detect increased resting muscle tension in patients diagnosed with tension-type headache. Muscle hardness (measured by external probing of resting muscle) has been found to be increased in the pericranial muscles of patients with chronic tension-type headache.[42] Abnormalities of cervical and masticatory muscle contraction are likely to exist, but the exact nature of any dysfunction has yet to be elucidated. Tender pericranial muscles during headache are not a universal finding in TTH, leading some investigators to postulate a central mechanism leading to peripheral pain in some patients.[43] Both muscular and psychogenic factors are believed to be associated with tension-type headache. A study by Kiran et al. indicated that patients with chronic tension headaches for longer than five years tend to have lower cortisol levels.[44] They postulated this to be due to hippocampus atrophy resulting from chronic stress, a cause of chronic tension headaches. Further research suggests that nitric oxide may be the local mediator of tension-type headache.[45] Infusion of a nitric oxide donor reproduces tension-type headache in patients previously diagnosed with chronic tension-type headache.

Clinical Findings

The clinical presenting symptoms and signs of TTH include bilateral, holocephalic, band-like tightness and pressure with beginning usually in late morning and persisting throughout the day. Unlike migraine, nausea and vomiting are rare, occurring only in cases of severe pain in a minority of patients, and those patients are most likely manifesting a mixed headache syndrome with triggering of secondary migrainous headache by intense musculoskeletal pain. A thorough headache history should include questions about the type, amount, effect, and duration of self-treatment strategies. Patients typically self-treat their tension-type headaches with over the counter (OTC) analgesics, caffeinated products, massage, or chiropractic therapy for symptom relief. A headache history should also include discussion of any lifestyle changes (e.g., smoking) that may have preceded or exacerbated the headache. Patients who have chronic daily headache present with the typical pain characteristics of tension-type headache but have symptoms that occur daily or almost daily. A careful history will generally reveal that the daily tension-type headache was preceded by intermittent migraine-type headaches rather than intermittent tension-type headaches.[46] The progression of either migraine or tension-type headache into chronic daily headache can occur spontaneously but often occurs in relation to frequent use of analgesic medication. Repeated use of analgesics, especially ones containing caffeine or butalbital, can lead to "rebound" headaches as each dose wears off and patients then take another round of medication. Common features of chronic daily headache associated with frequent analgesic use are early morning awakening with headache, poor appetite, nausea, restlessness, irritability, memory or concentration problems, and depression.

Indications for imaging neuroimaging in patients with headache symptoms are summarized in Box 13-2.

TABLE 13-7	Preventive Drugs for Migraine	
First line	High efficacy	Beta blockers
		Tricyclic antidepressants
		Divalproex
		Topiramate
	Low efficacy	Verapamil
Second line	High efficacy	Methysergide
		Flunarizine
		MAOIs
	Unproven efficacy	Cyproheptadine
		Gabapentin

MAOIs, MONOAMINE oxidase inhibitors.

Box 13-2 Indications for Neuroimaging in Patients with Headache Symptoms

- Focal neurologic finding on physical examination
- Headache starting after exertion or Valsalva's maneuver
- Acute onset of severe headache
- Headache awakens patient at night
- Change in well-established headache pattern
- New-onset headache in patient >35 years of age
- New-onset headache in patient who has HIV infection or previously diagnosed cancer

Management

Effective treatment of TTH includes psychological, physiologic, and pharmacologic therapies. Treatment goals for patients with tension-type headache should include recommending effective OTC analgesic agents and discovering and ameliorating any circumstances that may be triggering the headaches or causing the patient concern. Tension-type headache is most commonly self-treated with OTC NSAIDs and acetaminophen. Psychological management includes simple counseling and hypnosis, whereas relaxation and biofeedback measures, including acupuncture, are helpful physiologic treatments.[47] TTH is most often effectively treated with over-the-counter analgesics, including NSAIDs, acetaminophen or aspirin. Tricyclic antidepressants including amitriptyline and nortriptyline are often used for prevention. Amitriptyline (Elavil) is the most researched of the prophylactic agents for chronic tension-type headache.[48] It is typically used in doses of 10–75 mg, one to two hours before bedtime to minimize grogginess on awakening. Anticholinergic side effects (dry mouth, blurred vision, orthostasis) and weight gain can limit its usefulness in some persons. The number of cigarettes smoked has been "significantly related" to the headache index score and to the number of days with headache each week. Medications to treat TTH are reviewed in Table 13-8.

CLUSTER HEADACHE

Cluster headache (CH), also known as histamine headache, is a primary neurovascular primary headache disorder, the pathophysiology and etiology of which are not well understood. There are both episodic and chronic types. As the name suggests, CH involves a grouping of headaches, usually over a period of several weeks. The episodic form is characterized by at least two cluster phases lasting seven days to one year separated by a cluster-free interval of one month or longer. The chronic form is characterized by the absence of sustained periods of remission and can transform from the episodic type in which the clusters occur more than once a year without remission or the cluster-free interval is shorter than one month.[49]

Epidemiology

Compared with classic migraine, CH is relatively uncommon, with an incidence equivalent to only 2%–9% of that of migraine (prevalence = 0.4% in men and 0.08% in women).[50] CH usually begins in middle adult life (e.g., in the 30s); however, it has been reported in patients as young as one year and as old as 79 years. Presentations in females may differ from those in males, according to data from the United States Cluster Headache Survey.[51] For example, women tend to develop CH at an earlier age and are also more likely to exhibit a second peak of CH incidence after the age of 50. Cluster is more common in males over the age of 25, and men are affected seven to eight times more than women. Alcohol provokes the attacks in 70% of cases initially but ceases to be provocative when the bout remits.

Pathophysiology

The etiology of cluster, although not fully understood, is classified as a trigeminal-autonomic headache disorder with features of both migraine and neuralgia. Although no consistent cerebral blood flow changes have been demonstrated with cluster attacks, the strongest evidence for a central mechanism includes the periodicity of attacks and the association with autonomic symptoms.[52] The periodicity of the attacks suggests the involvement of a biologic clock within the hypothalamus (which controls circadian rhythms), with central disinhibition of the nociceptive and autonomic pathways—specifically, the trigeminal nociceptive pathways.[53] Positron emission tomography (PET) and voxel-based morphometry have identified the posterior hypothalamic gray matter as the key area for the basic defect in CH.[54] Oxygen desaturation may lead to abnormal serotoninergic neurotransmission combined with hypersensitive chemoreceptors in the carotid body and neurogenic inflammation with elevations of CGRP, substance P, Vasoactive intestinal polypeptide (VIP), and other neuropeptides during attacks.[55]

Clinical Features

CH is unilateral among the most painful of all headache disorders. Attacks last from 30 minutes to 2 hours and have a nocturnal onset in half of cases, waking patients several hours after falling asleep. Several factors have been shown to provoke CH attacks. Subcutaneous injection of histamine provokes attacks in 69% of patients. Stress, allergens, seasonal changes, or nitroglycerin may trigger attacks in some patients. Alcohol induces attacks during a cluster but not during remission. About 80% of CH patients are heavy smokers, and 50% have a history of heavy ethanol use. Periorbital pain is commonly associated with autonomic symptoms, including ipsilateral lacrimation, reddening of the eye, nasal stuffiness, and nausea. Occasionally an ipsilateral Horner's syndrome is seen. In addition, 10%–20% of patients

TABLE 13-8   Medications Effective in Tension-Type Headache
Nonsteroidal anti-inflammatory agents
Acetaminophen
Aspirin
Diclofenac
Ibuprofen
Etodolac
Naproxen sodium
Combination analgesics
Acetaminophen plus butalbital
Acetaminophen plus butalbital plus caffeine
Aspirin plus butalbital
Aspirin plus butalbital plus caffeine
Prophylactic medications
Amitriptyline
Doxepin
Nortriptyline

report superimposed paroxysms of stabbing, ice pick–like pains in the periorbital region that last for a few seconds and may occur once or several times in rapid succession; this paroxysmal pain usually heralds the end of an attack. The symptoms often resolve in one to two minutes. The pain usually begins in, around, or above the eye or the temple; occasionally, the face, neck, ear, or hemicranium may be affected, and the pain can be confused with pain of odontogenic origin.

Management

Management of cluster headache includes use of medications to prevent cluster attacks as well as abortive therapies. Individual headaches are difficult to treat because they are short-lived. Abortive medications, including the use of 100% oxygen at the outset of an episode, are often useful in confirming a diagnosis of cluster. Oxygen inhalation (9 L/min) over a period of 20 minutes results in rapid resolution of symptoms in over 70% of cases. Intranasal sprayed lidocaine 4% is also effective in nearly half of cases.[52] "Triptan" therapy can be effective, although, typically, parenteral forms are required due to their more rapid absorption. Most cluster headaches occur repeatedly within a day and require more than just abortive therapy. Short courses of oral glucocorticoids are typically effective in aborting repeated clusters of headaches. For more chronic cluster, effective prophylactic medications include, methysergide, sodium valproate, and verapamil. Since cluster occurs as a series of episodes with a period of remission, preventive measures should be discontinued to see if remission has occurred.

TEMPORAL ARTERITIS

Epidemiology

Temporal (or giant cell) arteritis is a systemic inflammatory disorder that often involves the extracranial carotid circulation. This is commonly a disorder of elderly individuals, with an annual incidence of 77:100,000 individuals, usually over age 50. The average age at onset is 70 years, and women account for 65% of cases. This is a rare form of chronic daily headache with clinical importance because it is treatable. Failure to treat giant cell arteritis may lead to serious ischemic complications, including blindness, stroke, and myocardial infarction.

Pathophysiology

Temporal arteritis is classified as a systemic vasculitis, although it primarily affects the extracranial large and medium muscular arteries of the head and the neck. The exact etiology of temporal arteritis remains unknown, although it is T-cell dependent and antigen driven. Tumor necrosis factor (TNF) and, more recently, interleukin-6, have been recognized to may play a major role in the pathophysiology of temporal arteritis.[56] Inflammation of the temporal artery on biopsy is seen in over half of cases and can spread to arteries other than the temporal artery and extracranial vessels. The inflammatory process appears to be similar to both an acute immune-mediated vasculitis and chronic noncaseating granulomatous inflammation similar to that seen in sarcoid. Blindness occurs when the posterior ciliary artery is affected, which supplies the optic disk, leading to ischemic optic neuropathy.[57]

Clinical Features

Temporal arteritis often manifests in an insidious manner with vague constitutional symptoms such as malaise, weight loss, fever, and fatigue. The classic manifestations are fever, anemia, headache, and an elevated erythrocyte sedimentation rate (ESR). Symptoms of diffuse unilateral headache (along with chest pain, jaw pain and claudication, fever, and weight loss) initially are low grade; progress in severity and duration, increasing in the evening when the patient reclines; and are sometimes reported as a bitemporal constant dull ache. Most patients are able to recognize that their pain is superficial and extracranial and associated with scalp tenderness that interferes with hair brushing, resting the head on a pillow or wearing a hat. Pain in the temporal and masseter muscles on chewing is virtually pathognomonic of temporal arteritis, making it easily confused with other causes of facial pain (e.g., myofascial pain and TMDs) in a clinical setting. Erythrocyte sedimentation rate and C-reactive protein levels are frequently, although not always, elevated, and patients may be anemic. At the time of diagnosis, the ESR typically ranges from 60 to 100 mm/h. Hepatic enzyme levels, particularly alkaline phosphatase, are elevated in 20%–30% of cases.[58] A bilateral temporal artery biopsy should be performed to confirm the diagnosis; with a positive predictive value of greater than 90%, temporal artery biopsy stands out as the definitive test for temporal arteritis.[59]

Management

Medical care for temporal arteritis (TA) is supportive and symptom specific. Approximately half of patients with untreated temporal arteritis develop blindness due to involvement of the ophthalmic artery.[60] This significant complication can be prevented by immediate initiation of glucocorticoid therapy. An initial dose of 40–60 mg/d of prednisone (or equivalent) as a single or divided dose is generally found to be adequate in the vast majority of the cases. It is usually given for two to four weeks until all reversible signs and symptoms have resolved and levels of acute-phase reactants are back to normal.[61] The dose is then gradually reduced every one to two weeks by a maximum of 10% of the total daily dose. Most patients are treated for one to two years, but some with a prolonged or relapsing course may require low doses of glucocorticoids (GCs) for several years. Clinical flares may occur when the prednisone is reduced to 5–10 mg/d.

CHRONIC PAROXYSMAL HEMICRANIA

Chronic paroxysmal hemicrania (CPH) is a vascular headache disorder that is frequently confused with odontogenic pain, TMD, or regional pathology of structures of the face and head. It has features similar to migraine headache and may share some etiology and pathophysiology.[62] The short-lasting primary headache syndromes may be divided into (1) headaches with autonomic activation and (2) headaches without autonomic activation. Headaches with autonomic activation include chronic and episodic paroxysmal hemicrania, CH, and short-lasting unilateral neuralgiform headache with conjunctival injection and tearing (SUNCT syndrome).[62]

Epidemiology

CPH is a rare syndrome, but the number of diagnosed cases is increasing. The prevalence of CPH is not known, but the relative frequency compared with cluster is reported to be approximately 1%–3%. Although the precise prevalence of CPH is unknown, it is estimated to be 1 in 50,000. In contrast to cluster headache, CPH has a distinct female predominance, with a gender ratio of 2:1.[63] The condition usually begins in adulthood during the fourth decade and can last several years to decades.

Clinical Features

CPH has a rapid onset and is associated with severe, consistently unilateral head pain (oculofrontotemporal location) lasting a few minutes to an hour. It differs from cluster in its high frequency and shorter duration of attacks, but they have numerous overlapping characteristics. Most often, the temporal and orbital regions are the site of pain, with the jaw and face also affected. Episodic attacks are more frequent than cluster and can number greater than five per day during acute periods of recurrence. Like cluster, there are associated symptoms, including conjunctival injection, lacrimation, rhinorrhea or nasal stuffiness, and swelling of the painful areas (e.g., eyelid edema).[63] No confirmatory diagnostic test exists, diagnosis is made via the patient history and confirmation of symptoms and signs during attacks. The treatment of choice for chronic paroxysmal hemicrania (CPH) is indomethacin, which has an absolute effect on the symptoms. Episodic cluster headache (CH) and CPH respond well to this agent. The clinician must take precautions to prevent serious gastrointestinal and renal complications secondary to long-term use of this nonsteroidal anti-inflammatory.[64]

Over the past 35 years, there have emerged several rare headache disorders that respond selectively to indomethacin. Often referred to as "indomethacin responsive headaches", including CPH, cough or exertional headache, and the ice-pick headache syndrome. Other headaches also may be sensitive to indomethacin, and a trial of this drug should be considered in patients in whom these headache syndromes are suspected.[65]

OTHER CAUSES OF HEADACHES

Brain Tumor

Headache associated with intracranial masses is usually nondescript. Approximately 30% of patients with brain tumors consider headache to be their chief complaint or first presenting symptom.[66] However, headache is the presenting symptom in < 0.2% of patients with a brain tumor. Intermittent deep, dull, and aching pain of moderate intensity that worsens with physical exertion or position change and is associated with nausea and vomiting is the symptom most commonly described in migraine but is also seen in brain tumor headaches. Sleep disturbances occur in 10% of patients, and vomiting preceding headaches by weeks is highly characteristic of tumors of the posterior cranial fossa.[67] Tumors should be suspected in patients with progressively severe new "migraine" headaches that are solely unilateral.

Intracranial Hemorrhage

Most vascular disorders associated with headache require immediate medical or surgical intervention. Severe, acute headaches associated with a stiff neck in the absence of fever are highly suggestive of subarachnoid hemorrhage (SAH). Sudden onset of the "worst headache of life" is a medical emergency, and aneurysmal SAH must be excluded by a CT scan, which is approximately 90% sensitive for SAH, and a lumbar puncture if the CT scan is negative.[68] Other causes of severe acute headache can include rupture of an arteriovenous malformation, or intraparenchymal hemorrhage.

Lumbar Puncture

Headache following lumbar puncture usually begins within two days following the procedure. It is relatively common, with an incidence of 10%–30%, and is associated with head pain that worsens with an upright posture and is relieved when recumbent. Nausea, neck pain, vertigo, photophobia, tinnitus, and blurred vision are frequent complaints. Loss of cerebrospinal fluid (CSF) decreases the brain's supportive cushion, resulting in dilation and traction on pain-sensitive dural structures when patients are upright. Intracranial hypotension often occurs, but severe lumbar puncture headache can be present in patients with normal CSF pressure.[69,70] Spontaneous CSF leaks can also occur due to exertion, minor trauma such as a fall or following surgical procedures near the dura and are also characterized by positional modulation.

Idiopathic Intracranial Hypertension

Headache resembling that of brain tumor is a common presenting symptom of raised intracranial pressure, usually resulting from impaired CSF absorption by arachnoid villi. This disorder, also called pseudotumor cerebri, is most commonly seen in young, obese adult females and is associated with daily headaches that worsen with coughing or straining. Severe increases in intracranial pressure can result in unilateral of bilateral sixth nerve palsies. Patients may have a history of exposure to precipitating agents such as tetracycline, vitamin A, or glucocorticoids. Intracranial hypertension is diagnosed by lumbar puncture, which can also provide temporary relief. Chronic management includes acetazolamide, diuretics or rarely surgical implantation of a ventriculoperitoneal shunt.[71] Ophthalmologic evaluation with formal visual field testing is required in patients with idiopathic intracranial hypertension. High intracranial pressure is transduced along the optic nerve resulting in an enlarged blind spot and constriction of the peripheral visual fields.

Headaches after Head Injury

Many patients report symptoms such as headache, dizziness, vertigo, behavioral changes, and impaired memory after seemingly trivial head injuries. Symptoms may resolve after a few weeks or can persist months to years after injury. In nearly all cases, clinical neurologic examination and radiographic and imaging studies are normal. Although the etiology of this headache is poorly understood, it does not appear to be entirely psychogenic, and symptoms usually persist after a pending legal settlement. These headaches may be part of a TMD also related to direct or indirect trauma to the temporomandibular complex.[72–75]

Suggested Readings

De Rossi SS. Orofacial pain: a primer. *Dent Clin North Am.* 2013;57(3):383–392.

Headache classification committee, International Headache Society. Classification and diagnostic criteria for headache disorders, cranial neuralgias, and facial pain. *Cephalalgia.* 2004;24(suppl 1):1–160.

Hainer BL, Matheson EM. Approach to acute headache in adults. *Am Fam Physician.* 2013;87(10):682–687.

Abrams BM. Factors that cause concern. *Med Clin North Am.* 2013;97(2):225–242.

Charles A. The evolution of a migraine attack–a review of recent evidence. *Headache.* 2013;53(2):413–419.

Tfelt-Hansen PC, Koehler PJ. One hundred years of migraine research: major clinical and scientific observations from 1910 to 2010. *Headache.* 2011;51(5):752–778.

Benoliel R, Eliav E. Primary headache disorders. *Dent Clin North Am.* 2013;57(3):513–539.

Smitherman TA, Walters AB, Maizels M, Penzien DB. The use of antidepressants for headache prophylaxis. *CNS Neurosci Ther.* 2011;17(5):462–469.

Bender SD. Temporomandibular disorders, facial pain, and headaches. *Headache.* 2012;52(suppl 1):22–25.

Gonçalves DA, Camparis CM, Franco AL, et al. How to investigate and treat: migraine in patients with temporomandibular disorders. *Curr Pain Headache Rep.* 2012;16(4):359–364.

For the full reference lists, please go to http://www.pmph-usa.com/Burkets_Oral_Medicine.

CHAPTER 14

Diseases of the Respiratory Tract

Patrick Vannelli, MD

Frank A. Scannapieco, DMD, PhD

Sandhya Desai, MD

Mark Lepore, MD

Robert Anolik, MD

Michael Glick, DMD, FDS RCSEd

❏ **UPPER AIRWAY DISEASES**
  Viral Upper Respiratory Tract
    Infections
  Allergic Rhinitis and Conjunctivitis
  Otitis Media
  Sinusitis
  Laryngitis and Laryngotracheobronchitis
  Pharyngitis and Tonsillitis

❏ **LOWER AIRWAY DISEASES**
  Acute Bronchitis
  Pneumonia
  Bronchiolitis
  Asthma
  COPD
  Cystic Fibrosis
  Pulmonary Embolism
  Pulmonary Neoplasms

Given the fact that the oral cavity is contiguous with the trachea and lower airway, it is biological plausible that conditions within the oral cavity might influence lung function. Respiratory infections are commonly encountered among dental patients. Commonalities between chemotherapeutic options and the anatomic proximity with the oral cavity lead to much interplay between oral and respiratory infections. Recent studies have reported on oral bacteria as causative pathogens in respiratory diseases and conditions associated with significant morbidity and mortality. Furthermore, some respiratory illnesses, such as asthma, may have an effect on orofacial morphology or even on the dentition. This chapter discusses the more common respiratory illnesses and explores the relationship between these conditions and oral health.

UPPER AIRWAY DISEASES

There are several major oral health concerns for patients with upper respiratory infections. These concerns are about infectious matters, such as the possible transmission of pathogens from patients to health-care workers and reinfection with causative pathogens through fomites such as toothbrushes and removable oral acrylic appliances. Furthermore, antibiotic resistance may develop because of the use of similar types of medications for upper respiratory infections and odontogenic infections. Lastly, oral mucosal changes, such as dryness due to decongestants and mouth breathing, and increased susceptibility to oral candidiasis in patients using long-term glucocorticosteroid inhalers, may be noticed.

Viral Upper Respiratory Infections

The most common cause of acute respiratory illness is viral infection, which occurs more commonly in children than in adults. Rhinoviruses account for the majority of upper respiratory infections in adults.[1] These are ribonucleic acid (RNA) viruses, which preferentially infect the respiratory tree. At least 100 antigenically distinct subtypes have been isolated. Rhinoviruses are most commonly transmitted by close person-to-person contact and by respiratory droplets. Shedding can occur from nasopharyngeal secretions for up to three weeks, but seven days or less is more typical. In addition to rhinoviruses, several other viruses, including coronavirus, influenza virus, parainfluenza virus, adenovirus, enterovirus, coxsackievirus, and respiratory syncytial virus (RSV), have also been implicated as causative agents. Infection by these viruses occurs more commonly during the winter months in temperate climates.

Pathophysiology

Viral particles can lodge in either the upper or lower respiratory tract. The particles invade the respiratory epithelium, and viral replication ensues shortly thereafter. The typical incubation period for rhinovirus is two to five days.[2] During this time, active and specific immune responses are triggered, and mechanisms for viral clearance are enhanced. The period of communicability tends to correlate with the duration of clinical symptoms.

Clinical and Laboratory Findings

Signs and symptoms of upper respiratory tract infections are somewhat variable and are dependent on the sites of inoculation.[3] Common symptoms include rhinorrhea, nasal congestion, and oropharyngeal irritation. Nasal secretions can be serous or purulent. Other symptoms that may be present include cough, fever, malaise, fatigue, headache, and myalgia.[4] A complete blood count (CBC) with differential may demonstrate an increase in mononuclear cells, lymphocytes, and monocytes ("right shift"). Laboratory tests are typically not required in the diagnosis of upper respiratory infections. Viruses can be isolated by culture or determined by rapid diagnostic assays. However, these tests are rarely clinically warranted.

Diagnosis

A diagnosis is made on the basis of medical history as well as confirmatory physical findings. Diagnoses that should be excluded include acute bacterial rhinosinusitis, allergic rhinitis, and group A streptococcal pharyngitis.

Management

The treatment of upper respiratory infections is symptomatic as most are self-limited. Analgesics can be used for sore throat and myalgias. Antipyretics can be used in febrile patients, and anticholinergic agents may be helpful in reducing rhinorrhea. Oral or topical decongestants, such as phenylephrine and pseudoephedrine, are an effective means of decreasing nasal congestion. Adequate hydration is also important in homeostasis, especially during febrile illnesses.

Antimicrobial agents have no role in the treatment of acute viral upper respiratory infections.[5] Presumptive treatment with antibiotics to prevent bacterial superinfection is not recommended.[6] Any excessive use of antibiotics can result in the development of drug-resistant bacteria.[7]

Antiviral compounds have not been found to provide significant benefit for viral upper respiratory infections.[8]

Prognosis

As most patients recover in 5–10 days, the prognosis is excellent. However, upper respiratory infections can put patients at risk for exacerbations of asthma, acute bacterial sinusitis, and otitis media; this is especially so in predisposed patients, such as children and patients with an incompetent immune system.

Oral Health Considerations

The most common oral manifestation of upper respiratory viral infections is the presence of small round erythematous macular lesions on the soft palate. These lesions may be caused directly by the viral infection, or they may represent a response of lymphoid tissue. Individuals with excessive lingual tonsillar tissue also experience enlargement of these foci of lymphoid tissue, particularly at the lateral borders at the base of the tongue.

Treatment of upper respiratory infections with decongestants may cause decreased salivary flow, and patients may experience oral dryness (see Chapter 10 for a discussion of the treatment of oral dryness).

Although there has been some discussion in the dental literature in regards to a relationship between dentofacial morphology and mouth breathing, this association has not been verified in prospective longitudinal studies.[9]

Allergic Rhinitis and Conjunctivitis

Allergic rhinitis is a chronic recurrent inflammatory disorder of the nasal mucosa. Similarly, allergic conjunctivitis is an inflammatory disorder involving the conjunctiva. When both conditions occur, the term *allergic rhinoconjunctivitis* is used. The basis of the inflammation is an allergic hypersensitivity (type I) to environmental triggers. Allergic rhinoconjunctivitis can be seasonal or perennial. Typical seasonal triggers include grass, tree, and weed pollens. Common perennial triggers include dust mites, cockroach, animal dander, and mold spores.

Allergic rhinitis is one of the most prevalent chronic medical conditions in the United States (US). It affects up to 58 million people in the US.[10] Allergic rhinitis is associated with a significant economic burden with a total of more than $11.2 billion (US) in direct costs due to this condition in 2005.[11] It is estimated that allergic rhinitis accounts for 3.5 million lost work days and 2 million missed school days each year.[12]

Pathophysiology

Patients with allergic rhinoconjunctivitis have a genetically predetermined susceptibility to allergic hypersensitivity reactions, known as atopy. Prior to the allergic response, an initial phase of sensitization is required. This sensitization phase is dependent on exposure to a specific allergen and on recognition of the allergen by the immune system. The end result of the sensitization phase is the production of specific immunoglobulin E (IgE) antibody and the binding of this specific IgE to the surface of tissue mast cells and blood basophils. Upon reexposure to the allergen, an interaction between surface IgE and the allergen takes place, which results in IgE cross-linking. The cross-linking of surface IgE triggers degranulation of the mast cell and basophils causing the release of preformed mediators. This is the early-phase allergic reaction. Histamine is the primary preformed mediator released by mast cells, and it contributes to the clinical symptoms of sneezing, pruritus, and rhinorrhea. Mast cells also release cytokines that permit amplification and feedback of the allergic response. These cytokines cause an influx of other inflammatory cells, including eosinophils, resulting in the late-phase allergic reaction. Eosinophils produce many proinflammatory mediators that contribute to chronic allergic inflammation and to the symptom of nasal congestion.

Clinical and Laboratory Findings

The symptoms of allergic rhinoconjunctivitis can vary from patient to patient and depend on the specific allergens to which the patient is sensitized. Conjunctival symptoms may include pruritus, lacrimation, crusting, and burning. Nasal symptoms may include sneezing, pruritus, clear rhinorrhea, and nasal congestion. Other symptoms can occur, such as postnasal drainage with throat irritation, pruritus of the palate and ear canals, and fatigue.

The clinical signs of allergic rhinoconjunctivitis include injection of the conjunctiva with or without cobblestoning; prominent infraorbital creases/folds (Dennie-Morgan lines), swelling, and darkening ("allergic shiners"); a transverse nasal crease; and frequent upward rubbing of the tip of the nose (the allergic "salute"). Direct examination of the nasal mucosa reveals significant edema and a pale blue coloration of the turbinates. A copious clear rhinorrhea is often present. Nasal polyps may also be visible. Postnasal drainage or oropharyngeal cobblestoning might be identified upon examination of the oropharynx. A high-arched palate, protrusion of the tongue, and overbite may be seen.

Laboratory investigations are usually kept to a minimum. Patients with allergic rhinitis might have elevated levels of serum IgE and an elevated total eosinophil count. These findings are not, however, sensitive or specific indicators of atopy. Microscopic examination of nasal secretions often demonstrates significant numbers of eosinophils. Blood tests, such as the traditional radioallergosorbent test (RAST), is a method of testing for specific allergic sensitivities that is based on circulating levels of specific IgE. Specific IgE levels are determined by using serum samples and are quantified by using radioactive markers. Although bloodwork is somewhat less reliable than skin testing (see below), it is a useful test in certain situations, such as pregnancy or severe chronic skin disorders, including atopic dermatitis.

Classification

There is no universal classification system for allergic rhinoconjunctivitis. Many authors make the distinction between perennial and seasonal illness, with the former being caused mainly by indoor allergens (e.g., house dust mites, cockroaches, pets) and the latter being triggered primarily by outdoor allergens (e.g., trees, grasses, weeds). Perennial allergic rhinitis sufferers might benefit more from specific environmental control measures than would seasonal allergic rhinitis sufferers.

Diagnosis

The diagnosis of allergic rhinoconjunctivitis is usually apparent, based on history and physical examination. Patients present with a history suggestive of allergic sensitivity, recurrent symptoms with specific exposures, or predictable exacerbations during certain times of the year. Symptoms that have recurred for two or more years during the same season are very suggestive of seasonal allergic disease. Alternatively, the history might indicate a pattern of worsening symptoms while the patient is at home, with improvement while the patient is at work or on vacation; this pattern is highly suggestive of perennial allergic disease with indoor triggers. The presence of the characteristic physical findings described above would confirm the presence of allergic rhinoconjunctivitis.

The preferred method of testing for allergic sensitivities is skin testing, which is performed with epicutaneous (prick/scratch) tests and this can be followed by intradermal testing if needed. Prick skin testing is the type most widely used. With prick testing, a small amount of purified allergen is inoculated through the epidermis only (i.e., epicutaneously) with a pricking device. Positive (histamine) and negative (saline) controls are used for comparison (Figure 14-1A and B). Reactions are measured at 15 minutes, and positive reactions (wheal and flare reactions) indicate prior allergen sensitization. Tests that yield negative results may be repeated intradermally to increase the sensitivity of the testing. All tests with positive results need to be interpreted carefully in the context of the patient's history and physical findings.

Management

Three general treatment modalities are used in the therapy of allergic rhinoconjunctivitis: allergen avoidance, pharmacotherapy (medication), and immunotherapy (i.e., allergy injections). The best treatment is avoidance of the offending allergen. This requires the accurate identification of the allergens implicated and a thorough knowledge of effective interventions that can minimize or eliminate the exposure. Complete avoidance is rarely possible.

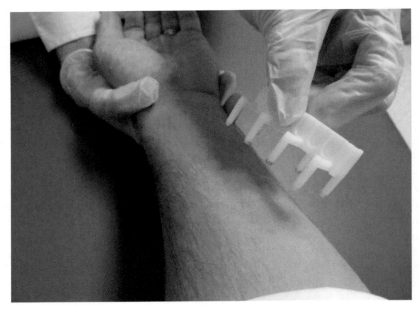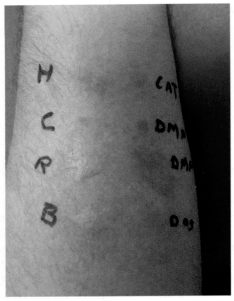

FIGURE 14-1 (A) Skin prick allergy testing about to be applied to the forearm of patient to a panel of allergens. (B) Positive sensitivities to multiple allergens from previous panel placed. Note the large wheals (bubble) and flare (redness) to Ragweed and Birch tree. Note: H, histamine; C, control; R, ragweed; B, birch; DM, dust mite.

Pharmacotherapy is often recommended for patients with incomplete responses to allergen avoidance and for patients who are unable to avoid allergen exposures. Many treatment options are available. For patients with prominent sneezing, pruritus, or rhinorrhea, antihistamines are an excellent treatment option. Second-generation antihistamines such as cetirizine, loratadine, and fexofenadine are now widely available. These medications deliver excellent antihistaminic activity with few side effects.[13] Oral decongestants can be added to oral antihistamines to relieve nasal congestion and obstruction. Combination medications are available in once-daily and twice-daily dosage forms for ease of administration. Leukotriene receptor antagonists may have additional benefit as well. Some studies have demonstrated that therapy with a leukotriene receptor antagonist plus antihistamine may have a greater effect than either agent administered alone.[13,14] For patients with daily nasal symptoms or severe symptoms that are not relieved with antihistamine-decongestants, topical anti-inflammatory agents for the nasal mucosa are available. These medications include corticosteroid, antihistamine and cromolyn sodium nasal sprays. The benefits of topical corticosteroids include relief of the total symptom complex and once daily dosing.

Immunotherapy is an effective means of treatment for patients with allergic rhinoconjunctivitis. Numerous studies have shown the efficacy of long-term allergen immunotherapy inducing prolonged clinical and immunologic tolerance.[15] Immunotherapy is available for a variety of airborne allergens, including grass, tree, and weed pollens; dust mites; animal dander; and mold spores. Excellent candidates for immunotherapy include those patients who are unable to avoid exposures, patients with suboptimal responses to pharmacotherapy,

patients who prefer to avoid the long-term use of medications, and women who are contemplating pregnancy.

Prognosis

Although allergic rhinoconjunctivitis is not a life-threatening disorder, it does have a significant impact on the patient's quality of life. With proper allergy care, most patients can lead normal lives, with an excellent quality of life.

Oral Health Considerations

The use of decongestants and first-generation antihistamines may be associated with oral dryness. There may also be an increased incidence of oral candidiasis in long-term users of topical corticosteroid-containing sprays.

It has been reported that dental personal are at risk for allergic respiratory hypersensitivity from exposure to dental materials such as methacrylates and natural rubber latex.[16] It is thus important for oral health-care professionals to minimize exposure to allergenic materials in the workplace.

Otitis Media

Otitis media is inflammation of the middle ear space and tissues. It is the most common illness that occurs in children who are 8 years of age or younger. Approximately 70% of children experience at least one episode of otitis media by age 3 years; of these, approximately one-third experience three or more episodes in this same time interval.[17]

Otitis media can be subdivided into acute otitis media, recurrent otitis media, otitis media with effusion, and chronic suppurative otitis media. The underlying problem in all types of otitis media is dysfunction of the eustachian tube. A poorly functioning eustachian tube does not ventilate the middle ear space sufficiently. This lack of proper ventilation results in pressure changes in the middle ear and subsequent fluid accumulation. The fluid frequently becomes infected, resulting in acute otitis media. The most common infectious causes are *Streptococcus pneumoniae, Haemophilus influenzae, Moraxella catarrhalis,* and viruses. In chronic infections, *Staphylococcus aureus* and anaerobic organisms may be causative pathogens while in young infants gram-negative bacilli may be isolated.[18]

Pathophysiology

There are several factors that influence the pathogenesis of otitis media. Nasopharyngeal colonization with large numbers of bacteria such as *S. pneumoniae, H. influenzae,* or *M. catarrhalis* and pathogenic viruses can increase the risk of otitis media. The likelihood of aspiration of these nasopharyngeal pathogens can be increased by nasal congestion or obstruction, negative pressure in the middle ear space, acute viral upper respiratory infections, and exposure to tobacco smoke.[19] For infants, breast-feeding can decrease the risk of otitis media, whereas impaired immune responsiveness can increase this risk.

Under normal circumstances, the eustachian tube acts to ventilate the tympanomastoid air cell system during the act of swallowing. Any process that impairs normal eustachian tube function can lead to negative pressure in the middle-ear space. Transient impairments of eustachian tube function are seen in conditions that cause nasopharyngeal mucosal edema and obstruction of the eustachian tube orifice, such as allergic rhinitis and viral upper respiratory infections. Chronic eustachian tube obstruction can be seen with several conditions, including cleft palate and nasopharyngeal masses, such as enlarged adenoids. Aspiration of nasopharyngeal pathogens can then occur due to negative pressure in the middle ear space, with subsequent infection by these pathogens. This leads to the clinical manifestations of otitis media.

Clinical and Laboratory Findings

The most common symptoms in acute otitis media are fever and otalgia. Other symptoms include irritability, anorexia, and vomiting. Parents may note their child pulling or tugging at one or both ears. Symptoms of a viral upper respiratory infection might also be present, preceding the development of otitis media. On physical examination, the tympanic membrane may appear erythematous and bulging, suggesting inflammation of the middle ear. Other otoscopic findings include a loss of landmarks and decreased mobility of the tympanic membrane as seen by pneumatic otoscopy.

In otitis media with effusion, patients often complain of "clogged" ears and "popping." Otoscopic examination reveals serous middle-ear fluid, and air-fluid levels may be present. The mobility of the tympanic membrane is usually diminished, and mild to moderate conductive hearing loss may be demonstrated. In chronic suppurative otitis media, otorrhea is present and can be visualized either from a tympanic membrane perforation or from surgically placed tympanostomy tubes.

Investigations that can aid in the diagnosis or management of otitis media include tympanometry and myringotomy with aspiration. Tympanometry is a technique that measures the compliance of the tympanic membrane by using an electroacoustic impedance bridge. Decreased compliance of the tympanic membrane indicates a middle-ear effusion. Myringotomy with aspiration can be useful in situations when culture of the middle ear fluid is needed, such as with immunocompromised hosts or with patients who have persistent effusions despite medical management.

Classification

Acute otitis media is defined as middle-ear inflammation with an infectious etiology and a rapid onset of signs and symptoms. Otitis media with effusion is defined as a middle ear effusion (often asymptomatic) that can be either residual (3–16 weeks following acute otitis media) or persistent (lasting more than 16 weeks). Recurrent otitis media is defined as three or more new episodes of acute otitis media in six months' time or four or more new episodes in a 12-month period. Chronic suppurative otitis media is defined as persistent otorrhea lasting longer than six weeks.

Diagnosis

The diagnosis of otitis media is made on the basis of the history and physical examination. The most useful tool for diagnosing otitis media is pneumatic otoscopy, which allows the clinician not only to visualize the tympanic membrane but also to assess its mobility. As stated above, an immobile tympanic membrane probably represents the presence of middle ear fluid, and (in the context of a confirmatory medical history) the diagnosis of otitis media is made in such a case.

Management

Recent practice guidelines in the management of otitis media without significant signs and symptoms, have suggested that observation with close follow up is justified.[20] There is evidence that suggests that antibiotics may be more beneficial in certain children, specifically those aged less than 2 years with bilateral acute otitis media and in those with both acute otitis media and otorrhea.[21,22] If antibiotics are indicated, initial antibiotic therapy is directed toward the most common middle-ear pathogens. Common choices include amoxicillin, azithromycin, and trimethoprim-sulfamethoxazole. In recalcitrant cases, treatment is directed toward β-lactamase–producing organisms and antibiotic-resistant strains of *S. pneumoniae.* Common choices for this situation include high-dose amoxicillin, amoxicillin-clavulanate, second- or third-generation cephalosporins, and clindamycin. The duration of therapy varies from 3–14 days.[23]

Multiple surgical modalities currently are used for the management of otitis media, including myringotomy with or without tympanostomy tube insertion, tympanocentesis, and adenoidectomy. Insertion of tympanostomy tubes is indicated when a patient experiences more than six acute otitis media episodes during a six-month period or has recurrent otitis media in addition to otitis media with effusion or persistent bilateral effusions for longer than three months.[24] A trial of antibiotic prophylaxis is commonly carried out prior to surgical consultation.[25]

Antihistamines and decongestants are ineffective for otitis media with effusion and are not recommended for treatment.[26] The management of chronic suppurative otitis media often includes parenteral antibiotics to cover infection by *Pseudomonas* species and anaerobic bacteria.

Prognosis

The prognosis for acute otitis media is excellent. Studies show that over 80% of children in the United States who were treated symptomatically for acute otitis media without antibiotics had complete resolution of otitis without suppurative complications.[27] However, complications can occur, more commonly in patients younger than 1 year of age. The most common complication is conductive hearing loss related to persistent effusions. Serious complications, including mastoiditis, cholesteatoma, labyrinthitis, extradural or subdural abscesses, meningitis, brain abscess, and lateral sinus thrombosis, are uncommon.[28]

Oral Health Considerations

Many children with recurrent otitis media are treated frequently (and sometimes for extensive periods) with various antibiotics. Included in the antibiotic armamentarium are medications that are also used for odontogenic infections. Oral health-care providers need to be aware of what type of antibiotics the patient has taken within the previous four to six months, to avoid giving the patient an antibiotic to which resistance has already developed. It has been demonstrated that antibiotic regimens used for the treatment of otitis media promote the emergence of antibiotic-resistant bacteria.[29] Furthermore, the extended use of antibiotics may result in the development of oral candidiasis.

Sinusitis

Sinusitis is defined as an inflammation of the epithelial lining of the paranasal sinuses. The inflammation of these tissues causes mucosal edema and an increase in mucosal secretions. The most common trigger is an acute upper respiratory infection, although other causes, such as exacerbations of allergic rhinitis, dental infections or manipulations, and direct trauma can be implicated. If blockage of sinus drainage occurs, retained secretions can promote bacterial growth and subsequent acute bacterial sinusitis.

Acute sinusitis is a very common disorder, affecting about 31 million Americans per year.[30] Sinusitis accounts for about $5.8 billion (US) in costs with about 73 million days of restricted activity per year.[31]

Pathophysiology

The paranasal sinuses are air-filled cavities that are lined with pseudostratified columnar respiratory epithelium.

The epithelium is ciliated, which facilitates the clearance of mucosal secretions. The frontal, maxillary, and ethmoid sinuses drain into an area known as the ostiomeatal complex. Rhythmic ciliary movement and the clearance of secretions can be impaired by several factors, including viral upper respiratory infections, allergic inflammation, and exposure to tobacco smoke and other irritants. In addition, foreign bodies (accidental or surgical) or a severely deviated nasal septum can cause obstruction. If blockage of the sinus ostia or obstruction of the ostiomeatal complex occurs, stasis of sinus secretions will allow pooling in the sinus cavities, which facilitates bacterial growth.

The most common organisms found in acute bacterial sinusitis are *S. pneumoniae*, *H. influenzae*, and *M. catarrhalis*. Organisms that are commonly associated with chronic sinusitis are *Staphylococcus aureus* and anaerobic bacteria such as *Bacteroides* spp. and *Fusobacterium* spp. Sinusitis due to a fungal infection rarely occurs, usually in immunocompromised patients and in patients who are unresponsive to antibiotics.[32]

Clinical and Laboratory Findings

The symptoms of acute sinusitis include facial pain, tenderness, and headache localized to the affected region. Sinusitis affecting the sphenoid sinuses or posterior ethmoid sinuses can cause headache or pain in the occipital region. Other symptoms that are commonly described include purulent nasal discharge, fever, malaise, and postnasal drainage with fetid breath. Occasionally, there may be toothache or pain with mastication. Patients with chronic sinusitis often present with other symptoms that are often vague and poorly localized. Chronic rhinorrhea, postnasal drainage, nasal congestion, sore throat, facial "fullness," and anosmia are common complaints.

Physical examination reveals sinus tenderness and purulent nasal drainage. On occasion, erythema and swelling of the overlying skin may be evident. The nasal mucosa can appear edematous and erythematous, and nasal polyps might also be visible.

In routine cases of suspected acute bacterial sinusitis, imaging studies are not required.[33] When there are more persistent symptoms as in chronic sinusitis or an incomplete response to initial management, imaging studies may become appropriate. Plain-film radiography is not helpful for establishing ostiomeatal complex disease.[34] Computed tomography (CT) is the study of choice for documenting chronic sinusitis with underlying disease of the ostiomeatal complex and is superior to magnetic resonance imaging (MRI) for the identification of bony abnormalities. CT can also accurately assess polyps, reactive osteitis, mucosal thickening, and fungal sinusitis.[35]

Classification

Sinusitis is classified as either acute, subacute, or chronic, based on the duration of the inflammation and underlying infection. Acute sinusitis is defined as inflammation of less than four weeks, subacute as four to eight weeks, and chronic as either longer than 8–12 weeks in duration.[36]

Diagnosis

The diagnosis of acute sinusitis is made on the basis of history and physical examination. As previously noted, radiologic evaluations may be helpful in certain situations. Patients with recurrent disease need to be evaluated for underlying factors that can predispose patients to sinusitis. Allergy evaluation for allergic rhinitis is often helpful. Chronic sinusitis may be the presentation of an underlying systemic disease, such as Wegener granulomatosis or Churg-Strauss vasculitis.[36] Other predisposing factors, such as tobacco smoke exposure, immunodeficiency, cystic fibrosis, primary ciliary dyskinesia, and septal deviation, should be considered.[36,37]

CT usually aids the diagnosis of chronic sinusitis. Evaluation of the ostiomeatal complex is crucial in the management of these patients. In addition, rhinoscopy may be helpful for direct visualization of sinus ostia.

Management

Initial medical treatment consists of antibiotics to cover the suspected pathogens, along with topical or oral decongestants to facilitate sinus drainage. First-line antibiotics such as amoxicillin are often effective, although second-generation cephalosporin, azithromycin, and amoxicillin-clavulanate can be helpful in resistant cases. Comprehensive treatment of bacterial sinusitis may also include adequate hydration, sinus rinses, steam inhalation, and pharmacologic measures intended to treat underlying disease, such as rhinitis, and to restore ostial patency. Nasal glucocorticosteroids are thought to be potentially effective adjuncts to antibiotic therapy, but available objective data have not unequivocally demonstrated effectiveness.[38] Acute frontal or sphenoid sinusitis can be serious because of the potential for intracranial complications. Intravenous antibiotics are indicated, and surgical intervention is considered, based on the condition's response to medical management.[39]

The management of chronic sinusitis involves antibiotics of a broader spectrum, and a prolonged treatment course may be required.[40] Topical corticosteroids or short courses of oral corticosteroids may help reduce the swelling and/or obstruction of the ostiomeatal complex.[41] Avoidance of exacerbating factors such as allergens or tobacco smoke should be emphasized. Patients with histories suggestive of allergy should undergo a thorough allergy evaluation.

Patients who have chronic sinusitis with evidence of disease of the ostiomeatal complex who fail medical management often require surgical intervention. Functional endoscopic sinus surgery (FESS) involves the removal of the ostiomeatal obstruction through an intranasal approach. This procedure can be performed with either local or general anesthesia and without an external incision. The recovery time from this procedure is short, and morbidity is generally low.

Prognosis

Patients treated for acute sinusitis usually recover without sequelae. Children with sinusitis, particularly ethmoid and maxillary sinusitis, are at risk for periorbital or orbital cellulitis. Periorbital cellulitis is most often treated on an outpatient basis with broad-spectrum antibiotics and rarely leads to complications. Orbital cellulitis, on the other hand, requires hospital admission with broad-spectrum intravenous antibiotics. Further treatment is tailored on a case-by-case basis and may entail surgical or endoscopic drainage of the infection.[42]

Frontal sinusitis can extend through the anterior wall and present as Pott's puffy tumor. Sinusitis can also spread intracranially and result in abscess or meningitis. These complications, although uncommon, are more likely to occur in male adolescent patients.

Patients with chronic sinusitis are more likely to require a prolonged recovery period, with a resultant decrease in quality of life. Chronic medication use can lead to side effects or other complications, such as rhinitis medicamentosa from prolonged use of topical decongestants. Surgical intervention and underlying-factor assessment will often reverse the chronic process, leading to an improvement in quality of life.

Oral Health Considerations

Patients with sinus infections who present with a complaint of a toothache are commonly encountered in a dental office. The oral health-care professional evaluating the patient must be able to differentiate between an odontogenic infection and sinus pain. On history, sinus infections usually present with pain involving more than one tooth in the same maxillary quadrant, whereas a toothache usually involves only a single tooth. Ruling out odontogenic infections by a dental examination and appropriate periapical radiography strengthens a diagnosis.

Chronic sinus infections are often accompanied by mouth breathing. This condition is associated with oral dryness and (in long-time sufferers) increased susceptibility to oral conditions such as gingivitis.[43]

As with other conditions for which the prolonged use of antibiotics is prescribed, the potential development of bacterial resistance needs to be considered. Switching to a different class of antibiotics to treat an odontogenic infection is preferable to increasing the dosage of an antibiotic that the patient has recently taken for another condition.

The use of decongestants may be associated with oral dryness, which may need to be addressed.

Laryngitis and Laryngotracheobronchitis

The upper airway is the site of infection and inflammation during the course of a common cold, but respiratory viruses can affect any portion of the respiratory tree. Laryngitis is defined as an inflammation of the larynx, usually because of a viral infection. Laryngotracheobronchitis (also termed viral croup) involves inflammation of the larynx, trachea, and large bronchi. Although these illnesses have distinct presenting features, both result from a similar infectious process and the reactive inflammation that follows. Laryngitis can present at any age, although it is more common in the adult population.[44] In contrast, laryngotracheobronchitis is an illness seen primarily in young children and has a peak incidence in the second and third years of life. These infections are most common during the fall and winter months, when respiratory viruses are more prevalent.

The viruses most commonly implicated in laryngitis are parainfluenza virus, coxsackieviruses, adenoviruses, and herpes simplex virus (HSV). The viruses most commonly associated with laryngotracheobronchitis are parainfluenza virus, RSV, influenza virus, and adenovirus.[45]

Acute laryngitis can also result from excessive or unusual use of the vocal cords, gastroesophageal reflux, or irritation due to tobacco smoking.

Pathophysiology

The underlying infectious process is quite similar to that seen in viral infections of the upper respiratory tract (see above). After infection of the respiratory epithelium occurs, an inflammatory response consisting of mononuclear cells and polymorphonuclear leukocytes is mounted. As a result, vascular congestion and edema develop. Denudation of areas of respiratory epithelium can result. In addition to edema, spasm of laryngeal muscles can occur. Because the inflammatory process is triggered by a viral infection, the disease processes are usually self-limited.

Clinical and Laboratory Findings

Patients with laryngitis usually have an antecedent viral upper respiratory infection. Complaints of fever and sore throat are common. The most common manifestation of laryngitis is hoarseness, with weak or faint speech.[46] Cough is somewhat variable in presentation and is more likely when the lower respiratory tract is involved.

Children presenting with viral croup commonly have an antecedent upper respiratory tract infection, which may include fever. Shortly thereafter, a barking cough and intermittent stridor develop. Stridor at rest, retractions, and cyanosis can occur in children with severe inflammation. Neck radiography will demonstrate subglottic narrowing (a finding termed "steeple sign") on an anteroposterior view.

Classification

There is no universal classification system for these illnesses. The anatomic site mostly affected describes these diseases.

Diagnosis

The diagnosis of laryngitis is based on the suggestive history. There are no specific findings on physical examination or laboratory tests, although the presence of hoarseness is suggestive. The differential diagnosis includes other causes of laryngeal edema, including obstruction of venous or

lymphatic drainage from masses or other lesions, decreased plasma oncotic pressure from protein loss or malnutrition, increased capillary permeability, myxedema of hypothyroidism, and hereditary angioedema. Carcinoma of the larynx can also present with hoarseness.

The diagnosis of laryngotracheobronchitis is usually apparent and is based on a suggestive history. Radiologic evaluation may or may not aid physicians in the diagnosis. Only 50% of patients with laryngotracheobronchitis show the classic steeple sign on plain neck radiography (Figure 14-2).[47] With children, it is important to rule out other causes of stridor, including foreign-body aspiration, acute bacterial epiglottitis, and retropharyngeal abscess.[48]

Management

Most cases of laryngitis are mild and self-limited, so only supportive care need be prescribed. The use of oral corticosteroids in severe or prolonged cases can be considered, although their routine use is controversial.[49]

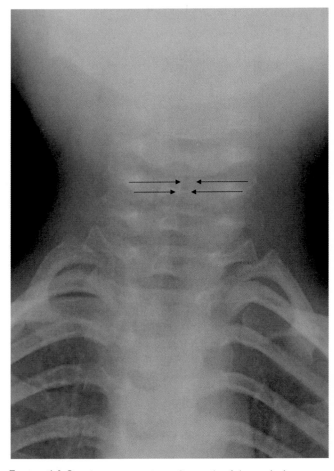

FIGURE 14-2 Anteroposterior radiograph of the neck show narrowing of the upper trachea that is most evident on the anteroposterior view (black arrows). This type of narrowing is typically present in croup and is known as the steeple sign on the anteroposterior radiograph given its similarity to a church steeple.

The most important aspect in the management of laryngotracheobronchitis is airway maintenance. The standard therapy includes mist therapy, corticosteroids, and racemic epinephrine. Any child with evidence of respiratory distress should be considered a candidate for steroid treatment. Less frequently, hospitalization and intubation or tracheotomy are necessary.[47]

Prognosis

As with viral upper respiratory infections, most cases of laryngitis and laryngotracheobronchitis are self-limited and require minimal medical intervention. Recovery within a few days to a week is expected. In some cases, laryngotracheobronchitis can recur, although the factors influencing this are not well understood.

Pharyngitis and Tonsillitis

Inflammation of the tonsils and pharynx is almost always associated with infection, either viral or bacterial. The vast majority of cases are caused by viral infections. These infections can be associated with fever, rhinorrhea, and cough. The major viral etiologies include rhinovirus, coronavirus, adenovirus, Epstein-Barr, para-influenza, HSV, and influenza.[50]

The most common bacterial cause of acute tonsillopharyngitis is group A β-hemolytic *Streptococcus* (GABHS) infection, specifically *Streptococcus pyogenes* infection. Proper diagnosis and treatment of this infection are extremely important in order to prevent disease sequelae, namely, acute rheumatic fever and glomerulonephritis. Less common bacterial causes include *Corynebacterium diphtheriae*, *Neisseria gonorrhoeae*, *Chlamydia*, and *Mycoplasma pneumoniae*.

Chronic mouth breathing, chronic postnasal drainage, and inflammation due to irritant exposure can also cause pharyngitis and tonsillitis.

Pathophysiology

Streptococcal infections are spread through direct contact with respiratory secretions. Transmission is often facilitated in areas where close contact occurs, such as schools and day-care centers. The incubation period is two to five days.

Clinical and Laboratory Findings

Sore throat is the predominant symptom. Associated clinical findings are based on the infectious etiology. Patients with Epstein-Barr virus infections develop infectious mononucleosis, a disease characterized by exudative tonsillopharyngitis, lymphadenopathy, fever, and fatigue. Physical examination can reveal hepatosplenomegaly. Common laboratory findings include leukocytosis, with more than 20% atypical lymphocytes on blood smear. Blood chemistries may reveal elevated liver enzymes.

Infection with coxsackievirus can cause several distinct illnesses, each associated with tonsillopharyngitis. Herpangina is a disease that is characterized by small ulcers that are 2 to 3 mm in size and located on the anterior tonsillar pillars and possibly the uvula and soft palate. Hand-foot-and-mouth disease is characterized by ulcers on the tongue and oral mucosa, in association with vesicles found on the palms and/or soles. Small yellow-white nodules on the anterior tonsillar pillars characterize ympho nodular pharyngitis; these nodules do not ulcerate.

Pharyngoconjunctival fever is a disorder characterized by exudative tonsillopharyngitis, conjunctivitis, and fever. Infection is due to adenovirus.

Measles is a disease with a prodromal phase that is characterized by symptoms of upper respiratory infection, tonsillopharyngitis, and small white lesions with erythematous bases on the buccal mucosa and inner aspect of the lower lip (Koplik's spots). These lesions are pathognomonic of early measles infection.

Streptococcal pharyngitis is characterized by exudative tonsillitis and fever. Physical examination often reveals a beefy red uvula, cervical adenitis, and oral petechiae. Laboratory evaluation should include testing for group A *Streptococcus*.[51]

Classification

Pharyngotonsillitis is classified on the basis of etiology and clinical presentation (see above).

Diagnosis

Diagnosis is based on a history of sore throat and is established by appropriate physical findings and results of testing. A rapid antigen detection test is available for diagnosing streptococcal pharyngitis. The test has a high specificity (95+%) and slightly lower sensitivity (80 to 90%).[52] The importance of confirmatory cultures is still controversial, with some studies concluding that culture confirmation of negative rapid antigen detection tests may not be necessary in all circumstances.[53]

Antistreptococcal antibody titers reflect past and not present immunologic events and are of no value in the diagnosis of acute GABHS pharyngitis. They are valuable for confirmation of prior GABHS infections in patients suspected of having acute rheumatic fever or post streptococcal acute glomerulonephritis.

Management

The viral causes of tonsillopharyngitis are treated symptomatically. Gargle solutions, analgesics, and antipyretics are often helpful. The course is self-limited.[5]

Acute streptococcal pharyngitis is treated with oral penicillin V, cephalosporins, macrolides, clindamycin, or an intramuscular injection of benzathine penicillin G. Failure rates for penicillin vary from 6% to 23%, so an additional antibiotic course may be necessary.[51] GABHS carriers appear unlikely to spread the organism to close contacts and are at a low risk of developing complications. Antimicrobial therapy is generally not indicated for the majority of GABHS carriers.[54]

Prognosis

The prognosis for viral tonsillopharyngitis is very good as the infections are self-limited. Late sequelae from group A streptococcal tonsillitis can be avoided by prompt diagnosis and treatment.[55] Other complications due to streptococcal tonsillitis are uncommon but include cervical adenitis, peritonsillar abscesses, otitis media, cellulitis, and septicemia.

Oral Health Considerations

The association between GABHS infection and the development of severe complications, such as rheumatic fever and its associated heart condition, is well known. Although failure to successfully treat GABHS infections was more common in the pre-penicillin era, there are some concerns today regarding reinfection in cases in which penicillin is unable to eradicate the organism. One study found a significant association between the persistence of GABHS on toothbrushes and removable orthodontic appliances and the recovery of GABHS in the oropharynx of symptomatic patients after 10 days of treatment with penicillin.[56] Interestingly, when toothbrushes were rinsed with sterile water, organisms could not be cultured beyond three days, whereas nonrinsed toothbrushes harbored GABHS for up to 15 days. Thus, patients with GABHS infections should be instructed to thoroughly clean their toothbrushes and removable acrylic appliances daily. It is also advisable to change to a new toothbrush after the acute stage of any oropharyngeal infection.

LOWER AIRWAY DISEASES

The association between oral health and respiratory diseases has received renewed attention. Several articles have suggested that dental plaque may be a reservoir for respiratory pathogens involved in pneumonia and chronic obstructive pulmonary disease (COPD).[57–62] Although this may not be a critical problem for ambulatory healthy individuals, deteriorating oral health may be a major factor for both morbidity and mortality among institutionalized elderly persons, as well as for patients in critical care units.

Acute Bronchitis

Acute bronchitis is an acute respiratory infection involving the large airways (trachea and bronchi) that is manifested predominantly by cough with or without phlegm production that lasts up to three weeks. In patients who are otherwise healthy and without underlying pulmonary disease, bronchitis is commonly caused by a viral infection.[63] The viruses most commonly implicated are influenza, parainfluenza, and RSV. Viruses that are predominantly associated with upper respiratory tract infections, including coronavirus, rhinovirus, and adenovirus, have also been implicated as causes of acute bronchitis.[64] Acute bronchitis due to bacterial infection is less common. Atypical bacteria including *Mycoplasma pneumoniae*, *Chlamydia pneumoniae*, and *Bordetella pertussis* are often important causes of bronchitis.[65] *Staphylococcus* and gram-negative bacteria are common causes of bronchitis among hospitalized individuals.

Pathophysiology

The pathophysiology of acute bronchitis is similar to that of other respiratory tract infections. Following infection of the mucosal cells, congestion of the respiratory mucosa develops. Inflammation causes an increase in secretory activity, resulting in increased sputum production. Polymorphonuclear leukocytes infiltrate the bronchial walls and lumen. Desquamation of the ciliated epithelium may occur, and spasm of bronchial smooth muscle is common.

Clinical and Laboratory Findings

Acute viral bronchitis usually presents with sudden onset of cough, with or without sputum expectoration and without evidence of pneumonia, the common cold, acute asthma, or an acute exacerbation of chronic bronchitis.[64] Chest discomfort may occur; this usually worsens with persistent coughing bouts.[66] Other symptoms, such as dyspnea and respiratory distress, are variably present. Physical examination may reveal wheezing. The presentation may closely resemble an acute asthma exacerbation. Symptoms gradually resolve over a period of one to two weeks. Patients with underlying chronic lung disease might also experience respiratory compromise, with a significant impairment in pulmonary function.

The presentation of acute bacterial bronchitis is very similar to that of bacterial pneumonia (see below). Symptoms may include fever, dyspnea, productive cough with purulent sputum, and chest pain. Bacterial bronchitis can be differentiated from pneumonia by the lack of significant findings on chest radiography.

Classification

Although there is no universal classification scheme, acute bronchitis can be differentiated on the basis of etiology. Viral bronchitis presents differently from bacterial bronchitis, as described above.

Diagnosis

Diagnosis of acute bronchitis is based on a suggestive history and a physical examination. Neither blood cell counts nor sputum analyses are particularly diagnostic in otherwise healthy patients. Routine testing for viruses is generally not obtained for bronchitis.[63] Chest radiography may be helpful in distinguishing bacterial bronchitis from pneumonia. Patients with recurrent bouts of acute bronchitis should be evaluated for possible asthma. This evaluation should include pulmonary function testing.

Patients with persistent symptoms in the course of presumed viral bronchitis should be evaluated to determine possible underlying etiologies. Sputum cultures might prove useful in these circumstances but are not performed routinely.[67]

Management

Viral bronchitis can be managed with supportive care only as most individuals who are otherwise healthy recover without specific treatment. If significant airway obstruction or hyperreactivity is present, inhaled bronchodilators, such as albuterol, may be useful. Cough suppressants, such as codeine, can also be considered for patients whose coughing interferes with sleep.

The treatment of bacterial bronchitis may include amoxicillin, amoxicillin-clavulanate, macrolides, or cephalosporins. For suspected or confirmed pertussis infection, treatment with a macrolide or trimethoprim-sulfamethoxazole is appropriate to decrease disease transmission. Although commonly used, inhaled β_2-agonist bronchodilators and mucokinetic agents, like expectorants, are not recommended for routine use in patients with acute bronchitis.[64]

Prognosis

Acute bronchitis carries an excellent prognosis for patients who are without underlying pulmonary disease, and recovery without sequelae is the norm. However, for patients with chronic lung disease and respiratory compromise, bronchitis can be quite serious and may often lead to hospitalization and respiratory failure. In other high-risk individuals, such as those with human immunodeficiency virus (HIV) infection or other immunodeficiencies, acute bronchitis may lead to the development of bronchiectasis.

Oral Health Considerations

Resistance to antibiotics may develop rapidly and last for 10–14 days.[68] Thus, patients who are taking amoxicillin for acute bronchitis should be prescribed another type of antibiotic, (such as clindamycin or a cephalosporin) when an antibiotic is needed to treat an odontogenic infection.

Pneumonia

Pneumonia is defined pathologically as an infection and a subsequent inflammation involving the lung parenchyma. Both viruses and bacteria are the causes, and the presentation is dependent on the causative organism. Pneumonias can be broadly classified as either nosocomial or community-acquired. Nosocomial infections are infections that are acquired in a hospital or health-care facility and often affect debilitated or chronically ill individuals. Community-acquired infections can affect all persons but are more commonly seen in otherwise healthy individuals. In the US, there were 52,000 deaths from community-acquired pneumonia in 2007 with 4.2 million ambulatory care visits for this condition in 2006.[69]

Formerly, bacterial pneumonia was categorized into several subtypes; community-acquired pneumonia, aspiration pneumonia, hospital-acquired (nosocomial) pneumonia, ventilator-associated pneumonia, and nursing home–associated pneumonia. In all cases, connections have been made with oral health status. However, in 2005, a new category was created called health care–associated pneumonia (HCAP).[70] HCAP was defined as pneumonia occurring in a diverse group of patients including those undergoing home-infusion therapy or wound care, chronic dialysis, recently hospitalized patients, or nursing home residents. Patients in these settings are often at high risk for pneumonia caused by multidrug resistant

organisms such as methicillin-resistant *Staphylococcus aureus* (MRSA) or resistant gram-negative bacilli. Thus, treatment guidelines for HCAP include broad-spectrum antibiotic therapy.

The most common bacterial cause of community-acquired pneumonia is *S. pneumoniae*, followed by *H. influenzae*. The organisms responsible for HCAP include aerobic gram-negative bacilli, such as *P. aeruginosa*, *Escherichia coli*, *Klebsiella pneumoniae*, and *Acinetobacter* species. Infections due to gram-positive cocci, such as *S. aureus*, particularly MRSA, have been rapidly emerging in the United States as well.[71] A related condition is aspiration pneumonia, which is typically caused by anaerobic organisms most often originating from the gingival crevice.[72] Aspiration pneumonia often occurs in patients with dysphagia, depressed consciousness, or others at risk for aspiration of oral contents into the lung including alcoholics. Aspiration pneumonia occurs both in the community and in institutional settings.

Atypical organisms commonly associated with pneumonia include *M. pneumoniae*, *Legionella*, and *Chlamydia*.[73] The atypical organisms may cause a pneumonia that differs in clinical presentation from that caused by the aforementioned bacteria (see below). Pneumonia can be caused by viruses, such as influenza, pararinfluenza, adenovirus, and RSV, as well as fungi such as *Candida*, *Histoplasma*, *Cryptococcus*, and *Aspergillus*. Pneumonia may also be caused by other organisms including *Pneumocystis jiroveci (carinii)*, seen in immunocompromised hosts, *Nocardia*, and *Mycobacterium tuberculosis*. Infection with these organisms can often be differentiated by chest radiography.

Pathophysiology

The pathophysiology of pneumonia is dependent on the causative infectious organism. In bacterial pneumonia caused by *S. pneumoniae*, for example, the bacteria first enter the alveolar spaces after inhalation. Once inside the alveoli, the bacteria rapidly multiply, and extensive edema develops. The bacteria cause a vigorous inflammatory response, which includes an influx of polymorphonuclear leukocytes. In addition, capillary leakage is pronounced. As the inflammatory process continues, the polymorphonuclear leukocytes are replaced by macrophages. Subsequent deposition of fibrin ensues as the infection is controlled, and the inflammatory response resolves.[74]

Other infections of the lung (i.e., viral, atypical, etc.) are interstitial processes. The organisms are first inhaled into the alveolar spaces. The organisms then infect the type I pneumocytes directly. As these pneumocytes lose their structural integrity and necrosis ensues, alveolar edema begins. Type II pneumocytes proliferate and line the alveoli, and an exudative cellular debris accumulates. An interstitial inflammatory response is mounted, primarily by mononuclear leukocytes. This process can occasionally progress to interstitial fibrosis, although resolution is the norm.

Clinical and Laboratory Findings

Pneumonia due to community-acquired bacterial infection typically presents acutely, with a rapid onset of symptoms.

A prodrome similar to that seen with acute infections of the upper respiratory tract is unusual. Common symptoms include fever, pleuritic chest pain, and coughing that produces purulent sputum.[66] Chills and rigors are also common. Pneumonia due to *H. influenzae*, which is seen more commonly in patients with COPD or alcoholism, presents with fever, cough, and malaise. Chest pain and rigors are less common.

Nosocomial pneumonia with *Staphylococcus* secondary to aspiration presents with fever, dyspnea, cough, and purulent sputum. In cases acquired hematogenously, signs and symptoms related to the underlying endovascular infection predominate. Otherwise, respiratory tract symptoms are mild or absent despite radiographic evidence of multiple pulmonary infiltrates. The classic clinical features of non-bacteremic *Enterobacteriaceae* or *Pseudomonas* pneumonia are abrupt onset of dyspnea, fever, chills, and cough in an older patient who is either hospitalized or chronically ill.[75]

Physical examination demonstrates crackles (rales) in the affected lung fields. Decreased breath sounds and dullness to percussion might also be noted. Signs of respiratory distress may be present in severely affected individuals, including retractions, use of accessory muscles and cyanosis.

With atypical pneumonia, symptoms usually develop over three to four days and initially consist of low-grade fevers, malaise, a nonproductive cough, and headache. Often systemic complaints are more prominent than the respiratory complaints. Sputum production, if present, is usually minimal. Findings on physical examination of the chest are usually unremarkable, with only scattered rhonchi. Infection due to *Mycoplasma* is common among younger patients. Pneumonias due to viral causes have a similar presentation but can have a more rapid onset.

Infection with *Legionella* spp. (Legionnaires' disease) begins with a prodrome consisting of fever and malaise and progresses rapidly to an acute phase of high fever, rigors, pleuritic chest pain, gastrointestinal complaints, and confusion. The cough is typically nonproductive and is only variably present. Elevated liver enzymes and proteinuria indicate renal and hepatic involvement. Hypoxia can also develop and progress rapidly. Legionnaires' disease was first described at an American Legion convention in Philadelphia in 1976. The causative organisms have a predilection for moist areas such as air-conditioning ducts and cooling towers. The infection tends to occur more commonly among middle-aged men with a history of tobacco smoking.

Classification

Pneumonia is initially classified on clinical presentation as either viral, bacterial, or atypical. Different classifications based on radiologic or pathologic manifestations are less commonly used.

Diagnosis

When a patient with probable pneumonia is being evaluated, the possible causative organism will be suggested by (1) the clinical presentation and course of the illness, (2) the degree of immunocompetency of the patient, (3) the presence or absence of underlying lung disease, and (4) the place of acquisition (hospital or community). Ultimately, the goal is rapid diagnosis to establish an etiology so that appropriate antimicrobial therapy can be initiated. With community-acquired pneumonia, the diagnosis should be based on a clinical history and physical examination findings. Chest radiography, laboratory studies, and blood cultures may be considered.[76]

In nosocomial infection, the presence of pneumonia is defined by new lung infiltrate on radiography plus clinical evidence that the infiltrate is of an infectious origin. The presence of a new or progressive radiographic infiltrate plus at least two of three clinical features (fever greater than 38°C, leukocytosis or leukopenia, and purulent secretions) represents the most accurate combination of criteria for starting empiric antibiotic therapy.[71] For diagnosis of ventilator associated pneumonia, quantitative microbiological cultures from bronchoalveolar lavage (BAL) samples are often employed, with pathogenic bacteria ≥10^4cfu/mL of BAL indicative of an infection.[77]

Sputum analysis is the traditional tool used for diagnosis and management. Spontaneously coughed or induced sputum is analyzed by Gram stain and allows for the identification of a select group of pathogens and thus a more directed antibiotic therapy. For example, gram-positive cocci in pairs (diplococci) are suggestive of pneumococcal infection. Gram-positive cocci in grape-like clusters suggest infection with *S. aureus*. Gram-negative pleomorphic rods are typical of *H. influenzae*, whereas *Klebsiella* is identified by its short plump gram-negative rod appearance. Numerous polymorphonuclear leukocytes are also often seen. This method, however, is limited since very often sputum contains bacteria of the normal flora that may be confused with pathogens.

Quantitative cultures for hospital-acquired infections can be performed on endotracheal aspirates or samples collected either bronchoscopically or nonbronchoscopically. These techniques may aid in diagnosis and management as well. Routine culture can identify *S. pneumoniae*, *H. influenzae*, *S. aureus*, and gram-negative rods. Specialized culturing techniques are needed to identify *Legionella*, *Mycobacterium*, *Nocardia*, *Mycoplasma*, and fungi. Tissue cultures are used to identify viruses and *Chlamydia*. In patients with nosocomial pneumonia, a lower respiratory tract culture should be collected before antibiotic therapy, but collection of cultures should not delay the initiation of therapy in critically ill patients.[71]

Chest radiography can be a valuable tool in the evaluation of the patient with pneumonia. The radiologic presentation is dependent on the infectious etiology and the underlying medical condition of the patient. A pattern of lobar consolidation and air bronchograms is seen most commonly in cases of pneumococcal pneumonia (Figure 14-3). The lower lobes and right middle lobe are most commonly involved. A pattern of patchy nonhomogeneous infiltrates, pleural effusion, and cavitary lesions is common with staphylococcal pneumonia. *Klebsiella* pneumonia typically involves multiple lobes and can also be associated with effusion and cavitation. Viral or atypical organisms usually present with an

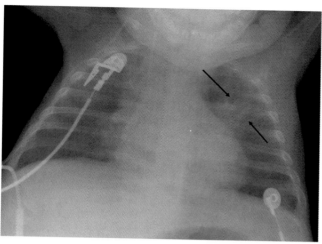

FIGURE 14-3 Anteroposterior radiograph of the chest in an infant shows an infiltrate in the left upper lobe (black arrows). Blood cultures obtained on this infant were positive for pneumococcus.

interstitial infiltrative pattern or patchy segmental infiltrates. Organisms such as *Nocardia*, *Mycobacterium*, and fungi often cause nodular or cavitary lesions, which are demonstrable on chest radiography. Rapid accumulation of pleural fluid or empyema is seen most often with bacterial infection.

The presence of cold agglutinins is suggestive of *Mycoplasma* infection. Cold agglutinins are antibodies (produced in response to *Mycoplasma* infection) that agglutinate red blood cells upon cold exposure. Titers reach maximal levels in three to four weeks but can be detected one week after the onset of disease. These antibodies can be found in 60%–70% of patients with *Mycoplasma* pneumonia but are not specific to this disease.

Legionella pneumonia can be diagnosed by a urine antigen assay and by culture of the organism, using specialized media, or by direct fluorescent antibody staining of sputum.

Management

Empiric treatment is started immediately upon diagnosis of pneumonia. Treatment options for outpatients with community-acquired pneumonia include β-lactams (e.g., amoxicillin-clavulanate), macrolides, and doxycycline. Patients who have received antimicrobial therapy within the previous three months are at increased risk for infection with antimicrobial-resistant *S. pneumoniae* and may require starting with a fluoroquinolone or a combination of antibiotics (e.g., β-lactam and macrolide).[78]

In the case of nosocomial pneumonia, patients with low risk of infection by an antibiotic-resistant organism should be treated with empiric therapy such as a third-generation cephalosporin or fluoroquinolone. However, more aggressive broad-spectrum therapy (such as an antipseudomonal cephalosporin, carbapenem, or fluoroquinolone, along with linezolid or vancomycin for MRSA), is required for high-risk patients, such as those with a prolonged duration of hospitalization (five days or more), admission from a health care–related facility, or recent prolonged antibiotic therapy.[71]

Nonspecific treatment for patients with pneumonia includes aggressive hydration to aid in sputum clearance. Chest physiotherapy is advocated by many clinicians, although evidence of efficacy is lacking. If hypoxia is present, supplemental oxygen is given.[79]

A pneumococcal vaccine is available for active immunization against pneumococcal disease. The vaccine is effective for preventing disease from of the most common pneumococcal serotypes. It is effective for adults and for children older than 2 years of age and is recommended for all individuals over the age of 65 years and selected high-risk patients with certain medical conditions.[78] A conjugate pneumococcal vaccine has been part of the US childhood immunization schedule since 2000 and has led to a sustained reduction in hospitalizations for childhood pneumonia.[80]

Prognosis

Mortality due to community-acquired pneumonia is low. The risk of mortality is higher for older patients, patients with underlying pulmonary disease, patients with immunodeficiency (i.e., asplenia), and patients with positive blood cultures. Most deaths occur within five days of the onset of disease.

Mortality due to staphylococcal pneumonia is high, and patients who do recover often have residual pulmonary abnormalities. Mortality due to atypical pneumonia is low, with the exception of *Legionella* pneumonia, which has a 15% mortality rate if left untreated.

Oral Health Considerations

The aspiration of salivary secretions containing oral bacteria into the lower respiratory tract can cause aspiration pneumonia. Numerous periodontally associated oral anaerobes and facultative species have been isolated from infected pulmonary fluids.[81] Although most reports suggest increased susceptibility to the development of nosocomial pneumonia from periodontal pathogens, other oral bacteria (such as *Streptococcus viridans*) have been implicated in community-acquired pneumonia.[82]

The connection of oral health to pneumonia involves aspiration of a pathogen from a proximal site, for example, the oral-pharyngeal cavity, into the lower airway. The teeth or dentures have nonshedding surfaces upon which oral biofilms, that is, dental plaque, form, which are susceptible to colonization by respiratory pathogens. Indeed, intensive care subjects were found to harbor greater levels of dental plaque than nonhospitalized control patients, and bacterial pathogens known to cause pneumonia were found to be prevalent in the dental plaque from the intensive care subjects.[59] In some cases, up to 100% of the aerobic flora was found to be *S. aureus*, *P. aeruginosa*, or several enteric species. In contrast, the control dental patients were only rarely colonized by respiratory pathogens. Poor oral hygiene therefore may predispose high-risk patients to oral colonization by respiratory pathogens and therefore increase the risk for lung infection. In addition, the host response to oral biofilms results in inflammation of the periodontal tissues.[83] Thus, inflammatory products from the gingival tissues as well as pathogenic bacteria shed from oral biofilms into the secretions can be aspirated into the lower airway to promote lung infection.[81]

Elderly individuals residing in nursing homes also have an increased prevalence of poor oral health, including increased plaque retention.[84] Studies have evaluated the occurrence of pneumonia in cohorts of elderly individuals who were receiving and not receiving oral care. In one such study, the relative risk of developing pneumonia increased 67% in the group without access to oral health interventions compared with individuals who had access to oral care.[85] These data support the benefit of increased awareness and increased oral health interventions in hospitalized and institutionalized individuals. More intervention studies are needed to assess the impact of oral pathogens on the incidence of pneumonia, but at present, there is ample evidence that poor oral health status is a risk indicator for the development of pneumonia.

These and other studies support the notion that institutionalized subjects, especially those in hospital intensive care and nursing home settings, have a greater risk for dental plaque colonization by respiratory pathogens than do community-dwelling subjects. This suggests that oral intervention to reduce or control dental plaque may serve as a simple, cost-effective method to reduce pathogen colonization in high-risk populations. Several systematic reviews of the literature have examined the evidence for oral interventions to reduce the risk of pneumonia in hospital and nursing home patients. The weight of the evidence supports the notion that interventions that improve oral hygiene significantly reduce the incidence of pulmonary infection, however, mortality seems unaffected.[86–88]

Interventions tested to date include topical disinfections using chlorhexidine[89–91] and supervised mechanical plaque control augmented with topical agents.[92] Taken together, the available evidence suggests that there is a relationship between poor oral hygiene and bacterial pneumonia in special care populations, including those in hospital and nursing home settings. Interventions designed to improve oral hygiene may reduce the risk of pneumonia in these populations. This raises the question "what is the present status of oral hygiene practice in hospitals and nursing homes". A recent paper described clinical practice guidelines for oral hygiene in critically ill patients based upon a systematic literature review followed by prospective consideration of the evidence at a consensus development conference.[93] From this, several recommendations were offered to guide clinicians in the care of vulnerable patients. These recommendations were:

1. Provision of effective oral care is an important strategy in reducing nosocomial pneumonia.
2. The use of a designated oral care protocol.
3. Systematic clinical assessment of the oral cavity using standardized methods (to include the condition of the teeth, gums, tongue, mucous membranes and lips).
4. The use of a soft bristled brush can remove debris and subsequent plaque.
5. Mouth swabs (foam and cotton) should be used where there is a contraindication to brushing (e.g., bleeding gums associated with thrombocytopenia).
6. The use of one oral rinse over another was considered questionable (with the exception of chlorhexidine gluconate 0.12% in individuals undergoing cardiac surgery).
7. Tap water should not be used for oral hygiene in the critically ill (as it is often contaminated with potential respiratory pathogens).
8. Subglottic suctioning in mechanically ventilated patients to limit aspiration of contaminated secretions.
9. Although the optimal frequency for oral hygiene has never been evaluated, brushing at least twice a day was suggested.
10. Although the optimal duration for oral care has never been evaluated brushing, oral cleansing for 3–4 minutes using a brush that allows access to all areas of the mouth was suggested.
11. While there is no evidence available to support the use of individual, clean storage devices for oral hygiene tools, however, the guideline committee recommends the use of designated containers.

Other measures for consideration for intubated patients may include removal of all dental appliances upon admissions to the critical care unit, periodic repositioning the tube or deflation of the cuff. Removal of hard deposits (e.g., tartar/calculus) from the teeth should be considered if possible prior to admission (for example in the case of elective surgery). Placement the patient's head to the side or place in semi-fowlers (semi-reclined body position) will also minimize inadvertent aspiration.

Bronchiolitis

Bronchiolitis is a disease that affects children under the age of 2 years; it is most common among infants aged 2–12 months. It is characterized by infection of the lower respiratory tract, with the bronchioles being most affected. The inflammatory response can be caused by various pathogens, including RSV, human metapneumovirus, parainfluenza virus, influenza virus, adenovirus, and M. pneumoniae.[94–96]

Pathophysiology

Infection of the bronchioles leads to a marked inflammatory response with a prominent mononuclear cell infiltrate. This inflammatory response results in edema and necrosis of epithelial cells lining small airways, mucosal thickening and mucus hypersecretion, plugging, and bronchospasm.[96] Bronchiolar spasm is an occasional feature. Due to these changes, the lumina of the bronchioles are critically narrowed, leading to areas of microatelectasis and emphysema.

Respiratory compromise is common, with decreased blood oxygen saturation, hypercarbia, respiratory acidosis, and, in severe cases, respiratory failure.

Clinical and Laboratory Findings

Infants first develop signs and symptoms of an infection of the upper respiratory tract, with low-grade fever, profuse clear rhinorrhea, and cough. Signs of infection in the lower respiratory tract soon follow, including tachypnea, retractions, wheezing, nasal flaring, and on occasion, cyanosis. Crackles can be audible, and thoracic hyperresonance can be noted on percussion. Associated findings can include conjunctivitis, otitis media, and pharyngitis. Pulse oximetry can be used to determine oxygen saturation levels.

Chest radiography may show peribronchial cuffing, flattening of the diaphragms, hyperinflation, increased lung markings or areas of atelectasis.

Laboratory studies reveal a mild leukocytosis with a prominence of polymorphonuclear leukocytes ("left shift").

Classification

Bronchiolitis can be classified by the causative agent, as is the case with acute bronchitis.

Diagnosis

The diagnosis is clinical, based on the history and physical examination. Laboratory and radiologic studies for diagnosis are not generally required. The etiology can be determined (and the diagnosis confirmed) by performing a nasopharyngeal culture for RSV and other respiratory viruses. Rapid viral diagnostic assays are also available.

The differential diagnosis includes many other causes of wheezing and respiratory distress in this age group, such as asthma, congenital heart disease, and cystic fibrosis.

Management

Clinical treatment of these infants is generally limited to supportive care. Infants may be placed in cool-mist oxygen tents, where continuous oxygen administration can be given. Due to an increase in insensible water losses, hydration must be ensured. Aerosolized bronchodilators should not be used routinely in the management of bronchiolitis, although a carefully monitored trial may be attempted if there is a documented positive clinical response. Corticosteroid medications are generally not indicated.[97]

Antiviral therapy with ribavirin is rarely used, although it may be considered for use in highly selected situations involving documented RSV bronchiolitis with severe disease or in those who are at risk for severe disease (e.g., immunocompromised and/or hemodynamically significant cardiopulmonary disease).[96] Ribavirin is delivered by aerosol on a semicontinuous basis for up to one week.[98]

Mechanical ventilation is required in the infant with respiratory failure. Very young infants (less than 1 month of age) are at risk for apnea due to RSV infection, so close observation is required.

An intramuscular monoclonal antibody to the RSV-F protein, palivizumab, is effective in preventing severe RSV disease in high-risk infants when given before and during the RSV season. This prophylaxis is currently recommended only for high-risk patient populations such as those with chronic lung disease, a history of prematurity, or congenital heart disease.[99]

Prognosis

Although mortality due to bronchiolitis is not uncommon, most patients recover without sequelae. Epidemiologic studies with a several-year follow-up of index and control children show a higher incidence of wheezing and asthma in children with a history of bronchiolitis, unexplained by family history or other atopic syndromes. It is unclear whether bronchiolitis incites an immune response that manifests as asthma later or whether those infants have an inherent predilection for asthma that is merely unmasked by their episode of RSV.[99]

Asthma

Asthma is a chronic inflammatory disorder of the airways. It is characterized by recurrent and often reversible airflow limitation due to an underlying inflammatory process. The etiology of asthma is unknown, but allergic sensitivity is seen in most patients with asthma.[4] There is a significant hereditary contribution, but no single gene or combination of genes has yet been identified as causative. Multiple risk factors for the development of asthma have been indentified, including family history of asthma, atopy, respiratory infections, inhaled pollutants in indoor and outdoor air and in the workplace, allergens, food sensitivities, and other exposures, such as tobacco smoke.[100]

In the US, asthma affects about 19 million adults and 7 million children.[101] In addition, asthma represents a significant economic and social burden with about $56 billion (US) spent on medical costs, lost school/work days and early deaths.[102] It accounted for 3400 deaths in the US in 2010. Overall, trends do not appear to be declining despite advances in our understanding of asthma and newer pharmacologic modalities.

Pathophysiology

The clinical features of asthma are due to the underlying chronic inflammatory process. Although the etiology is not known, certain histopathologic features provide insights into the chronic process. Infiltration of the airway by inflammatory cells such as activated lymphocytes and eosinophils, denudation of the epithelium, deposition of collagen in the subbasement membrane area, and mast cell degranulation are often features of mild or moderate persistent asthma. Other features seen, include mucus hypersecretion, smooth muscle hypertrophy, and angiogenesis.[103]

Airway inflammation contributes significantly to many of the hallmark features of asthma, including airflow obstruction, bronchial hyperresponsiveness, and the initiation of the injury-repair process (remodeling) found in some patients. Bronchial smooth muscle spasm is instrumental in the excessive airway reactivity. Resident airway cells, including mast cells, alveolar macrophages, and airway epithelium, as well as migrating inflammatory cells, secrete a variety of mediators that directly contract the bronchial smooth muscle. These same mediators, such as histamine, cysteinyl leukotrienes, and bradykinin, increase capillary membrane permeability to cause mucosal edema of the airways.[104]

Atopy is the strongest risk factor associated with the development of asthma. Persistent exposure to relevant allergens in a sensitized individual can lead to chronic allergic inflammation of the airways. Although atopy is seen more commonly in childhood-onset asthma, it can also play an important role in asthma in adults.

Clinical and Laboratory Findings

The hallmark clinical features of asthma are recurrent reversible airflow limitation and airway hyperresponsiveness. These factors lead to the development of the signs and symptoms of asthma, which include intermittent wheezing, coughing, dyspnea, and chest tightness. Symptoms of asthma tend to worsen at night and in the early morning hours. In addition, well-defined triggers may precipitate asthma symptoms. These triggers include allergens, gastroesophageal reflux, exercise, cold air, respiratory irritants, nonsteroidal anti-inflammatory drugs, emotional extremes, and infections, particularly viral infections. Symptoms can progress slowly over time, or they may develop abruptly.[2,105–107]

Historical points that suggest the diagnosis of asthma include chronic coughing with nocturnal awakenings, dyspnea, or chest tightness with exertion, recurrent "croup" or "bronchitis" associated with infections of the upper respiratory tract, and wheezing that occurs on a seasonal basis. Physical examination of patients with mild disease often shows no abnormalities. However, common findings in patients with more severe disease include an increased anteroposterior chest diameter, a prolonged expiratory phase, wheezing, and diminished breath sounds. Digital clubbing is rarely seen. Concurrent allergic disease such as allergic rhinitis may be present. During acute exacerbations, patients may show signs of respiratory distress, with tachypnea, intercostal retractions, nasal flaring, and cyanosis.

Pulmonary function testing or spirometry is recommended in the initial assessment of most patients with suspected asthma. These tools can often be useful to monitor the course of asthma and a patient's response to therapy. The technique involves a maximal forced expiration following a maximal inspiration (see Figure 14-4). The key measurements are the forced vital capacity (FVC), which is the amount of air expired during the forced expiration, and the forced expiratory volume in 1 second (FEV_1), which is the volume of air expired during the first second of expiration; FEV_1 is a measure of the rate at which air can be exhaled. Given the FEV_1 and the FEV_1/FVC ratio, an objective determination of airflow limitation is

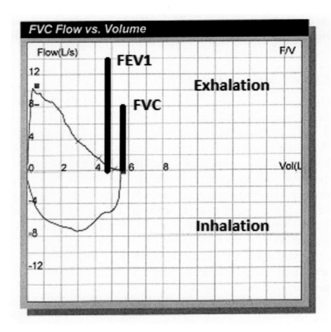

FIGURE 14-4 Spirometric Flow-Volume Curve demonstrating FEV1 and FVC along with exhalation and inspiration phases.

possible. Reversibility can be demonstrated after administration of a short-acting bronchodilator, such as albuterol, and repeating spirometry to demonstrate significant improvement in the FEV_1. In patients with normal baseline spirometry values, a demonstration of bronchial hyperresponsiveness is useful. This is performed by bronchoprovocation, using nonspecific triggers such as histamine or methacholine. When delivered by aerosol, these agents allow the determination of bronchial hyperreactivity by triggering a decrease in the FEV_1 immediately following inhalation. Subsequent measurements of peak expiratory flow rate (PEFR) at home may also be helpful to assess symptoms, to alert to worsening of airflow obstruction, and to monitor therapeutic responses.[104] The PEFR is easy to determine, and durable metering devices are available at little cost. Newer diagnostic tests like exhaled nitric oxide levels (FE_{NO}), are becoming useful in detecting eosinophilic airway inflammation.[108]

Allergen skin testing is another valuable tool. This testing allows the accurate identification of allergic triggers, which can translate into more specific therapies, such as allergen avoidance and immunotherapy (see "Allergic Rhinitis and Conjunctivitis," above). Chest radiography may be useful, especially as a means of excluding other diseases from the diagnosis.

Classification

Asthma is classified according to its severity taking into consideration impairment and risk. Although there is no universal classification scheme, the guidelines set forth by the National Asthma Education and Prevention Program (NAEPP) and updated in 2007 are widely used in the United States.[103,109] Asthma patients are classified as having intermittent, mild-persistent, moderate-persistent, or severe-persistent disease. The categories are defined by both subjective (historical) and objective (spirometric) points. Follow-up visits determine asthma is control thus classification can change over time. Asthma may also be classified by the underlying trigger (e.g., exercise-induced asthma and occupational asthma).

Diagnosis

The diagnosis of asthma is made on the basis of a suggestive history, confirmatory physical findings, and the demonstration of reversible airflow limitation. This can be documented during hospitalizations, by outpatient use of spirometry or PEFR determinations, or by clinical assessment after therapeutic trials.

The differential diagnosis of asthma includes other causes of chronic coughing and wheezing. The diseases that are usually considered are chronic rhinitis or sinusitis, cystic fibrosis, gastroesophageal reflux disease, airway narrowing due to compression (i.e., masses), and COPD (chronic bronchitis). Factors favoring the diagnosis of asthma include intermittent symptoms with asymptomatic periods, complete or nearly complete reversibility with bronchodilators, the absence of digital clubbing, and a history of atopy.

Management

The goals of asthma management include the patient having little or no chronic symptoms, few or no exacerbations requiring oral steroids, no hospitalizations, and minimal or no activity limitation. This is to be achieved using the least amount of medication. Ideal control would include no need for short-acting bronchodilators, normal PEFRs, no PEFR variability, and no adverse effects from controller medications. All patients with asthma, regardless of its severity, should have an asthma control plan to aid in understanding the underlying process and treatment options and to effectively treat asthma exacerbations. Regular monitoring of asthma is important; spirometry, PEFR measurement, FE_{NO} levels, and validated questionnaires may be useful tools for this purpose. Avoidance control measures are regularly emphasized, focusing on allergen and irritant triggers. Treatment for concomitant diseases that may exacerbate asthma (such as allergic rhinitis, gastroesophageal reflux disease, and chronic sinusitis) should be instituted.[110]

Pharmacotherapy of asthma is based on the severity of disease. NAEPP guidelines[103] provide a stepwise approach for increasing and decreasing medications (Figure 14-5). Patients with mild-intermittent disease usually require short-acting bronchodilators on an as-needed basis. These medications (such as albuterol) are preferably administered by inhalation. In addition to relaxing airway smooth muscle, β-agonists enhance mucociliary clearance and decrease vascular permeability.[111]

Patients with mild-persistent asthma usually require routine therapy for control of underlying airway inflammation. Inhaled corticosteroids are the most widely used and most effective asthma anti-inflammatory agents.[112] Inhaled corticosteroids are the most potent and consistently effective long-term control medication for asthma.[98] Patients with mild to moderate persistent asthma treated with inhaled steroids have improved symptom scores, decreased exacerbations, less β_2-agonist use, fewer oral steroid courses, and less hospitalizations.[113] Inhaled corticosteroids have an excellent safety profile at conventional doses, although high-dose therapy can put patients at risk for corticosteroid side effects. These medications have been used for decades in both children and adults without significant long-term side effects in most patients. Although there is the potential for a decreased growth-velocity effect, evidence suggests that the use of inhaled corticosteroids at recommended doses does not have long-term, clinically significant, or irreversible effects.[103] Alternative medications include the nonsteroidal anti-inflammatory agents nedocromil and cromolyn, leukotriene receptor antagonists (LTRAs), or sustained-release theophylline.

Patients with moderate and severe persistent disease require more intensive therapy. Long-acting bronchodilators such as salmeterol and formoterol have been shown to have an additive effect when used with inhaled corticosteroids and are useful additions to inhaled corticosteroid therapy.[114] LTRAs also are often a helpful addition to inhaled corticosteroids. A minority of patients might require long-term corticosteroids; these patients are difficult to manage, but adequate symptom control while minimizing the dose is of paramount importance.[115] Omalizumab, a recombinant humanized monoclonal anti-IgE antibody, currently indicated for perennial atopic patients with moderate to severe asthma, has been shown to improve asthma symptom scores, decrease exacerbations, and decrease inhaled corticosteroid dosese.[116] Other therapies that are also currently under investigation include PDE4 inhibitors[117] and anti-tumor necrosis factor (TNF) biologic agents. Anti-TNF biologic agents have been shown to result in a marked improvement in asthma symptoms, lung function, and bronchial hyperresponsiveness.[118,119] Bronchial thermoplasty involves administering thermal energy during bronchoscopy to decrease smooth muscle mass. It has been shown to decrease exacerbations, emergency room visits and days missed from school/work.[120] Patients with allergic triggers may benefit from allergen immunotherapy. Many studies have now documented improvement from following a three- to five-year course of specific immunotherapy.[121] This is an excellent means of minimizing medications while maintaining control for many patients.

Prognosis

Although asthma is not a curable disease, it is a controllable disease. Asthma education programs are extremely important in making early diagnosis and interventions possible. Despite an increase in our knowledge of the underlying pathophysiology, asthma mortality rates have not declined. With early diagnosis and a comprehensive management plan, patients with asthma can experience a normal life expectancy with good quality of life.

STEPWISE APPROACH FOR MANAGING ASTHMA LONG TERM

The stepwise approach tailors the selection of medication to the level of asthma severity (see page 5) or asthma control (see page 6). The stepwise approach is meant to help, not replace, the clinical decisionmaking needed to meet individual patient needs.

ASSESS CONTROL:
STEP UP IF NEEDED (first, check medication adherence, inhaler technique, environmental control, and comorbidities)
STEP DOWN IF POSSIBLE (and asthma is well controlled for at least 3 months)

At each step: Patient education, environmental control, and management of comorbidities

0–4 years of age

	STEP 1	STEP 2	STEP 3	STEP 4	STEP 5	STEP 6
	Intermittent Asthma	Persistent Asthma: Daily Medication — Consult with asthma specialist if step 3 care or higher is required. Consider consultation at step 2.				
Preferred Treatment†	SABA* as needed	low-dose ICS*	medium-dose ICS*	medium-dose ICS* + either LABA* or montelukast	high-dose ICS* + either LABA* or montelukast	high-dose ICS* + either LABA* or montelukast + oral corticosteroids
Alternative Treatment†‡		cromolyn or montelukast				

If clear benefit is not observed in 4–6 weeks, and medication technique and adherence are satisfactory, consider adjusting therapy or alternate diagnoses.

Quick-Relief Medication
- SABA* as needed for symptoms; intensity of treatment depends on severity of symptoms.
- With viral respiratory symptoms: SABA every 4–6 hours up to 24 hours (longer with physician consult). Consider short course of oral systemic corticosteroids if asthma exacerbation is severe or patient has history of severe exacerbations.
- Caution: Frequent use of SABA may indicate the need to step up treatment.

5–11 years of age

	STEP 1	STEP 2	STEP 3	STEP 4	STEP 5	STEP 6
	Intermittent Asthma	Persistent Asthma: Daily Medication — Consult with asthma specialist if step 4 care or higher is required. Consider consultation at step 3.				
Preferred Treatment†	SABA* as needed	low-dose ICS*	low-dose ICS* + either LABA,* LTRA,* or theophylline* OR medium-dose ICS	medium-dose ICS* + LABA*	high-dose ICS* + LABA*	high-dose ICS* + LABA* + oral corticosteroids
Alternative Treatment†‡		cromolyn, LTRA,* or theophylline*		medium-dose ICS* + either LTRA* or theophylline*	high-dose ICS* + either LTRA* or theophylline*	high-dose ICS* + either LTRA* or theophylline* + oral corticosteroids

Consider subcutaneous allergen immunotherapy for patients who have persistent, allergic asthma.**

Quick-Relief Medication
- SABA* as needed for symptoms. The intensity of treatment depends on severity of symptoms: up to 3 treatments every 20 minutes as needed. Short course of oral systemic corticosteroids may be needed.
- Caution: Increasing use of SABA or use >2 days/week for symptom relief (not to prevent EIB*) generally indicates inadequate control and the need to step up treatment.

≥12 years of age

	STEP 1	STEP 2	STEP 3	STEP 4	STEP 5	STEP 6
	Intermittent Asthma	Persistent Asthma: Daily Medication — Consult with asthma specialist if step 4 care or higher is required. Consider consultation at step 3.				
Preferred Treatment†	SABA* as needed	low-dose ICS*	low-dose ICS* + LABA* OR medium-dose ICS*	medium-dose ICS* + LABA*	high-dose ICS* + LABA* AND consider omalizumab for patients who have allergies††	high-dose ICS* + LABA* + oral corticosteroid** AND consider omalizumab for patients who have allergies††
Alternative Treatment†‡		cromolyn, LTRA,* or theophylline*	low-dose ICS* + either LTRA,* theophylline,* or zileuton‡‡	medium-dose ICS* + either LTRA,* theophylline,* or zileuton‡		

FIGURE 14-5 Updated stepwise approach for managing asthma in children and adults. (Reproduced with permission from National Heart, Lung and Blood Institute; National Institutes of Health; U.S. Department of Health and Human Services. http://www.nhlbi.nih.gov/guidelines/asthma/asthma_qrg.pdf.)

Oral Health Considerations

The main concern when treating any medically complex patient is to avoid exacerbation of the underlying condition. Several protocols suggesting appropriate procedures for dental treatment of asthmatic patients have been put forth.[122–125] However, few studies assessing the respiratory response of patients to dental care have been performed. One recent study indicated that although 15% of asthmatic pediatric patients will have a clinically significant decrease in lung function, no clinical parameter or historical data pertaining to asthma can predict this phenomenon.[126]

However, numerous dental products and materials, including toothpaste, fissure sealants, tooth enamel dust, and methyl methacrylate, have been associated with the exacerbation of asthma, whereas other items (such as fluoride trays and cotton rolls) have not been so associated.[122,127–131]

There is still no consensus regarding the association between asthma and dentofacial morphology.[132,133] Although nasal respiratory obstruction resulting in mouth breathing has been implicated in the development of a long and tapered facial form, an increased lower facial height, and a narrow maxillary arch, this relationship has never been substantiated with unequivocal evidence.

Oral manifestations of asthma include candidiasis, decreased salivary flow, increased calculus, increased gingivitis, increased periodontal disease, increased incidence of caries, and adverse effects of orthodontic therapy.[134–138]

It is possible that prolonged use of β_2-agonists may cause reduced salivary flow, with a resulting increase in cariogenic bacteria and caries and an increased incidence of candidiasis.[139] The increased incidence of caries is further accelerated by the use of cariogenic carbohydrates and sugar-containing anti-asthmatic medications.[140]

Dental treatment for asthmatic patients needs to address the oral manifestations of this condition, as well as its potential underlying systemic complications. Elective dental procedures should be avoided in all but those whose asthma is well controlled. The type and frequency of asthmatic attacks, as well as the type of medications used by the patient, indicate the severity of the disease.

The following are considerations and recommendations for administering dental care to patients who have asthma:

1. Fluoride supplements should be instituted for all asthmatic patients, particular those taking β_2-agonists.
2. The patient should be instructed to rinse his or her mouth with water after using inhalers.
3. Oral hygiene should be reinforced to reduce the incidence of gingivitis and periodontitis.
4. Antifungal medications should be administered as needed, particularly in patients who are taking inhaled corticosteroids.
5. Steroid prophylaxis needs to be used with patients who are taking long-term systemic corticosteroids (see Chapter 20).
6. Use stress-reducing techniques. Conscious sedation should be performed with agents that are not associated with bronchoconstriction, such as hydroxyzine. Barbiturates and narcotics should be avoided due to their potential to cause bronchospasm and reduce respiratory functions. Nitrous oxide can be used for all but patients with severe asthma as it may irritate the airways.[141]
7. Avoid dental materials that may precipitate an attack. Acrylic appliances should be cured prior to insertion. Dental materials without methyl methacrylate should be considered.
8. Schedule these patients' appointments for late morning or later in the day to minimize the risk of an asthmatic attack.[142]
9. Have oxygen and bronchodilators available in case of an exacerbation of asthma.
10. There are no contraindications to the use of local anesthetics containing epinephrine, but preservatives such as sodium metabisulfite may contribute to asthma exacerbation in susceptible patients.[143] Nevertheless, interactions between epinephrine and R_2-agonists may result in a synergistic effect, producing increased blood pressure and arrhythmias.
11. Judicious use of rubber dams will prevent reduced breathing capability.
12. Care should be taken in the positioning of suction tips as they may elicit a cough reflex.
13. Up to 10% of adult asthmatic patients have an allergy to aspirin and other nonsteroidal anti-inflammatory agents.[144] A careful history concerning the use of these types of drugs needs to be elicited. Although the use of acetaminophen has been proposed as an alternative to the use of aspirin, recent data suggest caution because these types of drugs have also been associated with more severe asthma.[145]
14. Drug interactions with theophylline are common. Macrolide antibiotics may increase the level of theophylline, whereas phenobarbital may reduce the level. Furthermore, drugs such as tetracycline have been associated with more accentuated side effects when given together with theophylline.
15. During an acute asthmatic attack, discontinue the dental procedure, remove all intraoral devices, place the patient in a comfortable position, make sure the airway is opened, and administer a β_2-agonist and oxygen. If no improvement is noted, administer epinephrine subcutaneously (1:1,000 concentration, 0.01 mg/kg of body weight, up to a maximum of 0.3 mg) and alert emergency medical assistance.

COPD

COPD is a disease state characterized by airflow limitation. The airflow is usually both progressive and associated with an abnormal inflammatory response of the lungs to noxious particles or gases.[146] COPD includes emphysema, an anatomically defined condition characterized by destruction and enlargement of the lung alveoli; chronic bronchitis, a clinically defined condition with chronic cough and phlegm; and small airways disease, a condition in which small bronchioles are narrowed. COPD is present only if chronic airflow obstruction occurs; chronic bronchitis without chronic airflow obstruction is not included within COPD.[147]

The prevalence and burden of COPD are projected to increase in the coming decades due to continued exposures to risk factors and the aging population.[146] The diagnosis should be considered in any patient with symptoms of cough, sputum production, or dyspnea and/or a history of exposure to risk factors for the disease.

Risk factors for the disease can include environmental exposures and host factors, such as a rare hereditary deficiency in the enzyme α_1-antitrypsin. This enzyme is responsible for inhibiting the activity of trypsin and other proteases in the serum and tissues. The characteristic panlobular emphysematous changes that are seen in α_1-antitrypsin deficiency are related to the loss of alveolar walls. More commonly, risk factors for the disease include environmental exposure to tobacco smoke, heavy exposure to occupational dusts and chemicals (vapors, irritants, fumes), and indoor/outdoor pollution.[146]

The clinical course of patients with COPD is quite varied. Most patients display some degree of progressive dyspnea, exercise intolerance, and fatigue. In addition, patients are susceptible to frequent exacerbations, usually caused by infections of the upper or lower respiratory tract. Most patients with COPD have little respiratory reserve. Therefore, any process that causes airway inflammation can lead to clinical deterioration.

Pathophysiology

Three processes are thought to be important in the pathogenesis of COPD: chronic inflammation throughout the airways, parenchyma, and pulmonary vasculature; oxidative stress; and an imbalance of proteases and antiproteases in the lung. These pathologic changes lead to the physiologic changes characteristic of the disease, including mucus hypersecretion, ciliary dysfunction, airflow limitation, pulmonary hyperinflation, gas exchange abnormalities, pulmonary hypertension, and cor pulmonale.[146]

Expiratory airflow limitation is the primary physiologic change in COPD. Airflow limitation results from fixed airway obstruction mainly. Patients with COPD may also have airway hyperresponsiveness overlapping with asthma.[147] Mucus hypersecretion and ciliary dysfunction lead to chronic cough and sputum production. In advanced COPD, peripheral airway obstruction, parenchymal destruction, and pulmonary vascular abnormalities reduce the lung's capacity for gas exchange, leading to hypoxemia and hypercapnia.[146]

Many toxins in tobacco smoke can cause a vigorous inflammatory response. In humans, chronic exposure to tobacco smoke results in an increase in the number of goblet cells because of hyperplasia and metaplasia. Acrolein, for example, causes both impairment of both ciliary and macrophage activities, as well as increases mucin hypersecretion.[148] Nitrogen dioxide causes direct toxic damage to the respiratory epithelium. Hydrogen cyanide is responsible for the functional impairment of enzymes that are required for respiratory metabolism. Carbon monoxide causes a decrease in the oxygen-carrying capacity of red blood cells by associating with hemoglobin to form carboxyhemoglobin. Lastly, polycyclic hydrocarbons have been implicated as carcinogens.

Hypoxemia is the result of the ventilation-perfusion mismatch that accompanies airway obstruction and emphysema. Portions of the lung that are not aerated due to obstruction cannot oxygenate the blood. This causes a decrease in overall oxygen concentrations. In addition, emphysema causes a decreased diffusion capacity because of a loss of air-space capillary units. Hypercarbia also develops and is often progressive

and asymptomatic. Pulmonary hypertension can result from chronic hypoxia due to vasoconstriction of pulmonary vessels.

Patients with emphysema alone have less ventilation-perfusion mismatching early in the course of the disease; this is due to the loss of both air space and supplying blood vessels. Severe hypoxia, pulmonary hypertension, and cor pulmonale are generally not seen until late in the disease process. Emphysema manifests as loss of the elastic recoil of the lungs, making the lungs more compliant. The work of breathing is therefore not significantly increased. However, the decrease in recoil allows the easy collapse of the peripheral airways, leading to further airway obstruction and airflow limitation.[149]

Clinical and Laboratory Findings

Patients with COPD have symptoms of dyspnea, cough, and sputum production. An increase in the production of purulent sputum is a sign of exacerbation due to respiratory infection. Physical findings include diffuse wheezing, possibly associated with signs of respiratory distress, including the use of accessory muscles of respiration (retractions) and tachypnea.[150] Liver enlargement due to congestion, ascites, and peripheral edema can develop as the disease progresses to pulmonary hypertension and cor pulmonale. This leads to the characteristic clinical patient presentation termed the *blue bloater*.

Patients with emphysema present primarily with dyspnea. Patients can be adequately oxygenated in the early stages of the disease and thus can have fewer signs of hypoxia; the term *pink puffer* has been used to describe these patients. Physical findings include an increase in chest wall size. Wheezing is present to varying degrees.

Chest radiography may show evidence of an increase in lung compliance, with flattened diaphragms, hyperexpansion, and an increase in anteroposterior diameter (Figure 14-6). Spirometry will show evidence of airflow limitation. A post bronchodilator FEV_1/FVC ratio of <0.7 confirms the presence of airflow limitation that is not fully reversible.[151] Complete

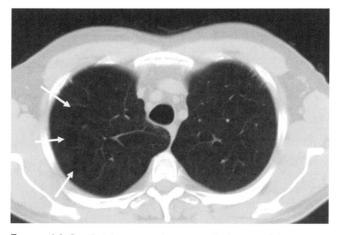

FIGURE 14-6 Axial computed tomography image of the upper chest demonstrates decreased attenuation of the lung tissue bilaterally, especially on the right (white arrows) where there is evidence of centrilobular emphysema.

pulmonary function studies will also indicate an increase in residual volume and total lung capacity.[150] Pulmonary diffusion capacity will be decreased due to a loss of gas-exchanging units.

Classification

COPD is now classified into five stages: at risk, mild, moderate, severe, and very severe. The at-risk stage is defined by normal spirometry, but patients have chronic symptoms of cough and sputum production. Mild, moderate, and severe COPD has evidence of increasing airway obstruction on spirometry in each progressive stage. Finally, very severe COPD is defined by severe airway obstruction with chronic respiratory failure. Patients with severe COPD are at more risk for other systemic diseases including cardiovascular disease, osteoporosis, lung cancer, and depression.[152]

Diagnosis

The diagnosis is suggested by the history and physical findings. Patients often have cough, dyspnea, and sputum production and/or a history of exposure to risk factors. Alternative diagnoses, such as asthma, CF, and congestive heart failure, should be considered. Complete pulmonary function tests are a valuable means of assessing airflow limitation and any reversibility. For patients with more severe disease, assessment of oxygen status with pulse oximetry is a valuable office procedure. A determination of arterial blood gases is important for patients who are clinically deteriorating and for the management of hospitalized patients.[153] Chest radiography can be helpful to exclude alternative diagnoses but is rarely diagnostic in COPD.

Management

There are no curative treatments for chronic bronchitis and emphysema. Smoking cessation is the single most important intervention to stop the progression of COPD. Reduction of exposures to occupational dusts and chemicals and indoor/outdoor pollution can also decrease the progression of disease.[146] Influenza and pneumococcal vaccines are recommended.

Management focuses on reducing symptoms and exacerbations. The most recent Global Initiative for Obstructive Disease guidelines gives management recommendations after patients have been assessed combining symptom scores, airflow limitations, and exacerbations (Figure 14-7).[146] Maintenance therapy includes trials of inhaled bronchodilators such as β-agonists and ipratropium bromide. Long-acting bronchodilators, such as formoterol or salmeterol, may be added as well as mucolytics. Theophylline products have also been used with some efficacy as well as phosphodiesterase-4 inhibitors. Long-term monotherapy with oral or inhaled corticosteroids is not recommended[146] as inhaled steroids with long acting β-agonists are more effective.

Chest physiotherapy has not been proven to be of value in the management of COPD.

The long-term administration of oxygen therapy to patients with chronic respiratory failure increases survival. Additionally, during exacerbations, oxygen therapy is often required. Caution must be used when administering oxygen to patients with COPD as their ventilatory drive will often be diminished. This is the result of chronic retention of carbon dioxide and subsequent insensitivity to hypercarbia. As a result, patients with COPD are sensitive to increases in oxygen tension, which provides the major stimulus for respiratory drive. Oxygen therapy during sleep can also be a useful means of limiting hypoxemia and subsequent pulmonary hypertension. An option for some patients involves lung-volume reduction which removes severely emphysematous tissue from the both upper lobes allowing the remaining tissue to expand and function more effectively.[152]

Antibiotics are often used during exacerbations of COPD. The presence of purulent sputum during an exacerbation generally requires treatment with 7–10 days of an oral antibiotic chosen based on local bacterial resistant patterns. The primary pathogens in COPD exacerbations include *S. pneumoniae*, *H. influenzae*, and *M. catarrhalis*.

Prognosis

The prognosis is poor for patients who are frequently symptomatic due to COPD. The need for hospital admission for an exacerbation, especially if intensive care is required, is an ominous prognostic sign in COPD as about half of such patients admitted to the intensive care unit do not survive a year after admission.[154]

Oral Health Considerations

The association, if any, between oral disease and lung disease was analyzed by the National Health and Nutrition Examination Survey I (NHANES I).[155] Of 23,808 individuals, 386 reported a suspected respiratory condition (as assessed by a physician) categorized as a confirmed chronic respiratory disease (chronic bronchitis or emphysema) or acute respiratory disease (influenza, pneumonia, acute bronchitis), or not to have a respiratory disease.

Significant differences were noted between subjects having no disease and those having a chronic respiratory disease confirmed by a physician. Individuals with a confirmed chronic respiratory disease had a significantly greater oral hygiene index (OHI) than subjects without a respiratory disease. Logistic regression analysis was performed to simultaneously control for multiple variables, including gender, age, race, OHI, and smoking status. The results of this analysis suggest that for patients having the highest OHI values, the odds ratio for chronic respiratory disease was 4.5.

Another study of elderly subjects (aged 70–79) found that, after controlling for smoking status, age, race, and gender, there was a significant association between periodontal health and airway obstruction in former smokers.[156] A more recent study, however, suggested that cigarette smoking may be a cofactor in the relationship between periodontal disease and COPD.[157] Further longitudinal epidemiologic studies and clinical trials are necessary to determine the role of oral health status in COPD.

These results were supported by a subsequent study that measured associations between poor oral health and chronic

	TABLE 4 Pharmacologic Therapy for Stable COPD*			
Patient Group	Recommended First Choice	Alternative Choice	Other Possible Treatments**
A	SA anticholinergic prn *or* SA beta₂-agonist prn	LA anticholinergic *or* LA beta₂-agonist *or* SA beta₂-agonist and SA anticholinergic	Theophylline
B	LA anticholinergic *or* LA beta₂-agonist	LA anticholinergic and LA beta₂-agonist	SA beta₂-agonist *and/or* SA anticholinergic Theophylline
C	ICS + LA beta₂-agonist *or* LA anticholinergic	LA anticholinergic and LA beta₂-agonist *or* LA anticholinergic and PDE-4 Inhibitor *or* LA beta₂-agonist and PDE-4 Inhibitor	SA beta₂-agonist *and/or* SA anticholinergic Theophylline
D	ICS + LA beta₂-agonist *and/or* LA anticholinergic	ICS + LA beta₂-agonist and LA anticholinergic ICS + LA beta₂-agonist and PDE-4 Inhibitor LA anticholinergic and LA beta₂-agonist LA anticholinergic and PDE-4 Inhibitor	Carbocysteine SA beta₂-agonist *and/or* SA anticholinergic Theophylline

*Medications in each box are mentioned in alphabetical order and therefore not necessarily in order of preference.

**Medications in this column can be used alone or in combination with other options in the First and Alternative Choice columns

Glossary:
SA: short-acting
LA: long-acting
ICS: inhaled corticosteroid
PDE-4: phosphodiesterase-4
prn: When necessary

FIGURE 14-7 Pharmacologic options for patients with COPD based on assessment. (Reproduced with permission from the Global Initiative for Obstruction Lung Disease (GOLD); At-A-Glance Outpatient Management Reference for Chronic Obstructive Pulmonary Disease (COPD); http://www.goldcopd.org/uploads/users/files/GOLD_AtAGlance_2011_Jan18.pdf.)

lung disease, and this study was able to carefully control for a number of potentially confounding variables. Data from NHANES III, which documented the general health and nutritional status of randomly selected United States subjects from 1988 to 1994, were analyzed.[158] This cross-sectional, retrospective study of the NHANES III database included a study population of 13,792 subjects 20 years of age and older having at least six natural teeth. A history of bronchitis and/or emphysema was recorded from the medical questionnaire. Lung function was estimated by calculation of the ratio of FEV1/ FVC. Oral health status was deduced from the Decayed Missing Filled System (DMFS/T) index, gingival bleeding, gingival recession, gingival pocket depth, and periodontal attachment level. Subjects with COPD had, on average, more periodontal attachment loss (clinical attachment loss [CAL] 1.48 ± 1.35—mean ± SD) than those without COPD (mean CAL 1.17 ± 1.09). The risk for COPD appeared to be significantly elevated when mean attachment loss (MAL) was found to be severe (MAL ≥ 2.0 mm) compared with periodontal health (<2.0 mm MAL: odds ratio 1.35, 95% CI: 1.07–1.71). Furthermore, the odds ratio was 1.45 (95% CI: 1.02–2.05) for those who had ≥ 3.0 mm

MAL. A trend was also noted in that lung function appeared to diminish as the amount of attachment loss increased. No such trend was apparent when gingival bleeding was considered.

Another study examined the relation between airway obstruction and periodontal disease in a cohort of 860 community dwelling elders enrolled in the Health, Aging, and Body Composition Study (Health ABC).[159] Results showed that, after stratification by smoking status and adjustment for age, race, gender, center, and number of pack-years, those with normal pulmonary function had significantly better gingival index (P .036) and loss of attachment (P .0003) scores than those with airway obstruction. Thus, a significant association between periodontal disease and airway obstruction was noted, especially in former smokers.

A recent meta-analysis explored the relationship between periodontal disease and COPD.[160] Fourteen observational studies including 3,988 COPD patients were included in the analysis. A significant association between PD and COPD was identified. There is thus great need for randomized controlled trails to determine if periodontal interventions prevent the initiation and/or progression of COPD.

Apart from the periodontal pathogens mentioned above, *streptococci* have been shown to be the causative pathogen of exacerbation in 4% of individuals with COPD.[161] One prospective study suggested that oral colonization with respiratory pathogens in patients residing in a chronic care facility was significantly associated with COPD.[57] The relationship between oral pathogens and exacerbations of COPD clearly deserves serious consideration. It is essential that elderly individuals (particularly institutionalized patients) receive adequate oral hygiene in order to minimize respiratory complications.

Drug interactions with theophylline may arise (see above), and a change of medications by the oral health-care provider may be appropriate.

As mentioned above, increased oxygen tension may diminish respiratory function in patients with COPD. Extreme caution must be exercised when administering supplemental oxygen in emergencies.

Cystic Fibrosis (CF)

CF is a multisystem genetic disorder that is characterized chiefly by chronic airways obstruction and infection and by exocrine pancreatic insufficiency, with its effects on gastrointestinal function, nutrition, growth, and maturation.[162]

The disorder is caused by numerous mutations in the gene that encodes the cystic fibrosis transmembrane conductance regulator (CFTR) that helps regulate ion flux at epithelial surfaces. The disease is characterized by hyperviscous secretions in multiple organ systems. Thickened secretions affect the pancreas and intestinal tract, causing malabsorption and intestinal obstruction. In the lungs, viscid mucus causes airway obstruction, infection, and bronchiectasis. Pulmonary complications are the major factors affecting life expectancy in patients with CF. This section focuses on the pulmonary manifestations of CF.

CF is an autosomal recessive trait resulting from mutations at a single gene locus on the long arm of chromosome 7. The incidence of CF among Caucasians is approximately 1 in 2000–3000 births; the incidence is lower among those of other races.[163]

Pathophysiology

The primary defect in the *CFTR* gene results in a defective chloride transport system in exocrine glands. As a result, mucus production occurs without sufficient water transport into the lumen. The resultant mucus is dry, thick, and tenacious and leads to inspissation in the affected glands and organs. In the airways, the viscid secretions impair mucociliary clearance and promote airway obstruction and bacterial colonization. Most airway injury in CF is believed to be mediated by neutrophil products, including proteases and oxidants, liberated by the abundance of neutrophils in the CF airway at almost all ages.[164] Bacterial superinfection is common and can lead to respiratory compromise.

Clinical and Laboratory Findings

Patients with CF may present in infancy with extrapulmonary manifestations such as meconium ileus or failure to thrive. Pulmonary manifestations include cough, recurrent infections of the lower respiratory tract, refractory lung infiltrates, and bronchospasm. Tachypnea and crackles can be found on physical examination. As the disease progresses, digital clubbing, and bronchiectasis (Figure 14-8) may become apparent. Most of the nonpulmonary pathology in CF occurs in the gastrointestinal tract and related organs.

Spirometry and pulmonary function testing are useful tools for documenting and monitoring airflow limitation. Airway obstruction tends to worsen with disease progression, although some patients with CF have mild pulmonary disease. CT analysis of the remarkable lung structural changes may be another potential outcome measure to monitor disease progression.[164]

Classification

There is no universally accepted classification system for CF.

Diagnosis

The diagnosis of CF is based on the presence of pulmonary or extrapulmonary symptoms, as described above. A sweat test can be performed to confirm the diagnosis. The procedure involves the collection of sweat after stimulation with pilocarpine. Samples containing > 60 mEq/L chloride are considered positive. Patients with indeterminate values (40–60 mEq/L) can be further assessed by using deoxyribonucleic acid (DNA) mutation analysis. Characteristic nasal epithelial bioelectric abnormalities can also serve as laboratory evidence of CFTR dysfunction and be used to diagnose CF when phenotypic clinical features are present.[162] Due to

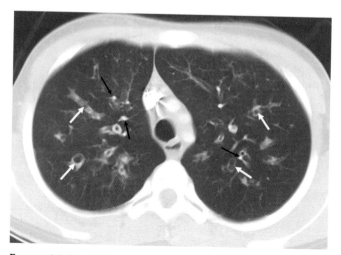

FIGURE 14-8 Axial computed tomography scan shows thickening of the bronchial walls in the upper lobes and bronchiectasis (dilation of the bronchi) bilaterally (white arrows). The bronchi should be approximately the same size as its associated pulmonary artery (black arrows).

the importance of early diagnosis, all states have now implemented newborn screening for CF.

Management

Treatment of CF includes antibiotics, bronchodilators, anti-inflammatory agents, chest physiotherapy with postural drainage, and mucolytic agents. In addition to oral and parenteral antibiotics, inhaled antibiotics such as tobramycin are used to help minimize systemic effects.[165,166] Long-term macrolide antibiotics have been used to effectively treat diffuse panbronchiolitis as well.[162] The use of anti-inflammatory agents in young patients with mild disease may help slow the decline of lung function.[167] Recombinant enzyme deoxyribonuclease therapy has also been shown to offer benefit to some patients with purulent airway secretions.[168,169] Finally, proper nutrition and exercise are essential. Approximately 90% of patients with CF require mealtime pancreatic enzymes,[154] and vitamin and caloric supplementation is essential as well. Exercise is generally considered beneficial for patients with CF and should be encouraged, except for those with the most severe lung disease and hypoxemia.[170]

Prognosis

Although the mortality rate is high, the most recent statistics from the Cystic Fibrosis Foundation indicate that 50% of patients can now be expected to survive beyond the age of 37 years.[162] The severity of lung disease often determines long-term survival. Lung transplantation has become an accepted treatment for respiratory failure secondary to CF.[171] New treatment modalities that are being investigated to help prolong survival include pharmacologic interventions targeted to improving CFTR functioning (potentiators) and trafficking (correctors).[172]

Oral Health Considerations

It has been suggested that patients with CF may have the same type of dentofacial morphology as other mouth-breathing patients.[173] However, larger prospective studies are need to confirm this.

Several studies have reported that the number of decayed, missing, and filled teeth and plaque, calculus, and gingival bleeding of CF patients is lower than that of non-CF control subjects and those heterozygous for CF.[174,175] This finding may be due to more antibiotic use by CF patients.

It has also been reported that the tongue, buccal mucosa, dental plaque, and saliva serve as a reservoir of colonization by both mucoid and nonmucoid strains of *P. aeruginosa*, an important bacterial pathogen for CF patients.[176,177] This suggests that oral hygiene strategies may help reduce the level of these pathogens in the mouth and thus reduce potential lung infection.

As with other patients with chronic lower respiratory infections, improved oral hygiene may minimize exacerbation of the underlying condition.

Pulmonary Embolism

Pulmonary embolism (PE) is a result of an exogenous or endogenous material traveling to the lung and causing blockage of a pulmonary arterial vessel. The embolus may originate anywhere, but it is usually due to a thrombosis in the lower extremities.[178] Other substances, such as septic emboli, venous gas, fat emboli, and intravascular foreign bodies are potential causes of pulmonary emboli.[179] Risk factors for PE include prolonged immobilization (such as in a postoperative state), lower extremity trauma, a history of deep venous thromboses, and the use of estrogen-containing oral contraceptives (especially in association with tobacco smoking).[180] The most common reversible risk factor for PE is obesity, an increasing problem in the US.[181]

Pathophysiology

PE causes occlusion of pulmonary arterial vessels, which results in a ventilation-perfusion mismatch. Massive PE causes right-sided heart failure and is rapidly progressive. Local bronchoconstriction may occur due to factors released by platelets and mast cells at the sites of occlusion. Pulmonary hypertension due to vessel occlusion and arterial vasospasm is a common finding.

Clinical and Laboratory Findings

Patients usually present with dyspnea. Other features that are variably present include chest pain, fever, diaphoresis, cough, hemoptysis, and syncope. Physical findings can include evidence of a lower extremity deep venous thrombosis, tachypnea, crackles, or rub on lung auscultation, and heart murmur.

Hypoxemia is common in acute PE. Measurements of arterial blood gases are helpful as patients may demonstrate a decrease in partial pressure of arterial oxygen (PaO_2) and partial pressure of arterial carbon dioxide ($PaCO_2$), with an increase in hydrogen ion concentration (pH). However, normal arterial blood gases do not rule out the possibility of PE.

Classification

Four separate PE syndromes have been described: (1) massive PE, (2) PE with pulmonary infarction, (3) PE without infarction or cor pulmonale, and (4) organized emboli in central arteries. There is significant overlap among these syndromes.[182]

Diagnosis

The diagnosis is made on the basis of history and physical findings. The diagnostic utility of plasma measurements of circulating D-dimer (a specific derivative of cross-linked fibrin) has been found to have a high negative predictive value of 99.5%.[183] However, in patients with a high clinical probability of a PE, a D-dimer test should not be used since the negative predictive value of this test is low.[184]

Chest radiography is often not helpful but may reveal suggestive signs such as elevated hemidiaphragm, pleural effusions, and pulmonary artery dilatation. Troponin levels may be elevated, the echocardiogram may be abnormal with increased right ventricular volume, and electrocardiography may help establish or exclude alternative diagnoses, such as acute myocardial infarction.

Although the ventilation-perfusion scan has historically been the most common diagnostic test used when PE is suspected, spiral (helical) CT scanning has replaced it at many centers.[184] The use of pulmonary angiography has declined and is typically reserved for cases in which catheter-based treatment would be an option.[184]

Management

Heparin, both unfractionated and low molecular weight, remains the mainstay of therapy. For most patients with PE, systemic thrombolytic therapy (such as streptokinase, urokinase, and tissue-type plasminogen activator) is not required unless the patient is hemodynamically unstable. Pulmonary embolectomy may be indicated in select patients who are unable to receive thrombolytic therapy or whose critical status does not allow sufficient time to infuse thrombolytic therapy.[185] Oxygen is administered as necessary, and the need for intubation and mechanical ventilation in massive PE is considered. Patients with recurrent disease may be candidates for vena caval interruption by placement of an inferior vena cava filter.

Prognosis

Although many patients with PE die before medical attention is received, the rate of mortality due to PE once adequate anticoagulation therapy is initiated is less than 5%.

Oral Health Considerations

The main concern in the provision of dental care for individuals with PE is the patient who is being managed with oral anticoagulants. As a general rule, dental care (including simple extractions) can safely be provided for patients with prothrombin times of up to 20 seconds or an international normalized ratio of 2.5. However, it is recommended that any dental care for these patients be coordinated with their primary medical care provider.

Pulmonary Neoplasm

Lung cancer is the leading cause of cancer deaths in both men and women. About 160,000 people in the United States died from lung cancer in 2012.[186] Men and women who are over the age of 45 years and who have a long history of tobacco smoking are at highest risk.[187] Non-small cell types of lung cancers account for about 85% of lung cancers and these include squamous cell, adenocarcinomas, and large cell.[188]

Squamous cell carcinomas account for about one-fourth of lung cancers. The neoplasm derives from bronchial epithelial cells that have undergone squamous metaplasia. This is a slow-growing neoplasm that invades the bronchi and leads to airway obstruction.

Adenocarcinomas are the most common type of lung cancer accounting for about 40%. These neoplasms are of glandular origin and develop in a peripheral distribution. They grow more rapidly than squamous cell carcinomas and tend to invade the pleura. The bronchoalveolar tumor (a type of adenocarcinoma) is derived from bronchiolar or alveolar epithelium. This cancer is not associated with exposure to tobacco smoke.[189]

Large cell carcinomas account for about 10% of lung cancers. They are poorly differentiated tumors that resemble neither squamous cell carcinomas nor adenocarcinomas. They can grow and spread quickly.

Small cell carcinomas account for approximately 15% of all lung cancers. This type of lung cancer has the highest association with smoking, almost never arising in the absence of a smoking history. These derive from neuroendocrine cells in the airways and metastasize rapidly. Most small cell tumors have metastasized prior to diagnosis.

Pathophysiology

Metaplasia of the respiratory epithelium occurs in response to injury, such as that induced by tobacco smoking. With continued injury, the cells become dysplastic, with the loss of differentiating features. Neoplastic change first occurs locally; invasive carcinoma usually follows shortly thereafter.[190]

Clinical and Laboratory Findings

A chronic nonproductive cough is the most common symptom. Sputum production may occur, usually associated with obstructive lesions. Hemoptysis is present in up to 30% of patients.[191] Dyspnea is variably present. Facial edema, cyanosis, and orthopnea indicate the possibility of superior vena cava syndrome, caused by compression of the superior vena cava by tumor. The acute onset of hoarseness may signal tumor compression of the recurrent laryngeal nerve. Shoulder and forearm pain might suggest the presence of Pancoast's tumor, which is found in the apical region of the lungs below the pleura.

Metastatic and paraneoplastic effects are also common. The symptoms of metastasis depend on the sites involved and on the size of the tumor. The bones, the brain, and the liver are common sites of metastasis. Paraneoplastic effects include endocrine abnormalities that are due to tumors that secrete hormones such as antidiuretic hormone, adrenocorticotropic hormone, and parathyroid hormone–related peptides.[192]

Classification

The World Health Organization has differentiated pulmonary neoplasms into histologic types. The major clinical distinction is between small cell types and non–small cell types; each type has different therapeutic implications. The above-mentioned four major pathologic categories are squamous cell carcinoma, adenocarcinoma, large cell carcinoma, and small cell carcinoma

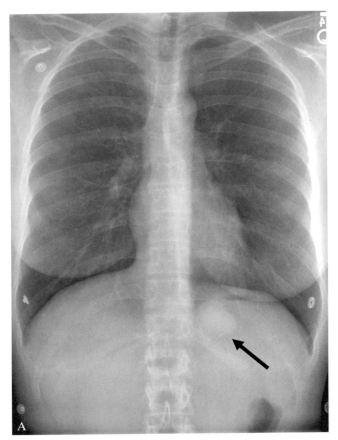
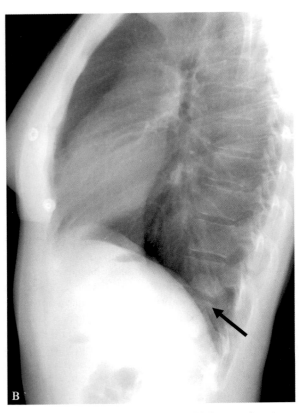

FIGURE 14-9   Anteroposterior (A) and lateral (B) chest radiographs demonstrate a rounded mass in the medial left costophrenic angle (black arrows) that is seen to be located in the posterior portion of the left lower lobe. This is best seen on the lateral view.

Diagnosis

Diagnosis is suggested by the history and physical examination. The method of diagnosis of suspected lung cancer depends on the type of lung cancer (i.e., small cell lung cancer or non–small cell lung cancer), the size and location of the primary tumor, the presence of metastasis, and the overall clinical status of the patient. CT scanning is the anatomic imaging modality of choice and is performed in virtually all patients with suspected or known lung cancer (Figure 14-9). Other diagnostic modalities include sputum or pleural fluid cytology, excisional biopsy, transthoracic needle aspiration, and bronchoscopy.[193]

Management

Complete surgical resection of localized lung cancer offers patients the best chance for cure. However, treatment is based on the stage of the disease and the patient's clinical status. In general, early-stage disease is surgically managed, locally advanced disease is managed with chemotherapy and radiotherapy, and advanced disease is managed with chemotherapy with supportive care or supportive care alone. Radiation therapy is an important palliative measure, especially for patients with superior vena cava syndrome, brain metastases, or bone lesions.

Prognosis

Despite the presence of developed modalities for treatment, the prognosis for patients with lung cancer has remained poor, with the overall five-year survival being approximately 15%. There is about a 50% five-year survival when lung cancer is detected. Unfortunately, most pulmonary cancers are found too late for a cure; only about 20% of patients undergo a radical surgical procedure, which is the only curative treatment.[194,195]

ACKNOWLEDGMENT

Douglas P. Beall, MD, chief of radiology, Clinical Radiology of Oklahoma, LLC. and associate professor of orthopedics, University of Oklahoma.

Selected Readings

Marik PE. Aspiration pneumonitis and aspiration pneumonia. *N Engl J Med.* 2001;344:665–671.

Ramsey BW, Pepe MS, Quan JM, et al. Intermittent administration of inhaled tobramycin in patients with cystic fibrosis; the Cystic Fibrosis Inhaled Tobramycin Study Group. *N Engl J Med.* 1999;340:23–30.

Reilly JJ, Silverman EK, Shapiro SD. Chronic obstructive pulmonary disease. In: Longo D, Fauci A, Kasper D, et al., eds. *Harrison's Internal Medicine.* 18th ed. New York, NY: McGraw-Hill Professional; 2011:2151–2160.

Sandler NA, Johns FR, Braun TW. Advances in the management of acute and chronic sinusitis. *J Oral Maxillofac Surg*. 1996;54:1005–1013.

Scannapieco FA. Role of oral bacteria in respiratory infection. *J Periodontol*. 1999;70:793–802.

Shi Z, Xie H, Wang P, et al. Oral hygiene care for critically ill patients to prevent ventilator-associated pneumonia. *Cochrane Database Syst Rev*. 2013;8:CD008367.

Simons D, Kidd EAM, Beighton D. Oral health of elderly occupants in residential homes. *Lancet*. 1999;353:1761.

Spurlock BW, Dailey TM. Shortness of (fresh) breath: toothpaste induced bronchospasm. *N Engl J Med*. 1990;323:1845–1846.

Zhu JF, Hidalgo HA, Holmgreen WC, et al. Dental management of children with asthma. *Pediatr Dent*. 1996;18:363–370.

For the full reference lists, please go to http://www.pmph-usa.com/Burkets_Oral_Medicine.

CHAPTER 15

Diseases of the Cardiovascular System

Peter B. Lockhart, DDS

Laszlo Littmann, MD

Cardiovascular disease (CVD) is the leading cause of mortality in the world. On the basis of 2010 mortality rate data, nearly 2150 Americans die of CVD each day, an average of one death every 40 seconds (Table 15-1).[1] More than 151,000 Americans who died from CVD in 2006 were <65 years of age.[2] Coronary heart disease mortality in 2010 was 379,559. It is estimated that in 2010 620,000 Americans had a new coronary attack, and 470,000 had a recurrent attack.[1] In addition, each year approximately 795,000 people in the United States experience a new or recurrent stroke.[1] According to the Centers for Disease Control and Prevention and the National Health and Nutrition Examination Survey (NHANES) III, the probability at birth of dying from CVD is 47%, compared to 22% from cancer, 2% from diabetes, and less than 1%

TABLE 15-1	Prevalence of Cardiovascular Disease in the United States, 2010 Data
Type of Cardiovascular Disease	No. of Patients
High blood pressure	77,900,000
Coronary artery disease	15,400,000
Myocardial infarction	7,600,000
Angina pectoris	565,000
Stroke	6,800,000
Heart failure	5,100,000
Total	83,600,000*

Reproduced with permission from American Heart Association.[1]
*Due to overlap among patients the added numbers will exceed the total.

from human immunodeficiency virus (HIV) disease. During the past decades, the age-adjusted death rate in the United States has declined overall. However, racial and ethnic disparities exist with African Americans exceeding that of whites by 32%.[1]

CVD includes hypertension, coronary artery disease (CAD), congestive heart failure (CHF), congenital cardiovascular defects, and stroke.[3] Although these diseases are associated with a high mortality, the associated morbidity affects all walks of life and has a great impact on the quality of life of affected individuals. This chapter presents an overview of common cardiovascular conditions and their implications for the practice of dentistry. Cerebrovascular accident (CVA), or stroke, will be discussed in chapter 24, Neuromuscular diseases.

Multiple guidelines exist to help dental practitioners with decision-making on assessment and management issues for specific cardiac patients, and some aspects of dental management are generic to several of the patient populations in this chapter.[4-12] For example, the determination of vital signs prior to dental care is an important preventive measure, to include: blood pressure, and pulse rate and rhythm; and any abnormal findings should be noted and described in the patient's chart. There are few prospective trials or large epidemiologic studies, and the vast majority of these guidelines are based on expert opinion from individuals and consensus groups. At the time this book was being published, a systematic review of guidelines for the dental management of cardiac patients was being conducted by the World Workshop on Oral Medicine VI, and scheduled to be published in 2014. This systematic review demonstrates the diversity of opinion on these clinical issues. Guidelines do not release the dental healthcare provider from the responsibility to use good clinical judgment, however, and they should be used in accordance with the dental provider's training, knowledge base, and experience.[8] For many of these patients, a consultation with the patient's primary care physician or cardiologist may be desirable for questions concerning sedation, exercise tolerance, or risks from invasive or stressful dental procedures, or anticoagulation and other medications.[13] Oral health care providers also need to be aware of medications that (1) may have systemic side effects that are of importance to the provision of dental care, (2) interact with medications used for dental care, and (3) cause intraoral changes, such as oral dryness, gingival overgrowth, or ulcerations. What follows is an overview of the demographics, diagnosis, medical management, and dental management considerations for the more common cardiovascular conditions seen in dental offices.

HYPERTENSION

General Description and Incidence

Data from NHANES 2011–2012 indicate that 29.1% of US adults ≥18 years of age have hypertension (Table 15-2).[14]

TABLE 15-2	Hypertension Among Persons Over 20 Years of Age, United States, 2001–2004[15]	
Age Category	Male	Female
20–34 years	6.4	*
35–44 years	16.8	14.0
45–54 years	30.2	32.6
55–64 years	45.8	54.6
65–74 years	58.5	74.3
75 years and over	68.8	81.7

*Unreliable estimate.

This amounts to an estimated 69,873,000 US adults with hypertension.[3] African-American adults have among the highest rates of hypertension in the world: 42.6% in black males, 47.0% in black females.[1] Among hypertensive adults, approximately 82% are aware of their condition, 76% are using antihypertensive medication, and nearly 52% of those treated had their hypertension controlled.[2,3,14-16]

Hypertension is defined as having systolic blood pressure (SBP) ≥ 140 mm Hg or diastolic blood pressure (DBP) ≥ 90 mm Hg or as having to use antihypertensive medications. Approximately every five years, the National Heart, Lung and Blood Institute (NHLBI), through its Joint National Committee on Prevention, Detection, Evaluation, and Treatment of High Blood Pressure, puts forth recommendations for the treatment of high blood pressure (BP). Its eighth and latest recommendations (JNC 8) was published in 2014.[17] JNC 7 defined cardiovascular risk stratification and also BP classifications for adults (Tables 15-3–15-5). The purpose of these guidelines is to reduce the morbidity and mortality associated with hypertension as several clinical trials have suggested that the lowering of BP reduces the risk of end-organ disease.[18,19]

Hypertension is classified as primary and secondary. Ninety-five percent of all hypertension is of unknown cause. There are many secondary causes, to include: renal disorders such as renal parenchymal disease, renovascular disease, renin-producing tumors, and primary sodium retention. Endocrinologic disturbances that may result in hypertension include thyroid disease, adrenal disorders, carcinoid, and exogenous hormones. Remaining causes include aortic coarctation, complications of pregnancy (such as preeclampsia), neurologic causes, acute stress, alcohol ingestion, nicotine use, increased intravascular volume, and the use of drugs such as cyclosporine or tacrolimus.

Risk Factor Modification

Hypertension is a well-recognized risk factor for CAD. There is an even greater relationship between hypertension and the risk of stroke; an elevated blood pressure is the single most important determinant of the risk of stroke.[20] Clinical trials have demonstrated that control of isolated systolic hypertension dramatically reduces stroke mortality.[21] A less than 5 mm Hg reduction in SBP reduces stroke mortality by almost 18%.

TABLE 15-3 Classification of Blood Pressure for Adults[16]			
Blood Pressure Classification	SBP		DBP
Normal	<120 mm Hg	and	<90 mm Hg
Prehypertension	120–139 mm Hg	or	80–89 mm Hg
Stage 1 hypertension	140–159 mm Hg	or	90–99 mm Hg
Stage 2 hypertension	>160 mm Hg	or	>100 mm Hg

TABLE 15-4 Cardiovascular Risk Factors[16]
Major Risk Factors
Hypertension
Age (older than 55 years for men, 65 years for women)
Diabetes mellitus
Elevated LDL (or total) cholesterol, or low HDL cholesterol
Estimated GFR <60 mL/min/1.73 m2
Family history of premature CVD (men <55 years of age or women <65 years of age)
Microalbuminuria
Obesity (BMI >30 kg/m²)
Physical inactivity
Tobacco use, particularly cigarettes
Target Organ Damage
Heart
LVH
Angina/prior MI
Prior coronary revascularization
Heart failure
Brain
Stroke or transient ischemic attack
Dementia
Chronic kidney disease
Peripheral arterial disease
Retinopathy

BMI, body mass index; CVD, cardiovascular disease; GFR, glomerular filtration rate; HDL, high-density lipoprotein; LDL, low-density lipoprotein; LVH, left ventricular hypertrophy; MI, myocardial infarction.

It is important to realize that hypertension is a chronic disease with long-term sequelae. Therefore, treatment focuses on prevention to reduce complications that eventually affect target organs such as the brain, heart, kidneys, eyes, and peripheral arteries (Table 15-4). Complications of hypertension include cerebral hemorrhage, left ventricular hypertrophy (LVH), CHF, renal insufficiency, aortic dissection, and atherosclerotic disease of various vascular beds.

Diagnosis

Because hypertension usually has a long, asymptomatic course, many patients are undiagnosed and/or have only a mild elevation in BP. The diagnosis is made only after an elevated BP has been recorded on multiple occasions. Stage 1 hypertension refers to a SBP of 140–159 mm Hg or a DBP of 90–99 mm Hg. Stage 2 hypertension is defined as an SBP of ≥ 160 or a DBP of ≥ 100 (Table 15-3). The BP level, as well as other clinical factors, determines the severity of hypertension. These other factors include certain demographic features (e.g., age, sex, race), the extent of the vascular damage induced by the high BP (i.e., target organ involvement), and the presence of other risk factors for premature CVD, especially diabetes (Table 15-4).

The three main goals of the medical evaluation of patients with hypertension are to identify treatable (secondary) or curable causes, to assess the impact of persistently elevated BP on target organs, and to estimate the patient's overall risk profile for the development of premature CVD. A routine history and physical examination should be performed. The history should focus on the duration of the hypertension and any prior treatment. Asking the patient about the duration of their high blood pressure may be misleading, as in many cases, the patient will not have had a BP measurement for many years prior to the discovery of hypertension. Symptoms of organ dysfunction, lifestyle habits, diet, and psychosocial factors should be included. It is important to note that making a diagnosis of hypertension is beyond the scope of practice of dentistry.

Physical Examination

The main goals of the physical examination are to identify signs of end-organ damage (Table 15-4) and a cause of secondary hypertension. Thus, the peripheral pulses should be palpated, and the abdomen should be auscultated for renal artery bruit that would indicate renovascular hypertension. The physical exam should include a funduscopic assessment. These types of examinations should only be performed by trained and experienced health care providers.

Laboratory and Additional Testing

Routine laboratory procedures include hemoglobin, urinalysis, routine blood chemistries (glucose, creatinine, electrolytes), and a fasting lipid profile consisting of total and high-density lipoprotein (HDL) cholesterol and triglycerides. Twelve-lead electrocardiography (ECG) should also be performed. Additional tests, outlined below, may be indicated in certain clinical settings.

TABLE 15-5   Lifestyle Modifications to Prevent and Manage Hypertension[16]

Modification	Recommendation	Approximate SBP Reduction
Weight reduction	Maintain normal body weight (BMI 18.5–24.9 kg/m2)	5–20 mm Hg/10 kg
Adopt DASH eating plan	Consume a diet rich in fruits, vegetables, and low-fat dairy products with a reduced content of saturated and total fat	8–14 mm Hg
Dietary sodium reduction	Reduce dietary sodium intake to no more than 100 mmol/d (2.4 g sodium or 6 g sodium chloride)	2–8 mm Hg
Physical activity	Engage in regular aerobic physical activity such as brisk walking (at least 30 min/d, most days of the week)	4–9 mm Hg
Moderation of alcohol consumption	Limit consumption to no more than two drinks (e.g., 24 oz beer, 10 oz wine, or 3 oz 80-proof whiskey) per day in most men, and to no more than 1 drink/d in women and lighter persons	2–4 mm Hg

DASH, Dietary Approaches to Stop Hypertension; SBP, systolic blood pressure; BMI, body mass index.

Electrocardiography

Electrocardiographic signs of hypertension frequently include signs of left atrial enlargement, left axis deviation, high QRS voltages, and ST-T abnormalities indicative of LVH. The width of the QRS complexes may also be increased. Cardiac arrhythmias, including premature atrial or ventricular complexes and atrial fibrillation are not uncommon. These dysrhythmias are associated with a further increase in the risk of stroke and mortality.

Echocardiography

Echocardiography can also reveal signs of left atrial enlargement and LVH. In addition, it provides information on left ventricular systolic and diastolic function, possible associated valvular abnormalities and the presence or absence of pulmonary hypertension. Echocardiography is a more sensitive method of detecting LVH than is routine ECG, and limited echocardiography offers a less expensive alternative to a complete echocardiographic examination when the sole question is whether the patient has LVH. Left ventricular hypertrophy is an independent predictor of mortality in patients with hypertension. This hypertrophy of the ventricle initially results in the impairment of left ventricular diastolic function and, if progressive, may impair systolic function as well, thus diminishing the normal function of pumping blood out of the heart through the aortic valve and into the aorta. This increase in left ventricular mass may result in increased myocardial oxygen demand, which can result in myocardial ischemia and ultimately myocardial fibrosis with CHF. Thus, the main indication for echocardiography is to detect possible end-organ damage to the heart in a patient with borderline elevated BP values.

Ambulatory Blood Pressure Monitoring

Ambulatory BP monitoring is indicated in patients with suspected "white-coat hypertension", in labile hypertension, resistant hypertension, and in those hypertensive patients who also experience hypotensive episodes.[22] Unfortunately, in the United States many insurers do not reimburse for this procedure.

The term "white-coat hypertension" is used to describe a phenomenon in which individuals present with persistent elevated BP in a clinical setting but present with non-elevated BP in an ambulatory setting. The relationship between white-coat hypertension and the development of essential hypertension has not been thoroughly elucidated, but it is estimated that about 20% of mild hypertensive individuals may present with white-coat hypertension. Since BP readings in the ambulatory BP setting reflect BP throughout the day, an accurate ambulatory measure would theoretically better predict end-organ damage than would occasional clinical or office BP readings; yet, it is not clear if white-coat hypertension is associated with end-organ damage.[23]

Radiologic Testing

Radiographic testing for renovascular disease is indicated only for patients whose history is suggestive and in whom a corrective procedure will be performed if significant renal artery stenosis is detected. Intra-arterial digital subtraction angiography has historically been the initial test when the history is highly suggestive; however, spiral computed tomography and magnetic resonance angiography are becoming the standard screening tests when renovascular hypertension is strongly suspected.[24] Recent evidence, however, suggests that revascularization in patients with atherosclerotic renovascular disease carries substantial risks but little evidence of worthwhile clinical benefit.[25] Renal ultrasonography is often used in a hypertensive patient with a family history of polycystic kidney disease.

Assessment of Cardiovascular Risk

Numerous aspects contribute to the detrimental association between hypertension and CVD.[26] Most studies have shown a strong correlation between long-term sustained elevated BP and the subsequent development of CVD. Recent prospective longitudinal studies suggest that BP that is even slightly elevated above normal is associated with increased mortality.[27] The underlying causes include the promotion of atherosclerosis and thrombogenesis, reduced coronary vasodilatory reserve, and LVH.[28–33]

The incidence of CVD increases stepwise with increasing BP. Studies have indicated that the risk of a cardiac event increases by 1.6 times in men and 2.5 times in women when BP increases from an normal level (<120/80 mm Hg) to a high normal level (130–139/85–89 mm Hg).[34] As is well defined by data from the Framingham Heart Study, a number of other risk factors interact with hypertension to affect the overall risk status of the individual patient.[35,36] These include hypercholesterolemia, diabetes mellitus, and smoking. Increased age of the patient may suggest a more detrimental effect conferred by an elevated systolic rather than diastolic pressure.[37] The presence or absence of other risk factors can influence the decision of whether to institute antihypertensive medications in a patient with borderline values.

Recently, two new hypertension guidelines were published, which establish a threshold of 140/90 and 150/90 mm Hg for initiating antihypertensive drug therapy in different age groups and disease categories.[17,38] These new thresholds which are somewhat higher than previously have already elicited considerable debate.[39]

Medical Management

Medical management should start with lifestyle modifications (Table 15-5). These include weight reduction, a Mediterranean diet, dietary sodium restriction, regular physical activity and moderation of alcohol consumption. Most patients, however, will also need to take antihypertensive medications.

The treatment of hypertension is among the leading indications for the use of drugs in the United States. A large number of agents exist, including diuretics, beta-blockers, calcium channel blockers, angiotensin-converting enzyme inhibitors (ACEIs), angiotensin II receptor blockers, direct vasodilators, and centrally acting agents. Each of the antihypertensive agents is roughly equally effective, producing a good antihypertensive response in 40%–60% of cases. Thus, the choice among the different antihypertensive drugs is not generally made on the basis of efficacy. There is, however, wide interpatient variability as many patients will respond well to one drug but not to another. The identification of the particular drug class to which a patient is more likely to respond is therefore one major criterion used in the choice of an antihypertensive agent.

The results of an increasing number of trials suggest that at the same level of BP control, most antihypertensive drugs provide similar degrees of cardiovascular protection. As an example, several major antihypertension drug trials found little overall difference in outcome between older (e.g., diuretics and beta-blockers) and newer (e.g., ACEIs and calcium channel blockers) antihypertensive drugs.[17,38,40,41] There is emerging evidence that beta-blockers, in general, confer less survival benefit and less reduction in the risk of stroke compared to other similarly effective antihypertensive agents such as calcium-channel blockers, diuretics, or ACEIs.[42] Beta-blocker therapy is an excellent choice for patients who have CAD and hypertension. An ACEI is usually first-line therapy for a diabetic patient with microalbuminuria since ACEIs retard the progression of diabetic nephropathy. Although the use of diuretics has been decreasing over the past 10 years, diuretics are still among the most frequently prescribed medications for treating hypertension, probably because they are effective, well tolerated, and inexpensive. In those with uncomplicated hypertension, beginning with a low dose of a thiazide diuretic (e.g., 12.5–25 mg of hydrochlorothiazide or 25–50 mg of chlorthalidone) has the advantages of very low cost and low risk of metabolic complications such as hypokalemia, lipid abnormalities, and hyperuricemia. If low-dose thiazide monotherapy is ineffective, an ACEI, a beta-blocker, or a calcium-channel blocker can be sequentially substituted. A calcium-channel blocker is likely to be most effective in African-American patients and in the elderly.

The role of education and the importance of patient contact are paramount in successfully treating hypertension. Self-recorded measurements and ambulatory BP monitoring aid in the physician's titration of medications and monitoring of the 24-hour duration of action of antihypertensive agents. The monitoring of BP by oral health care providers will therefore support the overall medical care of their hypertensive patients.

Dental Management Considerations for Patients with Hypertension

It is clear that patients with elevated blood pressure (BP) are at increased risk for adverse events in a dental office setting, particularly if their BP is poorly controlled or if there is target organ disease (e.g., brain or kidney) (Table 15-4). However, the absence of target organ disease does not mitigate a careful evaluation and treatment of patients within safe and appropriate parameters of care. The primary concern for these patients is precipitating a hypertensive crisis, stroke, or myocardial infarction (MI). Poor compliance with antihypertensive medications and diet is a common problem, and dentists can help by reinforcing the importance of compliance with these medications. Dental management guidelines have been proposed based on the medical model for assessment, risk stratification, and treatment of patients with hypertension (Table 15-6).[43–45]

TABLE 15-6	Blood Pressure Measurement in the Dental Setting[43]
Routine BP measurements	
Measure and record at initial visit	
Recheck:	
Every year for patients with BP < 130/85 mm Hg	
Every year for patients with BP of 130–139/85–89 mm Hg	
Every visit for patients with BP ≥ 140/90 mm Hg	
Every visit for patients with diagnosed hypertension	
Before initiating dental care:	
Assess presence of hypertension	
Determine presence of target organ disease	
After checking BP, determine treatment modifications	
Dental treatment for patients with elevated BP	
Asymptomatic, BP < 159/99 mm Hg, no target organ disease	
No dental modifications needed	
Can safely be treated in a dental outpatient setting	
Asymptomatic, BP = 160–179/100–109 mm Hg, no history of target organ disease	
Assessment on individual basis with regard to type of dental procedure	
BP ≥ 180/110 mm Hg, no history of target organ disease	
No elective dental care	
Target organ disease or poorly controlled DM	
Elective dental care only when BP is controlled, preferably < 140/90 mm Hg	

BP, blood pressure; DM, diabetes mellitus.

Side effects of antihypertensive medications vary and can include orthostatic hypotension, synergistic activity with narcotics, and potassium depletion. Additionally, beta-blockers will decrease the response to medications (e.g., epinephrine) used, for example, to treat anaphylaxis. The use of epinephrine in local anesthetics in this patient population is controversial.[46] Some authorities feel that the benefit of epinephrine in attaining a profound and more prolonged anesthesia outweighs, and perhaps reduces, the risk of systemic effects from endogenous epinephrine, such as stroke from an increased heart rate and blood pressure. Although largely opinion-based, concentrations of epinephrine greater than 1:100,000 are felt to be unnecessary and may carry a higher risk.[47] A small dose of low concentration epinephrine administered to the oral mucosa should not have a significant systemic effect. When using epinephrine, it is important to aspirate to determine if the needle entered a vein or artery. Due to the small diameter of dental anesthetic needles, however, aspiration does not insure that a negative aspiration will prevent intravascular injection.

Although safe limits for invasive dental procedures cannot be strictly defined, and they are largely based on an individual patients' overall medical condition, there are general guidelines depending on whether patients have prehypertension, stage one or stage two hypertension and target organ disease (Table 15-3 and 15-6).[5] Elective treatment should be avoided if the blood pressure is significantly above the patient's baseline or if > 180 mm Hg systolic or >100 mm Hg diastolic. It may be desirable to remove the source of infection (e.g., abscessed tooth) if the patient has mildly elevated blood pressures, but pain and infection can usually be controlled pharmacologically until the BP is brought under control. Patients with active infection may have somewhat elevated BP from pain and there may be some lowering of their pressures after local anesthesia, but this is unpredictable.

CORONARY ARTERY DISEASE

General Description and Incidence

Coronary artery disease (CAD) accounts for approximately 30%–50% of all cases of CVD[2] in the United States. Almost 8% of adults ≥20 years of age have CAD; this number is 9.1% for men and 7.0% for women. Approximately 12,400,000 Americans alive today have already suffered a MI or experienced angina pectoris (chest pain).[2] It is estimated that each year 620,000 Americans will have a new coronary attack, and 295,000 will have recurrent attacks.[1] In 2010, CAD caused about one of every six deaths in the United States.[1] CAD is the largest major killer of American males and females. Approximately every 34 seconds, an American will suffer a coronary event, and approximately every one minute 23 seconds, someone will die of one.[1]

Atherosclerosis, the most common cause of CAD, results from a wide variety of pathologic processes that interact with and disrupt the vascular endothelium. The result is plaque formation, with compromise of effective arterial luminal area. In the coronary circulation, this process may cause a chronic reduction in coronary blood flow and ensuing myocardial ischemia or it may cause acute plaque rupture, with intracoronary thrombus formation and subsequent MI. Atherosclerosis may affect any vascular bed, including the coronary, cerebral, renal, mesenteric, and peripheral vascular systems. When end-organ blood flow is compromised, the resulting ischemia can cause subsequent organ dysfunction.

Etiology

Atherosclerosis begins with a fatty streak, first seen in early adolescence; these lesions progress into plaques in early adulthood and may result in thrombotic occlusions and coronary events in middle age and later life. Other lipid metabolism abnormalities, systemic hypertension, diabetes mellitus, and cigarette smoking contribute to the total atherosclerotic plaque burden although these factors differ in their impact on CAD in clinical subgroups. For example, diabetes and a low HDL cholesterol/total cholesterol ratio have a greater impact in women, cigarette smoking has more of an impact in men, and SBP and isolated systolic hypertension are major risk factors at all ages and in either sex.

Risk Factors

Risk factor assessment is useful as a guide to therapy for dyslipidemia, hypertension, and diabetes; multivariable prediction rules can be used to help estimate risks for subsequent coronary disease events. An emerging model uses the risk of cardiovascular events over a 10–20-year period as a basis for initiating risk factor–modifying therapy for lipid abnormalities.[48] Based on the increased risk conferred by the various CAD risk factors, concepts of "normal" have continued to evolve from "usual" or "average" to more biologically optimal values associated with long-term freedom from disease. As a result, acceptable BP, blood sugar, and lipid values have been continually revised downward in the past 20 years.[18,49,50]

Lipids

The total cholesterol concentration in serum is a major and clear-cut risk factor for coronary artery disease (CAD). In the Multiple Risk Factor Intervention Trial of more than 350,000 middle-aged American men, the risk of CAD progressively increased with higher values of serum total cholesterol.[51] The concentration of serum HDL cholesterol is inversely associated with CAD incidence, consistent with its suggested role in reverse cholesterol transport.[52] Data from the Framingham Heart Study suggest that the risk for MI increases by about 25% for every 5 mg/dL decrement below median values for men and women.[53]

The total cholesterol/HDL cholesterol ratio represents a simple and efficient way to estimate coronary disease risk. Data from the Lipid Research Clinics and the Framingham Heart Study show that among men, a ratio of ≥6.4 identified a group that was at a 2%–14% greater risk than that predicted from serum total or low-density lipoprotein (LDL) cholesterol; among women, a ratio of ≥5.6 or more identified a group at a 25%–45% greater risk than that predicted from serum total or LDL cholesterol.[54] In contrast, serum total or LDL cholesterol did not add an independent predictive value to the ratio.

Recommendations for lipid evaluation and therapy in adults were formulated by an expert committee of the National Cholesterol Education Program (NCEP) and were revised in 2004 as the Adult Treatment Panel (ATP) III,[55] and in 2006 for secondary prevention for patients with established coronary and other atherosclerotic vascular disease.[56] Recently published guidelines, however, recommended a shift from focusing on specific total cholesterol and LDL targets to recommending medium-intensity and high-intensity statin treatment based on clinical presentation rather than purely on the lipid levels (Table 15-7).[57] In general, high-intensity statin therapy with atorvastatin (Lipitor) 40–80 mg daily or rosuvastatin (Crestor) 20–40 mg daily is recommended for patients with established CAD or diabetes and to those with very high LDL levels. Moderate-intensity statin therapy is recommended for moderate-risk patients.[57] Routinely checking the LDL level during statin therapy is no longer recommended.

TABLE 15-7 Common Cholesterol-Lowering Medications

Drug	Trade Name	Side Effects
HMG CoA reductase inhibitors (statins)*		Myopathy; increased liver transaminases
Atorvastatin**	Lipitor	
Fluvastatin	Leschol	
Lovastatin	Mevacor	
Pravastatin	Pravachol	
Rosuvastatin**	Crestor	
Simvastatin	Zocor	
Bile acid sequestrants		Decreased absorption of other drugs
Cholestyramine	Colestipol	
Colesevelam	Welchol	
Nicotinic acid		Flushing; hyperglycemia; upper-GI distress; hepatotoxicity
Crystalline nicotinic acid	—	
Extended-release nicotinic acid	Niaspan	
Fibric acid derivatives		Dyspepsia; upper-GI distress; myopathy
Gemfibrozil	Lopid	
Fenofibrate	Tricor	
Clofibrate	—	

GI, gastrointestinal; HMG CoA, 3-hydroxy-3-methylglutaryl coenzyme A.
*Avoid use with macrolide antibiotics.
**High potency statins.

Hypertension

Hypertension and LVH are well-established risk factors for adverse cardiovascular outcomes, including CAD morbidity and mortality, stroke, CHF, and sudden death. Systolic blood pressure is as powerful a coronary risk factor as DBP, and isolated systolic hypertension is now established as a major hazard for CAD and stroke, especially in the elderly population.[37,58]

However, while controlled trials have demonstrated clear benefits with BP reduction in terms of stroke and heart failure risk, they have not consistently demonstrated a benefit in coronary events, particularly in patients with mild degrees of hypertension. The increased coronary risk associated with hypertension is primarily seen in subgroups that have other risk factors or underlying target organ damage, and individuals in these subgroups derive the greatest benefit from antihypertensive therapy. The recommendations of the Eighth Joint National Committee on Prevention, Detection, Evaluation, and Treatment of High Blood Pressure provide guidelines for therapy according to stratification based on BP level and the presence or absence of underlying target organ disease.[17]

Glucose Intolerance and Diabetes Mellitus

Insulin resistance, hyperinsulinemia, and glucose intolerance all appear to promote atherosclerosis. As diabetic individuals have a greater number of additional atherogenic risk factors (including hypertension, hypertriglyceridemia, increased cholesterol-to-HDL ratio, and elevated levels of plasma fibrinogen) than do nondiabetic individuals, the CAD risk for diabetic persons varies greatly with the severity of these risk factors. Thus, aggressive treatment of these additional risk factors may help reduce cardiovascular events in diabetic patients. For example, there is increasing evidence of the value of aggressive BP control in diabetic patients.[59] JNC VIII and other recent guidelines help to provide goals for aggressive risk factor modification in diabetic patients.[17,38] Whereas in type 2 diabetes intensive diabetes control has been shown to reduce microvascular complications, such as retinopathy, neuropathy and nephropathy, rather than atherosclerotic vascular disease, there is evidence that in "juvenile-onset" type 1 diabetes, tight glucose control also reduces the risk of adverse cardiovascular outcomes.[60]

Cigarette Smoking

Cigarette smoking is an important and potentially reversible risk factor for CAD and CAD events such as MI. For both men and women, the risk increases with increasing tobacco consumption.[61] For example, in one study, the risk of MI was sixfold increased for women and threefold increased for men who smoked at least 20 cigarettes per day, compared to nonsmoking control patients.[62]

Lifestyle and Dietary Factors

Dietary factors such as a high-calorie, high-fat, and high-cholesterol diet contribute to the development of other risk factors, such as obesity, hyperlipidemia, and diabetes, which pre-dispose to CAD. Red meat consumption too is associated with an increased risk of total, cardiovascular and cancer mortality.[63] Conversely, a diet that emphasizes fruit and vegetables, the increased intake of dietary fiber, and the so-called Mediterranean-style diet rich in olive oil and nuts is associated with a decreased risk of CAD.[64,65] Weight gain and obesity directly worsen the major cardiovascular risk factors whereas weight loss appears to improve them.[66] Epidemiologic data indicate that the moderate intake of alcohol has a cardioprotective effect.[67–69] Elevation of serum HDL levels appears to be the primary mechanism by which alcohol imparts this benefit. It should be stressed that the benefits of alcohol apply only to moderate consumption and is not seen in those who "abuse" alcohol. Furthermore, the protective effects of alcohol are not seen in regard to the risks of hemorrhagic stroke, death due to trauma, or cancer, all of which may be increased in individuals who consume greater amounts of alcohol.

Exercise

Even a moderate degree of exercise appears to have a protective effect against CAD.[70] In one study of middle-aged men, participation in moderately vigorous physical activity was associated with a 23% lower risk of death than that associated with a less active lifestyle, and this improvement in survival was equivalent and additive to other lifestyle measures such as smoking cessation, hypertension control, and weight control.[71] Mechanisms that could account for the benefits of exercise include elevated serum HDL cholesterol levels, reduced blood pressure, weight loss, and a lower incidence of insulin resistance.

Obesity

As stated above, obesity is associated with the development of a number of risk factors for CAD, including systemic hypertension, impaired glucose metabolism, insulin resistance, hypertriglyceridemia, reduced HDL cholesterol, and elevated fibrinogen. Data from the Framingham Heart Study, the Nurses' Health Study, and other studies have shown the risk of developing CAD that is associated with obesity.[72–74] The distribution of body fat appears to be an important determinant as patients with abdominal (central) obesity are at greatest risk for subsequent CAD.[75] Patients with central obesity, elevated levels of serum triglycerides and (to a lesser degree) LDL cholesterol, low HDL cholesterol, insulin resistance, and hypertension are classified as having atherogenic dyslipidemia (metabolic syndrome).[76] This syndrome is more difficult to treat and is associated with a worse prognosis than is an isolated increased LDL level.[77]

Inflammation and Endothelial Dysfunction

Endothelial dysfunction appears to be an early step in the atherosclerotic process and may result from dyslipidemia, hypertension, and diabetes. Recent studies have suggested that coronary artery endothelial dysfunction predicts the long-term progression of atherosclerosis and an increased incidence of cardiovascular events.[78] C-reactive protein (CRP) is an inflammatory biomarker; increased levels of high-sensitivity CRP predict cardiovascular events. The JUPITER Study has demonstrated that in apparently healthy persons without hyperlipidemia but with elevated high-sensitivity CRP levels, the potent anti-lipid agent rosuvastatin reduced the incidence of major cardiovascular events.[79]

Risk Factor Modification

When atherosclerosis is identified, the immediate goals are to relieve symptoms and to improve organ perfusion. Aggressive risk factor modification to retard or prevent ongoing atherosclerosis is among the most important parts of long-term management. Smoking cessation, meticulous control of hypertension and diabetes, weight management, and aggressive lipid-lowering therapy should all be advised. Lipid-lowering therapy with 3-hydroxy-3-methylglutaryl coenzyme A (HMG CoA) reductase inhibitors has been shown to reduce mortality in patients with CAD, even when total cholesterol and LDL are only modestly elevated.[80,81] A low-fat low-calorie diet may result in improved serum lipid levels as well as improved weight management, and a cardiovascular exercise program may result in reduced morbidity and mortality from CHD.[82]

Diagnosis

The diagnosis of chronic CAD is usually suspected from the clinical presentation. A history of exertional or resting symptoms including (but not limited to) chest tightness, jaw discomfort, left arm pain, dyspnea, or epigastric distress should raise the suspicion of CAD. Many patients deny "chest pain" per se, but the clinician should recognize subtle symptoms (such as dyspnea, diaphoresis, or epigastric distress) that may limit activity. Some patients with CAD have no symptoms that are identified during careful questioning but have "silent ischemia" that is demonstrated by noninvasive testing such as exercise testing or ambulatory ECG.[83] Careful attention should be directed to the risk factor profile for CAD since the probability of atherosclerosis is increased in these individuals.[84,85] A statistical extrapolation of the most recent NHANES data suggested that oral health care professionals can effectively screen and identify patients that are unaware of their risk for developing CHD.[86]

Diagnostic testing begins with baseline 12-lead electrocardiography. Unfortunately, this is neither sensitive nor specific for the presence of CAD or prior MI. The presence of abnormal Q waves on the ECG may suggest prior MI although these are not invariably present, and often only non-specific changes of the ST segments or T waves are observed in patients with chronic CAD. Even a normal ECG does not exclude the presence of severe or even life-threatening CAD. Exercise stress testing, often combined with nuclear or echocardiographic imaging modalities, remains the mainstay of a noninvasive diagnosis.[87] Exercise testing with electrocardiographic monitoring is associated with a relatively low sensitivity and specificity for the detection of CAD and should be performed only if the resting ECG is normal. In low-risk patients, however, a negative exercise ECG strongly predicts a favorable clinical outcome.[88] Even in patients with an intermediate-to-high clinical risk of CAD, achieving a relatively high work load during exercise with no ischemic ST depression in the ECG is also associated with a very low prevalence of significant ischemia.[89]

Myocardial perfusion imaging with agents such as thallium 201 and technetium 99m sestamibi is used to assess coronary perfusion at rest and with physical stress. Since the uptake of these agents into the myocardium is an active process, ischemic or infarcted cells exhibit a reduced or absent uptake. A 70%–90% stenosis of a coronary artery typically is associated with decreased myocardial perfusion on the stress images but with normal myocardial perfusion at rest. This reversible defect is the perfusion pattern associated with stress-induced myocardial ischemia. A fixed defect demonstrates reduced myocardial perfusion both at rest and on exercise. Stress echocardiography detects myocardial ischemia by demonstrating regional differences in left ventricular contractile function during stress. Both myocardial perfusion imaging and stress echocardiography offer greater sensitivity and specificity than does exercise ECG alone, and they provide important prognostic information as well. The sensitivity of either modality has been reported as between 85% and 90%, and specificity has been reported to be as high as 90%. Up to 5%–10% of referred patients will have technically inadequate resting images and will require a perfusion imaging study for diagnostic accuracy. Stress perfusion imaging offers a higher technical success rate, higher sensitivity for the detection of single-vessel CAD, and better accuracy when multiple resting left ventricular (LV) wall motion abnormalities are present.[90,91] The role of exercise testing in asymptomatic individuals is highly controversial.[92,93] Coronary angiography is often needed to define the anatomy and to assist in planning an appropriate management strategy for selected intermediate- to high-risk patients.

Management

The management of chronic, stable CAD depends on a number of clinical factors, including the extent and severity of ischemia, exercise capacity, prognosis based on exercise testing, overall LV function, and associated comorbidities such as diabetes mellitus. Patients with a small ischemic burden, normal exercise tolerance, and normal LV function may be safely treated with pharmacologic therapy. The front line of modern medical therapy includes the selected use of aspirin, beta-blockers, ACEIs, and HMG CoA reductase inhibitors. These agents have been shown to reduce the incidence of subsequent MI and death.[91,94] Nitrates and calcium channel blockers may be added to the primary agents to relieve angina in selected patients. Percutaneous coronary intervention (PCI) with percutaneous transluminal coronary angioplasty and intracoronary stenting relieves symptoms of chronic ischemia, improves mortality when used acutely in patients with MI, and may improve regional or global LV function.[95,96] There is no evidence that in patients with chronic stable angina PCI is superior to optimum medical management in the prevention of heart attack and death.[97–100] On the basis of available data, therefore, it seems appropriate to prescribe optimal medical therapy in most patients with CAD and stable angina, and reserve myocardial revascularization for selected patients with disabling symptoms despite optimal medical therapy.[101] Patients with complex multivessel CAD may not be completely revascularized with PCI because of technical limitations of the procedure and commonly require PCI with adjunct medical therapy or surgical revascularization. Early randomized trials in the 1970s, comparing then-current medical therapy to bypass surgery, demonstrated that patients with reduced LV function and severe ischemia, often associated with left main or multivessel CAD, are often best served by coronary artery bypass graft (CABG) surgery.[102–105] More recently, certain subgroups of patients, such as those with left main CAD, multivessel disease or patients with diabetes mellitus, have been shown to have improved clinical outcomes when treated with surgery as compared to treatment by PCI.[106–109]

Prognosis

Recent improvements in pharmacologic therapy, PCI, and surgical technique have resulted in significant improvements in morbidity and mortality in patients with CAD. Risk factor modification is a critical element of the therapy and may result in improved prognosis as well. Despite these improvements, over one million Americans die each year of CAD.

ACUTE CORONARY SYNDROMES

The sudden rupture of an atherosclerotic plaque, with ensuing intracoronary thrombus formation that acutely reduces coronary blood flow, causes the acute coronary syndromes (ACSs).[110,111] This results in myocardial ischemia and subsequent infarction if there is a prolonged and severe reduction in blood flow. Acute coronary syndromes represent a continuous spectrum of disease ranging from unstable angina (USA) to non-ST-elevation MI (NSTEMI) to acute ST-elevation MI (STEMI).

If the intraluminal thrombus following acute plaque rupture is not completely occlusive, the corresponding clinical presentation is that of USA or NSTEMI.[112] There is a sudden change in anginal pattern relating to the frequency or duration of the symptoms. In some cases, the patient may present with symptoms at rest. With a greater degree of obstruction of the epicardial coronary arterial lumen, a non-Q-wave MI (NQWMI) may develop. This presents with prolonged symptoms of resting ischemia, typically without ST-segment elevation or the development of pathologic Q waves. Electrocardiography in a NQWMI patient may show resting ST-segment depression or deep symmetric T-wave inversions, consistent with severe ischemia. If a large epicardial coronary artery becomes obstructed for a relatively long duration of time, a larger myocardial infarct results, and the electrocardiographic findings will be STEMI and, without prompt restoration of blood flow, the subsequent development of pathologic Q waves.

Diagnosis of Acute Coronary Syndromes

The American College of Cardiology Foundation and the American Heart Association (AHA) recently updated their guidelines for the management of patients with USA and NSTEMI.[113] The diagnosis of an ACS is usually made on the basis of clinical data. The patient's history suggests a change in anginal pattern or ischemic symptoms at rest. Acutely, the electrocardiogram is the most important diagnostic tool to risk-stratify the patient and to make decisions regarding treatment. A normal ECG does not exclude the presence of acute MI (AMI). If a STEMI is located at the posterior wall of the left ventricle (LV), it will typically not be well represented on the standard 12-lead ECG. Resting ST-segment depression or T-wave inversions in the distribution of an epicardial coronary artery often accompanies USA or NQWMI; however, ST-segment elevation is the hallmark of an acute STEMI. Patients presenting with a history suggestive of an AMI who have a left bundle branch block pattern on the 12-lead ECG are usually treated as if they had STEMI, given the difficulty of interpreting the ECG when this conduction delay is present.

Levels of cardiac serum markers, such as creatine phosphokinase (CPK) and the more cardiac-specific CPK MB fraction, can be used to establish myocardial injury and infarction. It is important to remember that these levels do not rise significantly until 8 to 12 hours following an MI. Newer, more sensitive and specific cardiac serum markers such as troponin T and troponin I can be used to risk-stratify patients with cardiac injury or infarction.[114] The serum levels become elevated approximately four to eight hours after the acute insult and persist for five to seven days following the event. As both markers can be normal in the early phases of USA or acute STEMI, neither CPK nor troponin is significantly useful in the acute management of patients who may be at the highest risk because of STEMI. Patients with ACS and positive troponin T or I have been shown to have an increased risk of recurrent cardiac events.[115,116] These patients are typically treated more aggressively and are referred for diagnostic and therapeutic cardiac catheterization.

Therapy for Unstable Coronary Syndromes

The treatment of the unstable coronary syndromes should focus on the relief of myocardial ischemia and the institution of pharmacologic therapy targeting the underlying thrombotic mechanism (Table 15-8).[117] Aspirin should be promptly administered to inhibit platelet function. The selective use of beta-blockers

TABLE 15-8	Common Antiplatelet and Antithrombin Medications
Drug	**Trade Name**
Antiplatelet medications	
Aspirin	
Clopidogrel	Plavix
Prasugrel	Effient
Ticagrelor	Brilinta
Glycoprotein IIb/IIIa receptor antagonists	
Abciximab	ReoPro
Eptifibatide	Integrilin
Tirofiban	Aggrastat
Antithrombin medications	
Indirect thrombin inhibitors	
Unfractionated heparin	Heparin
Low-molecular-weight heparin	Enoxaparin
Direct thrombin inhibitors	
Lepirudin	Hirudin
Dicumarols	
Warfarin	Coumadin

may relieve ischemia by lowering heart rate and BP, which subsequently decreases myocardial oxygen demand (MVO_2). Beta-blockers are also antiarrhythmic agents and reduce the risk of malignant ventricular arrhythmias. Beta-blockers should not be administered to those with acute decompensated heart failure, bradycardia, heart block, or severe bronchospasm. Sublingual or intravenous nitroglycerin results in venodilation with a resultant decrease in LV preload and MVO_2, thereby reducing myocardial ischemia. They may also contribute to reducing ischemia by their action as epicardial coronary vasodilators.[113]

In troponin positive high-risk patients, there is robust clinical evidence of improved outcome when in addition to aspirin, a second antiplatelet agent is administered. These include clopidogrel (Plavix), prasugrel (Effient) or ticagrelor (Brilinta). The choice of these agents depends on the relative degree of ischemic vs. bleeding risk. It is important to know that these are potent and long-acting antiplatelet agents whose use is associated with major bleeding risk if a patient is to undergo emergent surgery. Intravenous platelet receptor IIb/IIIa inhibitors (i.e., integrilin and tirofiban), on the other hand, are short-acting agents and usually do not interfere with CABG.[113]

High-risk patients with ACS should also receive intravenous unfractionated heparin or subcutaneous low-molecular weight heparin such as enoxaparin (Lovenox). The short-acting IV unfractionated heparin is preferred in high-risk patients who may need emergent cardiac catheterization and/or bypass surgery, whereas enoxaparin may have some advantage in all other patients with ACS. Procedural outcomes are improved when dual antiplatelet therapy and heparin are used during angioplasty and stenting (see Table 15-8 for a list of these agents).

In patients with STEMI, thrombolytic therapy with agents such as streptokinase, tissue plasminogen activator, and reteplase have all been shown to improve coronary blood flow and to reduce mortality.[118,119] This benefit has not been demonstrated in patients with USA or NQWMI. If PCI is available within 90 minutes of clinical presentation ("door-to-balloon time"), balloon angioplasty and stenting should be performed instead of thrombolytic therapy. Prospective randomized trials have shown that PCI with stenting in patients with STEMI is superior to thrombolytic therapy when it is completed within one to two hours of clinical presentation. Only if a patient with STEMI presents to a center that lacks the ability to perform emergent PCI is thrombolytic therapy the treatment of choice if immediate transfer to a PCI center cannot be arranged. All patients who received thrombolytic therapy, however, should be immediately transferred to a PCI center for emergent rescue angioplasty, if the thrombolysis was unsuccessful, or for non-emergent routine cardiac catheterization with PCI in all other patients. Patients with NSTEMI usually undergo cardiac catheterization and PCI within 24–48 hours of presentation.[113]

Dental Management Considerations for Patients with Coronary Artery Disease

Several considerations need to be addressed when treating dental patients with CAD.[4] The primary concern is to prevent ischemia or infarction. The risk for such an event is determined by numerous factors, including the degree and type of CAD (i.e., stable vs. USA, or history of MI). Patients with CAD are at increased risk of demand-related ischemia from an increased heart rate or BP, as well as for plaque rupture and acute unstable coronary syndromes. Anxiety can increase the heart rate and BP and can provoke angina or ischemia,[120] but this risk is low during outpatient dental procedures. Protocols to reduce anxiety should be considered according to the level of anticipated stress. Premedication with antianxiety medications are commonly used for this purpose. Nitrous oxide/oxygen analgesia can be used for cardiac patients, but the nitrous oxide content should not exceed 65%. The patient's nitroglycerin tablets or spray should be readily available during the procedure. If the patient has anginal attacks more than one per week, or if the procedure is expected to be stressful, the patient may benefit from nitroglycerin use just prior to the procedure.

There is a longstanding dogma in dental practice that patients who have had an MI within past six months should not have elective dental procedures, but this concern is largely based on reports of increased complications occurring during general surgery in the operating room environment, with patients under general, not local anesthesia.[121] Recent protocols suggest that patients may be safely treated in an outpatient dental setting 30 days after an MI unless the patient is suffering from uncompensated

CHF. Considerations for dental patients who have undergone CABG are similar to those who have had an M, that is, there are no data to support waiting as long as six months before resuming dental treatment following CABG surgery. Following a CABG, however, sitting in a dental chair may be painful, even several weeks after their surgery. Elective dental care should therefore be postponed for at least a month and until the patient can sit comfortable for the required time period.

Elective procedures, especially those requiring general anesthesia, should be avoided for at least four weeks following a MI as there is a small increased risk of reinfarction.[122] Limited data indicate that the acute risk of administering local anesthesia for dental procedures three weeks after an uncomplicated AMI is very low. Be cautious if using epinephrine as a vasoconstrictor in local anesthetics, and consider nitrous oxide analgesia.

Patients with a history of CABG, arrhythmia, and some cardiac medications are at increased risk for long or stressful dental procedures. Multiple short appointments may be preferable, unless perhaps the patient has to travel long distances. As with patients with hypertension, the use of local anesthetics with vasoconstrictors such as epinephrine is controversial and may be of concern with other cardiac conditions.[46] The benefits of vasoconstrictors (e.g., more profound and prolonged anesthetic effect) likely outweigh the risks except in unusual and specific cardiac conditions. Limited data indicate that the acute risk of administering local anesthesia without vasoconstrictor for three weeks after an uncomplicated AMI is low, but if epinephrine-containing local anesthetic is necessary, it may be desirable to discuss this with the patient's primary care physician or cardiologist. Concentrations of epinephrine > 1:100,000 are not thought to be of any value and may increase the risk.[47] Clearly, it is important to restrict the total volume of local anesthetics, and especially epinephrine. For restorative treatment on elderly patients, particularly for teeth with existing restorations, pulpal discomfort is likely to be minimal and anesthetic may be unnecessary.

Although there may be a weak association between periodontal disease and atherosclerosis, independent of common risk factors (e.g., smoking), a causal link has not been established.[123] Nevertheless, caries and periodontal disease result in more frequent bacteremia and this may lead to an acute pulpitis or abscess that can trigger angina or MI.[124]

Dental Management Considerations for Patients with Angina

From the standpoint of the patient's history, it is important to know if angina occurs at rest, and if there are precipitating factors such as exercise, climbing stairs, or emotional stress. Patients should be asked about these precipitating factors and the frequency, duration, timing, severity of attacks, and the response to medication. Many patients will have one or more coronary stents. The presence of other cardiac conditions important to the medical history include the presence of other vascular disease and whether or not the patient has a pacemaker or defibrillator. Patients with angina may be on one or more of the following drugs: nitrates or beta-blockers, which can cause conduction disturbances and fatigue; and calcium channel blockers, which have side effects including bradycardia, worsening heart failure, headache, and dizziness. Respiratory depressants such as opioids, barbiturates and other sedatives can worsen the cardiovascular status.

Elective dental treatment is reasonable if the angina is stable and well controlled by one to two nitroglycerin tablets, and if episodes are less frequent than one per week. It is best to avoid elective dental treatment if these limits are exceeded because the angina is considered unstable. Crescendo (increasing frequency) angina patients are at high risk for MI, and the patient's physician should be contacted before any dental treatment.

Numerous studies have indicated the influence of circadian variation on the triggering of acute coronary events.[125] Most such events occur between 6:00 am and noon. It has been proposed that sympathetic nervous system activation and an increased coagulative state may be precipitating factors.[126] Medications designed to prevent these events include beta-blockers, aspirin, and antihypertensives. Dental care for high-risk patients might ideally be provided in the late morning or the early afternoon.

In addition to taking routine vital signs prior to stressful dental procedures, it is also desirable for oral health care professionals treating patients with a history of ischemic heart disease to be certified in the AHA basic life support or advanced cardiac life support.[127]

Side effects from cardiac drugs may cause oral mucosal changes. For example, gingival overgrowth can occur with calcium channel blockers and oral dryness may result from antihypertensive drugs.

Anticoagulation Therapy and Invasive Dental Procedures

Many cardiac patients will have impaired hemostasis due to one or more medications (e.g., warfarin), which may dictate modifications in dental management.[10] Anticoagulant therapy is used both to treat and to prevent thromboembolism, and different medications are used based on the patient's underlying medical condition. Dental providers in an outpatient setting will almost exclusively treat patients who are using anticoagulation therapy for prophylactic purposes, which include, but are not limited to atrial fibrillation or atrial flutter (with and without concomitant systemic embolism), valvular heart disease, prosthetic heart valves, ischemic heart disease, cerebrovascular accidents, pulmonary embolism, and deep-vein thrombosis. Two major groups of medications are used for anticoagulation: drugs with antiplatelet activity and drugs with antithrombin activity.

The most common antiplatelet drug is aspirin, which is used chronically in low doses to prevent cardiovascular and cerebrovascular events. Aspirin irreversibly decreases platelet aggregation, and patients take between 81 and 325 mg of aspirin once a day. With regard to invasive dental procedures, the dose and duration of aspirin usage may be irrelevant, as it appears that one aspirin tablet essentially blocks platelet aggregation for the lifetime of the platelets.[128]

The most commonly used antithrombin medications are the dicumarols (warfarin), which inhibit the biosynthesis of vitamin K-dependent coagulation proteins (factors II [prothrombin], VII, IX, and X). The full therapeutic effect of warfarin is reached after 48–72 hours and lasts for 36–72 hours if the drug is discontinued. The efficacy of warfarin therapy is monitored by the International Normalized Ratio (INR). The INR is calculated on the basis of the international sensitivity index (ISI) of the specific thromboplastin used in the test (see Chapter 19, Bleeding and clotting disorders for more information on PT, INR, and normal hemostatic values). The therapeutic level of the INR is dependent on the underlying condition but is usually kept in the range of 2.0–3.0. In patients with mechanical prosthetic heart valves in the mitral position, the target INR is frequently from 2.5 to 3.5; some of these patients may also be on low-dose aspirin. For an accurate assessment of an individual's anticoagulation status, an INR measurement should be performed within several hours of surgery. Dental care for patients who are on anticoagulation therapy has been discussed in numerous dental and medical publications, and various protocols have been suggested.[12,129–133]

Newer anticoagulants are coming into widespread use but there is not enough known to about differences between the dental management of patients on these newer drugs by comparison with warfarin.[12,134] The debate surrounding invasive dental procedures centers on the potential risk for excessive bleeding during or after the procedures if anticoagulation therapy is not adjusted (i.e., lowered) versus the risk of a thromboembolic event if the anticoagulation therapy is altered.[129,135] There seems to be a consensus that the risk to the patient if these drugs are discontinued or reduced for any period of time far exceeds the problem of prolonged bleeding.[136] If the patient has other underlying medical conditions that predispose to impaired hemostasis (such as uremia or liver disease), and/or takes other anticoagulants (including nonaspirin, nonsteroidal anti-inflammatory drugs [NSAIDs]), the possibility of oral bleeding following oral surgical procedures increases.[9,10,131,132,137–140]

Patients with CAD may be on antithrombotic therapy with one or more antiplatelet drugs or anticoagulant drugs. In unusual situations, patients may be on two or more drugs that interfere with hemostasis. Antiplatelet drugs, such as clopidogrel, prasugrel, or ticagrelor, are frequently used in patients with ACS and in all patients after coronary artery stenting (Table 15-8). The combination of dual antiplatelet therapy (e.g., aspirin and clopidogrel) is usually continued for a minimum of four weeks after placement of a bare metal stent, and for a minimum of 12 months following the use of a drug-eluting stent. There are limited data addressing the risk from dental procedures performed following coronary stenting.[141] It is prudent to wait approximately one month after placement of a bare metal stent, and 6–12 months following placement of a drug-eluting ("coated") stent. These time periods are required to allow re-endothelialization of the stent to decrease the risk of subacute stent thrombosis. Premature discontinuation of antiplatelet therapy has been significantly associated with adverse cardiac events, such as MI and death.[142] As the risk of bleeding from anything other than highly invasive oral surgical procedures is small, and postextraction bleeding is relatively easy to manage, antiplatelet therapy should not be discontinued for elective dental procedures.[10,140,143,144] The patient's cardiologist should be contacted prior to carrying out invasive dental procedures if there are uncertainties in the patient medical history or current cardiac status and medications.[142] Data that address the risks of bleeding from dental extractions in patients who use antiplatelet drugs are limited.[138,145] These drugs are unlikely to increase significantly the risk of bleeding when used alone, and the risk during routine dental procedures has been exaggerated. When used in combination, dual antiplatelet therapy does increase the risk for surgical bleeding, and this risk increases further with the addition of antithrombotic therapy with warfarin or one of the newer oral anticoagulants. Such a triple combination can be expected in patients who underwent coronary stenting but who also have atrial fibrillation, atrial flutter, or a history of deep venous thrombosis or pulmonary embolism.

Although a bleeding time test is often recommended to evaluate a qualitative defect in platelets, this test has not been shown to have a good correlation with impaired intraoral hemostasis unless bleeding time is significantly longer than 15–20 minutes.[131,138,146,147] If emergency surgery needs to be performed and there is concern about aspirin therapy, 1-desamino-8-D-arginine vasopressin (DDAVP) can be instituted to improve hemostasis.[148] In routine dental practice, the need for DDAVP is extremely uncommon. Multiple suggestions for patient management have been proposed, but there are no guidelines to guide treatment in these cases. DDAVP may be administered parenterally at 0.3 μg per kilogram of body weight, with a maximum dose of 20–24 μg within one hour of surgery. A nasal spray containing 1.5 mg of DDAVP per milliliter can be given in a dose of 300 mg per kilogram body weight.

Ultimately, the core of the problem of developing a uniform protocol for anticoagulated patients is the ability to quantify risk, using parameters that can be applied to the majority of patients.[131,149,150] Several relevant issues need to be considered, including the underlying medical condition requiring anticoagulation therapy, the type of medications used to achieve anticoagulation, the level of anticoagulation, the timing of dental care, and the cost and convenience to the patient. There is little or no indication for altering anticoagulation therapy before minor oral surgical procedures when the patient's INR is < 3.5.[10,151] This conclusion is based on a minimally increased risk of clinically significant intraoral bleeding at this level of anticoagulation and the ease with which most intraoral bleeding can be stopped with local measures, and the potentially devastating consequences of thromboembolic events if warfarin therapy is reduced or withheld, especially for an embolic stroke.

Historically, three different protocols have been used to treat patients who require moderately or highly invasive dental procedures and who have an elevated INR. In the first protocol, warfarin is continued without a change in the dose. This approach minimizes adverse thromboembolic events but may increase the risk of intraoperative and postoperative oral bleeding. If local antihemostatic measures are inadequate to stop bleeding after surgery, antifibrinolytic mouth rinses can be instituted and, if necessary, vitamin K injections by a physician.[152] With the second protocol, warfarin therapy is discontinued for two to three days prior to surgery, and the patient is not placed on any alternative anticoagulation therapy. It takes an additional two to three days after surgery to regain the full therapeutic effect of the medication, during which, patients may be in a hypercoagulable state and at an increased risk for developing a thromboembolic event. For patients who are at the highest risk of thromboembolism, such as those with mechanical prosthetic heart valves, atrial fibrillation with a history of stroke, or recent deep vein thrombosis and/or pulmonary embolism, this second approach of holding warfarin without "bridging" heparin (see below) may be too risky. In the third protocol, warfarin therapy is discontinued, and the patient is placed on an alternative anticoagulation therapy. This protocol has both advantages and disadvantages. The greatest advantage is that the patient's risk for developing thromboembolic events is minimized by comparison with the second protocol above. When unfractionated heparin is used for bridging the warfarin-free period, the patient is typically admitted to a hospital, has their oral anticoagulation (warfarin) therapy discontinued, is administered vitamin K and started on parenteral (heparin) therapy. Heparin is continued until approximately six hours before surgery and is reinstituted after surgery in combination with oral anticoagulation therapy until a desirable INR has been reached. This is both a time-consuming and costly course of action which is rarely indicated for dental procedures. The advantages of using heparin are its short half-life of four to six hours and the availability of an antidote, protamine sulfate, that has an immediate effect. An alternative to using standard unfractionated heparin is to have the patient self-administer a subcutaneous injection of low molecular-weight heparin on an outpatient basis.[153] The most commonly used protocol is with 1 mg/kg enoxaparin (Lovenox) given subcutaneously twice a day. This is becoming the treatment of choice in most clinical practices.

VALVULAR HEART DISEASE

Valvular heart disease is usually accompanied by heart murmur. The characteristics of the murmur is usually a good indicator of the type of valvular abnormality and also of the etiology of the valve disease (Table 15-9).

Mitral Valve Disease

The most common types of mitral valve disease include mitral valve prolapse (MVP), mitral regurgitation (MR), and mitral stenosis. In addition to the hemodynamic alterations that are present in patients with these conditions, there are additional issues with regard to the prevention of bacterial endocarditis.

Definition and Incidence

Mitral valve prolapse typically occurs as a result of myxomatous degeneration of the mitral leaflets and their supporting apparatus. This results in abnormal movement or prolapse of the mitral leaflets posteriorly toward the left atrium during mechanical systole. Thus, there is abnormal coaptation of the valve with varying degrees of MR. A small percentage of those with MVP have significant MR and ensuing left atrial and left ventricular (LV) volume overload. Rarely, MVP can be accompanied by malignant dysrhythmias such as ventricular tachycardia or fibrillation. Typically, more benign atrial dysrhythmias are seen and manifest clinically as palpitations. Cardiac auscultation frequently reveals a midsystolic click, late systolic murmur, or the combination of click and murmur. The gold standard for diagnosing and risk-stratifying MVP is echocardiography.

Mitral regurgitation (MR) is the result of abnormal closure of the mitral leaflets.[154] MR has various causes, including MVP, rheumatic heart disease (RHD), endocarditis, and the use of anorectic agents such as fenfluramine and phentermine (fen-phen).[155–157] Another cause of MR is dilation of the base of the LV in patients with dilated cardiomyopathy. This can result in incomplete coaptation of the mitral leaflets and significant MR. Regardless of the mechanism, if MR is left untreated, the final common end point is LV volume overload, with subsequent eccentric hypertrophy of the LV and resultant progressive heart failure.

Mitral stenosis most often occurs as a result of RHD. In RHD, there is characteristic thickening and fusion of the mitral commissures as well as thickening and calcification of the leaflets and subvalvular apparatus. This results in a restriction to LV inflow, subsequent left atrial hypertension and enlargement, atrial arrhythmias, and secondary pulmonary hypertension.

The clinical diagnosis of mitral valve disease requires a careful history suggesting a previously heard heart murmur, exertional or resting dyspnea, or symptoms of heart failure such as orthopnea, paroxysmal nocturnal dyspnea, or peripheral edema. Auscultatory findings include a midsystolic click in MVP, a holosystolic murmur in rheumatic MR, and an opening snap and diastolic rumble in mitral stenosis. Ancillary findings such as pulmonary or peripheral edema may be present as well.

Transthoracic echocardiography (TTE) remains the main-stay of noninvasive diagnosis in patients with mitral valve disease, and Doppler techniques are extremely useful in establishing the severity of stenosis or regurgitation.[158] Transesophageal echocardiography (TEE) is occasionally needed to further define the mechanism of MR or stenosis and to better assess the severity of the hemodynamic lesion[159]; this is instrumental in planning appropriate percutaneous interventional or surgical therapy. TEE offers improved image quality due to the proximity of the transducer to the mitral valve and left atrium. Cardiac catheterization has a limited role in the diagnosis of mitral valve disease and is primarily reserved for those patients who are referred for cardiac surgery.[160] The main goal of cardiac cathetrization in these cases is to exclude coexisting significant CAD.

Treatment of Mitral Valvular Disease

The American College of Cardiology and the AHA have published guidelines for treating valvular heart disease that are based on the strength of available evidence in the medical literature.[161] Mitral valve prolapse with relatively minor degrees of MR can be observed with serial clinical and echocardiographic examinations to screen for worsening degrees of regurgitation. Symptomatic patients with significant degrees of MR or mitral stenosis are typically referred for operative or other mechanical intervention. Asymptomatic patients with MR can be observed with serial clinical and echocardiographic examinations. The development of symptoms or, in the asymptomatic patient, an increase in LV dimension or a decrease in the LV ejection fraction are important factors in determining the timing of surgical intervention. Unfortunately, ideal criteria for proceeding to intervention prior to irreversible LV enlargement and contractile decompensation do not exist.[162] MR can be treated by either repair of the mitral valve or replacement with a mechanical or biologic prosthesis. Mitral repair is usually accomplished with the resection of the prolapsing or flail segment of the mitral leaflets and the placement of an annuloplasty ring to decrease mitral annular dimension in order to improve mitral coaptation. If significant fibrosis or calcification of the mitral valve is present, replacement with either a biologic or mechanical prosthesis may be necessary. More recently, a technique for a catheter-based percutaneous mitral valve repair has been worked out.[163] Although percutaneous repair appears to be less effective at reducing MR than conventional surgery, the procedure is associated with superior safety and similar clinical improvements, at least in the short term.[163] Mitral stenosis can be treated with percutaneous balloon valvuloplasty (PBV) or mitral valve replacement. Patients with highly calcified valves or those with significant degrees of MR that accompanies mitral stenosis are typically referred for valve replacement.

Aortic Valve Disease

The three major causes of aortic stenosis (AS) are congenital, rheumatic, and senile calcific valve disease. The leaflet excursion is restricted, and a systolic pressure gradient develops between the LV and the aorta, causing subsequent LV pressure overload. This leads to concentric hypertrophy of the LV. The natural history of untreated AS is eventual LV failure due to afterload mismatch.

Aortic regurgitation (AR) results from a wide variety of processes that directly affect the aortic leaflets, including congenital abnormalities, rheumatic disease, infective endocarditis, senile calcific valve degeneration, and the use of anorexigens.[164] Additionally, abnormalities of the aortic root such as aneurysm or aortic dissection may dilate or disrupt the aortic annulus, resulting in malcoaptation and regurgitation. AR imposes an acute or chronic volume load to the LV, with subsequent eccentric hypertrophy, LV enlargement and eventual LV contractile failure if the regurgitation is not corrected.

Diagnosis

The clinical diagnosis of aortic valve disease requires a careful history suggesting a previously heard heart murmur, exertional or resting dyspnea, or symptoms of heart failure such as orthopnea, paroxysmal nocturnal dyspnea, or peripheral edema. Patients with AS may also experience angina or syncope. Severe AR too may produce angina due to impaired coronary filling, which results from a decrease in aortic diastolic pressure and an increase in LV diastolic pressure.

The auscultatory findings of AS include a harsh crescendo-decrescendo systolic murmur best heard over the right upper sternal border, and a diminished or absent aortic component of the second heart sound. The murmur of AS frequently radiates to the neck arteries. AR is manifest on physical examination by a high-pitched and decrescendo early diastolic murmur heard best at the left sternal border when the patient is sitting upright with breath held after exhalation. Chronic AR often yields findings of a hyperdynamic circulation with bounding or "water hammer" pulses, head bobbing (titubation), "to-and-fro" murmurs heard in the femoral arteries, and Quincke's pulse (visible in the nail beds). Acute AR may present with heart failure and acute pulmonary edema, without the characteristic murmur of AR (Table 15-9).

TTE remains the mainstay of noninvasive diagnosis in the vast majority of patients with aortic valve disease. Doppler techniques are useful in establishing the severity of stenosis or regurgitation.[165] TEE may be needed to define the mechanism of AR or AS, to evaluate the aortic root and ascending aorta, and to investigate the possibility of endocarditis.[166,167] A role exists for cardiac catheterization in the diagnosis of aortic valve disease as well; it is primarily reserved for both evaluating the possibility of coexisting CAD and determining the need for surgical revascularization in patients who are being considered for cardiac surgery.

TABLE 15-9 Diseases and Conditions Associated with Different Types of Heart Murmurs[266]

Type of Murmur	Associated Abnormality	Possible Associated Diseases or Conditions
Holosystolic	MR	A fib; LVH; SLE; CTD
	TR	A fib; JVD; CTD
	VSD	A fib; L-to-R shunt; CHF
Midsystolic	AS	A fib; LVH
	PS	R-sided CHF
Late systolic	MVP	CTD; Stickler; Trisomy 21
Early diastolic	AI	CHF
	PI	CHF
Mid-diastolic	Rheum. MS	A fib
Late diastolic	Rheum. MS	A fib
Continuous	Aortopulmonary and arteriovenous connection	CHF; LVH

A fib, atrial fibrillation; LVH, left ventricular hypertrophy; SLE, systemic lupus erythematosus; CTD, connective tissue disease; JVD, jugular vein distention; CHF, congestive heart failure.

Treatment of Aortic Valvular Disease

Aortic disease with relatively minor degrees of stenosis or regurgitation can be observed clinically, with serial clinical and echocardiographic examinations to monitor progression. In cases of AS, the development of symptoms and, to a lesser degree, the severity of AS determines the timing of surgery.[168] Both retrospective and prospective studies have demonstrated that the risk of sudden death is low in asymptomatic patients with even a severe degree of stenosis.[169]

In patients with AR, the key factors to observe are the development of symptoms and a worsening of LV enlargement.[161] Heart failure symptoms typically develop in the late or decompensated stages of LV volume overload. Symptomatic patients with significant degrees of AR are typically referred for surgery.

Severe AR or AS is usually treated with aortic valve replacement with either a mechanical or biologic valve prosthesis. AS can also be treated with PBV; however, minimal hemodynamic improvements postprocedure and rapid restenosis rates limit the usefulness of this procedure. PBV is usually reserved for patients who are not operative candidates but who require end-stage symptomatic palliation or temporary hemodynamic improvements to tolerate additional noncardiac surgery or to overcome acute illness.

Patients who have clinical indication for aortic valve replacement (AVR) but are at a high risk for perioperative complications including operative mortality, a percutaneous technique of transcatheter aortic valve implantation (TAVI) has been recently developed.[170,171]

Prosthetic Heart Valves

There are numerous types and models of prosthetic heart valves, each with their own unique characteristics. These valves are either mechanical or bioprosthetic. The mechanical valves, which are classified according to their structure, include the oldest type caged-ball (Starr-Edwards) valve,

the single tilting-disk (Bjork-Shiley) valve, and the currently most widely used bileaflet tilting-disk valves (i.e., St. Jude, Edwards-MIRA). Bioprosthetic valves are either (1) heterografts made from porcine or bovine tissue or (2) homografts from preserved human aortic valves. Patients with mechanical valves require chronic anticoagulation therapy (typically with warfarin) to prevent thromboembolism. The degree of anticoagulation varies according to the type of the mechanical heart valve. The thrombogenic potential is the highest for caged-ball valves, moderate for single tilting-disk valves, and the lowest for bileaflet tilting-disk valves. In patients with mechanical valves, the risk of systemic embolization is approximately 4% per patient per year without anticoagulation, 2.2% with aspirin therapy, and 0.7%–1.0% with warfarin therapy.[172] Patients with mitral valve prostheses are at approximately twice the risk of those with aortic valve prostheses.[173] The risk of thromboembolism is highest in the period following placement of the valve and decreases over time as the valve becomes endothelialized. Bioprosthetic valves have a lower thrombogenic potential and do not require long-term anticoagulation except for the early postoperative period. The duration of transient postoperative anticoagulation in patients who undergo bioprosthetic heart valve replacement is debated but typically lasts for three to six months.[174,175] The recommended anticoagulation therapy for each type of prosthetic valve is summarized in Table 15-10. It is important that although these recommendations serve as broad guidelines, the level of chronic anticoagulation should be individualized and based on the location, type, and number of prosthetic valves, as well as the patient's age, comorbidities, and additional thromboembolic risk factors such as a history of atrial fibrillation or stroke. Thus, the intensity of anticoagulation is determined by weighing the patient's risk of thromboembolic events against the risk of adverse anticoagulation consequences (bleeding risks).[176]

Prosthetic heart valves increase the risk for infective endocarditis, which typically manifests as fever and as

TABLE 15-10 Anticoagulation Therapy for Patients With Prosthetic Heart Valves[176]

Risk of Thromboembolism	Type of Valve	Recommended INR	Antiplatelet Therapy
Low	Mechanical		
	More than one prosthesis	4.0–4.9	Not indicated
	Caged-ball	4.0–4.9	Not indicated
	Single tilted-disk	3.0–3.9	Not indicated
	Bileaflet tilted-disk	2.5–2.9	Not indicated
	Bioprosthetic		
	Heterograft	2.0–3.0 (1st 3 mo)	ASA, 325 mg/d
	Homograft	Not indicated	Not indicated
High*	Mechanical	3.0–4.5	ASA, 80–160 mg/d
	Bioprosthetic		
	Heterograft	2.0–3.0	Not indicated
	Homograft	2.0–3.0	Not indicated

ASA, acetylsalicylic acid; INR, international normalized ratio.

*High risk patients are those with a history of atrial fibrillation, previous systemic embolism, left ventricular thrombus, or severe left ventricular dysfunction.

other systemic symptoms.[177] Although endocarditis within 60 days of surgery typically is caused by non-oral bacteria, the cause of endocarditis that occurs 60 days after valve surgery is similar to that of native-valve endocarditis.

Congenital Heart Disease

Congenital cardiovascular malformations can be cyanotic (dominant right-to-left shunting), non-cyanotic (dominant left-to-right shunting) or without shunting. Cyanotic defects include tetralogy of Fallot, transposition of the great vessels, anomalies of the tricuspid valve, pulmonary atresia, pulmonary stenosis, Eisenmenger's syndrome, and hypoplastic left heart syndrome (aortic atresia). Surgical correction of these defects is often accomplished in infancy and early childhood. Non-cyanotic defects include ventricular septal defect (VSD), atrial septal defect (ASD), patent ductus arteriosus, coarctation of the aorta, aortic valve stenosis, and MVP.

Dental Management Considerations

Patients with valvular disease need to be questioned carefully about their symptoms, and any ongoing medical management, to include current medications. The extent to which dental treatment must be altered is determined by the degree of compromise with regard to cardiac output and tolerance for stressful and or prolonged dental procedures. Patients who are without symptoms, and who have limited or no exercise intolerance, and are without arrhythmias, can undergo routine dental procedures without significant risk. Otherwise, they should be discussed with their primary care provider or cardiologist prior to dental treatment. Many of these patients have concomitant CAD and this is a separate consideration with regard to modifications for dental care.

Considerations Concerning Bacteremia from Dental Procedures

Infective endocarditis (IE) has been associated globally with 1.58 million disability-adjusted life years or years of healthy life lost due to death and non-fatal illness or impairment.[178] The possibility that bacteremia from the mouth could cause IE was first suggested over 100 years ago and was later reinforced by others who targeted viridans group streptococci from poor oral hygiene and dental extractions.[179,180]

Community-acquired infective endocarditis (CA-IE) is initiated by a bacteremia in a susceptible host (e.g., heart valve abnormality), and has an overall mortality rate of 20%–30% depending on several host factors and the bacterial species involved.[35,181] Health care–associated (HCA) IE, is largely due to staphylococci and its incidence has increased as cardiac and other surgical procedures such as the use of intravascular catheters and implanted cardiac devices have become more common.[182–184] Although the literature suggests a very wide incidence range (20%–60%) for cases of IE caused by oral bacteria[185] it is likely that between 30-45% of CA-IE cases originate from oral bacterial species[183,186–191] and it is likely that the mortality rate for oral bacteria-related IE is 10%–20%.[181,185,190,192,193]

It is likely that the origin of many cases of IE is transient bacteremia from the close approximation of oral bacterial plaque adjacent to the teeth. In patients with poor oral hygiene and periodontal disease, it is likely that these bacteria are able to traverse the inflamed and ulcerated periodontal pocket tissue to enter the circulation.[194] Dental office procedure-generated bacteremia may occur one to two times per year on average and therefore should far fewer, if any, cases of IE than activities of daily living, which may occur hundreds of times per year. There is a consensus among the experts, therefore, that bacteremia occurs far more frequently, in a dentate individual, from naturally occurring sources such as tooth brushing and chewing food, than from dental procedures.[194] They also agree that antibiotic prophylaxis (AP) may not have a clinically significant impact on the incidence of IE and that it likely puts patients at risk.[35,190,195–197] Guidelines from the AHA also do not support the use of antibiotic prophylaxis for dental procedures in patients after coronary stent placement since there is no evidence of a risk of infection of grafted coronary vessels from dental procedures.[11]

There is an ongoing shift in thinking away from AP for invasive dental procedures, due to: i) concerns over a lack of evidence for efficacy, ii) the potential development of antibiotic resistant strains of bacteria, and iii) costs associated with this practice, toward improved oral hygiene and resolution of periodontal inflammation as a means of reducing oral bacteria-related CA-IE.[35,196,198–204] Current (2007) AHA guidelines reflect the lack of evidence for safety or efficacy for the use of AP prior to invasive dental procedures as a means for preventing IE, and there is an evolving hypothesis that routine bacteremia from poor oral hygiene and periodontal disease are far more likely to cause CA-IE than invasive dental procedures.[196,202,205] It is important to emphasize that current U.S. guidelines focus on the AHA-defined "higher risk" groups of four cardiac populations who are at risk for a "bad outcome" from IE (higher morbidity and mortality), which include: prosthetic heart valve; history of heart transplant with an associated new valvular lesion; and a history of unrepaired congenital cyanotic heart disease (Tables 15-11, 15-12, and 15-13).[196] These four groups comprise only about 10% of patients at

risk for IE.[196,200] The AHA-defined "moderate risk" groups of cardiac patients represent about 90% of people covered with antibiotic prophylaxis prior to 2007. AP is no longer recommended for these people, but they remain at risk for CA-IE from oral bacteria.

HEART FAILURE

Definition and Incidence

Heart failure represents a clinical condition that is broadly defined as the inability of the cardiovascular system to meet the demands of the end organs.[206,207] Heart failure may be due to pericardial disease, valvular heart disease, and most commonly, myocardial disease resulting in abnormal contractile function (systolic dysfunction) or impaired relaxation (diastolic dysfunction) (Table 15-14 and 15-15). Diastolic dysfunction is characterized by clinical heart failure syndrome with normal LV systolic function on cardiac testing.[208,209] In many series, it represents one of the most common types of heart failure encountered in the general population.[210] Common causes of diastolic dysfunction include hypertension, CAD, long-standing diabetes, and advanced age. In addition, diastolic dysfunction is almost always present in patients with any type of advanced systolic heart failure.

Diagnosis

Dyspnea, orthopnea, and paroxysmal nocturnal dyspnea are classic symptoms, but nonspecific complaints such as chest discomfort, fatigue, palpitations, dizziness, and syncope are not uncommon. The onset of symptoms may be insidious, and symptoms may present for medical attention only when an acute decompensation occurs. For example, a patient with asymptomatic LV dysfunction develops rapid atrial fibrillation resulting in decompensated heart failure (Table 15-16). Asymptomatic patients are sometimes diagnosed when routine testing is performed for other reasons which reveal abnormalities on ECGs, chest radiographs, or echocardiograms.

The physical-examination findings in heart failure are numerous. A relative decrease in SBP (due to reduced cardiac output) and an increase in DBP (due to peripheral vasoconstriction) may result in a decrease in pulse pressure. Cardiac percussion and palpation reveal an enlarged heart with a laterally displaced and diffuse apical impulse. Auscultation may reveal an apical systolic murmur of MR and the lower parasternal murmur of tricuspid regurgitation. Third and fourth heart sounds can be heard, signifying evidence of systolic and diastolic dysfunction. Rales suggest pulmonary congestion secondary to elevated left atrial and LV end-diastolic pressures. Jugular venous distention, peripheral edema, and hepatomegaly are markers of elevated right-heart pressures and right ventricular dysfunction. In advanced heart failure, additional findings may include cool extremities with decreased pulses, generalized cachexia, muscle atrophy, and profound weakness.

TABLE 15-11 Cardiac Conditions Associated With the Highest Risk of Adverse Outcome From Endocarditis for Which Prophylaxis With Dental Procedures Is Reasonable[196]

1. Prosthetic cardiac valve or prosthetic material used for cardiac valve repair

2. Previous IE

3. Congenital heart disease (CHD)*

   Unrepaired cyanotic CHD, including palliative shunts and conduits

   Completely repaired congenital heart defect with prosthetic material or device, whether placed by surgery or by catheter intervention,
      during the first 6 mo after the procedure†

   Repaired CHD with residual defects at the site or adjacent to the site of a prosthetic patch or prosthetic device (which inhibit endothelialization)

4. Cardiac transplantation recipients who develop cardiac valvulopathy

*Except for the conditions listed above, antibiotic prophylaxis is no longer recommended for any other form of CHD.
†Prophylaxis is reasonable because endothelialization of prosthetic material occurs within 6 months after the procedure.

TABLE 15-12 Regimens for a Dental Procedure[196]

| Situation | Agent | Regimen: Single Dose 30–60 min Before Procedure | |
		Adults	Children
Oral	Amoxicillin	2 g	50 mg/kg
Unable to take oral medication	Ampicillin	2 g IM or IV	50 mg/kg IM or IV
	OR		
	Cefazolin or ceftriaxone	1 g IM or IV	50 mg/kg IM or IV
Allergic to penicillins or ampicillin—oral	Cephalexin*†	2 g	50 mg/kg
	OR		
	Clindamycin	600 mg	20 mg/kg
	OR		
	Azithromycin or clarithromycin	500 mg	15 mg/kg
Allergic to penicillins or ampicillin and unable to take oral medication	Cefazolin or ceftriaxone†	1 g IM or IV	50 mg/kg IM or IV
	OR		
	Clindamycin	600 mg IM or IV	20 mg/kg IM or IV

IM, indicates intramuscular; IV, intravenous.
*Or other first- or second-generation oral cephalosporin in equivalent adult or pediatric dosage.
†Cephalosporins should not be used in an individual with a history of anaphylaxis, angioedema, or urticaria with penicillins or ampicillin.

TABLE 15-13 Dental Procedures for Which Endocarditis Prophylaxis Is Reasonable for Patients[196]

All dental procedures that involve manipulation of gingival tissue or the periapical region of teeth or perforation of the oral mucosa*

*The following procedures and events do not need prophylaxis: routine anesthetic injections through noninfected tissue, taking dental radiographs, placement of removable prosthodontic or orthodontic appliances, adjustment of orthodontic appliances, placement of orthodontic brackets, shedding of deciduous teeth, and bleeding from trauma to the lips or oral mucosa.

TABLE 15-14 Heart Failure Etiologies

Coronary artery disease (ischemic cardiomyopathy)

Hypertension

Idiopathic dilated cardiomyopathy

Hypertrophic cardiomyopathy

Alcohol

Diabetes

Viruses (Coxsackie virus, Enterovirus, human immunodeficiency virus)

Infiltrative disorders (amyloidosis, hemochromatosis, sarcoidosis)

Toxins (chemotherapeutic agents)

Metabolic disorders (hypothyroidism)

Valvular heart disease

Pericardial disease

Incessant tachyarrhythmia

High output states (thyrotoxicosis, atrioventricular fistula, thiamine deficiency)

TABLE 15-15 Classification of Heart Failure

The New York Heart Association classification assigns patients with heart failure to one of the four functional classes, depending on the degree of effort needed to elicit

• Class I—symptoms of HF only at activity levels that would limit normal individuals

• Class II—symptoms of HF with ordinary exertion

• Class III—symptoms of HF with less than ordinary exertion

• Class IV—symptoms of HF at rest

Chest radiography may demonstrate cardiac enlargement, pulmonary congestion, and pleural effusions. The ECG is frequently abnormal in a nonspecific manner and may be the only indication of heart disease in asymptomatic individuals. Electrocardiography may reveal prolonged repolarization (i.e., Q–T interval), and nonspecific ST and T-wave abnormalities. Conduction disturbances such as atrioventricular block, bundle branch blocks, and fascicular blocks are also seen. Criteria for LV hypertrophy with a repolarization abnormality may suggest hypertension as an etiology. Electrocardiography may also reveal evidence of arrhythmias such as atrial fibrillation and atrial flutter as well as premature atrial or ventricular contractions. Supraventricular tachyarrhythmias and nonsustained ventricular tachycardia are also associated with heart failure, as is the development of ventricular fibrillation usually resulting in sudden cardiac death.

TTE is the most useful noninvasive diagnostic tool for the initial evaluation of a patient with heart failure.[211] TTE provides information not only on overall heart size and

TABLE 15-16 Etiologies of Atrial Fibrillation

Hypertension

Rheumatic valvular disease

Coronary artery disease (including acute MI and ischemic cardiomyopathy)

Atrial septal defects

Hypertrophic cardiomyopathy

Congenital heart disease (Ebstein's disease, patent ductus arteriosus, tetralogy of Fallot)

Dilated cardiomyopathy

Alcoholic cardiomyopathy

Holiday heart syndrome

Pulmonary embolism

Pericardial disease

Chronic obstructive lung disease, cor pulmonale

Peripartum cardiomyopathy

Sleep apnea

Thyrotoxicosis

Autonomic dysfunction

Postcardiac surgery and transplantation

Noncardiac surgery (thoracic and esophageal)

Medications (theophylline, caffeine, digitalis)

Familial

Pheochromocytoma

MI, myocardial infarction.

function but also on valvular structure and function, wall motion and thickness, LV mass, and the presence of pericardial disease. Doppler-derived hemodynamic measurements accurately predict the severity of valvular regurgitation seen in heart failure and give a noninvasive estimation of pulmonary artery pressures. Doppler techniques may also be used to evaluate LV diastolic abnormalities, which are frequently present in those with heart failure.

Nuclear imaging techniques such as perfusion heart scans with thallium 201 and technetium 99m sestamibi, radionuclide ventriculography with multiple gated acquisition scanning, and positron emission tomography (PET) scanning may be useful in evaluating cardiac size and function and in screening for coronary disease as a cause of heart failure (Table 15-14). However, because of the inability of these tests to answer important etiologic questions with absolute certainty and their inherent use of radiation, these tests are often unnecessary in the routine evaluation of patients with a known cause of heart failure.

Cardiac catheterization (with measurement of intracardiac pressures and cardiac output), along with coronary angiography, is useful in evaluating the etiology of heart failure when ischemic cardiomyopathy is suspected. In middle-aged and elderly patients, the most common cause of heart failure and cardiomyopathy is CAD (Table 15-14). In patients with heart failure, typical findings at catheterization

include elevated LV end-diastolic, wedge, pulmonary artery, and right-heart pressures; increased LV size with decreased overall systolic function; and MR. Regional wall motion abnormalities may be seen in either ischemic or dilated cardiomyopathy but are usually less prominent in patients who do not have ischemic heart disease.

Therapy

The optimum management of patients with chronic systolic heart failure is highly evidence-based and is associated with dramatic decreases in the risk of heart failure exacerbations, hospitalizations and death. Several reviews and society guidelines, therefore, provide specific recommendations for treating heart failure.[212–216]

The treatment of heart failure must be individualized to the etiology of the heart failure and to the patient (Table 15-14). Patients with CAD and heart failure should be evaluated for ischemia as well as viable but hibernating myocardium that would improve systolic and diastolic performance with revascularization.[217–219] Patients with alcoholic cardiomyopathy should be advised to abstain from alcohol, in addition to the usual therapeutic options, as this often leads to an improvement in LV performance.[220] Hypertension should be aggressively treated with pharmacologic intervention and dietary measures.

The initial treatment in decompensated heart failure is with intravenous or oral diuretics. The optimum dose of intravenous diuretic is debated, but there is no evidence that continuous infusion of furosemide is superior to intravenous bolus administration.[221] Intravenous vasodilators such as nitroglycerin may also be used. The majority of patients with symptomatic heart failure will need to stay on oral diuretic therapy. The dose of the diuretic must always be individualized. For patients with systolic heart failure, ACEIs are one of the mainstays of chronic drug therapy. These agents have clearly been shown to decrease mortality and to prolong survival. They also delay onset and reduce the symptoms of heart failure in patients with LV systolic dysfunction. When ACEIs cannot be tolerated, angiotensin receptor antagonists or the combination of hydralazine and nitrate derivatives may be substituted. Digoxin is effective in reducing morbidity and hospitalizations but has little effect on overall mortality. Loop diuretics control symptoms but have not been shown to affect mortality. Conversely, the RALES trial found that the aldosterone antagonist agent spironolactone improves survival in patients with advanced CHF[222] and the EMPHASIS-HF trial showed a marked improvement in all clinical measures of outcome in patients with systolic heart failure and mild symptoms who were treated with the more specific aldosterone antagonist eplerenone.[223] Today beta-blockers, which were previously contraindicated in patients with heart failure, became the most important component of therapy in patients with clinically stable heart failure regardless of severity. Beta-blockers improve symptoms, reduce hospitalizations, and markedly prolong survival. The mean reduction in one-year mortality associated with the use of any of the evidence-based beta-blockers is 35%.[224] Beta-blockers are the only class of medications that can significantly improve LV systolic function. This is not a class effect. Only those beta-blockers should be used that have been shown in clinical studies to improve outcome. In the United States, the most widely used beta-blockers in patients with heart failure include carvedilol (Coreg) and metoprolol succinate (extended-release metoprolol, Toprol-XL). Doses should be initiated at low levels and gradually titrated up over weeks to months. Symptoms of heart failure may initially worsen, and other medication doses may need to be adjusted during the initial stages of beta-blocker therapy.[222] The long-term benefits, however, are robust.[225,226]

Anticoagulation with warfarin (Coumadin) in patients with LV dysfunction may reduce morbidity and mortality from cardioembolic events that develop secondary to chamber enlargement and stasis of blood; however, the risks of bleeding need to be considered.[227] Routine anticoagulation in patients with systolic heart failure is generally not recommended.[228,229] Anticoagulation therapy is likely to be most beneficial for patients with atrial fibrillation or atrial flutter, in patients with severe systolic heart failure who experienced a transient ischemic attack (TIA) or stroke, and in patients in sinus rhythm who were found to have an intracardiac clot in the echocardiogram.

For those patients who remain highly symptomatic, despite optimum medical management, intravenous therapy with diuretics and inotropes may need to be initiated. Some patients respond well to this treatment, and oral therapy can subsequently be resumed rapidly; other patients require long-term intravenous therapy. Patients with systolic heart failure whose electrocardiogram shows wide QRS complexes due to left bundle branch block (LBBB) have markedly increased symptomatology, quality of life and even mortality compared to patients with similar left ventricular ejection fractions but no LBBB.[230] Cardiac resynchronization therapy with implanted biventricular pacemakers has been shown to have a significant beneficial effect on morbidity and mortality in this subgroup of patients with heart failure.[231] Implantable cardioverter-defibrillators (ICDs) are also increasingly used for primary prevention of sudden death in patients with chronic heart failure whose LV ejection fraction remains below 30%–35% despite optimum medical management.[232]

Aggressive Treatment of Advanced Heart Failure

For selected heart failure patients who continue to be highly symptomatic despite optimum medical, interventional, and device therapies, evaluation for cardiac transplantation may be indicated. The patient must be otherwise fit for surgery, and must be able to adhere to the intensive medical treatment and follow-up that are required postoperatively.[60] Left ventricular assist devices (LVADs) are increasingly used to treat end-stage heart failure not only as a bridge to heart transplantation, but also as definitive "destination" therapy.[233]

In patients with end-stage heart failure, one-year survival with medical management is approximately 20%, with the newer continuous-flow LVAD it is 60%–70%, whereas with heart transplantation the one-year survival exceeds 85%.[233]

Dental Management Considerations

Patients with heart failure will often have a history of CAD and they may be on multiple medications and dietary measures to control and balance cardiac function. Anticoagulation with warfarin (Coumadin) in these patients may reduce morbidity and mortality from cardioembolic events that develop. The risks of bleeding need to be considered.

It is important to understand the status and stages of the CHF. For well-compensated patients with heart failure, no special modifications are necessary for routine dental care.[234,235] However, for patients with decompensated CHF, it is prudent to inquire about the patient's ability to be placed in supine position as this may cause severe dyspnea. Stressful or prolonged dental procedures put an increased demand on the heart that may exacerbate the problem and result in further inability for ventricles to pump blood. Patients should be questioned about signs of poor compensation, which include: paroxysmal nocturnal dyspnea; orthopnea; shortness of breath or dyspnea on exertion; pedal edema; body weight fluctuations.

These patients may have orthostatic hypotension as a result of medication. They should be brought to a sitting position in several stages and over several minutes, after which they should sit with their feet on floor for at least two minutes before standing up. Patients may also have urinary urgency during morning appointments in response to a diuretic medication and may want to use the bathroom before the procedure.

ARRHYTHMIA

Definition and Incidence

Abnormalities of cardiac rhythm can be broadly defined as any deviation from the normal cardiac pacemaker and conduction mechanism. Tachyarrhythmias, when the heart rate is > 100 bpm, occur as a result of increased automaticity of cardiac pacemaker cells or due to a reentrant mechanism where the electrical impulse circulates rapidly in certain areas of the heart. Bradyarrhythmias occur as a result of sinoatrial node dysfunction or conduction block at any level of the conduction system, including the atrioventricular node, His-Purkinje system, or distal branches of the left and right bundles. Bradyarrhythmias are defined as heart rates of < 60 bpm. Both tachyarrhythmias and bradyarrhythmias may be hemodynamically well tolerated in patients with normal cardiac function, or they may result in cardiovascular collapse if cardiac output is significantly compromised.

Supraventricular Tachycardia

Reentrant supraventricular tachycardias such as atrioventricular nodal re-entrant tachycardia (AVNRT) occur commonly in the absence of structural heart disease and are usually well tolerated from a hemodynamic standpoint. AVNRT is the most common form where the atrioventricular (AV) node is functionally dissociated into two discrete electrical pathways.[236,237] These pathways have different refractory periods and conduction velocities, which are both prerequisites for re-entry. AVNRT is usually triggered by a fortuitously timed premature atrial or ventricular impulse and therefore may be observed in settings where there is increased atrial ectopy due to anxiety or other types of sympathetic stimulation.[238] Interrupting conduction within the re-entrant circuit in the AV node can terminate the tachycardia.[239] The surface ECG of a patient with Wolff-Parkinson-White (WPW) syndrome is characterized by a short P–R interval and the slurred onset of the QRS complex (called a delta wave), representing atrial-to-ventricular conduction via the accessory pathway. Patients with the WPW syndrome are prone to a variety of supraventricular tachycardias. The most common form is a narrow complex tachycardia with retrograde P waves on the surface ECG following each QRS complex. This type of SVT is due to a reentrant circle where the anterograde (atrium to ventricle) conduction is through the normal AV node-His bundle axis, and retrograde conduction from the ventricles to the atria is through the accessory pathway. A less common but more dangerous arrhythmia in WPW syndrome occurs when patients develop atrial fibrillation. Because the accessory pathway cannot filter atrial impulses as well as the AV node, this constellation of atrial fibrillation and WPW can result in excessive ventricular rates and may precipitate ventricular fibrillation. In clinically stable patients, intravenous procainamide can be used; unstable patients must undergo immediate electrical cardioversion.

Atrial Fibrillation

Atrial fibrillation is the most common sustained dysrhythmia that occurs both with and without structural heart disease (Table 15-16).[240] It represents rapid and chaotic atrial activity with an irregular and rapid ventricular response. Atrial fibrillation (AF) can be classified as valvular as it frequently accompanies mitral stenosis, MR, or prosthetic heart valves. Nonvalvular AF may accompany a structurally normal heart (lone AF), hypertensive heart disease, cardiomyopathy, and a wide variety of other clinical conditions. In AF, the chaotic atrial activity results in ineffective atrial contraction and in stasis of blood within the left atrium and left atrial appendage. This stasis may lead to thrombus formation and markedly increases the risk of embolic events, including cerebral and peripheral embolization. In patients with atrial fibrillation, embolic stroke occurs in 1.6 to about 18% of patients per year, and the risk increases with increasing age, comorbidities, and CVD.[241] The highest risk of embolic stroke is that of patients with valvular AF. In nonvalvular AF, a history of previous TIA or stroke, age above 75, significant hypertension, systolic heart failure, and diabetes are major clinical risk factors. Frequently, younger patients with

brief episodes of paroxysmal AF are treated with antiplatelet drugs such as acetylsalicylic acid (ASA) because the risk of stroke is low; however, anticoagulation with warfarin is typically used in older patients and in those who have one or more of the listed high-risk characteristics.[241] The CHADS2 and CHA2DS2-VASc scoring systems are most widely used to estimate individual risks of stroke in patients with AF, and to guide stroke prevention.[242–245] With scores ≥2, anticoagulation is indicated. A number of trials have shown that warfarin use is associated with a 45%–82% reduction in the risk of stroke in patients with chronic AF.[246,247]

In many patients with a first episode of atrial fibrillation, the cardiologist will usually make an attempt to restore and maintain normal sinus rhythm.[248,249] In patients who have had atrial fibrillation for more than 48 hours or uncertain duration, cardioversion can be performed either following three to four weeks of anticoagulation with warfarin at a therapeutic INR, or following a transesophageal echocardiogram that did not reveal a clot in the left atrium or left atrial appendage.[250] Following cardioversion, anticoagulation needs to be continued for at least four more weeks because clots can still form during this period. After the four-week period, the ongoing requirement for anticoagulation is dictated by the CHADS2 or CHA2DS2-VASc score.[245]

In patients with recurrent paroxysmal or persistent atrial fibrillation, there are two treatment options available. These include rate control vs. rhythm control.[251] The rate control strategy makes no attempt at restoration or maintenance of sinus rhythm but simply tries to achieve an asymptomatic or minimally symptomatic condition by controlling the heart rate with beta-blockers, calcium-channel blockers (verapamil, diltiazem) and/or digoxin.[252] Those patients are good candidates for the rate control strategy in whom the success rate of maintaining sinus rhythm is estimated to be relatively low because of advanced age, underlying structural heart disease or a long history of atrial fibrillation, and in those who are tolerating AF well without significant symptoms. In younger patients without significant structural heart disease ("lone AF") and in those patients who poorly tolerate even a rate-controlled AF, a rhythm control strategy is usually chosen. Several studies have shown an overall similar clinical outcome with rate control and rhythm control, especially in the elderly.[253] Younger patients probably have better outcomes with rhythm control.[253,254]

When a rhythm control strategy is chosen, maintaining sinus rhythm can be attempted with antiarrhythmic drug therapy or with "curative" catheter ablation. In experienced centers, catheter ablation for atrial fibrillation has been shown to be more effective than antiarrhythmic drug therapy, although this claim has been recently challenged.[255,256] In addition, the efficacy of this procedure is much lower than the success rate of ablation for other supraventricular tachycardias.[257] Catheter ablation for AF is typically a lengthy procedure that is associated with possible complications.[258]

Ventricular Tachycardia and Fibrillation

Ventricular tachycardia (VT) and ventricular fibrillation (VF) typically occur in patients with structural heart disease of the LV, such as those with CAD, various forms of dilated cardiomyopathy, and hypertrophic cardiomyopathy. Rarely, VT may occur as an idiopathic event in an individual with a structurally normal heart or may originate in the right ventricle as in the case of arrhythmogenic right ventricular dysplasia. VF may occur in the setting of acute ischemia and infarction, in dilated and hypertrophic cardiomyopathy, and as a result of a variety of drug and electrolyte effects. VF caused sudden death. The percentage of patients successfully resuscitated is very low.

Patients with sustained VT and resuscitated VF typically require a thorough evaluation for the underlying structural or functional abnormality. Prevention of subsequent episodes may be achieved by treating the underlying cause. If such a cause is found, patients with structurally normal hearts and a history of clinically stable VT may undergo antiarrhythmic drug therapy trials. Beta-blockers appear to be the safest and most effective class of medications for this indication.[259] Patients who had a hemodynamically unstable VT or resuscitated VF, on the other hand, typically undergo implantation of a cardioverter-defibrillator (ICD). ICDs are also frequently implanted for primary prevention in patients who never had a VT or VF event but who are at a high risk for sudden arrhythmic death. Patient populations who may be candidates for an ICD for primary prevention (prophylactic ICD) include those with a remote history of MI and a left ventricular ejection fraction of 30% or less, and patients with either ischemic or nonischemic cardiomyopathy and an EF of 30-35% despite optimum medical therapy.[260,261]

PERMANENT PACEMAKERS

Permanent cardiac pacing is used in a wide variety of cardiac conditions, including symptomatic heart block and bradycardia, brady-tachy syndrome, carotid hypersensitivity, neurocardiogenic syncope and, heart failure. Single (typically ventricular) or dual chamber (atrial and ventricular) models are typically employed. Guidelines for the implantation of cardiac pacemakers have been established by the American College of Cardiology and the AHA joint task force on the basis of available evidence in the medical literature.[262,263]

Dental Management Considerations for Patients with Heart Failure

Implanted devices, such as cardiac pacemakers and implantable cardioverter-defibrillators (ICDs), are increasingly important in the management of heart failure and the prevention of sudden death from arrhythmias. The severity and type of a patient's arrhythmia will govern dental care considerations.[264] For example, it's important to know the nature of the arrhythmia and if the arrhythmia is symptomatic. If the patient has syncope or near syncope, or sustained periods of irregular rhythm, the patient needs medical attention. In particular, patients with severe supraventricular tachycardia should only be treated after consultation with the patient's cardiologist. Patients with atrial fibrillation may have an associated heart murmur and be taking anticoagulant medications to prevent thromboembolic events. It is also important to know if the patient has an implanted device such as pacemaker or defibrillator. Dental treatment modifications for patients with defibrillators or pacemakers are of little concern. According to the AHA, no antibiotic prophylaxis is indicated for patients with pacemakers or other implantable cardiovascular devices, unless the patient presents with an acute odontogenic infection.[11] Furthermore, an in-vivo study suggested that modern pacemakers are not influenced by any type of dental equipment, including high-speed rotary instruments or even the proximity of ultrasonic baths.[265]

Dental Management Considerations for Cardiac Transplantation

The major concerns for this patient population are life-long immunosuppression and their current cardiac status. The impact of immune suppression on the risks for and from oral infection, and the risk for infections distant from the mouth from a bacteremia are unclear, but likely exaggerated. The focus for immunosuppression for these patients is on lymphocytes, rather than leukocytes, and lymphocytes have less to do with suppression of infection due to oral bacterial species. Immunosuppression is maintained at a higher level in the first 6 months following transplantation, during which there may be more of a concern for bacteremia from an invasive dental procedure.

Valve damage can result from catheterization for heart muscle biopsy for evidence of rejection and this places these patients in a group recommended for antibiotic prophylaxis for specific dental procedures (Tables 15-11–15-13).

Patients with a heart transplant may be anticoagulated with warfarin, and if so, they should be tested for INR to ensure that they are not above or below the intended therapeutic range. They are then managed similarly to other anticoagulated patients.

These patients might be best managed by having dental treatment after, rather than before cardiac transplantation, depending on their overall medical status and the nature of the indicated dental treatment. A severely compromised patient in cardiac failure is likely at greater risk from dental treatment of any kind before transplantation, in spite of the concern for post-transplant procedure-related bacteremia in the presence of immunosuppression. Avoid elective treatment with less stable patients, and any dental treatment during a rejection episode. These patients should also be watched for oral complications or side effects from medications, for example: xerostomia, oral candidiasis (secondary to steroids); and cyclosporine-induced gingival hyperplasia.

CASE #1

Nicolas Alejandro is a 57-year-old financial planner referred to our office by his cardiologist for evaluation of a longstanding toothache, and for comprehensive dental care. He has not taken his antihypertensive medication for "several weeks."

HPI: About two weeks ago, he had a gradual onset of pain in the right maxilla, which radiates to the temporal region on that side. The pain has increased since that time such that he has not slept in two days and has had nothing by mouth except liquids for the past 24 hrs. He is taking acetaminophen without any relief. He states that his face on the right side feels "puffy" this morning.

PMH: (1) Hypertension since age 25, poorly controlled due to suboptimal adherence to prescribed medications. (2) Coronary artery disease. Cardiac catheterization performed three years ago for atypical angina revealed a 60% occlusion of the proximal portion of the left anterior descending coronary artery. The left ventricular ejection fraction was normal at 55%. Medical management with aspirin, long-acting metoprolol, and simvastatin was recommended. He has been partially compliant with this regimen. Over the last two months, he experienced substernal chest pain radiating to the left arm and jaw after about two blocks of level walking. The chest pain is associated with mild shortness of breath and diaphoresis; it is relieved with sublingual nitroglycerin. He denies ever having resting chest pain.

PDH: The patient states that he has had infrequent and only emergent dental care in the past, most recently for extraction of three teeth about six months ago.

ROS: As outlined in his PMH. In addition, he complains of 3-pillow orthopnea and occasional paroxysmal nocturnal dyspnea for the last few months. He has occasional palpitations with dizzy spells. He denies syncope.

EXAMINATION

HR: 92/min, regular. BP: 175/105 mm Hg. He appears comfortable, in no acute distress. He is not diaphoretic.

Extra oral: The only significant finding is a mild, diffuse swelling in the right, mid-maxillary area, which is mildly erythematous and feels warm to the touch.

Intraoral: The tongue, hard and soft palate, labial and buccal mucosa, floor of mouth, and pharynx are all normal appearing and without lesions, masses, or other abnormalities. He has 25 remaining teeth, all with moderate to severe gingival swelling and erythema. He has plaque and calculus throughout. Multiple teeth have deep caries or are root tips.

ASSESSMENT

This 57-year-old man with CAD, recent-onset class 2-3 exercise-induced angina, and poorly controlled hypertension. He has an abscess of his maxillary right first molar, which now involves the temporal region. He will likely need multiple other teeth removed at some point in the future.

PLAN

1. Discussed Mr. Alejandro today with his cardiologist who would like to evaluate him before any elective dental treatment. He is likely to perform a stress tests and/or cardiac catheterization followed by a percutaneous coronary intervention (balloon angioplasty with stenting) if appropriate. He would also like to optimize Mr. Alejandro's medication regimen for a better control of hypertension. Hydrochlorothiazide (HCTZ) and an ACE-inhibitor will likely be added to the current regimen.
2. Penicillin 500 mg four times a day for seven days. Ibuprofen 600 mg every four to six hours as needed for pain for the next two to three days until his spontaneous pain resolves.
3. To return to our office for extraction of this tooth as soon as possible, when his BP is within target range and when he is cleared by his cardiologist. Will consider sedation for invasive or stressful procedures.

DISCUSSION

This patient clearly should not, at this time, have what is an elective procedure and one that is invasive and at least somewhat stressful. His infection and pain should be well controlled with antibiotics and analgesics until a more extensive medical workup can be performed. If his angina were a symptom of the past and his hypertension were well controlled, he could have all of his dental care performed now, in an outpatient office setting. On the other hand, uncontrolled or crescendo angina and hypertension above 170/100 mm Hg require medical stabilization prior to dental procedures or, if the dental procedure is urgent, treatment in a hospital setting.

CASE #2

Ian Lucas is a 52-year-old carpenter, recently retired, referred to me by his cardiologist for dental evaluation prior to receiving a prosthetic cardiac valve for severe, symptomatic mitral regurgitation.

HPI: Although he has no acute dental problems at this time, he lost a large restoration from a lower posterior tooth last week, and has not had his teeth cleaned in over a year.

PMH: Mr. Lucas was found to have a loud systolic murmur 5 years ago and was diagnosed with mitral regurgitation from rheumatic heart disease. Initially, he was completely asymptomatic with a normal left ventricular size and systolic function. In the last two to three months, he experienced progressive dyspnea on exertion, three-pillow orthopnea, and occasional paroxysmal nocturnal dyspnea. Cardiac catheterization revealed clean coronaries, and confirmed severe mitral regurgitation with reduced left ventricular systolic function and moderate pulmonary hypertension. The patient has no history of atrial fibrillation. Current medication regimen includes furosemide (a diuretic), lisinopril (an ACE-inhibitor), and carvedilol (a beta-receptor blocker frequently used in patients with heart failure). His symptoms have improved since initiation of this regimen and he has been clinically stable.

PDH: Mr. Lucas has had routine dental care up until one year ago when he became disabled from his cardiac condition.

ROS: As outlined in the PMH. In addition, he has occasional ankle swelling, nocturia, and fatigue. He experiences rare, fleeting palpitations.

EXAMINATION

HR: 82/min, regular. BP: 128/74 mm Hg. He appears to be slightly tachypneic when he talks, along with cyanosis. A cursory cardiac exam reveals a loud systolic murmur over the cardiac apex.

Extra oral: No swellings, lesions, or other abnormalities.

Intraoral: The tongue, hard and soft palate, labial and buccal mucosa, floor of mouth, and oropharynx are all normal appearing and without lesions, masses, or other abnormalities. He has 28 remaining teeth, all well restored with the exception with the maxillary left first molar that is missing a large amalgam restoration, and which has obvious recurrent caries. His gingivae are of normal size and coloration, with 4–5 mm pocketing in several of his posterior teeth.

ASSESSMENT

This 52-year-old man with minor and routine restorative and periodontal needs. Cardiac surgery (mitral valve replacement) is planned in the near future. He has been appropriately managed and has well compensated chronic heart failure. He is not anticoagulated at this time.

PLAN

Discuss Mr. Lucas's medical status with his referring cardiologist. We need to know the degree of cardiac compromise at this point with regard to completing his dental treatment now versus deferring until sometime after his valve replacement. From the medical history, it appears that his cardiac status is stable. If this is confirmed by the cardiologist, it may be preferable to complete the dental treatment before the implantation of a prosthetic heart valve. A delay in the dental procedure until after surgery, however, is also reasonable.

DISCUSSION

It is important to know if this patient will get a mechanical vs. biological valve. Most patients with biological heart valves are anticoagulated only for the first three months following surgery. Mechanical heart valves in the mitral position, however, typically require long-term and a relatively high degree of warfarin anticoagulation with target INR levels ranging from 2.5–4.0. Moderately invasive dental and oral surgical dental procedures can be safely performed at these INR levels if no other coagulopathies exist. Highly invasive oral surgical procedures in patients with INRs above 3.5 may require slight adjustment of the warfarin anticoagulation. This potential but rarely needed bridging of the surgical period with subcutaneous low molecular weight heparin should be discussed with the cardiologist. After implantation of a prosthetic heart valve, the patient will be at higher risk from infective endocarditis. Any invasive dental treatment will require antibiotic prophylaxis.

388 ■ Burket's Oral Medicine

Selected Readings

Anderson JL, Adams CD, Antman EM, et al. 2012 ACCF/AHA focused update incorporated into the ACCF/AHA 2007 guidelines for the management of patients with unstable angina/non-ST-elevation myocardial infarction: a report of the American College of Cardiology Foundation/American Heart Association Task Force on Practice Guidelines. *Circulation*. 2013;127(23):e663-e828.

Anderson JL, Halperin JL, Albert NM, et al. Management of patients with atrial fibrillation (compilation of 2006 ACCF/AHA/ESC and 2011 ACCF/AHA/HRS recommendations): a report of the American College of Cardiology/American Heart Association Task Force on Practice Guidelines. *J Am Coll Cardiol*. 2013;61(18):1935–1944.

Bonow RO. Chronic mitral regurgitation and aortic regurgitation: have indications for surgery changed? *J Am Coll Cardiol*. 2013;61(7):693–701.

Chatterjee S, Sardar P, Lichstein E, et al. Pharmacologic rate versus rhythm-control strategies in atrial fibrillation: an updated comprehensive review and meta-analysis. *Pacing Clin Electrophysiol*. 2013;36(1):122–133.

Chen S, Yin Y, Krucoff MW. Should rhythm control be preferred in younger atrial fibrillation patients? *J Interv Card Electrophysiol*. 2012;35(1):71–80.

Chinitz JS, Halperin JL, Reddy VY, Fuster V. Rate or rhythm control for atrial fibrillation: update and controversies. *Am J Med*. 2012;125(11):1049–1056.

Coppens M, Eikelboom JW, Hart RG, et al. The CHA2DS2-VASc score identifies those patients with atrial fibrillation and a CHADS2 score of 1 who are unlikely to benefit from oral anticoagulant therapy. *Eur Heart J*. 2013;34(3):170–176.

Cosedis NJ, Johannessen A, Raatikainen P, et al. Radiofrequency ablation as initial therapy in paroxysmal atrial fibrillation. *N Engl J Med*. 2012;367(17):1587–1595.

Deedwania PC, Carbajal E. Evidence-based therapy for heart failure. *Med Clin North Am*. 2012;96(5):915–931.

Desai CS, Bonow RO. Transcatheter valve replacement for aortic stenosis: balancing benefits, risks, and expectations. *JAMA*. 2012;308(6):573–574.

DeSimone DC, Tleyjeh IM, Correa de Sa DD, et al. Incidence of infective endocarditis due to viridans group streptococci before and after publication of the 2007 American Heart Association's endocarditis prevention guidelines. *Circulation*. 2012;126(1):60–64.

Douketis JD, Spyropoulos AC, Spencer FA, et al. Perioperative management of antithrombotic therapy: Antithrombotic Therapy and Prevention of Thrombosis, 9th ed: American College of Chest Physicians Evidence-Based Clinical Practice Guidelines. *Chest*. 2012;141(suppl 2):e326S-e350S.

Findler M, Elad S, Kaufman E, Garfunkel AA. Dental treatment for high-risk patients with refractory heart failure: a retrospective observational comparison study. *Quintessence Int*. 2013;44(1):61–70.

Go AS, Mozaffarian D, Roger VL, et al. Executive summary: heart disease and stroke statistics–2014 update: a report from the american heart association. *Circulation*. 2014;129(3):399–410.

Homma S, Thompson JL, Pullicino PM, et al. Warfarin and aspirin in patients with heart failure and sinus rhythm. *N Engl J Med*. 2012;366(20):1859–1869.

Hong C, Napenas JJ, Brennan M, et al. Risk of postoperative bleeding after dental procedures in patients on warfarin: a retrospective study. *Oral Surg Oral Med Oral Pathol Oral Radiol*. 2012;114(4):464–468.

Ionescu-Ittu R, Abrahamowicz M, Jackevicius CA, et al. Comparative effectiveness of rhythm control vs rate control drug treatment effect on mortality in patients with atrial fibrillation. *Arch Intern Med*. 2012;172(13):997–1004.

James PA, Oparil S, Carter BL, et al. 2014 evidence-based guideline for the management of high blood pressure in adults: report from the panel members appointed to the Eighth Joint National Committee (JNC 8). *JAMA*. 2014;311(5):507–520.

Lackland DT. Hypertension: Joint National Committee on Detection, Evaluation, and Treatment of High Blood Pressure guidelines. *Curr Opin Neurol*. 2013;26(1):8–12.

Lane DA, Lip GY. Use of the CHA(2)DS(2)-VASc and HAS-BLED scores to aid decision making for thromboprophylaxis in nonvalvular atrial fibrillation. *Circulation*. 2012;126(7):860–865.

Liu SS, Monti J, Kargbo HM, et al. Frontiers of therapy for patients with heart failure. *Am J Med*. 2013;126(1):6–12.

Lockhart PB, Blizzard J, Maslow AL, et al. Drug cost implications for antibiotic prophylaxis for dental procedures. *Oral Surg Oral Med Oral Pathol Oral Radiol*. 2013;115(3):345–353.

Lockhart PB, Bolger AF, Papapanou PN, et al. Periodontal disease and atherosclerotic vascular disease: does the evidence support an independent association?: a scientific statement from the American Heart Association. *Circulation*. 2012;125(20):2520–2544.

Lockhart PB. Antibiotic prophylaxis for dental procedures: are we drilling in the wrong direction? *Circulation*. 2012;126(1):11–12.

Lockhart PB. Outpatient management of the medically compromised patient. In: Lockhart PB, ed. *Oral Medicine and Medically Complex Patients*. 6th ed. Hoboken, NJ: Wiley-Blackwell; 2013:33–149.

Mason PK, Lake DE, DiMarco JP, et al. Impact of the CHA2DS2-VASc score on anticoagulation recommendations for atrial fibrillation. *Am J Med*. 2012;125(6):603.e1–603.e6.

Merie C, Kober L, Skov OP, et al. Association of warfarin therapy duration after bioprosthetic aortic valve replacement with risk of mortality, thromboembolic complications, and bleeding. *JAMA*. 2012;308(20):2118–2125.

Mitka M. Groups spar over new hypertension guidelines. *JAMA*. 2014;311(7):663–664.

Murray CJ, Vos T, Lozano R, et al. Disability-adjusted life years (DALYs) for 291 diseases and injuries in 21 regions, 1990–2010: a systematic analysis for the Global Burden of Disease Study 2010. *Lancet*. 2012;380(9859):2197–2223.

Pan A, Sun Q, Bernstein AM, et al. Red meat consumption and mortality: results from 2 prospective cohort studies. *Arch Intern Med*. 2012;172(7):555–563. Stergiopoulos K, Brown DL. Initial coronary stent implantation with medical therapy vs medical therapy alone for stable coronary artery disease: meta-analysis of randomized controlled trials. *Arch Intern Med*. 2012;172(4):312–319.

Raymond C, Cho L, Rocco M, Hazen SL. New cholesterol guidelines: worth the wait? *Cleve Clin J Med*. 2014;81(1):11–19.

Rimoldi SF, Scherrer U, Messerli FH. Secondary arterial hypertension: when, who, and how to screen? *Eur Heart J* 2014;35(19):1245-54.

Sawaya F, Stewart J, Babaliaros V. Aortic stenosis: who should undergo surgery, transcatheter valve replacement? *Cleve Clin J Med*. 2012;79(7):487–497.

Shah RU, Freeman JV, Shilane D, et al. Procedural complications, rehospitalizations, and repeat procedures after catheter ablation for atrial fibrillation. *J Am Coll Cardiol*. 2012;59(2):143–149.

Skaar D, O'Connor H, Lunos S, et al. Dental procedures and risk of experiencing a second vascular event in a Medicare population. *J Am Dent Assoc*. 2012;143(11):1190–1198.

van Diermen DE, van dW, I, Hoogstraten J. Management recommendations for invasive dental treatment in patients using oral antithrombotic medication, including novel oral anticoagulants. *Oral Surg Oral Med Oral Pathol Oral Radiol*. 2013;116(6):709–716.

Weber MA, Schiffrin EL, White WB, et al. Clinical practice guidelines for the management of hypertension in the community a statement by the american society of hypertension and the international society of hypertension. *J Hypertens*. 2014;32(1):3–15.

For the full reference lists, please go to http://www.pmph-usa.com/Burkets_Oral_Medicine.

CHAPTER 16

Diseases of the Gastrointestinal Tract

Michael A. Siegel, DDS, MS, FDS, RCSEd

Lynn W. Solomon, DDS, MS

Lina M. Mejia, DDS

This chapter is intended to review diseases affecting the gastrointestinal tract, with an emphasis on the medical aspects, the dentist's role as a primary health care professional in screening for undiagnosed conditions, and the dentist's role in monitoring patient compliance with recommended medical therapy for gastrointestinal conditions that are likely to be encountered in the general practice of dentistry. Oral health care professionals (OHCPs) are expected to recognize, diagnose, and treat oral conditions associated with gastrointestinal diseases, as well as provide dental care for afflicted individuals. To provide safe and appropriate dental care, dentists are typically concerned with the proper diagnosis of oral manifestations of gastrointestinal disorders, homeostasis, risk of infection, drug actions and interactions, the patient's ability to withstand the stress and trauma of dental procedures, and, when necessary, proper medical referral. These dental management issues are discussed, where appropriate, for each gastrointestinal disorder.

Both OHCPs and gastroenterologists have their primary focus within the alimentary canal. The embryologic origin of the oral cavity is from the ectoderm layer and the embryologic origin of the gastrointestinal tract is the endoderm layer; initially, they are separated by the buccopharyngeal membrane. However, their common function as the alimentary canal is occasionally reinforced for the clinician when a heterotopic gastric mucosal cyst is found in the oral mucous membranes or on the tongue.[1] However, in addition to these relatively rare anomalies, the paths of gastroenterologists and dentists cross quite frequently in clinical practice. The digestive tract is a long muscular tube that moves food and accumulated secretions from the mouth to the anus. As ingested food is slowly propelled through this tract, the gut assimilates calories and nutrients that are essential for the establishment and maintenance of normal bodily functions. Protein, fats, carbohydrates, vitamins, minerals, water, and orally ingested drugs (prescription and nonprescription) are digested in this tract. This digestive process depends on the hydrolysis of large nonabsorbable molecules into smaller absorbable molecules through secreted enzymes and the absorption of substances through the epithelial lining of the digestive tract. From there, digested substances are transported by blood vessels and lymphatic channels through the body. The remaining contents of undigested food, typically cellulose fiber, are excreted out of the digestive tract through the rectum and anus. The digestion and absorption of nutrient materials depend on (1) an optimal hydrogen ion concentration (pH) in the gut; (2) the presence of conjugated bile salts; (3) adequate concentrations of enzymes to split fats, proteins, and carbohydrates; (4) adequate intestinal mobility; and (5) a normal gut microbiome.

Some of the foods entering the blood from the digestive tract can be used by cells without being altered. However, the majority of the absorbed food passes to special organs, where it is changed into new substances that are needed by cells. One such special organ is the liver, where this intermediate metabolism takes place. Additionally, the gastrointestinal tract is a primary route for drug administration, absorption, biotransformation, detoxification, and excretion. Many dental patients require drug therapy in which pharmacokinetic parameters may be altered by gastrointestinal and hepatobiliary dysfunction. Consequently, OHCPs must have a comprehensive understanding of the gastrointestinal system and of how normal and abnormal function may affect the oral health care of patients.

Digestion normally begins with ingestion of material into the oral cavity, moistening with saliva, mastication, and swallowing of the bolus by coordinated muscular function of the tongue, pharynx, and epiglottis. The digestive system is composed of the esophagus, stomach, small intestine, and large intestine. Each of these components performs specific functions as ingested substances move through the different anatomic areas. Additionally, the exocrine functions of the salivary glands, pancreas, liver, and gallbladder combine to complete the assimilation of dietary calories and nutrients.

This chapter is organized such that disorders are presented under the following anatomic divisions: esophagus, stomach, small intestine, large intestine, and hepatobiliary tree. A final section on gastrointestinal syndromes introduces disorders that affect both the oral cavity and the gastrointestinal tract but that are not primarily of oral or gastrointestinal etiology.

DISEASES OF THE UPPER DIGESTIVE TRACT

Gastroesophageal Reflux Disease

Medical Aspects

Gastroesophageal reflux disease (GERD) is one of the most commonly occurring diseases affecting the upper gastrointestinal tract. The incidence of GERD is increasing in the developed world; upward of 10% of the population experience heartburn daily.[2] Symptoms can range from mild to severe.

There is no difference between the percentage of men and the percentage of women who are affected by GERD. GERD is a disease that has a significant effect on activities of daily living as well as an economic effect on individuals and society.

During gastroesophageal reflux, gastric contents (chyme) passively move up from the stomach into the esophagus. Although this can occur normally, it may be attributed to GERD if it is associated with symptoms. GERD is often considered a syndrome because it can present with a wide variety of symptoms. Patients may experience mild symptoms with an esophagus that appears to be clinically normal, or they may have severe symptoms with surface abnormalities that can be detected with an endoscope. A presumptive diagnosis of GERD may be made for any symptomatic condition that is the result of gastric contents moving into the esophagus. Functional bowel disease is also known as irritable bowel syndrome, may have similar symptoms and mimic GERD. It is unclear if these are manifestations of a single disease spectrum or an overlap of two different conditions.[2]

Heartburn is the cardinal symptom of GERD and is defined as a sensation of burning or heat that spreads upward from the epigastrium to the neck.[3] Although symptoms of GERD can be quite varied, they are primarily symptoms that are associated with the sequelae of mucosal injury. These resultant injuries include esophagitis, esophageal ulceration, stricture, and dysplasia. Chest pain is another important symptom that is related to disorders of the esophagus. Chest pain can mimic the symptoms of an acute cardiovascular disorder and is often the impetus for patients seeking medical care. Dysphagia is also a common presenting complaint that may serve to prompt the dentist to refer the patient to the patient's physician. Several studies have shown that a number of airway problems that were previously thought to be idiopathic, such as laryngitis, chronic cough, hoarseness, and asthma, are, in fact, the result of microaspiration of refluxate into the airway.[4,5] This constellation of symptoms is known as laryngopharyngeal reflux (LPR), or extraesophageal reflux disease (EERD). Alternatively, these symptoms may also arise from disorders of the upper or lower respiratory tracts. GERD complications include premalignant and malignant conditions of the esophagus.

Barrett's esophagus is a variant of GERD in which normal squamous epithelium is replaced by columnar epithelium.[6] Patients with this phenomenon show an increased incidence of adenocarcinoma. This condition may increase the incidence of carcinoma by as much as 10%.[7] However, it has become clear that the majority of patients with Barrett's esophagus die from causes not related to adenocarcinoma of the esophagus.[8,9] The major reason to evaluate patients with chronic symptoms of GERD is to recognize Barrett's esophagus. The factors of gender, race, and age can be used to determine the threshold for endoscopy in patients with GERD to screen for the presence of Barrett's esophagus. The highest yield of Barrett's esophagus would be expected in white men with chronic symptoms of GERD. Endoscopic screening is recommended for patients with multiple risk factors for cancer in Barrett esophagus, including chronic GERD, hiatal hernia, advanced age, male sex, white race, cigarette smoking, and obesity with an intra-abdominal body fat distribution. During the last decade, new techniques have been introduced for diagnosis of GERD and Barret's esophagus.[10]

The relaxation of the lower esophageal sphincter for the purpose of relieving pressure in the stomach (from gas and the ingestion of food) is called the "burp" mechanism. This phenomenon is a normal process and occurs only when a person is in an erect posture; gastric contents are thereby prevented from flowing into the esophagus and possibly being aspirated. The gastroesophageal junction, which prevents the regurgitation (retrograde or upward flow) of gastric contents, is composed of an internal lower esophageal sphincter. External pressure on the junction by the diaphragm also assists in this function. When this barrier fails, gastric contents may make their way into the esophagus and cause symptoms. The cause of lower esophageal sphincter incompetence is unknown; however, it does not appear to be mechanical. Hiatal hernia was historically recognized as a cause of GERD, but there is no correlation between sphincter pressure and the presence of a hiatal hernia, which leads to the widely accepted position that GERD is not caused by hiatal hernia. Surgery, scleroderma, and drugs such as anticholinergics, cardiac vasoconstrictors, and nicotine can also cause an incompetent sphincter. Estrogen-progesterone combinations used in contraceptives and during pregnancy also have been shown to decrease sphincter pressures.

Symptoms occur when refluxate proceeds through the junction. The severity of the symptoms depends on the amount of acid in the refluxate, the speed with which the esophagus can clear the refluxate, and the presence of buffering agents, such as swallowed saliva. An insufficient amount of alkaline fluid prohibits the esophagus from properly buffering the acid that has moved up from the stomach. Patients who smoke, take certain drugs, have had head and neck radiation, or suffer from diseases such as Sjögren's syndrome often do not produce enough saliva to protect the esophagus from the acid in the refluxate. Increased abdominal pressure as a result of obesity, pregnancy, or a large meal may predispose patients to gastric content reflux. Moving into or out of various positions (e.g., lying down too soon after eating) will also promote reflux.

Medical Management

Significant success in preventing or reducing the symptoms of GERD is seen with lifestyle modification. Weight loss reduces the pressure difference between the abdomen and the thorax, thereby reducing reflux. Smoking cessation will increase the production of saliva and therefore counteract the symptoms of GERD. Fatty meals slow down gastric emptying and produce distention and reflux. An increase in the fat content of meals may be an important factor in explaining the increase of reflux in the Western world in recent years. Eating large meals and reclining too soon after meals also predispose individuals to reflux disease. Sleeping with the head of the bed elevated may help empty the esophagus of any refluxate and may prevent symptoms.

Since the mid-1970s, H_2 receptor antagonists have been used to treat GERD and ulcer disease. In patients with GERD, H_2 receptor antagonists improve the symptoms of heartburn and regurgitation and heal mild to moderate esophagitis. Symptoms have been eliminated in up to 50% of patients by twice-a-day prescription dosages of H_2 receptor antagonists. Approximately 50% of patients require higher or more frequent doses to promote the healing of esophagitis. Only about 25% of patients will remain in remission while taking these agents only.

Proton pump inhibitors (PPIs) such as omeprazole, (also available OTC) esomeprazole, lansoprazole, pantoprazole and rabeprazole, are available by prescription, and have been found to heal erosive esophagitis more efficaciously than do H_2 receptor antagonists. PPIs provide not only symptomatic relief but also resolution of signs, including those that involve significant ulcers and/or esophageal damage.[11] Studies have shown that PPI therapy can provide complete endoscopic mucosal healing of esophagitis at six to eight weeks in 75%–100% of cases. Daily PPI treatment provides the best long-term reduction of symptoms for patients with moderate to severe esophagitis. Remission for as long as five years has been seen.

Once relatively rare and reserved for patients who had failed every form of medical treatment, antireflux surgical procedures are now common and are considered part of the regular armamentarium by those who treat this disease.[12–14] Patients with a good initial response to medical therapy but who have severe functional and anatomic abnormalities of the gastroesophageal junction are the ones who are most commonly treated with surgery.

Oral Health Considerations

Patients who experience GERD may complain of extra-esophageal symptoms including, laryngitis, asthma, cough, chest pain, dental erosion, dysgeusia(foul taste), halitosis, tongue sensitivity, burning sensations, dental sensitivity related to hot or cold stimuli, and/or pulpitis.[15] Erosion is the chemical dissolution of enamel which may lead to exposed dentin and thermal sensitivity. On occasion, if the erosion is severe, irreversible pulpal (nerve) damage may result that requires root canal therapy. Tooth wear is multifactorial, and it is rarely possible to identify a single etiology in a specific patient.[16] Occlusal function causes attrition and erosion may be exacerbated by inadequate oral hygiene, salivary adequacy, acidic beverages or foods, occupation, alcoholism, and eating disorders. The presence of erosion and attrition is particularly harmful and demands active intervention. Dentists should closely monitor GERD patients and be proactive at treating dental erosion. Patients with erosion on palatal and lingual surfaces should be questioned for a history of heartburn and reflux and, if they have not been evaluated regarding these symptoms, referred to their primary care physician. Factors that determine whether an individual with GERD will or will not develop dental erosion have not been clearly identified. The strength and prevalence of the association between dental erosion and GERD is highly variable.[17] No relationship between GERD and changes in the oral cavity can be established through the use of saliva tests. However, a significantly lower oral pH was found in patients with gastroesophageal reflux disease and bulimia nervosa as compared to healthy individuals.[18] Mild baking soda mouthrinses may be swished and expectorated to minimize dysgeusia due to acid reflux. Dental management should provide topical fluoride applications using custom-made occlusive tray delivery in order to ensure optimal dental mineralization and reduction of thermal sensitivity. The dentist can restore tooth structure destroyed by gastric acid erosion in order to provide comfort and esthetics and to minimize further hard tissue damage. It is preferable to institute oral preventive measures at the earliest possible time in order to minimize the need for extensive dental restoration.

Medical therapy can affect the dental management of patients with GERD in a number of ways. Patients taking cimetidine or other H_2 receptor antagonists may experience a toxic reaction to lidocaine (or other amide local anesthetics) if the anesthetic is injected intravascularly.[19] Cimetidine also has been shown to inhibit the absorption and, therefore, the blood concentration of azole antifungal drugs such as ketaconazole via the potent inhibition of the cytochrome P-450 3A4 (CYP3A4) enzyme system. Soft tissue changes such as esophageal stricture and fibrosis may complicate intubation if the patient requires general anesthesia for an oral maxillofacial procedure. Oral mucosal changes are minimal; however, erythema and mucosal atrophy may be present as a result of chronic exposure of tissues to acid. Mild sodium bicarbonate rinses may again be useful if mild signs of stomatitis are present.

H_2 receptor antagonists may also cause central nervous system effects in a continuum from fatigue and lethargy to confusion, delirium, and seizures. These effects are dose dependent; thus, they may be seen more commonly in elderly persons or in those with impaired kidney or liver function.

Hiatal Hernia

Medical Aspects

The esophagus passes through the diaphragmatic hiatus and into the stomach just inferior to the diaphragm. The hiatus causes an anatomic narrowing of the opening into the stomach and thus helps prevent reflux of stomach contents into the esophagus. Some patients have a weakened or enlarged hiatus, perhaps due to hereditary factors. It may also be caused by obesity, exercising (e.g., weight lifting), or chronic straining when passing stools. When a weakened or enlarged hiatus occurs, a portion of the stomach herniates into the chest cavity through this enlarged hole, resulting in a hiatal

hernia. Hiatal hernias are quite common; occurrence rates of between 20% and 60% have been reported in the medical literature.[20] The incidence of hiatal hernia increases with age, although the condition is also seen in infants and children. Because the diaphragm separates the thorax from the abdomen, symptoms of hiatal hernia often include chest pain, which may radiate in patterns similar to those of myocardial infarction pain. If the hiatal hernia is small, there may be no symptoms. On the other hand, if the area of the hiatus is very weak, the function of preventing reflux may be compromised, resulting in the entry of acidic digestive juices into the esophagus.

Hiatal hernias are classified into three major types.[20] The sliding type is the most common. In this type, the herniated portion of the stomach slides back and forth through the diaphragm into the chest. These hernias are normally small and often present with minimal (if any) symptoms. In the fixed type of hiatal hernia, the upper part of the stomach is fixed through the diaphragm into the chest. There may be few symptoms with this type as well. However, the potential for problems in the esophagus increases. The complicated type is the most serious and least common form of hiatal hernia. This form includes a variety of herniation patterns of the stomach, including those in which the entire stomach moves into the chest. The likelihood of significant medical problems with this type is high; its treatment requires surgery.

Infants with hiatal hernia usually regurgitate blood-stained food and may also have difficulty in breathing and swallowing. Adult patients with hiatal hernia may experience chronic acid reflux into the esophagus. Chronic gastrointestinal reflux can erode the esophageal lining, causing bleeding, which may lead to anemia. Additionally, chronic esophageal inflammation may produce scarring, resulting in esophageal narrowing. This narrowing causes dysphagia, and because food does not pass easily into the stomach, patients experience an uncomfortable feeling of fullness or "bloating." Adults typically present with heartburn that is exacerbated when bending forward or lying down. The pain may spread to the jaw and down the arms, similar to an attack of angina pectoris. Other symptoms include hiccups, a dry cough, and an increase in the contractile force of the heart. In contrast to abdominal hernias, hiatal hernias have no outward physical signs. Diagnosis is made through a combination of endoscopy and contrast radiography.

Medical Management

Defects present at birth may sometimes correct themselves. Until this occurs, however, the infant should sleep in a crib with the head raised and be given an altered diet consisting of food that has a thicker-than-normal consistency. With adults, anything that will increase abdominal pressure and cause reflux, such as bending, abdominal exercises, and tight belts and girdles, should be avoided. Because obesity increases intra-abdominal pressure, weight loss may be recommended to relieve symptoms. Sleeping with the upper body elevated will also prevent the symptoms of hiatal hernia. Antacids help relieve heartburn by neutralizing stomach acids. H_2 receptor antagonists are effective in inhibiting the action of histamine on parietal cells, which reduces the production of gastric acids.[11] Patients should also eat smaller and more frequent meals and should have their main meal at lunchtime. This should be followed by a light supper, with nothing being consumed within two to three hours of bedtime. Foods and habits that increase the reflux of acid should be avoided or significantly reduced. These foods or habits include nicotine (tobacco products), alcohol, caffeine, chocolate, fatty foods, and peppermint or spearmint oil flavorings.

Drug therapy usually allows patients to avoid all symptoms of hiatal hernia without significant inconvenience. The disadvantage to this approach is that many patients object to taking daily medications for the rest of their lives or find the process too onerous to carry out. When conservative medical measures fail to control the condition, the hernia is surgically corrected. However, surgical correction is complex, and nonsurgical remedies are preferable.[21] Surgery is currently considered to be a treatment of last resort, and some authors argue that surgery is never indicated for a hiatal hernia. Surgical access is gained either through the chest or through the abdomen. These approaches carry high risks of operative and perioperative morbidity. Recent surgical advances have made it possible to do the repair laparoscopically.[22]

Oral Health Considerations

If a hiatal hernia is treated with medications that cause xerostomia (dry mouth), the dose or drug type may need to be altered by the patient's physician. Various treatment modalities for dry mouth, such as artificial saliva, alcohol-free mouthwashes, or increased fluid intake, may need to be prescribed. Class V caries, or root caries, are sequelae of dry mouth, even in patients who have been relatively free of caries prior to developing the disease. If reflux into the oral cavity is present, oral manifestations that are the same as those of GERD may be present.

DISEASES OF THE LOWER DIGESTIVE TRACT

Disorders of the Stomach

The stomach serves primarily as a secretory organ and as a reservoir. The stomach secretes acid, mucus, pepsinogen, and intrinsic factor. The secreted hydrochloric acid is essential for killing swallowed bacteria while the mucus helps coat and lubricate the stomach's lining epithelium in order to propel the ingested contents through the digestive system. Pepsinogen is a proteolytic enzyme that helps digest protein, and intrinsic factor is a glycoprotein that permits the adequate absorption of dietary vitamin B_{12}. The stomach collects food that is often ingested in bursts and then slowly, over time, empties the chyme—the semifluid mass of partly digested food—into the duodenum.

Peptic Ulcer Disease

Peptic ulcer disease (PUD) is a common benign (nonmalignant) ulceration of the epithelial lining of the stomach (gastric ulcer) or duodenum (duodenal ulcer). When patients or physicians refer to stomach ulcers or ulcer disease, they are usually referring to a gastric or duodenal ulcer. PUD is highly associated with *Helicobacter pylori* and the use of nonsteroidal anti-inflammatory drugs (NSAIDs) and aspirin; in populations without these risk factors the incidence of PUD is very low.[23] In the United States, PUD has a significantly negative effect on patients quality of life, activity, and overall work productivity; although it is uncommonly a direct cause of mortality, estimated at 2,956 deaths in 2008.[24] Since PUD includes both gastric (stomach) and duodenal ulcers, a general discussion of PUD is presented first, followed by specific information on gastric and duodenal ulcers, under the corresponding anatomic region.

PUD represents a serious medical problem largely because of its frequency; there are approximately 500,000 new cases and 4,000,000 recurrences each year in the United States, responsible for 2.7 million physician office visits.[25] The total estimated annual cost for treatment of patients with PUD is US$3.1 billion).[26] Beginning in the 1970s, the frequency of inpatient and ambulatory care for PUD declined 51%, and from 1993–2005 the rate declined 68%.[26] However, it is likely that the growing geriatric population in the United States, coupled with the increasing use of NSAIDs that have inherent damaging effects on the gastroduodenal mucosa, will contribute to increasing costs of this disease.

Data indicate that the lifetime prevalence of peptic ulcers ranges from 11%–14% for men and 8%–11% for women. The one-year point prevalence of active gastric and duodenal ulcers in the United States is about 1.8%.[27] Genetic factors appear to play a role in the pathogenesis of ulcers. The concordance for peptic ulcers among identical twins is approximately 50%. In first-degree relatives of ulcer patients, the lifetime prevalence of developing ulcers is about threefold greater than that in the general population.[27]

Within the last two decades, it has become accepted that gastric ulcers primarily result from altered mucosal defenses, whereas duodenal ulcers are associated with increased acid production. It has become clear that *H. pylori* plays a vital role in peptic ulcer development at both sites. A complex relationship exists between host defense mechanisms, the presence of elevated acid, pepsin levels, and *H. pylori*. Paradoxically chronic infection with H. pylori is common, occurring in approximately half of the world's population. Infection is typically acquired early in life, especially among those in lower socioeconomic groups.[28] Although H. pylori infection results in chronic inflammation of the underlying gastric mucosa, the vast majority of infected patients do not experience any clinically significant symptoms.

The incidence of duodenal ulcers increases in cigarette smokers, patients with chronic renal disease, and alcoholics. *H. pylori* is observed in the gastric mucosa in 90%–100%

of patients with duodenal ulcers and 70%–90% of patients with gastric ulcers. Consequently, it has been proposed that the bacteria may be the cause of both the gastritis and the reduced mucosal resistance that leads to ulcer formation in the stomach. It is noteworthy that healing of peptic ulcers of either the stomach or duodenum is usually facilitated by specific antimicrobial treatment and by the elimination of this bacterium.[29]

Many patients with duodenal ulcers have demonstrable hyperacidity, and it is thought that this is the dominant factor in the development of ulcer disease. Concomitant inflammation and chronic infection with *H. pylori* are noted in the non–acid secreting gastric antrum causing increased gastrin release, which in turn induces excess acid secretion from the fundic mucosa and damage and ulceration of the duodenal mucosa.[28] In gastric ulcers, however, the relative importance of the two major factors of acid amounts and mucosal resistance is reversed. Typically, the concentration of gastric acid is normal or reduced, and prior injury (mucosal) from other causes appears to be a prerequisite for the development of gastric ulcers.

Most patients with the disease have recurrent pain and consult their physician periodically for relief of symptoms and to prevent recurrence. About 10%–20% of these patients have a life-threatening complication (i.e., hemorrhage, perforation, or obstruction).[30] Failure to recognize and manage these patients properly on these occasions can have grave consequences. Since about 6% of the patients attending a dental office will have a peptic ulcer, it is essential that dentists (1) recognize the morbidity associated with peptic ulcers and the symptoms associated with undiagnosed or poorly managed PUD and (2) make a referral to the primary care physician or gastroenterologist when these symptoms are recognized.

It is important to discuss gastric and duodenal ulcers separately because each has implications for dentists and the patients they treat.

Medical Aspects

Gastric ulcers are only one-tenth to one-fourth as frequent as duodenal ulcers. They are also more common in lower socioeconomic groups. Gastric ulcers occur more often after 50 years of age and are seen at a male to female ratio of 3:1. Gastric ulcers are generally of more concern because approximately 3%–8% of gastric ulcers represent malignant ulceration of the gastric mucosa.[30] In addition, gastric ulcers with *H. pylori* infection are associated with increased risk for mucosa-associated lymphoid tissue lymphomas (MALT). Some patients with early-stage MALT lymphoma may experience remission after use of antibiotics to eradicate the bacteria.[31]

Therefore, accurate diagnosis requires multiple biopsies and brush specimens for cytologic examination. These additional diagnostic tests are often performed by a gastroenterologist. In general, the diagnostic procedures are the same as those performed in cases of duodenal ulcers, except that the diagnosis is more urgent and additional diagnostic studies

other than gastroscopy are warranted. It is essential to ascertain gastric acidity levels with ulcers of the stomach because a stomach ulcer in the presence of histamine-fast achlorhydria has a very high chance of being a malignant ulcer rather than a peptic ulcer.

Patients with gastric ulcers often present with epigastric pain radiating to the back. In contrast to the symptoms of duodenal ulcers, the pain is aggravated by food. The management and the treatment of gastric ulcers are similar to those of duodenal ulcers, except that gastric ulcers are usually diagnosed and treated more vigorously. Follow-up studies to document the healing process are essential for gastric ulcers. Nevertheless, the standard medical treatment of gastric ulcers involves antacid compounds, antibiotics to eradicate *H. pylori*, H_2 blocking agents, and other protective drugs. Additional information about PUD and management in the dental office is presented in the following section on duodenal ulcers.

Disorders of the Intestines

The small intestine comprises the duodenum, jejunum, and ileum. The duodenum is the principal site of digestion and absorption. When chyme enters the duodenum, it stimulates the pancreas to secrete sodium bicarbonate (to neutralize the gastric acid) and to secrete digestive enzymes for normal digestion of food. Additionally, chyme in the duodenum stimulates the gallbladder to discharge stored bile through the common bile duct. Vitamin B_{12} in the presence of intrinsic factor is absorbed in the distal small intestine (ileum). The bile acids that promote fat absorption in the duodenum are themselves also reabsorbed in the small bowel, returned to the liver, and resecreted into the bile. The motor activity of the small intestine propels the chyme forward to the large intestine. The major role of the large intestine is to receive the ileal effluent, absorb most of the water and salt, and thus produce solid feces.

Duodenal Ulcer Disease

Medical Aspects

A duodenal ulcer represents a break through the mucosa into the submucosa or deeper. The base of the ulcer is necrotic tissue consisting of pus and fibrin. When the ulcer erodes into an adjacent blood vessel, there is hemorrhage. If erosion continues through the serous outer layer of the duodenum, involvement of adjacent organs or perforation into the peritoneal cavity occurs. When conditions are favorable, the ulcer heals, with granulation tissue and new epithelium. If the ulcer is present for prolonged periods, it becomes associated with scar tissue and possible deformity.

The incidence of duodenal ulcer is thought to be declining, but it is still a common disorder developing in about 10% of the US population. Of all peptic ulcers, 80%–85% are duodenal, and duodenal ulcers occur at a male to female ratio of 4:1. The most common primary cause is *H. pylori* infection, but NSAID use can also be an associated etiologic factor. Less commonly, factors such as stress, exogenous glucocorticosteroids, parathyroid disease, malignant carcinoid, cirrhosis, gastrinoma of the pancreas (Zollinger-Ellison disease), polycythemia vera, and chronic lung disease have been associated with duodenal ulcers.[28] The ulceration is usually located in the first part of the duodenum because the acidic chyme ordinarily becomes alkaline after pancreatic secretions enter the intestines in the second part of the duodenum.

The most common symptom of an uncomplicated ulcer is epigastric pain. The pain is often perceived as a burning or gnawing sensation sometimes associated with nausea and vomiting and usually occurs when the stomach is empty or when not enough of a meal remains in the stomach to adequately buffer the acid stimulated by the meal. Therefore, the pain often begins one or more hours after eating and when the patient is asleep. The pain is characteristically relieved within a few minutes by buffering or diluting the gastric acid with ingestion of an antacid, milk, food, or even water. Once an individual has had a duodenal ulcer, the chance of recurrence is high. Frequently, these attacks will occur with a change of season, especially in spring or autumn. When an ulcer perforates and hemorrhages, the patient often vomits gross blood. When the blood interacts with acid, it can appear as coffee grounds. Also, the stools can appear black or tar-like or may sometimes contain gross blood. The blood loss can lead to iron deficiency anemia, and if the blood loss is acute, the patient may be weak, lightheaded, and short of breath.

Physical examination is usually of little use in the diagnosis of duodenal ulcers. The early diagnostic cues are based on the history of a periodic pain pattern. Duodenal ulcers usually feel better postprandially, and the pain of gastric ulcers is frequently exacerbated by meals. The mainstay of the diagnosis of a duodenal ulcer is an upper gastrointestinal radiologic examination, which will demonstrate the presence of an ulcer in up to 85% of patients. In this procedure, the patient swallows a barium salt that outlines the lumen and mucosal surface of the gastrointestinal tract and thereby demonstrates any disruption of the mucosal surface. Endoscopy is an acceptable and sometimes preferable means of diagnosis. If the ulceration is too superficial to be detected by a gastrointestinal radiologic examination or if a gastric ulcer with the possibility of malignancy is suspected, endoscopy is recommended.[32] The presence of H. pylori can be demonstrated by biopsy if endoscopy is used. Serologic tests and tests that detect the presence of labeled carbon dioxide in the breath after oral administration of labeled urea are available.[28]

In cases of Zollinger-Ellison syndrome caused by a gastrinoma of the pancreas, specific determination of the etiology is necessary because this disease is treatable and is particularly severe, causing multiple ulcers and debilitating diarrhea. The tumor of Zollinger-Ellison syndrome secretes gastrin, a potent acid producer, and the diagnosis is made on the basis of extremely high levels of gastric acid and elevated levels of serum gastrin.[33] The usual laboratory tests include a complete blood count for detecting anemia and leukocytosis, an examination of the stool for occult blood, and a serum calcium test for detecting an occasional elevation from an associated hyperparathyroidism or endocrine tumors with Zollinger-Ellison syndrome.

Medical Management

In the absence of complications such as massive bleeding, obstruction due to scarring, and perforation, medical rather than surgical treatment is preferred. Obviously, foods that cause discomfort to the patient should be avoided. Substances or drugs that have potent acidogenic properties with little ability to neutralize acid should be avoided; among these are alcohol, tobacco, aspirin, and NSAIDs. If NSAIDs cannot be avoided, the patient should also be treated with misoprostol. Attempts to eradicate H. pylori are necessary in all patients with a peptic ulcer in which the organism can be demonstrated. Bismuth, metronidazole, amoxicillin, and tetracycline have been shown to be effective.[32] In addition to the drugs used to eliminate H. pylori, medical treatment involves the following six other classes of drugs: (1) sedatives to reduce mental stress if anxiety is thought to be etiologic; (2) antacids to neutralize acid; (3) drugs that act by covering and protecting the ulcer; (4) anticholinergic drugs to decrease the production of acid by the gastric mucosa; (5) histamine H_2 receptor antagonists (cimetidine, famotidine, nizatidine, or ranitidine), which block the action of histamine on the gastric parietal cells, thus reducing food-stimulated acid secretion up to 75%; and (6) omeprazole, which also suppresses gastric acid secretion but which has a different mechanism of action from that of anticholinergics or H_2 receptor antagonists. Antacids and dietary changes are the mainstays of therapy. Anticholinergics are sometimes prescribed, particularly for reducing acid production at night. However, limited effectiveness and side effects such as mouth dryness make anticholinergics less attractive than histamine H_2 receptor antagonists. In most patients, the pain is controlled within one week, and most ulcers heal by the sixth week. Intractable symptoms or complicated duodenal ulcers may require surgery.[33]

Oral Health Considerations

If a patient presents with symptoms of epigastric pain, as described previously, the dentist should refer this person to the primary care physician for diagnostic workup. Oral manifestations of PUD are rare unless there is severe anemia from gastrointestinal bleeding or persistent regurgitation of gastric acid as a result of pyloric stenosis that leads to dental erosion, typically of the palatal aspect of the maxillary teeth. Vascular malformations of the lip have been reported and range from a very small macule to a large venous pool.[34,35] H. pylori has been islolated from dental plaque implicating the oral cavity as a potential source of this organism which is responsible for both PUD and gastric cancer.[36] A study of patients with recurrent aphthous stomatitis (RAS) who tested positive for H. pylori showed that eradication therapy was effective in reducing the number and intensity of RAS recurrences.[37] Oral health status may play a role in PUD of the stomach as low salivary secretion may contribute to the decrease in efficacy of *H. pylori* eradication from the stomach in some patients treated with certain drug regimens.[38]

Aggravation of the PUD might be minimized by avoidance of actions that increase the production of acid. Thus, lengthy dental procedures should be avoided or spread out over shorter appointments to minimize stress. To avoid aspirations, patients should not be left in a supine or subsupine position for lengthy periods during dental appointments. Dentists should avoid administering drugs that exacerbate ulceration and cause gastrointestinal distress such as aspirin and other NSAIDs. Instead, acetaminophen products should be recommended. Additionally, because many of the antacids contain calcium, magnesium, and aluminum salts that bind antibiotics, such as erythromycin and tetracycline, dentists should remember that administering one of these drugs within one hour of antacid therapy may decrease the absorption of the antibiotic as much as 75%–85%. Consequently, erythromycin and tetracycline should be taken one hour before or two hours after ingestion of antacids. Exogenous steroid administration is likely to exacerbate the ulcer because of the increased production of acid caused by the steroid and should be avoided. Although it is generally good policy to prescribe penicillin V instead of penicillin G (because of the destruction of penicillin G by gastric acid), it is essential with patients who have peptic ulcers.[39]

Hyposalivation and dry mouth (xerostomia) are common complaints in patients taking anticholinergic drugs. Patients who wear either complete or partial dentures are particularly troubled by oral dryness. Denture adhesives and artificial saliva may aid in the retention of their dental prostheses. Dentate patients are at an increased risk of dental caries if the hyposalivation is prolonged or if the patient places sugar-containing candies or antacids into the mouth in an effort to stimulate saliva flow. In these cases, dental management is prudent to ensure that appropriate preventive measures are instituted. Medical management of PUD often includes the use of medications that may cause xerostomia. If the patient specifically complains of dry mouth, it may be possible to alter the specific drug type or dosage in consultation with the patient's physician. Various therapeutic modalities for dry mouth are available, such as artificial saliva, alcohol-free mouth rinses, or increased fluid intake. Class V (root) caries are sequelae of dry mouth, even in patients who have been relatively caries free prior to the disease. Commonly used sialogogues, such as pilocarpine or cevimeline, may be contraindicated due to their parasympathomimetic action. If reflux into the oral cavity is present, referral to the dentist for restorative dental therapy is indicated.[19,40]

Prior to extensive oral surgical or periodontal procedures, physicians should be consulted in order to ascertain the patient's serology, especially if the patient has had a history of ulcer perforation and subsequent hemorrhage resulting in anemia. Delayed healing and risk of bacterial infection, particularly anaerobic bacterial infection due to tissue hypoxia, and the potentially grave side effects of respiratory depression induced by narcotic analgesics are examples of such associated oral surgical risks in the chronically anemic gastrointestinal patient. Cimetidine and ranitidine, drugs commonly prescribed for duodenal ulcer patients, have occasionally been associated with thrombocytopenia and may compete with antibiotics or antifungal medications.[19]

Inflammatory Bowel Disease

Inflammatory bowel disease (IBD) is a general classification of inflammatory processes that affect the large and small intestines. Ulcerative colitis and Crohn's disease together make up IBD. Since many other intestinal diseases with known etiologies also have an inflammatory basis, it has been suggested that Crohn's disease and ulcerative colitis should more appropriately be designated as idiopathic IBD. Ulcerative colitis involves the mucosa and submucosa of the colon. Crohn's disease or regional enteritis is an inflammatory condition involving all layers of the gut. The precise etiology and pathogenesis of ulcerative colitis and Crohn's disease are unknown, and the two diseases share many features. Accordingly, the diagnostic separation of these two disorders often depends on the results of the radiographic, endoscopic, and histologic examinations. The two conditions are presented separately in this chapter since the management and prognosis of each may be different.

The medical and dental literature is replete with articles describing extra-abdominal and oral signs of IBDs, including pyostomatitis vegetans, chronic stomatitis, aphthous ulcerations, cobblestone appearance of the oral mucosa, oral epithelial tags and folds, gingivitis, persistent lip swelling, lichenoid mucosal reactions, granulomatous inflammation of minor salivary gland ducts, candidiasis, and angular cheilitis.[41–53] Current dental literature focuses on the oral status of IBD patients with regard to the potential use of thalidomide and biologics such as infliximab against tumor necrosis factor α (TNFα) for the treatment of recalcitrant oral granulomatous lesions, caries rate, salivary antimicrobial proteins, and infections of bacterial and fungal origins.[54–63] In fact, it is accepted that oral manifestations of IBD may precede the onset of intestinal radiographic lesions by as much as one year or more.[47,64] Both diseases are of interest to the dentist because of their associated oral findings and the impact of their medical management, particularly the use of glucocorticosteroids on dental management.

Once IBD is established, patients may suffer episodic acute attacks during the chronic disease progression. As a result, the patient is likely to suffer from disabling disease for decades. The annual incidence of ulcerative colitis in North America is 19.2 cases per 100,000 person-years; for Crohn's disease the annual incidence is 20.2 cases per 100,000 person-years.[65] Incidence rates for both diseases are higher in urban areas than in rural areas. Crohn's disease occurs less frequently than ulcerative colitis, but both are slightly on the rise.[23–33,65] In North America, the prevalence of ulcerative colitis is 249 per 100,000 person-years and the prevalence of Crohn's disease is 319 per 100,000 person-years.[65] Overall, both diseases show three peak prevalence rates. The first and highest peak occurs between the ages of 20 and 24 years, the second at ages 40–44 years, and the third at ages 60–64 years. By the age 60 years, the incidence of ulcerative colitis far exceeds that of Crohn's disease. Northern European and English women appear to have a 30% increased risk of developing ulcerative colitis or Crohn's disease. IBD more frequently affects Caucasians, and Ashkenazi Jews, especially those originating in Middle Europe, Poland, or Russia, exhibit a particularly high IBD risk.[23–33]

Ulcerative Colitis

Medical Aspects

The inflammation in ulcerative colitis may affect all or part of the large intestine. Macroscopically, the mucosa may have a granular appearance if the disease is mild. When fulminant, the disease may include stripping of the mucosa, with areas of sloughing, ulceration, and bleeding. As the superficial mucosal lesions enlarge, they may be perpetuated by secondary bacterial invasion.[23–33] Ulcerative colitis remains a disease of unknown etiology. Despite intense interest in possible bacterial, viral, immunologic, and psychological factors, there has been no firm etiology established. Although much has been written about psychological factors associated with IBD, most gastroenterologists no longer accept the idea that the disease is primarily a psychiatric disorder. Rather, the frequent psychiatric problems experienced by patients are a result of the disease, not the cause of it. The accumulating body of experimental and clinical evidence strongly suggests that IBD results from a dysregulated immune response to components of the normal gut flora in genetically susceptible individuals, with sensitization and destruction of the colonic mucosa.[62]

The hallmark of ulcerative colitis is rectal bleeding and diarrhea. The frequency of bowel movements and the amount of blood present reflect the activity of the disease. Typically, the diarrhea is severe, possibly five to eight bowel movements in 24 hours. Patients usually complain of pain that is in both abdominal quadrants and that is crampy in nature and exacerbated prior to bowel movement. Along with the change in the pattern of bowel movements, the patient may have nocturnal diarrhea. Extraintestinal manifestations may be prominent. Erythema nodosum, characterized by red swollen nodules that are usually on the thighs and legs, may be present. Eye changes such as episcleritis, uveitis, corneal ulcers, and retinitis may cause pain and photophobia. Joint symptoms occur in up to 20% of patients with the disease, usually affecting the ankles, knees, and wrists. Perhaps the most pernicious complication of ulcerative colitis is liver disease. Although other extraintestinal manifestations usually undergo remission with control of the colon inflammation, liver disease may continue, and the dentist must recognize this risk. Anemia is commonly associated with ulcerative colitis. It is most likely caused by blood loss and is typically a microcytic hypochromic anemia of iron deficiency. Leukocytosis occurs in active disease and is usually associated with intra-abdominal abscess. Electrolyte imbalances, hypoalbuminemia, and low serum magnesium and potassium levels may occur because of the severe diarrhea.[23–33]

Medical Management

Diagnosis of ulcerative colitis is made on the basis of careful history, physical examination, gastrointestinal radiography, and endoscopy, which involves direct visualization of the intestinal mucosa. Most important is the sigmoidoscopic examination, which usually reveals the characteristic picture of multiple tiny mucosal ulcers covered by blood and pus. Lacking any specific markers, the diagnosis of ulcerative-colitis is essentially one of exclusion.[26]

The therapy for ulcerative colitis is aimed at reducing the inflammation and correcting the effects of the disease. Sulfasalazine is used to initiate and maintain a remission in ulcerative colitis. Its active moiety, 5-aminosalicylate, has a direct anti-inflammatory effect on intestinal tissues without altering the colon flora. Corticosteroids and corticotropin (adrenocorticotropic hormone [ACTH]) are used in patients who have not responded satisfactorily to sulfasalazine. They are administered in high doses (e.g., 40–60 mg of oral prednisone daily initially and then maintenance doses of 10–20 mg of prednisone daily). Immunosuppressive agents such as azathioprine, cyclosporine, and mercaptopurine are being used, with varying results. Because of the risk of hematologic suppression and superinfection in patients taking these medications, they are reserved for patients who have not responded to traditional medical therapy. Approximately 15%–20% of patients will receive surgery for intractable disease. Proctocolectomy combined with ileostomy is a curative procedure for ulcerative colitis. With the new disposable ileostomy equipment available today, most patients can look forward to an active lifestyle and normal life expectancy.[23,26] Recent advances in understanding of the human gut microbiota in health and disease have led to investigation of fecal and synthetic microbiome transplants as promising therapies for intestinal dysfunctions associated with perturbation of the gut microbiome.[62,63]

Oral Health Considerations

Due to the symptoms of severe frequent diarrhea and abdominal pain or cramping, it is unlikely that a patient will be seeking routine dental care with undiagnosed ulcerative colitis. Nonetheless, should an undiagnosed patient attend a dental office for care, then the risks associated with anemia, such as delayed healing, an increased risk of infection, the side effects of narcotic analgesics, and depression of respiration, may collectively contraindicate surgical treatment until the disease is under control. Obviously, following a history and a thorough examination, signs and symptoms of ulcerative colitis and/or anemia would warrant a referral to the patient's primary care physician. More likely is the situation of a diagnosed and medically managed patient attending a dental office for routine or episodic oral health care. The following section addresses those issues an OHCP should be knowledgeable about when treating patients with ulcerative colitis.

The oral changes that occur in ulcerative colitis cases are nonspecific and uncommon, with an incidence of less than 8%. Aphthous stomatitis of the major and minor variety has been reported in patients with active ulcerative colitis. There is nothing unique about these lesions, and it has been suggested that their appearance is coincidental.[35] However, they may result from nutritional deficiencies of iron, folic acid, and vitamin B_{12} due to poor absorption in the gut and/or blood loss directly related to the ulcerative colitis. In addition, anti-inflammatory medications such as the 5-aminosalicylates, which often represent the mainstay of therapy for IBD patients and which are excreted in saliva, are known to cause recurrent aphthous ulcers in some patients.[66–68] In patients who are prone to develop aphthous ulcers, the appearance of a new crop of oral ulcers often heralds a flare-up of the bowel disease. Other nonspecific forms of ulceration associated with skin lesions have been reported. Pyoderma gangrenosum may occur in the form of deep ulcers that sometimes ulcerate through the tonsillar pillar.[44] Pyostomatitis vegetans, a purulent inflammation of the mouth, may also occur. These oral lesions are characterized by deep tissue vegetating or proliferative lesions that undergo ulceration and then suppuration. As the lesions disappear with a total colectomy, it is speculated that these manifestations are due to the effects of circulating immunocomplexes induced by antigens that are derived from the gut lumenor the damaged colonic mucosa.[44] Finally, ulcerative colitis patients also can develop hairy leukoplakia, a lesion more commonly associated with human immunodeficiency virus (HIV) disease. This lesion probably serves as a marker of severe immunosuppression and may result from the use of corticosteroids or other immunosuppressive agents.[69] Medical management for ulcerative colitis may necessitate alterations of dental therapy or special precautions. Sulfasalazine interferes with folate metabolism, and supplemental folic acid may be needed, especially if a macrocytic anemia is revealed in a complete blood count.

Medical management of ulcerative colitis may necessitate alterations of dental therapy. A number of oral health care considerations are related to the therapeutic use of glucocorticosteroids. These are the many side effects associated with the use of corticosteroids and ACTH, including hypertension and hyperglycemia. Obtaining a blood pressure reading and a blood glucose measurement by finger prick in the office and/or consultation with the treating physician to understand the patient's current medical status is highly recommended. Long-term glucocorticosteroid therapy may also cause osteoporosis and vertebral compression fractures; thus, carefully positioning the patient in the dental chair and encouraging the patient to take dietary calcium supplements may help prevent fractures.

Chronic use of glucocorticosteroids can also result in adrenal suppression. Major operative or surgical procedures can precipitate adrenal insufficiency if the glucocorticosteroid dosing is not adjusted properly. Patients undergoing surgery may require supplemental glucocorticosteroids before and after the procedure because their own adrenal response to stress is blunted. Patients who were formerly on glucocorticosteroid therapy may also experience adrenal suppression. Routine maintenance dental therapy such as cleanings or simple restorations should be unaffected by steroid or immunosuppressive therapy.[19] Consultation with the patient's physician is warranted prior to surgical procedures.

Ulcerative colitis can be associated with chronic bleeding. Prior to dental procedures, blood studies that include hemoglobin, hematocrit, and a red blood cell count should be undertaken to rule out the presence of anemia. Patients taking the immunosuppressive agent azathioprine may suffer from additional side effects that impact dental management. Patients on azathioprine might be expected to have changes in white and red blood cell counts, and total and differential white blood cell counts should be ascertained before embarking on surgical procedures. Suppression of the liver can be expected, and liver function tests should be completed in those patients who will receive dentist-prescribed medications that are metabolized in the liver. Abnormal liver function tests should be discussed with the attending dentist who might need to prescribe analgesic or antibiotic medications that are metabolized in the liver. Typically, patients taking an immunosuppressive agent such as azathioprine are monitored by their primary care physician with liver function tests. Consequently, consultation with the patient's physician will help the dentist determine the patient's liver function. Obviously, toxic doses of the same drugs may be reached if reduced drug metabolism is not taken into consideration. Patients who have extensive bowel surgery may suffer from malabsorption of vitamin K, vitamin B_{12}, and folic acid. Before any surgical procedures are completed, these patients should be evaluated for both macrocytic and microcytic anemia and bleeding disorders from insufficient levels of vitamin K (fibrin clot formation). Clotting factors II, VII,IX, and X are all dependent on vitamin K. A prothrombin time/international normalized ratio (INR) and a partial thromboplastin time will provide information about the patient's ability to form a blood clot.

Crohn's Disease
Medical Aspects

Crohn's disease is an inflammatory disease of the small or large intestine. The inflammation involves all the layers of the gut. Gross examination may reveal mucosal ulceration (aphthous ulcers within the mucosa that appear normal, deep ulcers within areas of swollen mucosa, or long linear serpiginous ulcers). Recent epidemiologic evidence suggests that there are two forms of Crohn's disease: a non-perforating form that tends to recur slowly and a perforating or aggressive form that evolves more rapidly. Patients with the aggressive perforating type are more prone to develop fistulae and abscesses, whereas the more indolent non-perforating type tends to lead to stenotic obstruction.[23-33] With the involvement of either the colon or small intestine, microscopic examination reveals inflammatory infiltrate in all layers of affected bowel, with plasma cells and lymphocytes predominating in the lamina propria.

Crohn's disease shares many epidemiologic features with ulcerative colitis. There has been a steady rise in the incidence and prevalence of Crohn's disease, but no clear correlation exists between the increased incidence and environmental or lifestyle changes. Crohn's disease affects all ages and both sexes and occurs most frequently in urban women aged 20–39 years. The prevalence of Crohn's disease among first-degree relatives is 21 times higher than that among non-relatives. Evidence for familial association in Crohn's disease includes increased incidence in Jewish populations, strong familial aggregation, and increased concordance among monozygotic twins or triplets.[23-33]

The cause and evolution of Crohn's disease are unknown. The single strongest risk factor for Crohn's disease, overpowering any influences of diet, smoking, stress, or hygiene, is having a relative with the disease. The fact that first-degree relatives of Crohn's disease patients exhibit increased intestinal permeability supports the theory of an inheritable permeability defect in Crohn's disease. This abnormal intestinal barrier could result in the increased uptake of injurious materials and/or enhanced immune reaction to intestinal antigens. Other theories have included vascular disease, lymphatic obstruction, and emotional stress. Whatever the process, tiny erosions of the overlying normal mucosal lymphoid tissues eventually coalesce to form small aphthous-like ulcers or more diffuse ulceration of the mucosa. With progression, there is marked hyperplasia of the lymphoid tissue extending through the wall, fibrosis, and muscular hypertrophy leading to constrictures, and inflammatory tracts. Granulomas are present in about 50% of patients.[23-33]

The clinical presentation of Crohn's disease depends on the extent of inflammation and on the site of intestinal involvement. The usual presentation is that of a young person in the late teens or twenties who has been ill for an indefinite period and whose disease suddenly worsens. The history often reveals intermittent episodes of abdominal distress, fever, and crampy abdominal pain accompanied by loose stools. Although bleeding is a prominent feature of ulcerative colitis, it is rare in cases of small bowel Crohn's disease.[26]

Inflammation of the small intestine may impair its absorption of vital nutrients. Calcium, iron, and folate are absorbed in the duodenum, and their decreased absorption due to inflammation can lead to deficiencies. Disease in the terminal ileum may interfere with the absorption of bile salts and vitamin B_{12}. Inflammation of the small or large intestines may impair the absorption of fat, fat-soluble vitamins, salt, water, protein, and iron.

The absorptive function of the small bowel is more likely to be altered in patients with Crohn's disease than in those with ulcerative colitis. Electrolyte abnormalities and low albumin levels commonly occur in cases of severe diarrhea. Anemia, usually resulting from an iron or folate deficiency, may also be present. Leukocytosis, cell counts of $>15,000/cm^3$, is suggestive of abscess or perforation.

The signs and symptoms of Crohn's disease are often more subtle than those associated with ulcerative colitis, frequently delaying the diagnosis. However, the diagnosis can usually be made on the basis of a careful history, physical examination, and diagnostic testing. The most reliable and sensitive method for differentiating between ulcerative colitis and Crohn's disease is a colonoscopy with endoscopically directed colonic biopsies. The following features distinguish Crohn's disease from ulcerative colitis: (1) involvement of the small intestine or the upper part of the alimentary canal; (2) segmental disease of the colon, with "skip" areas of normal rectum; (3) the appearance of fissures or sinus tracts; and (4) the presence of well-formed sarcoid-type granulomas.[23-33]

In the case of ulcerative colitis, the signs and symptoms of disease are rather dramatic, and it is unlikely that a patient would attend a dentist's office with untreated disease. The probabilities are greater that someone with undiagnosed Crohn's disease could visit the dentist. Consequently, a thorough history and examination may uncover signs and symptoms of this inflammatory bowel disease, in which case, a referral to the primary care physician is warranted. The associated risks of proceeding with dental care in a patient with undiagnosed Crohn's disease are essentially the same as those described for patients with ulcerative colitis. Anemia, vitamin K–dependent blood clotting disorders, and general nutritional deficiencies may occur if the diagnosis and treatment of Crohn's disease are delayed.

Oral Health Considerations

Oral lesions, both symptomatic and asymptomatic, affect 6%–20% of Crohn's disease patients. Most oral manifestations of Crohn's disease occur in patients with active intestinal disease, and their presence frequently correlates with disease activity. Recurrent aphthous ulcers are the most common oral manifestation of Crohn's disease.[35,48] It is not clear whether these oral manifestations are true expressions of Crohn's disease, preexisting and/or coincidental findings, direct results of medical treatment, or manifestations of an associated problem, such as anemia. Certainly, pyostomatitis vegetans, cobblestone mucosal architecture, and minor salivary gland duct pathology represent granulomatous changes that constitute the hallmark of Crohn's disease. Biopsy specimens of these multiple small nonhealing aphthous ulcers reveal granulomatous inflammation. Less often, Crohn's disease patients develop diffuse swelling of the lips and face, inflammatory hyperplasias of the oral mucosa with a cobblestone pattern, indurated polypoid tag-like lesions in the vestibule and retromolar pad area, and persistent deep linear ulcerations with hyperplastic margins. Granulomatous lesions have also been observed in the salivary glands, where they may cause rupture of the ducts and localized mucocele formation.

Numerous medications, including anti-inflammatory and sulfa-containing preparations that are commonly used to manage IBD patients, have been reported to cause oral lichenoid drug reactions.[70,71] Superinfection with *Candida albicans* is often associated with IBD and may represent a primary manifestation of the disorder, a reaction to the bacteriostatic effect of sulfasalazine, or an impaired ability of neutrophils to kill this granuloma-provoking organism.[72] Of interest is the possibility that oral lesions may precede the radiologic changes of the disease by up to one year. This underscores the sometimes subtle signs and symptoms of Crohn's disease and the possibility that a dentist may encounter a patient with undiagnosed Crohn's disease. Frequently, patients will complain of pain associated with ulcerative lesions in the oral cavity. Palliative rinses, ointment, and topical steroids may be helpful. There appears to be an increased risk of dental caries that is probably related to dietary changes in patients with IBD.[54,55] The causes of the dental caries and increased incidence of bacterial and fungal infections are multifactorial but appear to be related to either the patient's altered immune status or diet.[54–59]

Oral effects of malabsorption may also be seen. Pallor, angular cheilitis, and glossitis, all oral manifestations of anemia, may occur, particularly in undiagnosed or poorly controlled disease. Nutritional deficiencies that are directly related to the section of the bowel affected by the disease can occur. Malnutrition is often a problem, and monitoring the patient's compliance with dietary supplementation is essential.[35,48]

As with ulcerative colitis, the medical management of a patient with Crohn's disease may require modifications to standard oral health care routines. The underlying assumption of this management change is that patients with IBD are at increased risk for the development of oral infections, including dental caries. Consequently, dental management of patients with IBD should include frequent preventive and routine dental care to monitor oral health and to prevent the destruction of hard and soft tissue. If the patient is taking a systemic glucocorticosteroid, monitoring of blood pressure and evaluation of blood glucose are necessary. A determination needs to be made regarding the need for glucocorticosteroid replacement therapy. This is based on the dosages and length of time of taking glucocorticosteroids and the type of planned dental procedure. Screen, diagnose, and treat any oral inflammatory, infectious, or granulomatous lesions as necessary. Palliative rinses and topical steroid therapy, such as fluocinonide 0.05% gel, may be helpful. Topical steroid therapy should be short term and monitored because of the side effect of mucosal atrophy and systemic absorption. To completely comprehend the medical management of the patient, knowledge of the effects, side effects, and drug interactions of any medications the patient is taking is important and may necessitate a consultation with the patient's physician.

Depending on the results of the consultation with the patient's physician, the following laboratory studies may be indicated before surgical procedures are performed: (1) complete blood count; (2) hematocrit level; (3) hemoglobin level; (4) platelet count; (5) coagulation studies (prothrombin time/INR, and partial thromboplastin time); (6) liver function test; and (7) blood glucose level. Coordination and collaboration with the patient's primary care physician will enhance the overall outcome for the patient.

OHCPs are responsible for treatment of oral manifestations of IBD, particularly if the lesions are symptomatic. Palliative sodium bicarbonate mouthrinses (one-half teaspoon of baking soda in 8 ounces of water) may be used as swish and expectorate. Moderate-potency topical steroid preparations, such as 0.05% fluocinonide, desoximetasone, and triamcinolone, or ultra-potency preparations, such as clobetasol and halobetasol, can be topically applied to the lesions, four times daily (not to exceed two continuous weeks).[19,40] Ointments and creams are useful when the lesions are localized and direct topical application is possible. In cases when lesions are disseminated or oropharyngeal in distribution, dexamethasone elixir 0.5 mg/5 mL can be used as a rinse or gargle for one minute, four times daily, and expectorated. The patient must be advised that prolonged use of topical steroids will result in mucosal atrophy, systemic glucocorticosteroid absorption (especially with the ultra-potency preparations), and an increased incidence of mucosal candidiasis.

IBD patients appear to be at an increased risk of dental caries as well as bacterial and fungal infections. These are multifactorial in etiology but appear to be related to either the patient's altered immune status or diet.[54–59] Oral manifestations of anemia may be noted in patients with ulcerative colitis, especially in undiagnosed or poorly controlled disease. The oral manifestations include pallor, angular cheilitis, and glossitis.

Antibiotic-Induced Diarrhea and Pseudomembranous Enterocolitis

Medical Aspects

In patients who are receiving antibiotic therapy, diarrhea may occur as a result of an alteration of the colonic flora. Often, this condition is mild and subsides when antibiotic therapy is discontinued. Occasionally, a severe disease results with the development of a thick mucosal exudate that has the appearance of a membrane and is termed pseudomembranous enterocolitis. This condition is extremely serious and demands aggressive treatment. Practically, all antibiotics can be associated with this condition. Patients who are debilitated or who have renal failure seem to be at a higher risk of contracting the disease. Recent studies have shown a major role for *Clostridium difficile* in the pathogenesis of antibiotic-produced pseudomembranous enterocolitis. Infections with *C. difficile* account for 10%–25% of cases of antibiotic-associated diarrhea and virtually all cases of antibiotic-associated pseudomembranous colitis.[73]

The type of antibiotic and the route of its administration influence disease incidence. More cases occur when the drug is given orally than when it is administered parenterally. Clindamycin, ampicillin, and the cephalosporins are most commonly associated with antibiotic-associated pseudomembranous colitis, but virtually any antibiotic may produce this disorder. Symptoms typically occur during antibiotic treatment, with the majority occurring within 14 days of antibiotic administration. However, cases have been documented to occur up to three months after antibiotic exposure.[73] Pseudomembranous colitis is known to follow the administration of clindamycin, amoxicillin, or the cephalosporins, all of which are now recommended for antibiotic prophylaxis of infective endocarditis and late prosthetic joint infections. Presumably, the normal colonic flora is inhibited when antibiotics are administered, allowing *C. difficile* to proliferate and produce a cytopathic toxin. The precise mechanism is not known but probably involves both the cytotoxic and vasoconstrictive effects of toxins. The timing is highly variable, with some cases appearing after a single dose and about one-third of cases occurring after the medicine is stopped. About 1–3 of 100,000 individuals who take antimicrobial agents develop *C. difficile* colitis.[26,73] Diarrhea is present in all cases and is associated with colitis and hemorrhage in 20% of cases. Bowel movements may occur every 15–20 minutes. The patient may be febrile and may have lost considerable fluid, electrolytes, and protein. Sigmoidoscopy may reveal mild or severe inflammation, along with yellow raised membranous plaques of exudate. Stool cultures may demonstrate *C. difficile* or may be tested for the enterotoxin.[23–33]

Pseudomembranous colitis is a life-threatening disease, and individuals must be treated aggressively with fluids and electrolyte replacement. Vancomycin, given orally in dosages of 125–500 mg four times daily for 10–14 days, is effective in eliminating *C. difficile* infection. Metronidazole, in doses of 250–500 mg three times daily, is also effective and is less expensive.[23–33] Fecal microbiota transplantation is becoming increasingly accepted as an effective and safe intervention in patients with recurrent disease, likely due to the restoration of a disrupted microbiome. Cure rates greater than 90% are being consistently reported from multiple centers.[74]

Oral Health Considerations

The primary role of the dentist is to recognize the signs and symptoms of antibiotic-associated diarrhea and pseudomembranous colitis in patients who either are taking an antibiotic or have a recent history of an antibiotic regimen. Cessation of the antibiotic and prompt referral to the patient's physician are necessary for definitive diagnosis.

Diseases of the Hepatobiliary system

In this section, the liver, biliary tract, and pancreas are considered together due to their interrelated functions with regard to the digestive system. The liver dominates this group of structures in size and multiplicity of roles. Consequently, the majority of this section focuses on liver disease and dental management in patients with disease or dysfunction.

The liver serves as the major locus of synthetic, catabolic, and detoxifying activities in the body. The intermediary metabolism of all foodstuffs occurs here. The liver is essential in the excretion of heme pigments, and it participates in the immune response. Impairment of the hepatocyte will interfere with the liver's ability to synthesize and store glycogen, a major source of glucose. Should glycogen stores be depleted, liver gluconeogenesis from amino acids is initiated to maintain glucose levels. Lipids are metabolized in the liver to form cholesterol and triglycerides. Cholesterol is the major building block of cell membranes, steroids, and bile salts. Bile salts are essential in the absorption of fat in the small intestine. Proteins, albumin, and clotting factors are synthesized and stored in the liver; specifically, clotting factors I, II, V, VII, IX, and X are synthesized in the liver. Since some of the clotting factors are also dependent on vitamin K (e.g., II, VII, IX, and X), coagulopathy can occur from hepatocyte dysfunction and/or vitamin K malabsorption due to biliary problems. The metabolism of drugs is principally performed by the cytochrome P-450 microsomal enzyme system in the hepatocyte. Local anesthetics, analgesics, sedatives, antibiotics, and antifungals are all metabolized in the liver. Consequently, cautious use of these drugs in a person with liver dysfunction is essential. Lastly, the liver inactivates or metabolizes hormones such as insulin, aldosterone, antidiuretic hormone, estrogens, and androgens. Clearly, liver dysfunction can express itself through multiple signs and symptoms. Liver disease commonly manifests itself through jaundice, and the disease process can lead to liver failure and cirrhosis.[75–83] Accordingly, jaundice and cirrhosis are considered separately below.

Liver disease may be systemic in etiology or due to traumatic injury. Causes of abnormal liver function tests include trauma, viral or chemically induced hepatitis, alcohol intake, nonalcoholic fatty liver disease, autoimmune liver diseases and hereditary diseases such as hemochromatosis, α_1-antitrypsin deficiency, and Wilson's disease. Many patients with liver disease are treated with multi-drug regimens, compounding the problem of liver toxicity. Knowledge of liver involvement in systemic diseases is important for the accurate diagnosis of liver injury and to avoid unnecessary examination and treatment.[84]

Jaundice

Jaundice (or icterus), which is a sign rather than a disease, results from excess bilirubin in the circulation and the accumulation of bilirubin in the tissues. Jaundice is a yellow discoloration most often seen in the skin, in mucous membranes, and in the sclera of the eye. This excess bile pigment may be caused by (1) excess production of bilirubin by hemolysis of red blood cells (hemolytic jaundice); (2) obstruction in the biliary tree, preventing the excretion of bilirubin (obstructive jaundice); or (3) liver parenchymal disease (hepatocellular jaundice). Each of these three processes is briefly reviewed in this section, and the role of the dentist is discussed with regard to dental management.

Hemolytic Jaundice

Hemolytic jaundice is not a gastrointestinal disease. Hemolytic anemias are the most common cause of this disorder, so it is critical to understand the implications of hemolytic jaundice. Excessive destruction of erythrocytes will lead to mild hyperbilirubinemia. This excess destruction is often due to an inherent abnormality in the cells (e.g., sickle cell disease, hereditary spherocytosis, thalassemia, and glucose-6-phosphate dehydrogenase deficiency). Additionally, drugs and poisonous agents (e.g., nitrobenzene, toluene, and phenacetin), as well as acquired immune disease (e.g., systemic lupus erythematosus), can lead to hemolytic jaundice. Even with a thorough history and examination, it would be difficult for a dentist to make a diagnosis of hemolytic jaundice with only a presenting sign of jaundice. Referral to the patient's primary care physician is necessary to elucidate the source of the excess pigmentation of the tissues. Medical diagnosis of jaundice by a hemolytic process is based on laboratory studies demonstrating the presence of anemia with a high reticulocyte count, a decreased level of serum haptoglobins, and elevated serum bilirubin. The specific cause of the increased hemolysis of red blood cells is determined by studies such as hemoglobin electrophoresis, erythrocyte fragility studies, and Coombs' test for antibodies to red cells. Typically, once a proper diagnosis is made and the underlying disorder (excessive hemolysis) is controlled, the jaundice resolves as the liver functions normally to remove bilirubin. Since the liver has enormous reserve capacity, the dentist should anticipate little to no residual damage to the liver unless liver function tests indicate otherwise.

Obstructive Jaundice (Cholestasis)

As its name implies, this form of jaundice is caused by a partial or complete stoppage in bile flow. The causes of this disorder are obstructions of the extrahepatic biliary tree and those associated with intrahepatic abnormalities. In either case, the flow of bile through the liver and out of the common bile duct can be impeded, resulting in an increase in bilirubin in the tissues. Gallstones and malignancies are the causes of most cases of extrahepatic cholestasis. Tumors of the pancreatic head are the most common malignant cause of extrahepatic cholestasis, and adenocarcinoma is the most frequent. The causes of intrahepatic cholestasis include neoplasms (e.g., metastatic carcinomas, lymphomas), toxic drugs and chemicals (e.g., phalloidin, the toxic component of mushrooms), hepatitis, IBD, and metabolic derangements.[76]

Exploration of biliary obstruction may involve multiple imaging modalities and multiple specialties. Radiologists, hepato-gastroenterologists and surgeons may examine using ultrasound, CT, MRI, endoscopic ultrasonography, and percutaneous, intraoperative or endoscopic retrograde cholangiography. Interpreting radiological examinations and choosing an optimal strategy can be difficult.[77] Evaluation of obstructive jaundice may include magnetic resonance cholangiopancreatography which is a relatively quick, accurate, and non-invasive imaging modality for the assessment of this disorder. This strategy rules out correctable underlying causes and reduces unnecessary invasive interventions.[78]

The OHCP's primary function is recognition of the clinical signs of jaundice and timely referral to a primary care physician for appropriate diagnosis and treatment. Once successful disease management is achieved, routine dental care can continue. Consultation with the patient's physician to ascertain the patient's liver function and ability to undergo dental treatment is necessary. Oral surgical procedures in the jaundiced patient should be deferred whenever possible. The main danger in surgery on the patient with obstructive jaundice is excessive bleeding resulting from vitamin K malabsorption. If surgery is essential, vitamin K should be given parenterally at a dose of 10 mg daily for several days. General anesthesia in a severely jaundiced patient can lead to renal failure.

Hepatocellular Jaundice

Hepatocellular jaundice can be caused by hepatitis and cirrhosis. Alcoholic hepatitis and drug-induced hepatotoxicity are discussed in this section, along with cirrhosis.

Alcoholic Hepatitis

Medical Aspects

Alcoholic hepatitis is a term used to describe the clinical presentation of alcoholic patients with jaundice. Alcoholic hepatitis is a form of toxin-induced liver disease that runs a wide clinical spectrum from subclinical disease to cirrhosis and fulminant hepatic failure. Excessive use of alcohol remains the most important cause of cirrhosis in the Western world and a leading cause of death and mortality during midlife. Although alcoholic hepatitis is somewhat dose related, the variability and extent of injury are remarkable. Clearly, it is a matter not only of how much alcohol is ingested but by whom. Ingestion of at least 40–60 g of ethanol per day for more than 15 years is necessary for development of alcoholic cirrhosis; this is equal to about six 12-ounce beers per day, four glasses of wine, or three 2-ounce shots of whisky. Hepatocyte injury from alcohol develops predominantly as a consequence of the direct cellular toxicity of acetaldehyde, the major metabolite of alcohol. However, there are important contributions from the associated nutritional deficiencies that often accompany alcoholism. There is compelling evidence that the tendency to alcoholism is inherited. Only 1 in 12 alcoholics develops evidence of severe liver injury. Genetic variation in the metabolism of ethanol may explain the higher prevalence of alcoholic liver injury in some populations. Clinicians from around the world are generally convinced that females are at greater risk of developing alcohol-induced liver disease than are males. The reasons for this observation remain obscure. However, women have lower levels of alcohol dehydrogenase (essential for metabolizing alcohol into acetaldehyde) in the gut; consequently, more alcohol reaches the liver.[83]

Due to the large number of individuals who have only mild symptoms, the true incidence of alcoholic hepatitis can only be estimated. In a US study involving veterans with liver disease who underwent liver biopsy, approximately 35% of subjects had changes consistent with alcoholic hepatitis. There have been numerous efforts to identify cofactors that may affect the progression of alcohol-induced injury. Nutrition, genetics, cytokines, hepatitis B and C, and therapeutic drugs all have been implicated. However, the evidence to date is only suggestive.[83]

There is a broad spectrum of clinical manifestations of alcoholic liver disease. Often there is little correlation and sometimes considerable disassociation between the apparent severities of injury as based on clinical findings and as based on evidence found on liver biopsy. Alcoholic hepatitis is often found superimposed on cirrhosis that is already established. Alcoholic hepatitis is considered to be at least partially reversible. The earliest indication of alcoholic liver disease is an enlarged liver. The patient may also exhibit signs of both acute hepatitis (jaundice, fever, anorexia, and malaise)and more chronic liver disease, which may include spider angiomas, gynecomastia, jaundice, ascites, and ethanol intoxication.[76,83]

The clinical problems associated with alcoholic hepatitis reflect the disordered metabolism and circulation in the liver. Jaundice reflects the inability of the hepatocyte to conjugate and excrete bilirubin, and bleeding is secondary to decreased synthesis of clotting factors by the hepatocytes. Also, there can be an associated thrombocytopenia in cases of alcoholic jaundice. Mental confusion results from failure of the liver cells to metabolize and excrete toxins such as ammonia. Spider angiomas and gynecomastia result from elevated levels of estrogen, which is normally metabolized by hepatocytes.[77,83]

Medical Management

Alcoholic hepatitis requires consideration in the case of any patient who has a history of regular alcohol use. Treatment may include abstinence and enteral nutrition. Pharmacotherapy using corticosteroids either with or without N-acetylcysteine may be indicated for patients with severe alcoholic hepatitis. Pentoxifylline was found to reduce the risk of hepatorenal syndrome, but data on mortality are limited.[84]

Severe alcoholic hepatitis is still associated with high mortality and presence of liver failure manifested by jaundice, coagulopathy, and encephalopathy is a poor prognostic indicator. The management of these patients includes at first hand several supportive measures as treatment of alcohol withdrawal, administration of fluid and vitamins and admission to an intensive care unit in the unstable patient.[85]

Confirmation of the diagnosis and assessment of the extent of injury is best done by performing a liver biopsy. There are no biochemical tests that have proven to be sufficiently helpful in establishing a diagnosis of alcohol-induced injury. Even with a liver biopsy, one can only guess the extent of reversible injury. However, the severity of alcoholic hepatitis can be objectively measured by using the laboratory criteria of prothrombin time and bilirubin. This measure is called a Maddrey discriminate function or Child-Pugh classification. Values of >32 in this measure indicate severe disease and poor prognosis with significant mortality.[83,85]

Abstinence is the mainstay of the treatment of alcoholic hepatitis. However, this is difficult to achieve. Nutritional support for the malnourished patient is also important. Although medications such as corticosteroids, anabolic steroids, propylthiouracil, colchicine, and insulin/glucagon show promise, there is insufficient evidence to support their general use. In those patients with alcoholic hepatitis without liver cirrhosis, the disease is reversible.[83]

Glucocorticoids have been the most intensively studied therapy in alcoholic hepatitis and are effective in certain subgroups. Indication for such a therapy is usually defined on a Maddrey Discriminant Function >32. The Lille score at day 7 is used to decide whether corticosteroid therapy should be stopped or continued for a one-month course. Nutritional supplementation is also likely to be beneficial. The main progress in better understanding its pathophysiology has come from cytokine studies. Various proinflammatory cytokines such as TNFα or interleukin-1 (IL-1) have been proposed to play a role in this disease. This advancement has recently led to pilot studies investigating anti-TNF drugs such as pentoxifylline, infliximab (anti-TNF antibody), or etanercept in the treatment of this disease. These studies revealed besides for pentoxifylline rather negative results. Despite this fact, targeting of certain cytokines such as IL-1 remains an attractive treatment concept for this devastating disorder in the future.[84]

Oral Health Considerations

The oral lesions that may be seen in patients with alcoholic hepatitis are primarily related to dysfunction of the hepatocyte. Jaundice (yellow pigmentation) may be observed on the mucosa and may be accompanied by cutaneous and scleral jaundice. Jaundice usually occurs when total serum bilirubin reaches levels ≥3 mg/dL. There may be extraoral and/or intraoral petechiae and ecchymosis, gingival crevicular hemorrhage due to the deficient clotting factors associated with dysfunctioning hepatocytes, and thrombocytopenia associated with alcohol. Additional oral findings can include manifestations of malnutrition, such as vitamin deficiencies and anemia. Consequently, pallor, angular cheilitis, and glossitis may be exhibited as expressions of related problems. Additionally, the sweet ketone breath, indicative of liver gluconeogenesis, should raise the suspicion of hepatotoxicity. The presentation of the above clinical signs, as well as a history or symptoms suggestive of alcohol abuse, should warrant a referral to the patient's primary care physician for evaluation. Liver impairment would necessitate specific dental management procedures before proceeding with dental treatment.[75] Adverse interactions between alcohol or resultant alcoholic liver disease and medications used in dentistry include but are not limited to acetaminophen, aspirin, ibuprofen, some cephalosporins, erythromycin, metronidazole, tetracycline, ketoconazole, pentobarbital, secobarbital, diazepam,lorazepam, chloral hydrate, and opioid analgesics.[86]

The prevalence of dental disease is usually extensive because of disinterest in performing appropriate oral hygiene techniques and a decrease in salivary flow.[86] Obviously, elective dental treatment should not be carried out in a patient who has ingested a large amount of alcohol. Conversely, routine dental treatment of a patient with a history of alcoholic liver disease is not contraindicated unless there is significant cirrhosis. Cirrhotic changes due to alcoholism are not reversible, whereas noncirrhotic changes generally are. Consequently, the dentist must determine the functioning level of the liver through consultation with the patient's physician and through appropriate liver function tests. To obtain the appropriate information from the physician, the dentist must be familiar with the laboratory tests used in evaluating the patient's status.[75,83,87]

Drug-Induced Hepatotoxicity

Medical Aspects

Drug-induced liver disease can mimic any acute or chronic liver disease. Patients may present with fulminant hepatic-failure from an intrinsic hepatotoxin such as acetaminophen or may simply have had an abnormal liver function test result on a laboratory screening panel. Ingested drugs are absorbed into the portal circulation and pass through the liver en route to distant sites of action. The liver is responsible for the conversion of lipid-soluble drugs, which are difficult to excrete, into polar-soluble metabolites that are easily excreted through the kidneys. This solubilization and detoxification may paradoxically produce toxic intermediates. Fortunately, death from drug-induced hepatic injury is uncommon. Nevertheless, the dentist's role in recognizing the potential for drug-induced hepatotoxicity from drugs prescribed by the dentist, other medications (either prescribed or over the counter[OTC]) being taken by the patient, and drug interactions are critical. Herbal and other alternative (nontraditional) drugs, which are increasing in popularity, have been reported to elicit hepatocellular toxicity as well.[76]

Drugs may be conjugated, oxidized, or reduced through the cytochrome P-450 system. This system can be induced by the long-term use of alcohol, barbiturates, or other drugs. With some hepatotoxic drugs, the relative activity of the cytochrome P-450 system is crucial; a drug that exerts its toxic actions through the generation of cytochrome P-450 metabolites may be relatively more toxic in a patient whouses alcohol or other agents that are capable of inducing

cytochrome P-450. An example is the enhanced toxicity of acetaminophen in chronic alcoholics.[76,83]

Most drug reactions occur in one of two general patterns: dose-dependent drug toxicity and idiosyncratic drug reaction. In dose-dependent drug toxicity, a particular agent may be expected to produce hepatic injury in virtually all persons who take a large enough dose. A classic example of this type of toxicity is associated with acetaminophen. Toxicity usually occurs with weeks or months of use, is usually reversible, and recurs at approximately the same dose if stopped and then reintroduced.[76]

Idiosyncratic drug reactions occur at an unpredictable dose, recur at lower doses if stopped and reintroduced, and are occasionally associated with features suggesting involvement of the immune system. Sulfonamides and phenytoin are examples of drugs associated with this type of drug-induced hepatotoxicity. Because of the nature of the reaction, a small dose is as likely to produce a serious reaction as is a full therapeutic dose. Consequently, death may occur upon rechallenge, even at low doses. Idiosyncratic hypersensitivity reactions make up the most common type of drug-induced hepatotoxicity.[76,82]

Regardless of the mechanism involved, drug-induced hepatotoxicity can result in hepatocellular injury, cholestatic drug reactions, abnormal lipid storage, cirrhosis, and vascular injury. Hepatocellular injury and cholestatic drug reactions account for the majority of drug reactions encountered in dentistry. Hepatocellular injury is the most commonly recognized drug-induced injury, with acetaminophen toxicity probably being the most frequent risk in the practice of dentistry. Nonetheless, there are many categories of drugs that are known to have demonstrated hepatotoxicity that are not covered in this chapter.

Oral Health Considerations

As stated previously, drug-induced liver disease can present as any acute or chronic disorder. Also, since idiosyncratic reactions often have an immunoallergic basis, the patient can present not only with jaundice and other features of chronic liver disease but also with fever, dermatitis, arthralgia, and eosinophilia. Regardless of clinical presentation, referral to the patient's primary care physician is necessary should the dentist suspect drug-induced hepatotoxicity. It is simplistic to recommend that, since any drug may produce hepatotoxicity, the drug in question should be stopped. Rather, consultation with the physician is necessary to weigh the relative risks of stopping or changing therapy. Fortunately, most of the drugs that dentists might use or prescribe that are known to be hepatotoxic have safe and effective alternatives, and stopping the most likely offending drug is a prudent course of action. Nonetheless, coordination of dental therapy and medical therapy is critical. For example, the alternative agent in the case of NSAID toxicity would be a drug from a different subclass. However, after starting the alternative agent, the patient should be followed for at least four to eight weeks with biochemical tests in order to ensure that the original drug reaction has resolved.

Since many drugs produce idiosyncratic drug toxicity, there is no way to predict or prevent such reactions. A patient who experiences an abrupt episode of hepatocellular injury should be considered to have an idiosyncratic drug reaction and should not be challenged again. For patients who take drugs associated with dose-dependent drug reactions, the obvious precaution is to keep the dose to a minimum. Since it is possible to take a toxic dose of acetaminophen without greatly exceeding the recommended doses, patients with chronic pain should be warned of the potential toxicity of acetaminophen. Also, patients who are taking large doses of acetaminophen should be advised to avoid alcohol and to ensure adequate nutrition.

Because most drug reactions are hepatocellular and may lead to hepatocyte failure and death, patients with a history of drug-induced hepatotoxicity should be evaluated with serial liver function tests. There may be cell death to the extent that drug metabolism and homeostasis are affected and that the patient's ability to undergo dental care is significantly affected.

Liver Cirrhosis

Cirrhosis can be classified into several categories, including infectious (commonly viral), metabolic, vascular disturbances, toxicologic, immunologic, biliary disease, and obstruction. The result of persistent hepatocellular necrosis is the end result of these multiple etiologic factors. Depending on the case-specific etiology, the incidence of cirrhosis shows considerable social and geographic variability. Although alcohol has been known as the principal cause of cirrhosis in the United States and elsewhere in the Western world, chronic viral hepatitis (mainly type C) has now emerged as the world's leading cause of both chronic hepatitis and cirrhosis.[81]

Medical Aspects

Cirrhosis is neither a single process nor a single disease; rather, it is the end result of a variety of conditions, primarily alcoholism, that produce chronic inflammatory change and liver cell injury. The progressive scarring leads to abnormal fibrosis and nodular regeneration. Alcohol-induced liver disease is either the first or second commonest specific indication for liver transplant throughout Europe and the United States.[80] Symptoms are the result of hepatocellular dysfunction, portal hypertension, or a combination of the two conditions. The most common symptoms include malaise, weakness, dyspepsia, anorexia, and nausea. One-third of the patients complain of abdominal pain, and 30%–78% of patients present with ascites. Approximately 65% of cirrhotic individuals are jaundiced at presentation. Increased pigmentation, particularly on overexposed surfaces, is seen in hemochromatosis, whereas xanthomas are suggestive of biliary cirrhosis. Less frequently seen are nonspecific findings of clubbing, cyanosis, and spider angiomas.[77,83]

Liver biopsy is the gold standard for diagnosing cirrhosis and can sometimes aid in identifying the etiology. For example, fat and Mallory bodies are typical in alcoholic liver injury, as compared with chronic inflammation and periportal necrosis, which are characteristics of cirrhosis resulting from chronic viral hepatitis.[82]

Medical Management

The medical management of liver cirrhosis is dependent on the underlying etiology. The main objective is to prevent further injury to the liver. Discontinuation of alcohol and other toxins is essential. Some patients may benefit from taking corticosteroids and other immunosuppressive agents, such as methotrexate. Phlebotomy to deplete iron stores and deferoxamine is used as an iron-chelating agent in patients with hemochromatosis. Liver transplantation is reserved for irreversible progressive liver disease.[76,83]

Oral Health Considerations

The oral cavity may show evidence of cirrhosis with the presence of hemorrhagic changes, petechiae, hematoma, jaundiced mucosal tissues, gingival bleeding, or icteric mucosal changes. Oral mucosa pigmentation is rarely observed in cases of hemochromatosis. Patients with cirrhosis have been reported to have impaired gustatory function and are frequently malnourished. Nutritional deficiencies can result in glossitis and loss of tongue papillae along with angular or labial cheilitis, which is complicated by concomitant candidal infection. Sialadenosis, a bilateral, painless hypertrophy of the parotid glands is a frequent finding in patients with cirrhosis. The enlarged glands are soft, nontender, and are not fixed. The condition appears to be caused by a demyelinating polyneuropathy that results in abnormal sympathetic signaling, abnormal acinar protein secretion, and acinar cytoplasmic swelling.[82]

Oral findings may be associated with vitamin deficiencies and anemia; these findings include angular cheilitis, glossitis, and mucosal pallor. Yellow pigmentation may be observed on the oral mucosa and may be accompanied by scleral and cutaneous jaundice. Salivary gland dysfunction secondary to Sjögren's syndrome may be associated with primary biliary cirrhosis. Pigmentation of the oral mucosa is only rarely observed in cases of hemochromatosis.

The dental patient who presents with a history of liver cirrhosis deserves special attention. First, patients with cirrhosis may have significant hemostatic defects, both because of an inability to synthesize clotting factors and because of secondary thrombocytopenia. These deficits can be overcome with replacement with fresh frozen plasma and platelets. Therefore, laboratory evaluation prior to any surgical or periodontal procedures should be directed at bleeding parameters; specifically, complete blood count, prothrombin time or INR, partial thromboplastin time, and platelet count should be obtained.[75]

Second, the ability to detoxify substances is also compromised in patients with hepatic insufficiency, and drugs and toxins may accumulate. Patients may become encephalopathic due to an ammonia buildup from the incomplete detoxification of nitrogenous wastes. Patients with encephalopathy are likely to be taking neomycin or lactulose. The use of sedatives and tranquilizers should be avoided in patients with a history of taking encephalopathy narcotics. Additionally, there may be an induction of liver enzymes, leading to a need for increased or decreased dosages of certain medications. Consequently, consultation with the patient's physician is essential to the proper management of the dental patient with liver cirrhosis. The patient with ascites may not be able to fully recline in the dental chair because of increased pressure on abdominal vessels. Lastly, liver transplantation patients who are on immunosuppressive therapy should be monitored for systemic infection of oropharyngeal origin, oral viral infection (herpes simplex virus, cytomegalovirus), and oral ulcers of unknown origin. Oral manifestations of acute graft-versus-host disease in the post-transplant patient can present as a mucositis, whereas chronic graft-versus-host disease may resemble oral lichen planus.[19]

GASTROINTESTINAL SYNDROMES

Eating Disorders: Anorexia and Bulimia

Medical Aspects

The two most common eating disorders are anorexia nervosa and bulimia.[88] A variety of specialists, including psychiatrists, psychologists, dentists, internists, clinical social workers, nurses, and dietitians, must provide the treatment of eating disorders.[89] Anorexia involves individuals who intentionally starve themselves when they are already underweight. People suffering from this disorder have an intense fear of becoming fat, even when they are extremely underweight (defined as body weight that is 15% or more below the recommended levels). Those who suffer from anorexia are unable to perceive their physical appearance accurately.

In contrast to those with anorexia, persons with bulimia nervosa consume large amounts of food during "binge" episodes in which they feel out of control of their eating. Bulimic individuals are also not as successful in dieting as are those with anorexia. They may successfully diet for a short time, but they often again lose the ability to restrict food intake, often as a result of some emotional trauma. They then try to prevent weight gain after such episodes by vomiting, using laxatives or diuretics, dieting, and/or exercising aggressively. Persons with bulimia, like those with anorexia, are very dissatisfied with their body shape and weight, and their self-esteem is unduly influenced by their appearance. To be diagnosed with bulimia nervosa, an individual must engage in bingeing and purging at least twice a week for three months; exhibit a feeling of lack of control over eating; regularly use self-induced vomiting, laxatives, or diuretics to prevent weight gain; and exhibit a persistent excessive concern with body shape and weight.

The diagnosis of anorexia or bulimia is not always clear. For example, some anorexic persons may binge and purge, whereas some bulimic persons may restrict food intake and overcompensate for overeating by exercising. If an individual eats through bingeing but is 15% or more below recommended weight, then anorexia nervosa is the appropriate diagnosis. Both of these disorders seem to be most prevalent in industrialized societies, particularly where thinness is espoused as the ideal. Eating disorders are predominantly adolescent females with prevalence rates of up to 5%.[90–93]

Anorexia usually develops in adolescence, between the ages of 14 and 18 years, whereas bulimia is more likely to develop in the late teens or early twenties. It is estimated that anorexia occurs in about 0.5% of adolescent girls and that bulimia occurs in about 1%–2% of adolescent girls. However, 5%–10% of young women may exhibit less severe signs and symptoms of these diseases. Anorexia affects 0.3%–0.7%, whereas bulimia affects 1.7%–2.5% of women.[66] Studies indicate that by their first year of college, 4.5%–18% of women and 0.4% of men have a history of bulimia and that as many as 1 in 100 females between the ages of 12 and 18 years have anorexia.

Anorexia and bulimia are both considered psychiatric disorders with physical complications.[94] Before diagnosing either of these eating disorders, other possible causes of significant changes in weight or appetite (e.g., tumors, immunodeficiency, malabsorption, and alcohol) must be ruled out. Symptoms of eating disorders can also be primary signs of depression and schizophrenia. Eating disorders can be differentiated from these other disorders by the presence of a distorted body image and preoccupation with losing weight. Because patients may develop a good rapport with their dentists, dentists may be the first health care providers to sense that a diagnosis of an eating disorder is appropriate.

Although many people with an eating disorder recover fully, relapse is common and may occur months or even years after treatment. An estimated 5%–10% of anorexic patients will die from the disorder; their deaths most commonly result from starvation, suicide, or electrolyte imbalance.

Oral Health Considerations

The cardinal oral manifestation of eating disorders is severe erosion of the enamel on the lingual surfaces of the maxillary teeth. Acids from chronic vomiting are the cause.[95–97] Examination of the patient's fingernails may disclose abnormalities related to the use of fingers to initiate purging. Mandibular teeth may be affected but not as severely as the maxillary teeth. Parotid enlargement may develop as a sequela of starvation. Rarely does one observe soft tissue changes of the oral mucosa because of trauma from gastric acids.

The dentist should be aware of a possible eating disorder when these symptoms are encountered and should take steps to arrange for referral to other practitioners.[70] Support of the patient both physically, by treatment of tooth desensitization and esthetics, and psychologically, by demonstrating a caring and compassionate attitude, is a part of the dental practitioner's treatment responsibility to these patients.

Dental erosion is the most common oral manifestation in patients with eating disorders. These patients practice self-induced vomiting that causes regurgitation of gastric contents into the oral cavity thereby making them more susceptible to enamel demineralization and erosion. Duration and frequency of purging incidents per day, oral hygiene habits (particularly after a vomiting incident), the degree of acid of water rinsing or drinking neutralizing liquids, such as milk and timings of tooth cleaning. A chronic insult of acidic gastric contents from purging may cause erosion of tooth surfaces particularly on the lingual/palatal and occlusal surfaces, in some cases extended into the dentin or close to dentinal exposure. In patients with anorexia nervosa who consume highly acidic foods such raw citrus fruits to maintain their low-calorie diets, present erosion of the buccal or facial surfaces of teeth. The location of enamel demineralization plays an essential role in making a differential diagnosis in patients with eating disorders.[90–92]

Salivary gland changes include dry and/or cracked lips, burning sensation in the mouth (particularly on the tongue) and parotid gland swelling uni-or bilateral, are common findings in patients with eating disorders. This imparts a negative effect on the salivary glands, possibly caused by frequent vomiting or starvation that resulted in hyposalivation. Enlargement anterior to the ear and at the anatomical region of the parotid gland, and occasionally the submandibular gland is well recognized in patients with bulimia nervosa. However, the secrecy with which patients with bulimia nervosa conceal their vomiting habits may complicate diagnosis of bulimia nervosa–associated parotid hypertrophy. It has been reported that salivary stones and reduced resting salivary flow rates are often observed in patients with bulimia nervosa. Patients with bulimia nervosa may harbor high proportions of aciduric organisms in the saliva due to acid regurgitation. High prevalence of salivary microbes including *Streptococcus* (*S.*) *mutans*, *S. sobrinus*, *lactobacilli*, and *yeasts* have been reported in patients with bulimia nervosa. An increased salivary colonization of *S. sobrinus* may be a marker for a history of vomiting in patients with bulimia nervosa.[90–92]

Dental caries have been reported in most people with eating disorders that consume high-sugar diets several times daily. This habit pattern may in turn provide a source of nourishment to the cariogenic microbes residing in the oral cavity. Additionally, those patients who are using anti-depressants may develop xerostomia. During an eating binge, individuals with bulimia nervosa consume fats and sugars. The fat in dairy products with regular diets may have a protective effect on dental caries; further studies needs to be done.[90–92]

Periodontal disease may be jeopardized by vitamin deficiency. It has been suggested that avitaminosis-C in patients with eating disorders may play a role in eliciting and aggravating periodontal disease in these individuals. Severe vitamin-C deficiency has been associated with the development of a periodontal syndrome called "scorbutic gingivitis" is characterized by rapid periodontal pocket development and ulcerative gingivitis. Vitamin-D plays an essential role in bone immunity and bone maintenance; for that reason, one could consider vitamin-D deficiency in patients with EDs may put at risk the periodontal apparatus including the alveolar bone.[90–92]

Disorders of the temporomandibular joint may manifest due to mechanical pressure exerted during frequent episodes of self-triggered vomiting. This damage is similar to those sustained during intubations for general anesthesia, such as dislocation or subluxation of the mandibular condyle/s caused by excessive mouth opening. Patient with eating disorders complain of symptoms, such as facial pain, headache, jaw tiredness, tongue thrusting and lump feeling in the throat as well as dizziness and sleep disturbances.[90]

Oral health might be affected even in patients with a relatively short history of eating disorders. Dry lips, burning tongue, and parotid gland swelling are common manifestations in patients with eating disorders; a critical oral-dental examination during routine dental check-ups may reveal valuable information regarding the presence or absence of eating disorders. Awareness on the part of dentists of how self-reported symptoms and clinical signs affect eating disorder patients will provide for early detection and diagnosis, which is fundamental for successful management, including the prevention of further psychiatric, somatic, and oral deterioration caused by the disease.[91]

Gardner's Syndrome

Gardner's syndrome consists of intestinal polyposis (which represents premalignant lesions) and multiple impacted supernumerary (extra) teeth. This disorder is inherited as an autosomal dominant trait, and few patients afflicted with this syndrome reach the age of 50 years without surgical intervention.[98–102] In a young patient with a family history of Gardner's syndrome, dental radiography (such as a panoramic radiograph) can provide the earliest indication of the presence of this disease process.[103]

Gardner's syndrome, a variant of familial adenomatous polyposis, is an autosomal dominant genetic disease characterized by the combined presence of multiple intestinal polyps (which represent premalignant lesions) and extraintestinal manifestations. The extraintestinal manifestations include multiple osteomas, multiple impacted supernumerary teeth, connective tissue tumors, thyroid carcinomas, and hypertrophy of the pigmented epithelium of the retina. Osteoma is a benign neoplasm of bone tissue characterized by slow continuous growth that usually affects the long bones and cranial bones and is a major symptom for Gardner syndrome. Dental abnormalities are present in 30%–75% and osteomas in 68%–82% of GS patients.[98,100]

Osteomas are generally located in the paranasal sinuses and mandible. They display slow growth, and vary from a slight thickening to a large mass. Osteomas predominantly affect the mandible and maxilla but can additionally affect the skull and long bones. Calvarium osteomas, maxillary osteomas, and dental hypercementosis also occur.[99,100] Osteomas are an essential component of Gardner's syndrome, forming a slight thickening to a large mass that may affect all parts of the skeleton. The frontal bones are the most frequent site for osteoma development.[98] Exostoses osteomas, also called peripheral osteomas can be palpable and be detected by routine radiography.[100–102] In the mandible, two types of osteomas occur, central or lobulated. Central osteomas are characteristically near the roots of the teeth, and lobulated types arise from the cortex and most commonly observed at the mandibular angle.[100,102]

Seventy percent of Gardner's syndrome patients display dental anomalies such as impacted or unerupted teeth, congenitally missing teeth, supernumerary teeth, hypercementosis, dentigerous cysts, fused molar roots, long and tapered molar roots, hypodontia, compound odontomes, and/or multiple carious lesions. Difficulties in extraction due to ankylosis have also been reported.[100–102]

In a young patient with a family history of Gardner's syndrome, dental radiography (such as a panoramic radiograph) can provide the earliest indication of the presence of this disease process.[103]

Plummer-Vinson Syndrome

Plummer-Vinson syndrome (also termed Paterson-Kelly syndrome), originally described as "hysterical dysphagia," is noted primarily in white middle-aged women, in the fourth to seventh decade of life. This syndrome has also been described in children and adolescents. The hallmark of this disorder is dysphagia resulting from esophageal stricture, causing many patients to have a fear of choking.[105–107] The etiopathogenesis is uncertain, although iron deficiency is a possible factor. Other possible factors include malnutrition, genetic predisposition, or autoimmune processes.[106]

Patients may present with a lemon-tinted pallor and with dryness of the skin, spoon-shaped fingernails, koilonychia, and splenomegaly. The oral manifestations are the result of an iron deficiency anemia. Oral findings include atrophic glossitis with erythema or fissuring, angular cheilitis, thinning of the vermilion borders of the lips, and leukoplakia of the tongue. Inspection of the oral mucous membranes will disclose atrophy and hyperkeratinization. These oral changes are similar to those encountered in the pharynx and esophagus. The syndrome can be treated effectively with iron supplementation and mechanical dilation.[106] Carcinoma of the upper alimentary tract has been reported in 10%–30% of patients.[105] Thorough oral, pharyngeal, and esophageal examinations are mandatory to ensure that squamous cell carcinoma is not present. Artificial saliva may reduce the sensation (and thereby the fear) of choking.[105,106]

Peutz-Jeghers Syndrome

Peutz-Jeghers syndrome is characterized by multiple intestinal polyps throughout the gastrointestinal tract but primarily in the small intestine. Malignancies in the gastrointestinal tract and elsewhere in the body have been reported in approximately 10% of patients with this syndrome. Pigmentation (present from birth) of the face, lips, and oral cavity is a hallmark of this syndrome.[108] Interestingly, the facial pigmentation fades later in life, although the intraoral mucosal pigmentation persists. No specific oral treatment is necessary.

Peutz-Jeghers syndrome is a rare hereditary disorder characterized by intestinal polyposis, mucocutaneous pigmentation and increased risk for cancer.[108–110] It is caused by a germline mutation in the serine/threonine-protein kinase 11 (STK11) and inherited in an autosomal dominant manner.[108] Prevalence of Peutz-Jeghers syndrome is approximately one in 200,000.[112]

The diagnosis of Peutz-Jeghers syndrome is the hamartomatous gastrointestinal polyp characterized histopathologically by the unique finding of mucosa with interdigitating smooth muscle bundles in a characteristic branching tree appearance. They can cause abdominal pain, anemia, and gastrointestinal bleeding by intussusception or obstruction.[110,112]

Pigmentation (present from birth) of the face, lips, and oral cavity is a hallmark of this syndrome.[108,109,111,113] Cutaneous hyperpigmented macules are rarely present at birth; they become pronounced in most individuals before the fifth year, but then may fade in puberty and adulthood. Intraoral mucosal and labial pigmentation persists.[108–111] Histologically, increased melanocytes are observed at the epidermal-dermal junction, with increased melanin in the basal cells. Malignancies in the gastrointestinal tract and elsewhere in the body have been reported in approximately 10% of patients with this syndrome.[108] No specific oral treatment is necessary.

Cowden's Syndrome

Cowden's syndrome (multiple hamartoma and neoplasia syndrome) is an autosomal dominant disease characterized chiefly by facial trichilemmomas, gastrointestinal polyps, breast and thyroid neoplasms, and oral abnormalities. Cowden's syndrome is considered to be a cutaneous marker of internal malignancies.[114–119] Pebbly papilloma-like lesions and multiple fibromas may be found widely distributed throughout the oral cavity.[115]

According to the International Cowden Consortium (2000), facial trichilemmomas, acral keratoses, mucosal lesions, and papillomatous papules constitute the pathognomonic criteria of the syndrome, whereas major criteria for the syndrome include breast cancer, thyroid cancer, endometrial cancer, and macrocephaly. Minor criteria of the syndrome include thyroid lesions, mental retardation, gastrointestinal hamartomas, fibrocystic breast disease, lipoma, fibroma, genitourinary tumor and malformations. Skeletal system, nervous system, cardiopulmonary system and ophthalmologic findings may accompany in some cases.[116,117] The diagnosis of Cowden syndrome is established in the presence of pathognomonic lesions that include (1) ≥6 facial papules of which ≥3 must be trichilemmomas; (2) cutaneous facial papules; (3) papillomatosis in oral mucosa; (4) acral keratosis; (5) ≥6 palmoplantar keratosis lesions; and (6) macrocephaly.[116–118] The responses of facial papules to different treatment modalities, including topical 5-fluorouracil, oral retinoids, curettage, electrosurgery, cryosurgery, laser ablation, and surgical excision, are variable.[116–119] Patients with Cowden syndrome require lifelong follow-up, and family members should be screened for the disease. Cases of Cowden syndrome are rarely encountered; early diagnosis would decrease the associated mortality and morbidity.[116–119]

CASE NUMBER 1: CROHN'S DISEASE

S: This 31-year-old Jewish white female presented for routine dental care with a chief complaint, "I have a rash in my mouth." This complaint had been present for one month and was coincident with an increase in the sulfasalazine therapy she was taking for her Crohn's disease. Past medical history is significant for inflammatory bowel disease (Crohn's disease) only. Her present medication regimen included sulfasalazine 500 mg four times daily for anti-inflammatory control of the Crohn's disease and diphenoxylate HCl with atropine for control of the attendant diarrhea.

O: Vital signs and extraoral examination were within normal limits. Intraorally, the patient was dentate and had bimaxillary arch integrity through the second molars. Inspection of the periodontium disclosed a "cobblestone architecture" frequently described in patients with Crohn's disease (Crohn's Figure 16-1). Inspection of the buccal mucosae disclosed white filamentous superficial plaques that were easily wiped away with gauze sponges (Crohn's Figure 16-2). The tongue was coated dorsally. There were no other significant abnormalities noted during the head and neck examination.

A: While a lichenoid drug reaction to sulfasalazine was considered based on the reticular appearance of the buccal mucosae, the coated tongue and superficial, wipeable plaques strongly suggested a diagnosis of oral candidosis (112.0). A number of factors were considered as predisposing this patient to candidal infection. Sulfasalazine contains a bacteriostatic sulfa moiety that would allow for fungal overgrowth. Atropine therapy causes xerostomia that reduces the naturally occurring antifungal activity of saliva (histatins).

P: The patient was instructed to perform good oral hygiene and uses gauze sponges to wipe her mucosal surfaces to mechanically remove the majority of her pseudomembranous plaques. Clotrimazole troches, five times daily for a two week period were prescribed with instructions to slowly dissolve the troches intraorally and not to chew them so as to prolong mucosal contact with this antifungal medication. The patient returned two weeks later and her condition had resolved. She was advised to continue utilizing the gauze wipes to help to prevent recurrence of the candidosis.

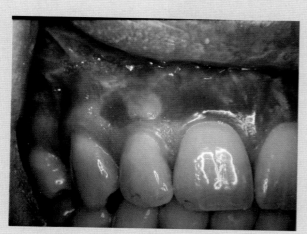

FIGURE 16-1 Cobblestone gingival architecture in a 31-year-old female patient with Crohn's disease.

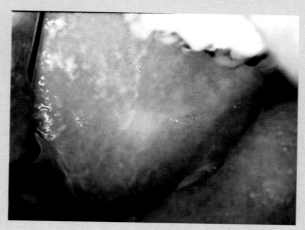

FIGURE 16-2 Pseudomembranous plaques of Candida albicans in a patient with Crohn's disease treated with sulfasalazine. The plaques were easily removed with wet gauze sponges.

CASE NUMBER 2: ULCERATIVE COLITIS

S: This 44-year-old Jewish white female presented for emergency dental care with a chief complaint, "I have a mouth full of ulcers that are killing me." This complaint had been present for three days and was coincident with a flare-up of her ulcerative colitis. She also complained about dysphagia and difficulty eating. Past medical history is significant for inflammatory bowel disease (ulcerative colitis) only. Her present medication regimen included sulfasalazine 500 mg four times daily and prednisone 10 mg daily for anti-inflammatory control of the ulcerative colitis.

O: Vital signs and extraoral examination were within normal limits. Intraorally, the patient was partially dentate due to missing maxillary and mandibular posterior teeth. She did not wear maxillary or mandibular removable prostheses. The periodontal tissues appeared healthy. Inspection of the soft palate disclosed three major aphthous-like ulcerations measuring greater than 1.0 centimeter in diameter (Ulcerative Colitis Figure 16-3). The tongue was normally papillated and was not coated dorsally. There was no palpable lymphadenopathy. There were no other significant abnormalities noted during the head and neck examination.

A: This is a relatively straightforward case of extra-abdominal ulcerative colitis resulting in oral ulceration (528.2). The oral ulcerations occurred simultaneously with an abdominal flare-up of the ulcerative colitis resulting in diarrhea. The patient reported that she has had similar episodes of oral ulcers in the past but that they were not as severe as during this episode.

P: The patient's gastroenterologist was contacted and it was suggested that the prednisonedosage be increase from 10 mg daily to 40 mg daily for a 10-day period. This measure helped control the flare-up of the ulcerative colitis and resulted in the complete resolution of the oral lesions.

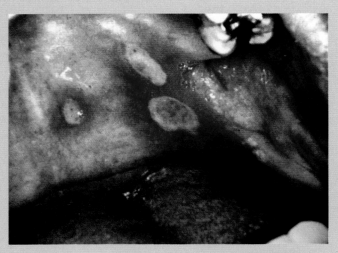

FIGURE 16-3 Major aphthous-like ulcerations of the soft palate in a 44-year-old female patient with ulcerative colitis.

Selected Readings

Aframian DJ, Ofir M, Benoliel R. Comparison of oral mucosal pH values in bulimia nervosa, GERD, BMS patients and healthy population. *Oral Dis.*2010;16:807–811.

Costa AG, Costa RO, de Oliveira LR, Grossmann S.Multiple oral radiopaque masses leading to Gardner's syndrome diagnosis. *Gen Dent.* 2013; 61(4):12–14.

Erickson K, Donovan T, Swift E. Dental Erosion. *J Esthet Restor Dent.* 2013;25:212.

Fatahzadeh M. Inflammatory bowel disease. *Oral Surg Oral Med Oral Pathol Oral Radiol Endod.* 2009;108:1–10.

Firriolo FJ. Dental management of patients with end-stage liver disease. *Dent Clin North Am.* 2006;50(4):563–590.

Glick M. Medical considerations for dental care of patients with alcohol-related liver disease. *J Am Dent Assoc.* 1997;128(8):61–70.

Golla K, Epstein JB, Cabay RJ. Liver disease: current perspectives on medical and dental management. *Oral Surg Oral Med Oral Pathol Oral Radiol Endod.* 2005;98(5):516–521.

Grossner-Schreiber B, Fetter T, Hedderich J, et al. Prevalence of dental caries and periodontal disease in patients with inflammatory bowel disease: a case-control study. *J Clin Periodontol.* 2006;33:478–484.

Lourenco SV. Hussein TP. Bologna SB, et al. Oral manifestations of inflammatory bowel disease: a review based on the observation of six cases. *J Eur AcadDermatolVenereol.* 2010;24:204–207.

Ruff JC, Koch MO, Perkins S. Bulimia: dentomedical complications. *Gen Dent.* 1992;40(1):22–25.

Siegel MA, Hupp WS. Oral considerations in patients with gastrointestinal disorders. In: Bayless TM, Diehl AM, eds. *Advanced Therapy in Gastroenterology and Liver Disease.* 5th ed. Chap 7. Burlington, Ontario, Canada: B.C. Decker, Inc.; 2005:43–48.

Siegel MA, Jacobson JJ. Inflammatory bowel diseases and the oral cavity. *Oral Surg Oral Med Oral Pathol Oral Radiol Endod.* 1999;87:12–14.

Wassenaar E, Oelschlager B. Effect of medical and surgical treatment of Barrett's metaplasia. *World J Gastroenterol.* 2010;16:3773–3779.

For the full reference lists, please go to http://www.pmph-usa.com/Burkets_Oral_Medicine.

CHAPTER 17

Renal Disease

Scott S. De Rossi, DMD
Matthew J. Diamond, DO, MS, FACP

❑ KIDNEY STRUCTURE AND FUNCTION

❑ FLUIDS, ELECTROLYTES, AND pH HOMEOSTASIS

❑ DIAGNOSTIC PROCEDURES IN RENAL DISEASE
Serum Chemistry
Urinalysis
Creatinine Clearance Test
Renal Ultrasonography
Computed Tomography
Magnetic Resonance Imaging
Intravenous Pyelography
Nuclear Medicine (Radionuclide Scintigraphy)
Biopsy

❑ RENAL FAILURE

❑ ACUTE KIDNEY INJURY
Prerenal Failure
Postrenal Failure
Acute Intrinsic Renal Failure

❑ CHRONIC RENAL FAILURE
Clinical Progression
Etiology and Pathogenesis

❑ MANIFESTATIONS OF RENAL DISEASE: UREMIC SYNDROME
Biochemical Disturbances
Gastrointestinal Symptoms
Neurologic Signs and Symptoms
Hematologic Problems
Calcium and Skeletal Disorders (Renal Osteodystrophy)
Cardiovascular Manifestations
Respiratory Symptoms
Immunologic Changes
Oral Manifestations

❑ MEDICAL MANAGEMENT OF CKD
Conservative Therapy
Renal Replacement Therapy

❑ HEMODIALYSIS

❑ PERITONEAL DIALYSIS

❑ OTHER APPROACHES TO SOLUTE REMOVAL

❑ ORAL HEALTH CONSIDERATIONS
AKI Patients
CKD and ESRD Patients

Diseases of the kidney are a major cause of morbidity and mortality in the United States, affecting close to 20 million Americans.[1] The kidneys are vital organs for maintaining a stable internal environment (homeostasis). The kidneys have many functions, including regulating the acid–base and fluid–electrolyte balances of the body by filtering blood, selectively reabsorbing water and electrolytes, and excreting urine. In addition, the kidneys excrete metabolic waste products, including urea, creatinine, and uric acid, as well as foreign chemicals. Apart from these regulatory and excretory functions, the kidneys have a vital endocrine function, secreting renin, the active form of vitamin D, and erythropoietin. These hormones are important in maintaining blood pressure, calcium metabolism, and the synthesis of erythrocytes.

Disorders of the kidneys can be classified into the following diseases or stages: disorders of hydrogen ion concentration (pH) and electrolytes, acute kidney injury (AKI), chronic kidney disease (CKD), and end-stage renal disease (ESRD) or uremic syndrome. Approximately 1 of 20 hospitalized patients develops AKI, most often related to the trauma of surgery. Death from AKI occurs in 30%–80%

of patients, depending on their underlying medical conditions.[2–5] Almost 1 in 10,000 persons develops end-stage renal failure annually, whereas mortality related to CKD accounts for more than 50,000 deaths each year in the United States (Figure 17-1). It is estimated that 10% of adults in the United States—more than 20 million people—may have CKD (United States Renal Data System Fact Sheet 2014).[1] The risk of developing CKD increases after 50 years of age and is most commonly found among adults older than 70 years. Oral health care professionals are frequently challenged to meet the dental needs of medically complex patients. This chapter reviews the etiology and pathophysiology of renal disorders and reviews considerations for the provision of dental care.

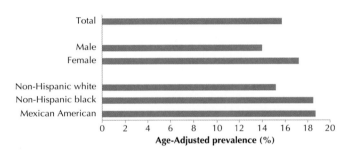

FIGURE 17-1   Age-adjusted prevalence of kidney disease among US adults aged 20 years and older from 1999 to 2010. Centers for Disease Control and Prevention (CDC). National Chronic Kidney Disease Fact Sheet: General Information and National Estimates on Chronic Kidney Disease in the United States, 2013. Atlanta, GA: US Department of Health and Human Services, Centers for Disease Control and Prevention; 2013[1]

KIDNEY STRUCTURE AND FUNCTION

The human kidneys are bean-shaped organs located in the retroperitoneum at the level of the waist. Each adult kidney weighs approximately 160 g and measures 10–15 cm in length. Coronal sectioning of the kidney reveals two distinct regions: an outer region called cortex and an inner region known as the medulla (Figure 17-2A). Structures that are located at the corticomedullary junction extend into the kidney hilum and are called papillae. Each papilla is enclosed by a minor calyx that collectively communicates with the major calyces to form the renal pelvis. The renal pelvis collects urine flowing from the papillae and passes it to the bladder via the ureters. Vascular flow to the kidneys is provided by the renal artery, which branches directly from the aorta. This artery subdivides into segmental branches to perfuse the upper, middle, and lower regions of the kidney. Further subdivisions account for the arteriole-capillary-venous network or vas recta. The venous drainage of the kidney is provided by a series of veins leading to the renal vein and ultimately to the inferior vena cava.

The kidney's functional unit is the nephron (Figure 17-2B), and each kidney is made up of approximately one million nephrons. Each nephron consists of Bowman's capsule, which surrounds the glomerular capillary bed; the proximal convoluted tubule; the loop of Henle; and the distal convoluted tubule, which empties into the collecting ducts. The glomerulus is a unique network of capillaries that is suspended between afferent and efferent arterioles enclosed within Bowman's capsule and that serves as a filtering funnel for waste. The filtrate drains from the glomerulus into the tubule, which alters the

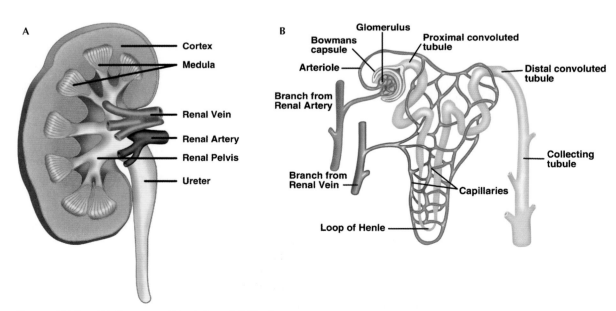

FIGURE 17-2   (A) Structure of the kidney. (B) Nephron.

concentration along its length by various processes to form urine. The glomerulus funnels ultrafiltrate to the remaining portion of the nephron or renal tubule. Following filtration, the second step of urine formation is the selective reabsorption and secretion of filtered substances, which occurs along the length of the tubule via active and passive transport processes.

Each day, the kidneys excrete approximately 1.5–2.5 L of urine; although the removal of toxic and waste products from the blood remains their major role,[6] the kidneys are also essential for the production of hormones such as vitamin D and erythropoietin and for the modulation of salt and water excretion. The major functions of the kidney are summarized in Table 17-1.

Once destroyed, nephrons do not regenerate. However, the kidney compensates for the loss of nephrons by hypertrophy of the remaining functioning units. This theory, often referred to as the intact nephron hypothesis, maintains that diseased nephrons are totally destroyed. Normal renal function can be maintained until approximately 50% of the nephrons per kidney are destroyed, at which point abnormal laboratory values and changes in the clinical course occur. This hypothesis is most useful in explaining the orderly pattern of functional adaptation in progressive renal failure.

FLUIDS, ELECTROLYTES, AND pH HOMEOSTASIS

With advancing nephron destruction, water and electrolyte regulation becomes increasingly more difficult. Adaptations to sudden shifts in intake occur slowly, resulting in wide swings in water and solute concentrations. The first clinical sign of diminished renal function is a decreased ability to concentrate the urine (isosthenuria). As a result of this inability to conserve water, dehydration ensues. With early renal insufficiency, sodium is also lost in the urine. This loss is often independent of the amount of water lost. As renal disease progresses, volume overload leading to hypertension and congestive heart failure can be serious sequelae. When glomerular filtration becomes markedly diminished, the distal tubule can no longer secrete sufficient potassium, leading to hyperkalemia.

In a healthy body, the acid–base balance is maintained via buffers, respiration, and the amounts of acid or alkaline wastes in the urine; this is because the daily load of endogenous acid is excreted into the urine with buffering compounds such as phosphates. As the glomerular filtration rate (GFR) progressively decreases, the tubular excretory capacity for positive hydrogen (H^+) ions is overwhelmed because renal ammonia production becomes inadequate. In its early phases, the resultant acidosis usually has a normal anion gap. As the kidney deteriorates, metabolically derived acids accumulate, leading to an increase in the anion gap. Clinically, this metabolic acidosis is manifested as anorexia, nausea, fatigue, weakness, and Kussmaul's respiration (a deep gasping respiration similar to that observed in patients with diabetic ketoacidosis).

DIAGNOSTIC PROCEDURES IN RENAL DISEASE

Serum Chemistry

In the presence of renal dysfunction, changes in homeostasis are reflected in serum chemistry. Sodium, chloride, blood urea nitrogen (BUN), glucose, creatinine, carbon dioxide, potassium, phosphate, and calcium levels provide a useful tool to evaluate the degree of renal impairment and disease progression. Serum creatinine and BUN are often important markers to the GFR. Both of these products are nitrogenous waste products of protein metabolism that are normally excreted in the urine, but they may increase to toxic levels in the presence

TABLE 17-1 Major Functions of the Kidneys

Nonexcretory functions

Degradation of polypeptide hormones

Insulin

Glucagon

Parahormone

Prolactin

Growth hormone

Antidiuretic hormone

Gastrin

Vasoactive intestinal polypeptide

Synthesis and activation of hormones

Erythropoietin (stimulates erythrocyte production by bone marrow)

Prostaglandins (vasodilators that act locally to prevent renal ischemia)

Renin (important in regulation of blood pressure)

1,25-Dihydroxyvitamin D3 (final hydroxylation of vitamin D to its most potent form)

Excretory functions

Excretion of nitrogenous end products of protein metabolism (e.g., creatinine, uric acid, urea)

Maintenance of ECF volume and blood pressure by altering Na^+ excretion

Maintenance of plasma electrolyte concentration within normal range

Maintenance of plasma osmolality by altering water excretion

Maintenance of plasma pH by eliminating excess H^+ and regenerating HCO_3^-

Provision of route of excretion for most drugs

Abbreviations: ECF, extracellular fluid; H^+, hydrogen; HCO_3^-, bicarbonate; Na^+, sodium; pH, hydrogen ion concentration.

TABLE 17-2 Laboratory Changes in Progressive Renal Disease

Laboratory Test	Normal Range	Level in Symptomatic Renal Failure
Glomerular filtration rate	90–120mL/min/1.73 m²	<15 mL/min
Creatinine clearance	85–125 mL/min (female)	10–60 mL/min (moderate failure)
	97–140 mL/min (male)	<15 mL/min (severe failure)
Serum creatinine	0.6–1.20 mg/dL	>5 mg/dL
Blood urea nitrogen	8–18 mg/dL	>50 mg/dL
Serum calcium	8.5–10.5 mg/dL	Depressed
Serum phosphate	2.5–4.5 mg/dL	Elevated
Serum potassium	3.8–5.0 mEq/L	Elevated

of renal dysfunction. A characteristic profile of changes occurs with advancing renal dysfunction, including elevations in serum creatinine, BUN, and phosphate, compared with low levels of serum calcium. Laboratory findings commonly seen in renal disease are summarized in Table 17-2.

Urinalysis

The most important aspects of urine examination in patients with renal disease include the detection of protein or blood in the urine, determination of the specific gravity or osmolality, and microscopic examination. The hallmarks of renal dysfunction detected by urinalysis are hematuria (the presence of blood in the urine) and proteinuria (the presence of protein in the urine). Hematuria can result from bleeding anywhere in the urinary tract. Rarely hematuria is a sign of clinically significant renal disease. Microscopic hematuria in patients younger than 40 years is almost always benign, and further workup is rarely indicated. Occasionally, significant underlying disease, such as a neoplasm or proliferative glomerulonephritis, can cause hematuria. However, the accompanying active sediment of proteins and red blood cell casts makes the diagnosis relatively straightforward. In older people, hematuria warrants further evaluation, including urologic studies to rule out prostatic hypertrophy and neoplasia, urine cultures to rule out infection, urine cytology, and advanced renal studies (such as renal ultrasound or noncontrasted computed tomography [CT] scan of the abdomen and pelvis) to rule out intrinsic abnormalities.

proteinuria is probably the most sensitive sign of renal dysfunction. The upper limit of normal urinary protein is 150 mg per day; anything greater should be considered pathologic and warrant further investigation. Patients who excrete >3 g of protein per day have, by definition, a glomerular pathology and carry a diagnosis of nephrotic syndrome (discussed below). However, many benign conditions (including exercise, stress, and fever) can produce transient elevated protein in the urine. Daily proteinuria estimation can be ascertained by measuring the total protein-to-creatinine ratio (expressed in grams of protein/grams of creatinine), which can be extrapolated to grams of proteinuria per day. Should any doubt still exist, or precise quantification is necessary, 24-hour urine collection can be performed. This procedure has fallen out

Cockcroft-Gault Equation:

$$eGER = \frac{[(140 - age) \times Mass(kg) \times (0.85 \text{ if female})]}{72 \times SCr (mg/dL)}$$

MDRD Formula:

$$eGFR = 170 \times SCr^{-0.999} \times Age^{-0.176} \times [0.762 \text{ if female}] \times [1.18 \text{ if Black}] \times BUN^{-0.170} \times Albumin^{0.318}$$

Cockcroft-Gault equation and MDRD formula. Adapted from Cockcroft and Gault (1976) and Levey et al. (1999).

of favor, as it is cumbersome and somewhat difficult for the patient to complete accurately. Specific gravity is measured to determine the concentration of urine. In chronic renal disease, the kidney initially loses its abilityto concentrate the urine and then loses its ability to dilute the urine, resulting in a relatively fixed osmolality near the specific gravity of plasma. This occurs when approximately 80% of the nephron mass has been destroyed.

Creatinine Clearance Test

The GFR assesses the amount of functioning renal tissue and can be calculated indirectly by the endogenous creatinine clearance test. Creatinine is a breakdown product of muscle, liberated from muscle tissue and excreted from the urine at a constant rate. This results in a steady plasma concentration of 0.7–1.5 mg/dL (often slightly higher in men because of increased muscle mass). Creatinine is 100% filtered by the glomerulus and is not reabsorbed by the tubule. Although a very small portion is secreted by the tubule, this test is an effective way to estimate the GFR. GFR is estimated by incorporating the serum creatinine into a formula, along with the patient's age, weight, and race, and is expressed in milliliter per minute of clearance (mL/min/1.73 m²). The two most common equations used are the Cockcroft–Gault Formula and the modified diet in renal disease formula.

In some instances, it is necessary to measure absolute GFR. To accomplish this, a 24-hour urine specimen and a blood sample in the same 24-hour period are required. This has fallen out of favor, as the test is cumbersome and inconvenient for the patient.

Renal Ultrasonography

Ultrasonography is the most commonly used and relied-upon radiologic examination of the kidneys. This diagnostic procedure uses high-frequency sound waves (ultrasound) directed at the kidneys to produce reflected waves or echoes from tissues of varying densities, thereby forming images (sonograms). Ultrasound is a noninvasive method to determine kidney size, presence of retained urine within the renal pelvis or calicies (hydronephrosis), identification and limited evaluation of vascular structures, and presence of fluid-filled cysts within the kidney parenchyma.[2–5] Renal ultrasonography is also utilized to localize the kidney during percutaneous biopsy. Because it is noninvasive, readily available in most imaging centers, does not use radiation or intravenous (IV) contrast, and is quick, renal ultrasonography is the imaging modality of choice for initial evaluation of the kidneys. Renal ultrasonography is the modality of choice for pregnant patients because it does not use radiation to obtain clinical images.

Computed Tomography

CT imaging is utilized when the entire genitourinary (GU) tract or retroperitoneum needs evaluation. It provides more information about the structures of the GU tract (ureters, bladder, urethra, prostate) and retroperitoneum, as well as surrounding structures that could contribute to renal pathology (tumors, lymphadenopathy, masses). Furthermore, because of technological advances over the years, CT scanners are far more cost-effective, quicker, and more readily available in hospitals or imaging centers. Like other CT scans, the procedure can be performed with or without IV contrast for vascular enhancement; with CKD, caution must be used with IV contrast media, as this can incur further renal decline (see section "Acute Kidney Injury" section). A noncontrasted CT scan of the abdomen and pelvis is the imaging modality of choice when investigating the presence of kidney stones. A newer modality of CT scan, dubbed CT-urography, can be used for a detailed, three-dimensional evaluation of the GU tract.

Magnetic Resonance Imaging

Magnetic resonance imaging (MRI) is not commonly utilized as the first imaging modality for the diagnosis of kidney disorders. This modality can give much of the same information as a CT scan, with far more detail and information about specific tissues and structures. The cost, time investment, and, to a lesser extent, patient comfort prohibit this modality from becoming mainstream in kidney disease evaluation. Furthermore, the contrast medium used for magnetic resonance angiography (MRA) is gadolinium-based. Gadolinium has been linked to cause a progressive skin fibrosis called nephrogenic systemic fibrosis, which is seen exclusively in patients with advanced kidney disease (GFR<30 mL/min/1.73 m²) or who are on dialysis. This condition carries a high morbidity and mortality burden; therefore, gadolinium-based contrast medium is generally not administered when the patient's GFR is <50 mL/min/1.73 m².

The primary nephrocentric indications for utilizing MRI/MRA is either the evaluation of the renal vasculature if significant renal artery stenosis is suspected or evaluation of a mass, solid or cystic, when radiocontrast cannot be used with a CT scan.

Intravenous Pyelography

Prior to ultrasonography and computed tomography, IV pyelography was the most commonly used and relied upon radiologic examination of the kidneys. Following the IV injection of a contrast medium, a plain-film abdominal radiograph is taken. Further films are exposed every minute for the first 5 minutes, followed by a film exposed at 15 minutes and a final film exposed at 45 minutes. Since various diseases of the kidney alter its ability to concentrate and excrete the dye, the extent of renal damage can be assessed. The location and distribution of the dye itself give information regarding the position, size, and shape of the kidneys. This examination has limited application, particularly in patients with severe azotemia(the building up of nitrogenous waste products in the blood) (whose BUN > 70 mg/dL), this test is deferred because there is sufficiently low glomerular filtration to prevent the excretion of the dye, rendering information about the kidney nondiagnostic.

Nuclear Medicine (Radionuclide Scintigraphy)

While the aforementioned imaging modalities can provide *structural* information, radionuclide scintigraphy can provide qualitative and quantitative *functional* information about the kidneys. Using radiolabeled tracers, information can be garnered about renal blood flow, glomerular filtration, or urinary excretion. Several compounds are available that incorporate Technetium-99 as the radioactive isotope; these include diethylenetriamine pentaacetic acid, mercaptoacetyl triglycine, and *o*-iodohippurate ([^{131}I]OIH). Measurement of these radiolabeled substances can be used to calculate true GFR or the presence/absence of renal blood flow. They can also be combined with captopril to investigate possible renal artery stenosis, or furosemide to uncover unilateral urinary obstruction. Radionuclide scintigraphy is the modality of choice to accurately measure GFR in patients who have undergone a spinal injury, as serum creatinine is linked to muscle mass, which may be disproportionately lower in this patient population. This modality is frequently used in renal transplant evaluation, as IV radiocontrast may be contraindicated and renal ultrasound may be equivocal.

Biopsy

The development and growing use of renal biopsy have considerably advanced the knowledge of the natural history of kidney diseases. Percutaneous needle biopsy guided by ultrasonographic or radiographic reference is usually performed by nephrologists, with the patient in the supine position. Intrarenal and perirenal bleeding may be common sequelae, with serious postprocedural bleeding and hematuria occurring in 5% of cases. Patients are placed on bed rest for at least six hours following the procedure while vital signs and abdominal changes are monitored.

RENAL FAILURE

The classification of renal failure is based on two criteria: the onset (acute vs. chronic failure) and the location that precipitates nephron destruction (prerenal, renal or intrinsic, and postrenal failure). CKD is a slow, irreversible, and progressive process that occurs over a period of years, whereas AKI develops over a period of days or weeks. The distinction between acute and chronic disease is important; acute disease is usually reversible if managed appropriately, whereas CKD is a progressive and irreversible process that leads to death in the absence of medical intervention. In both cases, the kidneys lose their normal ability to maintain the normal composition and volume of bodily fluids. Although the terminal functional disabilities of the acute and chronic diseases are similar, AKI has some unique aspects that warrant its separate discussion.

ACUTE KIDNEY INJURY

AKI is a clinical syndrome characterized by a rapid decline in kidney function over a period of days to weeks, leading to severe azotemia. It is very common in hospitalized patients; AKI occurs in up to 5% of all admitted patients and in as many as 30% of patients admitted to intensive care units. Sepsis, shock, medications, surgery, pregnancy-related complications, and trauma are the most common causes of AKI. Unlike patients who develop CKD, patients with AKI usually have normal baseline renal function, yet mortality from AKI (even with medical intervention including dialysis) can reach 80%, demonstrating the critical illness of these patients.[4] The clinical course of AKI most often progresses through three stages: oliguria (urine volume <400 mL per day), diuresis (high urine volume output >400 mL per day), and, ultimately, recovery.[5] The causes of AKI are often divided into three diagnostic categories: prerenal failure, postrenal failure, and acute intrinsic renal failure.

Prerenal Failure

Prerenal failure, defined as any condition that compromises renal function without permanent physical injury to the kidney, is the most common cause of hospital-acquired renal failure. This condition, often referred to as prerenal azotemia, results from reversible changes in renal blood flow and is the most common cause of AKI, accounting for more than 50% of cases.[4] Some etiologic factors commonly associated with prerenal failure include volume depletion, heart failure and cardiovascular shock, medications that perturb blood flow through the nephron, and changes in fluid volume distribution that are associated with sepsis and burns.[3–5]

Postrenal Failure

Postrenal causes of failure are less common (<5% of patients) than prerenal causes. Postrenal failure refers to conditions that obstruct the flow of urine from the kidneys at any level of the urinary tract and that subsequently decrease the GFR. Postrenal failure can cause almost total anuria, with complete obstruction or polyuria. Renal ultrasonography often shows a dilated collecting system (hydronephrosis). Obstructive uropathy is, most commonly, seen in older men as a result of the enlargement of the prostate gland. If present in females, a thorough pelvic examination is warranted to elicit the cause of the obstruction. Although postrenal failure is the least common cause of AKI, it remains the most treatable.

Acute Intrinsic Renal Failure

Glomerular disease, vascular disease, and tubulointerstitial disease comprise the three major causes of acute intrinsic renal failure and describe the sites of pathology. Glomerulonephritis is an uncommon cause of AKI and usually follows a more subacute or chronic course. However, when fulminant enough to cause AKI, it is associated with an active urinary sediment. Prominent clinical and laboratory findings include hypertension, proteinuria, microscopic hematuria, and red blood cell casts. Post infectious, membranoproliferative, and rapidly progressive glomerulonephritis, as well as glomerulonephritis associated with endocarditis, are the most common glomerular diseases to cause a sudden renal deterioration. The pathogenesis of glomerulonephritis appears to be related to the immuno complex and complement-mediated damage of the kidney.[7,8]

Vascular diseases that induce AKI cover the spectrum of vessel size from large (renal artery and vein) to the microscopic (afferent and efferent arterioles of the glomerulus). Large vessel occlusive processes such as renal arterial or venous thromboses present as a classic triad of severe and sudden lower back pain, severe oliguria, and macroscopic hematuria. Medium-to-small vasculature AKI is often caused by autoimmune vasculidities, thrombotic microangiopathies, or cholesterol crystal embolization.

By far, the most common causes of acute intrinsic failure are tubulointerstitial disorders (>75% of cases), including interstitial nephritis and acute tubular necrosis (ATN). Infiltrative diseases (such as lymphoma or sarcoidosis), infections (such as syphilis and toxoplasmosis), and medications are the leading causes of interstitial nephritis. With drug-induced interstitial nephritis, there are accompanying systemic signs of a hypersensitivity reaction, and the presence of eosinophils is a common finding in the urine. Although renal function usually returns to normal with the discontinuation of the offending drug, recovery may be hastened with corticosteroid therapy.[9] ATN is a renal lesion that forms in response to prolonged ischemia or exposure to a nephrotoxin.[10] ATN remains more of a clinical diagnosis of exclusion than a pathologic diagnosis. The period of renal failure associated with ATN can range from weeks to months, and the major complications of this transient failure are imbalances in fluid and electrolytes, as well as uremia. Serum levels of BUN and creatinine peak, plateau, and slowly fall, accompanied by a return of renal function over 10–14 days in most cases.[9-11]

Sudden renal failure in hospitalized patients is often very apparent from either oliguria or an increase in BUN and creatinine levels. However, renal dysfunction in the outpatient population is often more subtle. A patient can present to the dental office with vague complaints of lethargy and fatigue or entirely without symptoms. These patients can often go undiagnosed but for abnormal results on routine urinalysis, the most common test for screening for renal disease.[12,13]

CHRONIC RENAL FAILURE

CKD is defined by the National Kidney Foundation Kidney Disease Outcomes Quality Initiative as either of the following: (1) the presence of markers of kidney damage for >3 months, as defined by structural or functional abnormalities of the kidney with or without a decrease in GFR manifest either by pathologic abnormalities or other markers of kidney damage, including abnormalities in the composition of blood or urine, or abnormalities in imaging tests; (2) the presence of GFR < 60 mL/min/1.73 m² for >3 months, with or without other signs of kidney damage.[14-16]

CKD can be caused by many diseases that devastate the nephron mass of the kidneys. Most of these conditions involve diffuse bilateral destruction of the renal parenchyma. Some renal conditions affect the glomerulus (glomerulonephritis), others involve the renal tubules (polycystic kidney disease or pyelonephritis), whereas others interfere with blood perfusion to the renal parenchyma (nephrosclerosis). Ultimately, nephron destruction ensues in all cases unless this process is interrupted.

The United States Renal Data System has generated statistics showing that the most common primary diagnosis for CKD or ESRD patients is diabetes mellitus (DM), followed by hypertension, glomerulonephritis, and others (Figure 17-3). Despite the varying causes, the clinical features of CKD are always remarkably similar because the common denominator remains nephron destruction.

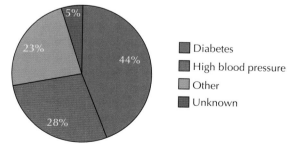

FIGURE 17-3 New cases of kidney failure by primary diagnosis in 2011. United States Renal Data System. Centers for Disease Control and Prevention (CDC). National Chronic Kidney Disease Fact Sheet, 2014. Atlanta, GA: US Department of Health and Human Services, Centers for Disease Control and Prevention; 2014[1]

The prognosis of the patient with renal disease has improved significantly during the last two decades. The improvement of antimicrobial therapy to combat increased susceptibility to infection, along with advances in dialysis and transplantation techniques, has provided patients with the opportunity for survival in the face of a complete loss of renal function. However, despite these advances, the current annual mortality rate for patients with ESRD in the United States is approximately 24%.[1,16]

Clinical Progression

CKD is divided into stages 1to 5 based on the current GFR (see Table 17-3). Patients with stage 1 and 2 generally have "normal" renal function (GFR > 60 mL/min/1.73 m²) with evidence of structural kidney dysfunction (proteinuria, glomerular hematuria, recovery from ATN, etc.). At stage 3 CKD, patients are usually referred to a nephrologist for evaluation and management. The extrarenal pathologies that accompany CKD (anemia, secondary hyperparathyroidism [HPTH], metabolic acidosis) may begin to manifest at this level of renal function (< 60 mL/min). Renally excreted medications generally need dose adjustment starting at this stage as well.

During late stage 4 (GFR < 30 mL/min/1.73 m²) disease or early stage 5 (GFR < 15 mL/min/1.73 m²) disease, patients often become symptomatic and may develop uremic symptoms, which include nausea, vomiting, weight loss, decreased appetite, or a metallic taste in the mouth. They may also manifest symptoms of excessive fluid retention, such as leg swelling, generalized edema, or shortness of breath due to pulmonary edema. Patients may also develop severe biochemical abnormalities, including severe anemia, hyperkalemia, metabolic acidosis, hyperphosphatemia, hypocalcemia, and increased parathyroid hormone levels. The complex biochemical changes, including anemia, hypocalcemia, hyperphosphatemia, and metabolic acidosis, together with systemic symptoms patients experience, are termed the "uremic syndrome." At this point in the disease process, renal replacement therapy or dialysis is a necessity or death is a certain consequence.[17]

Etiology and Pathogenesis

The progression of the varied renal diseases, culminating in CKD, ranges from a few months to 30–40 years. Currently, diabetes and hypertension account for 44.4% and 26.6%, respectively, of the total cases of ESRD. Glomerulonephritis is the third most common cause of ESRD (12.2% of cases). Interstitial nephritis, pyelonephritis, and polycystic kidney disease account for 7.2% of cases. The remaining 9.6% of the causes of ESRD include systemic lupus erythematosus (SLE) and relatively uncommon conditions such as obstructive uropathy.[1,16]

Age, race, gender, and family history have been identified as risk factors for the development of ESRD. The average age of a newly diagnosed patient with ESRD is 61.1

TABLE 17-3	Stages of Chronic Kidney Disease	
Stage	GFR (mL/min/1.73 m²)	Manifestation
1	>90	Asymptomatic; may have hematuria or proteinuria
2	60–90	Asymptomatic; may have hematuria or proteinuria
3	30–60	May develop anemia, SHPT
4	15–30	Start to prepare for dialysis or transplantation; significant development of anemia, SHPT, metabolic acidosis
5	<15	Initiate dialysis when patients exhibit signs or symptoms of uremia

Abbreviations: GFR, glomerular filtration rate; SHPT, secondary hyperparathyroidism.

years, and 53.1% of ESRD patients are male. White people, including Hispanics, account for 63.5% of ESRD patients; black people account for 28.7% of ESRD patients; and people of Asian ancestry make up 2.9%.[1,16,17] Family history is a risk factor for diabetes and hypertension, both of which adversely affect the kidneys and therefore constitute a risk for developing ESRD. Recent evidence suggests that smoking is a major renal risk factor, increasing the risk of nephropathy and doubling the rate of progression to end-stage disease.[18]

Nephritic Syndrome

The nephritic syndrome describes a constellation of kidney diseases, which manifest as inflammation of the glomerulus. The hallmark of these diseases is microscopic anemia and, typically, subnephrotic proteinuria (<3.5 g/d proteinuria). This subclass of kidney disease also, typically, consumes complement as part of the pathophysiology; complement deposition can be seen along the glomerulobasement membrane on microscopic examination of a kidney biopsy. Examples of glomerular diseases that display the nephritic syndrome include membranous nephropathy, lupus nephritis, membranoproliferative glomerulonephritis, IgA nephropathy, and post infectious glomerulonephritis. Some of these kidney diseases are aggressive and can lead to rapid deterioration of renal function over a period of days to weeks. Others such as IgA nephropathy is more insidious and can take decades to progress to end-stage kidney disease. The continuous nature of the immunologic injury is shown by the recurrence of disease in kidneys that have been transplanted to patients with some type of glomerulonephritis, even after their own kidneys had been removed.[19,20]

Glomerulonephritis represents a heterogeneous group of diseases of varying etiology and pathogenesis that produce irreversible impairment of renal function. Glomerulonephritis also may enter the chronic stage from a nephritic syndrome. The most typical examples are focal segmental glomerulosclerosis, idiopathic membranous glomerulonephritis, and membranoproliferative glomerulonephritis.[19,20] In most cases, the patients present with the features of CKD and hypertension or with a chance proteinuria that has progressed to chronic nephritis over a period of years.

Nephrotic Syndrome

Nephrotic syndrome is the clinical manifestation of anyglomerular lesion that causes an excess of more than 3.5 g of protein excretion in the urine per day. Nephrotic syndromeis caused by multiple diseases, all of which enhance the permeability of the glomerulus to plasma proteins. Excessive protein excretion leads to a decline of plasma osmotic pressure, with consequent generalized edema and serosal effusions. The differential diagnosis of nephrotic syndrome is vast but includes diabetic nephropathy, minimal change disease, focal and segmental glomerulosclerosis, multiple myeloma, lupus nephritis (certain subtypes), and membranous glomerulonephritis. Bacterial infections secondary to hypogammaglobulinemia have been described as a cause of death in children with nephrotic syndrome.

Pyelonephritis

Pyelonephritis refers to the effects of bacterial infection in the kidney, with Escherichia coli being the most frequent cause of infection.[21] Pyelonephritis may present in an acute form with active pyogenic infection or in a chronic form in which the principal manifestations are caused by an injury sustained during a preceding infection. The chronic form of bacterial pyelonephritis can be further subdivided into reactive and inactive forms, and one or both kidneys may be affected.

Any lesion that produces an obstruction of the urinary tract can predispose a patient to active pyelonephritis. Pyelonephritis also may occur as part of a generalized sepsis, as s een in patients with bacterial endocarditis orstaphylococcal septicemia.

The clinical picture of acute pyelonephritis is often characteristic, consisting of a sudden rise in body temperature (to 38.9°C–40.6°C), shaking chills, aching pain in one or both costovertebral areas or flanks, and symptoms of bladder inflammation. Microscopic evaluation of the urine reveals large numbers of bacteria and a polymorphonuclear leukocytosis. There are no signs of impaired renal function or acute hypertension as is sometimes seen in patients with acute glomerulonephritis. Patients with chronic active pyelonephritis often suffer from recurrent episodes of acute pyelonephritis or may have persistent smoldering infections that gradually result in end-stage renal failure secondary to destruction from the scarring of renal parenchyma. This process may continue for many years.

Polycystic Renal Disease

Autosomal dominant polycystic kidney disease (ADPKD) describes a kidney disease manifested by large (>15 cm), bilateral kidneys with multiple cysts that distort the expected beanshape of the kidneys. It is acquired through an autosomal-dominant inheritance,[22] with two gene expressions (PKD1 and PKD2), which produce a bimodal pattern of expression throughout life. The PKD1 phenotype presents with symptoms in the fourth decade of life, whereas the PKD2 phenotype presents much later (sixth or seventh decade). The disease causes renal insufficiency in 50% of individuals by age 70 years.[23] Most patients present with microscopic or gross hematuria, abdominal or flank pain, and recurrent urinary tract infections. Clinically, these patients have large, palpable kidneys, and the diagnosis is confirmed via renal ultrasonography or CT. Most patients develop hypertension during the course of their disease, and more than one-half of patients are hypertensive at the time of presentation. Although no preventive therapies have proven to be effective, treating the hypertension with angiotensin-converting enzyme inhibitors may help slow the progression of polycystic disease. Patients with ADPKD may develop cyst-like manifestations in other organ systems, including liver cysts, diverticular disease of the colon, or cerebral aneurysms.

Another form of "polycystic kidney disease" is an acquired, reactive process seen in about half of patients with longstanding ESRD. The kidneys of patients who receive hemodialysis or peritoneal dialysis for longer than three years will have multiple cysts present in small, shrunken kidneys. These atrophic, cystic kidneys are clinically important, as the development of adenocarcinomas is seen in approximately 5% of these multiple cysts throughout the remnant kidneys.

Hypertensive Nephrosclerosis

The association between the kidneys and hypertension is recognized, yet the primary disease often is not. Hypertension may be the primary disorder damaging the kidneys, but, conversely, severe CKD may lead to hypertension or perpetuate it through changes in sodium and water excretion and/or in the renin-angiotensin system.[24] Hypertension remains one of the leading causes of CKD, especially in nonwhite populations (see Chapter 15, "Diseases of the Cardiovascular System," for detailed discussion of hypertension). The heart, brain, eyes, and kidneys comprise four major target organs of hypertension. Long-standing hypertension leads to fibrosis and sclerosis of the arterioles in these organs and throughout the body. Benign nephrosclerosis results from arteriosclerotic changes due to long-standing hypertension. It is the

direct result of ischemia caused by narrowing of the lumina of the intrarenal vascular supply. The progressive closing of the arteries and arterioles leads to atrophy of the tubules and destruction of the glomerulus. "Malignant nephrosclerosis" refers to the structural changes that are associated with the malignant phase of essential hypertension.

Connective Tissue Disorders

Renal diseases are very prevalent among patients with connective tissue disorders, commonly referred to as collagen vascular diseases. Approximately two-thirds of patients with SLE and scleroderma or progressive systemic sclerosis (PSS) have clinical evidence of renal involvement. In rheumatoid arthritis, the prevalence of renal involvement is considerably less and is often related to complications of treatment with gold salts or D-penicillamine.

End-stage renal failure occurs in 25% of patients with SLE. Lupus nephritis, caused by circulating immune complexes that become trapped in the glomerular basement membrane, produces a clinical picture similar to that of acute glomerulonephritis or nephrotic syndrome.[25] PSS is characterized by the progressive sclerosis of the skin and viscera, including the kidneys and their vasculature, leading to changes resembling the nephrosclerosis seen in patients with long-standing hypertension.

Metabolic Disorders

The most common metabolic disorders that may lead to CKD include DM, amyloidosis, gout, and primary HPTH. By far, DM is one of the most important causes of CKD and accounts for nearly one-half of new ESRD patients (data from United States Renal Data System, 2014).[1,16] The type of diabetes the patient has affects the probability that the patient will develop ESRD. It has been estimated that about 50% of patients with type 1 DM develop ESRD within 15–25 years after the onset of diabetes compared with 6% for patients with type 2 DM. The term *diabetic nephropathy* refers to the various changes that affect the structure and function of the kidneys in the presence of diabetes. Glomerulosclerosis is the most characteristic lesion of diabetic nephropathy. Other lesions include chronic tubulointerstitial nephritis, papillary necrosis, and ischemia. The natural progression of diabetic nephropathy follows five stages, beginning with early functional changes (stage 1) and progressing through early structural changes (stage 2), incipient nephropathy (stage 3), clinical diabetic nephropathy (stage 4), and, finally, progressive renal insufficiency or failure (stage 5). The final stage is characterized by azotemia (elevated BUN and serum creatinine) resulting from a rapid decline in the GFR and leading to ESRD.

Toxic Nephropathy

The kidney is particularly exposed to the toxic effects of chemicals and drugs because it is an obligatory route of excretion for most drugs and because of its large vascular perfusion.[26] There are medications and other agents (referred toas "classic" nephrotoxins) whose use leads directly to renal failure. However, abuse of nonsteroidal anti-inflammatory drugs (NSAIDs) can also result in CKD. The renal protective effects of prostaglandins are inhibited by NSAIDs. Currently, abuse of analgesics accounts for 1%–2% of all ESRD cases in the United States.[1,16,26]

MANIFESTATIONS OF RENAL DISEASE: UREMIC SYNDROME

Two groups of symptoms are present in patients with uremic syndrome: symptoms related to altered regulatory and excretory functions (fluid volume, electrolyte abnormalities, acid–base imbalance, accumulation of nitrogenous waste, and anemia) and a group of clinical symptoms affecting the cardiovascular, gastrointestinal, hematologic, and other systems (Table 17-4).

Biochemical Disturbances

Metabolic acidosis is a common biochemical disturbance experienced by patients with renal failure. As kidney function fails, excretion of hydrogen (H^+) ions diminishes, leading to systemic acidosis that results in a lower plasma pH and bicarbonate (HCO_3^-) concentration. Ammonium(NH_4^+)excretion, decreased because of reduced nephron mass, is the most important factor in the kidney's ability to eliminate H^+ and regenerate HCO_3^- These patients often suffer from a moderate acidosis (serum bicarbonate level stabilized at 18–20 mEq/L). The symptoms of anorexia, lethargy, and nausea frequently observed in patients with uremia may be due partly to this metabolic acidosis. Kussmaul's breathing, a symptom caused by acidosis, is a deep sighing respiration aimed at increasing carbon dioxide excretion and reducing the metabolic acidosis. Disturbances in potassium balance are serious sequelae of renal dysfunction since only a narrow plasma concentration

(normal = 3.5–5.5 mEq/L) is compatible with life. As kidney function deteriorates, hyperkalemia ensues. Fatal dysrhythmias or cardiac standstill will occur when the potassium level reaches 7–8 mEq/L. The normally functioning kidney allows great flexibility, excreting, andconserving sodium in response to changing intake. Patients with CKD lose this adaptability, and small fluctuations often have serious consequences. Initially, patients experience osmotic diuresis and excess sodium excretion because of the polyuria. Sodium loss is more common in those conditions that are likely to affect the tubules (polycystic kidney disease and pyelonephritis). When oliguria develops in end-stage renal failure, sodium retention invariably occurs, resulting in edema, hypertension, and congestive heart failure.

Gastrointestinal Symptoms

The gastrointestinal system, particularly the esophagus, stomach, duodenum, and pancreas, shows a myriad of symptoms in cases of uremic syndrome. The more common symptoms are often the first signs of the disease and include nausea, vomiting, and anorexia. Dysgeusia often follows, with patients describing a "metallic" taste to all foods affecting quality of life and nutritional intake. Gastrointestinal inflammations such as gastritis, duodenitis, and esophagitis are common in late renal failure and can affect the entire gastrointestinal tract. Mucosal ulceration in the stomach, small intestine, and large intestine may hemorrhage, resulting in lowered blood pressure and a resultant lowered GFR. Digestion of hemorrhagic blood may lead to a rapid increase in BUN.[27]

Neurologic Signs and Symptoms

Some of the early signs and symptoms of advanced CKD are related to changes in the neurologic system.[28] Both central and peripheral nervous systems are involved, with diverse consequences. The degree of cerebral disturbance roughly parallels the degree of azotemia. The patient's electroencephalogram becomes abnormal, with changes that are commensurate with metabolic encephalopathy. As the disease progresses, asterixis and myoclonic jerks may become

Table 17-4 Systemic Disturbances in Renal Disease (Uremic Syndrome)	
Body System	**Manifestations**
Gastrointestinal	Nausea, vomiting, anorexia, dysgeusia, ammonia taste and smell, stomatitis, parotitis, esophagitis, gastritis, gastrointestinal bleeding
Neuromuscular	Headache, peripheral neuropathy, paralysis, myoclonic jerks, seizures, asterixis
Hematologic–immunologic	Normocytic and normochromic anemia, coagulation defect, increased susceptibility to infection, decreased erythropoietin production, lymphocytopenia
Endocrine–metabolic	Renal osteodystrophy (osteomalacia, osteoporosis, osteitis cystica, and adynamic bone disease), secondary hyperparathyroidism, impaired growth and development, loss of libido and sexual function, amenorrhea
Cardiovascular	Arterial hypertension, congestive heart failure, cardiomyopathy, pericarditis, arrhythmias
Dermatologic	Pallor, hyperpigmentation, ecchymosis, uremic frost, pruritus, reddish brown distal nail beds

evident; central nervous system irritability and eventual seizures may occur. Seizures also can occur secondary to hypertensive encephalopathy, electrolyte disturbances (such as hyponatremia), and hypocalcemia.

Along with neurologic hyperirritability, peripheral neuropathy is commonly present as a result of a disturbance of the conduction mechanism rather than a quantitative loss of nerve fiber. The clinical picture is dominated by sensory symptoms and signs. Impairment of vibratory sense and loss of deep tendon reflexes are the earliest, most frequent, and most constant findings. The predominant patient complaint is paresthesia or "burning feet," which may progress to eventual muscle weakness, atrophy, and, finally, paralysis; there is a tendency toward increasing incidence with decreasing renal function. This predominantly affects the lower extremities but can affect the upper extremities as well. Rarely, facial, oral, and perioral regions also can be affected. Restless leg syndrome is prevalent across all levels of CKD, occurring in about 20% of patients with some degree of CKD.[29] Severe uremic neuropathy is less commonly seen today because dialysis or transplantation is usually performed before uremic symptoms become prolonged or severe. Renal replacement therapy may halt the progress of peripheral neuropathy, but once these changes occur, sensory changes are poorly reversible, whereas motor changes are considered irreversible.

The treatment of renal failure also may lead to the development of neurologic abnormalities in the form of dialysis disequilibrium, which may be seen during the first or second dialysis treatments and is characterized by headache, nausea, and irritability that can progress to seizures, coma, and death. This is uncommon as precautions are taken in the first few treatments not to reduce the uremic toxins from the blood too rapidly.

Hematologic Problems

Patients with CKD often have an underlying anemia, which runs parallel to the degree of renal insufficiency. The anemia caused by renal dysfunction is multifactorial and impacts both the manufacture and longevity of erythrocytes. The nephron produces erythropoietin in response to hypoxic stress, which triggers increased production of erythrocyte from the bone marrow. As kidney disease progresses (often when GFR < 30 mL/min/1.73 m^2), erythropoietin production is likewise truncated, and a normocytic, normochromic anemia ensues (anemia of chronic disease). Nutritional deficiencies, iron metabolism abnormalities, and uremic toxins also inhibit erythropoiesis through various mechanisms. Erythrocyte lifespan is shortened by the suboptimal living environment created by the multiple metabolic abnormalities that manifest in CKD as well. Lower body pH, intravascular fluid hypertonicity, hypertension, and retention of uremic waste products all contribute to an accelerated destruction of erythrocytes. Another cause of anemia in many dialysis patientsis the frequent blood sampling and loss of blood in hemodialysis tubing and coils.

These patients may also have a microcytic hypochromic anemia that may be caused by deficiencies in iron stores. Previously, patients were given aluminum-containing medications, often given as phosphate-binding agents to control hyperphosphatemia, which could also contribute to the anemia. Aluminum also can be found in domestic tap water supplies or in nondealuminized dialysis water. This form of anemia is treated by chelation with deferoxamine.[30] This form of anemia is extremely rare in this modern era, andaluminum-containing medications are not used anymore in chronic dialysis patients.

Interestingly, these patients tolerate their anemia quite well. Red blood cell transfusions are usually unnecessary, with the exception of cases of significant surgical blood loss or when the patient exhibits severe symptoms of anemia. These symptoms and signs of anemia may include pallor, tachycardia, systolic ejection murmur, a widened pulse pressure, and angina pectoris (in patients with underlying coronary artery disease). Transfusions may further suppress the production of red blood cells. The risk of hepatitis B and C, HIV infection, and other blood-borne infections is increased with the number of transfusions, although blood screening techniques continue to minimize these risks.

Recombinant human erythropoietin (epoetin alfa) (Epogen Amgen, Procrit Ortho Biotech Products; Aranesp, Amgen) corrects the anemia of ESRD and eliminates the need for transfusions in virtually all patients.[31] A dosage of 50–150 U/kg of body weight IV three times a week produces an increase in hematocrit of approximately 0.01–0.02 per day.[32-34] Therapy with recombinant erythropoietin is not without its potential dangers. "Normalization" of the hemoglobin or hematocrit is not recommended, as this has been shown to increase overall mortality in dialysis patients[35] and rapid decline of renal function in non dialysis CKD patients.[36] Recombinant erythropoietin therapy in diabetic CKD patients doubles their likelihood in having a stroke.[37]

During early therapy, iron deficiency will develop in most patients. Therefore, it is initially essential to monitor the body's iron stores monthly.[38] With all patients, except those with transfusion-related iron overloads, prophylactic supplementation with ferrous sulfate (325 mg three times daily) or IV iron is recommended.[39,40] Onset or exacerbation of hypertension has been observed as a possible complication of recombinant human erythropoietin therapy for the anemia of ESRD.[41] This effect is attributed to an overly rapid increase in the hematocrit level in the accompanying increased hemoglobin, blood viscosity, and renal cell mass.[42]

Bleeding may be a significant problem in patients with end-stage renal failure, and it has been attributed to increased prostacyclin activity, increased capillary fragility, and a deficiency in platelet factor 3. The bleeding risk in renal failure results from an acquired qualitative platelet defect secondary to uremic toxins that decrease platelet adhesiveness. In addition, the low hematocrit levels commonly found in uremic patients negatively influence the rheologic component of platelet–vessel wall interactions. Platelet defects secondary to uremia are best remedied by dialysis but are also treated successfully by cryoprecipitate or 1-deamino-8-D-arginine vasopressin (DDAVP).[43] Platelet numbers affect bleeding, and mechanical trauma to the platelets during dialysis can cause a decrease of up to 17% in the platelet count. In addition to lowered platelet counts (which are usually not clinically significant) and qualitative platelet defects, the effects of medications on platelets contribute to bleeding episodes.

During dialysis, patients are given heparin to facilitate blood exchange and to maintain access patency. However, since the effects of heparinization during dialysis last only approximately three to four hours after infusion, the risk of excessive clinical bleeding because of anticoagulation is minimal in dentistry.[44] Some patients have a tendency to be hypercoagulable; for these patients, a regimen of warfarin sodium (Coumadin) therapy may be instituted to maintain a continuous anticoagulated state and to ensure shunt patency.

Calcium and Skeletal Disorders (Renal Osteodystrophy)

Renal osteodystrophy (RO) refers to the skeletal changes that result from chronic renal disease and that are caused by disorders in calcium and phosphorus metabolism, abnormal vitamin D metabolism, and increased parathyroid activity. In early renal failure, intestinal absorption of calcium is reduced because the kidneys are unable to convert vitamin D into its active form. Upon exposure to sunlight, 7-dehydroxycholesterol in the skin is converted to cholecalciferol (vitamin D3) and is subsequently metabolized in the liver to a more biologically active form, 25-hydroxycholecalciferol (25-HCC). Further conversion to either 1,25-dihydroxycholecalciferol (1,25-DHCC) or 21,25-dihydroxycholecalciferol (21,25-DHCC) then occurs in the kidney parenchyma.

When the serum calcium level is high, 25-HCC is metabolized to 21,25-DHCC; conversely, a hypocalcemic state initiates the conversion of 25-HCC to 1,25-DHCC. This form is the most biologically active for absorbing calcium from the digestive tract. Impaired absorption of calcium because of defective kidney function and the corresponding retention of phosphate cause a decrease in the serum calcium level. This hypocalcemia is associated with a compensatory hyperactivity of the parathyroid glands (parathyroid hormone production) that increases the urinary excretion of phosphates, decreases urinary calcium excretion, and augments the release of calcium from bone.

The most frequently observed changes associated with compensatory HPTH are those that involve the skeletal system. These changes can appear before and during treatment with hemodialysis. Although it is a lifesaving therapy, hemodialysis unfortunately fails to perform vital metabolic or endocrine functions and does not correct the crucial calcium–phosphate imbalance. In some cases, RO becomes worse during hemodialysis. Some of the changes that are accelerated are bone remodeling, osteomalacia, osteitis fibrosa cystica (a rarefying osteitis with fibrous degeneration and cystic spaces that result from hyperfunction of the parathyroid glands), and osteosclerosis.[45]

The bone lesions are usually in the digits, the clavicle, and the acromioclavicular joint. Other lesions that can be seen are mottling of the skull erosion of the distal clavicle and margins of the symphysis pubis, rib fractures, and necrosis of the femoral head.[45] The manifestations of metabolic RO of the jaws include bone demineralization, decreased trabeculation, a "ground-glass" appearance, loss of lamina dura, radiolucent giant cell lesions, and metastatic soft tissue calcifications.

In children, the predominant lesion is osteomalacia (a deficiency or absence of osteoid mineralization), which is associated with bone softening that leads to deformities of the ribs, pelvis, and femoral neck (renal rickets). Early stages of RO may be detected histologically or biochemically without the presence of definitive radiographic changes because dependable radiographic evidence of bone disease appears only after 30% of bone mineral contents have been lost.

Osteodystrophy patients are placed on protein-restricted diets and phosphate binders (calcium and noncalcium based) to keep the serum phosphorus within the normal range (between 2.5 and 4.5 mg/dL) (Table 17-2. They also are given vitamin D supplements (such as 1,25-DHCC) and medications to target the calcium receptor (Cinacalcet).[46] If these measures fail, a parathyroidectomy may be performed, whereby two or more of the four glands are removed, leaving residual parathyroid hormone–secreting tissue.[47]

Most recently, a newer form of renal bone disease termed a dynamic bone disease (ABD) has emerged as the most frequent finding on bone biopsy of patients who are on dialysis. ABD is a variety of RO characterized by reduced osteoblasts and osteoclasts, no accumulation of osteoid, and markedly low bone turnover. It has been found in a relatively high percentage of patients on dialysis, either peritoneal or hemodialysis, but also in CKD patients on conservative treatment. The histologic pattern of ABD is generally associated with low levels of PTH. However, PTH serum levels in CKD are generally higher than normal even when associated to ABD. Therefore, it is felt that, basically in uremia, bone tissue is resistant to PTH, so that a relative reduction of its levels is able to induce the emergence of a low turnover state.[48]

Cardiovascular Manifestations

Hypertension and congestive heart failure are common manifestations of uremic syndrome. Alterations in sodium and water retention account for 90% of cases of hypertension in CKD patients.[49] The association of circulatory overload and hypertension caused by disturbances in sodium and water balance contributes to an increased prevalence of congestive heart failure. In addition, retinopathy and encephalopathy can result from severe hypertension. Because of the early initiation of dialysis, the once frequent complication of pericarditis resulting from metabolic cardiotoxins is rarely seen.[50] Accelerated coronary artery disease is also seen in patients with ESRD and accounts for the largest cause of mortality in dialysis patients.[51-55]

Respiratory Symptoms

Kussmaul's respirations (the deep sighing breathing seen in response to metabolic acidosis) is seen with uremia. Initially, however, dyspnea on exertion is a more frequent and often overlooked complaint in patients with progressing disease. The other respiratory complications, pneumonitis and "uremic lung," result from pulmonary edema associated with fluid and sodium retention and/or congestive heart failure.

Immunologic Changes

The significant morbidity experienced by patients with renal failure can be attributed to their altered host defenses. Uremic patients appear to be in a state of reduced immunocapacity, the cause of which is thought to be a combination of uremic toxemia and ensuing protein and caloric malnutrition compounded by protein-restricted diets. Uremic plasma contains non dialyzable factors that suppress lymphocyte responses that are manifested at the cellular and humoral levels, such as granulocyte dysfunction, suppressed cell-mediated immunity, and diminished ability to produce antibodies.[54] In addition, impaired or disrupted mucocutaneous barriers decrease protection from environmental pathogens. Together, these impairments place uremic patients at a high risk of infection, which is a common cause of morbidity and mortality.

Oral Manifestations

With impaired renal function, a decreased GFR, and the accumulation and retention of various products of renal failure, the oral cavity may show a variety of changes as the body progresses through an azotemic to a uremic state (Table 17-5). The oral health care professional should be able to recognize these oral symptoms as a part of the patient's systemic disease and not as an isolated occurrence. In studies of renal patients, up to 90% were found to have oral symptoms of uremia. Some of the presenting signs were an ammonia-like taste and smell, stomatitis, gingivitis, decreased salivary flow, xerostomia, and parotitis.

As renal failure develops, one of the early symptoms may be a bad taste and odor in the mouth, particularly in the morning. This uremic fetor, an ammonia odor, is typical of any uremic patient and is caused by the high concentration of urea in the saliva and its subsequent breakdown to ammonia. Salivary urea levels correlate well with the BUN levels, but no fixed linear relationship exists. An acute rise in the BUN level may result in uremic stomatitis, which may appear as an erythemopultaceous form characterized by red mucosa covered with a thick exudate and a pseudomembrane or as

an ulcerative form characterized by frank ulcerations with redness and a pultaceous coat. In all reported cases, these intraoral lesions have been related to BUN levels >150 mg/dL and disappear spontaneously when medical treatment results in a lowered BUN level. Although its exact cause is uncertain, uremic stomatitis can be regarded as a chemical burn or as a general loss of tissue resistance and inability to withstand normal and traumatic influences. White plaques called "uremic frost" and occasionally found on the skin can be found intraorally, although rarely. This uremic frost results from residual urea crystals left on the epithelial surfaces after perspiration evaporates or as a result of decreased salivary

TABLE 17-5	Oral and Radiographic Manifestations of Renal Disease and Dialysis
Oral manifestations	
Enlarged (asymptomatic) salivary glands	
Decreased salivary flow	
Dry mouth	
Odor of urea on breath	
Metallic taste	
Increased calculus formation	
Low caries rate	
Enamel hypoplasia	
Dark brown stains on crowns	
Extrinsic (secondary to liquid ferrous sulfate therapy)	
Intrinsic (secondary to tetracycline staining)	
Dental malocclusions	
Pale mucosa with diminished color demarcation between attached gingiva and alveolar mucosa	
Low-grade gingival inflammation	
Petechiae and ecchymosis	
Bleeding from gingiva	
Prolonged bleeding	
Candidal infections	
Burning and tenderness of mucosa	
Erosive glossitis	
Tooth erosion (secondary to regurgitation associated with dialysis)	
Dehiscence of wounds	
Radiographic manifestations	
Demineralization of bone	
Loss of bony trabeculation	
Ground-glass appearance	
Loss of lamina dura	
Giant cell lesions, "brown tumors"	
Socket sclerosis	
Pulpal narrowing and calcification	
Tooth mobility	
Arterial and oral calcifications	

flow. A more common oral finding is significant xerostomia, probably caused by a combination of direct involvement of the salivary glands, chemical inflammation, dehydration, and mouth breathing (Kussmaul's respiration). Salivary swelling can occasionally be seen. Another finding associated with increased salivary urea nitrogen, particularly in children, is a low caries activity. This is observed despite a high sugar intake and poor oral hygiene, suggesting an increased neutralizing capacity of the urea arising from urea hydrolysis. With the increased availability and improved techniques of dialysis and transplantation, many of the oral manifestations of uremia and renal failure are less commonly observed.

Other oral manifestations of renal disease are related to RO or secondary HPTH. These manifestations usually become evident late in the course of the disease. The classic signs of RO in the mandible and maxilla are bone demineralization, loss of trabeculation, ground-glass appearance, total or partial loss of lamina dura, giant cell lesions or brown tumors, and metastatic calcifications (Figure 17-4). These changes appear most frequently in the mandibular molar region superior to the mandibular canal. The rarefaction in the mandible and maxilla is secondary to generalized osteoporosis. The finer trabeculae disappear later, leaving a coarser pattern. Small lytic lesions that histologically prove to be giant cell or brown tumors may occur.

The compact bone of the jaws may become thinned and eventually disappear. This may be evident as loss of the lower border of the mandible, the cortical margins of the inferior dental canal and floor of the antrum, and lamina dura. Studies have shown that the finding of decreasing thickness of cortical bone at the angle of the mandible correlates well with the degree of RO. Spontaneous and pathologic fractures may occur with the thinning of these areas of compact bone and may complicate dental extractions.

Although the skeleton may undergo decalcification, fully developed teeth are not directly affected; however, in the presence of significant skeletal decalcification, the teeth will appear more radiopaque. The loss of lamina dura is neither pathognomonic for nor a consistent sign of HPTH. A similar loss of lamina dura also may be seen in Paget's disease, osteomalacia, fibrous dysplasia, sprue, and Cushing's and Addison's diseases. Various studies indicate changes in lamina dura in only 40%–50% of known HPTH patients.

The radiolucent lesions of HPTH are called "brown tumors" because they contain areas of old hemorrhage and appear brown on clinical inspection. As these tumors increase in size, the resultant expansion may involve the cortex. Although the tumor rarely breaks through the periosteum, gingival swelling may occur. The brown tumor lesion contains an abundance of multinucleated giant cells, fibroblasts, and hemosiderin. This histologic appearance is also consistent with central giant cell tumor and giant cell reparative granuloma. Associated bone changes consist of a generalized osteitis fibrosa, with patches of osteoclastic resorption on all bone surfaces. This is replaced by a vascular

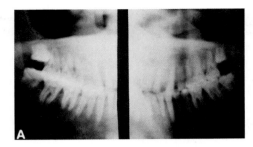
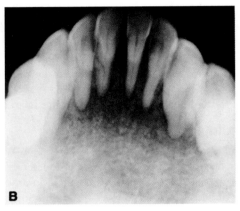
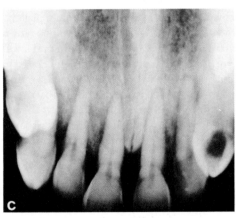
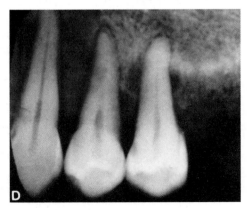

FIGURE 17-4 (A) Panoramic image showing trabecular changes. Also note erupted lower third molars without fully developed root formations. (B) Mandibular anterior loss of trabeculation. (C) Maxillary anterior loss of trabeculation. (D) Loss of lamina dura.

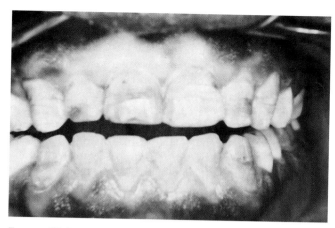

FIGURE 17-5   Enamel hypoplasia and tetracycline stains in a young patient with end-stage renal disease.

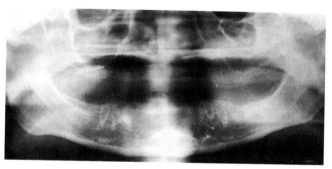

FIGURE 17-6   Panoramic radiograph of extraction sites representative of socket sclerosis. Teeth were extracted sixyears before the radiograph and twoyears before diagnosis of end-stage renal disease.

connective tissue that represents an abortive formation of coarse-fibered woven bone. This histologic picture also may be seen in fibrousdysplasia, giant cell reparative granuloma, osteomalacia, and Paget's disease.

Other clinical manifestations of RO include tooth mobility, malocclusion, and metastatic soft tissue calcifications. Increasing mobility and drifting of teeth with no apparent pathologic periodontal pocket formation may be seen. Periapical radiolucencies and root resorption also may be associated with this gradual loosening of the dentition. The teeth may be painful to percussion and mastication, and positive thermal and electric pulp test responses often willbe elicited. Splinting is a useful adjunct to prevent pain and further drifting, and the splint should be maintained until adequate treatment of the HPTH results in bone remineralization. Malocclusion may result from the advanced mobility and drifting of the dentition. Extreme demineralization and collapse of the temporomandibular and paratemporomandibular bones may also produce a malocclusion.

Metastatic calcification can occur particularly when the Ca × P is >55. In normal subjects, a relationship exists between plasma calcium and inorganic phosphate. When

expressed in terms of total calcium and inorganic phosphate (both as milligrams per deciliter), the ion product or calcium–phosphate solubility product (Ca × P) is normally an average of 35. An increase in the calcium–phosphate ion product in the extracellular fluid may cause metastatic calcifications because of the precipitation of calcium–phosphate crystals into the soft tissues, such as the sclera, corner of the eye, subcutaneous tissue, skeletal and cardiac muscle, and blood vessels. This also may occur in the oral and associated perioral soft tissues. These calcifications are often visible radiographically.

Abnormal bone repair after extraction, termed "socket sclerosis" and radiographically characterized by a lack of lamina dura resorption and by the deposition of sclerotic bone in the confines of the lamina dura, has been reported in patients with renal disease, although it is not unique to them (Figure 17-5).

Enamel hypoplasia (a white or brownish discoloration) is frequently seen in patients whose renal disease started at a young age. The location of the hypoplastic enamel on thepermanent teeth corresponds to the age at onset of advanced renal failure. Prolonged corticosteroid administration also may contribute to this deficiency (Figure 17-6). Another frequent dental finding is pulpal narrowing and calcifications. In some patients who are on dialysis, severe tooth erosionas a result of the nausea and extensive vomiting that often follows dialysis treatment may be seen. Because of the platelet changes with renal disease itself and with dialysis therapy, gingival bleeding may be a common patient complaint.

MEDICAL MANAGEMENT OF CKD

The treatment of CKD is often divided into (1) conservative therapy aimed at delaying progressive renal dysfunction and (2) renal replacement therapy, instituted when conservative measures are no longer effective in sustaining life.[56–58]

Conservative Therapy

Once the extent of renal impairment is established and reversible causes are excluded, medical management is devoted to the elimination of symptoms and the prevention of further deterioration.[59] Conservative measures are initiated when the patient becomes azotemic. Initial conservative therapy is directed toward managing diet, fluid, electrolytes, and calcium–phosphate balance and toward the prevention and treatment of complications.[59] Dietary modifications are initiated with the onset of uremic symptoms. Dietary regulation of protein (0.8 g per kg lean body weight daily) may improve acidosis, azotemia, and nausea. The restriction of protein reduces not only BUN levels but also potassium and phosphate intake and hydrogen ion production. Also, a low-protein intake reduces the excretory load of the kidney, thereby reducing glomerular hyperfiltration, intraglomerular pressure, and secondary injury of nephrons.[60,61] This restricted diet is often supplemented with multivitamins specific to the needs of the renal patient. Despite difficulties with hypertension, edema, and weight gain, salt and fluid excess and depletion must be avoided. For patients with early renal insufficiency, prevention of hyperphosphatemia by limiting the intake of phosphate-containing foods and by supplementing the diet with calcium carbonate (which prevents intestinal absorption) may potentially minimize the sequelae of uremic osteodystrophy.[62]

Recently, a practical clinical approach to the management of patients with CKD, using BEANS (blood pressure, erythropoietin, access to dialysis, nutritional status, specialty evaluation by a nephrologist), has gained popularity. To temper renal dysfunction, attenuate uremic complications and prepare patients for renal replacement therapy, medical care providers should "take care of the BEANS," as follows.[63] Blood pressure should be maintained in a target range lower than 130/80 mm Hg. Toward this end, the use of angiotensin-converting enzyme inhibitorsor angiotensin receptor blockers, because of their renal protective effects, has gained favor with many clinicians.[64] Hemoglobin levels should be maintained at 10–12 g/dL with erythropoietin-stimulating agents. Hyperlipidemia should be treated with a "statin" lipid-lowering medication.[65] Smoking cessation should also be encouraged.[66] Access to dialysis should be created when the serum creatinine reaches >4.0 mg/dL or the GFR decreases to <20 mL/min/1.73 m^2. This is also the appropriate time to refer patients for renal transplant evaluation. Close monitoring of nutritional status is important to avoid protein malnutrition, correct metabolic acidosis, prevent and treat hyperphosphatemia, administer vitamin supplements, and guide the initiation of dialysis therapy. Specialty evaluation by a nephrologist should be instituted when serum creatinine is >1.2 mg/dL in a female and >1.5 mg/dL in a male or in patients with stage 3 kidney disease or an estimated GFR <60 mL/min/1.73m^2.[67,68]

Renal Replacement Therapy

For patients with ESRD, dialysis has significantly decreased the mortality of this once invariably fatal disease. Long-term maintenance dialysis therapy has been a reality since 1961. In 1964, there were fewer than 300 patients in the United States receiving dialysis. Because of amendments to the Social Security Act in 1972 and the extension of Medicare benefits in 1973, dialysis therapy was made available to virtually everybody who developed ESRD. Although access to treatment is of less concern today, discrepancies between the morbidity and the mortality rates of for-profit and not-for-profit dialysis centers remain a source of controversy.[69,70] Today, more than 450,000 people are receiving treatment in more than 3000 dialysis facilities in the United States.[71]

There are no clear guidelines for determining when renal replacement therapy should begin. Most nephrologists base their decisions on the individual patient's ability to workfull time, the presence of peripheral neuropathy, and the presence of other signs of clinical deterioration or uremic symptoms.[72] Most nephrologists will initiate dialysis when the GFR is <15 mL/min/1.73m^2 and the patient is exhibiting hard uremic symptoms. There are a number of absolute clinical indications to initiate maintenance dialysis. These include pericarditis, fluid overload or pulmonary edema refractory to diuretics, accelerated hypertension poorly responsive to antihypertensive medications, progressive uremic encephalopathy or neuropathy (confusion, asterixis, myoclonus, wrist or foot drop, seizures), clinically significant bleeding attributable to uremia, and persistent nausea and vomiting. There are two major techniques of dialysis: hemodialysis and peritoneal dialysis. Each follows the same basic principle of diffusion of solutes and water from the plasma to the dialysis solution in response to a concentration or pressure gradient.

HEMODIALYSIS

Hemodialysis is the removal of nitrogenous and toxic products of metabolism from the blood by means of a hemodialyzer system. Exchange occurs between the patient's plasma and dialysate (the electrolyte composition of which mimics that of extracellular fluid) across a semipermeable membrane that allows uremic toxins to diffuse out of the plasma while retaining the formed elements and protein composition of blood (Figure 17-7). Dialysis does not provide the same degree of health as normal renal function provides because there is no resorptive capability in the dialysis membrane; therefore, valuable nutrients are lost, and potentially toxic molecules are retained. The usual dialysis systemconsists of a dialyzer, dialysate production unit, roller blood pump, heparin infusion pump, and various devices to monitor the conductivity, temperature, flow rate, and pressure of dialysate and to detect blood leaks and arterial and venous pressures.[73]

Dialysis therapy can be delivered to the patient in outpatient dialysis centers, where trained personnel administer therapy on a regular basis, or in the home, where family members trained in dialysis techniques assist the patient in dialysis therapy. It has been shown that patients who undergo dialysis at home fare better psychologically, have a better quality of life, and have lower rates of morbidity andmortality than patients who undergo dialysis in hospital.[74,75] Unfortunately, home dialysis may not be applicable for all patients because it is more difficult and requires a high degree of motivation.

The frequency and duration of dialysis treatments are related to body size, residual renal function, protein intake, and tolerance to fluid removal. The typical patient undergoes hemodialysis three times per week, with each treatment lasting approximately three to four hours on standard dialysis units and slightly less time on high-efficiency or high-flux dialysis units. Nocturnal dialysis and daily dialysis are newer forms of hemodialysis that are gaining acceptance due to improved control of both biochemical abnormalities and blood pressure and volume

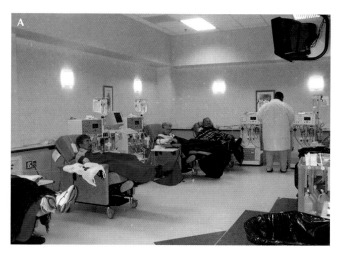

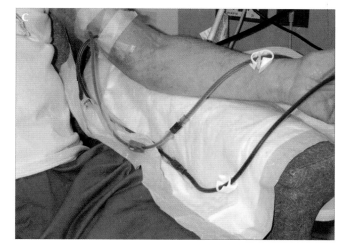

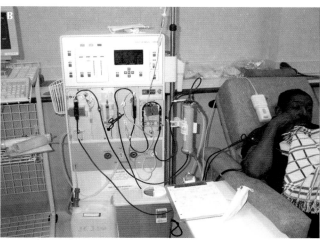

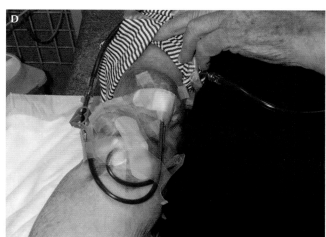

FIGURE 17-7 (A) Dialysate. (B) Dialysis unit. (C) Patient receiving dialysis. (D) Close-up of access.

status. During treatments and for varying amounts of time afterward, anticoagulants are administered by regional or systemic methods.

There are three major types of vascular access for maintenance hemodialysis: primary arteriovenous (AV) fistula, synthetic AV graft, and double-lumen, cuffed tunneledcatheters.[60] Vascular accesses for hemodialysis can be created by a shunt or external cannula system or by an AV fistula; the fistula is preferred for long-term treatment. The classic construction is a side-to-side anastomosis between the radial artery and the cephalic vein at the forearm. In patients with very thin veins, it can be technically impossible to create a direct AV fistula, and in some patients, fistulae have clotted in both arms, resulting in a demand for other forms of vascular access (sometimes the thigh is used as a site). A great advance in access capability was the introduction of subcutaneous artificial AV grafts, beginning with Gore-Tex heterografts (W.L. Gore, Flagstaff, AZ). Fistulae are now constructed between arteries and veins by means of saphenous vein, autografts, polytetrafluoroethylene grafts, Dacron, and other prosthetic conduits. Hemodialysis is performed

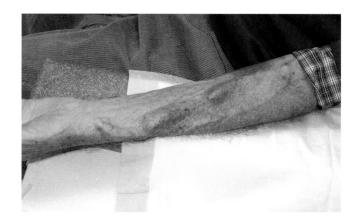

FIGURE 17-8 Vascular access site in the arm.

by direct cannulation of these grafts or vascular anastomoses (Figure 17-8).[76,77] There is an increasing trend toward the use of indwelling central venous catheters for maintenance hemodialysis.[78]

Despite optimal dialysis, these patients remain chronically ill with hematologic, metabolic, neurologic, and cardiovascular problems that are more or less permanent. Growth alterations may be seen in very young renal disease patients, particularly if they are maintained on hemodialysis. This growth deficiency has been attributed to the poor caloric intake of these patients and to the uremic state.[79] Dietary supplements have produced accelerated growth spurts, and successful kidney transplantation may restore a normal growth rate.[80] The major determining factor is the bone age. For patients older than 12 years, it is doubtful that significant growth would be attained.

PERITONEAL DIALYSIS

Peritoneal dialysis accounts for only 10% of dialysis treatments. During peritoneal dialysis, access to the body is achieved via a catheter through the abdominal wall into the peritoneum. One to two liters of dialysate is placed in the peritoneal cavity and is allowed to remain for varying intervals of time. Substances diffuse across the semipermeable peritoneal membrane into the dialysate. Compared with the membranes used for hemodialysis, the peritoneal membrane has greater permeability for high molecular weight species. The Tenckhoff silastic catheter has made peritoneal puncture for each dialysis unnecessary. The Tenckhoff catheter is

apermanent intraperitoneal catheter that has two polyester felt cuffs into which tissue growth occurs. If used with a sterile technique, it permits virtually infection-free long-term access to the peritoneum (Figure 17-9).

Several regimens can be used with peritoneal dialysis. In one chronic ambulatory peritoneal dialysis, 2 L of dialysis fluid is instilled into the peritoneal cavity, allowed to remain for 30 minutes, and then drained out. This is repeated every 8–12 hours, 5–7 days per week. A popular variation of this is continuous cyclic peritoneal dialysis, in which 2–3 L of dialysate is exchanged every hour over a 6- to 8-hour period overnight, 7 days per week.[81]

Two of the benefits of peritoneal dialysis are that heparinization is unnecessary and that there is no risk of air embolism and blood leaks. It also allows a great deal of personal freedom; for this reason, it is often used as the primary therapy or a temporary measure. These features, along with its simplicity, make peritoneal dialysis safe for patients who are at risk when hemodialysis is used (e.g., the young, elderly patients, those with high-risk coronary and cerebral vascular disease, and those with vascular access problems).[82] Some of the problems encountered with peritoneal dialysis are pain, intra-abdominal hemorrhage, bowel infarction, inadequate drainage, leakage, and peritonitis (approximately 70% of

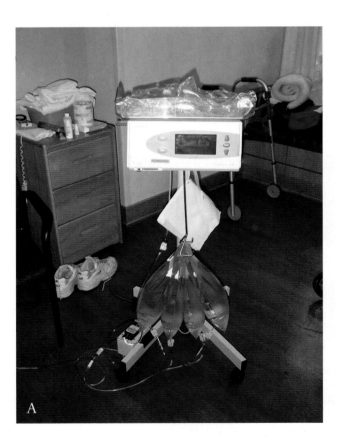

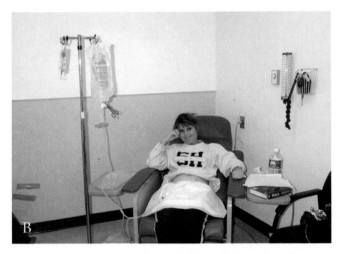

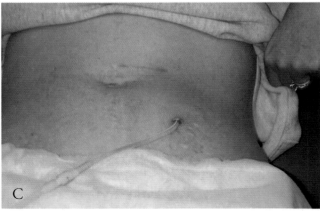

FIGURE 17-9 (A) Dialysate for chronic ambulatory peritoneal dialysis. (B) Close-up of patient receiving dialysis. (C) Close-up of peritoneal access.

which is caused by a single gram-positive microorganism that is indigenous to the patient's skin or upper respiratory tract and that infects the peritoneal cavity).[83] Recent studies have shown inferior mortality data in peritoneal dialysis versus hemodialysis patients, especially in patients with diabetes and coronary artery disease.[84,85]

Today, renal transplantation is the treatment of choice for patients with irreversible kidney failure. However, the use of transplantation is limited by organ availability. Renal transplantation and its specific dental management considerations are discussed in Chapter 21, "Transplantation Medicine."

OTHER APPROACHES TO SOLUTE REMOVAL

Many patients continue to have various disturbances in metabolic functions despite optimal dialysis, maintaining uremic metabolites (e.g., urea, creatinine, and phosphate) at nearly normal levels. These observations have led investigators to postulate that uremic toxins of a molecular weight between that of urea (<500 Da) and that of plasma proteins (>50,000 Da), effectively unfiltered by dialysis, account for these clinical abnormalities. This theory, termed the middle molecular hypothesis, has led to the development of two techniques: hemofiltration (HF) and absorbent therapy. HF is based on the principle of convection instead of diffusion and is based on the physiologic function of the glomerulus.[86] In HF, the standard dialysis technique is modified by sequentially prediluting the blood with an electrolyte solution that is similar to plasma and subsequently "ultrafiltering" it under high hydraulic pressures. This technique is more efficient than dialysis in removing solutes in the middle molecular range and results in patients who feel well and have little hemodynamic instability. Adjunctive techniques used with maintenance dialysis or for patients with significant residual renal function (a GFR of 5–10 mL/min/1.73 m^2) include the use of absorbent materials for solute removal. These absorbents may be used through direct action on the bloodstream (hemoperfusion), through regeneration of dialysate (REDY sorbent hemodialysis), or indirectly, through introduction into the gut. The REcirculating DialYsis System (REDY 2000, REDY Sorbent system), which was manufactured initially by Organon Teknika and now by Gambro Healthcare, Inc., differs from regular single-pass dialysis in that after passing through the dialyzer, the REDY dialysate fluid is regenerated, rather than discarded, by passing through a sorbent cartridge.

ORAL HEALTH CONSIDERATIONS

For the purposes of dental management, patients with renal disease can be categorized into two groups: patients with AKI and patients with chronic progressing renal failure or end-stage renal failure who are undergoing dialysis. The

dental management considerations for patients with renal disease are summarized in Table 17-6.

AKI Patients

AKI is most commonly observed in young healthy adults after injury to the renal tubules as a result of toxic agents, severe necrotizing glomerular disease, or complications of surgery, including hemorrhage and transfusion. Patients with AKI are not candidates for elective dental care, and some patients with AKI require the institution of dialysis therapy. In such cases, elective dental care should be deferred until the patient makes a complete renal recovery.

CKD and ESRD Patients

Oral disease is highly prevalent in the general population and represents a potential and preventable cause of poor health in dialysis patients.[87–95] The results of a study assessing the dental needs of hemodialysis patients showed that 64% of these patients needed dental treatment and that the majority of these patients were not aware of the possible complications of dental neglect while on hemodialysis.[89] Oral disease may be increased in patients treated with dialysis due to their lower uptake of public dental services, as well as increased malnutrition and inflammation, although available exploratory data are limited by small sample sizes and few studies evaluating links between oral health and clinical outcomes for this group, including mortality and cardiovascular disease. Recent data suggest that periodontitis may be associated with mortality in dialysis patients and well-designed, larger studies are now required. Because most dialysis centers refer their patients to general practitioners for most forms of treatment, it is important that more general dentists become familiar with the management problems associated with patients with ESRD who are undergoing dialysis. A study by Ioannidou et al. showed that tooth loss independently predicts low-energy and low-protein intake, as well as serum albumin levels, a biomarker of malnutrition in CKD.[91]

A systematic review by Ruospo et al. evaluating the prevalence and severity of oral disease in adults with CKD looked at 88 studies in 125 populations comprising 11,340 adults. They reported that edentulism affected one in five adults with CKD stage 5D (dialysis) (20.6% [95% confidence interval {CI}, 16.4–25.6]). Periodontitis was more common in CKD stage 5D (56.8% [CI, 39.3–72.8]) than less severe CKD (31.6% [CI, 19.0–47.6]), although data linking periodontitis with premature death were scant. One-quarter of patients with CKD stage 5D reported never brushing their teeth (25.6% [CI, 10.2–51.1]) and a minority used dental floss (11.4% [CI, 6.2-19.8]); oral pain was reported by one-sixth (18.7% [CI, 8.8-35.4]), while half of patients experienced a dry mouth (48.4% [CI, 37.5–59.5]). Data for kidney transplant recipients and CKD stages 1–5 were limited.[93]

Recently, periodontal disease (PD) has been looked at as a marker for CKD.[94] Periodontal pathogens cause both local infection and bacteremia, eliciting local and systemic

TABLE 17-6 Drug Therapy for Renal Disease

Drug	Normal	Adjustments for Renal Failure	
		Moderate (GFR = 10–50 mL/min/1.73 m²)	Severe (GFR < 10 mL/min/1.73 m²)
Antifungal agents			
Amphotericin	q24h	Avoid if possible	Avoid if possible
Fluconazole	q24h	Unchanged	Unchanged
Miconazole	q8h	Unchanged	Unchanged
Aminoglycosides			
Gentamicin	q8h	Avoid if possible	Avoid if possible
Tobramycin	q8h	Avoid if possible	Avoid if possible
Streptomycin	q12h	Avoid if possible	Avoid if possible
Other antimicrobials			
Penicillin G	q6–8h	q8–12h	q12–18h
Penicillin V	q6h	q6h	q6h
Erythromycin	q6h	Unchanged	Unchanged
Ampicillin	q6h	q6–12h	q12–16h
Amoxicillin	q8h	q8–12h	q12–16h
Cephalothin	q6h	Unchanged	q8–12h
Carbenicillin	q4h	q8–12h	Avoid if possible
Clindamycin	q8h	q8h	q8h
Metronidazole	q8h	q8h	q12–16h
Vancomycin	q6h	q72–240h	q240h
Tetracycline	q6h	q6h	q6h
Doxycycline	q12–24h	q12–24h	q12–24h
Analgesics			
Acetaminophen	q4h	q6h	q8h
Acetylsalicylic acid	q4h	q4–6h	Avoid
Ketorolac	q6h	Avoid	Avoid
Phenacetin	q6h	Avoid	Avoid
Ibuprofen	q6h	Avoid	Avoid
Local anesthetics	Unchanged	Unchanged	Unchanged
Narcotics			
Codeine	q4h	Unchanged	Unchanged
Meperidine (Demerol)	q4h	Unchanged	Unchanged
Morphine	q4h	Unchanged	Unchanged
Pentazocine (Talwin)	q4–6h	Unchanged	Unchanged
Propoxyphene (Darvon)	q4h	Unchanged	Unchanged
Naloxone (Narcan)	Bolus	Unchanged	Unchanged
Sedatives, hypnotics, barbiturates, and tranquilizers			
Chlordiazepoxide (Librium)	q6–8h	Unchanged	Unchanged
Diazepam (Valium)	q8h	Unchanged	Unchanged
Flurazepam (Dalmane)	q24h	Unchanged	Unchanged
Meprobamate (Miltown)	q6h	q9–12h	q12–18h
Methaqualone (Quaalude)	q8h	Unchanged	Unchanged
Amitriptyline (Elavil)	q8h	Unchanged	Unchanged
Secobarbital	q8h	Unchanged	Unchanged
Phenobarbital	q8h	Unchanged	Unchanged
Pentobarbital	q8h	Unchanged	Unchanged

TABLE 17-6 Drug Therapy for Renal Disease

Antihistamines			
Chlorpheniramine(Chlortrimeton)	q4–6h	Unchanged	Unchanged
Diphenhydramine (Benadryl)	q6h	q6–9h	q9–12h
Corticosteroids			
Cortisone	q8h	Unchanged	Unchanged
Hydrocortisone	q8h	Unchanged	Unchanged
Prednisone	q8h	Unchanged	Unchanged
Neurologic agents			
Phenytoin (Dilantin)	q8h	Unchanged	Unchanged
Lidocaine	—	Unchanged	Unchanged

Abbreviation: GFR, glomerular filtration rate.

inflammatory responses. PD is associated with the acute-phase reactant C-reactive protein, a major risk factor for CKD. Nonsurgical periodontal therapy has shown to improve periodontal health, endothelial function, and levels of C-reactive protein and other inflammatory markers. Evidence for the association of PD with CKD consists of a small body of literature represented mainly by cross-sectional studies. No definitive randomized-controlled trials exist, however, with CKD as primary endpoints.[94]

Little is known about the effect of CKD on the success of implants in dentistry. A recent study attempted to investigate whether CKD impairs the quality of the osseointegration of titanium implants.[95] This study provides substantial in vitro and in vivo data on the effects of CKD on implant osseointegration using an uremic mouse model. In this study, all implants reached osseointegration successfully in vivo, implying that dental implant treatment might be applicable for CKD patients, but special requirements in terms of bone healing time may need to be taken in consideration.[95]

Excessive bleeding and anemia are the two major hematologic conditions that most commonly affect patients with uremia and renal failure. Bleeding tendencies in these patients are attributed to a combination of qualitative and quantitative platelet defects, increased prostacyclin activity, intrinsic coagulation defects, and capillary fragility. This hemorrhagic tendency can be magnified in the presence of uremia. Hemorrhagic episodes in the gingiva are not uncommon. Ulcerations and purpural or petechial lesions may be noted throughout the oral mucosa. Bruising after trauma is common, and hematoma formation should be expected after alveolectomy or periodontal surgery. Adjunctive hemostatic measures should be considered for patients who are at risk. DDAVP, the synthetic analogue of the antidiuretic hormone vasopressin, has been shown to be effective in the short-term management of bleeding in patients with renal failure. The effects of conjugated estrogen, used for long-term hemostasis, commonly last for up to two weeks, compared with a few hours for DDAVP. Tranexamic acid (an antifibrinolytic agent) administered in the form of a mouthrinse or soaked gauze significantly reduces operative

and postoperative bleeding. Meticulous surgical technique, primary closure, and local hemostaticaids such as microfibrillar collagen and oxidized regeneratedcellulose should be used as the standards of care. Although rare, hemorrhagic effusions into the temporomandibular joint space presenting as pain and swelling have been reported in a patient who was on dialysis and systemic anticoagulant therapy.

The timing of dental care for the patient who is undergoing dialysis has long been a source of discussion in the literature. Since dialysis will return hydration, serum electrolytes, urea nitrogen, and creatinine toward normal levels, arguments have been made for treating patients in a dental setting on the day of dialysis treatment. This argument is countered by the facts that patients often do not feel well immediately after undergoing dialysis and that they a reheparinized. Ideally, elective dental procedures, as well as extractions and other surgery, should be done on nondialysis days as early as possible from the next dialysis treatment. At this point, the blood is free of uremic toxins, and the patient is far enough removed from dialysis to allow sufficient time after surgery for clotting before the next cycle and reheparinization. Also, it is less likely that the patient will have a clotting defect that is due to uremia-related platelet dysfunction, which develops because of retained urea metabolites. A platelet count and complete blood count are important guides for the dental practitioner with regard to the management of bleeding tendencies and anemic conditions. However, since patients are physically and emotionally exhausted and do not feel well following dialysis treatments, elective dental procedures should be scheduled on nondialysis days, when patients are more likely to tolerate care. Peritoneal dialysis generally poses no contraindications to dental treatment. The exceptions are in times of acute peritoneal infections, when elective care should be postponed.

Apart from serving as a potential site for infection, the AV site should never be jeopardized. The arm with the vascular access should be identified and noted on the patient's chart with instructions to avoid both intramuscular and IV injection of medication into this arm, and the access site should not be used as an injection site. The blood flow through the arm should not be impeded by requiring the patient to assume a cramped position or by using that arm to measure blood pressure. When the access site is located in a leg, the patient should avoid sitting for long periods. Obstructing venous drainage by compression at the groin or behind the knee must be avoided, especially because it tends to occur normally when the patient is in the sitting position. Such patients should be permitted to walk about for a few minutes every hour during a lengthy dental procedure.

Susceptibility to infection is a serious concern for patients with uremia or ESRD who are undergoing hemodialysis.[89,95–101] These patients have an increased susceptibility to bacterial infections that results from altered cellular immunity secondary to the effects of uremic toxins combined with malnutrition from protein-restricted diets. Oral diseases and dental manipulation create bacteremia that may lead to significant morbidity and potential mortality in patients with renal failure who are undergoing hemodialysis. A majority of septicemic infections have been attributed to the vascular access site, but oral diseases such as PD, pulpal infection, and oral ulcerations, along with dental treatment, may provide microorganisms with a convenient portal of entry into the circulatory system.[90,95] Therefore, every effort should be made to eliminate potential sources of infection. Meticulous oral hygiene, including good home care, frequent oral health maintenance, and routine use of antifungal and antimicrobial oral rinses, may reduce the risk of dentally induced infections.[90]

Infective endocarditis is a serious concern in hemodialysis patients.[96,97] Sepsis and bacterial endarteritis occur from infections at the access site by organisms seeded through punctures. Infective endocarditis has been reported in patients with access-site grafts on hemodialysis after receiving dental treatment. The incidence of infective endocarditis in patients undergoing hemodialysis is 2.7%. In those patients with a history of vascular access-site infection, the incidence increases to 9.0%. *Streptococcus viridans* accounts for almost one-third of the cases of infective endocarditis, whereas staphylococcal species such as *Staphylococcus epidermidis* and *Staphylococcus aureus* account for the majority of cases.[96,97] The cause of endocarditis in these patients is debatable but seems to be related to a combination of vascular access and intrinsic cardiovalvular pathology. The presence of an AV shunt or synthetic graft (fistula) sutured in place increases the risk for infective colonization at the suture lines or at the surface discrepancies between normal arterial intima and the so-called prosthetic pseudointima. These sites may provide a nidus for intravascular lodgment of bacteria, leading to the persistence of an otherwise transient bacteremia (such as one resulting from dental manipulation), with subsequent endarteritis, embolization, and possible endocardial infection.[97] A period of high susceptibility to infection is usually seen within the first three months after implantation (the risk is highest in the first three weeks), after which there is a gradual decline in risk.

This reduced risk is possibly caused by an "insulating effect" of the developing pseudointima and endothelialization.

Endocarditis infection is more likely to affect previously abnormal cardiac valves, yet there is a high incidence of endocarditis in hemodialysis patients with no previously demonstrated valvulopathy. A possible explanation may lie in the theory that changes in fluid volume with uremia and hemodialysis may affect blood flow through the heart and cardiac function, creating mechanical stresses on the valves that play a role in the development of infective endocarditis. Current American Heart Association Guidelines on the prevention of infective endocarditis should be followed to determine the need for prophylaxis. The choice of antibiotic depends on many variables but is primarily based on the type of microorganisms that have been cultured at the site of manipulation. In patients who were reported to have acquired infective endocarditis after dental treatment, either viridans streptococci or *Enterococcus* spp were the causative agents. This indicates a prophylactic regimen of either (1) amoxicillin or clindamycin or (2) a broad-spectrum antibiotic such as oral clarithromycin (as recommended by the American Heart Association) or IV vancomycin given at the time of dialysis in patients with hypersensitivity to penicillin or clindamycin. Limited insurance reimbursement for vancomycin infusion historically has limited many patients' access to this therapy.

Because these patients are exposed to a large number of blood transfusions and exchanges and also because of their renal failure–related immune dysfunction, they are at a greater risk of hepatotropic viral infections (such as hepatitis B and C), HIV infection, and tuberculosis. Many patients with renal disease may have viral hepatitis without clinical manifestations. In these patients, the disease tends to run a chronic and persistently active (although subclinical) course. With the advent of prophylactic immunoglobulin and the hepatitis B vaccine, the number of dialysis unit outbreaks of hepatitis has decreased; however, the dialysis patient should still be considered to be in a high-risk group. The prevalence of hepatitis C virus infection in dialysis patients ranges from 3.9%–71%.[98,99] Patients undergoing dialysis should be encouraged to undergo periodic testing for hepatitis infectivity. Hemodialysis patients with accompanying conditions such as HIV disease, viral hepatitis (and associated liver dysfunction), and tuberculosis have complicating issues that affect the provision of dental care. CKD patients who are on hemodialysis have been reported to be at an increased risk of developing tuberculosis.[100] (The dental management of patients with infectious diseases is discussed in Chapter 22, "Infectious Diseases.")

As a result of changes in fluid volume, sodium retention, and the presence of vascular access, these patients are commonly affected by a host of cardiovascular conditions. Often, hypertension, postdialysis hypotension, congestive heart failure, and pulmonary hypertension can be seen in patients who are undergoing hemodialysis.[101] Hypertension in the presence of ESRD can lead to accelerated atherosclerosis. Although the medical management of these patients includes the aggressive use of antihypertensive agents, the dental practitioner should obtain blood pressure readings at every visit, prior to and during procedures. Avoiding excessive stress in the dental chair is important to minimize intraoperative elevations of systolic pressure. The use of sedative premedication should be considered for patients who are to undergo stressful procedures. Hypotension resulting from fluid depletion is a common complication of hemodialysis and occurs in up to 30% of dialysis sessions. Cerebrovascular accidents, angina, fatal dysrhythmias, and myocardial infarction are less common but serious sequelae of hemodialysis and most commonly present during or immediately following dialysis. Therefore, elective dental care should be performed on nondialysis days, when the patients are best able totolerate treatment.

Pharmacotherapeutics are a serious concern for dentists treating patients who have renal disease. Most drugs are excreted at least partially by the kidney, and renal function affects drug bioavailability, volume of drug distribution, drug metabolism, and rate of drug elimination. The dentist can obviate problems of drug reactions and further renal damage by following simple principles related to drug administration and by altering dosage schedules according to the amount of residual renal function. Many ordinarily safe drugs must not be administered to the uremic patient, and many others must be prescribed over longer intervals (Table 17-7). The plasma half-lives of medications that are normally eliminated in the urine are often prolonged in renal failure and are effectively reduced by dialysis. Even drugs that are metabolized by the liver can lead to increased toxicity because the diseased kidneys fail to excrete them effectively. Theoretically, a 50% decrease in creatinine clearance corresponds to a twofold increase in the elimination half-life of any medication excreted fully by the kidneys. For drugs that are partially excreted by the kidneys, the change in plasma

half-life is proportionally less. For most drugs, it is proper to give a loading dose similar to that given to patients without renal disease; this provides a clinically desirable blood concentration that can be sustained by the necessary dosage

TABLE 17-7 Drugs to Limit or Avoid When Treating Dialysis Patients

Indication	Drug
Magnesium content	Antacids (Maalox, Milk of Magnesia), laxatives
Potassium content	IV fluids
	Salt substitutes
	Massive penicillin therapy (1.7 mEq/million U)
Sodium content	Carbenicillin (4.7 mEq/g), Alka Seltzer (23 mEq tablet), IV fluid
Acidifying effects	Ascorbic acid, ammonium chloride (in cough syrup), nonsteroidal anti-inflammatory agents
Catabolic effects	Tetracyclines, steroids
Nephrotoxicity	Phenacetin, ketorolac
	Cephalosporins[a]
Alkalosis effect	Absorbed antacids
	Carbenicillin (large doses), penicillin (large doses)

Abbreviation: IV, intravenous.
[a]Long term, especially when combined with gentamicin.

TABLE 17-8 Summary of Dental Considerations and Management of the Patient With Renal Disease

Before treatment

Determine hemodialysis schedule and treat on day after hemodialysis. No such concerns with peritoneal dialysis.

Consult with the patient's nephrologist for recent laboratory tests and discussion of antibiotic prophylaxis in presence of prior infective endocarditis.

Identify arm with vascular access and type; notate in chart and avoid taking blood pressure measurement/injection of medication on this arm.

Evaluate patient for hypertension/hypotension routinely.

Institute preoperative hemostatic aids (DDAVP, conjugated estrogen) when appropriate.

Determine underlying cause of renal failure (underlying disease may affect provision of care, e.g., diabetes mellitus, hypertension).

Obtain routine annual dental radiographs to establish presence and follow manifestations of renal osteodystrophy.

Consider routine serology for HBV, HCV, and HIV antibody.

Consider antibiotic prophylaxis when appropriate according to current AHA guidelines.

Consider sedative premedication for patients with dental anxiety and elevated BP or history of unstable angina. Discuss with patient medication adherence counseling.

During treatment

Perform a thorough history and physical examination for the presence of oral manifestations.

Aggressively eliminate potential sources of infection/bacteremia.

Use adjunctive hemostatic aids during oral/periodontal surgical procedures.

Maintain the patient in a comfortable uncramped position in the dental chair.

Allow the patient to walk or stand intermittently during long procedures.

After treatment

Use postsurgical hemostatic agents.

Encourage meticulous home care and hygiene.

Institute therapy for xerostomia/salivary gland hypofunction when appropriate.

Consider use of postoperative antibiotics for traumatic procedures if uremic.

Cautious use of respiratory-depressant drugs in the presence of severe anemia.

Adjust dosages of postoperative medications according to the extent of renal failure.

Ensure routine recall maintenance.

Abbreviations: DDAVP, 1-deamino-8-D-arginine vasopressin; HBV, hepatitis B virus; HCV, hepatitis C virus.
Source: Adapted from De Rossi SS, Glick M (1996).[90]

adjustments. Whenever reliable blood drug level measurements are available, they can be used to monitor therapy. In the absence of precise blood levels, the best guide to therapy is carefully obtained data on biologic half-lives of drugs in humans with varying degrees of renal failure.

Certain drugs are themselves nephrotoxic and should be avoided. Particular medications may be metabolized to acid and nitrogenous waste or may stimulate tissue catabolism. NSAIDs may induce sodium retention, impair the action of diuretics, prevent aldosterone production, affect renal artery perfusion, and cause acidosis. Tetracyclines and steroids are antianabolic, increasing urea nitrogen to approximately twice the baseline levels. Other drugs, such as phenacetin, are nephrotoxic and put added strain on an already damaged kidney (Table 17-8). The challenge for dentists in prescribing medications is to maintain a therapeutic regimen within a narrow range, avoiding subtherapeutic dosing and toxicity.

The safety of a fluoridated community water supply for patients undergoing hemodialysis has been questioned in regard to whether such water is a contributing factor to the incidence of RO, fluoride toxicity, and fluorosis. There is no satisfactory evidence that the fluoride content of fluoridated drinking water is harmful to patients with severe renal disease. Dialysis patients, however, should receive dialysates that are water purified and deionized. No studies have been reported on the dental use of topical fluoride in patients with renal disease or on any related problems. If a patient with renal disease needs fluoride supplements for caries control (particularly because of diminished salivary flow), the preferred route should be fluoride rinses until more definitive studies are carried out.

Selected Readings

Besarab A, Bolton WK, Browne JK, et al. The effects of normal as compared with low hematocrit values in patients with cardiac disease who are receiving hemodialysis and epoetin. *N Engl J Med.* 1998;339(9):584–590.

Centers for Disease Control and Prevention (CDC). *National Chronic Kidney Disease Fact Sheet: General Information and National Estimates on Chronic Kidney Disease in the United States, 2013.* Atlanta, GA: US Department of Health and Human Services, Centers for Disease Control and Prevention; 2013.

Chonchol M. Neutrophil dysfunction and infection risk in end-stage renal disease. *Semin Dial.* 2006;19:291–296.

Cockcroft DW, Gault MH. Prediction of creatinine clearance from serum creatinine. *Nephron.* 1976;16(1):31–41.

Collins AJ, Kasiske B, Herzog C, et al. Excerpts from the United States Renal Data System 2004 annual data report: atlas of end-stage renal disease in the United States. *Am J Kidney Dis.* 2005;45(1 suppl 1):A5-A7.

de Francisco AL. Medical therapy of secondary hyperparathyroidism in chronic kidney disease: old and new drugs. *Expert Opin Pharmacother.* 2006;7:2215–2224.

De Rossi SS, Glick M. Dental considerations for patients with renal disease receiving hemodialysis. *J Am Dent Assoc.* 1996;127:211–219.

El-Kishawi AM, El-Nahas AM. Renal osteodystrophy: review of the disease and its treatment. *Saudi J Kidney Dis Transpl.* 2006;17:373–382.

Fishbane S. Iron supplementation in renal anemia. *Semin Nephrol.* 2006;26:319–324.

Ganesh SK, Hulbert-Shearon TE, Port FK, et al. Mortality differences by dialysis modality among incident ESRD patients with and without coronary artery disease. *J Am Soc Nephrol.* 2003;14:415–428.

Ledebo I, Lamiere N, Charra B, et al. Improving the outcome of dialysis—opinion vs scientific evidence. *Nephrol Dial Transplant.* 2000;15:1310–1316.

Lee J, Nicholl DD, Ahmed SB, et al. The prevalence of restless legs syndrome across the full spectrum of kidney disease. *J Clin Sleep Med.* 2013;9(5):455–459.

Levey AS, Bosch JP, Lewis JB, et al. A more accurate method to estimate glomerular filtration rate from serum creatinine: a new prediction equation. Modification of Diet in Renal Disease Study Group. *Ann Intern Med.* 1999;130(6):461–470.

Liu J, Kalantarinia K, Rosner MH. Management of lipid abnormalities associated with end-stage renal disease. *Semin Dial.* 2006;19:391–401.

Maggiore Q, Pizzarelli F, Dattolo P, et al. Cardiovascular stability during hemodialysis, hemofiltration, and hemodialfiltration. *Nephrol Dial Transplant.* 2000;15(suppl 1):68–73.

Orth SR. Effects of smoking on systemic and intrarenal hemodynamics: influence on renal function. *J Am Soc Nephrol.* 2004;15(suppl 1):S58-S63.

Pereira BJ. Optimization of pre-ESRD care; the key to improved dialysis outcomes. *Kidney Int.* 2000;57:351–365.

Singh AK, Szczech L, Tang KL, et al.; CHOIRInvestigators. Correction of anemia with epoetin alfa in chronic kidney disease. *N Engl J Med.* 2006;355(20):2085–2098.

St Peter WL, Obrador GT, Roberts TL, Collins AJ. Trends in intravenous iron use among dialysis patients in the United States (1994–2002). *Am J Kidney Dis.* 2005;46:650–660.

Strippoli GF, Palmer SC, Ruospo M, et al. Oral disease in adults treated with hemodialysis:prevalence, predictors, and association with mortality and adverse cardiovascular events: the rationale and design of the ORAL Diseases in hemodialysis (ORAL-D) study, a prospective, multinational, longitudinal, observational, cohort study. *BMC Nephrol.* 2013;14:90.

Trial to Reduce Cardiovascular Events With Aranesp Therapy (TREAT) Investigators. Erythropoietic response and outcomes in kidney disease and type 2 diabetes. *N Engl J Med.* 2010;363(12):1146–1155.

For the full reference lists, please go to http://www.pmph-usa.com/Burkets_Oral_Medicine.

CHAPTER 18

Hematologic Diseases

Michaell A. Huber, DDS
Vidya Sankar, DMD, MHS, FDS RCSEd

PROCESS OF HEMATOPOIESIS

Hematopoiesis has long been thought of as a hierarchal linear process. Long-term hematopoietic stem cells (LT-HSCs) located in the adult bone marrow are pluripotent, can self-replicate, and are the progenitors from which all blood cell lineages arise.[1] Short-term HSCs (ST-HSCs) are derived from LT-HSCs, exhibit limited self-replication capacity, and generate multipotent progenitors (MPPs). MPPs further differentiate into the lineage-committed oligopotent progenitors: the common lymphoid progenitor (CLP), common myeloid progenitor (CMP), megakaryocyte–erythrocyte progenitor (MEP) and granulocyte–monocyte progenitor (GMP). CLPs give rise to B lymphocytes, T lymphocytes, and Natural killer cells. CMPs undergo further differentiation to GMPs and ultimate maturation to the following cell types: monocytes, eosinophils, neutrophils, and basophils. MEPs become committed to megakaryocytic cells that mature to platelets or erythroid cells that mature to red blood cells (RBCs)(Figure 18-1).[1] It is now acknowledged that the process of lineage commitment is not strictly unidirectional, but more plastic and flexible.

The process of hematopoiesis is adaptive and capable of responding to metabolic, infectious, and inflammatory challenges to maintain homeostasis. Perturbations of the system lead to disease.[2,3] Regulation of hematopoiesis is complex and only partially understood. It entails signaling through external factors such as, cytokines and intracellular factors such as transcriptional signaling factors and microRNAs.[4] The primary cytokines governing erythrocyte, platelet, and granulocyte production have been identified and are erythropoietin, thrombopoietin, and granulocyte colony-stimulation factor (G-CSF), respectively.[2,5,6]

A healthy human produces approximately 10^9 RBCs, 10^8 white blood cells (WBCs), and 4 billion platelets every hour. Different cell types have different normal life spans (e.g., 120 days for erythrocytes, 5–10 days for platelets, 6–8 hours for neutrophils, day to years for lymphocytes). Senescent or otherwise damaged erythrocytes are recognized and removed by the reticuloendothelial system. At least half of senescent RBCs are destroyed in the spleen by splenic macrophages and the remaining RBCs are destroyed in the liver, bone marrow, or other sites of the mononuclear phagocyte system. Aging platelets are also sequestered in the

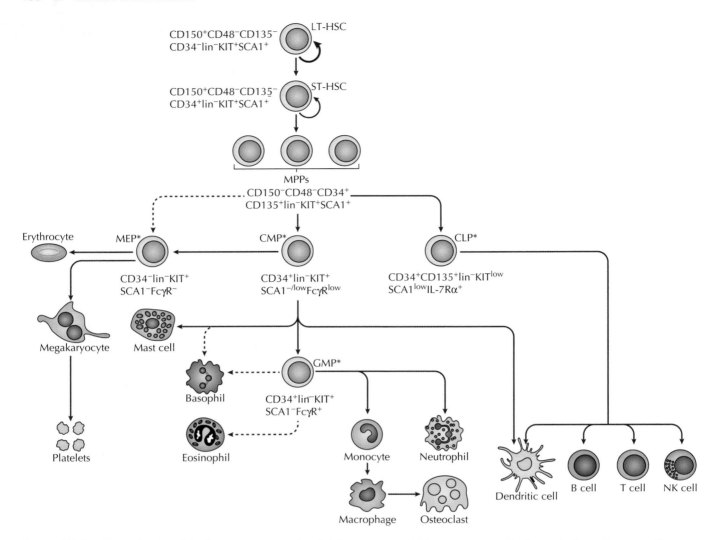

FIGURE 18-1 Hierarchical model of hematopoiesis in the adult bone marrow. All hematopoietic cells ultimately derive from a small population of hematopoietic stem cells (HSCs), which is separable into at least two subsets: long-term reconstituting HSCs (LT-HSCs) and short-term reconstituting HSCs (ST-HSCs). LT-HSCs maintain self-renewal and multilineage differentiation potential throughout life (represented by the bold arrow). ST-HSCs derive from LT-HSCs and, although they maintain multipotency, they exhibit more limited self-renewal potential. Further differentiation of ST-HSCs generates multipotent progenitors (MPPs) and then oligopotent progenitors, which are marked with asterisks. Hematopoietic progenitor cells lose their differentiation potential in a stepwise fashion until they eventually generate all of the mature cells of the blood system (these are depicted at the bottom of the schematic). Several potentially distinct subsets of MPPs have been described, but MPPs are shown here as a condensed population for simplicity. Lineage-committed oligopotent progenitors derived from MPPs include the common lymphoid progenitor (CLP), common myeloid progenitor (CMP), megakaryocyte–erythrocyte progenitor (MEP), and granulocyte–monocyte progenitor (GMP) populations. HSC and progenitor populations can be discriminated by flow cytometry, using antibodies that recognize unique combinations of cell surface markers. Some commonly used profiles for identifying these cells are shown adjacent to the HSC and progenitor populations. Dotted arrows denote a proposed lineal connection. CD135, also known as FLK2 and FLT3; IL-7R, interleukin-7 receptor; lin, lineage markers (which are a combination of markers found on mature blood cells but not on HSCs or progenitors); NK, natural killer cells; SCA1, surface cell antigen 1.

spleen and are subject to phagocytosis by macrophages. The death and removal of neutrophils and lymphocytes is less well understood.

The initial laboratory test to assess hematopoietic health is the complete blood count with differential (CBC) (see Table 18-1). When necessary more specific testing to include a peripheral blood smear, bone marrow biopsy (BM), molecular/cytogenetic analysis, and functional assessments may be ordered to further assess the patient. Virtually all hematopoietic malignancies are associated with specific chromosomal translocations and aberrations of hematopoietic transcription factors.[2]

TABLE 18-1　Key Laboratory Tests for Red Cell Disorders

Test Name	Normal Range (SI units)	Increased	Decreased	Oral Findings
Red blood cell (RBC)	Adult male: 4.5–9.0×106/μL	Polycythemia; erythrocytosis; fluid loss due to dehydration, diuretics, diarrhea, burns	Anemia	Pale, atrophic oral mucosa; in chronic anemia, possible large trabecular pattern on dental radiographs from hypertrophic marrow
	Adult female: 4.5–5.1×10⁶/μL			
RBC indices				
Mean corpuscular volume	Adult: 80–93 fL	Vitamin B$_{12}$ & folate deficiency	Iron deficiency anemia; thalassemia	
Mean corpuscular hemoglobin	27.5–33.2 pg	Hyperchromia	Hypochromic anemia	
Mean corpuscular hemoglobin concentration	33.4%–35.5% (concentration fraction 0.334–0.355)	Hyperchromia	Hypochromic anemia	
Hemoglobin	Adult male: 14.0–17.5 g/dL	Same as RBC results	Same as RBC results	Same as RBC results
	Adult female: 12.3–15.3 g/dL			
Hematocrit	Adult male: 41.5–50.4%	Same as RBC results	Same as RBC results	Same as RBC results
	Adult female: 35.9–44.6%			

APLASTIC ANEMIA

Aplastic anemia (AA) is a rare heterogenous and potentially fatal blood dyscrasia characterized by pancytopenia and hypocellular bone marrow.[7-9] The estimated incidence of AA is 2 new cases per 1 million persons per year.[10] AA is classified as nonsevere (NSAA), severe (SAA), or very severe (VSAA) based on the extent of peripheral blood cytopenia.[7,11] The pathophysiologically linked disorders myelodysplastic syndrome and paroxysmal nocturnal hemoglobinuria (PNH) commonly arise in patients with AA.[10] Etiologically, AA is classified as either inherited or acquired.

Inherited conditions predisposing to AA include Fanconi anemia, Shwachman-Diamond syndrome, dyskeratosis congenital, congenital amegakaryocytic thrombocytopenia, and Diamond-Blackfan anemia.[12] The genetic defects associated with these disorders result in altered DNA damage repair mechanisms, telomerase dysfunction, and altered ribosomal function.[7] Acquired AA may occasionally be attributed to a known trigger such as drugs (e.g., chloramphenicol, quinine), benzene, pregnancy, or seronegative hepatitis; however, most cases of acquired AA are ultimately classified as idiopathic. In acquired AA, contraction of the stem cell compartment occurs as a consequence of apoptosis of hematopoietic stem/progenitor cells.[9] It is postulated by oligoclonally expanded self-reactive T cells that induce the apoptosis with further mediation through the Fas/Fas-ligand pathway or cytokines such as TNF-α and IFN-γ.

Clinical and Oral Manifestations

Patients with NSAA may have mild symptoms and need no therapy, whereas patients with severe disease may present with life-threatening pancytopenia.[7] A serendipitous abnormal hematologic profile may be the first and only clue to the presence of mild AA. Potential signs and symptoms of AA are nonspecific and include fatigue, dyspnea on exertion, headache, fever, easy bruising, epistaxis, gingival hemorrhage, and heavy menses.

The oral manifestations of AA reflect the underlying hematologic aberrations of the disease. In a case-control study of 79 patients with AA, the most commonly observed findings attributed to AA were petechiae, spontaneous gingival bleeding, herpetic infection.[13] Gingival hyperplasia was noted in 13 patients and was attributed to prior cyclosporine use. In a study of 12 children with AA followed over a period of 5 years, 29 hemorrhagic episodes, 10 episodes of oral candidiasis, and 10 episodes of oral herpetic infection were reported.[14] The hemorrhagic events were associated with platelet counts <25 × 10⁹/μL.

Diagnosis

A hypocellular BM along with evidence of depression of at least blood cell lineages is required to establish the diagnosis.[7,15] Classification of severity (NSAA, SAA, VSAA) is determined by the peripheral blood values. SAA is diagnosed when two of three blood lineages are depressed: absolute neutrophil count <500/μL, absolute reticulocyte count <60,000/μL, and platelet count <20,000/μL. Very severe AA is established when the absolute neutrophil count <200/μL. Further cytogenetic testing is useful to distinguish inherited from acquired forms of AA. Peripheral blood flow cytometry to detect cells missing glycosylphosphatidylinositol-anchored proteins (GPI-AP), bone marrow karyotyping, and fluorescence in situ hybridization (FISH) to help exclude hypoplastic myelodysplastic syndromes should be performed on all suspected patients. GPI-AP deficiency is a hallmark of PNH.[7] For NSAA, the laboratory values remain below the threshold of SAA and are often discovered serendipitously as part of routine checkup.

Treatment

The course, treatment, and outcome are related to the severity of the quantitative reduction in peripheral blood cell counts, particularly the neutrophil number. Patients with NSAA should be monitored for progression to SAA. Supportive therapy with blood transfusions to correct anemia and thrombocytopenia in severe disease can be lifesaving. Transfusions from family members should be avoided to prevent sensitization to potential bone marrow donors.[7]

Immunosuppressive therapy (IST) with antithymocyte globulins and cyclosporine is effective for restoring blood cell production for 60% to 75% of patients, but relapse occurs in about 30% to 40% of cases.[11] More troublesome is the potential clonal evolution to myelodysplasia and subsequent progression to high-grade myelodysplasia and leukemia. For children and young adults with AA, hematopoietic stem cell transplantation (HSCT) is potentially curative and the treatment of choice.[11] The best outcomes occur when the patient is young, has minimal comorbidities, and there is a human leukocyte antigen (HLA)-matched sibling donor. Transplant-related mortality doubles if the donor is not an HLA-matched sibling. As consequence, unrelated or mismatched HSCT is typically reserved for patients who fail to respond to IST.[7]

The most serious fatal complication of AA is infection and patients with SAA are at increased risk for viral, fungal, and bacterial infections. There are no standard guidelines to manage these patients, but a proactive approach to prescribe prophylactic antibiotics (when deemed clinically appropriate), antivirals, and antifungals in this patient population is imperative.[7]

Oral Health Considerations

The goal of dental therapy is to establish and maintain good oral health, thus reducing the risk of an oral sourced infection. Patients with NSAA can generally tolerate routine care and the need for prophylactic antibiotic prophylaxis in this AA cohort remains unanswered. Patients with SAA or very severe AA are at a high risk for hemorrhagic and infectious (both oral sourced and nosocomial) events. They should be managed in a hospital setting to ensure appropriate perioperative and follow-up management. For patients who are severely neutropenic (neutrophil count <200/μL), prophylactic antibiotics and antifungals should be used and foods that may be contaminated with bacteria or fungal pathogens avoided.[16]

Attention to details of oral hygiene and hand washing and avoidance of minor injuries or casual exposure to infectious agents can reduce the risk of serious complications.

RED BLOOD CELL DISORDERS

Erythrocytosis

Erythrocytosis occurs when the red-cell mass exceeds 125% of the predicted value for body mass of the patient.[17] It is typically characterized by an elevated hemoglobin (Hb) level (185 mg/dL for males, >165 mg/dL for females) or an elevated hematocrit (HCT) level (>52% males, >48% females). As these tests are surrogate indicators of true red-cell mass, specific testing (e.g., radioisotope RBC studies) may be necessary to distinguish absolute erythrocytosis from apparent or relative erythrocytosis.[18]

Apparent erythrocytosis is diagnosed when individuals have an elevated venous HCT but whose RBC mass falls below 125% of predicted value. Relative erythrocytosis generally only occurs with significant dehydration, use of diuretics, diarrhea, or burns, such that the RBC mass is in the normal reference range but the plasma volume is below the reference range. Absolute erythrocytosis is diagnosed when an individual's measured RBC mass exceeds 125% of the predicted value. Once an absolute erythrocytosis has been confirmed, it is desirable to identify the underlying etiology, which may be classified as either primary or secondary.[17]

Primary erythrocytosis is a condition in which the erythropoietic compartment is expanding independently of extrinsic influences or by responding inadequately to them. The predominant form of primary erythrocytosis is polycythemia vera (PV). Primary familial and congenital polycythemia is a rare primary form of erythrocytosis caused by mutations of the erythropoietin (Epo) receptor gene.[19]

Secondary erythrocytoses are driven by factors extrinsic to the erythroid compartment. Increased Epo production most frequently occurs as a consequence of a physiologic response to tissue hypoxia.[5] Common causes of hypoxia include chronic lung disease, high altitude habitat, smoking, and renal artery stenosis. Tumors such as cerebellar hemangiomas or parathyroid adenomas may secrete Epo and rare genetic mutations to the oxygen-sensing pathway may result in dysregulation of Epo synthesis.[20]

The term idiopathic erythrocytosis (IE) is reserved for cases in which all primary and secondary causes of increased red-cell mass have been ruled out. As a consequence of increased recognition of primary and secondary causes of erythrocytosis, patients classified as having IE are on the decline.

Polycythemia Vera

PV is a clonal disorder characterized by independent proliferation of a single erythroid cell line.[20] An acquired Janus kinase 2 (*JAK2*) V617F mutation in exon 14 accounts for 95% to 97% of PV cases, while a similar mutation of *JAK2* in exon 12 accounts for 3% of PV cases. The incidence of PV is estimated at 1.9 to 2.3 cases per 100,000 persons/year and there is a slight male predominance. PV shares several features with two other forms of myeloproliferative neoplasia: essential thrombocytosis and primary myelofibrosis. Collectively, these three conditions exhibit relatively normal cellular maturation, phenotypic and genotypic mimicry, *JAK2* gene mutations, and a tendency to evolve into each other or develop myelofibrosis.[21]

Clinical and Oral Manifestations

PV is usually asymptomatic and often only discovered incidentally. PV should be suspected in patients with elevated Hb or HCT levels, splenomegaly, or portal venous thrombosis. When symptoms occur, they may include pruritis, vertigo, gastrointestinal pain, headache, paresthesias, fatigue, weakness, visual disturbances, tinnitus, plethora, and bleeding gums. It is postulated that the paradoxical increased bleeding risk results from an altered degradation and function of von Willebrand factor.[22] Pruritis following a bath or shower is often the predominant complaint and has been attributed to mast cell degranulation.[20]

Major complications of PV (e.g., stroke, venous thromboembolism) are attributable to blood hyperviscosity and the qualitative and quantitative platelet alterations observed in the disease.[20] Factors associated with higher thrombotic risk include age >60 year, a prior history of thrombosis, and the presence of concurrent cardiovascular disease. Factors associated with shortened survival include history of thrombosis, leukocytosis, and advanced age (>60 years).[23] The median survival rate for the patient with PV in the absence of advanced age and leukocytosis is about 23 years. In contrast, the median survival rate for the patient with PV with advanced age and/or leukocytosis is about 9 years.

PV can manifest intraorally with erythema (red–purple color) of mucosa, glossitis, and erythematous, edematous gingiva.[24] Spontaneous gingival bleeding can occur because the principal sites for hemorrhage, although rare, are reported to be the skin, mucous membranes, and gastrointestinal tract.

Diagnosis

The diagnostic criteria for PV were updated by the World Health Organization (WHO) in 2008 and consist of both major and minor criteria.[20] Major criteria are: (1) Hb >18.5g/dL for males, >16.5 g/dL for females, or other evidence of increased red-cell mass and (2) presence of *JAK2* V617F mutation or similar mutation such as *JAK2* exon 12 mutation. Minor criteria are: (1) BM showing hypercellularity with trilineage growth (panmyelosis) with prominent erythroid, granulocytic, and megakaryocytic proliferation, (2) serum Epo level below the reference range for normal, and (3) endogenous erythroid colony formation in vitro. The presence of both major criteria plus one minor criterion or the first major criterion plus two minor criteria are required for the diagnosis.

Treatment

Contemporary PV therapy is focused on reducing vascular risks and tailored to the thrombotic risk stratification of the patient.[25] Patients with low or intermediate risk PV with a high HCT level are treated with phlebotomies to reduce the HCT (target: <0.45% for males and <42% for females) plus low-dose aspirin, if no contraindications are present.[26] Poorly compliant patients or those who manifest progressive myeloproliferation warrant myelosuppressive therapy. Hydroxyurea is the primary drug of choice, with anagrelide or peg-interferon-α as alternatives. All of these agents have potential side effects even when used properly. Hydroxyurea is a ribonuceotide reductase inhibitor and is an effective agent in managing PV, but is associated with leukemogenic potential. Radioactive phosphorus (^{32}P) has been used in the past, with a success rate of 80 to 90%; however, its association with an increased incidence of acute leukemic transformation severely restricts its usefulness to patients >75 years of age. The discovery of the *JAK2* gene mutations as the underlying cause of PV has prompted research to develop potential targeted inhibitors; however, to date no new agents or protocols have been approved.

Oral Health Considerations

There are no established guidelines addressing the delivery of dental care for the patient with PV. The delivery of routine dental care for the well-controlled patient with PV likely incurs minimal risk. Low-dose aspirin is rarely associated with hemorrhagic complications from dental extractions. Poorly controlled patients are at an increased risk for both thrombotic and hemorrhagic due to blood hyperviscosity and concurrent qualitative and quantitative platelet alterations.[27,28] Thus, a medical consultation to determine the current patient status should be obtained and referral is warranted for patients who are poorly controlled or who exhibit signs and symptoms of poor control.

Anemia

Anemia is a syndrome finding defined as a lower than normal Hb concentration (<13 g/dL for males and <12 g/dL for females).[29] The signs and symptoms of anemia occur as a consequence of the hypoxia and compensatory physiologic responses produced. Typical symptoms include fatigue and dizziness. The classic sign of anemia is pallor, which may be observed in the conjunctivae, face, nail beds, tongue, and palmar creases. Prevalence rates of 9.2% to 23.9% in males and 8.1% to 24.7% in females have been reported.[30] The prevalence of anemia is estimated at 36% in resource-poor underdeveloped countries compared to 8% in developed countries.[29] In the elderly, anemia is associated with decreased physical performance of daily activities, cognitive impairment, depression, diminished quality of life, increased hospital admissions, and impaired survival.[31]

The initial laboratory tests used to assess suspected anemia are the CBC and the blood smear. The blood smear is used to morphologically characterize the red cells (e.g., macrocytic, normocytic, microcytic, hypocytic). Once discovered, it is essential to determine the underlying cause of the anemia. While the potential causes of anemia are myriad, over 90% of cases are attributable to nutritional deficiencies, anemia of chronic inflammation (ACI), hemorrhage, and hemolytic anemia.[29]

Iron Deficiency Anemia (IDA) and Anemia of Chronic Inflammation (ACI)

Iron deficiency anemia (IDA) is defined as a reduction in total body iron to an extent that iron stores are fully exhausted and some degree of tissue iron deficiency is present. It may occur as a consequence of low dietary intake, impaired absorption, or excessive iron loss.[32] Globally, IDA is a serious health threat, resulting in an estimated 841,000 deaths and 35,057,000 disability-adjusted life years lost.[33] The most common cause of IDA in children is malnutrition, in adult males and postmenopausal women is bleeding, in women of childbearing age lactation or menstruation, and in the elderly bleeding.[29]

ACI, also known as anemia of chronic disease, mimics several clinical and laboratory features of IDA and is the second most frequent form of anemia observed in practice. Conditions in which ACI is frequently observed include autoimmune diseases, acute and chronic infection, malignancies, and chronic kidney disease.[32] Not surprisingly, ACI is more likely to be encountered in the elderly and inpatients. In ACI, the utilization of existing iron stores is impaired, resulting in iron sequestration. The mechanisms that underlie ACI are complex and center on the cytokine-stimulated overproduction of hepcidin. Hepcidin is a small peptide hormone that acts to inhibit iron flow into the plasma from macrophages participating in the recycling of senescent red blood cells, hepatocytes storing iron, and the absorption of dietary iron. Inflammatory cytokines such as interleukin-6 (IL-6) and signal transducer and activator of transcription-3 appear to play prominent roles in hepcidin production.

Clinical and Oral Manifestations

The most important clinical symptom of anemia is chronic fatigue. Outward signs may be subtle and include pallor of the conjunctivae, lips, and oral mucosa; brittle nails with spooning, cracking, and splitting of nail beds; and palmar creases that have traditionally been used by physicians in the diagnosis of anemia. Among 50 prospectively examined patients, a statistically significant correlation was noted between Hb concentration and the following: color tint of the lower eyelid conjunctiva, nail-bed rubor, nail-bed blanching, and palmar crease rubor.[34] As the assessed areas are all easily viewed by the oral health-care provider, these findings demonstrate the positive role the oral health-care professional can play in the early identification or suspicion of anemia. Other findings may include palpitations, shortness of breath, numbness and tingling in fingers and toes, and bone pain.

Glossitis and stomatitis are recognized oral manifestations of anemia. In a study of 12 patients oral signs and symptoms of anemia included angular cheilitis (58%), glossitis with different degrees of atrophy of fungiform and filliform papillae (42%), pale oral mucosa (33%), oral candidiasis (25%), recurrent aphthous stomatitis (8%), erythematous mucositis (8%), and burning mouth (8%) for several months to 1-year duration.[35] IDA or ACI should be suspected in every case of glossitis, glossodynia, angular cheilitis, erythematous mucositis, oral candidiasis, recurrent oral ulcers, and burning mouth when no other obvious causes are identified.[36-38] These findings are believed to be caused by the impaired cellular immunity, deficient bactericidal activity of polymorphonuclear leukocytes, inadequate antibody response, and epithelial abnormalities attributed to iron lack.[39] Clinically evident atrophic changes of the tongue, defined by a smooth red tongue appearance, in patients with iron deficiency anemia have been associated with a significant reduction in the mean epithelial thickness of the buccal mucosa as determined histologically.[40]

Diagnosis

The finding of a reduced Hb and HCT on the CBC is typically the first clue to IDA, which is classically characterized as a microcytic hypochromic anemia.[41] A definitive diagnosis of IDA requires evidence that iron stores are fully depleted and is usually based on the finding of low serum iron, low transferrin saturation, and low ferritin.[32,42] The most accurate initial diagnostic test for IDA is the serum ferritin level.[41,42] Serum ferritin levels <25 mcg/L are highly suggestive of IDA, while levels >100mcg/L are reflective of good iron stores. For intermediate results, attainment of the serum iron level, total iron-binding, and transferrin saturation is recommended to further refine the diagnosis. When the diagnosis remains ambiguous, further testing to include BM may be necessary.

Discrimination of ACI from IDA is frequently challenging. Serum ferritin levels are increased with chronic inflammatory conditions such as inflammatory bowel disease (IBD), infections, liver disease, malignancies, and chronic liver failure.[43] Indeed a patient with an inflammatory condition such as IBD may manifest both IDA and ACI. However, patients with ACI have normal transferrin receptor levels and high hepcidin levels, while patients with IDA have high transferrin receptor levels and normal or low hepcidin levels.[31,32]

Once the presence of IDA and/or ACI is determined, a medical evaluation to determine the cause is warranted. The various causes of IDA may be classified as either physiologic or pathologic. The most common physiologic cause of IDA affects premenopausal females in two ways. First, menstrual iron loss exceeds dietary intake. Second, dietary intake is insufficient to meet the demands of fetal development in the gravid or lactating female. Pathologic causes of IDA are more commonly observed in older adults and include gastritis, peptic ulcer disease, ulcerative colitis, GI carcinoma, achlorhydria, and Celiac disease.[41] Conditions commonly associated with ACI include autoimmune diseases, infections, chronic kidney disease, and non-GI malignancies.[32] Unfortunately, even after extensive medical assessment, up to one-third of patients will have unexplained anemia.[30]

Treatment

In addition to treating the underlying cause of the anemia, iron supplementation should be provided. Oral iron supplementation is safe, cost-effective and convenient. The goal is to raise serum Hb by 1–2 g/dL every 2 weeks, and ultimately restore iron stores in about 3–4 months. Ferrous sulfate and ferrous gluconate have good bioavailability and contain 20% and 12% of elemental iron for absorption, respectively.[43] The recommended dose for both is 325mg three times per day. To maximize absorption, they should be taken with orange juice, since iron is better absorbed in an acidic environment.[41] Foods and medications that inhibit iron absorption include tea, coffee, phosphate-containing carbonated beverages, antacids, proton-pump inhibitors, and H_2-blockers. Adverse effects of oral iron therapy are dose related, can adversely affect effect compliance and include nausea, epigastric discomfort, and constipation. For such cases a lower dosage regimen should be attempted.

When oral iron supplementation is ineffective due to poor patient compliance or intolerance, intravenous iron therapy is indicated. Other possible indications for intravenous iron therapy are: high iron requirements due to chronic uncorrectable bleeding or chronic hemodialysis; iron malabsorption secondary to a GI condition; IBD with ineffective erythropoiesis, poor iron absorption, and intolerance to oral iron supplementation; and the need for rapid restitution of iron stores (e.g., preoperative).[41] Intravenous iron products are made up of nanoparticles of iron oxyhydroxide gel in colloidal suspension held within a stabilizing carbohydrate shell.[43] Available products include high molecular weight iron dextran, low molecular weight iron dextran, iron sucrose, ferric gluconate, and ferumoxytol. Serious and potentially life-threatening hypersensitivity reactions may occur, with the highest risk associated with high molecular weight preparations.

Plummer-Vinson Syndrome

Plummer-Vinson syndrome, also called Paterson-Kelly syndrome, is a rare syndrome characterized by the classic triad of dysphagia, iron deficiency anemia, and upper esophageal webs or strictures.[44,45] It usually affects middle-aged white women in the fourth to seventh decade of life but has also been described in children and adolescents.

The dysphagia may be intermittent or progressive over years, is usually painless and limited to solids, and may be associated with weight loss. Symptoms resulting from anemia (weakness, pallor, fatigue, tachycardia) predominate the clinical picture. Other potential findings include glossitis, glossopyrosis, glossodynia, angular cheilitis, koilonychia, fragility, thinning of nails, and brittle hair. Radiologic examination of the pharynx shows the presence of webs.[46] The etiopathogenesis is unknown, but it is postulated that iron deficiency adversely affects iron dependent enzymes in the epithelium of the upper GI tract increasing free radical stress, DNA damage, and malignant transformation.[44]

Plummer-Vinson syndrome can often be treated effectively with iron supplementation. In cases of significant obstruction of the esophageal lumen by esophageal webs/strictures with persistent dysphagia despite iron supplementation, rupture and mechanical dilation of the web may be required. Since Plummer-Vinson syndrome is associated with an increased risk of squamous cell carcinoma of the pharynx and the esophagus, the patients should be monitored closely.[44]

Oral Health Considerations

For dental patients with extremely low Hb levels, physician consultation prior to surgical treatment is recommended. Patients with IDA or ACA whose Hb levels are above 11 g/dL and who are free from symptoms can tolerate routine dental care. Routine care should be deferred in those patients whose Hb is <11 g/dL or those who manifest signs and symptoms such as shortness of breath, abnormal heart rate, or oxygen saturation less than 91% (as determined by pulse oximetry) until their health status improves.[47] Narcotic use should be limited for those with severe anemia, and dentists should be aware that anemia places a patient at increased risk for ischemic heart disease.

Macrocytosis

The term macrocytosis refers to a blood condition in which RBCs are larger than normal and is reported in terms of mean corpuscular volume (MCV). MCV, the average volume of RBCs, is calculated as HCT × 1,000 divided by RBC (millions/μL). Normal MCV values range from 80 to 100 femtoliters depending on gender, age, and reference laboratory. Macrocytosis is identified by reviewing peripheral blood smears and/or by automated RBC indices and is diagnosed when the MCV is >100 fL. It is a relatively common finding with a reported incidence ranging from 1.7% to 3.6%.[48] There are numerous causes, and approximately 60% of cases are not associated with anemia.[29,48] Potential causes include alcoholism, B_{12} and folate deficiency, hemolysis or hemorrhage, hypothyroidism, liver dysfunction, and myelodysplasia.[49] Medications that interfere with nucleic acid metabolism such as hydroxyurea, trimethoprim/sulfamethoxazole, methotrexate, metformin, zidovudine, stavudine, lamivudine, valproic acid, and phenytoin may result in macrocytosis. Measures to address the underlying cause often results in normalization of the MCV.

B_{12} and Folate Deficiency Anemia

Vitamin B_{12} (cobalamin) deficiency and/or folate deficiency are common causes of macrocytic anemia.[50] Both vitamins participate in critical enzyme reactions necessary for proper DNA synthesis. From hematological perspective, lack of either vitamin results in an essentially identical megaloblastic anemia. The underlying cause of either anemia may entail conditions of decreased intake, impaired absorption, and/or increased requirements. These vitamins are also essential for proper neurological development.

The predominant causes of folate deficiency involve scenarios of inadequate intake, such as may occur in malnutrition and alcoholism. The increased physiologic folate requirement associated with pregnancy, lactation, and conditions of chronic hemolysis or hemorrhage may lead to an anemic state.

Vitamin B_{12} deficiency occurs frequently (>20%) among the elderly, but it is often unrecognized because the clinical manifestations are subtle and many patients will not progress to severe deficiency.[50] Most of these cases are believed to be caused by conditions that impair, but do not totally eliminate B_{12} absorption for the diet and include atrophic gastritis, gluten-induced enteropathy, and the use of proton-pump inhibitors. Pernicious anemia is an autoimmune disease defined by autoantibodies directed against intrinsic factor (a substance needed to absorb vitamin B_{12} from the gastrointestinal tract) and gastric parietal cells. Severe B_{12} deficiency develops when physiologic absorption is totally negated, such as may occur with pernicious anemia, total gastrectomy, or ileal resection. The prevalence of pernicious anemia in adults over the age of 60 years is estimated at 2.7% for females and 1.4% for males.[51]

Clinical and Oral Manifestations

The typical nonspecific symptoms of IDA or ACI such as fatigue, decreased mental concentration, and weakness are characteristic of folate or B_{12} deficiency. B_{12} deficiency may present as neurological symptoms such as clumsiness, unsteady gait, and paresthesia. Prolonged severe B_{12} deficiency, as may be seen in pernicious anemia, may lead to demyelination of the dorsal columns of the spinal cord, resulting in more advanced signs and symptoms such as peripheral neuropathy and ataxia. Unfortunately, these advanced signs and symptoms are often not reversed with replacement therapy.

Oral signs of folate and B_{12} deficiency are similar to those observed with IDA or ACI and include a beefy red tongue with smooth or patchy areas of erythema. Symptom complaints include soreness or a burning sensation affecting the tongue, lips, buccal mucosa, and other mucosal sites. Paresthesia and taste alterations have been reported.[52]

Diagnosis

The diagnostic process begins by establishing the presence of vitamin B_{12} or folate deficiency and then determining the cause of deficiency. The primary laboratory investigations include a CBC, peripheral blood smear, serum vitamin B_{12} assay, and RBC and serum folate assays. A single serum measurement of folate levels is insufficient to discriminate between a transient drop and true deficiency.[49,50] The measurement of RBC folate levels provides a good indication of folate levels over time, but the test is complex and not widely available. Two surrogate tests to assess folate and B_{12} levels are the homocysteine and methylmalonic acid levels. Both folate and B_{12} are necessary for the normal metabolic disposal of homocysteine, while only B_{12} is necessary for the metabolic disposal of methylmalonic acid.[50] As such, folate deficiency is unlikely if the homocysteine levels are normal.

The diagnosis of vitamin B_{12} deficiency is complex. Serum levels of B_{12} <100 pg/mL likely indicate true deficiency. B_{12} levels of 100–400 pg/mL are considered equivocal and should be followed by measurement of serum methylmalonic acid and homocysteine levels, which are increased early in vitamin B_{12} deficiency. The diagnosis of pernicious anemia requires demonstration of atrophic body gastritis and intrinsic factor deficiency.[51] Use of the Schilling test (which measures cyanocobalamin absorption by increasing urine radioactivity after an oral dose of radioactive cyanocobalamin) for detection of pernicious anemia has been supplanted for most part by serologic testing for parietal cell and intrinsic factor antibodies.[51]

Treatment

Treatment strategies for folate or B_{12} deficiency are dictated by the underlying cause. Fortunately the routine fortification of foods with folate has greatly reduced the occurrence of deficiency in most populations. However, prescribed folate supplementation may still be necessary in scenarios of alcoholism and malnutrition. Previously ingrained protocols entailing intramuscular B_{12} injections to manage deficiency have been largely supplanted by more convenient oral supplementation regimens.[53] A recent evidence-based review of two studies suggests the oral administration of between 1000 μg–2000 μg of B_{12} initially daily and then weekly effectively raised serum B_{12} levels.[54] Even when intrinsic factor is not present to aid in the absorption of vitamin B_{12}, as in pernicious anemia or in other diseases that affect the usual absorption sites in the terminal ileum, oral therapy was still effective.

Hemolysis

The normal RBC life span is 110 to 120 days in the circulation.[55] Hemolytic diseases result in anemia if the bone marrow is not able to replenish adequately the prematurely destroyed RBCs. The hemolytic anemias are classified as either inherited or acquired.[56] Inherited forms include sickle cell anemia, thalassemia, hereditary spherocytosis, hereditary elliptocytosis, glucose-6-phosphate dehydrogenase (G6PD) deficiency, and pyruvate kinase deficiency. Acquired forms are immune hemolytic anemia, mechanical hemolytic anemia, paroxysmal nocturnal hemoglobinuria, and exposure to certain infections, toxins, or snake venom.

With acute hemolytic disease, the signs and symptoms depend on the mechanism that leads to red cell destruction. The release of free Hb occurring in intravascular hemolysis may present as acute flank pain, free Hb in the plasma and urine, and renal failure. In patients with chronic or progressive anemia, symptoms depend on the patients' age and adequacy of blood supply to critical organs. With moderate anemia, symptoms may include fatigue, loss of stamina, breathlessness, tachycardia, and, less commonly, jaundice and hemoglobinuria. Physical findings include jaundice of skin and mucosae, splenomegaly, and other findings associated with specific hemolytic anemia.

A careful history and physical examination provide important clues to the diagnosis of hemolytic anemia. Once a patient presents with clinical signs and symptoms of anemia, laboratory testing should be supported by a complete drug and toxin exposure history and the family history. Laboratory tests in the patient with anemia may be ordered initially to demonstrate the presence of hemolysis and define its cause. An elevated reticulocyte count is the most useful indicator of hemolysis, reflecting erythroid hyperplasia of the bone marrow. Assessment of RBC morphology, findings on the peripheral blood smear, and, rarely, BM may provide additional clues to support the specific diagnosis.

Oral signs indicating possible hemolytic anemia may include pallor or jaundice of oral mucosa, paresthesia of mucosa, and, for those with chronic conditions, hyperplastic marrow spaces in the mandible, maxilla, and facial bones.

Paroxysmal Nocturnal Hemoglobinuria.

PNH is a rare acquired condition characterized by bone marrow failure, hemolytic anemia, thrombosis, and smooth muscle dystonia.[57] Clonal expansion of hematopoietic stem cells harboring somatic mutations in an X-linked gene, called phosphatidylinositol glycan class A renders lineage cells vulnerable to compliment-mediated intravascular and extravascular hemolysis.[58] Intravascular hemolysis leads to release of free Hb, a potent scavenger of nitric oxide. The subsequent lack of tissue nitric oxide is believed to underlie many of the clinical manifestations of PNH, including fatigue, pain, esophageal spasm, erectile dysfunction, and, possibly platelet activation. Patients with classic PNH are at an increased risk for thrombosis and other complications of intravascular hemolysis. Without therapy the median survival rate is 10 to 20 years.[57] Allogeneic bone marrow transplantation is the only curative therapy available for PNH, with reported success rates of 50% to 70%. The human monoclonal antibody eculizumab blocks terminal complement activation at C5 and markedly reduces the risk of intravascular thrombosis, decreases or eliminates the need for transfusions, and improves the quality of life.[57]

Glucose-6-Phosphate Dehydrogenase Deficiency.

G6PD deficiency is inherited as an X-linked hemolytic anemia caused by mutations in the *G6PD* gene[59] and more

than 400 mutational variants have been defined.[60] Affected individuals are at risk for developing hemolytic anemia. The WHO classifies the different variants according to the magnitude of enzyme deficiency and severity of hemolysis: Class I is <1% of enzyme activity; Class II is <10%, Class III is 10%–60%, Class IV is 60%–90%, and Class V is >110%.[60] G6PD deficiency is the most common enzyme deficiency in the world and is estimated to affect 330 to 400 million people worldwide, primarily men.[59,61] The two most commonly observed variants are Class II and III.[62] The geographic areas of highest prevalence correlate well with areas where malaria is endemic, such as Africa, Mediterranean Europe, southeast Asia, and Latin America. It is widely believed that G6PD deficiency confers some level of protection against *Plasmodium falciparum* malaria.[59,62,63]

The *G6PD* enzyme acts via the hexose monophosphate shunt to catalyze the oxidation of glucose-6-phosphate to 6-phosphogluconate while concomitantly reducing the oxidized form of nicotinamide adenine dinucleotide phosphate (NADP+) to nicotinamide adenine dinucleotide phosphate (NADPH). NADPH, a required cofactor in many biosynthetic reactions, maintains glutathione in its reduced form. Reduced glutathione acts as a scavenger for dangerous oxidative metabolites in the cell.[59,64] While other cells may produce NADPH via alternate pathways, the RBC relies exclusively on G6PD activity. Hemolysis typically occurs when the RBCs undergo excessive oxidative stress, usually due to an external trigger such as drug exposure, fava bean ingestion, or infection.[64] Other potential triggering factors include diabetes, myocardial infarction, and strenuous exercise.[59]

Clinical Manifestations

The vast majority of individuals with G6PD deficiency remain clinically asymptomatic throughout their lives. If hemolysis occurs in an affected patient, characteristic signs and symptoms of fatigue, flank pain, anemia, and jaundice are evident. Patients with the most severe Class I variant of the disease (aka congenital nonspherocytic hemolytic anemia) typically experience chronic anemia, more severe hemolytic episodes requiring transfusion, reticulocytosis, gallstones, and splenomegaly.

About one-third of male newborns who manifest neonatal jaundice within the first 1–4 days of age are G6PD deficient.[59] The icterus of neonatal jaundice is not due to hemolysis, but the inability of the liver to adequately conjugate bilirubin.[63] A rare, but serious consequence of neonatal jaundice is kernicterus and possible permanent neurological damage. This is compounded when the infant also inherits the UDP glucuronosyl transferase promoter polymorphism that is observed in Gilbert disease.

Infection is likely the most common trigger of hemolysis in at-risk patients.[59,63] Common infectious triggers include Salmonella, *Escherichia coli*, β-hemolytic streptococci, rickettsia infections, hepatitis A and B, pneumonia, cytomegalovirus, and typhoid fever.[59,62] While the mechanism triggering hemolysis is unknown, it is postulated that leuko- cytes release oxidative stressors during phagocytosis.

Ingestion of fava beans is a recognized trigger. Toxic components of the bean are postulated to activate the hex- ose monophosphate shunt and promote hemolysis.[59] How- ever, the exact etiopathogenesis of this phenomenon remains unknown, since many G6PD patients can eat fava beans with no adverse consequence.[63] Patients with the Class II vari- ant G6PD deficiency are at greatest risk. Fava bean-related hemolysis occurs within the first 24 hours of ingestion, is usually severe, and often leads to acute renal failure.

Drug-induced hemolysis typically occurs within 24 to 72 hours of exposure and dark urine due to hemoglobinuria is characteristic.[59] The anemia progresses for about a week, followed by recovery over the next 8 to 10 days.

Diagnosis

The rapid fluorescent spot test is the most frequently employed test to determine G6PD activity.[59,62] A defin- itive diagnosis of G6PD deficiency entails assessment of enzyme activity, by quantitative spectrophotometric ana- lysis of the rate of NADPH production from NADP. Quantifying the specific percent activity is necessary to determine severity.

Treatment

Most cases of acute hemolysis are usually short-lived and resolve without complication.[59] Severe cases of hemolysis may require transfusion and possibly hemodialysis due to acute renal failure. Neonatal jaundice is usually treated with phototherapy and, when severe, with exchange blood trans- fusion. Once the diagnosis of G6PD deficiency is estab- lished, measures to reduce exposure to oxidative stressors are warranted.

Infections should be promptly treated and immunizations kept up-to-date. Patients susceptible to fava bean-induced hemolysis should avoid ingestion. Drug-induced hemolysis has been attributed to several medications. However, the validity of this association with many drugs has been ques- tioned.[63] It is likely that many drugs previously cited as caus- ing hemolysis were in fact administered to patients suffering from an infection-induced hemolytic episode.[63,65] In a recent review, the authors identified seven drugs clearly associated with drug-induce hemolysis: dapsone, methylene blue, nitro- furantoin, phenazopyridine primaquine, and toluidine blue. All other drugs previously associated with clinically significant hemolysis are likely safe when prescribed in therapeutic doses.

Oral Health Considerations

Patients with G6PD deficiency can tolerate the delivery of all necessary dental care. Medications known to induce a hemolytic crisis should be strictly avoided and oral infections should be promptly managed. G6PD patients should main- tain excellent oral hygiene and comply with routine recall visits so as to prevent oral and periodontal infection.

Hemoglobinopathies

Hb is made up of heme (the iron-containing portion of Hb) and globin (amino acid chains that form a protein). Normal Hb types include adult Hb A (HbA; about 95%–98%), HbA contains two α chains and two β chains, HbA$_2$ (2%–3%) has two α and two δ chains, and fetal Hb (HbF; up to 2%) has two α and two γ chains. HbF is the primary Hb produced by the fetus during gestation. Its production usually falls to a low level shortly after birth.

Hemoglobinopathies occur when point mutations or deletions in the globin genes cause changes in the amino acids that make up the globin protein, resulting in abnormal forms of Hb. The structure of the Hb may be abnormal in its behavior, production rate, and/or stability. Several hundred Hb variants have been documented; however, only a few are common and clinically significant. The majority of these are b chain variants that are inherited in an autosomal recessive fashion. Because a person inherits one copy of each β-globin gene from each parent, if one normal β gene and one abnor- mal β gene are inherited, the person is said to be a carrier or heterozygous for the abnormal Hb. The abnormal gene can be passed on to any offspring but does not cause symptoms or disease in the carrier. If two abnormal β genes of the same type are inherited, the person is considered to have the dis- ease and is homozygous for the abnormal Hb. A copy of the abnormal β gene will be passed on to any offspring. If two abnormal genes of different types are inherited, the person is doubly or compound heterozygous and one of the abnormal β genes will be passed on to each offspring.

Sickle Cell Disease.

Sickle cell disease (SCD), formerly known as sickle cell anemia, affects an estimated 70,000 people in the United States and the global annual incidence of SCD exceeds 300,000.[66,67] About 3 million individuals in the United States are carriers of the SC trait (SCT) and most are African American. Globally, there are over 300 million carriers of SCT. While the disease burden of SCD is irrefutable, there has been substantial debate within the medical community regarding the significance of SCT. Some consider SCT as a benign carrier state, while others believe it should be con- sidered an intermediate disease phenotype.[68] Patients with SCT appear to be at increased risk of developing renal dis- ease, exertional rhabdomyolysis, venous thromboembolism, and exercise-related sudden death.

SCD occurs as a consequence of a Hb gene mutation, leading to a glutamic acid-to-valine substitution in the sixth position on the β-hemoglobin chain.[69] Under normal physiologic conditions, the altered Hb (HbS) polymerizes resulting in the formation of distorted rigid sickle cells. Sickle cells are prone to hemolysis and lose their ability to effectively transport oxygen to the microcirculation which in turn leads to end organ ischemia and necrosis.[66] While vaso-occlusive events clinically characterize SCD, the etiopathogenesis of SCD is far more complex and involves ongoing hemolysis;

increased RBC dehydration and adherence to endothelium; vascular instability due to nitric oxide deficiency; proinflammatory events; and activation of the complement cascade.[70] HbF acts to retard sickling and is considered to be a major modulator of SCD activity and patients with higher levels of HbF tend to experience milder disease.[71]

Endothelial activation, induced directly or indirectly by the proinflammatory behavior of sickle erythrocytes, is the most likely initiating step toward vaso-occlusion.[72] Stressors that can lead to vaso-occlusion typically include viral and bacterial infection, hypoxia, dehydration, iron overload, and cell and fluid phase–related causes. Microvascular occlusion arises predominantly in localized areas of marrow, leading to necrosis. Inflammatory mediators activate nociceptive afferent nerve fibers, evoking the pain response. Commonly affected areas are the long bones, ribs, sternum, spine, and pelvis, often with multiple-site involvement.

Clinical and Oral Manifestations

Target organ manifestations of SCD are wide-ranging and vary from acute to chronic, symptomatic to asymptomatic, and episodic to progressive.[66] Acute complications of SCD include acute chest syndrome, aplastic crisis, fever/sepsis, osteomyelitis, pain, priapism, splenic sequestration, and stroke.[73] Chronic conditions of SCD include asthma, avascular necrosis, gall bladder disease, hepatic dysfunction, leg ulcers, nephropathy, pulmonary hypertension, and silent infarcts.

Pain is characteristic of SCD and the most common reason for hospitalization.[74,75] The most frequently affected sites are the lower back, knee/shin area, and hips. Four phases of the pain event have been described: prodromal, initial infarctive, postinfarctive, and resolving. During the prodromal phase the patient experiences mild localized pain and there are no hematologic aberrations. The initial infarctive is characterized by increasing pain intensity, increased anxiety or irritability, and laboratory evidence of decreased Hb. Pain intensity peaks during the post infarctive phase, often driving the patient to seek emergency services. Laboratory findings include elevated reticulocytes, lactate dehydrogenase, and C-reactive protein. The resolving phase occurs when the pain intensity is decreased, usually as a result of appropriate care.[75]

Acute chest syndrome is the leading cause of death in young adults with SCD.[76] It can be defined as a *new* infiltrate in at least one segment of the lung, along with fever and respiratory symptoms. The impaired immune function associated with SCD places children at risk of developing life-threatening infections, especially from *Streptococcus pneumonia* and *Haemophilus influenzae*.[77] An estimated 25% of patients with SCD experience cerebral infarction.[78] Avascular necrosis of the hip may affect up to 40% of patients.[66] Other common sites of osseous involvement include the humerus, vertebra, and the phalanges and metatarsal bones.[79] Patients with SCD are at a greater risk of osteomyelitis than

controls, and the most frequently implicated pathogenic agents are *Salmonella* and *Staphylococcal aureus*.[78,79] Overall, osseous events in SCD are far more likely to be caused by infarction than osteomyelitis.

Numerous nonpathognomonic oral findings have been described in SCD and include mucosal pallor, delayed eruption, discolored and depapillated tongue, and increased periodontitis.[80] In radiographic assessment of 21 patients with SCD, findings included a "stepladder" trabeculae pattern (70%), enamel hypomineralization (24%), calcified canals (5%), increased overbite (30%–80%), and increased overjet (56%).[81] Vaso-occlusive events affecting the oral cavity have been reported to cause pain, paresthesia, or swelling.[82-84] In a case-control study of 36 patients with SCD, orofacial and dental pain with no obvious cause was detected in 83% of patients, 67% had deteriorated quality of the bone tissue, 22% had radiographic evidence of cortical thinning and irregularity in the mandible, and 6% of teeth with no restorations or a history of trauma were determined to be nonvital.[85]

Diagnosis

The National Sickle Cell Anemia Control Act of 1972 was passed to addresses a variety of SCD-related issues ranging from early diagnosis to comprehensive management.[77] Statewide universal screening of newborns for SCD has been in place since 2006. A definitive diagnosis requires confirmatory testing such as high-performance liquid chromatography, electrophoresis using cellulose acetate or acid citrate agar, or isoelectric focusing. Prenatal screening by deoxyribonucleic acid (DNA) analysis of amniotic fluid at 14 to 16 weeks can be ordered to investigate alterations and mutations in the genes that produce Hb components.[86]

Treatment

Improved medical therapies have dramatically improved the lifespan of patients with SCD and it is now considered a chronic adult disease characterized by poor quality of life with end organ failure.[66] Common causes of death in this patient cohort include cardiopulmonary causes such as cardiac arrest, heart failure, and pulmonary embolism, infections, stroke, and multiorgan failure.[77] General measures to provide palliation and reduce the myriad of SCD complications require a multidisciplined approach and comprehensive patient education.

Adequate pain management remains a persistent challenge and is essentially centered on using NSAIDs, opioids, and maintaining hydration. Many vaso-occlusive pain episodes are managed at home with a combination of anti-inflammatory and analgesic drugs, often with opioids. Severe pain episodes may require hospitalization for intravenous morphine, hydration, and supplemental oxygen therapy. Chronic sickle cell pain develops as a consequence of certain disease complications, such as leg ulcers and avascular necrosis and intractable chronic pain may be due to central sensitization.[74] Management of chronic pain entails a multidisciplinary approach.

Penicillin prophylaxis for children with SCD under the age of 5 years reduces the infection-related morbidity and mortality, as has appropriate vaccination against pneumonia and influenza.[77,87] Vaccination with both the 13-valent pneumococcal-conjugated vaccine starting at age 2–6 months and the 23-valent polysaccharide vaccine from age 2 years should be accomplished.

The risk of stroke in a child with SCD is 1% per year. Annual transcranial Doppler screening to assess cerebral blood flow in children between 2–16 years of age and prophylactic transfusions when indicated significantly reduces the risk.[66,76] The goal of prophylactic transfusions is to reduce the level of HbS to under 30% in patients who demonstrate persistently raised velocity measurements.

Acute chest syndrome is the leading cause of death in young adults with SCD.[76] Therapy is intensive and expansive and possible interventions include transfusion, supplemental oxygen, continued respiratory therapy, antibiotics, bronchodilators, pain management, fluid management, corticosteroids, and mechanical ventilation.

Medical management of osseous necrosis is site specific.[79] Core decompression remains the most common intervention for femoral head necrosis, but patients will often need total hip arthroplasty. Early and late complications rates are high and the failure rate within the first 6 years of placement exceeds 10%. Humeral/vertebral infarcts and dactylitis are typically managed with pain control and rest. While heat therapy may prove beneficial, cold therapy is generally avoided, as it may initiate vaso-occlusive crisis. Therapy of osteomyelitis requires surgical debridement, prolonged antimicrobial therapy, and possible orthotic support.

Existing and emerging therapies to modulate the underlying disease processes include induction of HbF, modulation of erythrocyte hydration, augmentation of nitric oxide (NO), chronic transfusion, stem cell transplantation, and gene therapy.[66,70] Hydroxyurea is the only FDA-approved drug for use in SCD and is a known inducer of HbF. Additional beneficial effects of hydoxyurea include improving RBC hydration, increasing NO production, and reducing the WBC, RBC, platelet count. Other potential inducers of HbF under investigations include 5-azacytidine, decitabine (an analogue of 5-azacytidine), butyrate, and erythropoietin. Agents to improve RBC hydration include ICA-17043 (Senicapoc) and magnesium pidolate. Agents under investigation to improve NO-mediated vasodilation include inhaled NO, arginine, sildenafil, and statins. An estimated 90% of SCD patients will undergo transfusion by adulthood. Hematopoietic stem cell transplantation (HSCT) is curative, but generally for patients with severe SCD.[69] Gene transfer therapy to induce a cure has entered Phase 1 trials.[66]

Oral Health Considerations

Measures to reduce oral disease burden and infection in patients with SCD are clearly indicated. Long-term penicillin prophylaxis in children with SCD under age 6 years inhibits acquisition of mutans streptococci, resulting in significantly lower caries rates in these children.[88] However, within 4 years of cessation of prophylaxis, the levels of mutans streptococci reached that of matched controls. While SCD is not associated with increased periodontal disease per say,[89] cases of periodontal infections[90] and mandibular osteomyelitis[91] precipitating a sickle cell crisis have been reported.

Given the wide variability in disease severity, it is essential a comprehensive history and medical consultation be obtained to determine the patient's status. During noncrisis periods, there are no contraindications concerning the delivery of routine dental care under local anesthesia with inhalational sedation.[82,92] The avoidance of using a local anesthetic agent without a vasoconstrictor is unwarranted. The need for providing antibiotic prophylaxis before rendering dental care is controversial and there exists no clear consensus or guidance.[82,93] A survey of 34 pediatric dentistry residency program directors and 72 pediatric hematologists revealed at least 50% recommended antibiotic prophylaxis of children with SCD for the following clinical situations: dental extractions, treatment under general anesthesia, and status postsplenectomy.[93] Amoxicillin was the most commonly chosen antibiotic, and the perceived risk of infectious complication was highest for extractions, followed by restorative treatment and tooth polishing.

For patients deemed low risk, simple surgical procedures may be accomplished in the outpatient setting. In a report of 21 patients with SCD undergoing extraction under local anesthesia with or without midazolam/fentanyl sedation, no complications were noted.[94] Pain management may be challenging and usually consists of anti-inflammatory agents, opioid/nonopioid analgesics, and proper hydration.[82] For patients deemed at moderate or high risk, dental therapy should be rendered in a hospital setting where appropriate medical support is readily available.[82]

Thalassemias

The thalassemias are a group of inherited autosomal recessive disorders of Hb synthesis characterized by a disturbance of either alpha (α) or beta (β) Hb chain production.[95,96] Worldwide, an estimated 1.7% of the population has α- or β-thalassemia trait (they carry only one β gene affected or one to two α genes affected). Thalassemia is estimated to occur in about 44 per 100,000 live births.[96] Historically, α-thalassemia is more prevalent in persons of African and Southeast Asian descent, and β-thalassemia is most common in persons of Mediterranean, African, and Southeast Asian descent. However, migration has greatly blurred these distinctions.[97]

Alpha Hb production is controlled by two genes on each chromosome. In α-thalassemia there is insufficient synthesis of α globin chains, resulting in excess β-like globin chains which form γ4 tetramers, termed Hb Bart's (in fetal blood) and β4 tetramers, termed HbH (in adult blood).[98] Mutations affecting one or two genes result in a trait status. Mutations affecting three of the four genes result in significant production of HbH and mild to moderate anemia called HbH disease. Mutations affecting all four genes result in significant production of Hb Bart's in the fetus and the typically fatal hydrops fetalis syndrome.

Beta hemoglobin production is controlled by one gene on each chromosome. In β-thalassemia insufficient β-globin synthesis, results in excess α Hb production. One gene defects result in β-thalassemia trait manifesting microcytosis and mild anemia. A variety of two gene defects may occur, resulting in either the β-thalassemia intermedia form or the more severe major form (aka Cooley's anemia). As β Hb synthesis is only activated after birth, the signs and symptoms of β-thalassemia usually do not develop until six months of age.[99]

Clinical and Oral Manifestations

Clinical signs and symptoms of thalassemia are dependent on the severity of the disease and range from none to life-threatening. Apart from mild to moderate microcytic hypochromic anemia (detected on a routine blood count), patients with α-thalassemia trait are asymptomatic.[98] Patients with HbH typically manifest anemia and splenomegaly, with possible jaundice, growth retardation in children, infections, leg ulcers, gall stones, folic acid deficiency, and drug-induced hemolysis. Infants with the Hb Bart's hydrops fetalis syndrome almost always either die in utero (23–38 weeks) or shortly after birth.

Patients with β-thalassemia trait are usually asymptomatic but may have mild anemia. Cooley's anemia patients develop signs and symptoms between 6 and 24 months to include failure to thrive, pallor, weakness, jaundice, protruding abdomen with enlarged spleen and liver, dark urine, abnormal facial bones, and growth retardation.[100] Compensatory hypertrophy of erythroid marrow with extramedullary erythropoiesis may result in deformities of the long bones and typical craniofacial changes (see below). Patients with β-thalassemia intermedia manifest variable signs and symptoms of anemia that are milder than and occur later than those observed in Cooley's anemia. However, patients with β-thalassemia intermedia are prone to experience thrombotic events, especially if splenectomized. Such events include deep vein thrombosis, stroke, portal vein thrombosis,+ and pulmonary embolism.

Significant oral manifestations related to thalassemia appear to occur more frequently in patients with β-thalassemia and are reflective of the underlying extramedullary erythropoiesis observed in the more severe phenotypes.[101] Characteristic craniofacial deformities include a Class II skeletal base relationship with a short mandible, a reduced posterior facial height, increased anterior facial proportions, and *chipmunk facies*.[102] Other reported potential findings include spiky-shaped and short roots, taurodontism, attenuated lamina dura, enlarged bone marrow spaces, small maxillary sinuses, absence of inferior alveolar canal, and thin cortex of the mandible.[103] Dental arch morphologic changes include a narrower maxilla and smaller incisor widths for the maxillary and mandibular arches.[104,105] Consistent with general growth retardation, the dental development of 31 of 39 patients with Cooley's anemia was delayed by a mean of 1.11 years and 0.81 years for boys and girls, respectively.[106]

Patients with thalassemia appear to experience similar rates of gingivitis and periodontitis as healthy controls.[107,108] An increased caries risk has been reported, which may be attributable to such factors as disease-induced immunological dysfunction, decreased access to care, and insufficient patient oral hygiene.[107,109] While the parotid salivary flow rates in patients with Cooley's anemia are similar to controls, quantitative changes consisting of reduced levels of phosphorus, IgA, and urea have been reported.[110,111] Increased oral cavity levels of *Streptococcus mutans* and Candida have also been reported.[110,112]

Diagnosis

Thalassemia is diagnosed using a battery of laboratory tests including a CBC, qualitative and quantitative Hb analysis, and molecular genetic testing.[98,100] Individuals with thalassemia have microcytic anemia, lowered Hb, and defects in α or β chains of Hb. The clinical signs and symptoms of severe thalassemia usually become apparent within the first 2 years of life. Anemia in children of Mediterranean origin or ancestry (Greek, Italian, Middle Eastern) and people of Asian and African descent is suggestive of β-thalassemia, and anemia in children of Southeast Asian, Indian, Chinese, or Filipino origin or ancestry may indicate α-thalassemia.

Treatment

The prognosis for patients with thalassemia has improved dramatically over the past decades, but medical management remains complex and multidisciplined.[98,100,113] Appropriate genetic counseling and screening should be affordable to all patients with thalassemia.[95] Patients with α- or β-thalassemia trait generally require no special medical management.

Patients with mild HbH may require intermittent transfusion therapy, mainly during intercurrent illness. More severely affected patients with HbH may require chronic transfusions and eventual splenectomy.[98] Management strategies for patients with Cooley's anemia usually entail periodic lifelong blood transfusions to maintain the Hb level above 13 to 14 g/dL to prevent growth impairment, organ damage, and bone deformities.[100] To meet this goal, transfusions are typically required every 2–4 weeks. The need for transfusions to manage patients with β-thalassemia is more episodic and dictated by the severity and potential progression of the disease.[96]

Regularly transfused patients require iron chelation to resolve the inevitable iron accumulation that leads to dysfunction, primarily involving the heart, liver, and endocrine system. In the United States, there are three FDA-approved iron chelators: deferoxamine (Desferal), deferasirox (Exjade), and deferiprone (L1).[114] The most commonly used agent is the oral dispersable agent deferasirox, likely due to its good oral bioavailability and convenient once-a-day dosing.

Common side effects include dose-related gastrointestinal symptoms (e.g., nausea, vomiting, diarrhea, abdominal pain) and mild skin rash. The most serious side effects with defer-asirox are potential kidney damage and renal tubular acidosis.

Bone marrow transplantation is the only available cure for thalassemia.[100] Success rates of 90% have been reported in scenarios involving an HLA-identical donor and a patient with minimal disease-related complications. Cord blood transplantation may be successful.[115] Future therapeutic strategies involving normal gene transfer via a suitable vector are being investigated.[116,117]

Infections are major complications and constitute the second most common cause of mortality and a main cause of morbidity in patients with thalassemia. Predisposing factors for infections in thalassemic patients include severe anemia, iron overload, splenectomy, and a range of immune abnormalities.[114,118] Major causative organisms of bacterial infections in thalassemic patients include *Klebsiella* spp in Asia and *Yersinia enterocolitica* in Western countries. It is important to recognize and presumptively treat infections in these patients as quickly as possible.

Oral Health Considerations

There are no contraindications for providing routine dental care for thalassemia patients under proper medical management. Splenectomized patients are more susceptible to developing postsplenectomy sepsis from encapsulated bacteria (e.g., *Streptococcus pneumoniae, Haemophilus influenzae* and *Neisseria meningitidis*). Prevention of postsplenectomy sepsis includes immunization against the above mentioned bacteria, antibiotic prophylaxis, and early antibiotic treatment for fever and malaise.[100] As such, consideration to provide antimicrobial prophylaxis (American Heart Association (AHA) regimen) for manipulative dental care is recommended by some authorities.[114] Patients with β-thalassemia intermedia may be on an antithrombotic.

WHITE BLOOD CELL DISORDERS

White blood cells (WBCs) are composed of granulocytes (neutrophils, eosinophils, and basophils) and agranulocytes (B and T lymphocytes, monocytes, and macrophages). The granulocytes are distinguished by their appearance under Wright's stain. The most abundant granulocyte is the neutrophil that has neutrally staining cytoplasmic granules. The granules in granulocytes contain hydrolases, elastase, myeloperoxidase, cathepsin G, cationic proteins, bactericidal/permeability-increasing protein, and *defensins*, with broad antimicrobial activity against bacteria, fungi, and certain enveloped viruses. WBC disorders can be either quantitative or qualitative in nature.

Leukocytosis is defined as a WBC count more than two standard deviations above the mean. Elevated WBC counts typically reflect a normal response to infection or inflammation and usually represent an increase in the number of neutrophils. In acute infections, leukocyte counts typically are 15,000–25,000/μL. Less often, leukocytosis is the sign of a primary bone marrow abnormality related to leukemia or a myeloproliferative disorder. Leukopenia is defined as an abnormally low WBC count. Neutropenia refers to a decrease in WBC count where the absolute neutrophil count (ANC) is <1,500/μL. ANC is calculated using the following equation: ANC=WBC × (%Segs + %Bands), where segs are fully mature neutrophils and bands are not. The normal ANC range is 1,500–8,000/μL. Table 18-2 outlines alterations in the WBC and differential cell count that occur clinically in various disorders.

Quantitative Leukocyte Disorders
Granulocytosis

Granulocytosis is an abnormally large number of granulocytes in the blood, most commonly associated with an increase in neutrophils. Neutrophilic leukocytosis (neutrophilia) is a total WBC count >11,000/μL with an ANC >7,700/μL. Common causes are infection, stress, smoking, pregnancy, and myeloproliferative disorders. Neutrophilia may exist, regardless of percentage, if the total number of neutrophils exceeds 7,000/μL (absolute neutrophilia), whereas a relative neutrophilia may exist if the percentage of neutrophils is greater than 70% and the total number of neutrophils is less than 7,000/μL.

Causes of neutrophilia are varied and include acute infections caused by cocci, bacilli, certain fungi, spirochetes, viruses, rickettsia, and parasites. Noninfectious causes include burns, postoperative states, acute myocardial infarction, acute gout, acute glomerulonephritis, rheumatic fever, collagen vascular diseases, and hypersensitivity reactions. Neutrophilia can also accompany metabolic conditions (diabetic ketoacidosis, preeclampsia, uremia), poisoning (with lead, mercury, digitalis, camphor, antipyrine, phenacetin, quinidine, pyrogallol, turpentine, arsphenamine, and insect venoms), rapidly growing neoplasms, and strenuous exercise. Table 18-3 summarizes the various conditions related to quantitative and qualitative neutrophil conditions.

Basophilia and eosinophilia are an excess number of basophils and eosinophils, respectively (Table 18-2). It is important to note that although patients may have adequate or elevated granulocytes, if they are immature (i.e., leukemia) they may not be functional and patients may present with features of neutropenia.

Agranulocytosis (Neutropenia, Granulocytopenia)

The terms *agranulocytosis, neutropenia,* and *granulocytopenia* are commonly used interchangeably to note a reduced quantity of leukocytes. Susceptibility to infectious diseases increases sharply when the ANC falls to <1,000/μL. When the ANC falls to <500/μL, control of endogenous microbial flora (e.g., mouth, gut) is impaired. Clinical symptoms of agranulocytosis include sudden onset of fever, rigors, and sore throat. When the ANC is <200/μL, the local inflammatory process is absent.[119]

TABLE 18-2 Key Laboratory Tests for White Cell Disorders

Test Name	Normal Range (SI units)	Increased	Decreased	Oral Findings
White blood cell (WBC)	4,400–11,000/µL	Infections Inflammation Cancer Leukemia	Hematologic neoplasia Early leukemia Drug-induced Cyclic neutropenia Viral infection Severe bacterial infections Bone marrow failure Congenital marrow aplasia	Enlarged gingival, oral ulcers, oral infection due to immune suppression from disease or therapy
Differential WBC				
Polymorphonuclear neutrophils[a]	41%–78%	See Table: 3	See Table: 3	
Band neutrophils[a]	0%–6%	Immature neutrophils; indicates rapid production of cell line often seen in infection		
Lymphocytes	23%–44%	Viral infections, mononucleosis, infectious lymphocytosis, hypoadrenalism, hypothyroidism	Immunodeficiencies, adrenal-corticosteroid exposure, severe debilitating illness, defects in lymphatic circulation	
Monocytes	0%–7%	Chronic infections (tuberculosis), bacterial endocarditis, granulomatous disease		
Eosinophils[a]	0%–4%	Parasitic diseases, certain allergic diseases, chronic skin diseases, various miscellaneous diseases (sarcoidosis, Hodgkin's disease, metastatic cancer)		
Basophils[a]	0%–2%	Chronic hypersensitivity states, no specific allergen, myeloproliferative disorders		

[a]Granulocytes.

The differential diagnosis of neutropenia (Table 18-3) depends upon the severity and duration of neutropenia, leukocyte and bone marrow morphology, and associated hematologic or congenital abnormalities. The most common underlying cause for a mild to moderate neutropenia is a transient marrow suppression associated with viral infections such as Epstein Barr virus (EBV) or respiratory syncytial virus.[120] Neutropenia may also be drug induced, either due to myelosuppression or antibody-mediated destruction. Many drugs, including antineoplastics alkylating agents, antimetabolites, antibiotics (chloramphenicol, sulfonamides, penicillins), anticonvulsants (carbamazepine), anti-inflammatories, antithyroid agents, mercurial diuretics, and phenothiazines, have been implicated. Other potential causes of neutropenia include antineutrophil antibodies and/or splenic trapping,

autoimmune disorders such as Felty's syndrome, rheumatoid arthritis, lupus erythematosis, and Wegener's granulomatosis. Antineutrophil antibodies may be detected by flow cytometry or agglutination assays to support the diagnosis of immune-mediated neutropenia. Congenital forms of neutropenia need to be considered in children and occasionally in adults presenting with low neutrophil counts. Bone marrow examination is indicated in cases of severe or persistent neutropenia or when other hematologic lineages are affected.[119]

Infection-mediated neutropenia requires only monitoring of blood counts until recovery. For potential drug-induced neutropenia, discontinuation of the suspected offending drug provides both the diagnosis and the cure. Neutropenia resulting from myelosuppression in patients on cytotoxic chemotherapy typically reaches a

TABLE 18-3 Neutrophil Disorders	
Quantitative Disorders	
Neutrophilia	**Neutropenia**
Primary	Primary
Hereditary	Cyclic neutropenia
Idiopathic	Familial benign
Inflammation	Myleokathexis
Cancer	Severe chronic
Leukemia	Glycogen storage disease
Colchicine	Failure to release
Sulfonamides	Secondary (Immunodeficiencies)
Down's syndrome	X-linked hyper IgM
Chronic Myelogenous	X-linked agammaglobunemia
Leukemia	Acquired AI
Polycythemia Vera	Drug induced
Leukocyte Adhesion	Clozapine
deficiency	Antithyroid
Secondary	Sulfasalazines
Infections	See text for others
Smoking	Destruction
Chronic inflammation	Hypersplenism
Stress	Felty's Syndrome
Exercise	Systemic lupus erythematosis
Steroids	Nutritional
Lithium	B12 and folate deficiencies
Marrow stimulation	Copper deficiency
Solid tumor	
Heat stroke	
Asplenia	
Sweet syndrome	
Qualitative Disorders	
Adhesion:	Granule Disorders:
Leukocyte adhesion	Myleoperoxidase deficiency
deficiency	Chediak-Higashi syndrome
(Types 1, 2 and 3)	Chronic granulomatous
Phagocyte Activation:	disease
Hyper immunoglobulin E	Neutrophil-specific granule
(Job's syndrome)	deficiencyImpaired
Chronic granulomatous	chemotaxis
disease	Shwachman-Diamond
Chediak-Higashi syndrome	syndrome

nadir between 7 and 14 days after chemotherapy has been delivered. Please see Chapter 9 for more details related to oral considerations related to cancer treatments.

Oral Health Considerations

There is a direct relationship between the onset and severity of oral complications and bone marrow status as expressed in peripheral blood counts.[121] Prophylactic antibiotics have historically been recommended by some for patients with a hematologic malignancy–caused ANC <1,000/μL prior to dental extractions.[122] Evidence from Cochrane reviews confirms that the provision of antibiotic prophylaxis in afebrile patients with neutropenia (ANC <1,000/μL) reduces mortality, febrile episodes, and bacterial infections, without apparent development of antibiotic resistance.[123,124] Recent studies assessing antibiotics of the quinolone class revealed fewer adverse events and better outcomes than other classes

of antibiotics. Hence, an oral fluoroquinolone plus amoxicillin/clavulanate (or plus clindamycin if penicillin allergic) is recommended as empiric therapy, unless fluoroquinolone prophylaxis was used before fever developed. Fluroquinolone regimens are routinely recommended for patients with acute leukemia, lymphoma, and solid organ tumors who are anticipated to receive regimens that cause severe neutropenia as defined as an ANC <100/μL.[125]

Physician consultation is warranted for guidance on the dental management of the patient with severe neutropenia. Patients with chronic neutropenia are at risk for *Staphylococcus aureus*, gram negative organism (*Klebsiella*), *Escherichia coli*, *Pseudomonas aeruginosa*, and fungal infections. Potential oral findings include gingivitis, thrush, stomatitis, and oral ulcers. These oral infections should be treated with the appropriate antimicrobial agents.

Cyclic Neutropenia

Cyclic neutropenia is a rare hematologic disorder, characterized by repetitive episodes of fever, mouth ulcers, and infections attributable to recurrent severe neutropenia. These patients manifest a distinctly cyclical pattern to episodes of neutropenia (<200/μL). Neutropenia recurs with a regular 21-day intervals, persists for 3 to 5 days, and is characterized by infectious events that are usually less severe than in severe chronic neutropenia. Cyclic neutropenia is an inherited autosomal dominant disorder due to mutations in the gene for neutrophil elastase (*ELA-2*, located at 19p13.3); thus affected patients also often have affected relatives.[126] Neutrophil elastase is synthesized in neutrophil precursors early in the process of primary granule formation. It is postulated that the mutant neutrophil elastase activity results accelerated apoptosis of the precursors, oscillatory production, and loss of a regulatory feedback loop.[127,128]

Clinical and Oral Manifestations

Periodic oscillations of neutrophil counts associated with fever and mouth ulcers are the key clinical hallmarks of this disease. A wide spectrum of symptom severity, ranging from asymptomatic to life-threatening illness, is seen in autosomal dominant cyclic neutropenia.[129] The phenotype changes with age, where children display typical neutrophil cycles with symptoms of mucosal ulceration, lymphadenopathy, and infections. Adults often have fewer episodes and milder chronic neutropenia without distinct cycles. The most severe consequences of cyclic neutropenia are gangrene, bacteremia, and septic shock due to perforating colonic ulcers and infections with *Clostridium septicum*. The occurrence of fever, abdominal pain, and a clinical picture of sepsis or a rapidly spreading area of cellulitis are critical and often life-threatening events in these patients. The oral manifestations of cyclic neutropenia include recurrent aphthous stomatitis (RAS), recurrent gingivitis, and periodontitis. RAS is one of the most common presenting symptoms in cyclic neutropenia; RAS arises during the nadir and resolves spontaneously as the neutrophil count improves. The finding of RAS with or without periodontal disease, particularly in a child, should raise the suspicion of cyclic neutropenia.[130,131] Diagnostic evaluation entails serial measurement of circulating neutrophils. The diagnosis may be established by demonstrating at least two cycles of neutropenia.[130]

Treatment

Hematopoietic growth factors, such as granulocyte colony-stimulating factor (G-CSF) (Neupogen [filgastrim], Amgen, Thousand Oaks, CA), reduce the number and severity of infectious episodes, prolong survival, and extend the time during which neutropenic patients remain free of life-threatening infections. Clinical trials and reports from international registries suggest that the majority of neutropenic patients (>90%) respond within 1 to 2 weeks to treatment with G-CSF at dosages lower than 30 μg/kg (2.4–2.6 μg/kg for patients with cyclic neutropenia) with a mean ANC increase of more than 1,500 to 2,000/μL.[132] Long-term, daily, or alternate-day administration reduces fever, mouth ulcers, and other inflammatory events associated with this disorder.[132]

Chronic Neutropenias

Chronic neutropenia can be congenital, acquired, or idiopathic and is defined as a low ANC for more than 6 months. The predominant types of chronic neutropenias are chronic benign idiopathic neutropenia and severe congenital neutropenia (SCN), also known as Kostmann's syndrome. In SCN, children typically have absolute neutrophil counts of <500/μL on a continuing basis. Chronic benign idiopathic neutropenia is characterized by prolonged non-cyclic neutropenia as the sole abnormality, with no underlying disease to which the neutropenia can be attributed.

SCN is a heterogeneous disease that results from mutations in a variety of genes (*ELANE, HAX1,* and *GFI1* mutation). Although generally seen as a monogenic disorder, a recent report has identified four SCN patients with mutations in multiple genes. While it is predicted that in these patients one genetic mutation is dominant disease causative, a second mutation could have a synergistic effect and worsen disease phenotype[128,133] Pathophysiologically, the expression of the mutant protein from some of these genetic mutations is that of accelerated apoptosis of developing myeloid cells.[126]

Clinical and Oral Manifestations

Clinical manifestations of chronic neutropenia vary according to type. Patients with SCN experience deep tissue infections with lung abscesses, liver abscesses, and severe skin infections. As a consequence, they are chronically ill soon after birth with secondary anemia, thrombocytosis, and onocytosis. A BM usually reveals *promyelocytic maturation arrest* with a paucity of mature cells but many early forms of the myeloid lineage. Other cells in the marrow generally appear normal.[126] Other manifestations include life-threatening bacterial infections, recurrent gingivitis, and even severe periodontitis, often starting in early childhood.[134,135] Patients with chronic benign idiopathic neutropenia tend to experience a more benign clinical course compared to SCN. In light of an otherwise unremarkable medical history, periodontitis of the primary dentition and early tooth loss may represent the sole manifestations of chronic benign idiopathic neutropenia affecting a juvenile patient.[136]

Treatment

Most patients with SCN respond to therapy with G-CSF, often at higher doses than required for cyclic neutropenia.[137] Prior to the G-CSF era, approximately half of SCN patients died of bacterial sepsis in the first year of life and the remainder in early childhood. Currently, these survivors are at an increased risk for development of acute myeloid leukemia or myelodysplastic syndrome and death from bacterial sepsis. G-CSF together with a dental care regimen resulted in resolution of neutropenic ulceration and periodontal breakdown within 2 weeks of treatment initiation in a patient with SCN, whereas normalized ANC levels were not sufficient to resolve chronic periodontal disease in other SCN patients. It is thought that this is possibly due to continued deficiency of the antibacterial peptide LL-37, normally produced by peripheral blood neutrophils and important to the destruction of periodontal disease–associated bacteria.[138] Patients with chronic benign idiopathic neutropenia typically require no specific treatment other than prompt recognition and institution of therapy for febrile infection. When indicated, G-CSF may be prescribed on a short-term basis to boost immune response.

Agranulocytes

Agranulocytes are mainly lymphocytes (B and T) and monocytes, which collectively make up about 20%–40% of all WBCs (Table 18-2). Lymphocytes determine and facilitate the body's humoral and cellular immunity response to foreign proteins and pathogens. A decrease in lymphocytes (lymphocytopenia) refers to a count of <1,000/μL of blood in adults. Causes of lymphocytopenia may be iatrogenic or due to infections, systemic diseases, or inherited (See Table 18-4).[139] Lymphocytopenias can vary in severity as well as duration. The treatment depends on its cause and severity. If an underlying condition is successfully treated, lymphocytopenias is likely to improve.

An increase in circulating lymphocytes (lymphocytosis) can be seen following infections such as infectious mononucleosis and pertussis, or in lymphoproliferative disorders such as acute and chronic lymphocytic leukemia (See Table 18-5). Evaluation of lymphocytosis begins with a search for a reactive cause, such as infection. Flow cytometry and a peripheral blood smear can help distinguish between clonal disorders and a nonclonal process (reactive lymphocytosis). Clonal

TABLE 18-4 Conditions Attributing to Lymphopenia

Infection	Iatrogenic	Systemic Disease	Other
Bacterial	Immunosuppressants	AI disorders	Congenital disorders
Viral	Glucocorticoids	SLE	Alcohol
Fungal	Antilymphocyte globulin	RA	Zinc deficiency
Parasitic	Rituximab	SS	Malnutrition
	Alemtuzumab	Lymphoma	Stress
	Chemotherapy	Sacroidosis	Exercise
	Radiation therapy	Renal failure	Trauma
		Aplastic anemia	
		Cushing's disease	

AI, autoimmune disorders;
RA, rheumatoid arthritis;
SLE, systemic lupus erythematosis;
SS, Sjogren's syndrome
Source: Reproduced with permission from UpToDate.[139]

TABLE 18-5 Conditions Contributing to Lymphocytosis

Polyclonal	Clonal
Viral infections	Malignant
Epstein Barr Virus	T-cell prolymphocytic
Cytomegalo Virus	leukemia
Human Immunodeficiency	T-cell leukemia or
Virus	lymphoma
Human T-lymphotropic	Chronic Lymphocytic
Virus 1	leukemia
Herpes Simples Virus	Large granular lymphocyte
Adeno Associated Virus	leukemia
Measles	T-cell non-Hodgkin's
Mumps	lymphoma
Rubella	Nonmalignant
Influenza	Thymoma
Hepatitis	Hereditary B cell
Enterovirus	lymphocytosis
Coxsackie B2	Monoclonal B cell
Polio	Sézary syndrome
Bacterial	
Tuberculosis	
Rickettsia	
Brucellosis	
Toxoplasmosis	
Syphilis	
Babesiosis	
Hypersensitivity	
Stress	
Drugs	
Hyperthyroidism	
Autoimmune diseases	
Polyclonal B cell	
Post splenectomy	

B-cell disorders can by diagnosed with immunophenotyping and possibly bone marrow or lymph node biopsy.

Leukemia

Leukemia results from the proliferation of a clone of abnormal hematopoietic cells with impaired differentiation, regulation, and programmed cell death (apoptosis). It is defined by a rapid disease course which progresses over weeks to months, ultimately culminating in bone marrow failure. Leukemia is classified based on clinical behavior (acute or

chronic) and the primary hematopoietic cell line affected (myeloid or lymphoid). The four principal diagnostic categories are: (1) acute myelogenous leukemia (AML), (2) acute lymphocytic leukemia (ALL), (3) chronic myelogenous leukemia (CML), and (4) chronic lymphocytic leukemia (CLL). Leukemic cells multiply at the expense of normal hematopoietic cell lines, resulting in marrow failure, altered blood cell counts, and, when untreated, death from infection, bleeding, or both.

For 2013, the American Cancer Society (ACS) estimated there were 48,610 new cases and 23,720 deaths attributable to leukemia[140] and there were 287,963 people living with leukemia in the United States.[141] Rates for new leukemia cases have been rising on average 0.1% each year over the last 10 years while death rates have been falling on average 1.0% each year over the same period. Five year survival rate is 56.0%. In 2010, leukemia was the 9th most common cancer to affect men of all races in the United States.[142] Leukemia is more common in adults than in children, with most chronic leukemia occurring in adults. Of acute leukemia, ALL is more common in children, whereas AML is more common in adults.

Leukemia is typically diagnosed via abnormal results on a full blood count. The peripheral granulocyte count is markedly elevated in chronic leukemia but may be increased (with numerous blast forms), decreased, or normal in acute leukemia. Confirmation is determined with identification of abnormal hematopoietic cells in bone marrow. Additional techniques that may be used to further classify the type of leukemia include flow cytochemical staining (myeloperoxidase, Sudan black B), cytometric immunophenotyping, and genetic analysis.[143]

Acute Leukemia
Acute Lymphocytic/Lymphoblastic Leukemia (ALL)

ALL is the most common malignancy in childhood. Overall, about one-third of ALL cases occur in adults. ALL is the clonal proliferation of lymphoid cells that have undergone maturational arrest in early differentiation. Although the contemporary survival rate approaches 90%, it remains the main cause of death from disease in children and young adults. An increased understanding of biological subtypes and higher quality of supportive care has led to improvement in the cure rate of ALL. The use of conventional technologies such as karyotype and polymerase chain reaction, combined with advanced methodologies such as gene expression profile, single nucleotide polymorphism (SNP) arrays, genome-wide analyses (GWA), and next-generation sequencing allows for the identification of virtually all of molecular aberrations underlying ALL (See Table 18-6).[144]

For 2013, the ACS estimated there were 6,070 new cases of ALL (3,350 males, 2,720 females) and 1,430 deaths from ALL (820 males, 610 females).[140] The risk for developing ALL is highest in children younger than 5 years of age. The risk then declines until the mid-20s, and rises again after age 50. ALL accounts for 10% to 15% of adult acute leukemia and 75% of childhood acute leukemia.[145]

Clinical and Oral Manifestations

Symptoms include fever, weight loss, muscle or joint pain, fatigue/malaise, anemia/pallor, mucosal bleeding, petechiae, and local infections. Fever and fatigue/malaise are the most common presenting symptoms in patients with all types of leukemia.[146] The most common manifestations or clinical signs of acute leukemia at initial presentation are lymphadenopathy (71.4% in ALL; 45% in AML), laryngeal pain (52.7% in ALL; 37.3% in AML), gingival bleeding (28.6% in ALL; 43.2% in AML), oral ulceration, and gingival enlargement.[147] In a study of 49 children with ALL, observed oral manifestations included gingivitis, 91.84%; caries, 81.63%; mucositis, 38.77%; periodontitis, 16.32%; cheilitis, 18.36%; recurrent herpes, 12.24%; and primary herpetic gingivostomatitis, 2.04%.[148] Other oral manifestations noted were dry lips, mucosal pallor, mucosal petechiae, ecchymoses, and ulcers. The prevalence of oral candidiasis was 6.12%. It was observed that high risk ALL and poor oral hygiene were important risk factors for the development of candidiasis and gingivitis. The type of leukemia, gender and phase of chemotherapy were apparently associated with the presence of candidiasis, gingivitis, and periodontitis and could be considered risk factors for the development of oral manifestations.

Treatment

While the treatment of pediatric ALL is a chemotherapy success story with long-term disease-free survival greater than 80%, survival statistics in adults remain poor at 40% due to relapse.[145] After risk stratification, treatment typically spans 2 years. Although most of the drugs used were developed before 1970, adjustments have been made in dosage, schedule, and treatment combinations based on leukemic-cell biological features to optimize treatment. This has resulted in higher survival rates. Central nervous system (CNS)-directed treatment helps prevent relapse from sequestered leukemia cells.

TABLE 18-6   WHO Classification of ALL
Precursor Lymphoid Neoplasms (Acute Lymphoblastic Leukemias)
B lymphoblastic leukemia not otherwise specified
B lymphoblastic leukemia with recurrent genetic abnormalities
• t(9;22)(q34;q11.2) (Philadelphia chromosome/BCR-ABL fusion gene)
• t(v;11q23) (Rearrangements of MLL gene with various partner genes)
• t(12;21)(p13;q22)
• t(5;14)(q31;q32)
• t(1;19)(q23;p13.3)
• hyperdiploid
• hypodiploid
T lymphoblastic leukaemia[a]
Mature B-cell neoplasms
Burkitt's lymphoma presenting as an acute leukemia

[a]Common genetic abnormalities seen in T-ALL include rearrangements with T-cell receptor loci resulting in altered transcription factor gene expression, rearrangements of TAL1 and mutations of NOTCH1 and hCDC4 genes.
Source: Reproduced with permission from the *Internal Medicine Journal*.[144]

Allogeneic hematopoietic stem cell transplantation is also an option for patients at very high risk. Cytogenetic and molecular abnormalities provide prognostic information and are used to guide therapy.

The most frequent structural cytogenetic abnormality (15%–30%) in adult ALL is the Philadelphia (Ph) chromosome (t[9;22][q34;q11]) resulting in the *BCR-ABL* fusion gene. With the advent of specific tyrosine kinase inhibitors (TKIs) used in combination with chemotherapy, treatment results are improving in Ph-positive adults. However, allogeneic stem cell transplant (SCT) is still usually recommended in suitable patients with a well matched donor. The use of the molecule kinase inhibitor imatinib and chemotherapy is considered frontline therapy,[149] and there is emerging evidence to support the use of the newer more potent TKI dasatinib, due to its greater CNS penetration.[150] The monitoring for minimal residual disease (MRD) after induction and during consolidation is a powerful predictor of disease recurrence and is used in current trials to stratify standard-risk patients.

The mainstays of induction therapy are vincristine, anthracyclines, corticosteroids, and L-asparaginase, although the latter is poorly tolerated in adults. Consolidation includes a complex series of cytotoxic treatments including cytarabine, high-dose intravenous methotrexate and cyclophosphamide. Although intensification improves outcomes in children, there are concerns that higher rates of toxicities in adults results in reduced compliance. Thus, the two key features of adult ALL management are the use of CNS prophylaxis and prolonged maintenance chemotherapy. Without CNS prophylaxis, the rates of CNS relapse are 30%–50%.[151] Maintenance therapy is a unique feature of ALL treatment and consists of 2 to 3 years of postconsolidation therapy, usually administered orally with antimetabolites. A commonly used maintenance regimen is oral weekly methotrexate and daily mercaptopurine. Other regimens include thioguanine, dexamethasone, and vincristine.

Allogeneic SCT still benefits several subgroups of patients, such as Ph+ ALL (even when treated with a TKI), those with a poor initial response to treatment, and adults with *MLL* gene rearrangements (e.g., t[4;11]). However, the selection of patients and the timing of allogeneic SCT in ALL remain controversial. A recently published large multicenter trial concluded that standard-risk patients in first complete remission benefit more from matched sibling allogeneic SCT than from chemotherapy.[152] This conclusion contrasts with that of previously published studies in which allogeneic SCT did not favor standard-risk patients.

Acute Myeloid Leukemia (AML)

AML subtypes are defined on the basis of morphological, cytogenetic, and molecular criteria. The median age of onset is 66 years with approximately 70% occurring over the age of 55 years. AML in the elderly has a less favorable outcome with few long-term survivors. For 2013, the ACS estimated there were 14,590 new cases of AML and 10,370 deaths attributable to AML.[140] In younger adults (<60 years), overall cure rates approach 40%–45%. Acute promyelocytic leukemia (APL) is a specific subset of AML which occurs most often in adults but has a much more favorable cure rate. Disseminated intravascular coagulation is a major feature of APL, and until recently, the early death rate exceeded 20% because of hemorrhage.[144] With current management regimens, the overall survival rate for APL approaches 90%–95%, especially in those <60 years.[153]

Clinical and Oral Manifestations

See section under ALL for clinical and oral manifestations. For precancer treatment–related oral health considerations, treatment recommendations as well as oral treatment–related side effects during and after treatment, please refer to Chapter 9.

Treatment

Prognosis of AML is based on stratification by chromosomal abnormalities in leukemic blasts (Table 18-7).[144] Specific treatment protocols are based on type risks associated with age (Table 18-8). The treatment approach in the younger and/or fitter patient is to achieve remission with an intensive induction course of cytotoxic therapy. Subsequent treatment is guided by pretreatment determinants and response to initial therapy. In poorer risk groups, when age, comorbidities, and donor availability permit, an allogeneic SCT is also a consideration.

A proportion of these patients will be cured by chemotherapy alone; however, determining which patient is likely to relapse and hence benefit from allogeneic SCT in first remission has not been easily defined. Generally, there is a reluctance to employ intensive induction chemotherapy in older patients due to toxicity and side effects and their

inability to survive treatment.[144] For the APL patient, therapy is aimed at reversing coagulopathy, with aggressive plasma and platelet support, and a distinct treatment regimen of all-trans retinoic acid (ATRA), in combination with anthracycline-based chemotherapy with intensification during consolidation with intermediate or high dose cytarabine and addition of arsenic trioxide during both induction and consolidation.

Chronic Leukemia

Chronic Myelogenous Leukemia (CML)

Chronic leukemia presents with less pronounced marrow failure than acute leukemia. They have an indolent course that usually lasts several years. For 2013, the ACS estimated there were 5,920 new cases of CML (3,420 men, 2,500 women) with about 610 deaths (340 men, 270 women).[140] The average age at diagnosis of CML is around 65 years.[154] Most cases of CML occur in adults, but it can occur rarely in children. Risk factors include older age, male gender, and exposure to ionizing radiation and benzene. CML is a clonal disorder resulting in myeloid marrow hyperplasia and myeloid cells in the blood displaying the t (9;22) chromosome translocation. This translocation produces the *Bcr-Abl* abnormal gene that produces Bcr-Abl tyrosine kinase, an abnormal protein that causes the excess WBCs typical of CML.[155]

Clinical and Oral Manifestations

CML typically follows a chronic and indolent course for 3 to 5 years, followed by an accelerated phase and blast crisis resembling acute leukemia. In the acute or blast

TABLE 18-7	Prognostic Stratification of AML	
Risk Profile	**Type**	**Defect**
Favorable	APLa	t(15;17)(q22;q22)
	CBFLb	t(8;21)(q22;q22)
	Normal karyotype	inv(16)(p13.1;q22)
		t(16;16)(p13.1;q22)
		Mutated NPM1 w/o
		FLT3 ITD mutation
		Biallelic mutated CEBPA
Intermediate	Trisomy 8	t(9;11)(p22;Q23)
Poor	Normal karyotype	FLT3 ITD mutation−5 or
	Complex karyotype	del(5q)−7
	(>3 abnormalities)	
	Monosomal karyotype	
	Abnormalities 17p	
	11q23 abnormalities	
	(other than t(9;11),	
	inv(3)(q21;q26.2)	
	T(3;3)(q21;q26.2)	
	T(6;9)(q23;34)	

aAPL, Acute promyelocytic leukemia.
bCBFL, Core binding factor leukemias.
Source: Adapted with permission from the Internal Medicine Journal.[144]

TABLE 18-8 Treatment Protocols for AML & APL

		Targeted Treatment	Induction	Intensification	Chemo Consolidation
AML	APL	Tyrosine kinase inhibitors FLT3 inhibitors	ATRA combo Arsenic trioxide	Anthracycline	Intermediate or high dose cytarabine Arsenic trioxide
	<60 yrs of age		Cytarabine/anthracyclines Alternative anthracyclines	Cytarabine daunarubicin and/or idarubicin	HiDAC
	>60 yrs of age		Avoid intensive chemo Azacitidine Decitabine		

Source: Reproduced with permission from the *Internal Medicine Journal.*[144]

phase, the most common manifestations are fever, weakness, fatigue, anorexia, weight loss, splenomegaly, anemia, and infection.[156] In the blast phase, there are excess immature WBCs (more than 30%) in the blood and bone marrow. Diagnostic confirmation is established by karyotype demonstration of the Philadelphia chromosome, visualization of *BCR-ABL1* fusion genes by FISH or amplification of *BCR-ABL1* fusion transcripts by reverse transcriptase polymerase chain reaction (RT-PCR). CML rarely has oral presentations.

Treatment

Preblast phase treatment is palliative. Subsequently, first-line therapy involves the newest drug, imatinib, a TKI with potent activity against *BCR-ABL*. Imatinib competitively occupies the adenosine triphosphate-binding site required for *BCR-ABL* to phosphorylate its substrates; consequently, signal transduction is inhibited, and the leukemic cells, which are "addicted" to *BCR-ABL* kinase activity, die.[156] The emergence of imatinib resistance has stimulated the development of second-generation TKIs for initial therapy of chronic phase CML. In comparison with imatinib in phase III randomized trials, both nilotinib[149] and dasatinib[150] have achieved more rapid and deeper molecular responses. They were also associated with less disease progression. However, neither can inhibit *BCR-ABL T315I*. Several other TKI are also in development, including bosutinib and ponatinib; the latter is the first TKI with activity against the *T315I* mutation. Other drugs that are active against *T315I* include omacetaxine mepesuccinate (homoharringtonine), a protein synthesis inhibitor that induces apoptosis through its effect on *MCL1*, a member of the BCL2 family of antiapoptotic proteins; and aurora kinase inhibitors. Allogeneic SCT is reserved for the following situations: (1) patients who do not respond to a second-generation TKI, especially those that develop *T315I* mutations, (2) patients who progress from chronic phase to accelerated or blast phase, and (3) patients who present in accelerated or blast phase (after initial cytoreduction with TKI chemotherapy).[156]

Chronic Lymphocytic Leukemia (CLL)

CLL results from the slow accumulation of clonal B lymphocytes in 95% of patients. For 2013, the ACS estimated there were 15,680 new cases of CLL with 4,580 deaths.[140] The median age at diagnosis of CLL is 65 years. There are two kinds of CLL. One grows very slowly, rarely needs to be treated and is associated with a 15-year or more survival rate.[157] The other kind of CLL grows faster, is more serious, and the average survival rate is 8 years. Lab tests look for proteins called ZAP-70 and CD38. Patients whose CLL cells contain low amounts of ZAP-70 and CD38 have a better prognosis. Most patients with CLL, including approximately 50% of those with early-stage disease, eventually die of disease progression or disease-related complications, including infection or a second malignant condition.

Lymphocytosis >5,000/μL for a month, with at least 30% of nucleated marrow granulocytes being well-differentiated lymphocytes, in an adult is diagnostic for CLL. Staging is based on the extent of lymph node, liver, or spleen involvement and anemia, thrombocytopenia, or both. The Rai and Binet clinical staging systems are commonly used in the United States and Europe, respectively (See Table 18-9).[158,159]

Clinical and Oral Manifestations

Historically, CLL was frequently recognized when patients presented for evaluation of constitutional symptoms (fever, night sweats, weight loss, fatigue), lymphadenopathy, anemia, or thrombocytopenia.[159] With the widespread use of automated blood counters, 70% to 80% of patients with CLL are diagnosed by incidental findings on CBC. Most of these individuals have early-stage disease (Rai stage 0 or I or Binet stage A) at diagnosis. However, about 10% to 20% will be symptomatic and require prompt evaluation by a hematologist and initiation of therapy. Oral manifestations at presentation of CLL are infrequent and generally involve bleeding or infection.[147,160] The oral lesion incidence rate increases once chemotherapy is initiated for treatment. Please see Chapter 9 for more on oral complications of cancer treatment.

TABLE 18-9 Prognostic Stages of Chronic Lymphocytic Leukemia (CLL)

CLL Stage		Characteristic[a]	Frequency (%)	Median Survival (yr)
Binet				
A			63	>10
B			30	5
C			7	1.53
Rai				
	Low/early			
	0	Lymphocytosis only	30	>10
	Intermediate			
	I	Lymphadenopathy	60	7
	II	Organomegaly (liver or spleen)		
	High/late			
	III	Anemia (hemoglobin <110 g/L)	10	1.5
	IV	Thrombocytopenia (platelet <100 × 10⁹cells/L)		

[a]Patients are categorized according to the worst characteristic present.
Source: Adapted from *Blood*[158] and the *Annals of Internal Medicine*.[159]

Treatment

Treatment decisions are guided by clinical staging using the systems of Rai and Binet. Patients with early stage disease may be monitored every 6 to 12 months (thorough medical history review, physical examination, and CBC) until constitutional symptoms, decreased performance status, or symptoms of complications from hepatomegaly, splenomegaly, and lympadenopathy, occur. Standard therapy consists of introduction of purine analogues (fludarabine in particular) and the use of monoclonal antibodies, which have significantly altered the management paradigm for the younger and fitter patients who require therapy. The current "gold standard" of FCR (fludarabine, cyclophosphamide, and the anti-CD20 monoclonal antibody rituximab [FCR]) has been shown to result in a significant increase in complete remission and progression free survival, when compared to traditional alkylating agent–based therapy.[156] For elderly patients unable to take FCR, oral chlorambucil is extensively used. Ongoing randomized trials include fludarabine monotherapy, the addition of a monoclonal anti-CD20 antibody (rituximab, obinutuzumab, or ofatumumab), and the newly available agent bendamustine, either alone or in combination with an anti-CD20 monoclonal antibody. Agents in various stages of development include novel monoclonals against CD20 (ofatumumab and GA-101), CD19 and bi-specific CD19/CD3 (blinatumomab), and anti-CD52 (alemtuzumab); BCR downstream signaling tyrosine kinases such as Btk (ibrutinib), Syk (fostamatinib), Src (dasatinib); leukemic microenvironment agents (plerixafor, lenalidomide); apoptosis and cell cycle agent Bcl-2 (navitoclax); and cyclin-dependent kinases (flavopiridol, dinaciclib).[156] There is currently little enthusiasm for autologous transplants.

Oral Health Considerations

CLL is a relatively indolent chronic hematologic malignant disease that often has a prognosis compatible with relatively normal dental treatment planning.[160] Patients in late-stage disease, with severe thrombocytopenia (<50,000/µL), should be considered for platelet supplementation prior to dental surgery.

Lymphoma
Hodgkin's Lymphoma

Lymphomas are solid tumors of the immune system. Hodgkin's lymphoma (HL) accounts for about 10% of all lymphomas and the remaining 90% are referred to as non-Hodgkin lymphoma. For 2013, the ACS estimated there were 9,290 new HL diagnoses (4,220 females, 5,070 males) and 1,180 deaths (660 males, 520 females).[140] HL has a bimodal age distribution at diagnosis, with the first peak in the third decade in life and a second smaller peak after the age of 55 years.[161] Because of advances in treatment, survival rates have improved in the past few decades. The 1-year relative survival rate for all patients diagnosed with Hodgkin disease is now about 92% and the 5-year and 10-year survival rates are about 85% and 80%, respectively. It occurs more frequently in men than in women, and peaks in incidence are noted in young adults and in people older than 60 years. HL is most common in the United States, Canada, and northern Europe, and is least common in Asian countries. Brothers and sisters of young people with the disease have a higher risk for Hodgkin disease but a family link is still uncommon (5% of all cases). It is not clear why family history might increase risk but it may be because family members have similar childhood exposures to certain infections (i.e., Epstein-Barr virus), inherited gene changes that make them more susceptible, or some combination of these factors. The risk of Hodgkin disease is greater in people with a higher socioeconomic background.

The WHO classification of lymphoid neoplasms distinguishes between two major subtypes of HL (classic and nodular lymphocyte predominant) and four subtypes (Nodular sclerosis [60%–80%], mixed cellularity [15%–30%], lymphocyte depletion [<1%], and lymphocyte-rich [5%]), which differ in presentation, sites of involvement, epidemiology, and association with Epstein-Barr virus.[162,163] Approximately 95% of patients with HL will have the classic HL histology, which is characterized by the presence of rare malignant Hodgkin's Reed-Sternberg cells among an overwhelming number of benign reactive cells.[164]

The etiology of HL is unknown; however, both genetic and environmental factors, including EBV are postulated to play a role.[163] It is thought such factors may lead to DNA changes in B lymphocytes, leading to the development of the Reed-Sternberg cell and Hodgkin disease. The pathognomic morphologic features used to establish the diagnosis of HL include an effacement of the involved lymph node with destruction of its normal architecture; an inflammatory cellular infiltrate consisting of lymphocytes, histiocytes, plasma cells, and fibroblasts; and the presence of the malignant cell, the Reed-Sternberg cell.

Clinical and Oral Manifestations

The first sign of HL is typically an asymptomatic enlargement of a supradiaphragmatic lymph node, often in the neck, which may wax and wane over a period of a few months.[163] Mediastinal lymph node involvement is common, occurring in 80% of cases. When mediastinal disease is bulky, patients may complain of chest pain, cough, and dyspnea. Systemic symptoms of drenching night sweats, fever which comes and goes over several days to weeks, and weight loss (about 10% of body weight over 6 months) are reported in approximately 30% of patients. Less common symptoms are generalized pruritus and alcohol-induced pain localized over the involved lymph node. Lymph node involvement of infradiaphragmatic sites such as the inguinal, pelvic, or retroperitoneal regions is rare. HL rarely presents as an extranodal mass in the head and neck region. However, physical examination may reveal involvement of Waldeyer's ring structures. The English language literature contains only nine reports of primary HL arising in the oral mucosa in the absence of nodal disease; most were cases of tongue involvement and soft tissue masses.[165,166]

The staging system for HL is known as the *Cotswold system*, which is a modification of the older Ann Arbor system (See Table 18-10).[163] It is currently used along with pathology and other prognostic factors to guide treatment choice. Approximately 70% of patients with HL present with stage I or II disease. The location and size of lymph node masses should be documented. Imaging tests are the key to defining the anatomic extent of disease and include the use of computed tomography of the head and neck, thorax, abdomen, and pelvis and positron emission tomography with ^{18}fluorodeoxyglucose (^{18}F-FDG PET).[163] ^{18}F-FDG PET is being used for staging, end of treatment and interim assessments, as well as follow-up surveillance. The use of ^{18}F-FDG PET during workup, has resulted in upstaging of 13%–24% more patients than did CT.[167] There is great interest in the potential use of ^{18}F-FDG PET for interim assessment after initial cycles of chemotherapy, with the aim to identify patients cured and those who need escalation of treatment.[163]

Treatment

Initial therapy for HL patients is based on the histology of the disease, the anatomical stage, and the presence of prognostic features. Patients with early stage disease are treated with combined modality strategies utilizing abbreviated courses of combination chemotherapy followed by involved-field radiation therapy (IFRT), while those with advanced stage disease receive a longer course of chemotherapy often without radiation therapy.[168] Chemotherapy regimens are (1) ABVD (Adriamycin [doxorubicin], bleomycin, vinblastine, dacarbazine); (2) Stanford V (doxorubicin, [Adriamycin], mechlorethamine [nitrogen mustard], vincristine, vinblastine, bleomycin, etoposide, prednisone); and BEACOPP (bleomycin, etoposide, doxorubicin, cyclophosphamide [Cytoxan], oncovin [vincristine], procarbazine, prednisone).[161] Concerns about the late effects of radiotherapy, especially the increased risk of secondary malignancies, have led some groups to recommend chemotherapy alone in carefully selected patients with early-stage disease when the risk of secondary malignancies is deemed high. Such patients might include women younger than 35 years or those who have a family history of breast cancer for whom the radiation field would incorporate breast tissue.

For refractory cases, high-dose chemotherapy (HDCT) followed by an autologous stem cell transplant (ASCT) is the standard of care for most patients who relapse following initial therapy. For patients who fail HDCT with ASCT, brentuximab vedotin, an anti CD-30 antibody conjugated to an antimicrotubule drug, shows promise.[169] Promising new drugs undergoing investigation include the immunomodulatory agent enalidomide, the mammalian target of rapamycin inhibitor everolimus, and the pandeacetylase inhibitor panobinostat. Bortezomib (a proteasome inhibitor) has poor activity when used alone, but could have a role in combination with other drugs.[163]

TABLE 18-10 Ann Arbor Staging Classification and Cotswold Modifications for Hodgkin's Lymphoma

Stage	
I	Involvement of one lymph node region or lymphoid structure (e.g., spleen, thymus, or Waldeyer's ring)
II	Involvement of two or more lymph node regions on the same side of the diaphragm
III	Involvement of lymph node regions on both sides of the diaphragm
	1. Splenic hilar, coeliac, or portal nodes
	2. Para-aortic, iliac, or mesenteric nodes
IV	Involvement of extranodal sites other than one contiguous or proximal extranodal site
Modifying features:	
A	No symptoms
B	Fever, drenching night sweats, loss of >10% bodyweight over 6 months
X	Bulky disease (mediastinal mass >1/3 of thoracic diameter or any nodal mass >10 cm in diameter)
E	Involvement of one contiguous or proximal extranodal site

Source: Reproduced with permission from the *Lancet*.[163]

Oral Health Considerations

The radiation fields for HL that involve bilateral cervical nodes have the potential to result in damage to the salivary glands. These include (1) IFRT when lymphoma involves the oral structures or Waldeyer's ring, (2) mantle, and (3) mini or modified mantle. Of these, the mantle field is the largest and involves radiation therapy to all supradiaphragmatic lymph node regions including the following groups bilateral cervical, supraclavicular, bilateral axillae, mediastinal, and bilateral lung hilar, treated in contiguity. Mini or modified mantle typically refers to radiation therapy covering bilateral cervical, supraclavicular, and axillary lymph nodes. Because the parotid glands are usually not in the field of radiation for these patients, the risk of radiation-induced caries is minimal; however, topical fluoride varnish, gel, or 1,000 parts per million fluoride toothpaste can be used for caries prevention if the patient's mouth appears to be dry or the caries rate appears elevated. The risk of osteoradionecros is very low due to low radiation doses delivered (30–40 Gy) and is limited to the inferior border and angle of the mandible. HL survivors who received mediastinal radiation 10 to 20 years earlier may suffer from late-onset heart disease characterized by heart valve pathology and accelerated atherosclerosis.

For patients undergoing chemotherapy please refer to Chapter 9 for treatment-related oral health considerations and related side effects during and after treatment.

Non-Hodgkin's Lymphoma

Non-Hodgkin's lymphoma (NHL) is one of the most common cancers in the United States, accounting for about 4% of all cancers. For 2013, the ACS estimated there were 69,740 new diagnoses of NHL (37,600 males, 32,140 females) and about 19,020 NHL deaths (10,590 males and 8,430 females).[140] The average American's risk of developing NHL during his or her lifetime is about 1 in 50. NHL incidence has risen steadily over the past several decades, not only in the United States, but in the United Kingdom, Brazil, India, and Japan as well. Immunosuppression (i.e., organ transplant recipients, chemotherapy, and stem cell transplant patients) and the emergence of HIV may have contributed to this increase. Conversely, 5-year survival rates have also improved.[170] NHL is known to be associated with chronic inflammatory diseases such as Sjögren's syndrome, celiac disease, and rheumatoid arthritis. Certain chronic infections are also associated with certain lymphomas such as the association between *Helicobacter pylori* infection and mucosa-associated lymphoid tissue lymphoma, human T-cell leukemia/lymphoma virus and adult T-cell lymphoma, EBV and Burkitt's lymphoma, *Clamydia psittaci* and ocular adenexal lymphomas, and hepatitis C and splenic or large cell lymphomas.[171]

The initial evaluation of the individual suspected of NHL includes a history and physical examination, laboratory studies, a bone marrow aspirate and biopsy, nodal biopsy, computed tomography, positron emission tomography, and lactate dehydrogenase levels to measure tumor proliferation. The wide range of clinical features as well as histologic appearances in the classification of NHL make the diagnosis difficult. Approximately 85% to 90% of cases arise from B cells (e.g., Burkitt lymphoma, chronic lymphocytic leukemia, diffuse large B-cell lymphoma [DLBCL], follicular lymphoma, mantle cell lymphoma) and the remaining arise from T cells (e.g., mycosis fungoides, anaplastic large cell lymphoma, precursor T-lymphoblastic lymphoma).[172] Several different classification systems have been proposed according to their histological characteristics. The most recent system is the fourth edition of the WHO classification of tumors of hematopoietic and lymphoid tissues, published in 2008 (See Table 18-11).[170] Classification is based on a combination of morphology, immunophenotype, genetic, molecular, and an expanded concept on clinical features such as age and tumor location, as defining criteria in several newly recognized categories.[173]

Clinical and Oral Manifestations

Clinical manifestations include lymphadenopathy, swollen abdomen, shortness of breath, fever, weight loss, night sweats, fatigue, severe or frequent infections.[170] Bone marrow involvement in indolent lymphomas is common and is sometimes associated with cytopenias, easy bruising, or bleeding. More aggressive B-cell lymphomas present with large abdominal or mediastinal masses.

Primary NHL of the oral region is rare[174] and may present as a gingival or mucosal tissue swelling or mass.[175] NHL may also manifest intrabony involvement characterized by osseous rarefaction around the roots of the symptomatic teeth, mimicking toothache.[176] In such a case, extraction of the associated tooth is followed by rapid growth of the tumor from the nonhealing extraction site. Nerve invasion can lead to paresthesia or anesthesia of related oral mucosal tissue. NHL may also present as a nonhealing mucosal ulceration with ill-defined borders, a benign-appearing gingival lesion, and a mucosal lesion resembling a vesiculobullous disease. Involvement of the oral mucosa in cutaneous T-cell lymphoma (mycosis fungoides) is uncommon and is usually associated with a poor prognosis.

A record review in Canada of 88 consecutive patients with extranodal maxillofacial NHL, with age at diagnosis ranging from 22 to 94 years (median 60 years), revealed the affected anatomic site distribution to be the maxillary sinus (22), nasal cavity (8), maxilla (13), mandible (8), salivary glands (14), and other sites (23). Although most presented as nonpainful masses, 72 patients had associated dental symptoms, including intraoral swelling, pain, and loose teeth.[177]

Treatment

NHL is a radiosensitive tumor, thus radiotherapy is used within all subtypes and stages.[172] Patients with NHL are classified into two groups: indolent lymphoma, grade I according to

TABLE 18-11 Subtypes of Non-Hodgkin Lymphoma According to the 2008 WHO Classification	
B-Cell Lymphomas	
Precursor B cell	Precursor B-cell lymphoblastic leukemia or lymphoma
Mature B cell	Chronic lymphocytic leukemia/small lymphocytic lymphoma; lymphoplasmacytic lymphoma; splenic marginal-zone lymphoma; extranodal marginal-zone B-cell lymphoma of mucosa-associated lymphoid tissue; nodal marginal-zone B-cell lymphoma; follicular lymphoma; mantle-cell lymphoma; diff use large B-cell lymphoma; Burkitt's lymphoma
B-cell proliferations of uncertain malignant potential	Lymphomatoid granulomatosis; post-transplantation lymphoproliferative disorders (polymorphic)
T-Cell and NK-Cell^a Lymphomas	
Precursor T cell	Precursor T-cell lymphoblastic leukemia or lymphoma
Extranodal mature T cell and NK cell	Mycosis fungoides; cutaneous anaplastic large-cell lymphoma; extranodal NK-cell or T-cell lymphoma; enteropathy-type lymphoma; hepatosplenic lymphoma; subcutaneous panniculitis-like lymphoma; primary cutaneous CD8-positive lymphoma; primary cutaneous γ/δ T-cell lymphoma; primary cutaneous CD4-positive lymphoma
Nodal mature T cell and NK cell	Peripheral T-cell lymphoma, not otherwise specified; angioimmunoblastic lymphoma; anaplastic large-cell ALK-positive lymphoma; anaplastic large-cell ALK-negative lymphoma; adult T-cell leukemia/lymphoma

^aNK, natural killer.
Source: Reproduced with permission from the *Lancet*.[170]

the British National Lymphoma Investigation (BNLI) (low-grade, mainly follicular lymphoma); or aggressive lymphoma, BNLI grade II (high-grade, mainly diffuse large B-cell lymphoma). Patients with indolent lymphoma may be cured with radiotherapy; for those with aggressive lymphoma, radiotherapy is used after or to consolidate chemotherapy and for palliative treatment.[171] The optimal radiation dose in indolent and aggressive lymphoma still remains unclear. Adults with NHL who were treated either with standard high dose (HD) radiation (40–45 Gy in both indolent and aggressive NHL) or low dose (LD) radiation (24 Gy in indolent NHL or 30 Gy in aggressive NHL) experienced the same efficacy with both radiation schemes. While safety was not statistically significantly reduced with the lower radiation dose, the lower dose might influence long-term outcomes positively. Chemotherapy of NHL differs between indolent or aggressive lymphoma. Additionally, the International Prognostic Index influences the therapy option (such as watch and wait, chemotherapy, radiotherapy, or combined modality treatment). Treatment with CHOP (cyclophosphamide, doxorubicin, vincristine, and prednisone) improves overall survival (OS), is associated with reduced toxicity, and is the mainstay of the treatment of aggressive and indolent NHL. The addition of a monoclonal antibody such as rituximab to CHOP (R-CHOP) is associated with increased OS.[172]

DLBCL accounts for approximately 40% of all NHL cases. Trials have demonstrated a beneficial effect of the R-CHOP regimens without increasing the secondary malignancy rate for young patients with a good prognosis. There was also improvement in patient-related outcomes such as

increased tolerability to toxicity. Similarly, R-ACVBP (doxorubicin, cyclophosphamide, vindesine, bleomycin, prednisone) regimens statistically significantly prolonged OS in patients with untreated, low-intermediate–risk DLBCL compared with standard R-CHOP but resulted in more serious adverse events.

Follicular lymphoma (FL) accounts for 25% of all NHL and follows an indolent course so patients are usually in advanced stages at diagnosis. For such patients, R-CHOP is standard therapy. Patients suffering from indolent B-cell NHL also receive chemotherapy because it is regarded to be highly effective. In patients with advanced-stage indolent B-cell NHL and FL grade 3B, there is currently no standard therapy, but R-CHOP shows promising results as well.[172] There is no evidence that HD radiation therapy improves OS in newly diagnosed or relapsed FL patients but its prolongation of increased progression-free survival favors its use.

Primary cutaneous T-cell lymphomas are a clinically and histologically distinct group of T-lymphocyte malignancies that manifest primarily in the skin. Cutaneous T-cell lymphomas remain incurable by conventional therapies. Although initial response rates on mono- or poly-chemotherapeutic regimens are high, remissions are often short-lived and the prolongation of lifespan is questionable. Furthermore, there are considerable toxicities associated with these regimens. Therefore, therapies focus on the effect of allogeneic stem cell transplantation as an alternative to conventional therapy for advanced primary cutaneous T-cell lymphoma.[172]

Oral Health Considerations

Acute complications of chemotherapy include mucositis, viral and bacterial infections, and hemorrhagic lesions related to bone marrow suppression. Please refer to Chapter 9 for more information on oral health considerations after cancer treatments.

Burkitt's Lymphoma

Early in the 20th century, Sir Albert Cook, a missionary doctor in Uganda, and other medical staff working in west, east, and central Africa noted the high frequency of jaw tumors and childhood lymphomas. Years later, Denis Burkitt, a surgeon working in Africa further described these jaw swellings which have come to be known as Burkitt's lymphoma (BL). BL is a highly aggressive, small, noncleaved cell lymphoma and has played an important role in the understanding of tumorigenesis as it was the first human tumor to be associated with EBV and one of the first tumors shown to have a chromosomal translocation that activates an oncogene.[178]

According to the 2008 WHO classification of BL, there are three clinical variants: endemic, sporadic (predominant type found in nonmalarial areas), and immunodeficiency-related.[173,179] These types are similar in morphology, immunophenotype, and genetic features. In present-day Africa, endemic BL continues to account for most childhood malignancies and is almost always associated with EBV. In adult Africans, BL is categorized as the immunodeficiency-related type when associated with HIV. Immunodeficiency-associated BL also occurs in organ transplant recipients after a relatively long interval posttransplantation and individuals with congenital immunodeficiency. The sporadic type occurs mainly throughout the rest of the world (predominantly North America and Europe), with no special climatic or geographical links, and only rarely associated with EBV infection.[179]

Diagnosis of Burkitt's lymphoma should be confirmed by microscopy and immunocytological analysis. The recommended approach is to remove and examine the most accessible disease-containing tissue. Surgical biopsy is preferable to fine needle aspiration as the later yields insufficient sample.[179] Flow cytometry, chromosome analysis using Giemsa banding or FISH, and immunostains are performed. The disease is staged according to blood smear, CSF, BM biopsy and presence/absence of HIV infection. Histopathology consists of intermediate-sized B cells (12 μ) with high nuclear-to-cytoplasmic ratio. Nuclear contours are round to oval without cleaves or folds, a key feature in the distinction from diffuse large cell lymphoma. Nucleoli are typically multiple, small-to-intermediate in size, and the nuclear chromatin is relatively immature, being finely granular.[180] The characteristic *starry-sky* is due to scattered tingible-body-laden macrophages that contain apoptotic tumor cells. The cells are always of B-cell lineage (CD20 positive and CD79a positive). CD10 and Bcl-6 are commonly coexpressed, but the cells are generally negative for Bcl-2.[178] A defining feature of BL is the presence of a translocation between the c-*myc* gene (the first oncogene described in lymphoma) and the *IgH* gene (found in 80% of cases [t (8;14) (q24;q32)]) or between c-*myc* and the gene for either the kappa or lambda light chain (*IgL*) in the remaining 10%–15% [t(2;8) (p12;q24) or t(8;22)(q24;q11)], respectively.[178] Deregulated expression arises as a result of juxtaposition of *MYC* to the enhancer elements of one of the following immunoglobulin genes: the heavy chain at 14q32; the kappa light chain at 2p12; or the lambda light chain at 22q11.

Clinical and Oral Manifestations

Endemic (African) BL refers to cases occurring in African children, usually 4 to 7 years old, with a male to female ratio of 2:1, nearly all EBV associated, involving primarily the bones of the jaw and other facial bones, as well as the kidneys, gastrointestinal tract, ovaries, breast, and other extranodal sites. Endemic BL is rare in the United States. Sporadic (American) BL is an uncommon form of NHL in the United States, with approximately 1,200 new cases reported per year. According to the 2007 National Cancer Institute Surveillance, Epidemiology and End Results (SEER) database, it suggests that *older* adult patients (age >40 years) account for roughly 59% of all adult BL cases in the United States. The abdomen, especially the ileocecal area, is the most common site of involvement. Patients may have malignant pleural effusions or ascites and involvement of the lymph nodes, jaws, ovaries, kidneys, breasts, omentum, Waldeyer's ring, and other sites.

Oral manifestations include clinically evident jaw tumors that may result in tooth mobility and pain, intraoral swelling of the mandible and maxilla, and anterior open bite.[181] Mobile teeth may be present even in the absence of clinically detectable jaw tumors.[182] Radiographic features on panoramic images include resorption of alveolar bone; loss of lamina dura; enlargement of tooth follicles; destruction of the cortex around tooth crypts; displacement of teeth and tooth buds by the enlarging tumor, resulting in the impression of "teeth floating in air;" and sun-ray spicules as bone forms perpendicular to the mandible from subperiosteal growth.[181] In a retrospective study of 661 BL patients from Malawi during 2005 through 2007, the maxilla was the most common site for oro-facial BL (13.7%) followed by the mandible (7.2%), cheeks (5.7%), maxilla and mandible (4.5%), and cervical lymph nodes (4.1%). The male to female ratio was 1.6:1. Generally the trend of BL occurrence had decreased from 2005 to 2007 possibly due to better access to health services, increased use of bed-treated mosquito nets for malaria prevention and knowledgeable health-care workers.[183]

Treatment

Management of BL can be divided into three broad groups of patients. Children with localized disease that has been completely removed surgically need only two cycles of moderately intensive chemotherapy such as cyclophosphamide, vincristine, prednisolone, and doxorubicin. Children with residual or stage III disease need at least four cycles of dose-intensive chemotherapy, such as two cycles of cyclophosphamide, vincristine, prednisolone, doxorubicin, and high-dose methotrexate, followed by two cycles of cytarabine and high-dose methotrexate with concurrent intrathecal treatment. Children with CNS or bone-marrow involvement are given similar treatment to the second group, but receive up to eight courses of dose-intensive treatment. The use of rituximab in primary therapy has been assessed, with encouraging results.[178]

No randomized therapeutic trials have been done for adult BL. Adults present with rapidly developing disease, commonly in the abdomen, and symptoms such as weight loss, night sweats, and unexplained fever. Extranodal disease is common, especially in bone marrow (70%) and the CNS (40%). Diagnosis and staging are urgent because treatment should be started as soon as possible. Aggressive high-dose therapy (cyclophosphamide, vincristine, doxorubicin, and high-dose methotrexate alternating with ifosfamide, etoposide, and high-dose cytarabine) is needed for adult BL and has yielded an 89% 2-year survival in younger individuals, and about a 70% 2-year survival rate in those >65.[184] With improved molecular profiling and understanding of the cause of BL, targeted therapy will be developed that still has excellent cure rates but has reduced toxic effects. Potential targets could include the MYC oncogene, DNA methyltransferase inhibitors, cyclin-dependent kinase inhibitors, and proteasome inhibitors. As further biological factors are identified, more targeted therapies will probably be developed.[178]

Multiple Myeloma

Multiple myeloma (MM) is a neoplastic plasma cell disorder that is characterized by clonal proliferation of malignant plasma cells in the bone marrow microenvironment, monoclonal protein in the blood or urine, and associated organ dysfunction. It accounts for approximately 1% of neoplastic diseases and 13% of hematologic cancers. In Western countries, the annual age-adjusted incidence is 5.6 cases per 100,000 persons.[185] For 2013, the ACS estimated there were 22,350 adults (12,440 men, 9,910 women) diagnosed with MM and 10,710 deaths (6,070 men, 4,640 women) attributable to MM.[140] The median age at diagnosis is approximately 70 years; 37% of patients are younger than 65 years, 26% are between the ages of 65 and 74 years, and 37% are 75 years of age or older.[186] In recent years, the introduction of ASCT and the availability of agents such as thalidomide, lenalidomide, and bortezomib have changed the management of myeloma and extended overall survival in patients presenting at an age under 60 years where 10-year survival is approximately 30%.[187]

Several genetic abnormalities that occur in tumor plasma cells play major roles in the pathogenesis of myeloma. Primary early chromosomal translocations occur at the immunoglobulin switch region on chromosome 14 (q32.33), which is most commonly juxtaposed to MAF (t[14;16][q32.33;23]) and MMSET on chromosome 4p16.3. This process results in the deregulation of two adjacent genes, MMSET in all cases and FGFR3 in 30% of cases. Secondary late-onset translocations and gene mutations that are implicated in disease progression include complex karyotypic abnormalities in MYC, the activation of NRAS and KRAS, mutations in FGFR3 and TP53, and the inactivation of cyclin-dependent kinase inhibitors CDKN2A and CDKN2C. Other genetic abnormalities involve epigenetic dysregulation, such as alteration in microRNA expression and gene methylation modifications. Gene-expression profiling allows classification of multiple myeloma into different subgroups on the basis of genetic abnormalities.[185]

Clinical and Oral Manifestations

Symptoms include fatigue, weakness, weight loss, bone pain, and recurrent infections. MM is characterized by a high capacity to induce focal osteolytic bone lesions, diffuse osteopenia, and pathologic fractures. Osteolytic bone lesions in MM result from increased osteoclast formation, osteoblast inhibition induced by MM cells, and activity that occurs in close proximity to myeloma cells.

Although rare, oral manifestations may be the sole presenting sign or part of a group of signs of disease progression. Clinical presentations of patients with oro-facial MM lesions can mimic common dental pathologies such as periapical or periodontal abscess, gingivitis, periodontitis, or other gingival enlargement or masses.[188] This mimicry can lead to delays in diagnosis and treatment. Initial signs and symptoms of MM may involve pain, paresthesia of the inferior alveolar and mental nerves, swelling, tooth mobility, and radiolucency.[189] Radiographic changes in patients with MM include typical "punched-out" lesions in the skull from the focal proliferation of plasma cells inside the bone marrow and jaw bone (mandible > maxilla) involvement, ranging from asymptomatic osteolytic lesions to pathologic fracture.

Diagnosis

The diagnosis of symptomatic MM requires ≥10% clonal plasma cells on BM proven plasmacytoma; and evidence of end-organ damage, the so-called CRAB criteria (hypercalcaemia, renal insufficiency, anemia, or bone lesions) that is felt to be related to the underlying plasma cell disorder. The tests to help determine whether MM is symptomatic or not include detection of the monoclonal (M-) component by serum and/or urine protein electrophoresis, nephelometric quantification of IgG, IgA, and IgM immunoglobulins, characterization of the heavy and light chains by immunofixation, serum-free light-chain measurement, BM plasma cell infiltration using cytogenetic/FISH studies, lytic bone lesions on radiological skeletal bone survey (spine, pelvis, skull, humeri, and femurs) and CBC with differential serum creatinine and calcium levels.[190]

Treatment

Asymptomatic (smoldering) myeloma requires clinical observation, since early treatment with conventional chemotherapy has shown no benefit. Symptomatic (active) disease should be treated immediately. The treatment strategy is mainly related to age. Current data support the initiation of induction therapy with thalidomide, lenalidomide, or bortezomib for any age group. In patients under the age of 65 years who do not have substantial heart, lung, renal, or liver dysfunction, HSCT is added. Investigational trials are currently evaluating the efficacy of immunomodulatory drugs to delay the progression from asymptomatic to symptomatic myeloma. Less intensive approaches that limit drug-induced should be considered in patients over 75 years of age or in younger patients with coexisting conditions.[185]

To manage focal bone lytic lesions, patients with MM frequently require radiation therapy, surgery, and analgesic medications. Bisphosphonates, inhibitors of osteoclastic activity have reduced the skeletal complications among patients with MM and are now a mainstay of myeloma therapy.

Oral Health Considerations

Osteonecrosis of the jaw, resulting in symptomatic exposed nonhealing areas of the maxilla and mandible, is increasingly recognized as a serious complication of long-term intravenous antiresorptive (e.g., bisphosphonate) therapy. Please refer to Chapter 9 for additional information. Another consideration for MM patients requiring dental surgery is the risk of hemorrhage.[191] Patients with MM and other disorders associated with high-titer serum paraproteins can manifest unique hemostatic disorders, predisposing the patient to hemorrhage, especially following surgical procedures. Predental surgical assessments should include radiographic assessment for plasma cell tumors of the jaw and CBC and coagulation studies. Prevention of hemorrhage should be managed by consultation with the patient's hematologist regarding the status of treatment of the underlying disease and, depending on clinical circumstances, the need for additional therapies that might include plasmapheresis with appropriate factor replacement, desmopressin acetate (Stimate), fibrinolysis inhibitors ε-aminocaproic acid (Amicar) and tranexamic acid (Cyclokapron), and splenectomy.[192]

Selected Readings

American Cancer Society. Leukemia–Acute Lymphocytic (Adults). http://www.cancer.org/acs/groups/cid/documents/webcontent/003109-pdf.pdf. Updated July 2013. Accessed November 30, 2013.

American Cancer Society. Leukemia–Acute Myeloid (Myelogenous). http://www.cancer.org/acs/groups/cid/documents/webcontent/003110-pdf.pdf. Updated July 2013. Accessed November 30, 2013.

American Cancer Society. Leukemia—Chronic Myeloid (Myelogenous). http://www.cancer.org/acs/groups/cid/documents/webcontent/003112-pdf.pdf. Updated September 2013. Accessed November 30, 2013.

American Cancer Society. Leukemia–Chronic Lymphocytic. http://www.cancer.org/acs/groups/cid/documents/webcontent/003111-pdf.pdf. Updated November 2013. Accessed November 30, 2013.

American Cancer Society. Hodgkin Disease. http://www.cancer.org/acs/groups/cid/documents/webcontent/003105-pdf.pdf. Updated January 2013. Accessed November 30, 2013.

American Cancer Society. Non-Hodgkin Lymphoma. http://www.cancer.org/acs/groups/cid/documents/webcontent/003126-pdf.pdf. Updated November 2013. Accessed November 30, 2013.

American Cancer Society. Multiple Myeloma. http://www.cancer.org/acs/groups/cid/documents/webcontent/003121-pdf.pdf. Updated February 2013. Accessed November 30, 2013.

Cardoso RC, Gerngross PJ, Hofstede TM, et al. The multiple oral presentations of multiple myeloma. *Support Care Cancer.* 2014;22(1):259–267.

Centers for Disease Control. National Program of Cancer Registries (NPCR), United States Cancer Statistics (USCS), Top Ten Cancers 2010. http://apps.nccd.cdc.gov/uscs/toptencancers.aspx. Updated 2013. Accessed November 30, 2013.

Dong A, Rivella S, Breda L. Gene therapy for hemoglobinopathies: progress and challenges. *Transl Res.* 2013;161(4):293–306.

Flowers CR, Seidenfeld J, Bow EJ, et al. Antimicrobial prophylaxis and outpatient management of fever and neutropenia in adults treated for malig nancy: American Society of Clinical Oncology clinical practice guideline. *J Clin Oncol.* 2013;31(6):794–810.

Gude D, Bansal D, Malu A. Revisiting plummer vinson syndrome. *Ann Med Health Sci Res.* 2013;3(1):119–121.

Gibson J, Iland HJ, Larsen SR, et al. Leukaemias into the 21st century. Part 2: the chronic leukaemias. *Intern Med J.* 2013;43(5):484–494.

Hattab FN. Patterns of physical growth and dental development in Jordanian children and adolescents with thalassemia major. *J Oral Sci.* 2013;55(1):71–77.

Kammerer PW, Schiegnitz E, Hansen T, et al. Multiple primary enoral soft tissue manifestations of a Hodgkin lymphoma–case report and literature review. *Oral Maxillofac Surg.* 2013;17(1):53–57.

Little JW, Falace DA, Miller CS, Rhodus NL. *Dental Management of the Medically Compromised Patient.* 8th ed. St. Louis, MO: Elsevier Mosby—USA; 2013.

Moreau P, San Miguel J, Ludwig H, et al. Multiple myeloma: ESMO Clinical Practice Guidelines for diagnosis, treatment and follow-up. *Ann Oncol.* 2013;24 Suppl 6:vi133–vi137.

National Heart Lung and Blood Institue. Types of Hemolytic Anemia. http://www.nhlbi.nih.gov/health/health-topics/topics/ha/types.html. Updated April 2011. Accessed November 30, 2013.

National Cancer Institute. *SEER Stat Fact Sheets: Leukemia.* http://seer.cancer.gov/statfacts/html/leuks.html. Updated 2013. Accessed November 30, 2013.

Northern California Comprehensive Thalassemia Center. Standards of Care Guidelines for Thalassemia 2012. http://www.thalassemia.com/documents/SOCGuidelines2012.pdf. Accessed November 30, 2013.

Olivieri NF, Brittenham GM. Management of the thalassemias. *Cold Spring Harb Perspect Med.* 2013;3(6):a011767.

Piel FB, Hay SI, Gupta S, et al. Global burden of sickle cell anaemia in children under five, 2010-2050: modelling based on demographics, excess mortality, and interventions. *PLoS Med.* 2013;10(7):e1001484.

Rancea M, Will A, Borchmann P, et al. Fifteenth biannual report of the Cochrane Haematological Malignancies Group–focus on non-Hodgkin's lymphoma. *J Natl Cancer Inst.* 2013;105(15):1159–1170.

Siegel R, Naishadham D, Jemal A. Cancer statistics, 2013. *CA Cancer J Clin.* 2013;63(1):11–30.

Stanley AC, Christian JM. Sickle cell disease and perioperative considerations: review and retrospective report. *J Oral Maxillofac Surg.* 2013;71(6):1027–1033.

UpToDate. Causes of lymphocytopenia. http://www.uptodate.com/contents/image?imageKey=HEME%2F58469&topicKey=HEME%2F8387&source=see_link&utdPopup=true. Updated 2013. Accessed November 30, 2013.

Younes M, Dagher GA, Dulanto JV, et al. Unexplained macrocytosis. *South Med J.* 2013;106(2):121–125.

For the full reference lists, please go to http://www.pmph-usa.com/Burkets_Oral_Medicine.

CHAPTER 19

Bleeding and Clotting Disorders

Joel J. Napeñas, DDS, FDS RCSEd
Lauren L. Patton, DDS, FDS RCSEd

OVERVIEW AND EPIDEMIOLOGY

Oral health-care professionals are increasingly called upon to provide care to individuals whose bleeding and clotting mechanisms have been altered by acquired or inherited mechanisms. This provides an opportunity for the dentist who is trained in the recognition of oral and systemic signs of altered hemostasis to assist in the screening and monitoring of the underlying condition. Invasive dental procedures resulting in bleeding can have serious consequences for the patient with a bleeding disorder, including severe hemorrhage or even death. Safe dental care may require consultation with the patient's medical provider, institution of systemic management, and dental treatment modifications.

Acquired coagulation disorders can result from drug actions or side effects of underlying systemic disease or their treatment. The use of coumarin anticoagulants (i.e., warfarin) is commonplace as a result of their demonstrated effectiveness in the treatment of atrial fibrillation and venous thromboembolism and control of thrombosis in the presence of a mechanical heart valve,[1] with usage in the United States in excess of 1 million patients.[2] Other commonly prescribed medications for the prevention of thromboembolic events for cardiac and stroke patients include antiplatelet medications such as acetylsalicylic acid (ASA), clopidogrel, and ticlopidine; heparins; and the new generation of anticoagulant medications (e.g., dabigatran, rivaroxaban, apixaban). A stratified household sample of 4,163 community residents aged 65 years or older living in a 5-county area of North Carolina revealed 51.7% to be taking one or more medications (aspirin, warfarin, dipyridamole, nonsteroidal anti-inflammatory drugs [NSAIDs], or heparin) with the potential to alter hemostasis.[3]

Patients with liver disease may have impaired hemostasis due to thrombocytopenia and/or lack of coagulation factors, whereas renal failure may result in qualitative disorders in platelet function. Patients with hematologic malignancies may have thrombocytopenia as a result of overgrowth of malignant cells in the bone marrow that leaves no room for platelet precursors (megakaryocytes). In addition, cancer patients may have thrombocytopenia as a result of the cytotoxic effects of chemotherapeutic agents to treat their disease.

Of the inherited coagulopathies, von Willebrand disease (vWD) is the most common, affecting about 0.8% to 1% of the population,[4] followed by hemophilia A and hemophilia B. Application to the US population resulted in an estimated national prevalence of 13,320 cases of hemophilia A and 3,640 cases of hemophilia B, with an incidence rate of 1 per 5,032 live male births. The age-adjusted prevalence of hemophilia in 6 surveillance states in 1994 was 13.4 cases in 100,000 males (10.5 for hemophilia A and 2.9 for hemophilia B).[5]

PATHOPHYSIOLOGY

Basic Mechanisms of Hemostasis and Their Interactions

Hemostasis is the process of blood clot formation at the site of tissue injury. Multiple processes occur either simultaneously or in rapid sequence (Figure 19-1). When specific elements of these processes are dysfunctional, abnormal bleeding or nonphysiologic thrombosis (i.e., thrombosis not required for hemostasis) occurs.

Hemostasis can be divided into four general phases: the vascular phase, the platelet phase, the coagulation cascade phase, and the termination and fibrinolytic phase. The first three phases are the principal mechanisms that prevent or diminish the loss of blood following vascular injury, whereas fibrinolysis is the process by which the clot is dissolved.

When vessel integrity is disrupted, platelets are activated, adhere to the site of injury, and form a platelet plug that reduces or temporarily arrests blood loss.[6] Platelets begin to aggregate at the wound site almost immediately following vascular contraction. The exposure of collagen and activation of platelets also initiates the coagulation cascade, which leads to fibrin formation and the generation of an insoluble fibrin clot that strengthens the platelet plug.[6] The coagulation cascade is under way within 10 to 20 seconds of injury; an initial hemostatic plug is formed

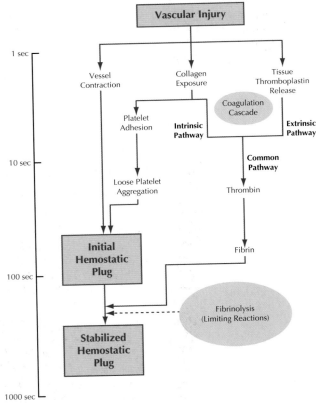

FIGURE 19-1 Mechanisms of hemostasis following vascular injury.

in 1 to 3 minutes; and fibrin has been generated and added to stabilize the clot by 5 to 10 minutes. Fibrinolysis is the major means of disposing of fibrin after its hemostatic function has been fulfilled, and it can be considered the rate-limiting step in clotting. It leads to fibrin degradation by the proteolytic enzyme plasmin.

Vascular Phase

After tissue injury, there is an immediate reflex vasoconstriction that alone may be hemostatic in small vessels. Reactants such as serotonin, histamine, prostaglandins, and other products are vasoactive and produce vasoconstriction of the microvascular bed in the area of the injury.

Platelet Phase

When circulating platelets are exposed to damaged vascular surfaces (in the presence of functionally normal von Willebrand factor (vWF), endothelial cells, collagen or collagen-like materials, basement membrane, elastin, microfibrils, and other cellular debris), platelets are activated to experience physical and chemical changes (Figure 19-2).[6] These changes produce an environment that causes the platelets to undergo the aggregation and release phenomenon and form the primary vascular plug that reduces blood loss from small blood vessels and capillaries. These platelet plugs adhere to exposed basement membranes. As this reaction is occurring, the release reaction is under way, involving the intracellular release of active components for further platelet aggregation as well as promotion of the clotting mechanism. In addition,

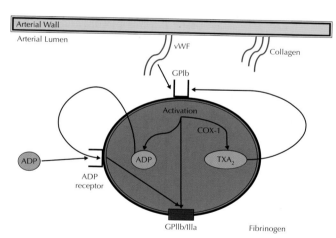

FIGURE 19-2 Platelet activation. Platelet adhesion occurs immediately (1–2 seconds) to the exposed collagen fibers and involves von Willebrand factor (vWF) and its receptor platelet membrane glycoprotein Ib (GPIb). Adherent platelet becomes activated with events such as secretion of adenosine diphosphate (ADP), which recruits additional platelets to form the primary plug. Platelets also secrete the prostaglandin thromboxane A2 (TXA$_2$), a potent platelet aggregator to enhance the clotting mechanism. Platelets provide surface membrane glycoproteins such as IIB/IIIa, which attach to other platelets via fibrinogen. Platelet aggregation begins 10 to 20 seconds following vascular injury.

the platelet plug, intermixed with fibrin and cellular components such as red and white cells, contracts to further reduce blood loss and to seal the vascular bed.

Platelet stimuli include adenosine diphosphate (ADP), epinephrine, thrombin, and collagen. Integrin glycoproteins GPIa/IIa and GPVI are important collagen receptors, involved in adhesion and activation, respectively.[7] ADP is a potent nucleotide that binds to receptors P2Y1 (which leads to calcium mobilization, platelet shape change, and aggregation) and P2Y12 (responsible for platelet secretion and stable aggregation), in effect activating and recruiting other platelets in the area and adding to the size of the plug. Platelet factor 3 is the intracellular phospholipid that activates F X and subsequently results in the conversion of prothrombin to thrombin.

There are four processes in the functional response of activated platelets: adhesion, aggregation, secretion, and procoagulant activity. Platelet adhesion primarily occurs through the binding of platelet surface receptor GP Ib/IX/V complex to vWF in the subendothelial matrix.[8] In addition, GP Ia/IIa on platelets bind to collagen fibrils in the matrix.[9] During platelet aggregation, GP IIb/IIIa binds activated platelets (e.g., activated by thrombin, collagen, or ADP) through binding of the receptor to fibrinogen. During the secretion phase, platelets secrete a number of substances to include: ADP and serotonin for platelet stimulation and recruitment; adhesive proteins bironectin and thrombospondin; fibrinogen; thromboxane A2 for vasoconstriction and further platelet aggregation; growth factors that stimulate smooth muscle cell mitosis; and other factors that enhance fibrin and platelet thrombus formation. In the platelet procoagulant phase, procoagulant phospholipids are exposed and enzyme complexes for the clotting cascade are assembled on platelet surfaces (discussed below).[10]

Coagulation Phase

The generation of thrombin and fibrin is the end product of the coagulation phase. This process involves multiple proteins, many of which are synthesized by the liver (fibrinogen; prothrombin; Factors (Fs) V, VII, IX, X, XI, XII, and XIII) and are vitamin K dependent (Fs II, VII, IX, and X) (Table 19-1).

Classical Coagulation Cascade Model

The blood clotting mechanism was originally outlined in 1903 by Markowitz as the prothrombin-to-thrombin and fibrinogen-to-fibrin conversion system. In 1964, the "cascade" or "waterfall" theory was proposed.[11,12] This offers the current traditional model of understanding this complex system, as well as the clinically important associated laboratory tests.

The coagulation of blood requires the presence of both calcium ions and exposed phospholipid on platelet surfaces. A sequence of interactions between the various clotting factors occurs following injury of tissue (Figure 19-3). The scheme of reaction is a bioamplification, in which a precursor is altered to an active form, which, in turn, activates the next

TABLE 19-1 Coagulation Factors

Factor (Name)	Coagulation Factor Affected		t1/2 (h)
	Intrinsic	Extrinsic	
XIII (fibrin-stabilizing factor)		✓	336
XII (Hageman factor)	✓		60
XI (plasma thromboplastin antecedent)	✓		60
X (Stuart factor)	✓	✓	48
IX (Christmas factor)	✓		18–24
VIII (antihemophilic factor)	✓		8–12
VII (proconvertin)		✓	4–6
V (proaccelerin)	✓	✓	32
IV (calcium)	✓	✓	—
III (tissue thromboplastin)		✓	—
II (prothrombin)	✓	✓	72
I (fibrinogen)	✓	✓	96

Abbreviation: t1/2, half-life.

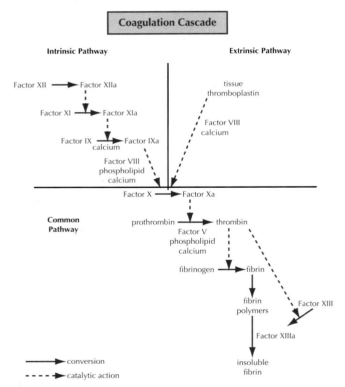

FIGURE 19-3 The coagulation cascade/waterfall model.

precursor in the sequence. Beginning with an undetectable biochemical reaction, the coagulation mechanism results in a final explosive change of a liquid to a gel. The traditional model of the cascade involves two separate pathways (intrinsic and extrinsic) that converge by activating a third (common) pathway.

The intrinsic pathway is initiated when F XII is activated by surface contact (e.g., with collagen or subendothelium), and it involves the interaction of F XII and F XI. The next step of intrinsic coagulation, the activation of F IX to F IXa, requires a divalent cation such as calcium.[13] Once activated, F IXa forms a complex with F VIII, in a reaction that requires the presence of both calcium ions and phospholipid, which, in turn, converts F X to an activated form—F Xa.

The extrinsic pathway is initiated by the release of tissue factor (TF), also called tissue thromboplastin, and does not require contact activation. TF binds to F VII in the presence of calcium, and this complex is capable of activating Fs IX and X, linking the intrinsic and extrinsic pathways.

The common pathway begins through the activation of F X. Once activated, F Xa converts prothrombin to thrombin in a reaction similar to the activation of F X by F IXa. The activation of prothrombin by F Xa requires the presence of calcium ions and phospholipid as well as F V, a plasma protein cofactor.[14] Once formed, thrombin converts fibrinogen, a soluble plasma protein, to insoluble fibrin. Fibrin polymerizes to form a gel, stabilizing the platelet plug. Finally, F XIII, which has been converted to an activated form by thrombin,[15] produces covalent cross-links between the fibrin molecules that strengthen the clot and make it more resistant to lysis by plasmin. Individuals deficient in this clotting factor experience poor wound healing.[16]

Updated Model of Coagulation

The aforementioned classical view of the coagulation cascade has been useful in the interpretation of laboratory clotting times and in vitro data; however, it may not be physiologically accurate in describing the process in vivo. This is demonstrated by a number of patterns. First, patients with deficiencies in components of the intrinsic pathway may have increased corresponding activated partial thromboplastin time (aPTT) without increased clinical bleeding tendencies.[17] Next, those with a deficiency of F XII, which is higher in the classical cascade, do have fewer bleeding tendencies than that with a deficiency of F VIII, which contradicts the stepwise, sequential cascade/waterfall model.[18] Conversely, patients who have deficiencies in other factors either in the intrinsic or in the extrinsic pathway have serious bleeding tendencies, even when the unassociated pathway is functional.[19,20]

The new accepted model has three overlapping phases: initiation, amplification, and propogation (Figure 19-4). It has been dubbed a "cell-based model" of coagulation because the activations and reactions of clotting factors occur on cell surfaces, and a number of different cells (e.g., monocytes, fibroblasts) are critical in the mechanism. It is now established that the primary initiating event in clotting is the generation or exposure of TF at the wound site, on TF-bearing cells, and its interaction with F VII.[21,22] This TF–FVII complex activates factor F X, which gives rise to a small amount of thrombin. The amplification phase occurs on the surface of platelets. In addition to activating platelets, the small amount of thrombin also activates F V, F VIII, and F XI, which participate in generating large amounts of thrombin.[23] In the propagation phase, procoagulant complexes assemble on platelet membrane surfaces in the presence of calcium. An extrinsic tenase (X-ase) complex consists of F Va and TF, which activates both F X and F IX. An intrinsic X-ase complex consists of F IXa and F VIIIa, which activates F X. The activated F X (F Xa) generated from either X-ases binds with F Va to form the prothrombase on the surface of the platelet, which then generates a large amount of thrombin through the conversion from prothrombin (F II) to thrombin (F IIa). This ultimately leads to the conversion of fibrinogen to fibrin.[23] In addition, the thrombin activates F XIII (fibrin-stabilizing factor), which cross-links the monomeric fibrin to stabilize the clot.

Termination and Fibrinolysis

The termination of the coagulation process involves two circulating enzyme inhibitors, antithrombin (AT) (formerly AT III) and TF pathway inhibitor, and the protein C pathway that is initiated by clotting. AT is a circulating plasma protease inhibitor, which neutralizes most of the enzymes (i.e., thrombin, F Xa, F IXa, F XIIa) in the coagulation cascade. Protein C is activated by thrombin after it binds to thrombomodulin during the process of clot formation, to form the protein C anticoagulant complex. Activated protein C, in association with protein S on phospholipid surfaces, inactivates F Va and VIII a, effectively inactivating the prothrombinase and intrinsic X-ase, respectively.[24,25]

Fibrinolysis is considered the major means of disposing of fibrin after its hemostatic function has been fulfilled (Figure 19-5). This is critical to the process of wound healing, to restore vessel patency and for tissue remodeling. Tissue plasminogen activator (tPA) is released from the endothelial cells and converts plasminogen to plasmin that degrades fibrinogen and fibrin into fibrin degradation products (FDPs). tPA is a proteolytic enzyme that is nonspecific and also degrades Fs VIII and V. Urokinase is also a plasminogen activator, which is responsible for extravascular fibrinolysis. Kallikrein, which is an intrinsic activator of plasminogen, is generated when prekallikrein is bound to kininogen, thereby becoming a substrate for F XIIa. Activation of the fibrinolytic system can be turned off by inhibition of plasmin activity by α_2-antiplasmin or by inhibition of plasminogen activators by plasminogen activator inhibitor (PAI) 1 and 2.[26,27]

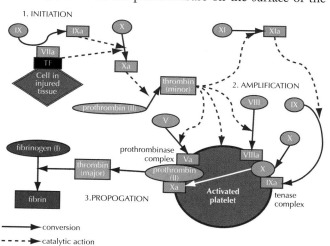

FIGURE 19-4 Cell-based model of coagulation cascade. Tissue factor (TF) complexes with factor VIIa (FVIIa) at the site of tissue injury. Activation of factor X (FX) produces small amounts of thrombin, which in turn activate platelets and factors V (FV) and VIII (FVIII), which assemble on the surface of platelets to form the prothrombinase and tenase complexes, respectively. The tenase complex activates FX, which forms on the prothrombinase complex that converts prothrombin to thrombin, which then converts fibrinogen to fibrin to form the stable clot.

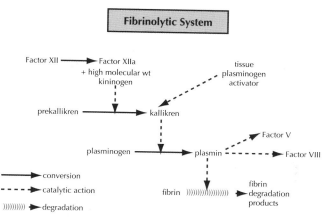

FIGURE 19-5 The fibrinolytic system.

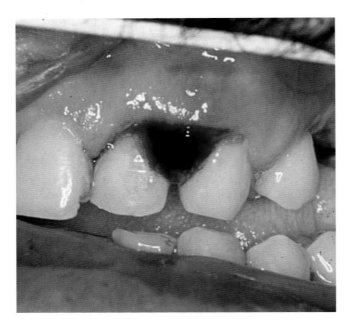

FIGURE 19-6 Spontaneous gingival bleeding between the upper left lateral incisor and canine and labial petechiae in a 38-year-old white male with idiopathic thrombocytopenic purpura.

CLINICAL AND LABORATORY FINDINGS

Clinical Manifestations

Clinical manifestations of bleeding disorders can involve various systems, depending on the extent and type of disease (Table 19-2). Individuals with mild disease may present with no clinical signs, whereas individuals with severe coagulopathies may have definite stigmata. When skin and mucosa are involved, individuals may present with petechiae, ecchymoses, spider angiomas, hematomas, or jaundice. Deep dissecting hematomas and hemarthroses of major joints may affect severe hemophiliacs and result in disability or death. Disorders of platelet quantity may result in hepatosplenomegaly, spontaneous gingival bleeding, and risk of hemorrhagic stroke (Figure 19-6). Specific clinical manifestations will be discussed in detail for the various conditions.

Laboratory Tests

There are a variety of laboratory tests that help identify deficiency of required elements or dysfunction of the phases of coagulation (Tables 19-3 and 19-4). Tests to evaluate primary hemostasis involving platelets are the platelet count and platelet function tests such as bleeding time (BT) and other new platelet function assays. Tests to evaluate the status of coagulation function include prothrombin time (PT)/international normalized ratio (INR), aPTT, thrombin time (TT), FDPs, specific coagulation factor assays (e.g., F VII, F VIII, F IX, fibrinogen), and coagulation factor inhibitor screening tests (blocking antibodies).

PLATELET COUNT

Normal platelet counts are 150,000 to 450,000/mm^3. Spontaneous clinical hemorrhage is usually not observed with platelet counts above 10,000 to 20,000/mm^3. Many hospitals have established a critical value of 10,000/mm^3 platelets, below which platelets are transfused to prevent serious bleeding sequelae, such as hemorrhagic stroke. Surgical or traumatic hemorrhage is more likely with platelet counts below 50,000/mm^3.

TESTS OF PLATELET FUNCTION

Bleeding Time

BT is thought to identify qualitative or functional platelet defects. The modified Ivy test involves a standardized incision on a forearm that has a blood pressure cuff placed at 30 mm Hg. The wound is blotted with filter paper and monitored until absorption of blood on the paper ceases. Normal range is between 1 and 6 minutes and is considered significantly prolonged when greater than 15 minutes. However, because of its technique sensitivity, it lacks specificity. The skin BT test has been shown to be a poor indicator of clinically significant bleeding at other sites, including oral postoperative bleeding after oral surgical procedures, and its use as a predictive screening test has been discouraged.[28,29]

TABLE 19-2 Clinical Features of Bleeding Disorders		
Feature	**Vascular or Platelet Disorders**	**Coagulation Disorders**
Bleeding from superficial cuts and scratches	Persistent, often perfuse	Minimal
Delayed bleeding	Rare	Common
Spontaneous gingival bleeding	Characteristic	Rare
Petechiae	Characteristic	Rare
Ecchymoses	Characteristic, usually small and multiple	Characteristic, usually large and solitary
Epistaxis	Common	Common
Deep dissecting hematomas	Rare	Characteristic
Hemarthrosis	Rare	Characteristic

TABLE 19-3   Laboratory Tests for Assessing Hemostasis

Test	Normal Range
Platelet count	150,000–450,000/mm³
Bleeding time	<7 min (by simplate); 1–6 min (modified Ivy's test)
PFA-100 closure time	CEPI<164 s; CADP<116 s (Ketesztes and Tazbir, 2005)
PT/INR	Control ± 1 s (e.g., PT: 11–13 s/INR 1.0)
Activated partial thromboplastin time	Comparable to control (e.g., 15–35 s)
Thrombin time	Control ± 3 s (e.g., 9–13 s)
Fibrin degradation products	<10 µg/dL
Fibrinogen assay	200–400 mg/dL
von Willebrand antigen	60%–150% vWF activity
Coagulation factor assays (e.g., F VIII assay)	60%–100% F VIII activity
Coagulation factor inhibitor assays (e.g., Bethesda inhibitor assay for F VIII)	0.0 Bethesda inhibitor units

Abbreviations: CADP, time it takes blood to block a membrane coated with collagen and adenosine diphosphate; CEPI, time it takes blood to block a membrane coated with collagen and epinephrine; F, factor; INR, international normalized ratio; PT, prothrombin time; vWF, von Willebrand factor.

TABLE 19-4   Results of Hemostatic Screening Tests for Selected Bleeding Disorders

Bleeding Disorder	Screening Laboratory Tests			BT
	Platelet Count	PT/INR	aPTT	
Thrombocytopenia / Leukemia / Liver disease	↓	N	N	↑
F VIII, IX, XI deficiency / Heparin anticoagulation / Dabigatran anticoagulation	N	N	↑	N
F II, V, X deficiency / Vitamin K deficiency / Intestinal malabsorption	N	↑	↑	N
F VII deficiency / Coumarin anticoagulation / Rivaroxaban anticoagulation / Liver disease	N	↑	N	N
von Willebrand disease	N, ↓	N	N, ↑	↑
DIC / Severe liver disease	↓	↑	↑	↑
F XIII deficiency	N	N	N	N
Vascular wall defect	N	N	N	↑

Abbreviations: ↑, increased; ↓, decreased; aPTT, activated partial thromboplastin time; BT, bleeding time; DIC, disseminated intravascular coagulation; INR, international normalized ratio; N, normal; PT, prothrombin time.

Platelet Function Analyzer

An in vitro system for the detection of platelet dysfunction, Platelet Function Analyzer (PFA-100; Dade-Behring, Deerfield, IL), is available at some laboratories.[30] Closure time (CT), measured by the PFA-100 device, is now reportable by many clinical laboratories as a possible alternative or supplement to the BT test.[31] This was found to be more sensitive to aspirin-induced platelet dysfunction and vWD and was more rapidly and cheaply performed than the BT.[32] However, because it is a global test system and also sensitive to low hematocrit, low platelet counts, and platelet dysfunction (both congenital and acquired), it is neither specific for nor predictive of any particular disorder (inclusive of vWD).[33] Consequently, international consensus opinion is that, although the PFA-100 CT is abnormal in some forms of platelet disorders, the test does not have sufficient sensitivity or specificity to be used as a screening tool for disorders of platelet function and is currently best restricted to research studies and prospective clinical trials.[31] Although one clinical trial has reported the use of the PFA-100 CT as a screening tool for oral surgery patients on antiplatelet therapy,[34] the role of the PFA-100 CT in routine therapeutic monitoring of platelet function remains to be established.

PROTHROMBIN TIME AND INTERNATIONAL NOMALIZED RATIO

The PT and INR tests evaluate the extrinsic and common coagulation pathways, screening for the presence or absence of fibrinogen (F I), prothrombin (F II), and Fs V, VII, and X. The normal range of PT is approximately 11 to 13 seconds. Because of individual laboratory reagent variability and the desire to be able to reliably compare the PT from one laboratory with that from another, the PT test is preferably commonly reported with the INR.[35,36] The INR, introduced by the World Health Organization in 1983, is the ratio of PT that adjusts for the sensitivity of the thromboplastin reagents, such that a normal coagulation profile is reported as an INR of 1.0, and higher values indicating abnormal coagulation.[37] Its most common use is to measure the effects of coumarin anticoagulants and reduction of the vitamin K–dependent Fs II, VII, IX, and X. It is not effective for hemophilia A and B, since it does not measure F VIII or F IX. Although most patients on coumarin anticoagulants are monitored by monthly venous blood draws and laboratory analysis, the CoaguChek system (Roche Diagnostics, Indianapolis, IN) allows Clinical Laboratory Improvements Amendments–waived point-of-care PT/INR testing of fingerstick blood in physicians' and dentists' offices.[38]

ACTIVATED PARTIAL THROMBOPLASTIN TIME

The aPTT is used to evaluate the intrinsic coagulation pathway, screening for deficiencies in F VIII, F IX, F XI, and F XII, in addition to prekallikrein and high-molecular-weight (HMW) kiningen. It is performed by calcifying plasma in the presence of a thromboplastic material (i.e., phospholipid tablet) and a contact activator that is a negatively charged substance (e.g., kaolin) in the absence of TF. It is considered normal if the control aPTT and the test aPTT are within 10 seconds of each other. Control aPTT times are usually 15 to 35 seconds. Normal ranges depend on the manufacturer's limits as each supplier varies slightly. As a screening test, the aPTT is prolonged only when the factor levels in the intrinsic and common pathways are less than approximately 30%. It is altered in hemophilia A and B and with the use of the anticoagulant heparin, which may result in clinical bleeding problems. However, elevated aPTT due to deficiencies in F XII, prekallikrein, and HMW kiningen do not correlate with clinical bleeding.

The precursor to the aPTT, the unactivated partial thromboplastin time (PTT), was originally described by Langdell et al. in 1953 as a simple one-stage assay for measuring F VIII.[39] In addition to the intrinsic pathway, it also checked elements of the common pathway (F V, F X, prothrombin, and fibrinogen).

THROMBIN TIME

The TT is used specifically to test the ability to form the initial fibrin clot from fibrinogen, by adding thrombin to plasma. It is considered normal in the range of 9 to 13 seconds, with values in excess of 16 to 18 seconds considered to be prolonged. It is used to measure the activity of heparin, FDPs, or other paraproteins that inhibit conversion of fibrinogen to fibrin. Fibrinogen can also be specifically assayed and should be present at a level of 200 to 400 mg/dL.

FIBRIN DEGRADATION PRODUCTS

The FDPs are measured using a specific latex agglutination system to evaluate the presence of the D-dimer of fibrinogen and/or fibrin above normal levels. Such presence indicates that intravascular lysis has taken place or is occurring. This state can result from primary fibrinolytic disorders or disseminated intravascular coagulation (DIC).

FACTOR ASSAYS

To further identify the factor deficiencies and their level of severity, specific activity levels of factors can be measured. Normal factor activity is usually in the 60% to 150% range. Inhibitor screening tests are essential when sufficient factor concentrate to correct the factor deficiency under normal conditions fails to control bleeding. To identify the specific type of vWD (types I–III and platelet type), additional studies, such as the ristocetin cofactor, ristocetin-induced platelet aggregation studies, and monomer studies are helpful.

TESTS OF CAPILLARY FRAGILITY

The tourniquet test for capillary fragility is useful for identifying disorders of vascular wall integrity or platelet disorders. Stasis is produced by inflating a sphygmomanometer cuff around the arm in the usual manner to a pressure halfway between systolic and diastolic levels. This moderate degree of stasis is maintained for 5 minutes. At 2 minutes following cuff deflation and removal, a 2.5-cm diameter (size of a quarter) of skin on the volar surface of the arm at 4 cm distal to the antecubital fossa is observed for petechial hemorrhages. This distal shower of petechiae is called the Rumpel–Leede phenomenon. Normally, petechiae in men do not exceed 5 in number, and in women and children, they do not exceed 10 in number in the skin region examined. The capillary fragility test is the only test to demonstrate abnormal results in vessel wall disorders.

VESSEL WALL DISORDERS

Vessel wall disorders can be due to structural malformation of vessels, and inherited or acquired disorders of connective tissue. They can result in hemorrhagic features, although bleeding is usually mild and confined to the skin, mucosa, and gingiva. Vascular purpura can result from damage to capillary endothelium, from abnormalities in the vascular subendothelial matrix or extravascular connective tissue bed, or from abnormal vessel formation.

Scurvy

Scurvy, resulting from dietary deficiency of water-soluble vitamin C, is found primarily in regions of urban poverty, among infants on nonsupplemented processed milk formulas, elderly who cook for themselves, or adults with alcohol or drug dependencies or the mentally handicapped.[40–42] Scurvy results when dietary vitamin C falls below 10 mg/d. Vitamin C is necessary for the synthesis of hydroxyproline, an essential constituent of collagen. Many of the hemorrhagic features of scurvy result from defects in collagen synthesis. One of the first clinical signs is petechial hemorrhages at the hair follicles and purpura on the back of the lower extremities that coalesce to form ecchymoses. Hemorrhage can occur in the muscles, joints, nail beds, and gingival tissues. Gingival involvement may include swelling, friability, bleeding, secondary infection, and loosening of teeth.[41] Implementation of a diet rich in vitamin C and administration of 1 g/d of vitamin C supplements provide rapid resolution.

Cushing's Syndrome

Cushing's syndrome, resulting from excessive exogenous or endogenous corticosteroid intake or production, leads to general protein wasting and atrophy of supporting connective tissue around blood vessels. Patients may show skin bleeding or easy bruising. Aging causes similar perivascular connective tissue atrophy and lack of skin mobility. Tears in small blood vessels can result in irregularly shaped purpuric areas on arms and hands, called purpura senilis. Other metabolic or inflammatory disorders resulting in purpura include Schönlein–Henoch or anaphylactoid purpura, hyperglobulinemic purpura, Waldenström's macroglobulinemia, multiple myeloma, amyloidosis, and cryoglobulinemia.

Ehlers–Danlos Syndrome

Ehlers–Danlos syndrome is an autosomal dominant inherited disorder of connective tissue matrix, generally resulting in fragile skin blood vessels and easy bruising. It is characterized by hyperelasticity of the skin and hypermobile joints. Eleven subtypes have been identified with unique biochemical defects and varying clinical features.[43] Type I is the classic form, with soft, velvety, hyperextensible skin; easy bruising and scarring; hypermobile joints; varicose veins; and prematurity. Type VIII, which was recently mapped to chromosome 12q13,[44] has skin findings similar to those in type I, with easy bruising following minor trauma mainly due to the resulting fragility of the oral mucosa and blood vessels and is characterized by early-onset periodontal disease with severe loss of alveolar bone and permanent dentition.[45,46] Children with type VII syndrome may present

with microdontia and collagen-related dentinal structural defects in primary teeth, in addition to bleeding after tooth brushing.[47] Other oral findings include fragility of the oral mucosa, gingiva, and teeth, as well as hypermobility of the temporomandibular joint (TMJ) and stunted teeth and pulp stones on dental radiographs.[48–50] Oral health may be severely compromised as a result of specific alterations of collagen in orofacial structures. A number of tissue responses (mucosa, periodontium, pulp) and precautions (e.g., prevention of TMJ dislocation) should be considered when planning dental treatment.[51]

Rendu–Osler–Weber Syndrome

Rendu–Osler–Weber syndrome, also called hereditary hemorrhagic telangiectasia (HHT), is a group of autosomal dominant disorders with abnormal telangiectatic capillaries, frequent episodes of nasal and gastrointestinal bleeding, and associated brain and pulmonary lesions.[52–54] Perioral and intraoral angiomatous nodules or telangiectases are common with progressive disease, involving areas of the lips, tongue, and palate that may bleed upon manipulation during dental procedures.[55] Diagnosis is facilitated by the history of nosebleeds and the observation of multiple nonpulsating vascular lesions representing small arteriovenous malformations.[54] These lesions blanch in response to applied pressure, unlike petechiae or ecchymoses. Mucocutaneous lesions may bleed profusely with minor trauma or on occasion, spontaneously.[56] Persistently bleeding lesions may be treated with cryotherapy, laser ablation, electrocoagulation, or resection.[57] Blood replacement and iron therapy may be necessary following dental extractions in involved areas.[56] It has also been suggested that antibiotic prophylaxis should be considered before dental care for patients with HHT and concomitant pulmonary arteriovenous malformation.[52]

PLATELET DISORDERS

Platelet disorders may be divided into two categories by etiology—congenital and acquired—and into two additional categories by type—thrombocytopenias and thrombocytopathies (Table 19-5). Thrombocytopenias occur when platelet quantity is reduced and are caused by one of three mechanisms: decreased production in the bone marrow, increased sequestration in the spleen, or accelerated destruction. Thrombocytopathies, or qualitative platelet disorders, may result from defects in any of the critical platelet reactions. Dysfunctional platelet mechanisms may occur in isolated disorders or in conjunction with dysfunctional coagulation mechanisms.

Congenital Platelet Defects

Congenital abnormalities of platelet function or production are rare, and the causes are quite diverse, ranging from defects in receptors critical to platelet adhesion and aggregation, to defects in signaling molecules or in transcription factors important for production of functional platelets.[58]

TABLE 19-5 Classification of Platelet Disorders
Congenital
Thrombocytopenic—quantitative platelet deficiency
May–Hegglin anomaly
Wiskott–Aldrich syndrome
Neonatal alloimmune thrombocytopenia
Nonthrombocytopenic—qualitative or functional platelet defect
Glanzmann's thrombasthenia
Platelet-type von Willebrand disease
Bernard–Soulier syndrome
Acquired
Thrombocytopenic—quantitative platelet deficiency
Autoimmune or idiopathic thrombocytopenia purpura
Thrombotic thrombocytopenic purpura
Cytotoxic chemotherapy
Drug induced (e.g., quinine, quinidine, gold salts, trimethoprim-sulfamethoxazole, rifampin)
Leukemia
Aplastic anemia
Myelodysplasia
Systemic lupus erythematosus
Associated with infection: HIV, mononucleosis, malaria
Disseminated intravascular coagulation
Nonthrombocytopenic—qualitative or functional platelet defect
Drug induced (e.g., by aspirin, NSAIDs, penicillin, cephalosporins)
Uremia
Alcohol dependency
Liver disease
Myeloma, myeloproliferative disorders, macroglobulinemia
Acquired platelet-type von Willebrand disease

Abbreviations: HIV, human immunodeficiency virus; NSAIDs, nonsteroidal anti-inflammatory drugs.

Bernard–Soulier syndrome results from identified absence in platelet membrane glycoprotein Ib from the platelet membranes, rendering the platelets unable to interact with vWF.[59] Platelet transfusions are the main treatment modality for Bernard–Soulier syndrome.

Glanzmann's thrombasthenia is a qualitative disorder characterized by a deficiency in the platelet membrane glycoproteins IIb and IIIa.[60–62] As a result, platelets cannot bind to fibrinogen and cannot aggregate with other platelets. Clinical signs include bruising, epistaxis, gingival hemorrhage, and menorrhagia. Treatment of oral surgical bleeding involves platelet transfusion and use of antifibrinolytics and local hemostatic agents. Treatment of bleeding episodes in the patient with Glanzmann's thrombasthenia is usually not warranted unless hemorrhage is life threatening.

Wiskott–Aldrich syndrome is a rare X-linked recessive disease characterized by cutaneous eczema (usually beginning on the face), thrombocytopenic purpura, and an increased susceptibility to infection due to an immunologic defect.[63] It is a quantitative and qualitative platelet disorder. Oral manifestations include gingival bleeding and palatal petechiae. Thrombocytopenia of Wiskott–Aldrich syndrome may be managed with platelet transfusions, splenectomy, or bone marrow transplantation.[63]

May–Hegglin anomaly is a rare hereditary condition characterized by the triad of thrombocytopenia, giant platelets, and inclusion bodies in leukocytes. Clinical features and the pathogenesis of bleeding in this disease are poorly defined.[64]

Acquired Platelet Defects

Two of the most commonly encountered platelet disorders, idiopathic or immune thrombocytopenic purpura (ITP) and thrombotic thrombocytopenic purpura (TTP), have clinical symptoms, including petechiae and purpura over the chest, neck, and limbs—usually more severe on the lower extremities. Mucosal bleeding may occur in the oral cavity and gastrointestinal and genitourinary tracts.

The age-adjusted prevalence of ITP in Maryland was 9.5 per 100,000 persons, with an overall female to male ratio of 1.9.[65] ITP may be acute and self-limiting (2–6 weeks) in children. In adults, ITP is typically more indolent in its onset, and the course is persistent, often lasting many years, and may be characterized by recurrent exacerbations of disease. In severe cases of ITP, oral hematomas and hemorrhagic bullae may be the presenting clinical sign.[66,67] Most patients with chronic ITP are young women. Intracerebral hemorrhage, although rare, is the most common cause of death. ITP is assumed to be caused by accelerated antibody-mediated platelet consumption. The natural history and long-term prognosis of adults with chronic ITP remain incompletely defined.[68] ITP may be a component of other systemic diseases. Autoimmune thrombocytopenia associated with systemic lupus erythematosus is often of little consequence but may be occasionally severe and serious, requiring aggressive treatment.[69] Immune-mediated thrombocytopenia may occur in conjunction with HIV disease in approximately 15% of adults, being more common with advanced clinical disease and immune suppression, although less than 0.5% of patients have severe thrombocytopenia with platelet counts below 50,000/mm^3.[70]

TTP is an acute catastrophic disease that, until recently, was uniformly fatal. The causative factors include metastatic malignancy, pregnancy, mitomycin C, and high-dose chemotherapy. If untreated, it still carries a high mortality rate. In addition to thrombocytopenia, clinical presentation of TTP includes microangiopathic hemolytic anemia, fluctuating neurologic abnormalities, renal dysfunction, and occasional fever. Microvascular infarcts occurring in gingival and other mucosal tissues are present in about 60% of the cases. These appear as platelet-rich thrombi. Serial studies of plasma samples from patients during episodes of TTP have often shown vWF multimer abnormalities.[71]

Although there are numerous therapeutic options, neither consensus among experts nor clear algorithms to treat ITP and TTP exist. Corticosteroids are indicated for ITP, with titration governed by the severity of hemorrhagic symptoms.[66,67] Splenectomy may be necessary in chronic ITP to prevent antiplatelet antibody production and sequestration and removal of antibody-labeled platelets.[67] Plasma exchange therapy combined with ASA/

dipyridamole or corticosteroids has recently lowered the mortality rate for patients with TTP over that previously obtained by treatment with fresh frozen plasma (FFP) infusions.[72,73] In addition, there is a role of newer therapies with diverse mechanisms of action, such as rituximab, anti-D, and thrombopoietin-like agents.[74]

Thrombocytopenia may also be a component of other hematologic disease, such as myelodysplastic disorders,[75] aplastic anemia,[76] and leukemia.[77] Thrombocytopenia and thrombocytopathy in liver disease are complicated by coagulation defects, as discussed below. Alcohol can, itself, induce thrombocytopenia in addition to qualitative platelet defects.[78] Renal disease can result in qualitative platelet defects resulting from uremia.[79]

Drug-Induced Platelet Defects

Medications can also reduce absolute numbers of platelets or interfere with their function, resulting in postsurgical hemorrhage.[80–82] Bone marrow suppression from cytotoxic cancer chemotherapy can result in severe thrombocytopenia, requiring platelet transfusions for prevention of spontaneous hemorrhage.

Antiplatelet agents are routinely used therapeutically for thromboembolic protection in patients with ischemic heart disease, prosthetic heart valves, coronary artery stents, and those at risk of ischemic cerebrovascular accidents. Antiplatelet therapy reduces the risk of death from cardiovascular causes by about one-sixth and the risk of nonfatal myocardial infarction and stroke by about one-third for patients with unstable angina or a history of myocardial infarction, transient ischemia, or stroke.[83] A science advisory panel consisting of the American Heart Association and American Dental Association recommends that 12 months of dual antiplatelet therapy is required after the placement of drug-eluting coronary artery stents.[84]

ASA, also known as aspirin, is an inexpensive and effective drug that is widely used. ASA induces a functional defect in platelets detectable as prolongation of BT and altered PFA-100 CTs. It inactivates an enzyme called prostaglandin synthetase, resulting in inactivation of cyclooxygenase (COX) catalytic activity and decreasing biosynthesis of prostaglandin and thromboxanes (such as thromboxane A2) that are needed to regulate interactions between platelets and the endothelium.[83] A single 100 mg dose of ASA provides rapid complete and irreversible inhibition of platelet COX activity and thromboxane production. This type of drug-related platelet disorder is compensated for within 7 to 10 days. Most NSAIDs have a similar but less significant antiplatelet effect and therefore are of mild concern to patients who have other disorders of hemostasis. The COX-2 inhibitors, such as celecoxib (Celebrex, Pfizer, New York, NY), generally do not inhibit platelet aggregation at indicated doses.

Other therapeutic antiplatelet medications work by different mechanisms affecting platelet adhesion, activation, and aggregation, which include the inhibition of ADP receptor (e.g., clopidogrel, ticlopidine, and prasugrel); adenosine reuptake (dipyridamole); phosphodiesterase (e.g., cilostazol); and GP IIb/IIIa (e.g., abciximab, eptifibatide, tirofiban). Clopidogrel bisulfate (Plavix, Bristol-Meyers Squibb-Sanofi Pharmaceuticals Partnership, New York, NY) alone carries less risk of prolonged bleeding than ASA, which is commonly used in dual antiplatelet therapy.[85]

Treatment of Platelet Disorders

Treatment modalities for platelet disorders are determined by the type of defect. The thrombocytopenias are primarily managed acutely with transfusions of platelets to maintain the minimum level of 10,000 to 20,000/mm³ necessary to prevent spontaneous hemorrhage (Table 19-6). This has also been indicated for thrombocytopenias secondary to liver disease, Glanzmann's thrombasthenia, and is the main therapy for Bernard–Soulier disease.[86] However, repeated platelet transfusions may carry the risk of development of antiplatelet isoantibodies thereby losing its effectiveness. As a consequence, transfusions are usually reserved for more acute bleeding episodes or for surgical procedures. Human leukocyte antigen (HLA)-matched platelets may be required after antibody development, to reduce the number of platelet transfusions needed for hemostasis. In the absence of satisfactorily compatible platelets, blood volume and constituents can be maintained with low-antigenicity blood products. Plasmapheresis to remove circulating isoantibodies is held in reserve for cases of severe thrombasthenia and life-threatening bleeding.

COAGULATION DISORDERS— CONGENITAL

Inherited disorders of coagulation can result from deficiency of a number of factors (Table 19-1) that are essential in the coagulation cascade or deficiency of vWF. Clinical bleeding can vary from mild to severe, depending on the specific clotting factor affected and the level of factor deficiency.

von Willebrand Disease

vWD is the most common inherited bleeding disorder. Described originally by Erik von Willebrand in 1926,[87] it can be due to quantitative or qualitative defects in vWF, a multimeric HMW glycoprotein.[88] vWF has two functions that qualify it as both a platelet disorder and a disorder affecting coagulation: (1) platelet adhesion to the injured vessel wall under conditions of high shear forces and (2) carrier of F VIIIc in plasma.[89] Normal plasma vWF level is 10 mg/L, with a half-life of 6 to 15 hours.

This disorder is usually transmitted as an autosomal dominant trait with varying penetrance. The common genetic profile suggests a heterozygous state, with both males and females affected. The uncovering of all of the biochemical, physiologic, and clinical manifestations of vWD has held experts at bay for many years. Because of the complexity of

TABLE 19-6   Principal Products for Systemic Management of Patients With Bleeding Disorders

Product	Description	Source	Common Indications
Platelets	"One pack" = 50 mL; raises count by 6000	Blood bank	<10,000 in nonbleeding individuals; <50,000 presurgical;<50,000 in actively bleeding individuals; nondestructive thrombocytopenia
Fresh frozen plasma	Unit = 150–250 mL 1 h to thaw Contains Fs II, VII, IX, X, XI, XII, XIII and heat-labile Fs V and VII	Blood bank	Undiagnosed bleeding disorder with active bleeding; severe liver disease; when transfusing >10 units blood Immune globulin deficiency
Cryoprecipitate	Unit = 10–15 mL Contains Fs VIII and XIII, vWF, and fibrinogen	Blood bank	Hemophilia A, von Willebrand disease, when factor concentrates/DDAVP are unavailable Fibrinogen deficiency
F VIII concentrate (purified antihemophilic factor)[a]	Unit raises F VIII level by 2% Heat-treated contains vWF	Pharmacy	Hemophilia A, with active bleeding or presurgical; some cases of von Willebrand disease
	Recombinant and monoclonal technologies are pure F VIII		
F IX concentrate (PCC)[a]	Unit raises F IX level by 1%–1.5% Contains Fs II, VII, IX, and X Monoclonal F IX is only F IX	Pharmacy	Hemophilia B, with active bleeding or presurgical PCC used for hemophilia A with inhibitor
DDAVP	Synthetic analogue of antidiuretic hormone 0.3 µg/kg IV or SQ Intranasal application	Pharmacy	Active bleeding or presurgical for some patients with von Willebrand disease, uremic bleeding, or liver disease
ε-Aminocaproic acid	Antifibrinolytic 25% oral solution (250 mg/mL) Systemic: 75 mg/kg q6h	Pharmacy	Adjunct to support clot formation for any bleeding disorder
Tranexamic acid	Antifibrinolytic 4.8% mouthrinse—not available in the United States Systemic: 25 mg/kg q8h	Pharmacy	Adjunct to support clot formation for any bleeding disorder

Abbreviations: DDAVP, desmopressin acetate; F, factor; IV, intravenously; PCC, prothrombin complex concentrate; SQ, subcutaneously; vWF, von Willebrand factor.
[a]See Table 19-7 for additional factor concentrate products.

the disease, diagnosis of vWD is one of the most challenging of any coagulation disorder.

vWD is classified into three primary categories.[88] Type 1 (85% of all vWD) includes partial quantitative deficiency, type 2 (10%–15% of all vWD) includes qualitative defects, and type 3 (rare) includes virtually complete deficiency of vWF. vWD type 2 is divided into four secondary categories. Type 2A includes variants with decreased platelet adhesion caused by selective deficiency of HMW vWF multimers. Type 2B includes variants with increased affinity for platelet glycoprotein Ib. Type 2M includes variants with markedly defective platelet adhesion despite a relatively normal size distribution of vWF multimers. Type 2N includes variants with markedly decreased affinity for F VIII. These six categories of vWD correlate with important clinical features and therapeutic requirements.[88]

A rare fourth type is called pseudo- or platelet-type vWD, and it is a primary platelet disorder that mimics vWD. The increased platelet affinity for large multimers of vWF results primarily in mucocutaneous bleeding. Due to familial genetic variants, wide variations occur in the patient's laboratory profile over time; therefore, diagnosis may be difficult.[90] Unlike the other types of vWD, the platelet type is rare and presents with less severe clinical bleeding.

As early as 1968, acquired vWD was noted to occur as a rare complication of autoimmune or neoplastic disease, associated mostly with lymphoid or plasma cell proliferative disorders and having clinical manifestations that are similar to congenital vWD.[91] The clinical features of vWD are usually mild and include mucosal bleeding, soft tissue hemorrhage, menorrhagia in women, and rare hemarthrosis.[92]

Hemophilia A

Hemophilia A involves a deficiency of F VIII, the antihemophilic factor, and accounts for 79% of all hemophiliacs. Forty-three percent of hemophiliacs have a severe factor deficiency (<1% F VIII), whereas 26% have a moderate deficiency (1%–5% F VIII) and 31% present with a mild deficiency (6%–30% F VIII).[5] It is inherited as an X-linked recessive trait that affects males (hemizygous), and the trait is carried in the female (heterozygous) without clinical evidence of the disease, although a few do manifest mild bleeding symptoms. Males with hemophilia transmit the affected gene to all their female offspring, yet their sons are normal, and the effects skip a generation unless their wives were carriers and their daughters received the maternal affected X chromosome as well. Only 60% to 70% of families with newly diagnosed hemophiliacs report a family history of the disease, suggesting a high mutation rate. There is no racial predilection.

Clinical symptoms and F VIII levels vary from pedigree to pedigree. Severe clinical bleeding is seen when the F VIII level is less than 1% of normal. In contrast to the more superficial signs of bleeding observed in individuals with platelet-associated disorders, individuals with hemophilia exhibit bleeds into more deep-seated spaces. The more common signs include hematomas, hemarthroses, hematuria, gastrointestinal bleeding, and bleeding from lacerations or head trauma or spontaneous intracranial bleeding that require factor replacement therapy.[93] Retroperitoneal and central nervous system bleeds, occurring spontaneously or induced by minor trauma, can be life threatening. Severe hemorrhage leads to joint synovitis and hemophilic arthropathies, intramuscular bleeds, and pseudotumors (encapsulated hemorrhagic cyst). Since 1965, replacement therapy, prophylaxis, and home treatment have been used with intensification of clotting factor consumption that has led to decreases in the risk of hemophilic arthropathy.[94] Moderate clinical bleeding is found when F VIII levels are 1% to 5% of normal. Only mild symptoms, such as prolonged bleeding following tooth extraction, surgical procedures, or severe trauma, occur if levels are between 6% and 50% of normal.

Hemophilia B

F IX (Christmas factor) deficiency is found in hemophilia B. The genetic background, factor levels, and clinical symptoms are similar to those in hemophilia A. The distinction was made only in the late 1940s between these two X-linked diseases. Concentrates used to treat F VIII and F IX deficiencies are specific for each state; therefore, a correct diagnosis must be made to ensure effective replacement therapy. Circulating blocking antibodies or inhibitors to Fs VIII and IX may be seen in patients with these disorders. These inhibitors are specific for F VIII or F IX and render the patient refractory to the normal mode of treatment with concentrates. Catastrophic bleeding can occur, and patients can survive only with supportive transfusions.

F XI Deficiency

Plasma thromboplastin antecedent (F XI) deficiency is clinically a mild disorder seen in pedigrees of Jewish descent; it is transmitted as an autosomal dominant trait. Bleeding symptoms do occur but are usually mild. In the event of major surgery or trauma, hemorrhage can be controlled with infusions of FFP.

F XII Deficiency

Hageman factor (F XII) deficiency is another rare disease that presents in the laboratory with prolonged PT and PTT. Clinical symptoms are nonexistent; therefore, treatment is contraindicated.

F X Deficiency

Stuart factor (F X) deficiency, also a rare bleeding diathesis, is inherited as an autosomal recessive trait. Clinical bleeding symptoms in the patient with levels less than 1% are similar to those seen in hemophilias A and B.

F V Deficiency

Proaccelerin (F V) deficiency, like F XI and F X deficiencies, is a rare autosomal recessive trait that presents with moderate to severe clinical symptoms. When compared with hemophilias A and B, this hemorrhagic diathesis is moderate, only occasionally resulting in soft tissue hemorrhage and only rarely presenting with hemarthrosis; it does not involve the devastating degenerative joint disease seen in severe hemophilias A and B.

Fs XIII and I Deficiencies

Fibrin-stabilizing (F XIII) deficiency and fibrinogen (F I) deficiency are very rare, and these diagnoses can be made only with extensive laboratory tests usually available only in tertiary care medical centers. Both are autosomal recessive traits. Most dysfibrinogenemias result in no symptoms, others lead to moderate bleeding, and a few induce a hypercoagulable state. F XIII deficiency appears to have different forms of penetrance and in some families appears only in the males.

Systemic Management of Coagulation Disorders

Tables 19-6 and 19-7 outline the various products for the systemic management of patients with bleeding disorders. Therapy for vWD depends on the type of vWD and the severity of bleeding. Type I is treated preferentially with desmopressin acetate (1-deamino-8-D-arginine vasopressin [DDAVP]), which provides transient increases in coagulation. Intermediate-purity F VIII concentrates, FFP, and cryoprecipitate are held in reserve for those nonresponsive to DDAVP.[95] Types II and III require intermediate-purity F VIII concentrates (i.e., Humate-P or Koate-HS) or rarely cryoprecipitate or FFP. Bleeding episodes in patients with platelet-type vWD are usually

TABLE 19-7 Coagulation Factor Concentrate Products

Product Category	Proprietary Name[a]	Manufacturer/Distributor	US Corporate Location
	High-purity F VIII concentrates		
Monoclonal	Hemofil-M Monoclate-P Monarc-M	Baxter Healthcare Corp. ZLB-Behring LLC Baxter Healthcare Corp.	Westlake Village, CA Kankakee, IL Westlake Village, CA
Recombinant	Kogenate-FS Recombinate Advate Helixate-FS Bioclate ReFacto	Bayer Healthcare LLC Baxter Healthcare Corp. Baxter Healthcare Corp. CSL Behring LLC CSL Behring LLC Wyeth Biopharma	Tarrytown, NY Westlake Village, CA Westlake Village, CA Kankakee, IL Kankakee, IL Andover, MA
	Intermediate-purity F VIII concentrates		
Pasturized	Humate-P	CSL Behring LLC	Kankakee, IL
Solvent/detergent	Koate-HP Alphanate	Kedrion Biopharma Grifols Biologicals, Inc.	Ft. Lee, NJ Los Angeles, CA
	High-purity F IX concentrates		
Monoclonal	AlphaNine-SD Mononine	Grifols Biologicals, Inc. CSL Behring LLC/BDI Pharma	Los Angeles, CA Columbia, SC
Recombinant	BeneFix	Wyeth Pharmaceuticals/Pfizer	New York, NY
	Prothrombin complex concentrates (PCC) and F IX activated PCCs		
	Profilnine-SD Proplex-T Bebulin-VH FEIBA-NF	Grifols Biologicals, Inc. Baxter Healthcare Corp. Baxter Healthcare Corp. Baxter Healthcare Corp.	Los Angeles, CA Westlake Village, CA Westlake Village, CA Westlake Village, CA
	F VIIa concentrate		
Recombinant	NovoSeven-RT	Novo-Nordisk	Plainsboro, NJ

Abbreviation: F, factor.
[a]Product availability changes periodically.

controlled with platelet concentrate infusions. Other therapy is used for site-specific bleeding, such as estrogens or oral contraceptive agents for menorrhagia and local hemostatic agents and antifibrinolytics for dental procedures. Occasionally, circulating plasma inhibitors of vWF are observed in multiply transfused patients with severe disease. Cryoprecipitate infusion can cause transient neutralization of this inhibitor.[96]

Therapy for hemophilias A and B is dependent on the severity of disease, type and site of hemorrhage, and presence or absence of inhibitors. Commercially prepared Fs VIII and IX complex concentrates, DDAVP, and, to a lesser extent, cryoprecipitate and FFP are replacement options.

Cryoprecipitate and FFP

Cryoprecipitate and FFP are rarely the treatment of choice for hemophilias A and B because of their disadvantages of potential viral transmission and the large volumes needed to raise factor levels adequately for hemostasis. Cryoprecipitate is the cold insoluble precipitate remaining after FFP is thawed at 4°C. A typical bag (1 unit) of cryoprecipitate contains about 80 units of F VIII and vWF and 150 to 250 mg fibrinogen in a 10 to 15 mL volume. Cryoprecipitate has been used to treat selected patients with vWD and hemophilia A. FFP contains all coagulation factors in nearly normal concentrations and may aid hemorrhage control in a patient with mild hemophilia B. In the average-size patient, one unit of FFP raises F IX levels by 3%. Postoperative bleeding in mild to moderate F X deficiency can be managed with FFP, and prothrombin complex concentrates (PCCs) may be held in reserve for severely deficient patients.[97]

DDAVP

DDAVP is thought to stimulate endogenous release of F VIII and vWF from blood vessel endothelial cell storage sites. This synthetic vasopressin analogue is now considered the treatment of choice for bleeding events in patients with responsive bleeding diatheses owing to its absence of viral risk and lower cost. It provides adequate transient increases in coagulation factors in some patients with mild to moderate hemophilia A and type I vWD, avoiding the need for plasma concentrates.[98] However, DDAVP is ineffective in individuals with severe hemophilia A.

DDAVP can be given at a dose of 0.3 μg/kg body weight by an intravenous or subcutaneous route prior to dental extractions or surgery or to treat spontaneous or traumatic bleeding episodes.[99] It results in a mean increase of a two- to fivefold (range 1.5–20 times) in F VIII coagulant activity, vWF antigen, and ristocetin cofactor activity, with a plasma half-life of 5 to 8 hours for F VIII and 8 to 10 hours for vWF.[98] Intranasal spray application of DDAVP (Stimate, Aventis Behring, King of Prussia, PA) contains 1.5 mL of desmopressin per milliliter, with each 0.1 mL pump spray delivering a dose of 150 μg. Children require one nostril spray, and adults require two nostril sprays to achieve a favorable response; correction of bleeding occurs in around 90% of patients with mild to moderate hemophilia A and type I vWD.[100] Time to peak levels is 30 to 60 minutes after intravenous injection and 90 to 120 minutes following subcutaneous or intranasal application.[98] DDAVP is hemostatically effective provided that adequate plasma concentrations are attained.[101] A DDAVP trial or test dose response may be indicated prior to extensive surgery to evaluate the level of drug effect on assayed F VIII activity in the individual patient. Prolonged use of DDAVP results in exhaustion of F VIII storage sites and diminished hemostatic effect, therefore antifibrinolytic agents are useful adjuncts to DDAVP therapy.

Factor Replacement Therapy

Since partially purified Fs VIII and IX complex concentrates prepared from pooled plasma were first used in the late 1960s and 1970s, multiple methods of manufacturing products with increased purity and reduced risk of viral transmission have been developed.[102,103] Current intermediate-purity products are prepared by heat or solvent/detergent treatment of the final product. In 1987, dry-heated concentrates constituted approximately 90% of the total F VIII concentrate consumption in the United States.[102] High-purity F VIII products, manufactured using recombinant or monoclonal antibody purification techniques, are preferred today for their improved viral safety.[104] However, their cost of up to 10 times more than dry-heated concentrates can be financially restrictive for uninsured patients.[103]

F VIII concentrates are dosed by units, with one unit of F VIII being equal to the amount present in 1 mL of pooled fresh normal plasma. The plasma level of F VIII is expressed as a percentage of normal. Since one unit of F VIII concentrate per kilogram of body weight raises the F VIII level by 2%, a 70-kg patient would require infusion of 3500 units to raise his factor level from <1% to 100%. A dose of 40 U/kg F VIII concentrate typically is used to raise the F VIII level to 80% to 100% for management of significant surgical or traumatic bleeding in a patient with severe hemophilia A. Additional outpatient doses may be needed at 12-hour intervals, or continuous inpatient infusion may be established.

Highly purified recombinant and monoclonal F IX concentrates were developed in the late 1980s and early 1990s and are the treatment of choice for hemophilia B patients undergoing surgery.[105–107] F IX complex concentrates also

referred to as PCCs, which contain Fs II, VII, IX, and X, are also widely used at present for patients with hemophilia B. One unit of PCC or higher purity F IX concentrates given by bolus per kilogram of body weight raises the F IX level by 1% to 1.5%. Thus, a dose of 60 U/kg of F IX concentrate typically is needed to raise the F IX level to 80% to 100% for management of severe bleeding episodes in a patient with a severe hemophilia B. Repeat outpatient doses may be needed at 24-hour intervals. Properly supervised home therapy, in which patients self-treat with factor concentrates at the earliest evidence of bleeding, is a cost-effective method offered to educable and motivated patients by some medical centers.[108]

Complications of factor replacement therapy include allergic reactions, viral disease transmission (hepatitis B and C, cytomegalovirus, and HIV), thromboembolic disease, DIC, and development of antibodies to factor concentrates. Hepatitis C has been a major cause of morbidity and mortality in the hemophiliac population, resulting in chronic active hepatitis and cirrhosis in a number of patients.[93] Hepatitis C and HIV infection have been the most common transfusion-related infections in hemophiliacs. By the end of 1986, some centers reported that 80% to 90% of hemophiliacs treated with F VIII concentrates, and around 50% of those who had received F IX concentrates were HIV seropositive.[109] Since 1987, with viral screening of donated plasma, there have been no transfusion-related HIV seroconversions in the United States.

Use of F IX complex concentrate can result in thrombotic complications, such as deep venous thromboses, myocardial infarctions, pulmonary emboli, and DIC. DIC is believed to occur as a consequence of high levels of activated clotting factors, such as Fs VIIa, IXa, and Xa, that cannot adequately be cleared by the liver. Concurrent use of systemic antifibrinolytics with these products may increase the risks.

Development of F VIII or F IX inhibitors is a serious complication. These pathologic circulating antibodies of the IgG class, which specifically neutralize F VIII or F IX procoagulant activity, arise as alloantibodies in some patients with hemophilia.[110] A systematic review found that the overall prevalence of inhibitors in unselected hemophiliac populations to be 5% to 7%.[111] The cumulative risk of inhibitor development varied (0%–39%), with incidence and prevalence being substantially higher in patients with severe hemophilia.[111] Inhibitors develop in at least 10% to 15% of patients with severe hemophilia A and less commonly in patients with hemophilia B.[112,113] Development is related to exposure to factor products and genetic predisposition.[110,112] Inhibitor level is quantified by the Bethesda inhibitor assay and is reported as Bethesda units (BU).

The inhibitor titer and responsiveness to further factor infusion (responder type) dictate which factor replacement therapy should be used. Patients with inhibitors are classified according to titer level—low (<10 BU/mL) or high (>10 BU/mL)—and also by responder type.[113] Low responders typically maintain low titers with repeated factor concentrate exposure, whereas high responders show a brisk elevation in titer due to the amnestic response and are the most challenging to manage.[113,114] Patients with low inhibitor titers are usually low responders and those with high titers are often high responders. Seventy-five percent of hemophilia A patients with inhibitors are high responders, whereas only 25% are low responders.[113]

For hemorrhages, hemophilia A patients with low-level, low-responding inhibitors are treated with F VIII concentrates in doses sufficient to increase plasma F VIII levels to the therapeutic range. Critical hemorrhages in patients with high-responding inhibitors may be treated with large quantities of porcine F VIII; however, routine hemorrhages are often managed initially with PCCs, which provoke anamnesis in a few patients.[110] PCCs can bypass the F VIII inhibitor and are effective about 50% of the time.[115] Activated PCCs show slightly increased effectiveness (65%–75%). Highly purified porcine F VIII product use can be advantageous in patients with less than 50 BU since human F VIII inhibitors cross-react less frequently with porcine products.[109] However, because of the risk of hemostatic failure, surgery should be performed under coverage of F VIII.[116] Treatment of the patient with low-level (<10 BU) F IX inhibitors requires higher doses of F IX complex concentrates to achieve hemostasis. Developed in the early 1990s, recombinant F VIIa is a novel product that provides an alternative treatment option for patients with hemophilia A or B with inhibitors by enhancing the extrinsic pathway.[117] It has been proven to effectively control bleeding in patients with high-titer inhibitors[118,119] and for dental extractions.[120,121]

Several methods have demonstrated temporary removal of high-titer inhibitors in both hemophilia A and B. Exchange transfusion or plasmapheresis produces a rapid transient reduction in antibody level, with a rate of 40 mL plasma per kilogram decreasing levels by half.[122] Although laborious, it may be attempted in cases of critical hemorrhage as an adjunct to high-dose F VIII concentrate therapy. Antibody removal by extracorporeal adsorption of the plasma to protein A Sepharose or a specific F IX–Sepharose in columns has also shown promise in hemophilias A and B.[123,124]

Prognosis

Advances in the treatment of hemophilia, from the use of cryoprecipitate in the 1960s to the introduction of plasma-derived factor concentrates in the 1970s, led to dramatic improvement in quality of life and raised the life span for hemophiliacs from 11 years in 1921 to 60 years in 1980.[125]

Before effective virucidal methods were used in the manufacturing of clotting factor concentrates in 1985, hemophiliacs were at a very high risk of contracting blood-borne viruses from factor concentrates that exposed them to the plasma of thousands of donors. Viral infections, such as hepatitis B, C, and G and HIV acquired from infected blood products, have altered the prognosis for some patients.[126–130] In a Dutch study of hemophiliacs from 1992 to 2001, age-adjusted mortality was 2.3 times higher in hemophilia patients than in the general male population, largely attributed to the consequences of viral infections.[131] AIDS and hepatitis C were the main cause of deaths, in 26% and 22% of instances, respectively.[131] In patients with severe hemophilia, life expectancy decreased from 63 (1972–1985) to 59 years (1992–2001). Exclusion of virus-related deaths resulted in a life expectancy at birth of 72 years.[131]

HIV seroprevalence increased to 60% to 75% of patients with hemophilia (85%–90% with severe hemophilia), with HIV-associated opportunistic infections and neoplasms contributing substantially to the morbidity and mortality of hemophiliacs.[126,127,129] Oral mucosal diseases were common in hemophiliacs with HIV, particularly in those with advanced immunosuppression.[130,132] HIV protease inhibitor–containing drug combinations that resulted in improved health of some HIV-infected patients in the late 1990s have shown significant clinical and laboratory benefits when used by HIV-infected hemophiliacs.[133] Major reductions in AIDS and death rates were observed from 1997 to 2003 in hemophiliacs, with survival improvements largely attributable to decreases in AIDS-related deaths yet accompanied by increases in liver disease death rates.[134]

COAGULATION DISORDERS—ACQUIRED—DRUG INDUCED

Heparin

Indications for heparin therapy include prophylaxis or treatment for venous thromboembolism, including prophylaxis in medical and surgical patients.[135] Heparin is a potent anticoagulant that binds with AT to significantly inhibit activation of clotting enzymes, thereby reducing thrombin generation and fibrin formation. The major bleeding complications from heparin therapy are bleeding at surgical sites and bleeding into the retroperitoneum.

Heparin has a relatively short duration of action of three to four hours and so is typically used for acute anticoagulation, whereas chronic therapy is initiated with coumarin drugs. For acute anticoagulation, intravenous infusion of 1000 units unfractionated heparin per hour, sometimes following a 5000-unit bolus, is given to increase the aPTT to 1.5 to 2 times the preheparin aPTT. Alternatively, subcutaneous injections of 5,000 to 10,000 units of heparin are given every 12 hours. The most common outpatient use of subcutaneous heparin is for the treatment of deep venous thrombophlebitis during pregnancy,[136] with the goal being regulation of the aPTT between 1.25 and 1.5 times control. Protamine sulfate can rapidly reverse the anticoagulant effects of heparin.

Newer biologically active low-molecular-weight heparins (LMWHs) (e.g., enoxaprin [Lovenox, Sanofi-Aventis, Bridgewater, NJ], tinzaparin [Innohep, Pharmion, Boulder, CO], dalteparin [Fragmin, Eisai, Inc., Woodcliff Lake, NJ]) administered subcutaneously once or twice daily are less likely to result in thrombocytopenia and bleeding complications. Fondaparinux (Arixtra, GlaxoSmithKline, Research Triangle Park, NC) is an injectable direct F Xa inhibitor, chemically related to the LMWHs, used to prevent deep venous thromboembolism and postoperative complications.

Coumarin Anticoagulants

Coumarin anticoagulants, which include warfarin and dicumarol (Coumadin, DuPont Pharmaceuticals, Wilmington, DE), slow thrombin production and clot formation by blocking the action of vitamin K, leading to decreased levels of vitamin K–dependent factors (Fs II, VI, IX, and X). They are routinely used for anticoagulation to prevent recurrent thromboembolic events, such as pulmonary embolism, venous thrombosis, stroke, and myocardial infarction. It is used commonly in patients with atrial fibrillation and in patients with prosthetic heart valves.[137]

Daily doses of 2.5 to 7.5 mg warfarin are typically required to maintain adequate anticoagulation. PT/INR is used to monitor anticoagulation levels, with target therapeutic ranges varying based on medical indication, with PT of 18 to 30 seconds or INR of 1.5 to 4.0, but seldom above 3.5. Patients with paroxysmal atrial fibrillation and porcine heart valves require minimal anticoagulation (INR target 1.5–2.0), and venous thrombosis is managed with intermediate-range anticoagulation (INR 2.0–3.0), whereas mechanical prosthetic heart valves and hypercoagulable states require more intense anticoagulation (INR target 3.0–4.0).[137]

Coumarin therapy requires continual laboratory monitoring, (i.e., typically every 2–8 weeks) as fluctuations can occur. It has a longer duration of action, with coagulant activity in blood decreased by 50% in 12 hours and 20% in 24 hours of therapy initiation. Coagulation returns to normal levels in approximately two to four days following discontinuation of coumarin drugs.

Coumarin drugs are particularly susceptible to drug interactions. Drugs that potentially increase warfarin potency (i.e., elevate the INR) due so either by inhibiting the cytochrome P450 enzymes in the liver that break down the drug or by altering gut bacterial flora that affects gastrointestinal absorption of the drug. Such drugs that increase potency include metronidazole, penicillin, erythromycin, cephalosporins, tetracycline, fluconazole, ketoconazole, chloral hydrate, and propoxyphene. Those that reduce its potency (i.e., decrease the INR) include barbiturates, ascorbic acid, dicloxacillin, and nafcillin.[138] In addition, a synergistic antihemostatic effect is seen when coumarin drugs are used in combination with ASA or NSAIDs.

Warfarin is among the top 10 drugs with largest number of serious complications including death, as reported to the United States Food and Drug Administration, with intracranial hemorrhage (ICH) being the most feared complication due to its morbidity and mortality.[139] An observational study of over 100,000 outpatient adults on warfarin therapy showed an overall rate of 3.8% of bleeding episodes that required a hospital visit.[140] Intramuscular injections are avoided in anticoagulated patients because of increased risk of intramuscular bleeding and hematoma formation. The anticoagulant effect of coumarin drugs may be reversed immediately by infusion of FFP or PCC, or over a longer period of time by administration of vitamin K.

New Oral Anticoagulants

New oral anticoagulant medications (e.g., dabigatran, rivaroxaban, apixaban) have been recently recommended for atrial fibrillation over warfarin mainly due to its equivalent efficacy, its predictable and stable anticoagulant effect at regular fixed dosages thereby eliminating the need for regular monitoring, and the significantly decreased incidence of ICH.[141] Dabigatran (Pradaxa, Boehringer Ingelheim, Ingelheim am Rhein, Germany) is a competitive and reversible direct thrombin (F IIa) inhibitor, with incidence of major bleeding episodes that are decreased or similar to that of warfarin.[142,143] Although not routinely monitored, elevated TT, accompanied by an elevated aPTT, is consistent with therapeutic levels of the drug.

The new orally active direct factor Xa inhibitors include rivaroxaban (Xarelto, Janssen Pharmaceuticals Inc, Titusville, NJ) and apixaban (Eliquis, Bristol-Myers Squibb Co., Princeton, NJ) and are desirable due to their rapid onset of action. Although the PT/INR may be prolonged in patients treated with rivaroxaban, it is not useful for apixaban. Moreover, aPTT is not useful in detecting the therapeutic level of these drugs.

The main drawback to these medications is the lack of specific antidotes, which are currently in the development stages. PCC has been shown to reverse the prolongation of PT/INR in those treated with rivaroxaban, but not dabigatran,[144] and there is some data supporting the use of recombinant FVIIa to reverse the effects of dabigatran and rivaroxaban.[145] Current recommended algorithms for management of severe bleeding episodes due to these new oral anticoagulants include cessation of the drugs, local hemostatic measures at the source of bleeding, volume replacement, and transfusion of blood products if needed.[146]

COAGULOPATHIES—ACQUIRED—DISEASE ASSOCIATED

Liver Disease

Patients with liver disease may have a wide spectrum of hemostatic defects depending on the extent of liver damage, which affects both the platelet and the coagulation phases of hemostasis.[147] Owing to impaired protein synthesis, important factors and inhibitors of the clotting and the fibrinolytic systems are markedly reduced. Acute or chronic hepatocellular disease may display decreased vitamin K–dependent factor levels, with other factors still being normal. In addition, abnormal vitamin K–dependent factor and fibrinogen molecules have been encountered. Thrombocytopenia due to platelet sequestration in the spleen and thrombocytopathy are also common in severe liver disease.

Liver disease that results in bleeding from deficient vitamin K–dependent clotting factors (Fs II, VII, IX, and X) may be reversed with vitamin K injections for three days, either intravenously or subcutaneously. Infusion of FFP may be employed when more immediate hemorrhage control is necessary, such as prior to dental extractions or other surgical procedures.[148] Cirrhotic patients with moderate thrombocytopenia and functional platelet defects may benefit from DDAVP therapy.[149] Antifibrinolytic drugs, if used cautiously, have markedly reduced bleeding and thus reduced need for blood and blood product substitution.[147] Platelet transfusions may be required for liver disease patients who are thrombocytopenic.

Renal Disease

Patients with renal disease have thrombocytopathies due to the effects of accumulated urea on platelets. In uremic patients, dialysis remains the primary preventive and therapeutic modality used for control of bleeding, although it is not always immediately effective.[150] Hemodialysis and peritoneal dialysis appear to be equally efficacious in improving platelet function abnormalities and clinical bleeding in the uremic patient. The availability of cryoprecipitate[151] and DDAVP[152] offers alternative effective therapy for uremic patients with chronic abnormal bleeding who require shortened BTs acutely in preparation for urgent surgery. Conjugated estrogen preparations[153] and recombinant erythropoietin[154] have also been shown to be beneficial.

Vitamin K Deficiency

Vitamin K is a fat-soluble vitamin that is absorbed in the small intestine and stored in the liver. It plays an important role in hemostasis by activating various coagulation factors. Vitamin K deficiency is associated with having poorly functioning vitamin K–dependent Fs II, VII, IX, and X.[155] Deficiency is rare but can result from inadequate dietary intake, intestinal malabsorption, or loss of storage sites due to hepatocellular disease. Biliary tract obstruction and long-term use of broad-spectrum antibiotics, particularly the cephalosporins, can also cause vitamin K deficiency. Although there is a theoretic 30-day store of vitamin K in the liver, severe hemorrhage can result in acutely ill patients in 7 to 10 days. A rapid fall in F VII levels leads to an initial elevation in INR and a subsequent prolongation of aPTT. When vitamin K deficiency results in coagulopathy, supplemental vitamin K by injection restores the integrity of the clotting mechanism within 12 to 24 hours.

Disseminated Intravascular Coagulation

DIC is a process that causes both thrombosis and hemorrhage, occurring in approximately 1% of hospital admissions.[156] DIC is triggered by potent stimuli that activate both F XII and TF to initially form microthrombi and emboli throughout the microvasculature.[157] Thrombosis results in rapid consumption of both coagulation factors and platelets while also creating FDPs that have antihemostatic effects. The most frequent triggers for DIC are obstetric complications, metastatic cancer, massive trauma, and infection with sepsis. Clinical symptoms vary with disease stage and severity. Most patients have bleeding at skin and mucosal sites. Although it can be chronic and mild, acute DIC can produce massive hemorrhage and be life threatening.

In acute DIC, it is important to expeditiously identify the underlying triggering disease or condition and deliver specific and vigorous treatment of the underlying disorder if long-term survival is to be a possibility. Diagnosis is made by laboratory studies that confirm increased thrombin generation (e.g., decreased fibrinogen, prolonged PT/INR, and aPTT) and increased fibrinolysis (e.g., increased FDPs and D-dimer). For chronic DIC, diagnosis is based on the evidence of microangiopathies on the peripheral blood smear, and creased FDPs such as D-dimer. The dentist may be called upon to provide a gingival or oral mucosal biopsy specimen for histopathologic examination to confirm the diagnosis of DIC by the presence of microthrombi in the vascular bed.

Although somewhat controversial, active DIC is usually treated initially with intravenous unfractionated heparin or subcutaneous LMWH to prevent thrombin from acting on fibrinogen, thereby preventing further clot formation.[158–160] Infusion of activated protein C, anti-thrombin III, and agents directed against TF activity are being investigated as new therapeutic approaches.[161] Replacement of deficient coagulation factors with FFP and correction of the platelet deficiency with platelet transfusions may be necessary for improvement or prophylaxis of the hemorrhagic tendency of DIC prior to emergency surgical procedures. Elective surgery is deferred due to the volatility of the coagulation mechanism in these patients.

Fibrinolytic Disorders

Disorders of the fibrinolytic system can lead to hemorrhage when clot breakdown is enhanced or to excessive clotting and thrombosis when clot breakdown mechanisms are retarded. Primary fibrinolysis typically results in bleeding and may be caused by a deficiency in α_2-antiplasmin or PAIs, natural proteins that turn off activation of the fibrinolytic system. Laboratory coagulation tests are normal with the exception of decreased fibrinogen and increased FDP levels. Impaired clearance of tPA may contribute to prolonged bleeding in individuals with severe liver disease. As discussed earlier, deficiency of F XIII, a transglutaminase that stabilizes fibrin clots, is a rare inherited disorder that leads to hemorrhage. Patients with primary fibrinolysis are treated with FFP therapy and antifibrinolytics.

Differentiation must be made from the secondary fibrinolysis that accompanies DIC, a hypercoagulable state that predisposes individuals to thromboembolism. Dialysis patients with chronic renal failure show a fibrinolysis defect at the level of plasminogen activation.[162] Reduced fibrinolysis may be responsible, along with other factors, for the development of thrombosis, atherosclerosis, and their thrombotic complications. Activators of the fibrinolytic system (tPA, streptokinase, and urokinase) are frequently used to accelerate clot lysis in patients with acute thromboembolism, for example, to prevent continued tissue damage in myocardial infarction or treat thrombotic stroke. tPA has been used with great success in therapeutic doses to lyse thrombi in individuals with thromboembolic disorders associated with myocardial infarction, with effectiveness limited to the first six hours postinfarction.[163]

IDENTIFICATION OF THE DENTAL PATIENT WITH A BLEEDING DISORDER

Identification of the dental patient with or at risk for a bleeding disorder begins with a thorough review of the medical history.[164,165] Patient report of a family history of bleeding problems may help identify inherited disorders of hemostasis. In addition, a patient's history of bleeding following surgical procedures, including dental extractions, can help identify a risk. Identification of medications with hemostatic effect (e.g., oral anticoagulants, heparin, ASA, NSAIDs, and cytotoxic chemotherapy) is essential, in addition to identification of medications that may enhance their effect (e.g., antibiotics, antifungal medications). In addition, one must identify medical conditions (e.g., liver disease, renal disease, hematologic malignancy, cancer patients on chemotherapy, thrombocytopenia) that may predispose patients to bleeding problems. In addition, a history of heavy alcohol intake is a risk factor for bleeding consequences.

A review-of-systems approach to the patient interview can identify symptoms suggestive of hemostatic abnormalities (see Table 19-2). Although the majority of patients with underlying bleeding disorders of mild to moderate severity may exhibit no symptoms, symptoms are common when disease is severe. Symptoms of hemorrhagic diatheses reported by patients may include frequent epistaxis, spontaneous gingival or oral mucosal bleeding, easy bruising, prolonged bleeding from superficial cuts, excessive menstrual flow, and hematuria. When the history and the review of systems suggest increased bleeding propensity, laboratory studies are warranted.

ORAL COMPLICATIONS AND MANIFESTATIONS

Platelet deficiency and vascular wall disorders result in extravasation of blood into connective and epithelial tissues of the skin and mucosa, creating small pinpoint hemorrhages called petechiae and larger patches called ecchymoses. Platelet or coagulation disorders with severely altered hemostasis can result in spontaneous gingival bleeding, as may be seen in conjunction with hyperplastic hyperemic gingival enlargements in leukemic patients. Continuous oral bleeding over long periods of time fosters deposits of hemosiderin and other blood degradation products on the tooth surfaces,

turning them brown. A variety of oral findings are illustrated in Figures 19-7 and 19-8.

Hemophiliacs may experience many episodes of oral bleeding over their lifetime. One report includes an average 29.1 bleeding events per year serious enough to require factor replacement in F VIII–deficient patients, of which 9% involved oral structures.[166] The location of oral bleeds was as follows: labial frenum, 60%; tongue, 23%; buccal mucosa, 17%; and gingiva and palate, 0.5% (Figure 19-9). Bleeding

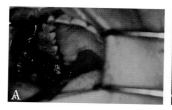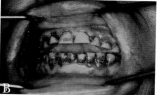

FIGURE 19-7 A 68-year-old woman with acute myelogenous leukemia and a platelet count of 9000/mm³. Platelet transfusion and e-aminocaproic acid oral rinses were used to control bleeding. A, Buccal mucosa and palatal ecchymoses. B, Extrinsic stains on teeth from erythrocyte degradation following continual gingival oozing.

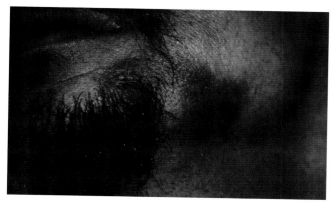

FIGURE 19-8 A 46-year-old man with severe liver cirrhosis due to hepatitis C infection. Shown is purpura of facial skin 1 week after full-mouth extractions.

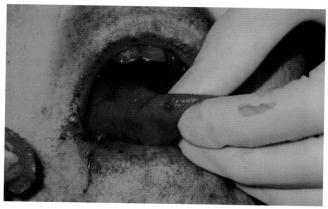

FIGURE 19-9 A 27-year-old man with type III von Willebrand disease and a 2-week duration of bleeding from the tongue that reduced his hematocrit to 16%. Hemorrhage control was obtained with cryoprecipitate.

occurrences were most frequent in patients with severe hemophilia, followed by moderate and then mild hemophilia. They most often resulted from traumatic injury. Bleeding events may also be induced by poor oral hygiene practices and iatrogenic factors. The frequency of oral hemorrhage by location in people deficient of F VIII and F IX has been reported as follows: gingiva, 64%; dental pulp, 13%; tongue, 7.5%; lip, 7%; palate, 2%; and buccal mucosa, 1%.[167] Many minor oral bleeds, such as those from the gingiva or dental pulp, can be controlled by local measures.

Evaluation of dental disease patterns in children with severe hemophilia revealed a significantly lower prevalence of dental caries and lower plaque scores compared with matched, healthy controls.[168]

Hemarthrosis is a common complication in hemophiliacs' weight-bearing joints, yet it rarely occurs in the TMJ. One case involved an acute TMJ hemarthrosis associated with F IX deficiency that was resolved with factor replacement without aspiration.[169] A second case involved a patient with F XI deficiency who had an associated TMJ arthropathy that was treated with arthrotomy, arthroscopic adhesion lysis, factor replacement, splint therapy, and physical therapy.[170]

DENTAL MANAGEMENT CONSIDERATIONS

Dental modifications required for patients with bleeding disorders depend on both the type and invasiveness of the dental procedure and the type and severity of the bleeding disorder. Thus, less modification is needed for patients with mild coagulopathies in preparation for dental procedures anticipated to have limited bleeding consequences. When significant bleeding is expected, the goal of management is to preoperatively restore the hemostatic system to an acceptable range while supporting coagulation with adjunctive and/or local measures. For reversible or acute hemostatic disorders, it may be best to treat the primary illness or defect to allow the patient to return to a manageable bleeding risk for the dental treatment period. With respect to therapeutic alterations in hemostasis due to medications, local hemostatic measures usually suffice; however, there are limited instances in which drug discontinuation and alteration may be required after physician consultation. For irreversible coagulopathies, the missing or defective element may need to be replaced from an exogenous source to allow control of bleeding (e.g., factor replacement therapy for hemophilia). Assessment of the coagulopathy and delivery of appropriate therapy prior to dental procedures are best accomplished in consultation with a hematologist and may involve treatment in specialized hospital facilities.[171]

Local Hemostatic Measures

Local hemostatic agents and techniques include pressure, surgical packs, vasoconstrictors, sutures, surgical stents, topical thrombin, and use of absorbable hemostatic materials.

Although having no direct effect on hemostasis, primary wound closure aids patient comfort, decreases blood clot size, and protects clots from masticatory trauma and subsequent bleeding.[172] Sutures can also be used to stabilize and protect packing, with resorbable and nonresorbable suture materials proven to be equally effective. Microfibrillar collagen fleeces (e.g., Avitene [Davol Inc., Cranston, RI], Helitene [Integra Life Sciences, Plainsboro, NJ]) aid hemostasis when placed against the bleeding bony surface of a well-cleansed extraction socket. It acts to attract platelets, causing the release phenomenon to trigger aggregation of platelets into thrombi in the interstices of the fibrous mass of the clot.[173] Surgifoam (Ethicon Inc., Somerville, NJ) and Gelfoam (Pfizer, New York, NY) are absorbable gelatin compressed sponges with intrinsic hemostatic properties. A collagen absorbable hemostat manufactured as a 3 × 4–inch sponge (INSTAT, Ethicon Inc.) or fabricated as a nonwoven pad or sponge (Helistat, Integra Life Sciences; Gelfoam, Pharmacia & Upjohn Co., Kalamazoo, MI; Ultrafoam, Davol Inc.) are also useful adjuncts.

Topical thrombin (Thrombogen, Ethicon Inc.), which directly converts fibrinogen in the blood to fibrin, is an effective adjunct when applied directly to the wound or carried to the extraction site in a nonacidic medium on oxidized cellulose. Surgical acrylic stents may be useful if carefully fabricated to avoid traumatic irritation to the surgical site. Diet restriction to full liquids for the initial 24 to 48 hours, followed by intake of soft foods for 1 to 2 weeks, will further protect the clot by reducing the amount of chewing and resultant soft tissue disturbances.

Fibrin sealants or fibrin glue has been used effectively in Europe since 1978 as an adjunct with adhesive and hemostatic effects to control bleeding at wound or surgical sites.[174] In the United States, extemporaneous fibrin sealant can be made by combining cryoprecipitate with a combination of 10,000 units of topical thrombin powder diluted in 10 mL saline and 10 mL calcium chloride. When dispensed over the wound simultaneously from separate syringes, the cryoprecipitate and calcium chloride precipitate almost instantaneously to form a clear gelatinous adhesive gel. The first proprietary formulation, Crosseal Fibrin Sealant (Human; Ethicon Inc., Israel, distributed by Johnson & Johnson Wound Management, Somerville, NJ), was approved in the United States in 2003 for patients undergoing liver surgery and is derived from human plasma, so it is not completely without risk of viral transmission.

Susceptibility to Infection

Susceptibility to infection among patients with congenital bleeding disorders is not a significant concern. However, due to bleeding into weight-bearing joints, hemophiliacs may have had joint replacement for which antibiotic prophylaxis should be considered.[175] Should a hematoma form as a result of an anesthetic injection or other dental trauma or spontaneously, use of a broad-spectrum antibiotic is indicated to prevent infection during resolution. If bleeding results from bone marrow–suppressive systemic disease or chemotherapeutic drug use, antibiotics may be used to prevent infection from bacteremia-inducing dental procedures when production of mature functional neutrophils is substantially diminished.

Pain Control

The use of ASA and other NSAIDs for pain management is generally avoided in patients with bleeding disorders due to their inhibition of platelet function and potentiation of bleeding episodes.

Ability to Withstand Care

Patients with bleeding disorders, appropriately prepared preoperatively, are generally as able to withstand dental care as well as unaffected individuals. Consultation with the patient's physician is recommended for guidance on medical management required for higher risk surgical dental procedures.

Dental treatment in the operating room under general anesthesia may be indicated to maximize treatment accomplishments and minimize the risk and cost because of the expense of some medical management approaches to severe bleeding disorders (e.g., coagulation factor replacement for severe hemophiliacs, the warfarin withdrawal—heparinization approach for patients at high risk of thrombosis), when patient cooperation or anxiety prohibits outpatient clinic or office treatment, or the patient has extensive treatment needs. Although oral endotracheal intubation provides access challenges for the dental operator, it is preferred over nasal endotracheal intubation, which carries the risk of inducing a nasal bleed that can be difficult to control.

Preventative and Periodontal Therapies

Periodontal health is of critical importance for the patient with coagulopathies because hyperemic gingiva contributes to spontaneous and induced gingival bleeding, and periodontitis is a leading cause of tooth morbidity, necessitating extraction. Individuals with bleeding diatheses are unusually prone to oral hygiene neglect due to fear of toothbrush-induced bleeding; however, regular oral hygiene can be accomplished without risk of significant bleeding. Periodontal probing and supragingival scaling and polishing can be done routinely. Careful subgingival scaling with fine scalers rarely warrants replacement therapy. Severely inflamed and swollen tissues are best treated initially with chlorhexidine oral rinses or by superficial gross débridement with ultrasonic or hand instruments to allow gingival shrinkage prior to deep scaling.[170] Deep subgingival scaling and root planing should be performed by quadrant to reduce gingival area exposed to potential bleeding. Locally applied pressure and posttreatment antifibrinolytic oral rinses are usually successful in controlling any protracted bleeding.[176,177]

Restorative, Endodontic, and Prosthodontic Therapy

General restorative, endodontic and prosthodontic procedures do not result in significant hemorrhage. Rubber dam isolation is advised to minimize the risk of lacerating soft tissue in the operative field and to avoid creating ecchymoses and hematomas with high-speed evacuators or saliva ejectors. Care is required to select a tooth clamp that does not traumatize the gingiva. Matrices, wedges, and a hemostatic gingival retraction cord may be used with caution to protect soft tissues and improve visualization when subgingival extension of cavity preparation is necessary.

Endodontic therapy is often the treatment of choice over tooth extraction for patients with severe bleeding disorders, due to the higher risk of hemorrhage from the latter. Instrumentation and filling beyond the apical seal should be avoided.[178] Application of epinephrine intrapulpally to the apical area is usually successful in providing intrapulpal hemostasis. Endodontic surgical procedures or implant placement surgeries require the same factor replacement therapy as do oral surgical procedures.

Removable prosthetic appliances can be fabricated without complications. Denture trauma should be minimized by prompt and careful postinsertion adjustment.

Pediatric Dental Therapy

The pediatric dental patient occasionally presents with prolonged oozing from exfoliating primary teeth. Administration of factor concentrates and extraction of the deciduous tooth with curettage may be necessary for patient comfort and hemorrhage control. One suggestion is the extraction of mobile primary teeth using periodontal ligament anesthesia without factor replacement after two days of vigorous oral hygiene to reduce local inflammation.[179] Hemorrhage control is obtained with gauze pressure, and hemostasis is achieved in 12 hours. Pulpotomies can be performed without excessive pulpal bleeding. Stainless steel crowns should be prepared to allow minimal removal of enamel at gingival areas.[180]

Orthodontic Therapy

Orthodontic treatment can be provided with little modification. Care must be observed to avoid mucosal laceration by orthodontic bands, brackets, and wires. Bleeding from minor cuts usually responds to local pressure. Properly managed fixed orthodontic appliances or use of transparent aligners are preferred over removable functional appliances for the patient with a high likelihood of bleeding from chronic tissue irritation. The use of extraoral force and shorter treatment duration further decrease the potential for bleeding complications.[181]

Platelet Disorders

For thrombocytopenic patients (primary or secondary to systemic disease or treatment), platelet transfusions may be required prior to dental extractions or other oral surgical procedures with the ideal target of increasing platelet counts above 50,000/mm³. The therapeutically expected increment in platelet count from infusion of one unit of platelets is approximately 10,000 to 12,000/mm³. Six units of platelets are commonly infused at a time. Patients who have received multiple transfusions may be refractory to random donor platelets as a result of alloimmunization. These individuals may require single-donor apheresis or leukocyte-reduced platelets.

The thrombasthenic patient needing dental extractions may be successfully treated with the use of local hemostatic measures and antifibrinolytic drugs.[182,183]

Patients on single or dual antiplatelet therapy have been shown to have no clinically significant risk of postoperative bleeding complications from invasive dental procedures, as indicated by a systemic review of multiple studies.[184] The risks of thromboembolic events due to discontinuation of the medications far outweighs that of postoperative bleeding complications, which can be usually prevented by or treated with local hemostatic measures. For minor oral surgery, adjunctive local hemostatic agents alone are useful in preventing postoperative oozing. One suggestion for patients on ASA when extensive surgery is indicated is to use DDAVP for preoperative prevention or to treat postoperative bleeding.[185]

Discontinuation or alteration of antiplatelet medications should only be considered, after physician consultation, for one or a combination of the following: patients with additional risk factors for postoperative bleeding (e.g., other anticoagulant medications or systemic conditions that may alter hemostasis), procedures with high risk of inducing significant bleeding, and patients with low medical risk (e.g., healthy patient with no history of underlying cardiovascular disease). In the case of ASA, discontinuation 1 week prior to extensive oral surgical procedures is typical since its effects remain for the 8- to 10-day lifetime of platelets.

Chemotherapy-associated oral hemorrhages, most frequently related to thrombocytopenia, are best managed by transfusions of HLA-matched platelets and FFP, together with topically applied clot-promoting agents.[77] A pilot study suggests a possible benefit of DDAVP for the prevention or treatment of bleeding in patients with thrombocytopenia associated with hematologic malignancy.[186]

Hemophilia A, Hemophilia B, and vWD

Block injections used in dentistry (i.e., inferior alveolar, posterior superior alveolar, infraorbital, lingual, long buccal) require minimal coagulation factor levels of 20% to 30%. These injections place anesthetic solutions in highly vascularized loose connective tissue with no distinct boundaries, where formation of a dissecting hematoma is possible, with development of hematomas in 8% of hemophilic patients not treated with prophylactic factor replacement prior to mandibular block injection.[187,188] Extravasation of blood into the soft tissues of the oropharyngeal area in hemophiliacs can produce gross swelling, pain, dysphagia, respiratory

obstruction, and grave risk of death from asphyxia (Figure 19-10).[189–191] Intramuscular injections should also be avoided due to the risk of hematoma formation.

Hemorrhagic problems after extractions have drastically declined over the last 10 years such that only an estimated 2% of hemophilic patients experience one or more delayed bleeding episodes.[192] Appropriate precautionary measures now allow surgery to be performed safely with no significantly greater risk of bleeding than in nonhemophiliacs.[193]

Determination of factor replacement requirements should be accomplished in consultation with the patient's hematologist and are dependent on the invasiveness of the procedure. Canadian clinical practice guidelines recommend, for surgical hemostasis, target replacement factor levels of 40% to 50% of F VIII (dose 20–25 U/kg) and F IX (dose 40–50 U/kg), in conjunction with antifibrinolytics.[194] Recommended minimum factor level during healing phases

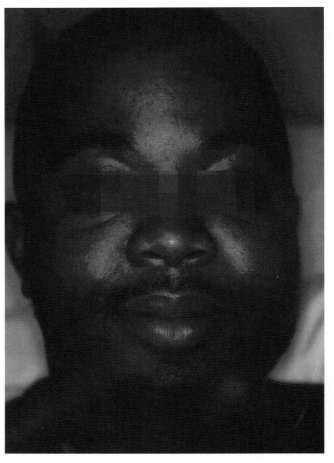

FIGURE 19-10 A 24-year-old man with severe hemophilia A and low-titer inhibitor, 3 days after inferior alveolar block–induced parapharyngeal hemorrhage. Patient presented with difficulty swallowing and pending airway compromise eight hours after nerve block. Subsequent treatment with prothrombin complex concentrates over three days controlled the bleeding and began the resolution of facial swelling.

is 20%. Higher hemostatic factor levels are needed for large wound cavities created by extraction of multiple or multi-rooted teeth or when gingival inflammation, bleeding, tooth mobility, or apical lesions are present.[167] Deficient factor activity levels required for postextraction hemostasis have been reported to vary from 3.5% to 25% for deciduous teeth and 5.5% to 20% for permanent teeth.[167] Gingival or dental bleeding unresponsive to antifibrinolytics requires 20% to 30% clotting F VIII or F IX.[194]

Three methods of replacement therapy have been employed to maintain circulating factor levels during surgical and healing phases. These include intermittent replacement therapy, continuous intravenous factor infusion therapy, and a single preoperative factor concentrate infusion combined with an antifibrinolytic mouthwash.[187] When single-bolus infusion is used for outpatient treatment, transfusion recommendations generally aim for replacement of missing coagulation factors to levels of 50% to 100%. This accounts for possible failure of factor activity to increase to target levels, and variable plasma half-lives (8–12 hours for F VIII and 18–24 hours for F IX). F VIII levels may be sufficiently raised by DDAVP in some patients with moderate to mild hemophilia A and vWD to allow dental extractions without transfusion. For extensive surgery, additional postoperative factor maintenance may be indicated, accomplished by infusion of factor concentrates, DDAVP, cryoprecipitate, or FFP.

Postsurgical bleeding due to fibrinolysis commonly starts three to five days after surgery and can usually be controlled by local measures and use of antifibrinolytics. Continual oozing from unstable fibrinous clots (i.e., "liver clots") may require their removal and the repacking of the extraction socket with local hemostatic agents. The use of fibrin sealants has allowed reduction in factor concentrate replacement levels in hemophiliacs undergoing dental surgeries when used in combination with antifibrinolytics.[195–197] However, the use of fibrin glue does not obviate the need for factor concentration replacement in severe hemophiliacs.[196]

Antifibrinolytic drugs such as ε-aminocaproic acid (EACA) (Amicar 25% syrup, VersaPharm Inc., Marietta, GA) and tranexamic acid (AMCA) (Cyclokapron, Pharmacia Corp, Peapack, NJ) inhibit fibrinolysis by blocking the conversion of plasminogen to plasmin, resulting in clot stabilization.[198] Postsurgical use of EACA has been shown to significantly reduce the quantity of factor required to control bleeding when used in conjunction with presurgical concentrate infusion sufficient to raise plasma F VIII and F IX levels to 50%.[187,199,200] A regimen of 50 mg/kg of body weight EACA given topically and systemically as a 25% (250 mg/mL) oral rinse every 6 hours for 7 to 10 days appears adequate as an adjunct. Tranexamic acid (4.8%) oral rinse was found to be 10 times more potent than was EACA in preventing postextraction bleeding in hemophiliacs, with fewer side effects, but it is not routinely available in the United States.[201,202] Systemic antifibrinolytic therapy can be given orally or intravenously as EACA 75 mg/kg (up to

4 g) every six hours or AMCA 25 mg/kg every eight hours until bleeding stops.[194] For the treatment of acute bleeding syndromes due to elevated fibrinolytic activity, it is suggested that 10 tablets (5 g) or 4 teaspoons of 25% syrup (5 g) of Amicar be administered during the first hour of treatment, followed by a continuing rate of 2 tablets (1 g) or 1 teaspoon of syrup (1.25 g) per hour. This method of treatment would ordinarily be continued for about eight hours or until the bleeding situation has been controlled.

Periodontal surgical procedures warrant elevating circulating factor levels to 50% and use of posttreatment antifibrinolytics. Periodontal packing material aids hemostasis and protects the surgical site; however, it may be dislodged by severe hemorrhage or subperiosteal hematoma formation.

Patients on Anticoagulant Therapy
Management of the dental patient on anticoagulant therapy involves consideration of the degree of anticoagulation achieved as gauged by the laboratory values, the dental procedure planned, and the level of thromboembolic risk for the patient.[203] In general, higher INRs result in higher bleeding risk from surgical procedures.[204]

Coumarin Anticoagulants
It is generally held that nonsurgical dental treatment can be successfully accomplished without alteration of the anticoagulant regimen, provided that the PT/INR is not grossly above the therapeutic range and trauma is minimized.[205–208] Some controversy exists over the management of anticoagulated patients for oral surgical procedures.[138,209–211] Patients who discontinue warfarin preoperatively are exposed to three to four days at subtherapeutic anticoagulation levels postoperatively after immediate resumption of therapy. Risks of a life-threatening thromboembolic event are three- to fivefold greater than that of significant uncontrollable postoperative bleeding.[212] The American Heart Association and American College of Cardiology scientific statement recommends that for patients undergoing dental procedures, tranexamic acid or EACA (Amicar) mouthwash can be applied without interrupting anticoagulant therapy.[213] The Ninth American College of Chest Physicians (ACCP) Antithrombotic Guidelines made similar recommendations, with the addition that coumarin therapy be discontinued two to three days before undergoing dental procedures for patients who are considered to be at high risk for bleeding.[214] A systematic review and meta-analysis of randomized controlled trials examined the bleeding potential in dental practice of patients on warfarin therapy.[215] Among all patients, there were no major bleeding episodes, and there were no differences in incidence of clinically significant minor bleeding episodes between those who continued their regular dose of warfarin and those who discontinued or altered their dose of warfarin.

Preparation of the anticoagulated patient for surgical procedures depends on the extent of bleeding expected. For surgical procedures, physician consultation is advised to determine the patient's most recent PT/INR level and the best treatment approach based on the patient's relative thromboembolic and hemorrhagic risks. When the likelihood of sudden thrombotic and embolic complications is small and hemorrhagic risk is high, warfarin therapy can be discontinued briefly at the time of surgery, with prompt reinstitution postoperatively.[203,216,217] Warfarin's long half-life

of 42 hours necessitates dose reduction or withdrawal 2 days prior to surgery to return the patient's PT/INR to an acceptable level for surgery.[203,218] For patients with moderate thromboembolic and hemorrhagic risks, warfarin therapy can be maintained in the therapeutic range with the use of local measures to control postsurgical oozing.[219,220]

The flow chart shown in Figure 19-11 graphically outlines an algorithm for assessment and management of the dental patient on coumarin therapy. No surgical treatment is recommended for those with an INR of >3.5 to 4.0 without

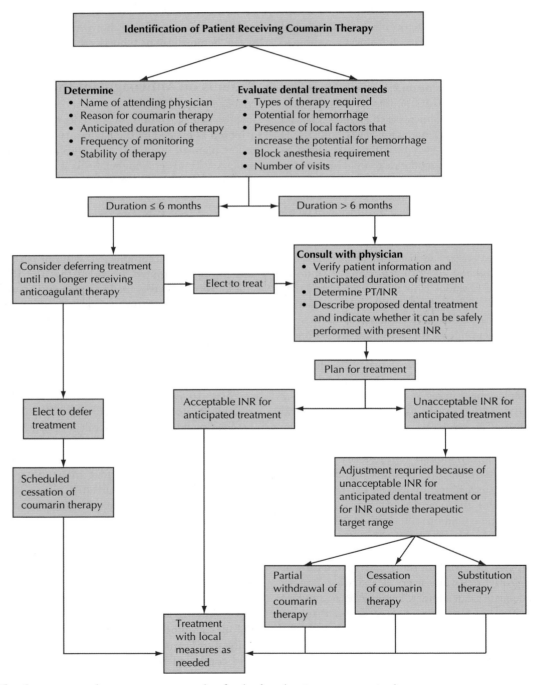

FIGURE 19-11 Assessment and management approaches for the dental patient on coumarin therapy.

coumarin dose modification.[138,208] With an INR <3.5 to 4.0, minor surgical procedures with minimal anticipated bleeding require local measures but no coumarin modification. At an INR of <3.5 to 4.0, when moderate bleeding is expected (multiple extractions or removal of wisdom teeth), local measures should be used, and INR reduction should be considered. When significant bleeding is anticipated, as from full-mouth or full-arch extractions, local measures are combined with reduction of anticoagulation to an INR of <2.0 to 3.0.[138,221] Extensive flap surgery or multiple bony extractions may require an INR of <1.5.[138]

High-risk cardiac patients undergoing high-bleeding-risk surgical procedures may be managed safely with a combination unfractionated heparin–warfarin method,[216] which requires hospitalization at additional cost. The main advantage is that it allows maximal hemostasis with minimal nonanticoagulated time (14–18 hours for a 2-hour surgery, as opposed to 3–4 days with the warfarin discontinuation method). Warfarin is withheld 24 hours prior to admission. Heparin, which has a four-hour half life, is instituted on admission and stopped six to eight hours preoperatively. Surgery is accomplished when the PT/INR and aPTT are within the normal range. Warfarin is reinstituted on the night of the procedure and may require two to four days to effectively reduce the patient's procoagulant levels to a therapeutic range. Heparin is reinstituted six to eight hours after surgery when an adequate clot has formed. Heparin reinstitution by bolus injection (typically a 5000 U bolus) carries a greater risk of postoperative bleeding than does gradual reinfusion (typically 1000 U/h).

As a less costly alternative to intravenous heparin substitution therapy that does not require hospital admission is LMWHs (e.g., enoxaparin). Using this management technique, a LMWH given once or twice daily is substituted for warfarin a few days before surgery, and it is withheld from the patient for only a few hours on the day of the surgery.[222] This is also referred to as anticoagulant "bridging" therapy.

Use of additional local hemostatic agents such as microfibrillar collagen, oxidized cellulose, or topical thrombin is recommended for anticoagulated patients. Fibrin sealant has been used successfully as an adjunct to control bleeding from oral surgical procedures in therapeutically anticoagulated patients with INRs from 1.0 to 5.0, with minimal bleeding complications.[223] Use of antifibrinolytics may have value in control of oral wound bleeding, thereby alleviating the need to reduce the oral anticoagulant dose.[224] In Europe, 4.8% tranexamic acid solution used as a mouthwash has proven effective in control of oral surgical bleeding in patients with INRs between 2.1 and 4.8 and is slightly superior when compared to an autologous fibrin glue preparation.[223,225,226] As previously discussed, the use of medications that interact with and alter warfarin's anticoagulant effectiveness is to be avoided.

Heparin

Continuous intravenous unfractionated heparin, which has the greatest hemorrhagic potential among the heparin techniques, is discontinued six to eight hours prior to surgery to allow adequate surgical hemostasis. In general, oral surgical procedures can be carried out without great risk of hemorrhage when local hemostatics are used in a patient receiving LMWH subcutaneously; however, on consultation, the patient's physician may recommend withholding the scheduled injection immediately prior to the operation. One small retrospective study found no postoperative bleeding events after invasive dental procedures for patients on LMWH alone, with several instances in patients who were concurrently on LMWH and warfarin.[227] If a bleeding emergency arises, the action of heparin can be reversed by protamine sulfate. Dosage for unfractionated heparin reversal is 1 mg protamine sulfate intravenously for every 100 units of active heparin. If given within eighth hours of the LMWH injection, then the maximum neutralizing dose of 1 mg protamine/100 units of LMWH given in the last dose is used.

New Oral Anticoagulants

Currently, there is no data on the risk of postoperative bleeding complications after invasive dental procedures for patients on the new oral anticoagulant medications. One recent case report describes a high-risk cardiovascular patient on dabigatran who required extensive oral surgical procedures (e.g., multiple surgical tooth extractions, alveoloplasty, and tuberosity reduction).[228] Dabigatran was discontinued on the night before surgery and resumed on the day after surgery. Postoperative bleeding and cardiovascular complications were not observed perioperatively or in a seven-month postoperative period. It is suggested that the short half-life and quick therapeutic response of dabigatran allows for a minimal risk of exposure to thromboembolic events due to subtherapeutic anticoagulant levels.[229]

Selected Readings

Beirne OR. Evidence to continue oral anticoagulant therapy for ambulatory oral surgery. *J Oral Maxillofac Surg*. 2005;63:540–545.

Bolton-Maggs PH, Pasi KJ. Haemophilias A and B. *Lancet*. 2003;361:1801–1809.

Brewer AK, Roeubek EM, Donachie M, et al. The dental management of adult patients with haemophilia and other congenital bleeding disorders. *Haemophilia*. 2003;9:673–677.

Greer JP, Foerster H, Lukens JN, et al, eds. *Wintrobe's Clinical Hematology*. 11th ed. Philadelphia, PA: Lippincott Williams & Wilkins; 2004.

Hemophilia and von Willebrand's disease: 1. Diagnosis, comprehensive care and assessment. Association of Hemophilia Clinic Directors of Canada. *CMAJ*. 1995;153:19–25.

Hemophilia and von Willebrand's disease: 2. Management. Association of Hemophilia Clinic Directors of Canada. *CMAJ*. 1995;153:147–157.

Herman WW, Konzelman JL Jr, Sutley SH. Current perspectives on dental patients receiving coumarin anticoagulant therapy. *J Am Dent Assoc*. 1997;128:327–335.

Liew A, Eikelboom JW, O'Donnell M, Hart RG. Assessment of anticoagulation intensity and management of bleeding with old and new anticoagulants. *Can J Cardiol*. 2013;29:S34–S44.

Lockhart PB, Gibson J, Pond SH, et al. Dental management considerations for the patient with an acquired coagulopathy. Part 2: coagulopathies from drugs. *Br Dent J*. 2003;195:495–501.

Mannucci PM. Treatment of von Willebrand's disease. *N Engl J Med.* 2004;351:683–694.

Martinowitz U, Schulman S, Horoszowski H, et al. Role of fibrin sealants in surgical procedures on patients with hemostatic disorders. *Clin Orthop.* 1996;328:65–75.

Napeñas JJ, Oost FC, DeGroot A, et al. Review of postoperative bleeding risk in dental patients on antiplatelet therapy. *Oral Surg Oral Med Oral Pathol Oral Radiol.* 2013;115:491–499.

Romney G, Glick M. An updated concept of coagulation with clinical implications. *JADA.* 2009;140:567–574.

Shopnick RI, Brettler DB. Hemostasis: a practical review of conservative and operative care. *Clin Orthop Relat Res.* 1996;328:34–38.

Todd DW. Evidence to support an individualized approach to modification of oral anticoagulant therapy for ambulatory oral surgery. *J Oral Maxillofac Surg.* 2005;63:536–539.

van Diermen DE, van der Waal I, Hoogstraten J. Management recommendations for invasive dental treatment in patients using oral antithrombotic medication, including novel oral anticoagulants. *Oral Surg Oral Med Oral Pathol Oral Radiol.* 2013;116:709–716.

For the full reference lists, please go to http://www.pmph-usa.com/Burkets_Oral_Medicine.

CHAPTER 20

Immunologic Diseases

Jane C. Atkinson, DDS

Niki Moutsopoulos, DDS, PhD

Stanley R. Pillemer, MD

Matin M. Imanguli, MD, DDS

Stephen Challacombe, BDS, PhD, FDS RCSEd, FRCPath

GENERAL PRINCIPLES OF IMMUNOLOGIC DISEASE

A large number of the inflammatory conditions treated by Oral Medicine clinicians are either autoimmune in nature or are influenced by the immune response. Immunology, once a small branch of microbiology, has evolved into a major field of biomedical research. Completion of human genome project and advances in genetically modified mice led to an explosion of knowledge about immunological pathways. This, coupled with developments in biotechnology, ushered in a new age of targeted therapies. Basic immunological concepts are reviewed in the next few sections of this chapter. The reader is referred to numerous excellent texts of immunology and reviews for a more in-depth treatment of the subject.[1]

Immunity: Protection Against Disease

The immune system's primary function is protection against infection.[1] It neutralizes foreign or *nonself*-antigens that are expressed by a large variety of microbial agents as well as some tumors. This coordinated system must be able to perceive antigens as foreign, generate activation signals, produce a variety of effector proteins that neutralize pathogens or activate other cells, and downregulate the inflammatory process once the foreign agent is eliminated.

Immune responses of vertebrates frequently are classified into two functional systems: (1) the innate system and (2) the specific or adaptive system. These two systems are highly coordinated with cross-talking signals. The biological advantage of having two systems of defense is that innate immunity eliminates foreign entities in a nonspecific manner, whereas the adaptive immune response is highly specific and targeted. However, the adaptive response takes several days to develop after antigen recognition, whereas the innate response is immediate.

Innate Immunity

Examples of the innate immune system are physical barriers, such as the skin or mucosa, the variety of secreted antimicrobial and inflammatory peptides, and cells that express receptors recognizing a wide variety of pathogens. In the oral cavity, mucosa covered with a mucin layer is the physical barrier. In addition to blocking penetration of pathogens, oral mucosal cells can produce antimicrobial peptides, such as β-defensins that kill or limit growth of many organisms. Similarly, saliva plays a critical role in innate immunity of the oral cavity. Several salivary proteins have antimicrobial, immunomodulatory, and anti-inflammatory properties, including histatins, cystatins, cathelicidin, lactoferrin, lysozyme, and mucins.[2] Many of these proteins are highly conserved between distant species, pointing to their ancient origin and evolutionary importance.[3]

The major cells of the innate immune system are the phagocytic cells and granulocytes (neutrophils, eosinophils, basophils, monocytes, and macrophages), mast cells, natural killer (NK) cells, and dendritic cells. Certain T cells with restricted specificity such as γδ T cells and NKT cells (T cells expressing both NK and T cell receptors) as well as certain B cells are sometimes included in this category. Over 70 types of leukocytes have now been characterized and defined by their *cluster of differentiation* (CD) surface antigens. The primary phagocytic cells are tissue macrophages and neutrophils, which are derived from a common myeloid precursor in the bone marrow. The phagocyte internalizes and neutralizes foreign material by creating an endosome, where the potential pathogen is degraded by hydrolytic enzymes. This process is enhanced when the material is bound by specific antibody and/or complement, a process known as opsonization. Another major function of foreign material internalization is antigen processing and presentation to lymphocytes to initiate the adaptive immune response. This is predominantly performed by dendritic cells (DCs) that originate from hematopoietic precursors and migrate into the tissues, but also macrophages and B cells. Cells performing this function are collectively known as antigen-presenting cells (APCs).[1] APCs not only process and present antigens to cells of adaptive immunity but also direct their differentiation through secretion of cytokines.

Neutrophils constitute about 75% of the circulating white blood cells. They are activated by bacterial products and cytokines released during inflammation. To function appropriately, neutrophils similar to all the other circulating immune cells must possess appropriate receptors such as adhesion molecules (selectins and integrins) and chemokine receptors that allow them to leave the circulation and migrate to sites of inflammation. Their life span is short (on average 24–48 hours), and the bone marrow releases increased numbers of neutrophils in response to certain infections. NK cells account for 10%–15% of peripheral blood lymphocytes. They lack a T- or B-cell receptor and are concentrated in the peripheral blood, spleen, and mucosal epithelia. Their primary function is to induce cytolysis of tumor or virus-infected cells and secrete cytokines that direct DC maturation and promote T- and B-cell functions. Their cytotoxic reactions are independent of antigen presentation in the context of the major histocompatibility complex (MHC). Another major arm of innate immunity is the complement system, which is a compilation of at least 30 proteins[1] with multiple functions, including pathogen lysis, opsonization of microorganisms for phagocytosis, chemotaxis and activation of leukocytes, clearance of immune complexes, and enhancement of antigen presentation. The primary components act in a particular order and sequentially activate each other. The complement system is highly regulated to minimize tissue damage from inflammation in the host.

ADAPTIVE (ACQUIRED) IMMUNITY

Antigen Presentation

A highly specific immune response develops after specific lymphocytes recognize nonself-antigens, are activated, and start proliferating. As a result of this process, clonal T- and B-cell populations are generated. Antigen presentation and recognition are central to the process. Antigen must be processed and bound to a Class I or Class II MHC molecule on the surface of the APC for the T cell to recognize it via the T-cell receptor (TCR). MHC molecules, expressed by most human cells, present both self and nonself-antigens to T cells. The T cell recognizes the MHC molecule as *self* and is not activated (T-cell tolerance). In addition to the primary signal through the specific receptor (TCR on T cells or surface immunoglobulin on B cells), T and B cells must receive costimulatory signals from coreceptors and cytokines that guide their differentiation.

Cell-Mediated Immunity

After production in the bone marrow, T-cell precursors migrate to the thymus where a functional T-cell repertoire is selected through positive selection and clonal deletion. After that, T cells populate the paracortical areas of lymph nodes and the white pulp of the spleen, and constitute 70%–80% of lymphocytes in the peripheral blood. When activated, T cells produce multiple cytokines, which are pluripotential proteins that both upregulate and downregulate inflammation. There are two major T-cell subsets, which bear either CD8 or CD4 coreceptors on their surface. Certain antigens (notably viral and tumor) are processed in the cytoplasm by the proteasome and presented on the MHC Class I molecules to CD8 T cells.[1] These cells then proliferate and become cytotoxic T lymphocytes, eventually leading to lysis of the infected or transformed host cell. The CD4 coreceptor binds exclusively to a MHC Class II molecule of an APC, and these cells develop into T-helper cells. T-helper cells can be further subdivided into various subtypes based on their distinctive cytokine secretion profile. Two major T helper subtypes are Th-1 and Th-2 cells, originally distinguished based on production of signature cytokines interferon γ (IFN-γ) and IL-4, respectively. IFN-γ produced Th-1 T cells activate macrophages and lead to elimination of phagocytosed intracellular organisms such as mycobacteria and certain fungi. In addition, Th-1 cells provide crucial help to cytotoxic CD8 cells. Both Th-1 and Th-2 cells provide help to B cells resulting in production of specific antibodies. Th-1 cells specifically induce production of IgG2a subclass, and Th-2 cells stimulate IgG1 production. Multicellular organisms, such as helminthes, are eliminated primarily through the action of Th-2 cells that attract and activate eosinophils (via the action of IL-5) and induce IgE class switching. Because Th-2 cells induce IgE production, they are key cells in the pathogenesis of allergy. In the past several years several additional T-helper subtypes have been described, most notably Th-17 cells, distinguished by production of IL-17. It is believed that this subtype is crucial for immunity against certain bacteria. The role of Th-17 cells in autoimmunity is an area of active research.[4]

Regulatory T Cells

Just as effective recognition and elimination of harmful microorganisms is crucial for the immune response, tolerance to self is paramount for an organism's survival. One of the mechanisms by which this is achieved is via deletion of T-cell clones recognizing self-antigens during thymic development (central tolerance). However, not all self-antigens are expressed in the thymus, and significant numbers of peripheral T cells express potentially self-reactive antigen receptors. How are these self-reactive T cells prevented from attacking the normal tissues? A major breakthrough in our understanding of peripheral tolerance came with the description of a particular population of CD4 T cells that were shown to suppress proliferation of effector cells. Termed regulatory T cells (Tregs), these unique T cells are distinguished by expression of the FoxP3 nuclear marker, and control autoimmune inflammation via contact-dependent mechanisms and suppressive cytokine production.[5]

Antibody (Humoral Immunity)

B cells migrate from the bone marrow and populate follicles around germinal centers of lymph nodes, spleen, and tonsils. Efficient antibody production occurs after the B cell recognizes an antigen through the surface-bound immunoglobulin receptor and receives costimulatory signals from T-helper cells. Early in the humoral immune response, B cells differentiate into IgM producing plasma cells. Further development of the humoral response involves increased antibody affinity and diversity through the processes of affinity maturation and somatic hypermutation. In addition, after a series of gene rearrangements, the B cell undergoes *class switching* and produces only one of the other antibody isotypes (IgG, IgA, IgD, or IgE). IgG isotypes, with lesser amounts of IgA, IgM, and IgE are found in serum, whereas secretions such as saliva contain primarily IgA and IgM.

Each of these immunoglobulins has different chemical and biologic properties. IgM antibodies are macromolecules composed of five antibody monomers and are produced chiefly during the body's primary response to a foreign antigen. IgM also plays an important role in the activation of complement and in the formation of immune complexes, which are aggregates of antibody, antigen, and complement. Most IgM in the body is intravascular. IgG constitutes 75% of the serum immunoglobulins and is the major component of the secondary antibody response. IgG crosses the placenta, giving protection to the newborn. It is the main immunoglobulin in tissue fluid, and over 50% of IgG in the body is extravascular. Four primary subgroups of IgG have been identified (IgG1, IgG2, IgG3, and IgG4), each of which have different biological properties. Serum IgA is the next most predominant immunoglobulin and is mainly monomeric. IgE binds to mast cells and basophils, triggering the release of histamine during allergic reactions such as anaphylaxis, hay fever, and asthma.

Antibodies found in secretions, such as saliva or bronchial secretions, are usually IgA (or sometimes IgM) produced by resident plasma cells of mucosal tissues. The antibodies are linked to secretory component, which facilitates antibody transport through the secretory epithelium. Another important molecule of secretory immunoglobulins is the J chain, which binds together the terminal portions of IgM monomers or IgA monomers to prevent proteolysis of the immunoglobulin molecule by secretory enzymes. Mucosal IgA is mainly dimeric and induced independently from serum IgA. It protects by neutralization of virus or enzyme, by aggregation of bacteria, and by preventing adherence of pathogens to the host.

Primary and Secondary Responses

Initial antigen recognition and the subsequent adaptive immune response typically peaks at 7–10 days, with IgM being the primary antibody produced.[1] After this first response, the sensitized specific T- and B-cells clones become antigen-specific memory cells, which can mount an adaptive immune response much quicker when challenged by the same antigen a second time. This secondary response peaks at 3–5 days, and is characterized by higher titers of predominately IgG antibody.

The Immune System of the Oral Cavity

Homeostasis in the oral cavity is maintained by the innate and adaptive systems in conjunction with normal oral flora and an intact oral mucosa. Components contributing to oral defenses include saliva with its innate antimicrobial proteins and secretory IgA, gingival crevicular fluid, transudate plasma proteins, circulating white blood cells, oral mucosal keratinocyte products, and proteins from microbial flora. Mucosal integrity prevents penetration of microorganisms and macromolecules in the diet and environment that might be antigenic. Different systems protect specific sites in the mouth. The crown of the tooth is protected from caries by salivary secretions, although neutrophil number and function must be adequate to prevent aggressive periodontitis. The complexity of the oral defense system is best illustrated by studies of humans who are deficient in particular arms of the immune system, such as those lacking adhesion molecules that results in leukocyte adhesion deficiency.

IMMUNODEFICIENCY

An individual with an *immunodeficiency* is a person whose immune system is not capable of mounting a normal immune response. The immunodeficiency may be hereditary, secondary to an infection such as human immunodeficiency virus (HIV), secondary to other major diseases such as cancer, diabetes or alcoholism, or a consequence of immunosuppressive medications. The number of patients with significant immunodeficiencies is increasing as patients with once-fatal diseases are living longer. HIV infection, cancer therapy, treatments for various autoimmune diseases, and organ or hematopoietic stem cell transplantation are more common causes of mild to profound immunosuppression that one might encounter in patients treated in regular dental practice.

PRIMARY IMMUNODEFICIENCIES

Primary immunodeficiencies (PIDs) are a heterogeneous group of genetic, often hereditary diseases affecting various components of the immune system. Defining the genetic causes that underlie PIDs and documenting infectious susceptibilities associated with specific genotypes has furthered our understanding of the roles specific immune factors and pathways play in mediating immunity, particularly in mounting defenses against specific pathogens. In 2011, the International Union of Immunological Societies Expert Committee on Primary Immunodeficiencies updated the classification of PIDs.[6] The update was warranted because of the discovery of many new genetic mutations that cause PIDs and further elucidation of relevant immune pathways. The update contained 15 new PIDs since the last revision, reflecting the rapid growth of new knowledge in this field. It is now estimated that up to 1 in 1200 persons in the United States have a PID.[7] To enhance clinical research studies of these diseases, multicenter registries have been established to define current natural histories of PIDs in this era of treatments such as hematopoietic stem cell transplant (HSCT) and gene therapy[8] that have dramatically changed the clinical courses of several PIDs. Registries help overcome the problems of past PID literature, which included small sample sizes, the use of different criteria to diagnose PIDs, and the tendency to describe patients with the most dramatic features. The goal of a multi-institutional registry is to enroll all patients that meet predefined PID diagnostic criteria and follow them prospectively to collect important, predefined outcomes.

In general, susceptibilities to specific types of infections are observed in different immunodeficiencies (Table 20-1). Therefore, when evaluating a patient suspected of having an immunodeficiency, a clinical immunologist notes the microbiological agent and frequency of infection. For example, a physician would suspect a T-cell defect in a child presenting with recurrent viral infections and oral candidiasis. Examples of different categories of PIDs with prevalent oral manifestations are reviewed in this chapter, but this list of PIDs is not comprehensive.

DEFECIENCIES IN ADAPTIVE IMMUNITY

Combined Immunodeficiency

Severe Combined Immunodeficiency

Children born with severe combined immunodeficiency (SCID) are profoundly immunocompromised. Without treatment, most die of infection before the age of 1 year.[9] The diagnosis of classic SCID is based on profound deficiencies of T-lymphocyte numbers and function, which may occur in the presence or absence of B and NK lymphocytes. Decreased levels of serum immunoglobulins are common in many,[8] consistent with the genetic mutations causing the SCID. Affected children are susceptible to infection with

TABLE 20-1	Infectious Susceptibilities and Oral Complications in Specific Immunodeficiencies		
Infection Susceptibility	**Immune Cells Involved**		**Specific Mutations/Syndromes**
Recurrent herpetic infections Human papilloma viruses	• T-cell function		• Tapasin genes/ MHC I deficiency • MCH II transcription genes/MHC II deficiency • Deletion chromosome 22q11.2/DiGeorge • DOCK8 • WAS/Wiskott–Aldrich syndrome • SCID
Odontogenic infections with sepsis	• B cells • Neutrophils		• BTK/BTK deficiency • Select IgG deficiencies • ITG/LAD-1
Chronic mucocutaneous candidiasis	• Epithelial cells (recognition of Candida) • T cells—particularly Th17		• Dectin-1 deficiency • CARD9 deficiency • Stat3 (Th17 differentiation)- HIES/JOBS • IL-17RA mutations • IL17F mutations • Sydromes with antibodies to IL-17F/IL22 (APECED)
Aggressive Periodontitis in Children and Young Adults	• Neutrophils		• ELANE mutations/cyclic neutropenia and severe congenital neutropenia • WAS /X-linked neutropenia • COH1/Cohen sydrome • LYST/Chediak–Higashi syndrome • ITG/LAD-1 • CTSC/Papillon–Lefèvre syndrome • FPR1/LJP

multiple bacteria, viruses, and fungi. Many types of genetic defects can result in SCID, including adenosine deaminase (ADA) deficiency, mutations in the γc subunit of cytokine receptors that result in X-linked SCID, mutations in the recombination-activating gene 1 or 2 (*RAG1* or *RAG2*), JAK3 mutations, mutations in the IL-7 receptor, and mutations in the CD3δ and CD3ε chains.[8–10] Mutations of these genes block normal T maturation. HSCT is the standard treatment for these children[10] and is more successful if performed early in life. Newborns suspected of having SCID can be screened using a test that involves quantification of T-cell receptor excision circles, which are nonreplicative pieces of DNA formed during normal T-cell receptor gene rearrangement in the thymus.[11] *Ex vivo* gene therapy has been tested to correct the immunodeficiency in 20 children with SCID-X1 and 38 with ADA deficiency[12]. Though five of the children with SCID-X1 subsequently developed T-cell leukemia, gene therapy continues to be tested as a treatment for these patients, particular those who lack human leukocyte antigen (HLA)–compatible donors for HSCT.

Oral complications noted in children with SCID include aphthous-like ulcerations,[10,13] candidiasis, and herpetic infections.[14,15,16] Children treated with HSCT may present with multiple complications associated with transplant and graft-versus-host disease (GVHD) (see Chapter 21, Transplantation Medicine).

Wiskott–Aldrich Syndrome

Wiskott–Aldrich syndrome (WAS) is a rare X-linked disorder characterized by thrombocytopenia, microcytic platelets, eczema, recurrent infections, and an increased

incidence of autoimmune disease and malignancies.[17,18] Clinical manifestations of classic WAS that can occur shortly after birth include petechiae, bruising, bloody diarrhea, otitis media, skin infections, and pneumonia from bacteria, but manifestations may be delayed to a later age. Other complications such as autoimmune hemolytic anemia, autoimmune neutropenia, and vasculitis are found.[17] The central defect in WAS is a defect in the *WAS* gene, which causes production of abnormal WAS protein (WASp). WASp is involved in transduction of signals from the cell surface of immune cells to the actin cytoskeleton. The severity of the immune deficiency in WAS varies between families, depending on the location of the mutations in the *WAS* gene. Mutations can affect both T and B cells, as well as platelets. Children born with classic WAS initially may have normal numbers of T cells, but T-cell counts may decline as the child ages. B cells numbers may be decreased or normal. Although WAS patients produce some antibodies, they often have impaired responses to polysaccharide antigens. Other clinical problems include an increased incidence of malignancy, particularly lymphomas.[17] Reported oral manifestations include purpura, oral bleeding,[17] candidiasis,[15] and herpetic infections[19]. Patients may have undergone splenectomy to increase platelet numbers and reduce bleeding episodes; therefore, antibiotic prophylaxis may be indicated for more invasive procedures[18].

Ataxia Telangiectasia

Ataxia telangiectasia (AT) is an inherited, autosomal recessive degenerative disorder characterized by cerebellar degeneration. The classic form of AT results from mutations of the *ATM* gene, which encodes the ATM protein that is a serine/threonine protein kinase broadly involved in cellular responses to DNA double strand breaks and cell cycle control.[20-22] In genotype/phenotype studies, disease severity is related to levels of the ATM kinase activity.[22] It is estimated to occur in 1:40,000 to 1:300,000 births, affecting men and women equally. Early clinical presentation includes deterioration of the gait between 1 and 4 years of age, with continued ataxia. Other features are ocular and facial telangiectases and a varied immunodeficiency including sinopulmonary infections.[21,22] Telangiectases of the skin and eyes become apparent after infancy. Though not all patients with AT have immunodeficiency, cohort studies identified up to 69% have evidence of a T-cell deficiency,[21,22] with decreased serum IgA in 60%, and decreased IgG2 in 48%. Reduced immune repertoire formation and reduced memory B-cell formation is proposed as a mechanism for the immunodeficiency in this disease.[23] These reductions are believed to be the result of insufficient ATM activity during double-strand DNA repair, which impairs class switching and V(D)J recombination. Patients with recurrent infections are treated with intravenous (IV) pooled immunoglobulin. Over 15% of individuals with severe AT develop cancers, particular of lymphoid origin, which often occur in childhood.[22] Many develop infections consistent with their T-cell deficiency, including warts, herpes simplex, molluscum contagiosum, candidal esophagitis, and herpes zoster,[21] in addition to sinopulmonary infections.

T-Cell Deficiencies

Decrease in T-Cell Number

Chromosome 22q11.2 Deletion Syndrome (DiGeorge Syndrome; Velocardiofacial Syndrome)

Deletion of chromosome 22q11.2 is one of the most common human deletion syndromes,[24] now estimated to occur in approximately 1 of 4000 births. The majority of patients with DiGeorge syndrome and Velocardiac facial syndrome have monosomic deletions of chromosome 22q11.2. As more cases are identified and studied, the full, highly variable spectrum of clinical consequences associated with this deletion are being characterized through cohort studies such as the registry at the Children's Hospital of Philadelphia (CHOP).[24] Common features in 906 individuals enrolled in the CHOP study were cardiac anomalies (77%) such as tetralogy of Fallot (20%) or ventriculoseptal defect (21%), lower than normal IQ (82%), oropharyngeal defects such as velopharyngeal insufficiency (42%), hypocalcemia (49%), and immune dysfunction (77%) most likely secondary to thymic hypoplasia.

The common embryonic precursors for the thymus, parathyroid, and conotruncal regions of the heart are the pharyngeal arches and pouches.[25] The cardiac neural crest cells, critical cells of the embryo, are necessary for normal cardiovascular development.[26] It is believed that these cells must migrate correctly for normal development of craniofacial complex, pharynx, and heart. Abnormal migration of neural crest cells in 22q11.2 deletion syndrome is hypothesized to impair normal development of the organs involved in the syndrome, such as the heart, the thymus, the parathyroid glands, and pharyngeal tissues. The 22q11.2 deletion mouse model is expected to further define the molecular basis of this syndrome.[25,26]

Clinically, patients with 22q11.2 deletion syndrome may present with a small or absent thymus, which impairs T-cell development. Normally after production in the bone marrow, progenitors of T lymphocytes migrate to the thymus for further selection and differentiation.[1] Before entering the thymus, T lymphocytes do not express the T-cell receptor, CD4 or CD8 markers. During their time in the thymus, T cells acquire the CD4 or CD8 molecule, and autoreactive T cells are deleted through a process of negative selection. Inadequate thymic function can result in low numbers of circulating T cells (both CD4 and CD8), which creates an immunodeficiency characterized by an increased susceptibility to infections with viruses and fungi. The severity of the T-cell deficiency in this deletion syndrome varies widely and rarely includes decreased serum immunoglobulins.[25] Although children can present with infections associated with T-cell deficiencies such as florid candidiasis (Figure 20-1), some patients have absent or mild signs of immunosuppression.[25] The rare patient with complete absence of the thymus may be treated with thymic transplant or HSCT with varying degrees of success.[25] Other presumed long-term consequences of thymic hypoplasia include increased prevalence of autoimmune diseases such as immune thrombocytopenia, and a possible predisposition to malignancy.[27] The abnormal development of the parathyroid glands can cause hypocalcemia, present in almost half of the patients.[24]

Craniofacial features of 22q11.2 deletion syndrome include velopharyngeal insufficiency (42%), submucous clefts (16%), cleft palate (up to 11%), bifid uvula, oral candidiasis, short palpebral fissures, a small mouth, prominent forehead, enamel hypoplasia, and hypodontia.[24,27,28] Insufficiency of the muscle groups in the velopharyngeal portal can cause abnormal speech such as hypernasality, poor feeding, and nasal regurgitation when babies drink liquids. The behavioral and neuropsychiatric aspects of 22q11.2 deletion syndrome, such as attention deficit hyperactivity disorder, autism and schizophrenia, are being defined in larger groups that more adequately represent the spectrum of the disease.[24].

Qualitative T-Cell Defects

Defects in the Major Histocompatibility Complex

If genes encoding the essential MHC proteins are mutated or deleted, there can be an impairment of both cell-mediated and humoral responses. The immunodeficiency associated with these defects was originally called *bare lymphocyte syndrome*. Further studies established that this syndrome encompasses several diseases mediated by defects in the expression of MHC molecules. Patients unable to express MHC Class I antigens correctly lack adequate presentation

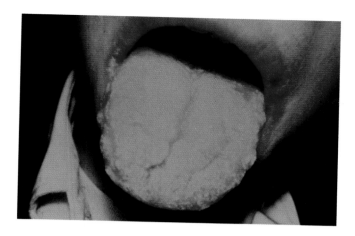

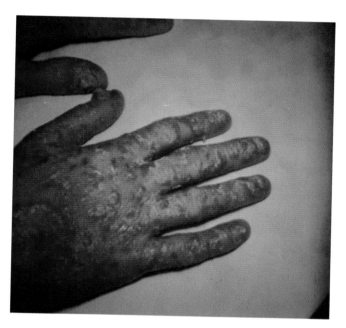

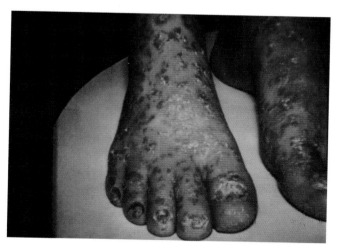

FIGURE 20-1 A, Chronic mucocutaneous candidiasis in patient with DiGeorge syndrome, with lesions of the tongue. B, Lesions of the same infection, on the hands. C, Lesions of the same infection, on the feet.

of antigenic peptides to CD8+ T cells and may have low CD8+ T-cell numbers.[6] This results in inadequate cytotoxic T-cell activation. Defects in MHC Class II expression ultimately lead to a decrease of CD4+ T cells that need these molecules for maturation.[29,30] Though B-cell numbers are normal in patients with MHC defects, serum immunoglobulin levels are decreased, as T cells fail to present antigen to B cells. *Cytomegalovirus*, *Salmonella*, and *Cryptosporidium* infections can occur, in addition to *Candida albicans*, herpes simplex viruses, and other opportunistic infections in the oral cavity. Many patients will die at a young age without HSCT.[31]

B-Cell Deficiencies

Inadequate B-cell number or function translates clinically into insufficient levels of circulating antibodies, termed hypogammaglobulinemia.[1] Extracellular bacteria often cause respiratory and sinus infections in patients with B-cell defects, demonstrating the importance of antibodies for defense of these tissues. Decreased resistance to bacterial infections is a major feature of patients with B-cell deficiencies, so patients may become septic from odontogenic infections. Recurrent aphthae occur.

Decrease in B-cell number

Bruton's X-linked Agammaglobulinemia and Other Immunodeficiencies Causing Profound Agammaglobulinemia

B-cell maturation and subsequent antibody production is a complex series of events with multiple steps. Initially, the precursor is produced in the bone marrow[32–34] where it develops into a pro-B cell. The pro-B cell must successfully transition through the pre-B-I and pre-B-II stages before leaving the bone marrow. A group of genetic PIDs caused by mutations in the genes involved with this process are Bruton's X-linked agammaglobulinemia and other immunodeficiencies causing agammaglobulinemia.

Bruton's X-linked agammaglobulinemia is a rare disorder (estimated to occur in 1 of 200,000 births) characterized by grossly depressed numbers of circulating B cells, normal numbers of pro-B cells, and little or no circulating immunoglobulin.[33–36] Newborns with this immunodeficiency are protected initially from infection by maternal antibodies, so diagnosis may be delayed for several months or even a few years. Clinical presentation is in a boy with recurrent pulmonary and sinus infections.[34,35] Patients have a high incidence of pneumonia, arthritis, and meningitis, and may also present with diarrhea and otitis media. Organisms often involved in these infections include streptococci, staphylococci, pseudomonas, and *Haemophilus influenzae*.[35,36] The primary defect in Bruton's X-linked agammaglobulinemia is a mutation of the *Btk* gene that is encoded in 19 exons at Xq22 and is expressed in all stages of B-cell maturation except for the plasma cell stage. Although over 800 mutations in *Btk* have been identified in families to date, it has been difficult to relate specific mutations to clinical phenotypes.[33] With aggressive antibiotic treatment and IV pooled immunoglobulin transfusions, patients with Bruton's X-linked agammaglobulinemia are surviving into middle age.[36] Many patients have adequate T-cell and phagocyte function, which provides protection from many viral and fungal infections once T-cell immunity develops. Although HSCT is not typically used for treatment,[36] inserting a functional *Btk* gene into stem cells using gene therapy techniques has been suggested as a future therapy for these patients.[33]

Individuals with other less common immunodeficiencies, such as μ heavy chain deficiency, λ5 deficiency, Igα deficiency, and Igβ deficiency, also present with normal numbers of pro-B cells, profound agammaglobulinemia, and the same clinical presentation as Bruton's. These patients may be men or women, and often have a homozygous recessive mutation in one of several genes involved with the maturation of pro-B cells to pre-B cells.[6] They do not have mutations involving *Btk*, but are managed similarly to Bruton's as they have the same clinical course and infectious susceptibilities.

DECREASES IN CERTAIN CLASSES OF IMMUNOGLOBULINS WITH NORMAL OR LOW NUMBER OF B CELLS

Common Variable Immunodeficiency Disorders

Common variable immunodeficiency (CVID) is a group of diseases characterized by an inability to produce sufficient levels of all classes of antibodies, particularly IgG and IgA.[6,37] Onset of clinical symptoms is varied, manifesting in both men and women sometime during early childhood to the second or third decade of life. The group is characterized by decreased immunoglobulins, the lack of significant antibody responses to protein antigens following immunization, and excludes those with other known causes of failure of immunoglobulin production as defined by the IUIS Primary Immunodeficiency Diseases Classification Committee.[6,38] Therefore, it is a diagnosis made by exclusion. Patients have the same infectious susceptibilities as those with Bruton's and to infections with particular organisms, including recurrent urinary tract infections due to *Ureaplasma urealyticum*, *Mycoplasma* species, and enteroviral infections. However, the spectrum of disease can be quite varied, from mild to severe. Other complications include development of autoimmune disease, the presence of multisystem granulomas, bronchiectasis, splenomegaly and hepatomegaly, and lymphoid malignancy such as non-Hodgkin lymphoma that are often in mucosal areas.[37,38] Patients may have immune thrombocytopenia.[39] The spectrum of disease is quite heterogeneous, as the group includes individuals with depressed immunoglobulin production secondary to several different impaired immune pathways. T-cell function is abnormal in some patients.[37]

Deficiency of ICOS, TACI, CD81, CD19 or BAFF Receptor

Genetic mutations in several immune pathways can cause the similar varied clinical spectrum of CVID infections.[39,40] Some of these genes regulate expression of cell surface ligands needed for T cell–B cell interactions. Without these interactions, B cells are not stimulated to make antibody. Two such examples are mutations of the inducible T-cell costimulator gene (ICOS) and mutations of TNFRSF13B, which encodes the transmembrane activator and calcium modulator and cyclophilin ligand interactor (TACI).[39,40] It is expected that future genetic studies will identify new mutations and functional deficiencies in many patients currently classified as having CVID.

Selective Immunoglobulin Deficiencies

Selective immunoglobulin deficiencies are characterized by an inability to produce a single class of antibody.[1] They are extremely varied in clinical presentation. Many patients have a fully functional immune system, and the deficiency is only noted if immunoglobulin levels are determined for another reason. Individuals may be healthy, as immunoglobulins of the other classes can provide adequate humoral defenses. Other patients present with recurrent respiratory infections, which leads to the diagnosis. Immunoglobulin isotypes, such as IgG subclasses, must be determined to make the diagnosis.

The most common immunodeficiency is selective IgA deficiency, occurring in 1 of 155 to 1 of 18,500 people,[41,42] with an estimated prevalence of 1 of 600 Caucasians. While some people are healthy, others have chronic respiratory or gastrointestinal infections.[41] Autoimmune diseases, such as systemic lupus erythematosus (SLE), rheumatoid arthritis (RA), and pernicious anemia, are more common in this deficiency.[41,42] Developmentally, B-cell maturation in IgA deficiency is impaired. As secretory IgA is the major immunoglobulin of saliva, the oral health of this patient group has been studied in detail. There is not sufficient evidence to conclude that patients with selective IgA deficiency have an increase in adult dental caries or periodontal disease,[43,44,45] though a small, unblinded study reported an increase in deciduous caries.[45] In one study, antistreptococcal mutans salivary IgM was higher in patients without salivary IgA, suggesting that IgM compensates for the loss of IgA in this population.[46]

HYPER-IGE SYNDROMES

The hyper-IgE syndromes (HIES) comprise a group of PIDs that are characterized by significantly elevated IgE levels and recurrent skin and pulmonary infections. Both autosomal dominant and autosomal recessive HIES form of the disorder have been described. Most autosomal dominant HIES (AD-HIES) are caused by mutations in STAT3 (signal transducer and activator of transcription 3; MIM#147060),[47] whereas DOCK8 (dedicator of cytokinesis 8) mutations have been identified in patients with autosomal recessive HIES (AR-HIES; MIM#243700).[47]

Autosomal Dominant Hyper-IgE Syndromes/ Job's Syndrome

First described in 1966, Job's syndrome is characterized by the triad of eczematoid dermatitis, recurrent skin and pulmonary infections.[48] Today AD-HIES is recognized as a multisystem disease with immunological and connective tissue features.[49] The link between the diverse array of manifestations was identified in 2007 when dominant-negative mutations in STAT3 were shown to underlie HIES.[50] STAT3 is integral to signal transduction for multiple cytokines and is widely expressed across tissue types. Oral, immunological, and skeletal findings are common in HIES.[47]

Oral Features of Immune Compromise

Patients with AD-HIES have increased susceptibility to fungal infection. Up to 80% are affected with chronic mucocutaneous candidiasis.[47] Defective STAT3-dependent differentiation of Th17 cells is thought to underlie fungal susceptibility in AD-HIES.[51] Defective IL-17 signaling has been linked to mucocutaneous candidiasis (see below). Importantly, the saliva of individuals with HIES has low levels of critical candidacidal peptides, including histatins and BD2 that are induced by IL-17.[52]

Craniofacial and Dental Features of HIES

Unique facial features are characteristic of AD-HIES. These features are noted in late childhood and early adolescence and become almost universal by late adolescence. They involve asymmetric facies with prominent forehead and chin, increased inter-alar width, wide-set eyes, and coarse skin.[53] In addition, craniosynostosis and Chiari I malformations have also been reported, although these are largely asymptomatic and do not usually require surgical intervention.[47]

Delayed exfoliation of primary teeth is also a frequent feature, with approximately 70% of patients reporting having delayed exfoliation of three or more teeth (Figure 20-2). Delay or absence of root resorption in primary teeth is observed, although the mechanism underlying

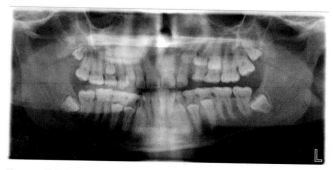

Figure 20-2 Panorex from a 22-year-old man with Job's syndrome demonstrating a generalized failure in primary tooth root resorption.

this phenomenon remains unclear.[47] Other intraoral findings include a high-arched palate with central ridges and fissures, and deep grooves and fissures on the tongue and buccal mucosa.[53]

AR-HIES/DOCK8 Deficiency

DOCK8 deficiency was identified in patients with an AR-HIES characterized by frequent, and often severe, viral and bacterial skin and respiratory tract infections, eczema, and malignancy.[54] Similar to AD-HIES these patients also exhibit cold abscesses and mucocutaneous candidiasis, but they lack the skeletal features of Jobs. The molecular defect is localized to DOCK8. DOCKs are a family of factors involved in actin cytoskeletal rearrangement and receptor-mediated signaling.[55] Immunologically, patients with DOCK8 deficiency have progressive B-cell, T-cell, and NK-cell lymphopenia, defects in CD8+ T-cell survival, NK-cell function and B-cell activation.[55] Intriguingly, the WASP, reduced or absent in WAS, functions downstream of DOCK8. WAS- and DOCK8-deficient patients share many clinical and laboratory findings.[55]

Reported oral manifestations in DOCK8 include persistent and often ulcerating *Herpes simplex* orolabial infections, oral associated abscesses, and orofacial squamous-cell dysplasia and carcinomas in patients with long-standing HSV infections.[54]

DEFECTS IN INNATE IMMUNITY
Chronic Mucocutaneous Candidiasis

T lymphocytes and epithelial cells appear to be most important for the control of mucocutaneous *Candida* infections. In recent years, human and animal studies have demonstrated the dominant role of IL-17 in anticandidal immunity.[56] *Candida* is typically recognized by Dectin-1 on epithelial and myeloid cells, and this initial interaction leads to CARD9-induced production of cytokines that promote Th17 differentiation through STAT3.[57] In turn, Th17 cells secrete IL-17A, IL-17F, and IL-22 that activate production of antimicrobial peptides and recruitment of neutrophils. Genetic defects associated with these pathways have been linked to chronic mucocutaneous candidiasis (CMC) with manifestations in the oral cavity. These include mutations in Dectin-1, CARD9, STAT3, IL-17RA, IL-17F, and syndromes with neutralizing antibodies against IL-17F and IL-22 (APECED).[57]

NEUTROPHIL DEFECTS

To function correctly, neutrophils and monocytes must migrate to sites of infection through a process known as chemotaxis, phagocytize bacteria, and have the capacity to kill engulfed pathogens. Recurrent infections with staphylococci, *Pseudomonas*, *Candida*, and other fungi occur if neutrophil number is severely decreased or phagocyte function is very abnormal.[58] Although secondary defects in neutrophil numbers and function will be covered in a separate section (see Chapter 18, Hematologic Diseases), this chapter will briefly review the PIDs that affect neutrophils and their oral consequences. The most recent classification of PIDs[6] has divided neutrophil disorders into those that affect neutrophil differentiation, defects of neutrophil motility, and defects in respiratory burst.

Disorders That Affect Neutrophil Differentiation

Defects of differentiation can attributed to various genetic defects. Mutations in the *ELANE* gene, which encodes neutrophil elastase, are involved in cyclic neutropenia and also in 40%–55% of cases of severe congenital neutropenia. Mutations in the *WAS* gene are linked to X-linked neutropenia, mutations in gene *COH1* are linked to Cohen syndrome, and mutations in the *LYST* gene lead to Chediak-Higashi syndrome. All syndromes result in neutropenia.[6] In the oral setting, many genetic forms of neutropenia are associated with severe forms of periodontitis in children and adults.[59]

Defects of Neutrophil Motility

Defects in neutrophil motility have been largely associated with severe early onset forms of periodontitis that manifests in children and adolescents. Some of the best characterized syndromes are LAD-1, an autosomal recessive disorder produced by mutations in the common β2 chain (CD18) of the β2 integrin family (ITGB2, 21q22.3)[60] that are required for tight adhesion and transmigration of neutrophils, and Papillon–Lefèvre syndrome caused by mutation in cathepsin C that leads to defective neutrophil chemotaxis.[6]

Defects of Respiratory Burst

Defects in the nicotinamide adenine dinucleotide phosphate (NADPH) oxidase are associated with autosomal and X-linked forms of chronic granulomatous disease (CGD), a rare genetic disease that predisposes individuals to recurrent life-threatening infections mostly caused by catalase-positive bacteria and fungi.[60] NADPH oxidase is assembled from six proteins in the secondary granule wall (p22phox and gp91phox), the cytosol (p40phox, p47phox, and p67phox), and the plasma membrane (Rac2). This complex is integral in the formation of superoxide and its downstream metabolites, which are pivotal for efficient microbial killing of engulfed bacteria. The gastrointestinal tract (including the oral cavity) of CGD patients is affected frequently by inflammatory and granulomatous manifestations.[60]

SECONDARY IMMUNODEFICIENCIES

Many disorders are associated secondarily with decreased numbers or function of the various components of the immune system, leading to increased incidence of infections. Just like PIDs, the type of infections suffered by patients with secondary immunodeficiencies depends on which particular component of the immune system is compromised, although frequently multiple defects are present. Secondary immunodeficiencies result either from decreased production or increased destruction of immune cells or loss of components of humoral immunity.

Cellular (Primarily Neutrophils)

Neutropenia can occur with several conditions, including hematologic malignancies, especially when the malignancy suppresses growth of myeloid precursors. Decreased neutrophil counts occur frequently during cancer chemotherapy, HSCT, aplastic anemia, and autoimmune neutropenia (see Chapter 18, Hematologic Diseases). There is a progressively increasing risk of infection in patients with low neutrophil count, which starts at an absolute neutrophil count (ANC) of 1000 cells/mm[3]. However, the majority of infections occur with counts below 500 cells/mm[3] and in particular below 100 cells/mm[3].[61,62] Although no published evidence exists regarding efficacy of prophylactic antibiotics before invasive dental procedures in neutropenic patients, many authorities recommend their use in patients with ANC below 500 cells/mm[3]. Whenever used, basic principles of antibiotic prophylaxis should be followed—antibiotics should be given in a single dose before the start of the procedure. Protocols recommended by the American Heart Association (AHA), which are designed to prevent bacteremia from oral sources, are the most commonly used.[63]

Complement

Acquired deficiency in complement components has been observed in advanced liver disease and is associated with an increased incidence of bacterial infections in these patients.[64] In addition, dysfunction of the complement pathway has been shown in some malignancies, such as chronic lymphocytic leukemia (CLL).[65] Individuals with inherited complement deficiencies may have infectious susceptibilities.[60]

Adaptive Immune System

Several conditions decrease T-cell numbers such as HIV infection, and/or function such as chronic GVHD, treatment with calcineurin inhibitors, treatment with antitumor necrosis factor-α (TNF-α) agents and other agents that block other immunomodulatory proteins. Clinically, patients often present with opportunistic infections. Specific aspects of these conditions are covered in the dedicated portions of this book. Infections with intracellular bacteria and fungi (*Pneumocystis carinii*), viruses (such as *Herpes* family viruses and papilloma viruses) (Figures 20-3 and 20-4), and parasites (*Toxoplasma* and *Cryptosporidium*) are typical of T-cell deficient states. Oral candidiasis is frequently the first sign of advanced HIV infection. *Herpes zoster* is common in patients with CLL.[65,66]

Humoral (Antibodies)

Secondary humoral immunodeficiency can be observed in conditions associated with increased loss (nephrotic syndrome)

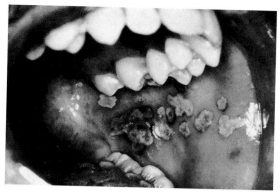

FIGURE 20-3 Extensive recurrent herpes simplex lesions of the buccal mucosa and palate of a patient receiving chemotherapy for leukemia.

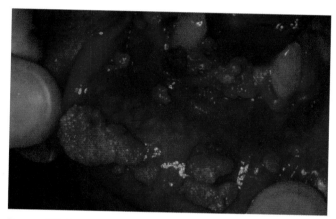

FIGURE 20-4 Extensive condyloma acuminatum from human papillomavirus infection in a patient receiving chemotherapy for non-Hodgkin's lymphoma.

or decreased production (multiple myeloma, CLL) of immunoglobulins. Antibodies are important in combating primarily extracellular bacterial infections and to a lesser degree viral infections before cell entry. Patients with decreased blood antibody concentrations are particularly susceptible to systemic infections with encapsulated bacteria such as *Streptococcus pneumoniae*, *Klebsiella*, and *Haemophilus influenzae*.[67]

AUTOIMMUNE DISEASES

The term *autoimmune disease* refers to a disorder in which there is evidence of an immune response against self.[1] Autoimmune diseases may be primarily due to either antibodies (autoantibodies) or immune cells, but a common characteristic is the presence of a lymphocytic infiltration in the target organ. Examples include type 1 diabetes mellitus, autoimmune thyroiditis, Sjögren's syndrome, SLE, and multiple sclerosis. Circulating antibodies can often be detected in vitro by tests that demonstrate antibody binding to appropriate human tissue substrates. In many cases, there is clear evidence that the autoantibodies are involved

in the disease pathophysiology (e.g., pemphigus). However, in other diseases autoantibodies have undefined roles and their presence is used primarily for diagnosis. In addition, autoantibodies are rarely specific for one autoimmune disease (Table 20-2). A common mechanism believed to be central to all autoimmune diseases is the failure of peripheral tolerance systems that normally control autoreactive T-cell clones.

Systemic Lupus Erythematosus

Systemic lupus erythematosus (SLE) is a multisystem autoimmune inflammatory disorder of unknown etiology. It is regarded as the archetypal autoimmune disease. An important feature is the formation of antibodies to DNA, which are associated with lupus nephritis. In the United States, SLE has a prevalence of approximately 1 in 2000 with a woman to man ratio of 9:1, and the prevalence is estimated to be two- to fourfold higher in non-Caucasian populations than in Caucasian populations.[68] In addition to systemic and isolated cutaneous lupus (chronic discoid lupus), a distinct syndrome of drug-induced lupus is recognized. Unlike SLE, drug-induced lupus rarely affects the kidney and is reversible on discontinuation of the offending agent.

Etiology and Pathogenesis

Although the exact etiology of SLE is unknown, a complex interplay of genetic and environmental factors that leads to a progressive loss of peripheral tolerance and production of autoantibodies is believed to be crucial for SLE initiation.[69] The genetic predisposition to SLE is demonstrated by twin studies. Concordance for SLE in dizygotic twins is 3%, whereas it is up to 34% for monozygotic twins.[70] The risk for SLE developing in a sibling of an affected person is up to 29 times higher than that in a general population. Genome-wide linkage and association studies have identified several gene groups strongly correlated with SLE. Genetic deficiency in complement components, although rare overall, are among the strongest risk factors for SLE. Ninety percent of persons with homozygous C1q deficiency and approximately 33% of those homozygous for *C2* deletion will develop SLE.[70] Our understanding of genetics and SLE has expanded greatly through genome-wide association studies (GWAS) that help define how common variants contribute to complex human diseases. Genome-wide studies have identified at least 29 SLE susceptibility loci that can be grouped by putative function into those involved in toll-like receptors (TLRs) and type I interferons (IFNs) signaling, TLR/IFN and lymphocyte signaling, lymphocyte development and signaling, and other/no known immune function.[70] At least three main immune pathways may be involved: aberrant clearance of nucleic acid–containing debris and immune complexes, excessive innate immune activation involving TLRs and type I IFNs, and abnormal T- and B-lymphocyte activation.[69] The importance of type I IFN genes in the pathogenesis of

TABLE 20-2 Autoantibody Profiles of Different Autoimmune Diseases

Autoantibody	Prevalence (% positive)					
	Systemic Lupus Erythematosus	Rheumatoid Arthritis	Sjögren's Syndrome	Systemic Sclerosis	Polymyositis/ Dermatomyositis	Mixed Connective Tissue Disease
Antinuclear antibodies[a]	95–100	30–60	90	90–96	60–80	>99
Anti-double-stranded DNA	40–80		5			
IgM rheumatoid factor	5–30	70–80	73	25	8	48
Anticyclic citrullinated antibody	13	65–80	1	11		
Anti-Sm	30–40	10	1	4		rare
Anti-U1 RNP	13–23	5	2	5–11	4	100
Anti-Ro/SS-A	24–60	3–15	54–80	11	21–30	24
Anti-La/SS-B	6–35	0–2	26–42	6	13	
Anti-Scl-70				84 (in diffuse form only)		8
Anti-centromere				70–80 (in CREST form only)		
Anti-Jo-1					23–36 (highest in DM)	

[a]Screening test that detects multiple autoantibodies
Sources: Adapted from Harris ED et al.[80]; Sherer Y et al.[92]; Zendman AJ et al.[160]; Rantapaa-Dahlqvist S[175]; Lee SJ, Kavanaugh A [176]; Lyons R et al.[200]; Sauerland U et al[201]; Ramos-Casals M et al[202]; Kyriakidis NC et al.[203]; Ghirardello A et al[204]; Piirainen HI.[205]

lupus has come to the fore and new treatments are in development based on this discovery.

As the concordance in monozygotic twins is less than 100%, factors other than genetic predisposition must play a role in the development of SLE. Environmental factors, including infections particularly with EBV and other viruses, exposure to pollutants, hormonal factors, ultraviolet light and smoking, and possibly diet have been linked to the development of SLE. In addition, over 80 drugs, classically hydralazine, isoniazide, and procainamide are associated with drug-induced lupus.[71]

Numerous immunologic abnormalities have been described in SLE.[72] Processes thought to be central to the pathogenesis are immune complex formation and deposition in target organs, complement activation, attraction of effector cells, and subsequent target tissue damage.[69] The innate immune system is activated by nucleic acids that are generated when cells normally break down, and must be cleared daily through a process that involves removal of the debris with minimal inflammation. The best studied innate cell in SLE is the plasmacytoid dendritic cell (pDC) that produces large amounts of type I IFNs when activated after exposure to cellular debris that is not cleared.[69] Other cytokines are produced, and the adaptive immune system becomes activated. B lymphocytes are involved at several stages in the development of lupus. Autoreactive B cells occur in normal individuals and are usually controlled by a variety of mechanisms

including clonal deletion, anergy, and Tregs.[73] Autoimmune disease tends to occur when the action of effector T cells is greater than that of Tregs. In SLE, Tregs appear to occur in lower numbers and function less than in healthy individuals.[73] In patients with SLE, autoreactive B cells escape peripheral control mechanisms and actively begin producing autoantibodies. Autoantibody production may precede clinical manifestations of SLE, sometimes by many years.[73]

Other components of the immune system may participate in the pathogenesis of SLE. Efficient antibody production cannot occur in the absence of appropriate T-cell help, and T cells become activated by the presentation of a peptide-MHC complex on the surface of an antigen-presenting cell.[70] There is evidence of a loss of T-cell and B-cell tolerance in SLE.[69] Other antigens, possibly from cytosolic RNA derived from viruses, may trigger some cases.[69] Complement plays a dual role in the pathogenesis of SLE. Although deficiencies in certain complement components are risk factors for SLE, complement activation following immune complex deposition is a major mechanism responsible for target tissue damage in SLE and decreases in complement components C3 and C4 correlate with flares of the disease.[69]

Clinical Manifestations

Lupus is known as *the great mimic*. Indeed, SLE can affect virtually every organ system and cause a wide spectrum of clinical symptoms. Skin is affected in up to 85% of SLE

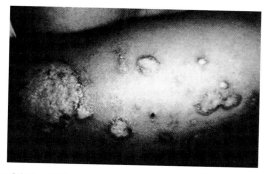

FIGURE 20-5 Skin lesions in a patient with systemic lupus erythematosus. (Courtesy of Dr. George Ehrlich.)

patients (Figure 20-5). In addition, cutaneous lupus can occur without multisystem involvement. Skin lesions of lupus can be classified into lupus-specific (having diagnostic clinical or histopathological features) and nonspecific lesions.

Three subtypes of lupus-specific skin lesions have been described: acute, subacute, and chronic.[75,76,77] Acute cutaneous lupus occurs in 30%–50% of patients and is classically represented by the butterfly rash—mask-shaped erythematous eruptions involving the malar areas and bridge of the nose but typically (as opposed to dermatomyositis) sparing nasolabial folds (Figure 20-6). Bullous lupus and localized erythematous papules also belong to the acute lupus category. Chronic cutaneous lupus occurs in 15%–20% of cases and affects the skin of the face or scalp in about 80% of cases (Figure 20-7). The least common subtype, subacute cutaneous lupus, occurs in 10%–15% of patients and includes papulosquamous (psoriasiform) and annular-polycyclic eruptions usually on the trunk and arms. Nonspecific but suggestive skin manifestations of lupus are common and include alopecia (both scarring, following discoid lesions and nonscarring), photosensitivity, Raynaud's phenomenon, livedo reticularis, urticaria, erythema, telangiectases, and cutaneous vasculitis.[75–77]

Renal

Kidney involvement occurs in up to 50%–60% of patients with SLE and is a primary cause of morbidity and mortality in this population.[78,79] Clinically, renal disease in SLE can range anywhere from asymptomatic proteinuria to rapidly progressive glomerulonephritis with renal failure. Several histological subtypes have been described. The severity of renal disease and its response to treatment are good predictors of overall prognosis in SLE.[79,80]

Musculoskeletal

Musculoskeletal manifestations occur in about 95% of patients with SLE, and arthralgia is the first presenting symptom in about 50% of cases.[80,81] Nonerosive symmetric arthritis most commonly affecting hands, wrists, and knees is typical of SLE. Fixed joint deformity (Jaccoud's arthropathy) can rarely occur and is due to ligamentous and tendon involvement. History of temporomandibular joint

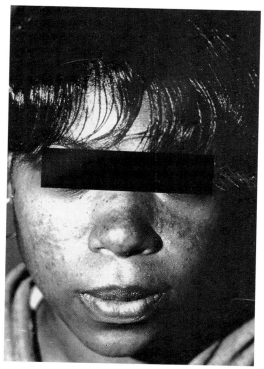

FIGURE 20-6 *Butterfly* rash on the face of a patient with systemic lupus erythematosus. (Courtesy of Dr. Robert Arm.)

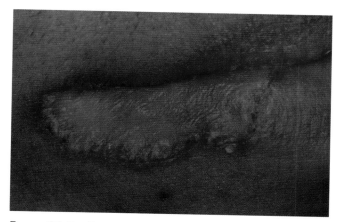

FIGURE 20-7 Discoid lupus lesions on the lower lip.

(TMJ)–related symptoms was reported in two thirds of SLE patients in one study.[82] Myalgias and myositis are also common. Avascular necrosis of the bones is a major cause of morbidity and is usually associated with corticosteroid therapy.[81]

Central Nervous System

Central nervous system (CNS) involvement occurs in about 20% of patients with SLE and is usually due to cerebral vasculitis or direct neuronal damage. CNS manifestations include psychosis, stroke, seizures and transverse myelitis and are associated with poor overall prognosis.[83]

Cardiovascular

Cardiovascular involvement in SLE is classically manifested by vasculitis and pericarditis.[84] In addition, endocardial damage (Libman–Sachs endocarditis and superimposed bacterial endocarditis), myocarditis, and conduction defects are commonly described. With increasing survival of lupus patients, accelerated atherosclerosis with coronary artery disease has become an important clinical problem.[84] In a community-based study, myocardial infarction (MI), heart failure, and stroke were 8.5, 13.2, and 10.1 (respectively) times more likely to occur in women with SLE than in the general population.[85] Multiple defects of blood coagulation pathways have been described in SLE. Abnormalities in fibrinolysis, decreases of anticoagulant proteins (protein S), and presence of antiphospoholipid antibodies contribute to increased tendency to thrombosis in SLE.[86] CNS and deep venous thromboses with pulmonary emboli are major causes of morbidity in these patients requiring high level of anticoagulation for prevention.

Other Manifestations

Fatigue, depression, and fibromyalgia-like symptoms are commonly present and can be debilitating.[80] Serositis manifested by pleuritic chest pain and auscultatory rub is one of the distinctive signs of SLE. Lupus pneumonitis, pulmonary hemorrhage, diffuse interstitial lung disease, and pulmonary hypertension occur infrequently but can have serious implications.[80] Gastrointestinal manifestations are uncommon but can include pancreatitis, hepatitis, peritonitis, and enteritis.[80] Premature ovarian failure is usually associated with cyclophosphamide therapy, and spontaneous abortions occur in patients with antiphospholipid syndrome. The most common ophthalmic manifestation of SLE includes keratoconjunctivitis sicca, present in up to a third of patients. Lupus retinopathy and optic neuritis are uncommon but can lead to blindness.[80] In addition to oral lesions, other head and neck manifestations of SLE include sensorineural hearing loss, nasal ulcerations sometimes complicated by septal perforation, auricular chondritis, laryngeal ulcerations and stenosis, and vocal cord paralysis.[80]

Oral Manifestations

The oral mucosa is affected in a significant percentage of lupus patients, with the predominant types of oral lesions being ulcerations, erythematous lesions, and discoid lesions. Estimates of prevalence vary from 9% to 45% in systemic disease and from 3% to 20% in localized cutaneous disease.[87,88] Oral ulcerations are listed among the criteria for SLE diagnosis (Figure 20-8). These ulcerations cannot be easily distinguished from other common oral conditions, such as aphthous ulcers, although they occur with increased frequency on the palate and in the oropharynx and are characteristically painless. Histologically, they are characterized by lymphocytic infiltrate at the base of the ulcer and in the perivascular distribution similar to that observed in discoid lesions.[89]

Discoid oral lesions are similar to those occurring on the skin and appear as whitish striae frequently radiating from the central erythematous area, giving a so-called *brush border*. Atrophy and telangiectases are also frequently present. Buccal mucosa, gingiva, and labial mucosa are the most commonly affected intraoral sites.[89,90] Isolated erythematous areas are also common, especially on the palate. It may be difficult to differentiate these lesions from other common mucosal disorders such as oral candidiasis or lichen planus, especially if there are few lesions and there is no systemic or cutaneous involvement. Histologically, subepithelial and perivascular infiltrate is usually present.[89,90] Disturbed keratinization with cellular atypia can also be observed. Direct immunofluorescent staining for immunoglobulins and complement C3 factor is a useful aid to diagnosis. Granular deposition of IgM, IgG, and C3 along the basement membrane is characteristic.[89,90]

Laboratory Findings

Anemia, leukopenia, and thrombocytopenia are among the most common manifestations of SLE.[91] Anemia of chronic disease is the predominant type, although autoimmune hemolytic anemia may occur. Leukopenia (neutropenia, lymphopenia or both) occurs in about 50% of patients. Autoimmune thrombocytopenia is also common and may be severe. Elevation of erythrocyte sedimentation rate with normal C-reactive protein levels is characteristic of SLE.[91] Although over 100 different autoantibody types are associated with SLE, the best studied are directed against various nuclear components and phospholipids.[92] Antinuclear antibodies (ANAs) are present in 98% of the SLE patients (Table 20-2) and are the most sensitive diagnostic test for this disease. However, the ANA test may be nonspecific, being present in many other autoimmune diseases and in low titers in up to a third of normal populations. In addition, some commonly used ANA assays have a substantial false-positive rate. The highest value of ANA, therefore, is the exclusion of SLE in those with a negative result. Anti-double-stranded DNA (anti-dsDNA)

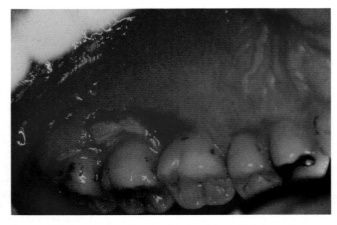

FIGURE 20-8 A chronic palatal lesion (the initial sign of systemic lupus erythematous in this patient).

antibodies are present in 50%–60% of SLE patients and are highly specific. Antibodies classically associated with Sjögren's syndrome, anti-Ro/SS-A and anti-La/SS-B, are present in SLE in 25%–40% and 10%–15% of cases, respectively. Other antibodies highly specific for SLE but found in a relatively small percentage of patients are antiribosomal P, anti-Smith antigen (anti-Sm), and antinuclear ribonucleoprotein (anti-nRNP).[93] Various autoantibody patterns are associated with distinct clinical presentations of SLE. For example, anti-Ro antibody is linked to subacute cutaneous lupus and neonatal heart block, and antiribosomal P antibody to lupus psychosis and nephritis.[92] Antiphospholipid antibodies (anticardiolipin and lupus anticoagulant) are causatively associated with many manifestations of SLE including thrombocytopenia, thrombotic complications and recurrent abortions (antiphospholipid syndrome), and endothelial damage with accelerated atherosclerosis.[93]

Diagnosis

Diagnosis of SLE is based on the compatible symptoms and signs in the presence of suggestive laboratory abnormalities. A standardized set of classification criteria, last modified in 2013, were proposed by the Systemic Lupus International Collaborating Clinics (SLICC) group. To enhance clinical relevance and account for new understanding of the immunology of SLE, they revised and validated the American College of Rheumatology (ACR) SLE classification criteria (Table 20-3).[94] Compared with previous versions of the criteria, more details are given about cutaneous lesions, dividing them into acute, subacute, and chronic. In addition, nonscarring alopecia, which had been removed from older versions of the criteria, is now included. The oral ulcer criterion specifies the exclusion of other causes including Behçet's disease, infections such as *Herpes* virus, inflammatory bowel disease, reactive arthritis, and acidic foods. In addition, low C3, C4, and CH50 complement have been added to the immunological criteria for the first time.[94] Low complement has long been known to accompany active SLE. Note that classification criteria are not diagnostic criteria, but are often used as such. An example of this is that patients with kidney biopsies that were pathognomic for lupus nephritis were considered to have SLE even if they did not meet the previous classification criteria. This is now included in the new SLICC-ACR criteria. The rule for classification is a patient classified with SLE if four of the clinical and immunologic

TABLE 20-3   The Systemic Lupus International Collaborating Clinics (SLICC) Group Proposed Revised American College of Rheumatology (ACR) Systemic Lupus Erythematosus (SLE) Classification Criteria

1. Acute cutaneous lupus (e.g., malar rash or photosensitivity and other)
2. Chronic cutaneous lupus (e.g., classic discoid lupus and other)
3. Oral ulcers or nasal ulcers
4. Nonscarring alopecia
5. Synovitis involving 2 or more joints, characterized by swelling or effusion
   OR tenderness in 2 or more joints and at least 30 minutes of morning stiffness
6. Serositis
7. Renal
   Urine protein greater than or equal to 500 mg protein/24 hours
   OR red blood cell casts
8. Neurologic disease (Seizures, psychosis, mononeuritis multiplex, myelitis, peripheral or cranial neuropathy, acute confused state).
9. Hemolytic anemia
10. Leukopenia (<4000/mm3 at least once)
    OR Lymphopenia (<1000/mm3 at least once)
11. Thrombocytopenia (<100,000/mm³) at least once

Immunologic criteria
1. ANA level above laboratory reference range
2. Anti-dsDNA antibody level above laboratory reference range
3. Anti-Sm: presence of antibody to Sm nuclear antigen
4. Antiphospholipid antibody positivity
5. Low complement
   Low C3
   Low C4
   Low CH50
6. Direct Coombs' test in the absence of hemolytic anemia

The proposed classification rule is as follows: classify a patient as having SLE if 4 of the clinical and immunologic criteria are satisfied, including at least one clinical and one immunologic criterions, OR if he or she has biopsy-proven nephritis compatible with SLE in the presence of antinuclear antibodies (ANAs) or anti-double-stranded DNA (dsDNA) antibodies. The criteria do not need to be present concurrently and other causes of a specific clinical finding such as oral ulcers should be excluded.
Source: Adapted from Petri M et al.[94]

criteria used in the SLICC classification criteria are satisfied, including at least one clinical and one immunologic criterion, or if there is biopsy-proven nephritis compatible with SLE in the presence of ANAs or anti-dsDNA antibodies. The presence of four positive findings has the sensitivity and specificity for SLE of 94%–97% and 84%–92%, respectively.[94]

Treatment

Corticosteroids remain the cornerstone of therapy in SLE and are especially useful for controlling disease flares. Although effective in a significant number of cases, long-term corticosteroid use is associated with several serious complications including opportunistic infections, steroid-induced diabetes, osteoporosis, avascular necrosis, and hypertension. Epidemiological studies have shown that it is important to strive for doses of prednisone of 10 mg per day or less to minimize the risk of cardiovascular complications.[95] Pulse IV cyclophosphamide regimen for remission induction followed by quarterly infusions for maintenance has been the mainstay of modern therapy of severe SLE, especially lupus nephritis.[79] Despite its high level of efficacy, cyclophosphamide is toxic, with a high frequency of complications such as hemorrhagic cystitis, bladder cancer, and ovarian failure. Recently, maintenance with other less toxic agents such as mycophenolate mofetil (MMF) and azathioprine have been shown to possess efficacy equivalent to that of quarterly cyclophosphamide with fewer side effects. Targeting of B cells with rituximab, a monoclonal antibody against CD20, was tested but results were not optimal in SLE.[96] Abatacept, targeting costimulation pathways, did not reach its primary or secondary clinical trial endpoints as a treatment for SLE, but the possibility that it may have a role in nonlife-threatening events was raised.[97] A major breakthrough was the approval of belimumab, a monoclonal antibody, for the treatment for SLE.[98] This was the first new drug specifically approved for SLE in 50 years. Belimumab is a monoclonal antibody that inhibits B-cell activating factor (BAFF), which has a role in the differentiation and proliferation of B cells. Currently, other biologics are in clinical trials for SLE including antibodies against other BAFF-related targets.

Nonsteroidal anti-inflammatory drugs (NSAID) are used frequently in SLE for symptomatic relief of arthritis but are of little benefit in more severe disease. Cyclosporine, tacrolimus, sirolimus, methotrexate, and IV immunoglobulins (IVIG) have also been used in SLE but data to support efficacy is scarce. Antimalarials, such as hydroxychloroquine, are effective in cutaneous lupus with fewer adverse effects.[99–101] Antimalarials are also important in managing the systemic manifestations of the disease.

Dental Management

The dental management of the lupus patient should take into account the complex pathologic manifestations of the disease, including oral aspects and complications of immunosuppressive treatment.

Risk of Infection

Daily treatment with higher doses of prednisone (over 7.5–10 mg/day) or other glucocorticoids, treatment with high doses of cyclophosphamide, and high disease activity are risk factors for infection in SLE patients.[102–104] Impaired immune function that is part of this disease is also felt to contribute to their increased susceptibility to infection. Treatment with other immunosuppressive medications such as mycophenolate mofetil and azathioprine does not appear to increase infection susceptibilities[104] beyond those associated with the disease. Respiratory bacterial infections, urinary tract infections, and infections with *Herpes zoster* and human papilloma viruses are reported to occur more frequently in SLE.[102,103] A baseline complete blood count should be obtained before dental treatment of SLE patients, as leukopenia, neutropenia, and/or thrombocytopenia can occur.[102,105] If possible, elective oral surgical procedures with the potential for bacteremia should be delayed until the absolute neutrophil count is over 1000 cells/mm³, as neutropenia may be transient and respond to treatment with glucocorticoids.[105] If an oral procedure cannot be postponed, prophylactic antibiotics can be considered. Although the evidence behind prophylactic antibiotics before dental management in neutropenic patients is scarce, current guidelines recommend prophylactic antibiotics when ANC falls below 500 cells/mm³. As no studies have been performed regarding efficacy of antibiotic prophylaxis in neutropenic patients before oral surgical procedures, the optimum regimen is unknown. AHA endocarditis prophylaxis guidelines are the most commonly recommended.[63]

Patients with prosthetic heart valves, who had prosthetic materials used to repair a cardiac valve, certain congenital heart diseases or history of previous infective endocarditis should be given antibiotic prophylaxis consistent with AHA recommendations.[63] Libman–Sachs endocarditis also may occur. This is a noninfectious valvular heart disease that can be associated in secondary infectious endocarditis. In planning the dental treatment of SLE patients on dialysis, the potential for increased bleeding, infection, and decreased renal clearance of medications should be taken into account (see Chapter 17, Renal Disease).[63,107]

Risk of Bleeding

Traditionally, platelet transfusions have been recommended in surgical patients with platelet counts below 50,000 per mm³. A recent retrospective review of dental extractions in individuals with platelets counts of 100,000 or less per mm³ found postoperative bleeding was more common in those with lower platelet levels.[108] However, opinions vary as to whether or not platelet transfusions should be given for minor invasive procedures.[109] The decision for preoperative transfusion should take into account the location and extent of the surgery, the potential risk if bleeding does occur, and the ability to control the bleeding by local measures rather than relying on a pre-set platelet count trigger.[109] Routine platelet transfusions are associated with risks such as alloimmunization and infection transmission. Dental postoperative bleeding can be readily controlled by local measures such as pressure, application of hemostatic agents, and aminocaproic acid rinses.[108]

For patients with lupus who are receiving anticoagulants, established guidelines should be followed. In general, oral surgical procedures are safe in patients taking warfarin with therapeutic international normalized ratio ranges (2–3.5) and do not require discontinuation of anticoagulation.[110,111]

Adrenal Suppression/Secondary Adrenal Insufficiency

The subject of perioperative corticosteroid replacement has been surrounded with controversy since early reports of adverse events in patients at risk for adrenal suppression undergoing surgery.[112] Although detailed discussion of the issue is beyond the scope of this text, several points are worth mentioning.

First, there are very few reported cases of adrenal crisis occurring in association with a dental procedure.[113] In one review of the literature, only six cases had been published in the last 66 years.[113] Second, it is very difficult to estimate the risk of adrenal suppression based on the dose, duration of therapy, or time since the last dose without formal testing such as the adrenocorticotropic hormone ACTH (cosyntropin) stimulation test.[112] Although, as a rule, a patient who has received a glucocorticoid in doses equivalent to at least 20 mg a day of prednisone for more than 5 days is at risk for hypothalamus–pituitary–adrenal (HPA) suppression, it is difficult to predict those patients with adrenal insufficiency. Studies found weak correlations between total dose, duration of glucocorticoid treatment and tests of HPA function.[112] Also, HPA suppression is more common in critically ill patients.[112]

Although older guidelines recommended routine doubling of the steroid dose in patients at risk for adrenal suppression undergoing surgical procedures, more recent studies have determined that normal cortisol secretory rate in response to general anesthesia and surgery is about 75–150 mg/day, rarely exceeding 200 mg of cortisol/day.[112] The cortisol secretory rate in patients undergoing minor surgery is approximately 50 mg/day.[112] As almost all oral surgical procedures fall in the category of minor surgery, replacement with over 50 mg of hydrocortisone a day (12.5 mg of prednisone) would be unnecessary. Although a recent Cochrane review concluded there was currently inadequate evidence to support or refute the use of supplemental perioperative steroids in patients with adrenal insufficiency, only two studies were available for analysis and the authors emphasized the need for high-quality randomized clinical trials in various surgical settings to further study this question.[114] The surgical duration of an oral surgery procedure, the use of general anesthesia, the presence of infection, whether or not additional glucocorticoids are administered to reduce postoperative swelling, and the underlying health of the patient should be considered when deciding if it is necessary to prescribe supplemental glucocorticoids.[113]

Oral Complications

There are no reported controlled studies specifically addressing management of oral mucosal involvement in SLE. Hydroxychloroquine is commonly used for discoid lesions on the skin and mucosa. Topical steroids with antifungal agents are recommended for discoid and ulcerative lesions, as well as topical tacrolimus ointment and intralesional injection of steroids for refractory lesions.

SLE can be found in conjunction with Sjögren's syndrome, which is usually termed secondary Sjögren's syndrome. The two rheumatic diseases share several immunologic features, including the presence of anti-Ro antibody, leukopenia, and the women:men distribution (nine times more common in women). It is estimated that up to 20% of SLE patients will have Sjögren's syndrome, and the prevalence is higher in SLE patients with anti-Ro antibody.[115] However, SLE patients can have anti-Ro without Sjögren's syndrome. Sjögren's syndrome increases the risk of caries and other oral complications, which should be managed accordingly (see Chapter 10, Salivary Gland Diseases).

Scleroderma

The term *scleroderma*, derived from the Greek words for hard and skin, describes a group of clinical disorders characterized by thickening and fibrosis of the skin. The generalized form, systemic sclerosis, is a multisystem connective tissue disease in which the fibrosis extends to the internal organs, including the heart, lungs, kidney, and gastrointestinal tract.[116] The prevalence is estimated to be between 18 and 20 per million, with women being affected three to four times as frequently as men.[116,117] There are two main forms, systemic sclerosis (SSc) and localized sclerodema.

SSc is further divided into limited cutaneous scleroderma (previously called CREST syndrome for calcinosis cutis, Raynaud's phenomenon, esophageal dysmotility, sclerodactyly, and telangiectasia) and diffuse cutaneous scleroderma.[80] Patients with limited scleroderma often have a long history of Raynaud's phenomenon before the appearance of other symptoms. They have skin thickening limited to hands and frequently have problems with digital ulcers and esophageal dysmotility. Although generally a milder form of disease than diffuse scleroderma, limited scleroderma can have life-threatening complications. Diffuse scleroderma patients have a more acute onset, with constitutional symptoms, arthritis, carpal tunnel syndrome, and marked swelling of the hands and legs. They also characteristically develop widespread skin thickening (progressing from the fingers to the trunk), internal organ involvement (including gastrointestinal and pulmonary fibrosis), and potentially life-threatening cardiac and renal failure.[116] Other possible variants are overlap syndromes with SLE, Sjögren's syndrome, RA, and dermatomyositis.[80]

Localized scleroderma refers to scleroderma primarily involving the skin, with minimal systemic features.[80] It is rare that patients with localized scleroderma progress to SSc. There are two major types of localized scleroderma: linear scleroderma and morphea. Linear scleroderma is characterized by a band of sclerotic induration and hyperpigmentation occurring on one limb or side of the face. This form of the disease develops as a thin band of sclerosis that may run the entire length of an extremity, involving underlying muscle, bones, and joints.[80] When the disease crosses a joint, limitation of motion is possible, along with growth abnormalities. The lesion of linear localized scleroderma of the head and face is called en coup de sabre, and these lesions may result in hemiatrophy of the face. Morphea is characterized by small violaceous skin patches or larger skin patches (guttate morphea) that indurate and lose hair and sweat gland function (Figure 20-9). Later in the disease, the lesion burns out and appears as a hypo- or hyperpigmented area depressed below the level of the skin.[80] A small number of patients develop numerous larger lesions that coalesce, and these patients are said to have generalized morphea. Scleroderma localized to the hands is called acrosclerosis.

Etiology and Pathogenesis

The etiology of SSc is unclear, but the pathogenesis is characterized by vascular damage and an accumulation

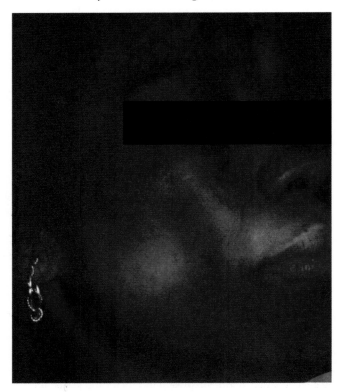

FIGURE 20-9 Morphea of the face.

of collagen and other extracellular matrix components at involved sites.[117] Biopsies of the skin in early stages show bundles of collagen in the lower dermis and upper subcutaneum in association with perivascular and interstitial mononuclear cell infiltrates. The inflammatory process precedes the deposition of collagen. Once in the tissue, T cells drive processes through secretion of cytokines such as IL-4 and IL-13 that result in vasculopathy and fibrosis.[116] These cytokines induce fibroblast production of transforming growth factor (TGF)-β1, which is the main profibrotic cytokine in SSc. As the disease progresses, the rete pegs are lost and the epidermis thins.[117]

Unregulated collagen deposition is a hallmark of this disease. Cultured fibroblasts from patients synthesize more collagen in vitro that is structurally normal, although collagen degradation pathways appear to be normal.[80] The excess collagen narrows small arteries and changes the microvasculature in early stages of the disease, causing eventual pulmonary hypertension, renal disease, myocardial dysfunction, and digital gangrene.

Recent GWAS studies have identified multiple susceptibility loci associated with SSc.[118] Environmental exposure to pesticides, benzene derivatives, and silica has been linked to the development of scleroderma-like conditions in miners and stonemasons. Viral triggers such as parvovirus B19 are proposed.[116]

Clinical Manifestations

Patients with SSc as opposed to limited scleroderma typically have rapid skin thickening and visceral organ involvement. Severe skin and kidney complications developed in 70% of a cohort of 953 patients with diffuse cutaneous systemic sclerosis followed for more than 20 years.[119] Forty-five percent to 55% also had serious heart, lung, and gastrointestinal tract disease. Visceral organ involvement was significantly associated with an increase in mortality.

Raynaud's Phenomenon

Raynaud's phenomenon is the most common initial finding of SSc.[120] Marked intimal hyperplasia of the digital arteries narrows the vessels. Stimuli such as cold that normally stimulate vasoconstriction can cause complete obstruction of the blood flow to the fingertips.[120] More than 95% of scleroderma patients eventually experience a more severe form of the digital cyanosis, numbness, and blanching found with Raynaud's phenomenon. In addition to pain, patients with severe Raynaud's can develop digital pitting scars, nail fold infarcts, or ulcers that occasionally cause loss of the digit.[120]

Cutaneous Manifestations

Skin thickening of SSc patients begins in the fingers and hands in almost all cases.[120] The neck and the face are usually the next sites to be involved. The changes begin with pitting edema that is replaced by tautness and hardening of the skin. This limits motion in affected areas. Hyperpigmentation, telangiectases, (Figure 20-10), and subcutaneous calcifications may also occur, leading to retrognathia (Figure 20-11).

Musculoskeletal Manifestations

Generalized arthralgias and morning stiffness are common in SSc, and may be confused with RA.[80] Clinically evident joint inflammation is uncommon, though erosions are reported in as many as 29% of patients.[80] Muscle weakness can occur from disuse atrophy or from primary myopathy that is accompanied by mild elevations of serum muscle enzymes.

Gastrointestinal Manifestations

Upper or lower gastrointestinal (GI) involvement is reported in up to 90% of scleroderma patients with either the progressive or limited cutaneous forms.[121] Patients may have disorders of motility and transit time, affecting any area from the esophagus to the anus. Esophageal motor dysfunction and gastroesophageal reflux disease occur in the majority of scleroderma patients. In severe forms, the intestinal fibrosis results in malabsorption.[121]

Cardiac Manifestations

Cardiac injury in scleroderma may occur secondary to the primary pathological processes of this disease.[122] The microvasculature is altered, and collagen production is increased in the infiltrated tissue. These processes lead to ischemic, fibrotic, and inflammatory lesions in the pericardium, myocardium, and cardiac conduction system. *Patchy fibrosis* is a term used to describe the myocardial lesions associated with SSc.[122] Hypertension, dysrhythmias, conduction disturbances, and left ventricular hypertrophy can develop.[122]

Pulmonary Manifestations

Pulmonary complications of scleroderma are now the leading cause of death in patients with scleroderma.[123] They can be insidious in onset and resist treatment. Progressive interstitial lung disease can lead to pulmonary arterial hypertension

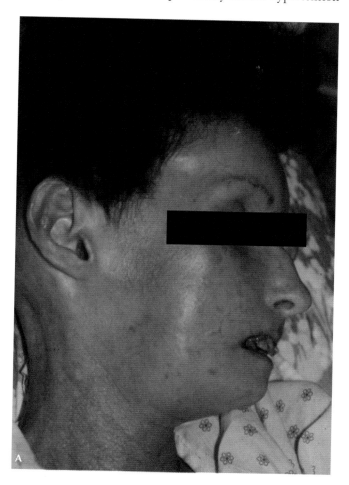

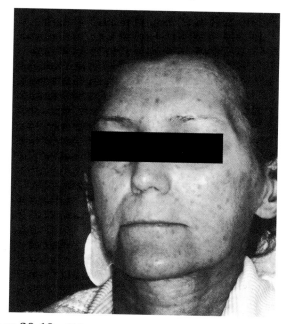

FIGURE 20-10   Telangiectases in a patient with scleroderma.

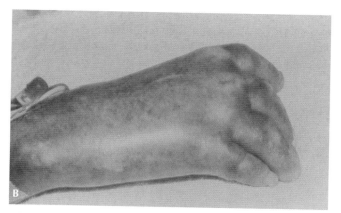

FIGURE 20-11   Manifestations of scleroderma. A, Severe tightening of the skin and narrowing of the oral aperture of a patient with scleroderma. B, Extensive involvement of the fingers and hand of the same patient causes a lack of mobility and the resorption of phalanges.

(PAH), which is estimated to occur in 10%–15% of patients. Longitudinal studies suggest that pulmonary deterioration tends to progress once the pathologic process is established.[123]

Renal Manifestations

Until recently, renal involvement was the most deadly complication of scleroderma.[80,119] *Scleroderma renal crisis* is a syndrome characterized by malignant hypertension, rapidly progressive renal insufficiency, hyperreninemia, and evidence of microangiopathic hemolysis.[123] Pathologic changes are present in the kidney that mimics other lesions characteristic of SSc. Profound decreases in hemoglobulin and platelet counts can occur.[80] Normotensive renal failure related to arteriolar thrombosis is associated with previous glucocorticoid therapy.[80]

Oral Manifestations

The clinical signs of SSc of the mouth and jaws are consistent with findings elsewhere in the body. The lips become rigid, and the oral aperture narrows considerably.[80] Skin folds are lost around the mouth, giving a mask-like appearance to the face. The tongue can also become hard and rigid, making speaking and swallowing difficult. Involvement of the esophagus may cause dysphagia.[121,124] Oral telangiectasia is equally prevalent in both limited and diffuse forms of SSc and is most commonly observed on the hard palate and the lips.[121]

When fibrosis involves the muscles of mastication, mandibular resorption can occur. One study reported that about one-third of patients had resorption of either the angle of the mandible, the condylar heads, the coronoid process, or the digastric region.[125] Mandibular movement may be restricted by muscular fibrosis, and linear localized scleroderma may cause hemiatrophy of face. Dental radiographic findings have been reported and widely described. Classic findings such as uniform thickening of the periodontal membrane, especially around the posterior teeth, are found in 10%–37% of patients (Figure 20-12).[126] Other characteristic radiographic findings include calcinosis of the soft tissues around the jaws. The areas of calcinosis will be detected by dental radiography and may be misinterpreted as radiographic intrabony lesions. A thorough clinical examination will demonstrate that the calcifications are present in the soft tissue.

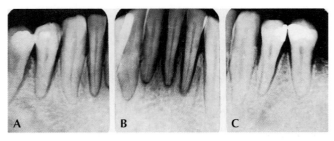

FIGURE 20-12 Radiographs showing thickening of the periodontal membrane in a patient with scleroderma.

Medications may reduce salivary flow rates, or patients with scleroderma may have secondary Sjögren's syndrome. Small studies have estimated the prevalence of secondary Sjögren's syndrome in patients with scleroderma to be between 21% and 44%.[124,125,127] Significant fibrosis was seen in the minor salivary gland biopsies of patients. Xerostomia results in an increased susceptibility to dental caries and *Candida* infections (see Chapter 10, Salivary Gland Diseases).

Manual dexterity is limited in scleroderma patients, which decreases their ability to maintain good oral hygiene.[128] Oral hygiene can be complicated further if opening is limited.

Laboratory Evaluation and Diagnosis

Circulating antinuclear autoantibodies are present in >90% of scleroderma patients (Table 20-2). Several are highly specific for the disease.[129] These include anti-centromere antibody(ACA), which is found in up to 50% of patients, anti-topoisomerase I (anti-topo I), anti–RNA polymerase I/III, and anti-Th/To2-36. Other autoantibodies not specific to scleroderma can be detected in serum, including anti-PM-Scl, anti-U3RNP, and anti-U1RNP.[129] Autoantibodies appear to have prognostic value for patients. ACAs are strongly associated with slowly progressive, limited disease, whereas anti-topo I and anti-RNA polymerase I/III are found more frequently in patients with progressive and diffuse disease.[130] Other abnormal laboratory findings include anemia, an elevated erythrocyte sedimentation rate, and hypergammaglobulinemia.

Although classification criteria are not diagnostic criteria, applying them is generally useful in diagnosis. In 2013, the ACR/European League Against Rheumatism (EULAR) classification criteria for systemic sclerosis were published.[131] These criteria supersede the 1980 ACR criteria for systemic sclerosis. The 2013 criteria include and apply various weights to the skin thickening, pulmonary manifestations, Raynaud's syndrome, telangiectases, and laboratory abnormalities (anti-centromere, antitopoisomerase I—also called anti-SCL70, anti-RNA polymerase III).[131]

Treatment

The treatment of SSc depends on the extent and severity of skin and organ involvement and on the clinical stage of the disease.[132] Early in the course of the disease, inflammation predominates, so treatment is focused on use of immunomodulatory agents to control inflammation.[132,133] Early diagnosis and treatment are advised. In the later stages of the disease, fibrosis predominates.[132] For Raynaud's phenomenon, avoidance of cold exposure is crucial. In addition, calcium channel blockers are prescribed for moderate to severe Raynaud's phenomenon. If these are inadequate, addition of another vasodilator, such as nitroglycerine, a phosphodiesterase inhibitor, or prostacyclin infusions may be considered. Endothelin inhibitors such as bosentan may be used.[132] Mild cutaneous disease may be observed. Progressive or severe cutaneous involvement may be treated initially with methotrexate alone as recommended by EULAR, or in combination with cyclophosphamide or mycophenolate.[132] Severe disease may be treated with cyclophosphamide initially, then mycophenolate for maintenance. Cyclophosphamide is used to treat early lung disease with alveolitis.[132] Epoprostinal, trepostenol, bosentan, and inhaled iloprost have been shown to improve PAH, whereas angiotensin inhibitors have greatly improved patient outcomes for those with scleroderma renal crisis.[133]

Dental Management

The most common problem in the dental treatment of SSc patients is the physical limitation caused by the narrowing of the oral aperture and rigidity of the tongue. Procedures such as molar endodontics, prosthetics, and restorative procedures in the posterior portions of the mouth become difficult, and the dental treatment plan may sometimes need to be altered because of the physical problem of access. Mechanical stretching devices are available or patients can try to stretch the aperture using tongue blades, but progressing disease limits the effectiveness of this approach.[128] Patients may have great difficulty with hygiene, and caries and plaque are associated with decreasing dexterity and strength.[134] Customized toothbrush handles should be provided for patients who cannot grip an ordinary toothbrush, and plaque control may improve with an electric toothbrush.

When treating a patient with diffuse scleroderma, the extent of the heart, lung, or kidney involvement should be considered and appropriate alterations should be made before, during, and after treatment. Patients with extensive resorption of the angle of the mandible are at risk for developing pathologic fractures from minor trauma, including dental extractions. Patients with Sjögren's syndrome and/or periodontal disease should apply topical fluorides daily such as 1.1% neutral sodium fluoride and have professional hygiene appointments 3–4 times/year (see Chapter 10, Salivary Gland Diseases).

IDIOPATHIC INFLAMMATORY MYOPATHIES

The idiopathic inflammatory myopathies (IIM) are a group of systemic rheumatic diseases that include adult polymyositis (PM), adult dermatomyositis (DM), juvenile dermatomyositis (juvenile DM), myositis associated with cancer or another connective tissue disease, and inclusion body myositis (IBM).[135] All are characterized by muscle weakness and nonsuppurative inflammation of the skeletal muscle. The true incidence and prevalence are difficult to ascertain because of the rarity of these diseases and the lack of consistent diagnostic criteria. However, identification of autoantibodies that are highly associated with certain clinical subtypes may lead to better classification of these diseases.[136] Most studies have found that the incidence

is higher in women, though males are reported to have a higher prevalence of IBM.[137]

The increased risk for malignancy in individuals with inflammatory myopathy has been confirmed in several studies. Cancer diagnosis can precede or occur after the diagnosis of the myopathy, and occurs primarily in adults.[137]

Subtypes

PM usually has an insidious onset characterized by symmetrical weakness of the limb-girdle muscles and anterior neck flexors, which develops into progressive muscle atrophy.[137] Characteristic histological changes that include necrosis of type I and II muscle fibers are present in a skeletal muscle biopsy. DM has most of the features of PM with additional characteristic skin lesions.[137] The most common cutaneous manifestation is a rash, termed Gottron's papules, which is a symmetric, palpable, erythematous eruption of the skin overlying the extensor surfaces of the metacarpophalangeal and interphalangeal joints of the fingers and other sites of the body (Figure 20-13).[137] This sign is considered pathognomonic for DM. The juvenile form typically occurs between ages 6 and 11 years, whereas the adult form develops in the fourth to sixth decades of life.[135] Another defined subset of the inflammatory myopathies is IBM. Clinically, patients have a unique pattern of weakness and lack a sustained response to immunosuppression, with the diagnosis made histologically.[137]

Etiology and Pathogenesis

The etiology and pathogenesis of inflammatory myositis is unknown. Evidence suggests roles for autoimmune injury, genetics, and the environment.[135] Most patients have autoantibodies to various antigens involved in protein translation. The types of cells found at the sites of inflammation differ in the various forms inflammatory myositis, suggesting each has a unique etiology.[135] In PM, the endomysial

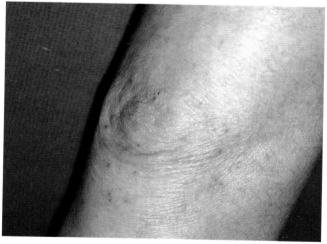

FIGURE 20-13   Gottron's papules on the knees of a patient with polymyositis. (Courtesy of Dr. Jaime Brahim.)

inflammation is primarily T cell, with very few NK cells, and no B cells. In DM, the muscle infiltrate has a high percentage of B cells and CD4+ T cells with loss of capillaries.[137,138]

Recent GWAS studies of a large patient cohort that included both children and adults with DM confirmed the MHC as the major genetic region associated with DM and identified genetic overlap with other autoimmune disorders.[139] Environmental factors suggested as cofactors for IIM are influenza, hepatitis, coxsackievirus infection, and infection with the protozoan *Toxoplasma gondii*. A registry report found that symptoms of rash and weakness often followed a history of respiratory or gastrointestinal complaints in juvenile DM, suggesting that the response to an infectious process is involved in its pathogenesis.[140]

No one malignancy is associated with the myositis of malignancy. Patients with ovarian, lung, pancreatic, non-Hodgkin lymphoma, stomach, and colorectal cancers have developed DM, whereas patients with non-Hodgkin lymphoma, lung and bladder cancers had the higher rates of PM.[137,140]

Clinical Manifestations

Most patients present with an acute or subacute onset of weakness of the proximal muscles that is symmetrical.[137] Patients may have difficulty raising their head while supine, climbing stairs, and dressing themselves. Muscle involvement may become severe enough to confine the patient to bed or to cause respiratory failure and death.

The primary classic skin lesion seen in DM is a violaceous macular erythema distributed symmetrically.[135] Pathognomonic skin manifestations, occurring in approximately 70% of patients, are Gottron's papules (described in Section Subtypes).[135–137] The symmetrical rash of DM is violaceous to dusky erythematous, sometimes with edema, involving the periorbital area and upper eyelids. Macular erythema over the lower neck, upper chest and the upper back in a shawl-like distribution, severe erythema of the palms, scaling scalp plaques, and hyperkeratosis of the palmar and lateral aspects of the fingers (mechanic's hands) are commonly seen. Periungual abnormalities including telangiectases and cuticular overgrowth, and gingival bushy loop formations may occur in juvenile DM. Other skin changes include telangiectases and Raynaud's phenomenon.

Skin calcinosis is most commonly seen in children or young adults.[140,141] Fibrosis of muscles can cause a retrognathia similar to scleroderma. Interstitial lung disease secondary to fibrosing alveolitis, cardiac conduction abnormalities, conjunctival edema, and renal damage also occur.

Oral Manifestations

A study of 34 patients with PM and DM found increased numbers of decayed, missing, and filled teeth, fewer teeth, poorer oral hygiene, and decreased masticatory forces in this patient group.[142] The most common mucosal lesion was telangiectasia, detected in seven cases. Fibrosis of the minor salivary glands was found in 12 patients and interstitial-perivascular infiltration was detected in eight cases. Dysphagia may complicate oral health. Calcinosis of the soft tissues is seen, especially in children. These calcified nodules may appear in the face and radiographs. The tongue may also become rigid because of severe calcinosis.

Gingival changes described as bushy loop formations have been noted in children with juvenile DM (Figure 20-14),[143,144] and was reported to be present in 16/26 children in a comprehensive study of oral and systemic changes.[144] Other findings in these 26 children were oral mucosa telangiectasias (23%), reduced mandibular mobility (50%), and reduced mouth opening (31%). Case reports exist of adults presenting with oral ulcerations, telangiectasia of oral mucosa, and systemic features of DM who were subsequently found to have malignancy.[145]

Laboratory Evaluation and Diagnosis (adapted from Harris et al.80)

Patients with PM show (1) symmetric weakness of the limb girdle muscles, progressing from weeks to months; (2) skeletal muscle biopsy showing necrosis of types I and II muscle fibers and other characteristic changes; (3) elevation of serum muscle enzymes (creatine kinase, aldolase, alanine aminotransferase, aspartate aminotransferase, and lactate dehydrogenase); and (4) electromyographic features of myopathy. The diagnosis of DM is made if a patient has the features of PM plus a cutaneous eruption that is typical of DM. *Ragged red* fibers, angulated atrophic fibers, and characteristic intracellular lined vacuoles are additional features in a muscle biopsy of IBM. Disease subsets may be identified by their autoantibodies, but more than one-third of patients with IIM will be autoantibody positive (Table 20-2).[80]

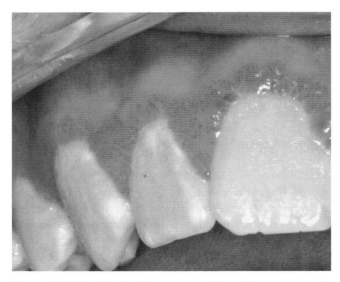

FIGURE 20-14 Gingival changes seen in juvenile dermatomyositis. Note the marked dilation of the capillaries of the attached gingiva.

Treatment

After exclusion of malignancy, patients are treated according to the extent of their disease. Initial therapy consists of high doses of systemic corticosteroids.[146,147] Other second-line treatments include cyclosporine, tacrolimus, leflunomide, and mycophenolate mofetil. Other treatments have been investigated in refractory disease, including the biologics rituximab, abatacept (a selective costimulation inhibitor of CD28 binding), alemtuzumab (humanized monoclonal anti-CD52 antibody), tocilizumab (a humanized anti-IL-6 receptor antibody), anakinra (a monoclonal IL-1 receptor antagonist), and MEDI-545 (an anti-INFα antibody).[147] Stem cell transplantation with autologous bone marrow–derived CD34+ cells and mesenchymal stem cells have been investigated. In extremely severe and refractory cases, gene therapy with follistatin, an inhibitor of myostatin, is under consideration as a treatment to be investigated to increase muscle size and strength.[147] Physical therapy should be included in any management plan.

Dental Management

Gingival lesions should be treated with standard hygiene therapy. However, they may continue to bleed and only resolve when the systemic disease responds to immunosuppressive therapy. The same precautions are necessary for all patients who are taking high-dose long-term steroids and other immunosuppressives (see *Dental management* under *Systemic Lupus Erythematosus*, above). Oral ulcerations of DM may be managed with topical steroids.

RHEUMATOID ARTHRITIS

RA is a disease characterized by symmetrical, inflammatory arthritis of small and large joints.[80] It is one of the most common autoimmune diseases, estimated to affect up to 2% of the population in the United States over the age of 60 years,[148] with a higher prevalence in women. Epidemiologic studies suggest that the incidence of RA is declining in younger age groups for unknown reasons.[149] In contrast to degenerative joint disease (osteoarthritis), RA is a systemic disease with constitutional symptoms, including fatigue, weight loss, morning stiffness, low grade fevers, and anemia.[80]

Subtypes

Juvenile arthritis (JA) is a term to describe any arthritis in children.[150] A subset, juvenile idiopathic arthritis (JIA) includes those children with chronic arthritis.[80,150] Some clinicians refer to this subset as juvenile RA. In general, symptoms of JIA include joint pain, swelling, tenderness, warmth, and stiffness for at least 6 weeks without another cause.[150] Similar to RA in adults, these children may have severe joint and organ damage. There are seven classifications of JIA: systemic arthritis, oligoarthritis, polyarthritis—rheumatoid factor (RF) negative, polyarthritis—RF positive, psoriatic arthritis, enthesitis-related arthritis, and undifferentiated arthritis.[150] It is estimated that approximately 300,000 children in the United States have some form of JA.[151] Long term, these patients may have failure to thrive secondary if treated with high-dose steroids. Recent data suggest growth hormone may reduce their deficiency in stature.[152] Etanercept, a TNF-blocking agent, has been used safely in these children.[153]

Felty's syndrome is characterized by neutropenia and splenomegaly in conjunction with RA. These patients have additional susceptibilities to bacterial infection if neutropenia is severe.[154]

Etiology and Pathogenesis

The etiology of RA is unknown, but there is substantial evidence that it is a complex genetic disease. However, other factors appear to either initiate or sustain RA, as the prevalence of RA overall in the United States has declined and is becoming a disease of older US adults.[151]

Genetic Factors

There is strong evidence from a body of work over the last two decades that certain genes increase the risk for RA. Over 100 risk loci have been identified to date, and there is evidence that certain genetic markers predict better responses to newer, targeted therapies for RA.[155]

Twin studies are used to calculate the contribution of genetics and environment to the development of diseases.[156] The finding of concordance in only 16% of monozygotic twins with RA suggests that the environment plays a significant role in the etiology of this disease. Smoking, environmental factors, diet, and infectious agents have all been suggested as triggers for RA.[156] A study examining the interactions of environment and genetics in RA found patients with specific HLA–DRB1 genotypes that conferred a genetic susceptibility to seropositive RA had a much greater risk of developing RA if they smoked. This study demonstrated a gene–environment interaction between smoking and HLA–DRB1 genotypes.[157] The finding that the disease is much more common in women (2:1 to 4:1 women: men ratio[157]) suggests there may be hormonal influences.

Immune Factors

The target organ of RA is the synovial tissue and the cartilage of the joint. Inflammatory cells, including T cells, infiltrate the synovium, causing an expansion of the tissue and formation of a *pannus* that overlays the articular surface of the cartilage and invades the bone.[80,158] Mediators of inflammation, such as the cytokine TNF-α, are released by invading cells and contribute to the destruction of the cartilage and bone. B cells, which can differentiate into plasma cells, are also found within the synovial infiltrate.[158] These cells may participate in the pathophysiology of RA by producing cytokines and autoantibodies. The most commonly found autoantibody in RA is RF, an antibody reactive against antigenic determinants on the Fc fragment of the IgG molecule.[159] Approximately 80% of RA patients will have circulating RF. Typically, either IgM RF or IgA RF is found in the circulation. Both severity and activity of RA is correlated with RF levels. A putative role for RF in the pathogenesis of RA is that it forms large immune complexes within the synovium that subsequently bind and activate other inflammatory molecules. Other autoantibodies described in RA that have aided in its diagnosis are anticyclic citrullinated antibodies, though these antibodies are also found in other autoimmune diseases such as SLE.[160]

Infectious Agents

The finding that many infections produce clinical symptoms similar to RA has generated interest in the role of infectious agents in this disease. These include parvovirus, rubella virus, Epstein–Barr virus, *Borrelia burgdorferi*, and others. However, epidemiology studies have not supported a role for any one agent.[161]

Clinical Manifestations

RA is a symmetric polyarthritis often involving the proximal interphalangeal joints of the fingers and metacarpophalangeal joints of the hands (Figure 20-15); the wrists, elbows, knees, and ankles also can be affected.[80] In some patients, all joints may be involved, including the TMJ and the cricoarytenoid joint of the larynx. Affected joints develop redness, swelling, and warmth, with eventual atrophy of the muscle around the involved area.

The clinical course and severity of RA varies greatly between patients.[80] Some patients may have a short course of nondisabling disease, whereas others have advancing disease that responds poorly to therapy. Those with progressive active disease develop joint destruction and deformity with time, including subcutaneous nodules and swan-neck deformities. Cervical spine disease may cause C1–C2 subluxation and spinal cord compression. Rheumatoid nodules may develop in the lungs, pleura, pericardium, sclera, and rarely the heart, the eyes, or the brain. RA can decrease life expectancy by as much as 5–10 years. One long-term complication of RA is a marked increase in cardiovascular disease.[162]

Oral Manifestations

The treatment of RA can cause oral manifestations. The long-term use of methotrexate and other antirheumatic agents such as NSAIDs can cause stomatitis with oral ulcerations. Minocyline may cause hyperpigmentation intraorally, whereas prednisone or TNF-α blocking therapy may predispose patients to the development of opportunistic infections (Figure 20-16).

Cohort studies suggest an increased prevalence of periodontal disease in patients with RA and a similar cytokine profile in patients with RA and aggressive periodontitis.[163] Both diseases exhibit inflammatory bone loss, and tooth loss is reported to be more common in RA patients when compared to controls. However, the increased dental and periodontal disease in the RA population may be related to a decreased ability to maintain proper oral hygiene because of limited manual dexterity. Unfortunately, most studies to date

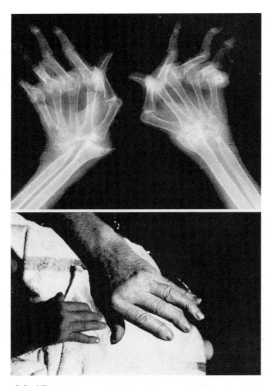

FIGURE 20-15 Characteristic involvement of the hands in a patient with rheumatoid arthritis. (Courtesy of Dr. George Ehrlich.)

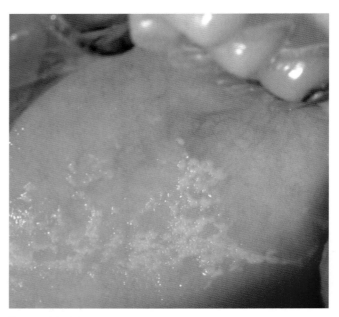

FIGURE 20-16 Oral candidiasis in a 24-year-old woman with rheumatoid arthritis and secondary Sjögren's syndrome treated with TNF-α blocking agents and prednisone.

have not controlled for plaque index. Sjögren's syndrome is common in RA, though reports vary from 25% to 65%.[164,165] This wide range is most likely because different diagnostic criteria were used to diagnose Sjögren's syndrome, and have based the diagnosis on the presence of nonspecific sicca symptoms. Tooth loss and increased caries may occur if an RA patient has significant decreased salivary flow (see Chapter 10, Salivary Gland Diseases), and patients with increased caries should be treated with additional topical fluorides such as neutral fluoride gel containing 1.1% sodium fluoride.

The TMJ is a synovial joint that can be affected by RA. Radiographic changes of the TMJ in RA patients may be detected commonly, but patients may be asymptomatic (see Chapter 11, Temporomandibular Disorders). Treatment is usually reserved for those with pain and/or dysfunction. In one study, 88 consecutive RA patients meeting ACR criteria for RA and 124 matched controls were evaluated using 1997 WHO criteria for TMJ examination.[166] Findings included increased TMJ pain complaints in the RA group (40.9% versus 8.1% of controls) and difficulty in opening the mouth (15.9% versus 2.4% of controls). The prevalence of TMJ destruction with dysfunction is believed to be much higher in children with JIA, though the reported range varies greatly.[167] In one retrospective study of 187 JIA patients who underwent MRI of the TMJ with IV contrast as part of a comprehensive evaluation, 43% had evidence of active or chronic TMJ arthritis.[168] A survey of 118 American and Canadian rheumatologists reported from 1% to 25% of their RA or JIA patients had TMJ arthritis.[169]

When TMJ arthritis is symptomatic, patients may present with pain on palpation, limited opening, deviation of the mandible on opening, ankylosis of the joint, and/or facial asymmetry. Only a few clinical trials have studied TMJ therapies, which include corticosteroid injections,[167] jaw rest, physiotherapy, NSAIDs, and occlusal splints[167] in RA patients. Most therapy is based on studies that tested TMJ treatments in individuals with osteoarthritis of the TMJ.[171] Systemic therapy such as anti-TNF-α agents also may improve pain and function.[172] When TMJ arthritis is advanced, the heads of the condyles can resorb, giving rise to mandibular and maxillary asymmetry. Treatment of these patients can be very complex, and involve surgical reconstruction of the joint, orthognathic surgery, and/or orthodontics.[170,173]

Laboratory Evaluation and Diagnosis

The initial diagnosis of RA is made primarily by observing clinical features. As with many autoimmune diseases, a list of diagnostic criteria developed by the ACR is used to evaluate patients (Table 20-4)[174] that considers the type and extent of joint involvement, the presence of rheumatoid factor, and other immunological findings.

RF and anti-CCP antibodies are present in approximately 80% of adult patients with RA, and antiperinuclear factor antibodies are present in up to 48.5% of patients (Table 20-2).[174,175] Several other autoantibodies may be

detected in these patients. Although these autoantibodies are not specific to RA and are found in patients who have other conditions such as SLE and scleroderma, a positive test for RF and anti-CCP antibodies adds considerable weight to the diagnosis of RA. RF, particularly in high titers, is associated with more destructive disease and a worse prognosis. Other associated laboratory findings include an elevated erythrocyte sedimentation rate and normochromic normocytic anemia.

Methotrexate is often used as initial therapy for symmetric polyarthritis involving three or more joints.[177,178] This drug reduces disease activity, joint erosions and is associated with a significant long-term reduction in mortality.[177] Patients with severe disease are usually treated with combination therapy, and early aggressive therapy has been shown to be advantageous.[179] Although high-dose prednisone therapy is not used as frequently as it was in the past, lower doses of prednisone (<10 mg/day) are still used commonly.[179] Many biological agents, typically antibodies that block receptors or mediators of inflammation, are being developed and used as treatments for RA. The most commonly prescribed at present are etanercept and infliximab, agents that block the actions of the cytokine TNF. Anti-TNF antibody therapy is associated with an increased risk of serious infections and a dose-dependent increased risk of malignancies in patients with RA.[180] Leflunomide, which inhibits pyrimidine synthesis and may inhibit T-cell activation, may cause diarrhea, abdominal pain, allergic reactions, and elevated serum transaminases.[181]

Dental Management

When treating an RA patient, it is imperative that the dentist understand the mechanism of action of the patient's current medications, their possible side effects, and their potential interactions with drugs commonly used in dentistry. Appropriate measures should be taken with these patients before dental care (see *Dental management* under *Systemic Lupus Erythematosus*, above).

Many patients with RA will take NSAIDs, which can cause gastric ulcerations and affect kidney function.[181] Older medications are rarely used today, but include aspirin, which inhibits platelet function; intramuscular doses of gold salts, which may cause stomatitis, blood dyscrasias, or nephrotic syndrome; azothiaprine, which is associated with bone marrow suppression, hepatitis, or pancreatitis; and D-penicillamine, a drug that may cause bone marrow depression, renal toxicity, heptotoxicity, or drug-induced pemphigus. However, any patient who is taking any of these drugs should have a complete blood count and serum chemistry studies before dental treatment.

Patients with cervical spine disease may have C1–C2 subluxation and spinal cord compression. Hyperextension of the neck must be avoided. Prolonged morning stiffness is common in RA, so later morning appointments may be best for patients. Patients with severe RA who have prosthetic joints may require prophylactic antibiotic therapy before

TABLE 20-4   American College of Rheumatology/European League Against Rheumatism Classification Criteria for Rheumatoid Arthritis

Rheumatoid arthritis: add score A through D; a score of ≥6 of 10 is needed for classification of a patient as having definite rheumatoid arthritis	
Classification	Score
A. Joint involvement[a]	
• 1 large joint (shoulders, elbows, hips, knees, ankles)	0
• 2–10 large joints	1
• 1–3 small joints[b] (with or without large joints)	2
• 4–10 small joints (with or without large joints)	3
• >10 joints (at least one small joint)	5
B. Serology (at least 1 test result is needed for classification)	
• Negative rheumatoid factor (RF) and negative anticitrullinated protein antibody (ACPA)	0
• Low-positive RF or low-positive ACPA	2
• High-positive RF or high-positive ACPA	3
C. Acute-phase reactants (at least 1 test result is needed for classification)	
• Normal C-reactive protein (CRP) and normal erythrocyte sedimentation rate (ESR)	0
• Abnormal CRP or abnormal ESR	1
D. Duration of symptoms	
• <6 weeks	0
• ≥6 weeks	1

The classification system is aimed at classifying newly presenting patients and is applied to those with at least one joint with synovitis that is not better explained by another disease. See full reference for complete details.
[a]Joint involvement refers to any swollen or tender joint on examination. Distal interphalangeal joints, first carpometacarpal joints, and first metatarsophalangeal joints are excluded from assessment.
[b]*Small joints* refers to the metacarpophalangeal joints, proximal interphalangeal joints, second through fifth metatarsophalangeal joints, thumb interphalangeal joints, and wrists.
Source: Adapted from Aletaha D et al.[174]

invasive dental procedures,[182] though the evidence for the practice is very limited.[183]

Patients with Sjögren's syndrome may require additional instruction in personal oral care and instruction on diet and dietary modifications (see Chapter 10, Salivary Gland Diseases). They should use topical fluorides such as 1.1% neutral sodium fluoride to prevent caries, and may need more frequent recall visits. Salivary stimulants such the cholinergic agonists pilocarpine or cevimeline can be prescribed for eligible patients. If the RA patient has Felty's syndrome, a complete blood count should be obtained before treatment as these patients may have neutropenia and thrombocytopenia.[154]

MIXED CONNECTIVE TISSUE DISEASE

The term *mixed connective tissue disease* (MCTD) was adopted in 1972 to describe a condition that has overlapping clinical features of SLE, PSS, and DM. The prevalence of MCTD is unknown, and there is some debate as to whether it is a distinct clinical entity.[184]

Etiology, Pathogenesis, and Clinical Manifestations

There are very few long-term studies of patients with this disease. Most patients with MCTD are women who develop symptoms in the second or third decade of life.[184] Initial presentation usually includes polyarthritis, myositis, Raynaud's phenomenon, puffy hands or mild sclerodactyly, interstitial lung disease, and esophageal dysmotility.[80] Other inflammatory manifestations of MCTD include serositis, rash, arthritis, aseptic meningitis, myocarditis, myositis, lymphadenopathy, anemia, trigeminal nerve sensory neuropathy, and leukopenia.[184] In addition, patients may have scleroderma-like features including esophageal involvement and pulmonary hypertension that can be unresponsive to corticosteroid therapy.[185] Peripheral neuropathies, nephrotic syndrome, and severe deforming arthropathy are also known to occur. GI manifestations of MCTD are similar to those in scleroderma. Pulmonary hypertension is the main cause of death in patients.[186]

Laboratory Findings and Diagnosis

The presence of autoantibodies against the U1–small nuclear ribonucleoprotein autoantigen (U1-snRNP) is an essential component of the classification criteria for MCTD (Table 20-2).[184] Other characteristic laboratory abnormalities in MCTD cases include high titers (>1:1000) of speckled ANAs.

Oral Manifestations and Dental Management

Little has been reported concerning the oral manifestations of MCTD. Focal sialadenitis and other salivary findings supporting the diagnosis of secondary Sjögren's syndrome was present in 14/15 patients with MCTD in one small study.[187] Patients receiving high-dose immunosuppression should be managed appropriately (see *Dental management* under *Systemic Lupus Erythematosus*, above).

WEGENER'S GRANULOMATOSUS

Wegener's Granulomatosus (WG) is a form of vasculitis.[188] The incidence is about 10 new cases per million population per year and the average age at diagnosis is 50 years.[189] It affects men and women equally, but men are more likely to have severe disease, whereas women tend to have limited disease. The great majority of affected individuals (approximately 90%) appear to be white.[189] WG is included among the antineutrophil cytoplasmic antibody (ANCA)–associated vasculitides, which also include microscopic polyangiitis, Churg–Strauss syndrome, and renal-limited vasculitis.[188] ANCAs are directed against granular and lysosomal components of neutrophils and monocytes.[188] Two fluorescent staining patterns may occur—cytoplasmic ANCA (C-ANCA) and perinuclear ANCA (P-ANCA). Generally, the target antigen of C-ANCA is proteinase-3 (PR3), and the target antigen of P-ANCA is myeloperoxidase (mPo).[188] PR3 is important in WG.[188]

Etiology, Pathogenesis, and Clinical Manifestations

Although the etiology of WG remains unclear, genetic and environmental factors have been found. Several genes including those on the short arm of chromosome 6 have been associated with WG, including: HLA-DPB1*0401 alleles, HLA-DR4, and HLA-DR13.[189] Environmental factors include exposure to silica dust exposure, infections, especially bacterial infections with *Staphylococcus aureus*, and drugs such as D-penicillamine, hydralazine, and minocycline. In addition, the drugs propylthiouracil and sulfasalazine may have a role.[189] ANCAs are thought to have a role in the pathogenesis of WG, but the relationship between ANCAs and disease activity remains controversial. In PR3 ANCA-associated WG, T effector cells are important in the pathogenesis.[189]

More than 90% of WG patients present with upper and lower respiratory tract symptoms.[189] Pulmonary manifestations include bronchial lesions, nodules, infiltrates, cavitary lesions, and alveolar hemorrhage, but the disease is systemic. Nasopharyngeal and oral manifestations include perforation of the nasal septum, saddle-nose deformity, subglottic stenosis, oral ulcers, and strawberry gingivitis.[188] Hearing may be affected, and conductive and sensorineural hearing loss can occur.[188] The ocular manifestations include anterior uveitis, scleritis, episcleritis, keratitis with potential for corneal melt, conjunctivitis, and orbital pseudotumor.[188] Renal involvement includes segmental necrotizing glomerulitis, which may progress to renal failure.[188] Cutaneous manifestations include palpable purpura and hemorrhagic, vesicular or ulcerative.[188] Cardiac valvular lesions and pericarditis may occasionally occur, and the nervous system can also be affected with aseptic meningitis and mononeuritis.[188]

Laboratory Findings and Diagnosis

The diagnosis of WG can be complex.[190] First, a clinical diagnosis of antibody-associated vasculitis (AAV) or polyarteritis should be made in a patient at least 16 years of age who has been followed for 3 months or more. Three criteria should be fulfilled before classification[190]: (1) symptoms and signs that are compatible or characteristic of primary vasculitis; (2) one or more of the following: (a) histological proof of vasculitis or granuloma formation (granuloma being defined according to the 1990 ACR Classification Criteria for Wegener's granulomatosus)[190]; (b) positive serology for ANCA; (c) specific investigations that are strongly indicative of vasculitis and/or granuloma, such as neurophysiology studies, angiography, magnetic resonance imaging, and other studies; (d) eosinophilia (>10% or 1.5 × 10⁹/L); (3) No other diagnosis that accounts for symptoms and signs, specifically: (a) malignancy; (b) infection; (c) drugs; (d) secondary vasculitis (e.g., rheumatoid vasculitis, Sjogren's syndrome); (e) Behçet's disease, Kawasaki's disease, Takayasu's arteritis, giant cell arteritis, Henoch–Schönlein purpura, anti-GBM disease, and essential mixed cryoglobulinemia; (f) vasculitis mimics (e.g., cholesterol embolism, atrial myxoma); (g) sarcoidosis and other nonvasculitic granulatomatous diseases.

The stepwise process of classification continues by excluding Churg–Strauss syndrome, followed by four ways to classify a case as WG[191]: (1) meets ACR criteria for WG; if not, (2) histology is compatible with Chapel Hill Consensus Conference (CHCC) definition for WG; if not, (3) histology is compatible with CHCC microscopic polyangiitis, and WG surrogate markers; if not, (4) no histology is available, but WG surrogate markers are present and there is positive serology for PR3 or myeloperoxidase.

Surrogate makers for WG address symptoms suggestive of granulomatous disease involving the upper and lower respiratory tract, after other causes have been excluded: (1) lower airway involvement as shown by radiographic evidence of fixed pulmonary infiltrates, nodules, or cavitations present for >1 month, or bronchial stenosis; (2) upper airway involvement as shown by bloody nasal discharge and crusting for >1 month, or nasal ulceration, chronic sinusitis, otitis media, or mastoiditis for >3 months, retro-orbital mass or inflammation (pseudotumor), subglottic stenosis, saddle nose deformity/destructive sinonasal disease. To support a diagnosis of WG, only one surrogate marker is necessary.

Treatment

Glucocorticosteroids and cyclophosphamide are often used as remission inducing therapies in WG, whereas rituximab appears to be as effective as cyclophosphamide.[189] In addition, treatments such as methotrexate may be used in combination with corticosteroids to treat limited disease. Azathioprine appears to be as effective as cyclophosphamide for maintenance of remission.[189] For refractory disease, TNF antagonists, deoxyspergualin, antithymocyte globulin, IVIG, and antibodies against B cells have been tried.[189]

ALLERGY AND HYPERSENSITIVITY REACTIONS

The modern dentist uses a wide variety of drugs to treat patients, including antibiotics, hypnotics, and anesthetics. All practitioners who use these medications must know how to manage adverse reactions triggered by these agents. A dental practitioner also uses a wide range of materials such as impression materials, adhesives, latex, and restorative and endodontic materials that contain potential allergens. These include preservatives, coloring agents, fixatives, binding agents, flavorings, and latex.

Hypersensitivity Reactions

Immunological reactions may be of several different types: type 1 IgE mediated (anaphylactic), type 2 antibody mediated, type 3 (immune complex mediated) and type 4 (cell-mediated or delayed hypersensitivity) (Table 20-5). Type 1 reactions are acute (e.g., penicillin, latex, or peanut allergy) and require immediate recognition and action. Type 2 reactions are not usually found in response to dental materials or drugs, but are found in autoimmune conditions affecting the oral cavity such as pemphigus. Such conditions are discussed in Chapter 4, Ulcerative, Vesicular and Bullous Lesions. Type 3 reactions can be seen in response to dental materials, but more commonly in response to viral infections such as recurrent herpes labialis, giving rise to erythema multiforme or Stevens–Johnson syndrome (clinical manifestations are discussed in Chapter 4). Delayed hypersensitivity (cell-mediated or contact sensitivity) reactions to dental materials are very common and are usually seen in the oral cavity where an amalgam or gold restoration is in direct contact with the buccal or lingual mucosa. Stomatitis associated with allergy is discussed in Chapter 4. In this section, acute allergic reactions and their management are discussed.

Acute allergic reactions are caused by an immediate-type hypersensitivity reaction mediated by IgE and are the most serious of allergies. Reactions can occur rapidly, and full-scale anaphylactic reactions may occur and be associated with local as well as systemic swelling. Type 1 reactions require the presence of mast cells with attached IgE. A patient previously exposed to a drug or other antigen has antibody (primarily IgE) fixed to mast cells. When the antigen (in the form of a drug, food, or an airborne substance) is reintroduced into the body, it will react with and cross-link the cell-bound antibody. This causes an increase in intracellular calcium and the release of preformed mediators including histamine, proteases, and newly synthesized lipid-derived mediators such as leukotrienes and prostaglandins. Cytokines are also released, which attract eosinophils and augment the inflammatory response. These substances cause vasodilation and increased capillary permeability, ultimately leading to fluid and leukocyte accumulation in the tissues and edema formation. Constriction of bronchial smooth muscle results when IgE is bound in the pulmonary region. The anaphylactic reaction may be localized producing urticaria and angioedema, or may result in a generalized reaction, causing anaphylactic shock.

Localized Anaphylaxis

A localized anaphylactic reaction involving superficial blood vessels results in urticaria (hives) (Figure 20-17). Urticaria begins with pruritus (itching) in the area where histamine and other active substances are released. Wheals (welts) then appear on the skin as an area of localized edema on an erythematous base. These lesions can occur anywhere on the skin or mucous membranes. There seems to be little doubt that the oral mucosa is well endowed with mast cells and

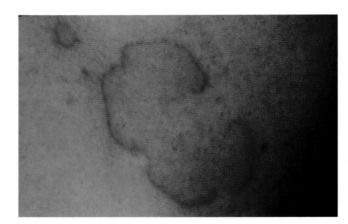

FIGURE 20-17 Urticaria resulting from use of a nonsteroidal anti-inflammatory drug.

TABLE 20-5 Immunological Reaction Classifications			
Type	**Mediator**	**Systemic Examples**	**Oral Examples**
1. Immediate	IgE	Hayfever, asthma	Penicillin anaphylaxis, oral allergy syndrome
2. Cytotoxic	IgG	Pemphigus	Mucous membrane pemphigoid
3. Immune complex	Complexes, complement	Serum sickness, SLE	Erythema multiforme
4. Delayed	Lymphocyte-Cell mediated	Contact sensitivity	Lichen planus, oral lichenoid reactions

that type 1 reactions can occur in the oral cavity. Urticaria of the lips and the oral mucosa occurs most frequently after food ingestion by an allergic individual. Common food allergens include chocolate, nuts, shellfish, and tomatoes. In the oral allergy syndrome (see below), it is thought that patients become sensitized by inhalation of allergens such as birch and then react orally to cross-reactive foods including apples. Drugs such as penicillin and aspirin may cause urticaria, and cold, heat, or even pressure may cause the reaction in susceptible individuals. Impression compounds, coloring agents, and preservatives, as well as ingredients of mouthwashes may all cause local swelling or even anaphylaxis.

Angioedema (incorrectly called angioneurotic edema in earlier literature) is characterized by rapid development of edematous swelling, particularly of the head and neck, sometimes accompanied by urticarial rashes. It occurs when blood vessels deep in the subcutaneous tissues are affected, producing a large diffuse area of subcutaneous swelling under normal overlying skin. This reaction may be caused by contact with a known allergen, but a significant number of cases are idiopathic. Many patients have short-term disfiguring facial swelling, but if the edema involves the neck and extends to the larynx, it can lead to fatal respiratory failure.

Angioedema most commonly occurs on the lips and tongue and around the eyes (Figure 20-18). It is temporary and not serious unless the posterior portion of the tongue or larynx compromises respiration. The patient who is in respiratory distress should be treated immediately with 0.5 mL of epinephrine (1:1000) subcutaneously or better intramuscularly. This can be repeated every 10 minutes until recovery starts. The patient should be given oxygen, placed in a recumbent position with the lower extremities elevated unless there is a danger of shortness of breath or vomiting, given fluids intravenously, and transported to hospital immediately. Patients may need intubation to maintain the airway.[192,193] When the immediate danger has passed, 50 mg of diphenhydramine hydrochloride (Benadryl [Pfizer, Parsippany, NJ]) should be given four times a day until the swelling diminishes.

Hereditary angioedema (HAE) is another life-threatening condition that is not associated with allergens.[194] It is a genetic disease with an autosomal dominant pattern of inheritance. The underlying defect is a failure to produce adequate levels of C1 esterase inhibitor (C1 inh), which normally acts as an inhibitor of the first component of complement and kallikrein. This inhibitor controls the degree of complement activation. Activation of kinin-like substances causes a sudden increase in capillary permeability. C4 is consumed and plasma levels fall, but C3 levels remain normal. An acquired form of angioedema in which antibody develops against C1 esterase inhibitor has also been described. Dental procedures can trigger attacks of HAE. These attacks do not respond well to epinephrine, and diagnosed patients are usually treated with the androgen danazol that increases C1 inh plasma levels. Fresh-frozen plasma may be given to patients before dental procedures or recombinant C1 inh

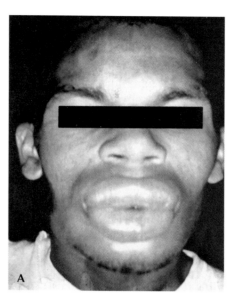

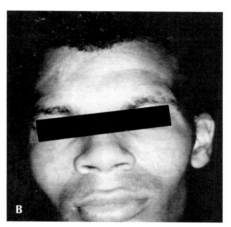

FIGURE 20-18 A, Angioedema of an allergic reaction to intramuscularly administered penicillin. B, Same patient 48 hours later, after therapy with epinephrine and antihistamine agents.

Generalized Anaphylaxis

Generalized anaphylaxis is an allergic emergency. The mechanism of generalized anaphylaxis is the reaction of IgE antibodies to an allergen causing the release of histamine, bradykinin, and SRS-A from mast cells and later eosinophils. These chemical mediators cause the contraction of smooth muscles of the respiratory and intestinal tracts, as well as increased vascular permeability. Within dentistry, penicillin is a frequently encountered cause, but muscle relaxants, cephalosporins, sulphonamides, vancomycin, radiographic contrast media, and vaccines may also cause anaphylaxis.

The following factors increase the patient's risk for anaphylaxis: (1) history of allergy to other drugs or food, (2) history of asthma, (3) family history of allergy (atopy), and (4) parenteral administration of the drug. Anaphylactic reactions may occur within seconds of drug administration or may occur 30–40 minutes later, complicating the diagnosis. Symptoms of generalized anaphylaxis should be known so that diagnosis and prompt treatment may be initiated. It is important to be able to differentiate anaphylaxis from syncope or a hypoglycemic event. The generalized anaphylactic reaction may involve the skin, the cardiovascular system, the GI tract, and the respiratory system. The first signs often occur on the skin and are similar to those seen in localized anaphylaxis (e.g., facial flushing, pruritis, parasthesia, or peripheral coldness). Pulmonary symptoms include dyspnea, wheezing, and asthma. GI tract disease, such as abdominal pain and vomiting, often follows skin symptoms. Symptoms of hypotension (loss of consciousness, pallor, and a cold clammy skin) appear as the result of the loss of intravascular fluid. The pulse becomes rapid, weak, and faint. If untreated, this leads to shock. Patients with generalized anaphylactic reactions may die from respiratory failure, hypotensive shock, or laryngeal edema.

Management

The most important therapy for generalized anaphylaxis is the administration of epinephrine. Clinicians should have a vial of aqueous epinephrine (at a 1:1000 dilution) and a sterile syringe easily accessible. For adults, 0.5 mL of epinephrine should be administered intramuscularly or subcutaneously; smaller doses of from 0.1 to 0.3 mL should be used for children, depending on their size. If the allergen was administered in an extremity, a tourniquet should be placed above the injection site to minimize further absorption into the blood. The absorption can be further reduced by injecting 0.3 mL of epinephrine (1:1000) directly into the injection site. The tourniquet should be removed every 10 minutes. Epinephrine will usually reverse all severe signs of generalized anaphylaxis. If improvement is not observed in 10 minutes, readminister epinephrine. If the patient continues to deteriorate, several steps can be taken, depending on whether the patient is experiencing bronchospasm or edema. For bronchospasm, slowly inject 250 mg of aminophylline intravenously, over a period of 10 minutes. Too rapid an administration can lead to fatal cardiac arrhythmias. Do not give aminophylline if hypotensive shock is a part of the clinical picture. Inhalation sympathomimetics may also be used to treat bronchospasm, and oxygen should be given to prevent or manage hypoxia. For the patient with laryngeal edema, establish an airway. This may necessitate endotracheal intubation; very rarely, a cricothyroidotomy may be necessary. Patients who have had an anaphylactic attack should carry self-injectable epinephrine.[193]

Latex Allergy

Latex allergy associated with undesirable cutaneous and mucosal reactions has been noticed with increasing frequency over the last few years, possibly related to the increased use of protective gloves. Although less than 1% of the general population is sensitized to latex, the US Occupational Safety and Health Administration estimates that over 8% of health care workers are sensitized.[195] Dental staff and students appear to be at high risk for latex sensitization and the overall prevalence of skin sensitization in dentists in several studies was about 10%, though this may be up to 30% in those reporting asthmatic symptoms. Much of the sensitization appears to have been by inhalation of the glove powder[195] and the rate of sensitization may be falling now that gloves are mainly powder-free.

The symptoms of latex allergy are usually those of type 1 hypersensitivity, but contact dermatitis to rubber chemicals is also well described. Sensitized individuals produce specific IgE antibody to at least 10 potent latex allergens, Hev b 1-Hev b 10, each of which differs in its structure, size, and net charge but testing for them is not yet routine. Cross-reacting antigens are found in banana, kiwifruit, avocado, and chestnuts. The important concept that latex allergy can induce clinical symptoms to specific foods (food allergy) is reinforced by the demonstration of amino acid sequence homology between latex antigens and proteins in kiwi fruit, avocado, tomatoes, and potatoes. Cross reacting IgE antibodies to 33 kd and 37 kd antigens shared between bananas and latex have been described.[197]

Testing

Recently a skin prick test reagent that contains most of the known clinically significant allergens for diagnosis of type 1 latex allergy has been standardized. The protein content of the gloves correlates with immunoreactivity and the ratio of the IgE to IgG response correlated positively with the severity of symptoms. In most studies, a history of atopy was a significant factor in latex allergy. There seems to be a reasonable correlation between in vitro IgE testing and in vivo skin prick tests.

Management

Patients with latex allergy may also show high levels of positive responses to certain foods, so a good medical history is imperative. Urticaria, rhinitis, and eyelid edema can be immediate manifestations of latex allergy. Severe systemic reactions (such as asthma and anaphylaxis), may result in permanent disability or even death. In the health care setting, the two major strategies for management are (1) the safe care of the latex allergic patient and (2) the prevention and treatment of occupational latex allergy in employees. In managing a patient with latex sensitivity,[197] the distinction between an immediate hypersensitivity reaction to latex and an allergic contact dermatitis because of other irritants must be established. At initial evaluation, latex allergy status should be established by the history and documented clearly on the medical record. Any history of an immediate hypersensitivity reaction to latex necessitates a latex-free environment for that person including *hypoallergenic* latex gloves. Latex-containing products (such as blood pressure cuffs and disposable tourniquets) should not be worn *or used in the vicinity* of persons who are allergic to latex. Premedication with antihistamines, steroids, and histamine H2 blocking agents is sometimes carried out in operating rooms, but anaphylactic reactions have occurred despite such pretreatment.

Workers who are irritated by gloves should change the type of gloves worn or change the type of soap used for scrubbing. In addition, the use of cotton liners and emollients may effectively prevent sensitivity reactions. In cases of true latex allergy, the avoidance of all latex products is the only measure that can avert a serious allergic reaction. All persons with latex hypersensitivity should carry an epinephrine auto-injection kit and wear MedicAlert identification. Acute systemic reactions to latex should be treated in the same manner as other anaphylactic reactions are treated (see above) (i.e., airway and circulation assessment, administration of oxygen, and administration of epinephrine and steroids as needed). In the course of resuscitation, all latex contact must be avoided.[198]

Oral Allergy Syndrome

Swelling of the lips, tongue and palate, and throat, along with oral pruritis and irritation, sometimes associated with other allergic clinical features including rhinoconjunctivitis, urticaria, and even anaphylaxis has been termed the oral allergy syndrome.[197] It seems to be precipitated by fresh foods including apples in people who have been sensitized to cross-reacting allergens in pollens, particularly birch.[199]

Immune Complex Diseases: Serum Sickness and Erythema Multiforme

Serum sickness is named for its frequent occurrence after the administration of foreign serum, which was given for the treatment of infectious diseases before the advent of antibiotics. It is a type 3 immune complex–mediated disease. The reaction is now uncommon but still occurs as a result of the susceptible patient being given tetanus antitoxin, rabies antiserum, or drugs that combine with body proteins to form allergens. The pathogenesis of serum sickness differs from that of anaphylaxis. Antibodies (usually IgG) form immune complexes in blood vessels with administered antigens. The complexes fix complement, which damage vessels and attracts leukocytes to the area, amplifying direct tissue injury. Serum sickness and vasculitis usually begin 7–10 days after the administration of the allergen, but this period can vary from 3 days to as long as 1 month. Unlike other allergic diseases, serum sickness may occur during the initial administration of the drug.

Major symptoms consist of fever, swelling, lymphadenopathy, joint and muscle pains, and rash. Less common manifestations include peripheral neuritis, kidney disease, and myocardial ischemia. Serum sickness is usually self-limiting, with spontaneous recovery in 1–3 weeks. Treatment is symptomatic; aspirin is given for arthralgia, and antihistamines are given for the rash. Severe cases should be treated with a short course of systemic corticosteroids, which significantly shortens the course of the disease. Although rare, the dentist who is prescribing penicillin should be aware of the possibility of serum sickness occurring days or weeks after use of the drug. It is thought that penicillin binds to host proteins to form a recognizable antigen and, as antibodies form, they meet across vessel walls and give a localized vasculitis.

Oral erythema multiforme is thought to be an immune complex disease where 7–10 days after a herpes simplex infection, IgG antibodies are formed and bind to remaining residual tissue-located herpes antigen giving rise to localized inflammation and ulceration. Similar oral appearances can sometimes occur after systemic therapy with antihypertensive drugs.

Delayed Hypersensitivity: Oral Lichenoid Reactions

Cell-mediated damaging immune reactions can occur in the oral cavity. Lichen planus is thought to be a cell-mediated autoimmune reaction against basal epithelial cells. Similarly, oral lichenoid reactions (OLRs) reflect cellular immunity to antigens found in dental restorations. These are usually associated with contact sensitivity to amalgam fillings, but similar OLRs can be found with gold, composite, or glass ionomer materials. They are important to recognize as there is increasing evidence of malignant potential of such lesions. The lesions usually present as chronic, unilateral, mixed red and white lesions in direct proximity to a restoration, which histologically appear very similar to lichen planus with a predominantly lymphocytic infiltrate. The combination of history, clinical appearance, and histology usually leads to the diagnosis.

Selected References

Al-Herz W, Alsmadi O, Melhem M, et al. Major histocompatibility complex class II deficiency in Kuwait: clinical manifestations, immunological findings and molecular profile. *J Clin Immunol* 2013;33(3):513–519.

Baldovino S, Montin D, Martino S, et al. Common variable immunodeficiency: crossroads between infections, inflammation and autoimmunity. *Autoimmun Rev*. 2013;12(8):796–801.

Ben-Mustapha I, Ben-Farhat K, Guirat-Dhouib N, et al. Clinical, immunological and genetic findings of a large tunisian series of major histocompatibility complex class II deficiency patients. *J Clin Immunol*. 2013;33(4):865–870.

Danza A, Ruiz-Irastorza G. Infection risk in systemic *Lupus* erythematosus patients: susceptibility factors and preventive strategies. Lupus. 2013;22(12):1286–1294.

Driessen GJ, Ijspeert H, Weemaes CM, et al. Antibody deficiency in patients with ataxia telangiectasia is caused by disturbed B- and T-cell homeostasis and reduced immune repertoire diversity. *J Allergy Clin Immunol*. 2013;131(5):1367–1375.e9.

Dvorak CC, Cowan MJ, Logan BR, et al. The natural history of children with severe combined immunodeficiency: baseline features of the first fifty patients of the primary immune deficiency treatment consortium prospective study 6901. *J Clin Immunol*. 2013;33(7):1156–1164.

Fernandez C, Bardin N, De Paula AM, et al. Correlation of clinicoserologic and pathologic classifications of inflammatory myopathies: study of 178 cases and guidelines for diagnosis. *Medicine (Baltimore)*. 2013;92(1):15–24.

Fillmore WJ, Leavitt BD, Arce K. Dental extraction in the thrombocytopenic patient is safe and complications are easily managed. *J Oral Maxillofac Surg*. 2013;71(10):1647–1652.

Fischer A, Hacein-Bey-Abina S, Cavazzana-Calvo M. Gene therapy of primary T cell immunodeficiencies. *Gene*. 2013;525(2):170–173.

Fortuna G, Brennan MT. Systemic lupus erythematosus: epidemiology, pathophysiology, manifestations, and management. *Dent Clin North Am*. 2013;57(4):631–655.

Hajishengallis E, Hajishengallis G. Neutrophil homeostasis and periodontal health in children and adults. *J Dent Res*. 2014;93:231–237.

Hernandez-Molina G, Zamora-Legoff T, Romero-Diaz J, et al. Predicting Sjogren's syndrome in patients with recent-onset SLE. *Rheumatology (Oxford)*. 2013;52(8):1438–1442.

Kaur S, White S, Bartold PM. Periodontal disease and rheumatoid arthritis: a systematic review. *J Dent Res*. 2013;92(5):399–408.

Khalaf MW, Khader R, Cobetto G, et al. Risk of adrenal crisis in dental patients: results of a systematic search of the literature. *J Am Dent Assoc*. 2013;144(2):152–160.

Kyriakidis NC, Kapsogeorgou EK, Tzioufas AG. A comprehensive review of autoantibodies in primary Sjögren's syndrome: clinical phenotypes and regulatory mechanisms. *J Autoimmun*. 2014;51:67–74. pii: S0896-8411(13)00145-5.

Massaad MJ, Ramesh N, Geha RS. Wiskott-Aldrich syndrome: a comprehensive review. *Ann N Y Acad Sci*. 2013;1285:26–43.

Mayes MD, Bossini-Castillo L, Gorlova O, et al. Immunochip analysis identifies multiple susceptibility loci for systemic sclerosis. *Am J Hum Genet*. 2014;94(1):47–61.

Miller FW, Cooper RG, Vencovsky J, et al. Genome-wide association study of dermatomyositis reveals genetic overlap with other autoimmune disorders. Arthritis Rheum. 2013;65(12):3239–3247.

Milner JD, Holland SM. The cup runneth over: lessons from the ever-expanding pool of primary immunodeficiency diseases. Nat Rev Immunol. 2013;13(9):635–648.

Mok CC, Kwok RC, Yip PS. Effect of renal disease on the standardized mortality ratio and life expectancy of patients with systemic lupus erythematosus. Arthritis Rheum. 2013;65(8):2154–2160.

Mok CC, Yap DY, Navarra SV, et al. Overview of lupus nephritis management guidelines and perspective from Asia. Nephrology (Carlton). 2014;19(1):11–20.

Newburger PE, Dale DC. Evaluation and management of patients with isolated neutropenia. Semin Hematol. 2013;50(3):198–206.

Newman K, Owlia MB, El-Hemaidi I, Akhtari M. Management of immune cytopenias in patients with systemic lupus erythematosus—old and new. Autoimmun Rev. 2013;12(7):784–791.

Norholt SE, Pedersen TK, Herlin T. Functional changes following distraction osteogenesis treatment of asymmetric mandibular growth deviation in unilateral juvenile idiopathic arthritis: a prospective study with long-term follow-up. Int J Oral Maxillofac Surg. 2013;42(3):329–336.

Okada Y, Wu D, Trynka G, et al. Genetics of rheumatoid arthritis contributes to biology and drug discovery. *Nature*. 2014;506(7488):376–381.

Qin X, Jiang LP, Tang XM, et al. Clinical features and mutation analysis of X-linked agammaglobulinemia in 20 Chinese patients. World J Pediatr. 2013;9(3):273–277.

Rethman MP, Watters W III, Abt E, et al. The American Academy of Orthopaedic Surgeons and the American Dental Association clinical practice guideline on the prevention of orthopaedic implant infection in patients undergoing dental procedures. J Bone Joint Surg Am. 2013;95(8):745–747.

Shah AA, Wigley FM. My approach to the treatment of scleroderma. Mayo Clin Proc. 2013;88(4):377–393.

Sidebottom AJ, Salha R. Management of the temporomandibular joint in rheumatoid disorders. Br J Oral Maxillofac Surg. 2013;51(3):191–198.

Svensson R, Hallmer F, Englesson CS, et al. Treatment with local hemostatic agents and primary closure after tooth extraction in warfarin treated patients. Swed Dent J. 2013;37(2):71–77.

Thanou A, Merrill JT. Treatment of systemic lupus erythematosus: new therapeutic avenues and blind alleys. Nat Rev Rheumatol. 2014;10(1):23–34.

van den Hoogen F, Khanna D, Fransen J, et al. 2013 classification criteria for systemic sclerosis: an American College of Rheumatology/European League Against Rheumatism collaborative initiative. *Arthritis Rheum*. 2013;65(11):2737–2747.

Watters W III, Rethman MP, Hanson NB, et al. Prevention of orthopaedic implant infection in patients undergoing dental procedures. *J Am Acad Orthop Surg*. 2013;21(3):180–189.

Yao CM, Han XH, Zhang YD, et al. Clinical characteristics and genetic profiles of 44 patients with severe combined immunodeficiency (SCID): report from Shanghai, China (2004–2011). *J Clin Immunol* 2013;33(3):526–539.

Yuen H, Hant F, Hatfield C, et al. Factors associated with oral hygiene practices among adults with systemic sclerosis. *Int J Dent Hyg*. 2014 Aug;12(3):180-6.

For the full reference lists, please go to http://www.pmph-usa.com/Burkets_Oral_Medicine.

CHAPTER 21

Transplantation Medicine

Thomas P. Sollecito, DMD, FDS RCS Ed

Andres Pinto, DMD, MPH

Ali Naji, MD, PhD

David L. Porter, MD

Transplantation is the treatment of choice for the restoration of function in end-stage organ disease. Innovative surgical techniques have played a major role in enhancing the success of organ transplants, leading to improved graft and patient survival. Advances in the biology of organ preservation have led to improved cold storage of the solid organs, improving the overall quality of the transplanted organs and diminishing the damage incurred by warm ischemia, allowing optimization of the medical conditions of the donor and the recipient.[1,2] Furthermore, insights into the biology of immune responses to transplanted tissues have aided the development of immunosuppressive techniques to prevent the rejection of the organ transplants while minimizing the morbidities associated with the chronic immunosuppression of the recipients. The main limitation to even greater use of transplantation as a treatment modality for end-stage organ damage remains the shortage of organ donors.

Attempts at organ and bone marrow transplantation date back to the 1800s. In more recent history, Dr. Joseph Murray performed the first successful human renal transplantation between identical twin brothers in 1954. This procedure was well tolerated as there was no rejection by the genetically identical recipient. The first successful allogeneic (not genetically identical) transplantation was a kidney transplant between fraternal twins performed in 1959 in which the recipient was "conditioned" (immunosuppressed to prevent rejection) by total-body irradiation. In 1962, a successful cadaveric donor renal transplantation was achieved, and in 1966, a pancreas transplantation was successfully performed. In the following year, the first human liver transplantation was performed, resulting in a 13-month survival. In the same year, a heart was transplanted. In 1968, a genetically related bone marrow transplantation (today referred to as hematopoietic cell transplantation [HCT]) was performed, and in 1973, a genetically unrelated HCT was performed. Lung transplantation has also been performed both as a single procedure and in combination with heart transplantation. The first heart–lung transplantation in the United States was performed in 1981, and the first single-lung transplantation in Canada was performed in 1983. Other organs that have been successfully transplanted include the small bowel, skin, various limbs, and components of the human eye.

In the past 20 years, significant advances, including tissue typing and the development of immunosuppressive medications and medication regimens, have increased the success of transplantation. Overall, long-term patient survival has also significantly increased over the past 30 years, both in solid organ and HCT recipients. Most transplant clinicians consider the discovery of the immunosuppressive agent cyclosporine A (CSA) to be the most significant advance in transplantation medicine. This medication was approved for use in 1983.[3] Both solid organ and non–solid organ transplantations are becoming more routine throughout the world. In November 2013, over 120,000 patients in the United States alone were waiting for a solid organ transplant. In 2012, 28,052 solid organs were transplanted (Table 21-1) approximately the same number as was seen in 2005.[3]

As the process of solid organ transplantation expands, there is a continued need to increase the supply of organs suitable for transplantation. The limitation of available donor organs will hopefully become less of an issue with increased awareness of organ donation and perhaps with collaborative sharing initiatives, alternative organ procurement methods, including xenografts or stem cell–derived tissue.

The likelihood of a dentist having the opportunity to treat a transplanted patient is increasing as many of these transplant recipients resume normal ways of life after the transplantation.

This chapter reviews different aspects of transplantation medicine pertinent for the oral health professional.

CLASSIFICATION

Most transplant clinical classification systems employ both the type of tissue transplanted and the genetic relationship of the tissue to the recipient. It is extremely important for the dental clinician to know exactly what type of transplantation was performed as both the management and the prognosis are intimately related. This will become evident as it is discussed later in this chapter.

Some authorities broadly divide clinical transplantations as being either a solid organ/tissue transplant or an HCT. Virtually all types of solid organs/tissues have been transplanted, including heart, lung, kidney, liver, stomach intestine, pancreas, skin, tendons, verves, veins, and eye components, as well as composite tissue transplants, including the face and limbs. Another type of transplantation frequently used to treat various hematologic and some nonhematologic malignancies, as well as other disorders, is known as HCT. HCT uses either an autologous "self" donor graft or a "non-self" donor (allogeneic graft); HCT poses special management concerns to the clinician, which are detailed later in this chapter.

Classification of transplants can also be based broadly on the genetic relationship of the recipient to the donor. For the purpose of this chapter, the transplanted cell, tissue, or organ is referred to as the graft. A transplant to and from one's self (autograft) is known as an autologous transplant. A transplantation from an identical twin (identical genetic make-up) is known as an isograft, with the process of this type of transplantation known as isogeneic or syngeneic transplantation. Most transplants are from donors that are not genetically identical to the recipient (allografts). These types of transplants are known as allogeneic transplants. Finally, transplants from donors of one species to recipients of another species (xenografts) are known as xenogeneic transplants.[4]

Because of the scarcity of isografts and the obvious limitations to autografts, allogeneic transplants are most commonly used today. The success of allogeneic transplantation relies on sophisticated mechanisms for identifying and matching specific genetic markers between the donor and the recipient, as well as suppressing the recipient's immune system to prevent transplant rejection. These are concepts that serve

TABLE 21-1 Waiting Lists (as of November 8, 2013) and Transplanted Solid Organs (2012ᵃ) in the United States		
Organ	Transplants Awaited	Transplants Performed
Liver	15,840	6,256
Kidney	98,611	16,486
Lung	1,609	1,754
Heart	3,661	2,378

ᵃNote that these numbers do not equal those cited in the text since other organs, including the small intestine and pancreas, are not included in this table.
Source: Based on Organ Procurement and Transplantation Network: optn.transplant.hrsa.gov. Accessed November 8, 2013.

as the basic foundation in transplantation medicine. In the future, these concepts may be extended and improved to allow transplantation across species. Tissue xenografts, which have been treated to reduce their immunogenicity, have been used as a successful treatment modality in some applications (i.e., porcine heart valves), but whole-organ xenografts have been unsuccessful. Research regarding genetically altered xenografts is ongoing. When the important immunologic barriers to xenogeneic transplantation are eliminated, the use of animal donors may possibly alleviate the relative paucity of available organs. Of course, significant ethical questions, as well as transplant longevity and transmissible infectious diseases from animals, are questions that must be entertained before these types of transplants become commonplace.[5] Bioengineered tissues that have been fabricated in vitro and transplanted back into the patient have also been successful including a trachea and a bladder.[6,7]

TRANSPLANTATION IMMUNOLOGY

Transplantation immunology encompasses most aspects of the human immune response to alloantigens expressed by the recipient as well as the donor organ/tissue. When donor and recipient genetic disparities exist, the recipient mounts a specific immune response to the alloantigens expressed by the donor grafted organ/tissue. In addition, donor T cells contained within the transplanted graft or organ can recognize foreign tissue in the host and mount a "graft-versus-host" reaction. Transplantation medicine would be grossly unsuccessful if this concept was not appropriately appreciated and manipulated. To appreciate the intricacies of organ transplantation, a basic understanding of immunologic concepts is helpful.

T lymphocytes are the primary though not the only cells which mediate graft rejection as well as graft versus host disease. T cells can become activated shortly after transplant by recognizing foreign major and minor human leukocyte antigen (HLA) molecules. The major histocompatibility complex (MHC), a genetic region found on the short arm of chromosome number 6 of all mammalian cells, codes for HLA molecules that allow immune cells to identify self from nonself. Although there are many other gene products, from more than 30 histocompatibility gene loci, that can stimulate graft rejection, it is the HLA system that produces the strongest immunologic response.[4]

MHC genes are inherited from each parent; every child has components of both the mother's and the father's HLAs on their cell surfaces. The MHC/HLA system is broadly divided into regions. MHC class I and class II regions are those significantly involved in rejection and graft-versus-host disease (GVHD). MHC class I regions include HLA-A, -B, -C, -E, -F, and -G. (The present role of the E, F, and G regions in transplantation is not well understood.) MHC class II regions include HLA-DR, -DQ, -DP, -DO, and -DN. MHC class II genes have two chains, allowing for four different gene products for each locus.

The MHC has extensive polymorphism, allowing remarkable diversity among genes of the HLA system.[8]

There are over 180 different class I alleles in the HLA-B region alone and over 220 class II alleles in just one loci of the HLA-DR region that have been recognized in humans. Today, deoxyribonucleic acid (DNA)-based typing (see below) has led to a more specific and detailed classification of the transplantation genes, such that the HLA alleles are related to their DNA sequences.[8]

HLA class I antigens are expressed on most nucleated cells and red blood cells, whereas class II antigens are expressed only on certain cells known as antigen-presenting cells (APCs). APCs include macrophages, B cells, dendritic cells, and some endothelial cells. The expression of these MHC gene products (antigens) on a cell's surface is regulated by various cytokines such as interferon (IFN) and tumor necrosis factor (TNF).

In the setting of solid organ transplantation, the transplanted foreign MHC molecules activate the immune response by stimulating the recipient's T cells to respond to foreign antigens. The interaction of the MHC of the donor cells with the recipient's T-cell receptor (TCR) initiates the immune reaction that can lead to rejection. T cells can be activated by either the donor's or the recipient's APCs, resulting in expression and production of lymphokines and cytokines that promote activation of cytotoxic T cells, activation of B cells, and activation of natural killer cell activity, as well as promote enhanced expression of MHC and increased macrophage activity. This, in turn, causes further immune reactions that result in direct tissue damage and damage to the vascular endothelium of the graft, which may ultimately result in graft rejection.

Despite the treatment of recipients with immunosuppressive drugs, the possibility of the immunologic rejection is not entirely eliminated. The rejection may evolve as an acute process occurring within days to weeks of the transplantation surgery. This acute process is related to the primary activation of T cells and usually can be reversed by modifying or intensifying the immunosuppressive regimen.

Chronic rejection of the transplanted organ is also a significant problem leading to organ failure. This type of rejection is slow and insidious and in most cases cannot be reversed by conventional immunosuppressive drugs. It probably occurs by continued, albeit muted, cell-mediated toxicity that results in vascular endothelial damage of the transplanted organ (as well as other actions, which have not been fully elucidated), ultimately leading to graft failure.[9]

Another type of rejection is known as hyper acute rejection; this occurs within minutes to hours after a transplantation procedure. This pattern of rejection occurs in patients who have undergone previous transplantations, patients who have had multiple pregnancies, and patients who have had multiple blood transfusions. It is caused by the presence of preformed antidonor antibodies in the recipient, which activate complement cascade, resulting in severe damage to the parenchymal constituents of the graft, which often cannot be reversed.[10,11]

Transplant immunology is even more complicated in the setting of allogeneic HCT.[12] Without proper immune suppression, residual host lymphocytes can mediate graft rejection leaving a patient aplastic. However unlike solid organ transplant, a hematopoietic stem cell graft has large numbers of mature lymphocytes capable of reacting against nonself antigens in the host in inducing graft versus host disease. Donor leukocytes tend to react against the skin, liver, and gastrointestinal tract. Occasional involvement of the lungs can be seen as well. GVHD varies from nonexistent in approximately 50% of patients to severe and life threatening. GVHD still remains one of the major limitations to successful HCT. Intensive therapies designed to minimize GVHD have resulted in higher rates of relapse from loss of the potential "graft versus tumor" effect and from higher rates of infection. Ultimately therapies that may limit GVHD and retain the important graft-versus-tumor (GVT) activity of the donor graft will be needed to improve the outcomes of HCT, and several strategies are in clinical testing.[13]

It should also be noted that in unusual cases after solid organ transplant, mature donor lymphocytes transplant with the organ can engraft and likewise cause GVHD.[14] This is particularly complicated and similar to "transfusion-associated GVHD" (TA-GVHD) that can lead to marrow aplasia without the support of a donor stem cell graft.[15] Similar to TA-GVHD, the prognosis is often poor, and treatment requires early recognition and intensive intervention with immune suppression.

CLINICAL INDICATIONS

The clinical indications for transplantation vary, but the disease outcome can be fatal without the transplant. The more common indications for transplantation are listed in Table 21-2.

TABLE 21-2 Major Indications for Transplantation[a]

Type of Transplant	Indications
Kidney	End-stage renal disease Diabetic nephropathy Glomerulonephritis Pyelonephritis Congenital abnormalities Nephrotic syndrome
Liver	End-stage liver disease Primary biliary cirrhosis Biliary atresia (children) Chronic hepatitis Sclerosing cholangitis
Pancreas	Severe diabetes leading to renal disease Severe hypoglycemic unawareness
Isolated pancreatic islets	Severe hypoglycemic unawareness
Intestinal	Massive short-bowel syndrome
Heart	Cardiomyopathy
	Severe coronary artery disease
	Congestive heart failure
Heart and lung	Multiorgan end-stage disease
	Congenital abnormalities
	Amyloidosis
Lung	Primary pulmonary hypertension
	COPD/emphysema
	Pulmonary fibrosis
	Cystic fibrosis
Hematopoietic cell transplantation (autologous)	Acute myelogenous leukemia Multiple myeloma and AL amyloidosis Lymphoma (Hodgkin and non-Hodgkin) Possibly solid tumors (germ cell, ovarian) SLE/autoimmune disorders
Hematopoietic cell transplantation (allogeneic)	Acute myelogenous leukemia Acute lymphoblastic leukemia Chronic myelogenous leukemia Aplastic anemia Primary immunodeficiencies Hemoglobinopathies (sickle cell, thalassemia)

Abbreviations: COPD, chronic obstructive pulmonary disorder; SLE, systemic lupus erythematosus.
[a]Partial listing only.

Other indications can also be added to this list when quality of life can be improved by transplantation. For example, autologous HCT may ameliorate the effects of systemic lupus erythematosus or other autoimmune disorders.[16–18] More recently, HCT has been cited as a possible treatment for the management of various metabolic disorders and solid tumors, germ cell tumors,[19] and neurobastoma.[20] Other potential uses for stem cell therapy in various other disorders, such as diabetes[21–24] and amyloidosis,[25,26] are also being researched.

MEDICAL MANAGEMENT

Medical management of the transplant candidate focuses on successfully preventing rejection. In solid organ transplantation, when the donor and recipient tissue are genetically identical (autologous or syngeneic), the outcome of the transplantation relies upon the surgical success of the procedure. For autologous HCT, success is largely dependent on the high-dose chemotherapy or radiation used to eradicate residual malignant cells prior to HCT. When tissue from genetically different sources is transplanted, a sophisticated means of preventing rejection must be instituted to ensure graft survival, and in the setting of allogeneic stem cell transplant, methods must be used to prevent both graft rejection and severe GVHD, as described latter. Transplantation surgeons and oncologists have improved the surgical procedures for various transplantations; medical management to achieve longer term successful grafts and longer term overall patient survival has been quite successful, yet it is still fraught with longer term complications. The success of an allogeneic transplantation relies on the ability to identify and match certain genetic markers between the donor and the recipient while suppressing the recipient's immune system to prevent rejection.

BLOOD AND TISSUE TYPING

Standard ABO and RhP blood typing is performed to prevent hyperacute rejection of the transplant based on isoagglutinin incompatibility. ABO matching is mandatory for solid organ transplant and directly impacts short-term graft survival. ABO matching does not appear to impact graft survival after allogeneic HCT[27]; the impact or patient outcomes such as relapse are controversial but are likely to be small and of unclear significance that may depend on graft source and disease.[28]

Cross-matching (crossing recipient serum with donor lymphocytes) is usually done to prevent hyperacute rejection in allogeneic solid organ transplants. This is a basic serologic test that is regarded as necessary particularly in those allogeneic transplant recipients who have previously experienced massive immune challenges such as a prior transplantation, multiple pregnancies, or multiple blood transfusions and have developed preformed anti-HLA antibodies. Currently, the existence of preformed alloantibodies is detected by single HLA bead (Luminex) technology.[29] Since transplantation of solid organs (heart, lung, liver) often requires some expediency, time-consuming complex cross-matching or tissue typing cannot be performed. Instead, absence of antibodies to a panel of cells (defined in advance and known as panel-reactive antibodies) is usually adequate for heart and lung transplantation.[30] Interestingly, MHC compatibility in liver transplantation seems negligible in achieving better outcomes.[31] This is fortunate because the timing of liver transplantation often precludes HLA typing.[32]

The most critical matching criteria for allogeneic hematopoietic stem cell transplantation (SCT) is tissue typing to determine and match histocompatibility antigens and alleles. HLA molecules are found on donor and recipient cells and in the setting of hematopoietic SCT are critical for determining engraftment and complications such as GVHD. HLA typing is much less critical in renal transplantations and for graft survival in liver or heart transplantations.[31] Tissue typing can be performed by serologic assays,[4] but more recently, most typing is performed using rapid DNA-based testing methods. Polymorphisms in HLAs are common, and it is now practical and routine to test not just for HLAs but for HLA alleles. In the setting of allogeneic HSCT, it is clear that allele level matching improves outcomes.[33] Matching at class I HLA-A, B, C and class II (HLA-DR) is critical in all cases. The role of matching at the HLA class II molecule DQ is less clear and a single DQ mismatch does not seem to impact the outcome after HCT.

IMMUNOSUPPRESSION

Immunosuppressive regimens vary among transplant centers and according to the type of the transplanted organ (intestines, liver, etc.). Since tissues in allogeneic transplants are not genetically identical, medications used to control the immune response are essential for graft survival.[34,35] All allogeneic transplantations initially require immunosuppression if the transplanted organs are not to be acutely rejected. Furthermore, most allogeneic solid organ transplant recipients require lifelong maintenance immunosuppression. This is usually not the case with allogeneic HCT (and no immunosuppression is required for autologous HCT). In addition, more intensive immunosuppressive regimens are employed later in the posttransplantation period in cases of acute rejection episodes.

Most immunosuppressive medications are nonspecific and cannot prevent a specific component of the immune response. More sophisticated and directed medications are being developed currently; these will allow for graft tolerance while allowing the body to still react to infectious and other detrimental antigens.

Arguably, the most significant advances in transplantation have been made in pharmacotherapeutic immunosuppression. As there is improved understanding of how graft rejection transpires, there is improvement in the specificity of the immunomodulator. The most frequently used contemporary medication classes are discussed in this chapter, with a brief review of some promising formulations (Table 21-3).

TABLE 21-3   Major Immunosuppressive Agents[a]

Drug	Type	Indications	Major Side Effects[b]	Dental Implications[b]
Cyclosporine	Macrolide immunosuppressant Calcineurin inhibitor	Prophylaxis against organ rejection	Hepatotoxicity Nephrotoxicity Elevation of blood pressure	Immunosuppressant[c] P-450 metabolized[d] Gingival hyperplasia Monitor CV system May effect renal elimination of some drugs Risk of neoplasm
Tacrolimus	Macrolide immunosuppressant Calcineurin inhibitor	Prophylaxis against organ rejection	Hepatotoxicity Neurotoxicity Nephrotoxicity Posttransplantation diabetes mellitus Elevation of blood pressure	Immunosuppressant[c] P-450 metabolized[d] Monitor CV system May effect renal elimination of some drugs Risk of neoplasm
Sirolimus	Macrolide immunosuppressant	Prophylaxis against acute and perhaps chronic organ rejection	Hyperlipidemia Hypertriglyceridemia	Immunosuppressant[c] P-450 metabolized[d] Monitor CV system May effect renal elimination of some drugs Risk of neoplasm
Azathioprine	Antimetabolite	Prophylaxis against organ rejection	Bone marrow suppression Hepatotoxicity	Immunosuppressant[c] Risk of neoplasm
Mycophenolate mofetil	Antimetabolite	Prophylaxis against organ rejection	Immunosuppressantc Leukopenia	Absorption is altered by antibiotics, antacids, and bile acid binders Risk of neoplasm
ATG/ALG	Polyclonal antibody	Conditioning agents used prior to transplantation Or reversal of established rejection	Leukopenia PTLD Pulmonary edema Renal dysfunction	Immunosuppressant[c]
Basiliximab	Monoclonal antibody	Reversal of acute organ rejection Induction immunosuppressant and prophylaxis against organ rejection	Pulmonary edema Renal dysfunction	Immunosuppressant[c] Risk of neoplasm
Corticosteroids	Nonspecific immunosuppressant	Reversal of acute organ rejection	Multiple Increases the incidence of glucose intolerance and diabetes	Broad nonspecific immunosuppressant[c] Avoid NSAIDs and ASA Monitor CV system Poor wound healing Risk of neoplasm Steroid supplement may be needed with stressful procedures

Abbreviations: ASA, acetylsalicylic acid; ATG/ALG, antithymocyte globulin/antilymphocyte globulin; CV, cardiovascular; NSAIDs, nonsteroidal anti-inflammatory drugs; PTLD, posttransplantation lymphoproliferative disease.
[a]Major mechanisms of action are outlined in the text.
[b]Partial listing only.
[c]Use of an immunosuppressant results in an increased risk of infection.
[d]Dental/oral pharmacotherapeutics that are metabolized by the liver's cytochrome P-450 3A system alter this drug's serum levels. This group of medications includes, but is not limited to, erythromycin, clarithromycin, "azole" antifungals, benzodiazepines, carbamazepine, colchicines, prednisolone, and metronidazole.

CYCLOSPORINE ANALOGUES

CSA is a cyclic polypeptide macrolide medication derived from a metabolite of the fungus *Beauveria nivea*. It is indicated for the prevention of graft rejection because of its immunosuppressive effects. It specifically and reversibly inhibits immunocompetent lymphocytes in the G0 and G1 phase of the cell cycle. CSA binds with an intracellular protein, cyclophilin, and inhibits calcineurin. Calcineurin activates a nuclear component of T cells that is thought to initiate gene transcription for the formation of interleukin (IL)-2. Presumably, CSA inhibits IL-2 by preventing the expression of its gene. CSA also reduces the expression of IL-2 receptors. T helper and, to some extent, T suppressor cells are preferentially suppressed.[36,37] This medication has some effect on humoral immunity but not on phagocytic function, neutrophil migration, macrophage migration, or direct bone marrow suppression. Absorption of this drug is variable, and blood levels must be drawn two hours after dosing to ensure that the drug is in the therapeutic range.[38]

TACROLIMUS

Tacrolimus (FK-506) (Prograf, Fujisawa Healthcare Inc., Deerfield, IL) is a macrolide immunosuppressant produced by *Streptomyces tsukubaensis* that is used to prevent organ rejection. This medication is similar to CSA in that it suppresses cell-mediated reactions by suppressing T-cell activation. Tacrolimus inhibits calcineurin by interacting with an intracellular protein known as the FK-binding protein. Consequently, T cells are not activated, and cell-mediated cytotoxicity is impeded.[37] There may be a lower incidence of rejection with the use of tacrolimus as compared with the use of CSA in liver, kidney, and lung transplantations. Overall graft and patient survival rates in kidney transplantations do not seem to differ significantly with the use of this medication.

SIROLIMUS

Sirolimus (Rapamycin) (Rapamune, Wyeth-Ayerst Pharmaceuticals, Philadelphia, PA) is another macrolide immunosuppressive agent; it was discovered more than 25 years ago in the soil of Easter Island (Rapa Nui) and is produced by *Streptomyces hygroscopicus*. It is used for prophylaxis against acute rejection of various organs and may be appropriate for use in chronic rejection.[38] Sirolimus's mechanism of action is somewhat unique. Sirolimus inhibits the activation of a particular cellular kinase (target of rapamycin), which then interferes with intracellular signaling pathways of the IL-2 receptor, thereby preventing lymphocyte activation. The response of T cells to IL-2 and other cytokines is inhibited. Specifically, the overall effect is interference of T-cell activation during the cells' G1 to S phase. Sirolimus is used in conjunction with CSA and tacrolimus but is associated with significant toxicity.[35]

AZATHIOPRINE

AZA is an antimetabolite that inhibits ribonucleic acid and DNA synthesis by interfering with the purine synthesis that results in decreased T- and B-cell proliferation. It does not interfere with lymphokine production but has significant anti-inflammatory properties. AZA can be bone marrow suppressive, leading to pancytopenia, and it can also cause significant liver dysfunction. Significant drug interactions with allopurinol[39] and angiotensin-converting enzyme inhibitors have been reported. AZA has been used for many years in conjunction with CSA and corticosteroids as triple immunosuppressive therapy. Today, mycophenolate mofetil (MMF), a newer purine analogue, is being used as an alternative to AZA as it may have a more specific action against T cells.

MYCOPHENOLATE MOFETIL

MMF, an ester of mycophenolic acid, is an antimetabolite that is used for prophylaxis against graft rejection and that may have some action in reversing ongoing acute rejection. It inhibits inflammation by interfering with purine synthesis. Both T and B cells, which are dependent on this synthesis for their proliferation, are prevented from reproducing. In addition, MMF interferes with intercellular adhesion of lymphocytes to endothelial cells. It does not inhibit IL-1 or IL-2. It is thought that this medication can replace AZA in kidney and heart transplantation.[35]

ANTITHYMOCYTE AND ANTILYMPHOCYTE GLOBULIN

Polyclonal antilymphocyte sera, antilymphocyte globulin, and antithymocyte globulin are part of the same medication class. These agents are produced by immunizing animals with human lymphoid cells; the animals then produce antibodies that then reduce the number of circulating T cells after infusion into transplanted recipients. Individually, these agents affect lymphocyte immunosuppression by reacting with common T-cell surface markers and then coating (opsonizing) the lymphocyte—marking it as foreign for phagocytosis. Polyclonal antibodies are used as conditioning agents prior to transplantation[40] as well as for reversal of steroid-resistant rejection.

BASILIXIMAB

Basiliximab are synthetic monoclonal antibodies used for reversal of acute organ rejection. These humanized antibodies also have a significant role during induction immunosuppression.[35] These monoclonal antibodies bind the CD25 receptor (IL-2 receptor) on the surface of activated T cells (IL-2 receptor antagonists), preventing the expansion of CD4 and CD8 lymphocytes. They may be effective in conjunction with MMF and corticosteroids to eliminate the need for CSA use in the early posttransplantation period.[41] Anti-CD25 agents have also been reported to be efficacious in treatment of corticosteroid-resistant GVHD.[42]

Other promising targets for monoclonal antibody immunomodulation are being studied currently. The target receptors vary in their function, but development of target-specific medications will probably aid in selected immunosuppression.

ALEMTUZUMAB

Alemtuzumab is a monoclonal antibody that binds to and depletes CD52, which is expressed on the surface of mature lymphocytes. It is used for the treatment of chronic lymphocytic leukemia, and in some conditioning regimens for bone marrow, kidney and islet transplantation.[43]

CORTICOSTEROIDS

Corticosteroids are consistently used in all allogeneic transplantations for prophylaxis against graft rejection and for reversal of acute rejection. The mechanism of action of this medication is nonspecific as it affects the immune system in many complex ways. Steroids have anti-inflammatory effects and are able to suppress activated macrophages. They also interfere with antigen presentation and reduce the expression of MHC antigens on cells. Steroids reverse the effect of IFN-γ and alter the expression of adhesion molecules on vascular endothelium. These medications also have significant effects on IL-1 activity and block the *IL-2* gene and its production.[4,38]

OTHER CYTOTOXIC AGENTS

Unlike solid organ transplant, HCT requires "conditioning" of the patient with cytotoxic chemotherapy. Traditional conditioning regimens were designed to take advantage of the dose: response activity against cancer cells. High doses of chemotherapy or radiation are used to eradicate residual tumor prior to infusion of the hematopoietic stem cell product. Typical myeloablative agents include cyclophosphamide in combination with busulfan, etoposide, fludarabine, or often total body irradiation (TBI). A "side effect" is myeloablation requiring the need to transplant additional donor hematopoietic stem cells. The conditioning therapy must also be sufficiently immunosuppressive to prevent graft rejection or patients would be left aplastic and die from complications of cytopenias and infections. It has been recognized for years, however, that the success of transplant is also related to the immunological activity of the donor graft, independent of the conditioning therapy. Donor T cells have the ability to react against and kill residual tumor cells and induce a "GVT" effect.[44] This observation led to the development of less intensive reduced intensity conditioning (RIC) regimens designed primarily for immunosuppression to allow donor cell engraftment, and to take advantage of the GVT activity

without the organ toxicity often associated with very high doses of chemotherapy and radiation. Typical regimens for RIC HCT include similar drugs and TBI as used in myeloablative transplant but as the name implies, often at reduced doses. Although treatment-related morbidity and mortality are less with these regimens, this is often offset by higher relapse rates. However, RIC HCT results in significant less mucositis, pneumonitis, and other organ toxicity, and outcomes for many diseases seem similar after RIC HCT appear similar to outcomes after more conventional myeloablative SCT.

NEWER IMMUNOSUPPRESSIVE STRATEGIES

Novel approaches to immunosuppression are currently being developed. The definitive immunosuppressive agent would be an agent that is able to destroy only the T cells that are involved with graft rejection while leaving the remainder of the T cells and the immune system intact. Other monoclonal antibodies are currently under development, with promising immune modulation targets, including more specific T cells and natural killer cells, as well as endothelium-activated cells.[38]

Another promising approach to induce immunosuppression is via a class of biologic agents called the T-cell co-stimulatory pathway modifiers. Studies have suggested that immune system function has significant self-regulatory capabilities. It is now well recognized that TCRs must recognize MHC-presented antigens to activate a T-cell response. However, it is also thought that TCR recognition requires two specific signals to stimulate T-cell activation—that is, recognition of both the TCR signal and a costimulatory receptor(s) such as CD28 and/or CD40 ligand, both mandatory for optimal T-cell activation. Blocking of the costimulatory signal is the basis of this novel approach to preventing rejection of an allogeneic transplant. An engineered monoclonal antibody (Belatacept, LEA29Y) with potent costimulation blockade has been rationally designed from CTLA4-Ig-binding site modification. This monoclonal antibody has been an effective costimulatory agent in the prevention of renal transplant rejection, allowing avoidance of calcineurin inhibitor agents (tacrolimus and CSA) that have nephrotoxicity.[45]

Another interesting finding that has been reported is that use of pravastatin during the early transplantation period may have some effect as an adjunct in immunosuppressive therapy via reduction in natural killer cell cytotoxicity.[46]

Although newer immunosuppressive agents have been developed and are being used, they have not shown any clear benefit in patient or organ survival over CSA or tacrolimus. The newer agents, however, have shown some promise in reducing the incidence and severity of rejection. These newer agents probably have a role in reducing the need for corticosteroids as well as reducing the toxic profiles of CSA or tacrolimus.[38]

Ultimately, graft and patient survival profiles coupled with side effects will determine the best antirejection "cocktail" to be used in various transplantations.

Similar immunosuppressive therapies are necessary and used in patients undergoing hematopoietic stem cell transplant. Immunosuppression in this setting is used not only to prevent graft rejection but also to prevent graft versus host disease. Approaches used for GVHD prevention and management include pharmacologic agents that inhibit T-cell function, antibody therapy directed against T cells, selection of stem cell grafts in ways that eliminate T cells prior to transplant, novel approaches to inhibit T-cell trafficking to sites where GVHD can be initiated, enhancement of suppressive mechanisms that can limit T-cell activity (such as infusion of regulatory T cells and mesenchymal stem cells), and the use of other novel compounds that may modulate T-cell function and activity. This is a rapidly changing landscape and has been reviewed in detail.[47]

ANTIMICROBIAL MEDICATION

In addition to immunosuppressive medication regimens, antimicrobial medication regimens are important in preventing infection in the transplant recipient. These regimens vary from center to center and from program to program. After transplant, patients are typically profoundly immunosuppressed for months. Many factors affect the pace of immune reconstitution, but it is common to use prophylactic antibiotics for bacterial, protozoan, fungal, and viral infections and antifungal and antiviral preparations. These medications may include sulfamethoxazole-trimethoprim, nystatin, fluconazole, acyclovir, ganciclovir, and others.

The Centers for Disease Control and Prevention (CDC) has published updated guidelines for preventing opportunistic infections among HCT recipients based on the quality of the evidence supporting the recommendation.[48] During the HCT process, prophylactic antibiotics can be used but it is mandatory to treat patients with empiric therapy in the setting of neutropenia and fevers. Prophylaxis against fungal and viral infections is recommended, and it is common to treat patients with an azole or echinocandin to prevent fungal infection, and acyclovir or similar therapy to prevent viral infections. After transplant, prophylaxis is standard against fungal and viral infections as well. Cytomegalovirus (CMV) infection after transplant is particularly concerning, but data suggest that sensitive screening for reactivation and preemptive rather than prophylactic therapy is a safe and reasonable strategy to avoid side effects from prolonged exposure to antibiotics such as ganciclovir. In some cases of transplant, there is also a risk of Epstein–Barr virus (EBV) reactivation and routine monitoring and preemptive therapy may be used in these cases as well.

Various protocols have been proposed based on the type of transplant, the time frame after transplantation, and the signs and symptoms that a transplant patient may experience.[49] Antimicrobial medication coverage has proven to be effective in prevention of some of the transplant-associated infections.[50] Some have questioned whether antimicrobial agents are overused during the perioperative period in renal transplants.[51]

The CDC also proposes guidelines for vaccination for HCT patients and for their family members/close contacts.[48] Vaccination against hepatitis B virus and varicella-zoster virus (VZV) is usually considered if the transplant recipient does not have antibodies to these diseases. Special consideration for vaccination must be taken into account in the pediatric population. It is of utmost importance for children to receive appropriate vaccination.

COMPLICATIONS

Complications with transplantation are still common and require close evaluation and management. General complications can be broadly characterized into those caused by rejection, side effects from medication, and those induced by immunosuppression. In addition, there are some organ-specific complications observed in certain types of transplantations.

REJECTION

As mentioned earlier, rejection of the transplanted organ remains a significant obstacle for long-term transplant graft and patient survival. The temporal relationship between the transplant and rejection episodes allows categorization of the particular rejection process. Rejection leads to end-organ damage and remanifestation of the various complications of a nonfunctioning organ. Clinically, rejection may be indicated in many ways, including an increased bleeding tendency (rejection of liver), a decreased metabolism of medications (rejection of liver/kidney), or even complete organ failure and death (rejection of lung/heart). In cases of end-organ disease (except those of kidney failure), retransplantation may be the only way to prevent death.

Rejection is continually monitored throughout the posttransplantation period. Most chronic rejections are insidious and are monitored by frequent laboratory analysis and by organ biopsy. Biopsy of tissue from the transplanted organ provides a reliable means to assess rejection. An alternative approach to monitoring rejection in a transplanted heart is the use of pacemakers to record changes in ventricular evoked response (VER). Subtle changes in VER have been correlated with rejection of heart transplants.[52]

MEDICATION-INDUCED COMPLICATIONS

The medications used to produce immunosuppression and prevent graft rejection have significant systemic side effects, which pose serious complications to the transplant recipient. Some of the major side effects are listed here; however, complete drug information can be obtained through an appropriate medication reference source.

CSA, a mainstay in immunosuppression, is nephrotoxic and may alter renal function. It is also associated with hypertension and hepatotoxicity. CSA is metabolized via the P-450 CYP 3A system of the liver; therefore, it has many drug interactions, including interactions with drugs frequently used in dentistry (see below).

Tacrolimus has also been associated with hypertension and hepatotoxicity. In addition, it is nephrotoxic and neurotoxic. There are many other side effects associated with the use of this medication, one of which is the development of insulin-dependent posttransplantation diabetes mellitus (PTDM). The incidence of PTDM appears to be higher with tacrolimus use than with CSA use in liver transplantations.[53] Tacrolimus is metabolized by the P-450 CYP 3A system in the liver. It is 99% protein bound and requires titration. Tacrolimus also has significant interactions with medications used in dentistry (see below).

Sirolimus is hepatotoxic and may cause liver dysfunction. Sirolimus is also associated with a high incidence of hyperlipidemia owing to elevated triglyceride and cholesterol levels.[38] Being a substrate for P-450 CYP 3A, sirolimus also interferes with the metabolism of other medications.

AZA may cause bone marrow suppression, resulting in pancytopenia, which leaves the patient not only susceptible to opportunistic infections but also at significant risk for bleeding.

MMF has significant drug interactions that are particularly important to the dentist. One interaction that is commonly cited occurs as a result of antibiotic regimens that can alter gastrointestinal flora, leading to dramatic changes in MMF drug levels. For example, if a patient is taking a broad-spectrum antibiotic for a dentoalveolar infection, the possibility and probability of an abnormal MMF level does exist. Other medications, such as antacids (containing magnesium or aluminum) and bile acid binders, may also interfere with absorption of MMF. MMF is usually well tolerated, without significant hepatotoxicity (although higher doses are associated with gastrointestinal symptoms of nausea, vomiting, and diarrhea) or nephrotoxicity, but hematologic alterations (mostly leukopenia) can be a side effect.

Monoclonal and polyclonal antibodies can be associated with a severe reaction known as cytokine release syndrome. Cytokines (including TNF-α) are rapidly released, resulting in significant medical issues, including fever, chills, nephrotoxicity, vomiting, pulmonary edema, and, in a few instances, arterial thrombosis.[54]

Both monoclonal and polyclonal antibodies have been associated with significant side effects (in addition to significant cytokine release), including a high risk of viral/fungal infection and an increased incidence of posttransplantation lymphoproliferative disorders (PTLDs).[42]

Corticosteroids, another mainstay used in transplantation immunosuppression, can have multiple detrimental side effects, causing various disorders (Table 21-4).

Cytotoxic agents such as cyclophosphamide, busulfan, and total body irradiation cause bone marrow suppression, resulting in pancytopenia.

IMMUNOSUPPRESSION-INDUCED COMPLICATIONS

Immunosuppression used to prevent rejection of a transplanted organ also can pose serious complications to the recipient, including life-threatening infections and cancer.

Infections after HCT are a significant problem.[55] The type of transplant and the time that transpires since the transplantation often predict the specific infection. For example, patients who have had an HCT usually have broad immunologic defects, either due to their underlying disease

Table 21-4   Corticosteroid Side-Effect Profile
Induces diabetes
Induces muscle weakness
Induces osteoporosis
Alters fat metabolism and distribution
Induces hyperlipidemia
Induces electrolyte imbalances
Induces central nervous system effects, including psychological changes
Induces ocular changes—cataracts, glaucoma
Aggravates high blood pressure
Aggravates congestive heart failure
Aggravates peptic ulcer disease
Aggravates underlying infectious processes (e.g., tuberculosis)
Suppresses the pituitary-adrenal axis, resulting in adrenal atrophy
Suppresses the stress response

or more likely from a combination of immunosuppressive drugs and delayed immune reconstitution. This impacts all components of the immune system. These patients are at a significantly higher risk of infection than are those patients transplanted with solid organs. In addition, transplants of certain organs are associated with a greater likelihood of a particular infection.

Timing following the transplantation may correspond with a specific infective process.[49] Bacterial infections are usually seen in the early postoperative period (immediately after transplantation) in solid organ transplantations. The type of bacteria varies with each specific organ. Infections may include both gram-positive and gram-negative bacterial species. Drug-resistant bacterial infections have been documented, such as staphylococcal infections associated with skin wounds, upper and lower respiratory infections (pneumonia), and tuberculosis. Infective endocarditis has also been seen in transplant recipients. In this population, endocarditis is often related to *Staphylococcus* or aspergillosis.[56]

Systemic viral infections are also a common problem in immunosuppressed patients. CMV and herpes simplex viruses (HSVs) are often the etiologic viral agents involved. Other viral agents, including adenovirus, hepatitis B and C viruses, VZV, EBV, and human parvovirus B19, have also common causes of disease in a transplant population.[57] Viral infections are also related to time following transplantation. HSV infections usually occur at 2 to 6 weeks after organ transplantation, whereas CMV infections usually occur at 1 to 6 months after transplantation, and VZV infections usually occur between 2 and 10 months posttransplantation.[58]

Patients who are immunosuppressed are susceptible to local and systemic fungal infections. These infections vary from those of *Candida* species to deep fungal infections caused by *Aspergillus, Cryptococcus neoformans, Fusarium,* and *Trichosporon*. Invasive fungal infections are usually seen later in the transplantation process. Systemic fungal infections are often difficult to treat in the immunosuppressed patient and require systemic antifungal agents.[50,59] Some have considered the role of macrophage colony-stimulating factor, a cytokine used to stimulate macrophages and monocytes, in the treatment of patients with fungal infections.[60–62]

Parasitic infections caused by *Toxoplasma gondii* and other parasites can be seen in immunosuppressed transplant recipients.[50]

In addition to, and perhaps directly related to, infectious complications, immunosuppression renders the patient at a higher risk for the development of secondary cancers. The immune system provides surveillance against antigens that may act as initiators or promoters of cancer. When the immune response is muted, so, too, is the surveillance system. Cancers most commonly associated with immunosuppression are squamous cell carcinomas of the skin,[63] lymphomas (mostly B-cell lymphomas including PTLDs), and Kaposi sarcoma.[63,64] Human herpes virus 8 has been implicated in Kaposi sarcoma[63] and EBV virus in PTLDs.[63]

The most important factors in the development of PTLD is the level of immunosuppression and the EBV serology status.[65] In addition, there seems to be a clinicopathologic difference between those transplant recipients who are diagnosed with PTLD early (within the first year of transplantation, which are EBV + PTLD) versus those diagnosed after the first year.[66] PTLDs have been treated with decreased immunosuppression, antilymphocyte agents, conventional chemotherapy, radiotherapy, and IFN-α therapy.[63]

SPECIFIC ORGANS/HCT COMPLICATIONS

A significant medical complication seen in patients receiving solid organ transplants is accelerated advanced cardiovascular disease, including coronary artery disease (CAD).[67] The cause of this rapid CAD is thought to be either infectious (CMV), medication induced, or, more likely, both. Many investigators have explored the etiologic role of hypertension in CAD. Probably in this population, CAD is multifactorial. For instance, steroids, CSA, and sirolimus have been associated with hyperlipidemia, a condition associated with CAD.

Hypertension is also a common posttransplantation problem, often related to the immunosuppressive medication regimen.[68] In many transplantation facilities, hypertension is treated by calcium channel antagonists. Some clinicians note that this group of medications may raise serum levels of CSA, thus decreasing the cost of immunosuppression.[69] Caution must be exercised with any drug affecting CSA metabolism; for this reason, most clinicians prefer to prescribe medications that do not alter CSA levels. Nifedipine is one such calcium channel antagonist, but it has adverse oral effects, such as gingival overgrowth (see below).

Another significant condition associated with transplantation is PTDM. This disorder is a frequent consequence of allogeneic organ transplantation. Both experimental and clinical observations suggest that this phenomenon is related to the immunosuppressive agents. PTDM may cause both macro- and microvascular changes, which affect both graft and patient survival.[70]

Neurologic complications, such as neuropathies, can also be noted in transplant recipients.[71] Reinfection with hepatitis C virus after transplantation is high in recipients of liver transplants. This reinfection is associated with a high mortality rate.[72]

The second most common long-term cause of morbidity and mortality (infection being the first) after lung transplantation is bronchiolitis obliterans.[73] This disorder is an inflammation and constriction in bronchioles. It is probably related to chronic rejection and infection and perhaps altered microvasculature.[73]

Heart transplantation is also fraught with complications. As mentioned earlier, posttransplantation CAD is common in all transplants, including heart transplants. In addition, early after transplantation, the heart is denervated such that symptoms of angina may be absent and the heart may have diminished vagal response. There is, however, evidence of sympathetic and possibly parasympathetic reinnervation later in the posttransplantation period, suggesting that angina and heart rate changes to stress are regained.[74,75] Care of patients with cardiac transplants must recognize these cardiac abnormalities. Mitral and tricuspid regurgitation has also been observed after heart transplantation.[76,77]

Perhaps the most significant complications are those observed after an allogeneic HCT. Allogeneic transplantation often involves both administration of intensive chemotherapy and/or radiation as well as the administration of immunosuppressive therapy. The major complications of allogeneic HCT include the following:

1. End-organ damage from pretransplantation conditioning therapy
2. GVHD
3. Infections

Major complications occur after HCT that are directly related to the conditioning regimen. Unlike solid organ grafting, HCT requires intensive chemotherapy and/or radiation to "condition" the recipient to accept the graft; the conditioning regimen must provide immunosuppression of the recipient to prevent rejection but typically has cytotoxic effects to kill any residual malignant cells. Direct organ toxicity appears to be higher after myeloablative conditioning then after nonmyeloablative or RIC but can occur with all types of HCT. One major complication is sinusoidal obstructive syndrome (SOS) or veno-occlusive disease (VOD) of the liver. SOS is felt to be initiated by endothelial injury that leads to nonthrombotic sinusoidal occlusion with an increase in sinusoidal pressures. This leads to cholestasis and ultimately can result in portal hypertension. There are associated hepatorenal abnormalities, with capillary leak, and ultimately can lead to multisystem organ failure, encephalopathy, and even death. Clinical manifestations of SOS/VOD include jaundice, hepatomegaly, and fluid retention. Treatment for this process is supportive, and severe VOD is associated with high mortality rates.[78] Another major complication is pulmonary toxicity manifested as interstitial pneumonitis or alveolar hemorrhage. Pulmonary complication of both solid organ and HCT has been reviewed in detail.[73] The use of RIC for allogeneic

transplantation appears to minimize direct organ toxicity and nonrelapsed mortality.

Perhaps the most frequently cited and unique complication associated with allogeneic HCT is GVHD, which is a complex immunologic phenomenon that occurs when immunocompetent cells from the donor are given to an immunodeficient host. The host, who possesses transplantation antigens foreign to the graft, stimulates an immune response by the newly engrafted immune cells. GVHD affects the entire gastrointestinal system, including the mouth, as well as the skin and the liver.[79] This reaction can be lethal and requires therapy with intensive immunosuppression. Mucosal ulceration seen in GVHD may serve as an entry port for other infectious pathogens. GVHD is also associated with a graft-versus-leukemia effect and may be protective against relapse.[44]

PROGNOSIS

Transplantation outcomes have improved over the past several decades. Outcomes of solid organ transplants are summarized and categorized by each specific organ. Data regarding clinical outcomes of solid organ transplantation must also be separated into graft survival as well as patient survival (Table 21-5). In the United States, total solid organ transplantation totaled just over 26,500 in 2004. In 2012 that number rose slightly to 28,052. The one-year graft survival of renal transplantations performed in 2002 to 2004 was approximately 95% for a living donor transplant and 89% for a cadaveric kidney transplant. The one-year graft survival for a liver transplant was 82%, while heart transplant graft survival was 87% for men and 86% for women. Lung graft survivals were 83% for either gender, and heart/lung graft survival for men and women were 56% and 72%, respectively.[3]

One-year patient survival was 98% for those receiving a living donor renal transplant, 86% for a cadaveric liver transplant, 87% for a heart transplant, and 83% for a lung transplant. Five-year graft and patient survival rates for solid organ transplants are lower. The five-year graft survival rate for cadaveric donor kidney transplants was 67%, whereas the rate for living donor kidney transplants was 80%. Five-year cadaveric liver graft survival was 65%, whereas heart and

TABLE 21-5 Outcomes of Solid Organ Transplantations					
	Type of Transplantation				
Type of Survival	Renal (Living Donor)	Renal (Cadaveric Donor)	Heart	Liver (Cadaveric)	Lung
1-yr graft survival (%)	95	89	87	82	83
5-yr graft survival (%)	80	67	69	65	46
1-yr patient survival (%)	98	94	87	86	83
5-yr patient survival (%)	90	82	71	72	47

Source: Based on OPTN data as of November 8, 2013.[3]

lung graft survivals were 69% and 46%, respectively. Patient survival rate at 5 years was 82% for cadaveric donor kidney transplant recipients and 90% for living transplant recipients. Five-year patient survival rates for liver, heart, and lung transplantations were 72%, 71%, and 47%, respectively.[3]

The number of patients on waiting lists for solid organ transplants continues to increase. The deaths of patients awaiting kidney transplants has increased in 2012 to 4521, whereas the death rates for patients awaiting heart and liver transplants in 2012 was 320 and 1512, respectively.

Current estimates of HCTs performed annually are greater than 50,000 worldwide.[80] The annual rate of growth of this procedure has been estimated to between 40% and 50%.[81] Improved HCT-related healthcare has resulted in less morbidity and lower mortality rates. Historically, HCTs for hematologic malignancies were undertaken as salvage therapy for refractory cancers, but outcomes are actually better for patients who are treated with HCT soon after diagnosis or in remission rather than after multiple relapses of hematologic disease. Outcomes have improved in both autologous and allogeneic HCTs. There are various reasons that the success of HCT has improved. In the setting of autologous HCT, changes in conditioning regimens hematopoietic growth factors and the use of peripheral blood stem cells rather than bone marrow stem cells have been credited in part with improving mortality by shortening the duration of neutropenia (and incidence of severe infections) after intensive chemotherapy or radiation. In addition, better supportive care, antibiotic use, and blood product support have all improved outcomes for autologous HCT. For allogeneic HCT, CSA was introduced in the 1980s as an immunosuppressive agent limiting the severity of GVHD, making allogeneic donor HCT practical. Currently, CSA is often used with other medications, including methotrexate or corticosteroids, in prevention of GVHD. Decrease in severe GVHD has improved outcomes in allogeneic HCT.[81] In addition, CMV accounted for high rates of mortality seen in patients treated with an allogeneic SCT. Viral transmission can be limited by using screened "CMV-free" blood products for CMV-negative patients or using leukocyte-reduced blood products for transfusions. CMV-positive patients are treated with a prophylactic or, more recently, "preemptive" strategy using new high-sensitivity assays for CMV reactivation. These procedures have decreased the mortality associated with CMV interstitial pneumonitis.[82,83] Posttransplantation cell growth factors have also been cited as improving outcomes in allogeneic HCT patients.[61] In allogeneic HCT, advances have led to a decrease in overall mortality.[84] There are many patients who have survived HCT for five years or greater, and the future holds even greater promise as the various transplantation techniques become further refined.

Outcomes of recipients who have received both bone marrow and solid organ transplantation have also been reviewed.[85] There are many clinical and immunologic considerations that are highlighted by reviewing this unique patient population. Further research regarding the concept of immunologic tolerance/chimerism in patients who have had both a solid organ and a HCT transplant may provide clues for future studies or for consideration of routine treatment regimens, including HCT with the transplanted solid organ. Close monitoring of these patients will allow a better understanding of the concept of chimerism and tolerance.[86]

ORAL HEALTH CONSIDERATIONS

Dental treatment of patients who are being considered for transplantation and those who have had a transplant must be coordinated with the surgeon performing the transplant. Patients who are being considered for transplant are often critically ill, requiring the dentist to consult with the patient's transplant physician to determine medical risk. Moreover, the transplant physician may consult the patient's general dentist before "listing" the patient for transplantation. The nature of this consultation is to ensure that the patient does not have an acute dental/oral infection that could complicate the transplantation process. Furthermore, there are specific oral lesions associated with transplantation. It is prudent for a transplant candidate to be examined by the dentist before and after transplant to avoid complications during transplantation.

Orofacial sequelae during and after transplantation are common, especially in HST patients. The Multinational Association of Supportive Care in Cancer (MASCC) has published several systematic reviews on the management of oncology patients.[87] A detailed overview of the epidemiology of oral complications and oral health management of this group is found in Chapter 9: "Oral Complications of Cancer Therapy."

Dental management of transplant patients may be divided into pretransplantation and posttransplantation periods (Table 21-6).

Orofacial Sequelae in Transplantation

Patients who have had organ transplantation may present to their health-care practitioner with oral complaints. These complaints can be related to oral mucosal lesions or masses, mucosal pain, osseous infection, dental pain, functional impairment including chewing and dysphagia, and oral malignancy.

A comprehensive oral examination in the transplant recipient is paramount, given the fact that the patient is more susceptible to, and therefore may exhibit, oral infections of bacterial, viral, and fungal origins. Signs of oral infection may be muted because of a decreased inflammatory response, or, occasionally, the signs of infection may be exaggerated.[88] The presentation of an oral infection is dependent on the patient's level of immunosuppression and his or her ability to mount an immune response. Oral infections must be diagnosed, and aggressively treated as local infections may spread quickly. Furthermore, systemic infections may manifest as changes in the oral tissues. It is important to remember that in severely

TABLE 21-6 Dental Management Considerations

Pre-transplantation considerations

Significantly ill patient with end-organ damage
Medical consultation required
Consider postponing elective treatment

Obtain laboratory information/supplemental information as needed: Complete blood count with differential, prothrombin time (PT), partial thromboplastin time (PTT), international normalized ratio (INR), metabolic panel, liver function tests, other organ specific panels
Become acquainted with specific management issues (e.g., blood products, prophylactic antibiotics, alternate medication regimens due to organ failure) that may need to be employed if treatment is rendered

Dental consultation prior to anticipated transplantation
Rule out acute dental infectious sources, stabilize oral disease
Remove sources of chronic infection that may lead to acute complications within the transplant process and immediate posttransplant period
Perform necessary treatment; this will require consultation with transplantation physician to determine medical risk:benefit ratio

Post-transplantation considerations

Immediately after transplant
No elective dental treatment performed
Emergency treatment only with medical consultation and consideration of specific management needs

Stable period after functioning transplant
Elective treatment may be performed after medical consultation with the transplantation physician
Issues of immunosuppression must be recognized
Oral mucosal disease must be diagnosed and treated
Evaluate oral hydration and salivary flow: supplement or treat with sialogogues as needed
Supplemental corticosteroids (steroid boost) may be necessary
Consideration for antibiotic prophylaxis due to immune suppression
Two grams of oral amoxicillin or 600 mg of clindamycin are suggested one hour prior to invasive dental care

Consideration of specific management needs
Chronic rejection period
Only emergency treatment

immunocompromised patients, infectious agents that are associated with oral ulceration may be caused by agents that are normally not associated with acute oral infection.[89,90] Culture and sensitivity testing of all types of infections is prudent in establishing therapy targeted to the microorganism involved. Dentoalveolar abscesses may not manifest in traditional patterns, and treatment of bacterial infections requires prompt antibiotic therapy with appropriate culture and sensitivity testing.

An increased incidence of caries in the posttransplantation period has been reported. Children who have undergone HCT for acute lymphoblastic leukemia have a higher incidence of caries and a higher decayed, missing, and filled (DMFT) index.[91] A recent age and gender, case-control matched study reported a significant increase in the prevalence of caries and periodontal disease in patients' status after liver transplantation compared to controls.[92] Other studies describe a relative decrease of salivary IgA levels as well as an increased pH in pediatric recipients after hepatic transplantation, and altered dental development post HCT.[93,94] In a retrospective study in a cohort of patients who developed chronic GVHD after allogeneic transplantation, 90% of patients developed mucosal disorders, 95% developed salivary gland involvement, and more than 50% developed extensive cervical caries at two years after transplantation.[95] These studies highlight the importance of dental caries as a severe complication of GVHD posttransplantation.

Periodontal health in the transplant population is also often compromised. Side effects of transplant-related medications have been associated with periodontal disorders, particularly gingival overgrowth. The medication-induced gingival overgrowth seen in the transplant recipient appears to be related to the immunosuppressive agent CSA (Figure 21-1). Furthermore, CSA-associated gingival overgrowth may be exaggerated by the coadministration of nifedipine, a calcium channel blocker often used to treat hypertension in this patient population. Nifedipine is often the drug of choice because it will not alter plasma levels of CSA, as do some other antihypertensive medications.

A biopsy/histopathologic analysis should be performed on the gingival overgrowth to rule out malignancy.[96,97] Impeccable oral hygiene has been noted to be helpful in preventing gingival overgrowth.[98] Partial reversal of CSA-induced overgrowth has been reported upon discontinuation of the medication.[99] Although treatment of severe gingival overgrowth usually requires gingivectomy, nonsurgical treatment of patients with gingival overgrowth has been effective in reducing bleeding on probing, plaque index, probing depth, and hypertrophy index in subsets of transplant patients.[100]

Viral infections are a common problem in immunosuppressed patients. HSV and other herpesviridae are the most common viral pathogens cultured from oral infections in HCT patients.[101] Recurrent herpes simplex infections can be of both

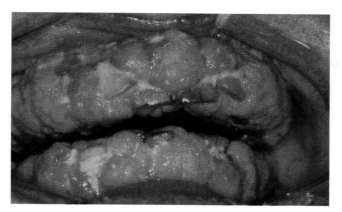

FIGURE 21-1 Gingival overgrowth in a kidney transplant recipient taking cyclosporine and nifedipine who also had poor oral hygiene.

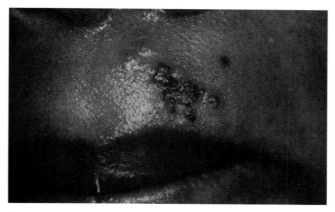

FIGURE 21-2 Recurrent herpes labialis.

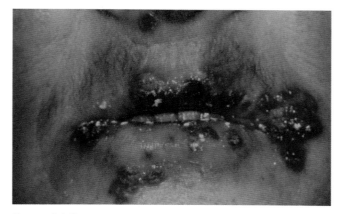

FIGURE 21-3 Recurrent herpes labialis in an immunocompromised patient.

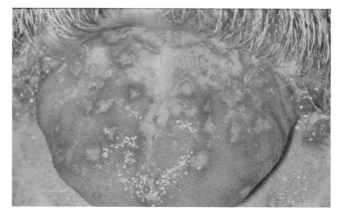

FIGURE 21-4 Recurrent intraoral herpes in a cardiac transplant recipient.

the labial and the intraoral varieties (Figures 21-2–21-4). Recurrent intraoral herpes may be chronic and difficult to diagnose solely on the basis of clinical appearance. VZV and EBV, as well as CMV, have been implicated in oral disease. Oral hairy leukoplakia (OHL) related to EBV has been reported in transplant recipients who are not infected with the human immunodeficiency virus.[102–106] In one case, OHL was identified as an earlier indicator of EBV-associated PTLD.[107] Treatment of viral infections requires administration of an appropriate antiviral agent. Occasionally, HSV not responsive to acyclovir will need treatment with foscarnet (an antiviral medication with a mechanism of action different from that of acyclovir).[106,108]

Patients who are immunosuppressed are more susceptible to fungal infections. These infections include members of the candida species, as well as deep fungal infections, such as aspergillosis, cryptococcosis, mucormycosis, and blastomycosis (Figures 21-5 and 21-6). These infections may manifest in various presentations in the oral cavity. Candidiasis can occur in the classic, pseudomembranous form, or it can be atrophic or even hyperplastic (see Figures 21-5, 21-7, and 21-8). Hyperplastic candidiasis cannot be removed by scraping the lesion and often requires biopsy for a definitive diagnosis. Occasionally, candidiasis is nonresponsive to the standard antifungal agents[109,110] and may need treatment with intravenous antifungal agents. It is interesting to note that candidal hyphae have been reported in CSA-induced gingival overgrowth.[111]

Deep fungal infections involving the upper respiratory tract and/or sinuses may manifest as necrotic plaques in the palatal areas of recipients of HCT (see Figure 21-6). These fungal infections are very difficult to treat and often require intravenous antifungal agents. In patients who are severely neutropenic, these infections may prove fatal, with the patient ultimately succumbing to a disseminated deep fungal infection.

Noninfectious oral lesions are also common in transplant recipients. Isolated cases of oral ulceration related to MMF and tacrolimus have been reported.[112,113] The advent of targeted therapy in oncology is an exciting therapeutic area developed in earnest in the last decade. Several of these interventions have reported oral side effects such as mucosal pain caused by the mammalian

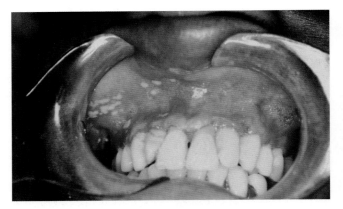

FIGURE 21-5   Pseudomembranous candidiasis.

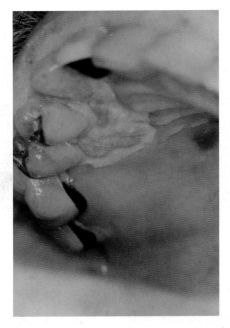

FIGURE 21-6   Deep fungal aspergillosis in a patient who underwent hematopoietic cell transplantation. The patient succumbed to disseminated aspergillosis shortly after this photograph was taken.

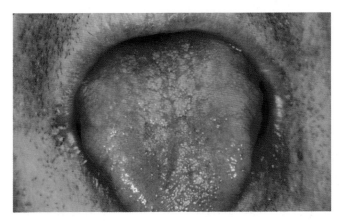

FIGURE 21-7   Atrophic candidiasis.

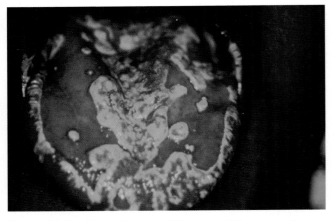

FIGURE 21-8   Hyperplastic candidiasis in a kidney transplant recipient. This infection did not respond to fluconazole.

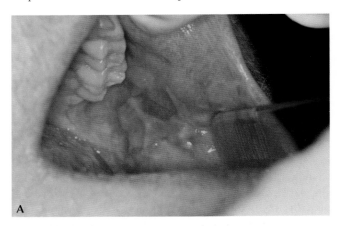

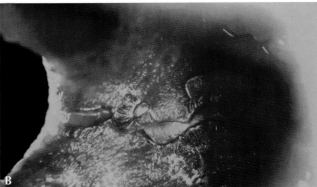

FIGURE 21-9   Graft-versus-host disease in a patient who had undergone hematopoietic cell transplantation. Note the clinical resemblance to erosive lichen planus.

target of rapamycin inhibitors (temsirolimus, everolimus, ridaforolimus) and ulceration associated to other phosphatidylinositol 3-kinase pathway inhibitors.[114] The descriptions of the oral lesions related to these agents have been reported as aphthous like in appearance, stomatitis, or frank oral mucositis (OM).[114] The pathophysiology and prevention of these lesions is still under scrutiny. Additional complications such as dysgeusia and dysphagia have been associated with the use of these novel therapies.[115]

Other oral lesions may represent neoplasms. The transplant recipient is at a higher risk of developing lymphoma and other cancers, like Kaposi sarcoma and squamous cell carcinoma of the skin. Lymphoma and Kaposi sarcoma can occur in the mouth,[96,116–118] whereas basal cell carcinoma often involves the lips.[119]

GVHD is a unique complication of HCT. In the oral cavity, this process clinically resembles lichenoid inflammation/lichen planus. Oral GVHD appears as an area of wispy hyperkeratosis on an erythematous base in various areas of the oral mucosa. In severe GVHD, the lesions may be eroded (Figure 21-9).[120] These ulcerations may serve as a port of entry for oral pathogens. There is also an increasing incidence of oral and esophageal squamous cell carcinoma in patients who have chronic GVHD after HCT.[121] GVHD not only affects the mouth but also the entire gastrointestinal system, as well as the skin and the liver. This reaction can be lethal, and *acute* disease requires urgent treatment. However, *chronic* GVHD may be considered somewhat beneficial if it functions as a graft-versus-leukemia reaction, an immunologic process that eliminates persistent leukemic cells. Oral GVHD is challenging to treat and may require a change in the immunosuppressive regimen and the implementation of systemic or topical mucosal therapy for effective management.[99,122,123] Some authors have used topical CSA or topical thalidomide gel in a bioadhesive base with good results.[124,125] Ultraviolet B irradiation as well as ultraviolet A irradiation with oral psoralen (PUVA) has also been reported to be effective.[126,127] A novel approach for treating oral GVHD involves the use of topical tacrolimus and AZA.[128,129] It appears that the progression of oral chronic GVHD may be predicted by the worsening of clinic erythema and lichenoid presentation. Superficial mucoceles form part of the clinical presentation of oral GVHD, and the presence of these salivary gland lesions is included in validated scoring systems for oral GVHD (Table 21-7).[130] The overall scores in the validation of the NIH scoring system for chronic oral GVHD correlate with pain levels and ulceration.[130]

In addition to GVHD, a patient who has had an allogeneic HCT may also experience a nongingival soft tissue growth, presumably related to the use of CSA. These lesions can be seen in the buccal mucosa, alveolar mucosa, and elsewhere (Figure 21-10).[131]

OM is a common complaint of patients who have had chemotherapy.[132] OM is a significant and dose-limiting complication of high-dose chemotherapy. Mucositis after HCT is usually related to the preconditioning regimen, and it is difficult to distinguish from an oral infection (Figure 21-11). Mucositis is often treated with palliative agents; a mixture of an anesthetic, an antihistamine, and a coating agent is commonly used. These agents tend to provide transient relief with no significant improvement in the mucositis. Palliative treatment with lidocaine for HCT-related OM has been associated with only minor systemic absorption.[133] The use of topical tretinoin prophylaxis has been advocated as an option to prevent HCT mucositis.[134] One product, Gelclair (OSI Pharmaceuticals, Melville, NY), is a bioadhesive gel that in a noncontrolled open-label trial

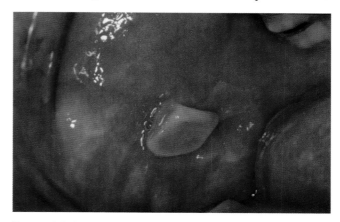

FIGURE 21-10 Nongingival soft tissue growth.

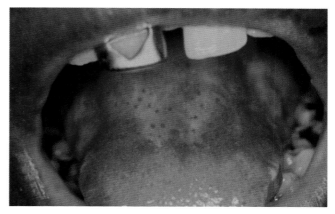

FIGURE 21-11 Mucositis shortly after induction chemotherapy for acute myelogenous leukemia.

TABLE 21-7 Main Components of the NIH Chronic GVHD Oral Mucosal Score (NIH OMS)[a]	
Erythema	Mild to moderate, severe depending on percentage of mucosal surface involved
Mucoceles	Mild to moderate, severe depending on number of mucoceles
Ulcers	Mild to moderate, severe depending on percentage of mucosal surface involved
Lichenoid	Mild to moderate, severe depending on percentage of mucosal surface involved

[a]Each item has a numerical score that combined provides a summary score of 0–15, reflective of the severity of oral GVHD.
Source: Adapted from Bassim et al.[149a]

reduced pain scores by 30% in persons with mucositis.[135] A comparison study on subjects with OM reported longer pain relief and better antibacterial properties of this intervention compared to other rinses.[136] The use of mucosal-protective agents such as misoprostol or carafate in head and neck oncology patients has also been described. Oral complications from oncologic treatment as well as their management is fully detailed in Chapter 9, "Oral Complications of Cancer Therapy."

Additional developments in mucositis prevention focus on the use of growth factors to shorten healing time. The use of granulocyte-macrophage colony-stimulating factor in preventing OM was found to have only a minor impact on the patients' quality of life and functional status.[137] Keratinocyte growth factor received Food and Drug Administration approval in 2004 for treatment of recurrent OM in patients undergoing autologous HCT with hematologic malignancies. The applicability of this intervention for OM secondary to other oncology treatments (chemotherapy or radiation; not HCT) is under investigation.[138] Treatments supported by recent MASCC recommendations are specific for head and neck radiation and include low-level laser therapy, with several studies published in 2013.[139,140]

A common staging system for OM is the World Health Organization scoring algorithm. This algorithm classifies OM as I through IV depending on the presence of mucosal ulceration and the patient's ability to consume solids (grade II), liquids (grade III), or nothing by mouth (grade IV). Grade I is defined by the presence of oral erythema and pain, and grade 0 is the absence of any clinical sign or symptom. The addition of a previously reported treatment for OM, cryotherapy, to low-level laser, appears to have synergistic effects on delaying the onset of OM.[141] This study reported a grade I OM in patients treated with the combined therapy versus grades III and IV in the control group.

The role of antibacterial topical agents, such as chlorhexidine rinses, in preventing OM is controversial and only recommended to decrease the risk of superinfection in extensive mucosal involvement (does not prevent or shorten the duration of OM).[142] As the understanding of the pathobiology of OM progresses, new targeted therapies will be developed to delay the onset and duration of this complication.

Salivary gland dysfunction is also quite common in patients after HCT and may be related to the toxic effects of chemotherapeutic regimens used to rid the bone marrow of leukemic cells. Patients who have chronic GVHD also have diminution of salivary flow, presumably from a lymphocytic infiltrate of salivary tissue (Figure 21-12).[143,144]

Developmental tooth defects such as altered root formation, hypodontia, and dentofacial growth alterations must also be considered as they have been reported in children who have undergone HCT (Figure 21-13).[145] Description and follow-up of late dental effects of HCT are limited to isolated case series and reviews.[146,147]

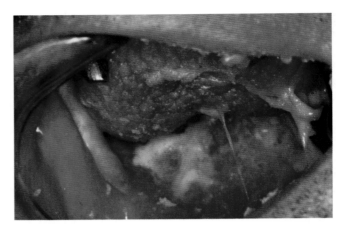

FIGURE 21-12 Salivary hypofunction.

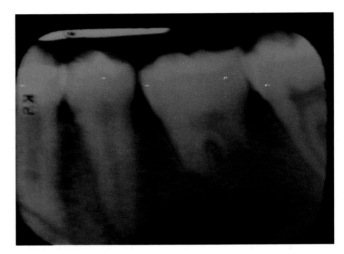

FIGURE 21-13 Dental root alteration as a result of childhood treatment for neuroblastoma and conditioning total body irradiation prior to HCT.

PRETRANSPLANTATION CONSIDERATIONS

When treating patients who are transplantation candidates, the dentist must be familiar with the underlying disorder as well as laboratory evaluations pertinent to the particular disorder. Consultation with the patient's physician is mandatory.

Pretransplantated patients are critically ill and have significant end-organ damage. Specific organ damage poses unique challenges. Patients with end-stage liver disease may have difficulties with excessive bleeding due to coagulopathy and often require changes in medications due to alterations in the hepatic metabolism (Table 21-8).

Patients awaiting a kidney transplant have end-stage renal disease and are usually receiving hemodialysis. These patients may be fluid overloaded and have hypertension; therefore, monitoring of the patient's blood pressure is necessary. When determining blood pressure, the cuff must not be placed on the arm used for dialysis access. Occasionally, electrolyte balance may be altered leading to metabolic

TABLE 21-8 Medication Considerations in Patients With Liver or Kidney Failure[a]

Drug	Dose Change Required	
	Kidney Failure[b]	Liver Failure
Acetaminophen	–	Avoid use
Acyclovir	+	–
Amoxicillin	+	–
Cephalexin	+	–
Clavulanic acid with amoxicillin	+	–
Clindamycin	–	+
Codeine	+	+
Diazepam	+	+
Erythromycin	–	+
Ibuprofen	–	Unknown
Ketoconazole	–	+
Lidocaine	–	–
Metronidazole	+	+
Minocycline	–	+
Naproxen	+	+
Penicillin	+	–
Salicylates	+/Avoid use	Avoid use
Tetracycline	+/Avoid use	Avoid use

+, May require a dose change and/or avoidance of use, depending on severity of renal or hepatic disease; –, No dose change required.
[a]Includes only drugs commonly used in dentistry.
[b]Degree of function of renal system must be considered before dose change is determined.
Source: Adapted from Byrne.[149b]

effects such as acidosis, and increased susceptibility to cardiac rhythm abnormalities. Changes in drug metabolism and excretion must also be considered in this population as changing of the dose of various medications, including those used in dentistry, may be required (see Table 21-8).[148] The dentist should be familiar with the radiographic signs of renal osteodystrophy and the oral signs and symptoms of uremia. Antibiotic prophylaxis of patients on hemodialysis is usually not required with the exception of central venous catheters.[149] Studies on the impact of oral microbiota on vascular site infections in hemodialysis patients, however, yield a very limited number of cases related to oral organisms, and further research on central venous catheters and bacteremia of oral origin in this population is warranted.

Patients awaiting a heart transplant are usually poor candidates for outpatient dental treatment. The majority of these patients have severe CAD or congestive heart failure. Both conditions can easily progress to life-threatening complications during invasive dental treatment. The sole effect of stress and pain can cause an adverse outcome in labile patients. The cardiovascular reserve of these patients is small, rendering them much better candidates for elective dental treatment after they have undergone transplantation. Some patients awaiting heart transplants may not be discharged from the hospital until they receive their new heart.

Patients awaiting lung transplants are also critically ill. Most are on oxygen therapy and have difficulty breathing. Dental treatment should preclude the use of combustible sources near the patient if he or she is using oxygen therapy. Inhaled anesthetics are contraindicated in these patients. Narcotic medications that cause respiratory depression are also contraindicated.

Patients awaiting pancreatic transplants have significant problems in glucose management; therefore, considerations of serum glucose levels prior to initiating treatment must be made. These patients may be poor wound healers and may have "brittle insulin-dependent diabetes"; that is, patients may experience sharp alterations in blood glucose levels and be prone to both ketoacidosis and insulin shock. Pancreatic dysfunction may be accompanied by hepatic failure. Hence, coagulation complications and medication/local anesthetic metabolism must be considered when performing dental procedures in these individuals.

HCT candidates are frequently significantly ill. Most have been through induction and have endured consolidation chemotherapy to treat a hematologic malignancy. Many of these patients are pancytopenic and are prone to infections and bleeding. They are therefore considered poor candidates for routine outpatient dental treatment. Other patients may have had a significant remission of their disease with normalizing blood counts, allowing emergency dental treatment prior to the HCT. Prompt consultation with the patient's oncologist is recommended.

A dentist caring for members of the pretransplantation population must not only consider providing/withholding care after evaluating the underlying disorders, but he or she must also consider the potential dental complications that can significantly impact the transplantation process. A detailed clinical examination of the dentition, periodontium, and oral mucosa as well as the head and neck areas, including the lymph nodes and salivary glands, is prudent. There has been some controversy as to the optimal radiographic examination regimen required to evaluate patients who will undergo HCT[150]; Some argue for full mouth series examination, while others prefer panoramic films and bitewings. However, there is consensus on the importance of having access to recent dental radiographs for the evaluation.

Once the evaluation has been performed, a medical/dental risk assessment should be formulated. Elective dental treatment in patients with end-stage disease should be postponed as the patient will be more "medically stable" after the transplantation. Whenever possible, it is important for the dentist to eliminate dental infections prior to the transplantation as the patient will be significantly immunosuppressed immediately and for some time after the transplantation. Therefore, dental treatment planning must take into account the patient's laboratory evaluation, including such parameters as complete blood cell and platelet counts, serum chemistry to determine the degree of organ dysfunction, and coagulation studies. In addition, other tests more specific for each particular organ to be transplanted must be obtained and reviewed. A medical risk assessment is necessary to determine whether a patient can systemically tolerate an extraction or other dental procedure. Some HCT and heart transplant candidates cannot withstand even emergency treatment. When risk assessment favors treatment, the most definitive treatment option should be considered (often extraction). Antibiotic coverage prior and after dental treatment (perioperative) is often warranted in patients awaiting HCT and in some patient's awaiting heart or kidney transplants and who undergo oral surgery. There are no evidence-based guidelines regarding antibiotic choice and dosing for dental perioperative care. In severely immunocompromised patients, the authors suggest in the absence of penicillin allergy, a pretreatment dose of 2 g amoxicillin one hour prior to procedure and a posttreatment infection dose (penicillin V 500 mg four times a day) for seven days. Patients awaiting HCT or liver transplants may need platelets, coagulation factors, or other supportive products prior to dental treatment.

POSTTRANSPLANTATION CONSIDERATIONS

Patients who have undergone transplantation also pose concerns to the treating dentist. The posttransplantation period can be divided into the immediate posttransplantation period, the stable period, and the chronic rejection period. The immediate posttransplantation period is the time when the patient is most susceptible to both rejection and severe infection. This period of time begins immediately posttransplantation and extends to when the grafted organ is functioning appropriately. Due to increased levels of immunosuppression used to foil rejection during this period, the dentist should not perform elective dental treatment, and emergency treatment should be provided only after consultation with the transplantation physician. However, the oral microbiome in HCT recipients does not change dramatically, with the exception of when there are concurrent respiratory complications.[151] Patients have shown some benefit from chlorhexidine mouthrinses during this period of time.[152]

The stable posttransplantation period occurs when the grafted organ is stable. It is during this time that the problems of chronic rejection, immunosuppression, and side effects of immunosuppressive medications may become apparent. Dental treatment planning must consider these important factors. The length of time that a patient remains in this stage is variable. Generally, this period is the best time to perform elective dental treatment since the organ is functioning appropriately. In general, there are no absolute contraindications to any type of dental procedure in patients after a successful HCT without medical or oral complications.[153] Consultation with the transplantation physician is essential due to the delicate balance of rejection/immunosuppression and their implications to medical/dental risk assessment. Since late dental effects of HCT include root stunting, hypodontia, or agenesis in young individuals,[144] stabilizing treatment and tooth replacement maybe needed.

Antibiotic coverage prior to dental treatment is often requested by the transplantation physician. This subject requires further evidence-based research. Corticosteroid supplementation may also be required due to adrenal suppression associated with higher dose chronic corticosteroid use. This supplementation may help avoid cardiovascular collapse during stressful procedures including general anesthesia, and it is recommended when the stress of the procedure or the patient's perception of the stress (pain) of the procedure is increased.[154] Some have questioned the need for supplementation when treating gingival overgrowth via gingivectomy under local anesthetic.[155]

Other considerations for the dental provider during the stable posttransplantation period involve medication interactions as several antirejection immunosuppressive medications have interactions with medications that a dentist may prescribe. For example, patients who are taking CSA may require the use of clindamycin instead of erythromycin. CSA levels are affected by anti-inflammatory drugs such as diclofenac, sulindac, and naproxen; antifungal medications such as itraconazole, fluconazole, and ketoconazole; and antibiotics such as clarithromycin and erythromycin. Reviewing potential interactions between the medications that the transplant patient is taking and those the dentist intends to prescribe is prudent. As the development and use of immunosuppressive agents evolve, the dentist will need to be familiar with the newer medications and the potential risk of interactions with the various medications used in dentistry.

The stable posttransplantation period ends when a grafted organ begins to fail, heralding the chronic rejection period. Laboratory parameters indicating organ function failure and biopsies are used to confirm this process. For dentists, these patients are often the most complicated to manage since the organ is failing and the patient remains immunosuppressed. Only emergency dental treatment is indicated, and the transplantation physician's input is essential. The treating dentist must consider the ramifications of organ failure and make appropriate provisions.

CONCLUSION

Oral considerations in the transplantation population are vast. The dentist needs a strong knowledge base in medicine to minimize adverse outcomes secondary to provision of oral healthcare. As this unique population grows, so does the need for qualified dental practitioners to treat them. It is essential that the dentist familiarize himself or herself with the special needs of these patients. Their oral and dental health is imperative; therefore, patients who have had a transplant need to have routine dental examinations. It is incumbent on the dental practitioner to expediently diagnose and treat any oral infection. Gingival health in this population is extremely important and must be monitored regularly, particularly because CSA may induce gingival overgrowth, which precludes adequate home care and encourages further periodontal breakdown.

Arguably, patients undergoing allogeneic HCT should be evaluated more frequently than the general population owing to decreased salivary flow, which may be associated with an increased caries rate.[156,144] Consideration should be given to prescribing supplemental topical fluoride applications and suggesting appropriate recall. These patients may also have oral ulcerations from GVHD. These ulcers can serve as a portal of entry for any oral pathogen to infect the immunocompromised host.

The patient's medical history should be updated with each dental appointment. Close communication and coordination with the transplantation physician is necessary as the patient's medical condition can change quickly.

As with all dental patients, excellent oral hygiene is difficult to achieve solely by the clinician's professional service. It is extremely important to provide oral hygiene instruction and to discuss with the patient, the need for appropriate hygiene to prevent oral infections. These patients can be at high risk of serious complications, even from initially innocuous oral infections. The patient should also be taught to perform a thorough oral examination and encouraged to perform it frequently at home. This procedure enables the patient to constantly monitor his or her own oral condition and to aid the health-care professional in early diagnosis of pathology.

Selected Readings

Alousi AM, Bolaños-Meade J, Lee SJ. Graft-versus-host disease: state of the science. Biol Blood Marrow Transplant. 2013;19:S102-S108.

Atsuta Y, Suzuki R, Yamashita T, et al.; Japan Society for Hematopoietic Cell Transplantation. Continuing increased risk of oral/esophageal cancer after allogeneic hematopoietic stem cell transplantation in adults in association with chronic graft-versus-host disease. Bone Marrow Transplant. 2013;48(8):1123-8.

Boers-Doets CB, Epstein JB, Raber-Durlacher JE, et al. Oral adverse events associated with tyrosine kinase and mammalian target of rapamycin inhibitors in renal cell carcinoma: a structured literature review. Oncologist. 2012;17(1):135-44.

Brennan MT, Elting LS, Spijkervet FKL. Systematic Reviews of oral complications from cancer therapies, oral care study group, MASCC/ISOO: methodology and quality of the literature. Support Care Cancer. 2010;18(8):979-984.

Castellarin P, Stevenson K, Biasotto M, et al. Extensive dental caries in patients with oral chronic graft-versus-host disease. Biol Blood Marrow Transplant. 2012;18(10):1573-9.

Castronovo G, Liani G, Fedon A, et al. The effect of nonsurgical periodontal treatment on the severity of drug-induced gingival overgrowth in transplant patients. Quintessence Int. 2014;45(2):115-24.

de Paula Eduardo F, Bezinelli LM, da Graça Lopes RM, et al. Efficacy of cryotherapy associated with laser therapy for decreasing severity of melphalan-induced oral mucositis during hematological stem-cell transplantation: a prospective clinical study. Hematol Oncol. 2014 Feb 11 doi: 10.1002/hon.2133. [Epub ahead of print].

Dey BR, Spitzer T. Major complications-cancer. In: Klein AA, Lewis, C.J., Madsen, J.C., eds. Organ Transplantation: A Clinical Guide. New York: Cambridge University Press; 2011. pp.31-37.

Fatahzadeh M, Schwartz RA. Oral Kaposi's sarcoma: a review and update. Int J Dermatol. 2013;52(6):666-72.

Fernandes LL, Torres SR, Garnica M, et al. Oral status of patients submitted to autologous hematopoietic stem cell transplantation. Support Care Cancer. 2014;22(1):15-21.

Furst D, Muller C, Vucinic V, et al. High-resolution HLA matching in hematopoietic stem cell transplantation: a retrospective collaborative analysis. Blood 2013;122:3220-3229.

Helenius-Hietala J, Ruokonen H, Grönroos L, et al. Oral mucosal health in liver transplant recipients and controls. Liver Transpl. 2014;20(1):72-80.

Hoffman KE, Pugh SL, James JL, Scarantino C, et al. The impact of concurrent granulocyte-macrophage colony-stimulating factor on quality of life in head and neck cancer patients: results of the randomized, placebo-controlled Radiation Therapy Oncology Group 9901 trial. Qual Life Res. 2014 Feb 4. [Epub ahead of print].

https://bethematchclinical.org

http://cibmtr.org

http://optn.tranplant.hrsa.gov

Hull KM, Kerridge I, Schifter M. Long-term oral complications of allogeneic haematopoietic SCT. Bone Marrow Transplant. 2012 Feb;47(2):265-70.

Mascarenhas S, Avalos B, Ardoin SP. "An update on stem cell transplantation in autoimmune rheumatologic disorders." Curr Allergy Asthma Rpts.2012;12(6):530-540.

Mickelson E, Petersdorf EW. Histocompatibility. In: Blume KG, Forman SJ, and Appelbaum FR, eds. Thomas' Hematopoietic Cell Transplantation, 3rd ed. Oxford, Malden (MA): Blackwell Publishing; 2004. p.31-42.

Ottaviani G, Gobbo M, Sturnega M, et al. Effect of class IV laser therapy on chemotherapy-induced oral mucositis: a clinical and experimental study. Am J Pathol. 2013;183(6):1747-57.

Petersdorf EW. The major histocompatibility complex: a model for understanding graft-versus-host disease. Blood 2013;122:1863-1872.

Porter D, Levine J, Kolb H. Adoptive immunotherapy in stem cell transplantation. In: Ferrara J, Cooke K, Deeg J, eds. Graft-vs-Host Disease: Immunology, Pathophysiology. Vol. 3. New York: Marcel Dekker; 2005:525-553.

Terasaki PI. A personal perspective: 100-year history of the humoral theory of transplantation. Transplantation 2012;93(8):751-6.

Tomblyn M, Chiller T, Einsele H, et al. Guidelines for preventing infectious complications among hematopoietic cell transplantation recipients: a global perspective. Biol Blood Marrow Transplant. 2009;15:1143-1238.

Treister N, Chai X, Kurland B, et al. Measurement of oral chronic GVHD: results from the Chronic GVHD Consortium. Ann Oncol. 2014;25(2):435-41.

Viswanathan C, Sarang S. Status of stem cell based clinical trials in the treatment for diabetes. Curr Diabetes Rev 2013;9(6):429-36.

www.transplantliving.org

For the full reference lists, please go to http://www.pmph-usa.com/Burkets_Oral_Medicine.

CHAPTER 22

Infectious Diseases

Michaell A. Huber, DDS

Spencer W. Redding, DDS, MEd

Vidya Sankar, DMD, MHS, FDS RCSEd

Sook-Bin Woo, DMD, FDS RCSEd

❑ BACTERIAL INFECTIONS
  Syphilis
  Chlamydia and Gonorrhea
  Actinomycosis
  Tuberculosis
❑ FUNGAL INFECTIONS
  Blastomycosis
  Histoplasmosis

Paracoccidioidomycosis
Aspergillosis
Cryptococcosis
Mucormycosis
❑ VIRAL INFECTIONS
  Viral Hepatitis
  Emerging Putative Viruses
  Human Immunodeficiency Virus

The goal of this chapter is to summarize a group of systemic infections that have manifestations in the head and neck and/or oral cavity or have significant issues for dental professionals. These will be divided into bacterial, fungal, and viral infections. More common oral infections are covered in other chapters.

BACTERIAL INFECTIONS

Syphilis

Syphilis is a bacterial infection caused by *Treponema pallidum* and is acquired primarily through sexual contact. Approximately 55,000 new cases of syphilis occur in the United States each year, and the average incubation period from contact to infection is 21 days. Syphilis lesions can develop on the external genitalia, the vagina, the anus, the rectum, and the oral cavity.[1,2]

There are typically three stages of syphilis infection. In the primary stage, the characteristic chancre develops at the point of inoculation. This lesion, which is typically painless, lasts for three to six weeks and heals even if not treated.[3] Without appropriate treatment, the infection enters the secondary stage to manifest as skin rashes and macular lesions affecting not only the area of inoculation but also other parts of the body such as the palms of the hands and the bottoms of the feet. Gray or white lesions may also occur in warm moist body sites including the mouth, the underarm, and the groin. Symptoms of secondary syphilis may include fever, lymphadenopathy, weight loss, hair loss, headache, sore throat, muscle ache, and fatigue.[3] As with primary syphilis, lesions of secondary syphilis resolve without treatment, but the disease will then progress to the tertiary stage or latent stage that can last for many years. Approximately 15% of patients with syphilis who are not treated through the secondary stage will develop tertiary syphilis which can occur up to 30 years after the initial infection. This is the most devastating form of syphilis and can cause multiple nervous system complications including paralysis and dementia. Multiple organ systems can also be involved leading to eventual death.[2] Syphilis may be passed from an infected mother to her child during pregnancy, and infected babies may suffer premature birth, low birth weight, and other long-term complications.[4]

The diagnosis of syphilis is best performed by using dark-field microscopy to identify organisms from lesion exudate or tissue. There are several screening blood tests that are positive to antibody formation to the *Treponema*. These include the nonspecific Venereal Disease Research Laboratory test and the more specific fluorescent treponemal antibody absorption test.[2,3]

Primary, secondary, and early tertiary stages of syphilis are treated with a single dose of 2.4 million units of benzathine penicillin G. Doxycycline or tetracycline can be used in patients with penicillin allergy. Late tertiary syphilis and syphilis with neurological symptoms requires treatment with much higher doses of penicillin over several weeks.[5]

Oral/Facial Considerations

Approximately 15% of patients with primary syphilis will present with highly infectious intraoral chancres, either as solitary or multiple lesions. Chancres typically present as painless, sometimes necrotic, ulcers with a rolled border and associated lymphadenopathy. Common sites of occurrence are the lips, tongue, palate, and nostrils. Lymphadenopathy commonly accompanies these lesions. As mentioned earlier, these lesions heal spontaneously without treatment.[6]

The typical oral lesion in secondary syphilis is described as a mucous patch that presents as thickened whitish plaque affecting the oral mucosa. Necrosis and sloughing may occur. Commonly affected sites include the tongue, lip, buccal mucosa, and palate. These patients may also present with mucosal ulcers and erythematous macular lesions.[7]

With tertiary syphilis, the typical lesion is the gumma. It primarily occurs on the hard palate but may also occur on the soft palate and the alveolus. The gumma begins as a swelling that eventually ulcerates and then goes through repeated phases of healing and breakdown. Bone destruction of the hard palate may occur with palatal perforation and in some cases, oral nasal fistula. A gumma may erode into underlying blood vessels.[8]

In congenital syphilis, infection is spread from a mother with primary or secondary syphilis to her developing fetus. In early congenital syphilis, from 0 to 2 years of age, infants may develop facial rashes. In late congenital syphilis, over two years of age, a number of complications develop including Hutchinson's notched incisors, mulberry-shaped molar teeth, corneal keratitis, deafness, frontal bossing, saddle nose, hard palate defects, and swollen joints.[4]

Chlamydia and Gonorrhea

Chlamydia and gonorrhea are the two most common sexually transmitted bacterial infections reported in the United States each year with over 2 million cases. However, less than half of these infections are reported. The infecting organisms are *Chlamydia trachomatis* and *Neisseria gonorrhoeae*, respectively, and since the infections often occur together, they will be discussed together. Infection is typically acquired through exposure through vaginal, anal, or oral sex with an infected partner. Groups at particular risk include sexually active teenagers, young adults, and African Americans. Symptoms of both infections include a burning sensation while urinating with a discharge of white, yellow, or green exudate in men. Infected women are usually asymptomatic. Anal infection can cause itching, soreness, bleeding, and painful bowel movements. Oral infection may result in pharyngitis.

Complications of these infections are particularly serious for women. Pelvic inflammatory disease may develop causing severe pain and fever and in some patients lead to a chronic pain condition. Damage to the fallopian tubes may occur, leading to ectopic pregnancies or sterility. Although rare, the infections may cause epididymitis in males. *N. gonorrhea* can result in disseminated infection of the skin, joints, and other systems. *C. trachomatis* can cause lymphogranuloma venereum, which is primarily observed in women from Africa, Southeast Asia, and India. It causes genital ulcers with adenopathy. Both chlamydia and gonorrhea can be passed to an infant during labor. Patients with chlamydia and gonorrhea are at greater risk of acquiring HIV, and indeed, HIV-positive patients commonly have these infections.[9–13]

Diagnosis of the infection involves taking a swab of the infected site and performing culture or identification of genetic material. More rapid testing is available that employs amplification techniques such as polymerase chain reaction (PCR) or deoxyribonucleic acid (DNA) probes.[9,11]

Treatment of these infections has changed in recent years. Co-infection with chlamydia and gonorrhea is very common, so treatment for both is recommended. Standard regimens usually include a parenteral cephalosporin plus oral azithromycin or doxycycline.[14–16] Infections resistant to standard therapy require susceptibility testing to guide further treatment.[17]

Oral/Facial Considerations

Both chlamydia and gonorrhea infections can cause pharyngitis secondary to oral sex. Oral infections are often asymptomatic, but fever and lymphadenopathy may occur. Tonsils typically manifest erythema with small punctate lesions. Lesions may also occur uncommonly in other locations in the mouth and are described as being erythematous, pustular, erosive, or ulcerated.[18–21]

Actinomycosis

Actinomycosis is an unusual bacterial infection caused primarily by *Actinomyces israelii* and occasionally by *Actinomyces bovis* and *Actinomyces naeslundii*. The infection tends to be chronic with the ability to move slowly but steadily through tissue and is characterized by swelling and inflammation, abscess formation, development sinus tracts, and scar formation. The four most common sites for occurrence are oral/cervical, thoracic, abdominal, and pelvic with the oral/cervical accounting for over 50% of all cases. Actinomycosis is a true opportunistic infection as the bacteria commonly colonizes mucosal linings without causing infection. With injury or disease, the organism can penetrate into body areas that are conducive of the anaerobic environment necessary for its growth and ability to cause infection.

An early stage infection may be difficult to diagnose, as the infection can mimic other conditions including cancer, appendicitis, pneumonia, and pelvic inflammatory disease. Most cases are diagnosed when a biopsy is performed to rule out other conditions. Aspiration of exudate from sinus tracts can also be examined for characteristic sulfur granules and branching filamentous bacteria. Actinomycosis is treated with parenteral penicillin for two to six weeks often followed by oral penicillin for up to a year. In some cases, surgery will be required to drain abscess formation and repair scar damage.[22-24]

Oral/Facial Considerations

Oral/cervical actinomycosis is characterized as a lumpy tender swelling, most often affecting the mandible. Development of sinus tracts is common as is the drainage of purulent exudate containing the characteristic sulfur granules. Occasionally a high fever will develop. Various disease states and trauma to the oral/facial tissues are felt to be prerequisites for actinomycosis and include periodontal disease, dental abscess, tooth extraction and/or jaw surgery, tonsillitis, and inner ear infection. In addition to penicillin, therapy includes incision and drainage and removal of any associated focus of dental infection.[25]

Tuberculosis

Tuberculosis (TB) is caused by the acid- and alcohol-fast mycobacterium, *Mycobacterium tuberculosis*. The organism is usually acquired by airborne transmission and grows in the pulmonary alveoli and macrophages with a local inflammatory response. In most cases, T helper cells activate macrophages through the secretion of cytokines and gamma interferon (IFN), and the infection is suppressed permanently or may remain latent to reactivate months or years later. If the immune response is compromised and cannot prevent replication of the bacteria, active disease begins. With active infection, the following symptoms are common: chronic cough, moderate fever, night sweats, fatigue, decreased appetite, and weight loss. Occasionally, TB can spread to other parts of the body by the lymph and blood systems. Miliary (blood infection) and meningeal TB are the most serious forms of the disease and area associated with high mortality rates.[26-30]

Although generally not considered a major health concern in the United States, at the international level, TB remains a leading killer of young adults, with some 2 billion people infected, one-third of the world's population. TB is a leading killer of those who have HIV infection.[30,31] The Centers for Disease Control and Prevention (CDC) estimates that worldwide, over 8 million people will develop active TB annually, resulting in over 1 million deaths. The potential for human to human transmission of TB through the respiratory route is extremely high.

Even in the United States, TB remains a persistent public health concern. The number of active cases has dropped from over 80,000 in 1953 to 9945 in 2012 (Table 22-1).[26] However, deaths from TB increased slightly from 2009 to 2010. Ethnic background is a strong risk factor for acquiring TB in the United States, affecting the following groups in descending order: Asians, Pacific Islanders, African Americans, Hispanics, Americans Indians, and Caucasians. Sixty-three percent of new TB cases in the United States affect foreign-born persons, and this group is 11 times more likely to be diagnosed with TB than native-born Americans.[31,32]

Several trends during the 1980s and 1990s contributed to the increased rate of TB infection in the United States. These factors continue to complicate the management of the disease today. People with HIV/AIDS are at significant risk of developing active TB after being exposed. As mentioned earlier, the increased immigration of foreign-born individuals from areas with high rates of TB, such as Asia, Africa, and Latin America, has contributed to the increase. Poverty, injection drug use, alcoholism, and homelessness has contributed to the spread of TB as large numbers of these individuals spend time in crowded shelters and/or prisons, where they are chronically exposed. Elderly people in nursing homes with declining health status are at risk for reactivating latent TB or acquiring a new infection when immunosuppressed. Finally, patients exposed to TB often do not comply with their TB medical treatment regimen, making them infectious longer and more likely to develop resistance to treatment.[28,32]

The diagnosis of latent disease is initiated by performing a tuberculin skin test (TST) on the forearm with purified protein derivative, a mycobacterial antigen. If a red welt forms within 72 hours, the patient is considered to have been exposed to *M. tuberculosis*. Another test, called the interferon-γ release assay (IGRA), is a blood test that detects

TABLE 22-1	Reported Cases of Tuberculosis in the United States by Year[26]
Year	**Total Number of Cases**
1953	84,304
1955	77,368
1960	55,494
1965	49,016
1970	37,137
1975	33,989
1980	27,749
1985	22,201
1990	25,701
1995	22,860
2000	16,337
2005	14,093
2010	11,163
2012	9,945

sensitization to *M. tuberculosis* by measuring IFN-γ release in response to antigens representing *M. tuberculosis*.[33] Compared to TST, IGRA tests are single-step tests that can be repeated several times, do not causes sensitization or boosting, and exhibit improved sensitivity.[34] However, IGRA tests are more expensive than TST.[35] Current recommendations prefer the IGRA test over TST to test patients who have had the Bacille Calmette-Guerin (BCG) vaccine or who cannot return to have the TST read (e.g., homeless persons, drug users). TB screening is recommended for certain high-risk populations (Table 22-2).[36]

The patient with a positive screening test or suspected of having active disease is evaluated to determine the presence of active TB disease. Signs and symptoms of active TB include productive cough, fever, chills, or night sweats. A chest radiograph often reveals pulmonary involvement. Confirmation of active TB involves collecting patient sputum to look for the infecting organism (aka acid-fast bacillus test).[27–29]

The patient diagnosed with a latent TB infection is typically treated with one of the following regimens for from four to nine months: isoniazid, isoniazid plus rifapentine, or rifampin.[37]

Active TB is curable in most patients, but patient compliance to complete the prescribed drug regimen is critical to prevent reactivation of the disease or the development of resistance. In this regard, the implementation of directly observed therapy has been extremely successful in curing poorly compliant patients and also in preventing the emergence of drug-resistant strains. The usual course of therapy is six to nine months and involves several drug regimens(Table 22-3).[37] If initial therapy fails, the patient may have multidrug-resistant TB (MDR-TB) or extensively drug-resistant TB (XDR-TB).

TABLE 22-2 High-Risk Groups Recommended for Purified Protein Derivative Testing[36]

1. People who have spent time with someone who has TB disease
2. People with HIV infection or another medical problem that weakens the immune system
3. People who have symptoms for TB disease (fever, night sweats, cough, and weight loss)
4. People from a country where TB disease is common (most countries in Latin America, the Caribbean, Africa, Asia, Eastern Europe, and Russia)
5. People who live or work somewhere in the United States where TB disease is more common (homeless shelters, prison or jails, some nursing homes)
6. People who use illegal drugs

Abbreviations: TB, tuberculosis.

TABLE 22-3 Treatment for Tuberculosis Infection[37]

Timing	Medications
Initial—Daily for 8 wk	Isoniazid, rifampin, ethambutol, pyrazinamide
Continuation—Daily for 18 wk	Isoniazid, rifampin

MDR-TB is defined as TB that is resistant to at least isoniazid and rifampicin, and XDR-TB is defined as MDR-TB with additional resistance to a fluoroquinolone and one of the second-line injectable therapeutic agents such as kanamycin, amikacin, or capreomycin.[38,39] Globally in 2012, there were an estimated 450,000 new cases of MDR-TB and 170,000 MDR-TB deaths. XDR-TB represents about 10% of the case burden of MDR-TB.[39] An estimated 70% of XDR-TB patients die within the first month of diagnosis.[40] MDR-TB and XDR-TB require special therapy with at least three drugs for up to two years. MDR-TB occurs in about 1% of active TB patients in the United States, of whom 86% are foreign born.[32]

Prevention programs have helped reduce the incidence of TB in the United States. Where there are large populations in close proximity, adequate ventilation is the most effective measure to prevent the spread of TB. High-risk groups are screened for latent TB and, if positive, managed as described above. Health-care facilities use ultraviolet light, special filters, special respirators, and masks to reduce the spread of TB. People with active TB are isolated in rooms with controlled ventilation until they are no longer infectious.[41]

The BCG vaccine is made from live weakened strain of *Mycobacterium bovis*. In countries where TB is common, this vaccine is administered to children and has an efficacy rate of 60% to 80%. However, the vaccine is much less effective in adults and often results in a positive TST. The vaccine is not routinely used in the United States.[42]

Oral/Facial Considerations

Oral manifestations may occur in up to 3% of patients with long-term active TB. Lesions may occur in the oral tissues and the neck lymph nodes. The latter is termed scrofula. The oral lesions are found in various soft tissues and supporting bone.[43]

The risk of a dental care provider acquiring TB from a patient is low, particularly in a conventional dental office. However, health-care settings serving patients listed in Table 22-2 put dental personnel at higher risk. Hospitals, nursing homes, prisons, and clinics that treat high-risk populations are of particular concern. Patients with active TB are isolated during initial therapy, and dental treatment should be deferred until the patient is no longer considered infectious. Patients are no longer considered infectious if they have two consecutive negative sputum cultures or have received TB treatment for at least two weeks. To identify health-care workers (HCWs) who have been exposed to TB, many hospitals require personnel to be skin tested annually. This appears to be a reasonable practice in settings with a significant high-risk population. Infected HCWs identified through screening are medically evaluated and considered for up to nine months of isoniazid (INH) therapy.[41,44,45]

FUNGAL INFECTIONS

Common endemic mycoses include blastomycosis, histoplasmosis, and paracoccidioidomycosis. Primary infection occurs through the respiratory track with dissemination to the skin and viscera via hematogenous and lymphatic spread. Nonendemic fungal infections such as aspergillosis, cryptococcosis, and mucormycosis often present as solitary oral ulcers. However, reactive epithelial and pseudoepitheliomatous hyperplasia may lead to heaped-up, exophytic mucosal lesions potentially misinterpreted as squamous cell carcinoma.

Blastomycosis

Blastomyces dermatitidis is a dimorphic organism that can grow as either a yeast or a mycelial form. It is a normal inhabitant of soil and agricultural and construction workers area at highest risk of infection, particularly those working in the Mississippi and Ohio River Valleys and around the Great Lakes and the St. Lawrence Seaway. This geographic distribution has led to the designation by some as "North American blastomycosis." However, infection by the same organism has been found in Mexico and Central and South America.[46] Immunosuppressed patients, such as HIV patients and solid-organ transplant patients, are at particular risk for developing blastomycosis. In addition, patients receiving tumor necrosis factor antagonists for autoimmune disease are at an increased risk.[47,48]

Infection with *Blastomyces* begins in a majority of cases by inhalation; this causes a primary pulmonary infection. Although an acute self-limiting form of the disease exists and some cases remain asymptomatic, the infection commonly follows a chronic course beginning with mild symptoms such as malaise, low-grade fever, and mild cough. If the infection goes untreated, the signs and symptoms may mimic TB and include dyspnea, weight loss, and production of blood-tinged sputum.[49] Some patients develop acute respiratory distress syndrome, with a mortality rate of 50% to 89%.[48] Infection of the skin, mucosa, and bone may also occur, resulting from spread of organisms from the pulmonary lesions through the lymphatic system. The skin lesions (usually on exposed surfaces) start as subcutaneous nodules, slowly progressing to well-circumscribed indurated ulcers.[50]

Blastomycosis is diagnosed using real-time PCR, antibody identification through enzyme immunoassay, biopsy, and culture on Sabouraud agar.[51–53] The organism is often identified in sputum or biopsy specimens characterized by the presence of granulomas with unipolar budding yeasts.[51]

Itraconazole therapy is used to manage mild cases of blastomycosis. More advanced cases infections are treated with amphotericin B.[49,54]

Oral/Facial Considerations

Oral lesions are rarely the primary site of infection. When oral lesions have been reported as a first sign of blastomycosis, they have occurred in patients with mild pulmonary symptoms that have been overlooked by the patient or physician. Most cases of oral involvement demonstrate concomitant pulmonary lesions on chest radiographs. The most common appearance of the oral lesions of blastomycosis is a nonspecific, painless ulcer with indurated borders and verrucous mucosal hyperplasia often mistaken for squamous cell carcinoma.[55–57]

Histoplasmosis

Histoplasmosis is caused by the fungus *Histoplasma capsulatum*, a dimorphic fungus with both yeast and mycelial forms that grows in the yeast form in infected tissue. Infection results from inhaling dust contaminated with droppings, particularly from infected birds or bats. An African form of this infection is caused by a larger yeast, *Histoplasma duboisii*, which is considered a variant of *H. capsulatum*.[46]

Histoplasmosis is the most common systemic fungal infection in the United States and presents primarily as pulmonary disease; in endemic areas such as the Mississippi and Ohio River valleys, serologic evidence of previous infection may be found in 75% to 80% of the population. Outbreaks of occupationally acquired histoplasmosis continue to be reported among agricultural workers and laborers in endemic areas. Particularly at risk are individuals working with aerosolized topsoil or dust with bat or bird droppings.[58–60]

In most cases, particularly in otherwise normal children, primary infection is mild, manifesting as a self-limiting pulmonary disease that heals to leave fibrosis and calcification similar to TB. In a small percentage of cases, progressive disease results in cavitation of the lung and dissemination of the organism to the liver, spleen, adrenal glands, and meninges. Patients with the disseminated form of the disease may develop anemia and leukopenia secondary to bone marrow involvement. Immunosuppressed or myelosuppressed patients are more likely to develop the severe disseminated form of the disease, and disseminated histoplasmosis is one of the infections that characterize AIDS.[59,61]

A rapid diagnosis may be made with the use of a smear of the lesion stained with methenamine silver or a biopsy of the lesion stained with periodic acid–Schiff or methenamine silver, which will reveal the presence of the fungi within granulomas. Cultures should be performed on a portion of tissue removed during the biopsy. Diagnosis of disseminated histoplasmosis occurs by antigen detection via enzyme immunoassay in serum and urine, antibody detection via immmunodiffusion, identification of histoplasma DNA via various PCR techniques, identification of the organism on biopsy, and culture.[51,62,63] There is some cross-reactivity with *Blastomyces* infection.

Immunocompromised patients with disseminated histoplasmosis are generally treated with amphotericin B and/or a triazole such as itraconazole; occasionally patients have also been treated with voriconazole and posaconazole.[46,60,64]

Oral/Facial Considerations

Oral involvement is usually secondary to pulmonary involvement and occurs in a significant percentage of patients with disseminated histoplasmosis. Most cases of oral histoplasmosis reported during the past two decades have been detected in HIV-infected individuals who live in or have visited endemic areas and may represent primary oral involvement or part of disseminated infection.[65] In one study, 3% of HIV-positive patients in an endemic area had oral lesions of histoplasmosis, and oral histoplasmosis had been reported as the first sign of AIDS.[66] Patients diagnosed with histoplasmosis should be tested for HIV infection.

Oral mucosal lesions begin as an area of erythema that becomes a papule and eventually forms a painful, granulomatous-appearing ulcer often with an indurated border, on the gingiva, palate, or tongue.[67] Some lesions are fungating. The cervical lymph nodes are often enlarged and firm. The clinical appearance of the lesions, as well as the accompanying lymphadenopathy, often resembles that of squamous cell carcinoma, other chronic fungal infections, or lymphoma. Ulcers present for weeks or months may represent other lesions of infectious etiology (other deep fungal, mycobacterial, treponemal, or parasitic), traumatic ulcerative granuloma, squamous cell carcinoma, lymphoma, or other malignancy.[68]

Paracoccidioidomycosis

Paracoccidioidomycosis, also called South American Blastomycosis, is produced by the organism, *Paracoccidioidomycosis brasiliensis*. It is an endemic disease from Mexico through Central America down to Argentina in South America. The niche for the organism is thought to be soil or wood and inhalation is the route of infection. Most patients are asymptomatic after initial infection, but the organism can be dormant within lymph nodes for many years and then reactivate when the patient experiences some types of immunosuppression. The disease affects primarily men (15:1 ratio men to women) older than 30 years. When activated, the infection involves primarily the oral mucosa, lungs, and skin. Other potential sites of involvement are the gastrointestinal (GI) tract, liver, bones, central nervous system (CNS), and male genitourinary tract. In severe cases, signs and symptoms may mimic those of TB and include fever, weight loss, and productive cough with bloody sputum.

The diagnosis is accomplished by direct examination of sputum, biopsy material from ulcers, or pus draining from lymph nodes. Establishing the diagnosis may be difficult as the organism occurs in the mold form and/or the yeast form. It is necessary to observe the yeast form, and this can be seen in a 10% potassium hydroxide (KOH) preparation. The specimen is then isolated in culture.[69–71]

Paracoccidioidomycosis is treated with azole antifungals, with itraconazole being preferred due to lower relapse rates. Amphotericin B may be given with the azoles, and maintenance therapy for up to five years is often necessary.[72]

Oral/Facial Considerations

Oral mucosal lesions are a prominent feature of paracoccidioidomycosis and present as ulcers, and oral complaints are often the presenting symptoms of these patients. Lesions of the gingival mucosa are most common followed by the palate and lips. The lesions are frequently painful. Ulcerative lesions with crusting also occur on the facial skin and may infiltrate subcutaneously.[73]

Aspergillosis

Organisms of the fungal genus *Aspergillus* cause multiple infections including pulmonary infections, invasive aspergillosis, and allergic bronchopulmonary reactions. Commonly found in soil, on plants, in decaying organic matter, and in dust from houses and building materials, *Aspergillus* species are ubiquitous in the environment and colonization of the respiratory tract is common in humans. The two most common infecting organisms are *Aspergillus fumigatus* and *Aspergillus flavus*. However, invasive infections are uncommon. Patients with a compromised immune system tend to be at risk for aspergillosis, particularly those receiving chemotherapy for malignancy. In addition to the lungs, invasive aspergillosis can involve the CNS, bones, eye, heart, and kidneys.[74,75]

Aspergillus infections are diagnosed using direct examination of clinical specimens on 10% KOH and then isolated with specific culture techniques. Invasive aspergillosis has a high mortality rate, but early diagnosis improves prognosis. Assay for galactomannan antigen (an exoantigen of *Aspergillus*) in the blood is often used as an effective screen for early diagnosis in patients at risk.[75]

Treatment of invasive aspergillosis is accomplished with several systemic antifungal medications including voriconazole, amphotericin B, itraconazole, posaconazole, caspofungin, and micafungin. Antifungal prophylaxis may be employed in certain high-risk groups (e.g., transplant).[76,77]

Oral/Facial Considerations

Oral colonization with *Aspergillus* species is common, although oral infections are rare. In contrast, allergic bronchopulmonary aspergillosis of the sinuses is fairly common. Patients present with a lingering chronic sinusitis of the maxillary sinuses that is not responsive to standard antibacterial medication. Standard medical therapy consists of corticosteroids and itraconazole, with some cases requiring surgery to clear the condition.[74,76]

Cryptococcosis

Cryptococcosis is a worldwide infection that develops after the fungal spores are inhaled from soil contaminated from bird droppings, primarily with two species, *Cryptococcus neoformans* and *Cryptococcus gattii*. The infection is common in patients with a compromised immune system such as with HIV, steroid exposure, transplantation, diabetes, and pregnancy; but otherwise healthy people may become infected. The incidence is particularly high in patients with HIV. In some cases, the patient presents with symptoms of pneumonia including cough, fever, chest pain, and weight loss. In others, the patient remains asymptomatic but develops a latent infection that remains dormant. The most serious infection involves the CNS and causes meningoencephalitis. Symptoms include fever, head-ache, lethargy, and mental changes and can lead to permanent neurologic damage.[78–80]

Cryptococcosis is diagnosed by microscopic examination and/or culture of tissue or body fluids. A cryptococcal anti-gen test may provide a rapid diagnosis when done on blood or cerebrospinal fluid.[81]

Severe cryptococcal infections, particularly those of the CNS, are treated with amphotericin B with flucytosine. Less severe infections are treated with fluconazole or itraconazole. Treatment requires long courses of medication of at least six months or longer. Maintenance therapy may be permanent in patients with cryptococcal meningoencephalitis.[78,79,82]

Oral/Facial Considerations

Oral lesions of cryptococcosis may occur in patients with disseminated disease and immunosuppression. They have been described as ulcers and tumor-like nodules occurring on the gingiva and tongue.[81]

Mucormycosis

The term mucormycosis describes an infection that is caused by the class of fungi known as the mucorales with the most common infecting organism being *Rhizopus arrhizus*. The order is Mucorales (from which is derived the terminology "mucormycosis"), and Rhizopus, Mucor, and Lichtheimia (formerly Absidia) can all cause mucormycosis.[83] The term zygomycosis has also been used for these infections, but cur-rently mucormycosis is the preferred term. These organisms are typically found in the soil and decaying organic matter. These fungi are nonpathogenic for healthy individuals and are opportunistic pathogens; they are regularly cultured from the human nose, throat, and oral cavity of healthy asymptomatic individuals. The two most common forms of mucormycosis are pulmonary/sinus and cutaneous. In pulmonary/sinus mucormycosis, spores are inhaled from the environment. For the cutaneous disease, spores enter traumatic wounds to the skin, such as those occurring from impact injuries contacting the ground.[84–86]

Mucormycosis is characterized by arterial invasion and a fulminant course, frequently resulting in death. The hallmark of infection is the formation of emboli with resulting nec-rosis of involved tissue. Mucormycosis may present as a pul-monary, sinus, rhinocerebral, skin, or disseminated infection. Infection occurs in patients with decreased host resistance such as those with poorly controlled diabetes; hematologic malignancies; post-solid-organ transplantation; post-hema-topoietic cell transplantation; patients with severe trauma or burns; and patients on deferoxamine therapy.[87,88]

Early diagnosis is essential for improved survival and reduced morbidity from extension of disease and dissemina-tion. Negative cultures do not rule out mucormycosis because the fungus is frequently difficult to culture; instead, a biopsy for culture and direct examination must be performed. The histopathology shows necrosis and nonseptate hyphae,

which are best demonstrated by a periodic acid–Schiff stain or the methenamine silver stain. Necrosis and occlusion of vessels are also frequently present. Newer techniques of iden-tification include the use of PCR.[89]

First-line therapy consists of surgical debridement and amphotericin B, whereas second-line treatment includes other antifungal chemotherapeutic agents such as posa-conazole and caspofungin.[90–92] The mortality rate is 50% to 100% in spite of therapy, compared with 35% to 45% for aspergillosis, and an increasing number of case has been noted in immunocompetent patients.[83]

Oral/Facial Considerations

The rhinomaxillary form of the disease, a variant of the rhino-cerebral form, begins with the inhalation of the fungus by a susceptible individual. The fungus invades blood vessels and causes damage secondary to thrombosis and ischemia. The fungus may spread from the oral and nasal region to the brain, causing death in a high percentage of cases. The most com-mon symptoms of the rhinomaxillary form include proptosis, loss of vision, nasal discharge, sinusitis, and palatal necrosis.

The most common oral sign of mucormycosis is ulceration of the palate, which results from necrosis due to invasion of a palatal vessel. The lesion is characteristically large and deep and may lead to exposure of underlying bone. Ulcers from mucormycosis have also been reported on the gingiva, lip, and alveolar ridge. Similar to other invasive fungal infections, sol-itary mucosal ulcers of several weeks and months duration may represent lesions of other infectious etiology, traumatic ulcerative granuloma, squamous cell carcinoma, lymphoma, or other malignancy. The initial manifestation of the disease may be confused with pain from an odontogenic infection or conventional bacterial maxillary sinusitis. More advanced dis-ease with ulcer and palatal perforation may suggest an anti-neutrophil cytoplasmic antibody–associated vasculitis (e.g., Wegener granulomatosis).[84,85,91,93]

VIRAL INFECTIONS
Viral Hepatitis

Approximately 80% of viral hepatitis infections are caused by hepatitis A virus (HAV), hepatitis B virus (HBV), hep-atitis C virus (HCV), hepatitis D virus (HDV), or hepatitis E virus (HEV) (Table 22-4).[94] However, the etiologic viral agent remains unidentified in an estimated 20% of acute hepatitis cases, 10% of fulminant hepatitis cases, and 5% of chronic hepatitis cases.[95] For these equivocal cases of hepat-itis, several emerging candidate viruses have been proposed as the etiologic agent and are briefly discussed at the end of this section.

HAV and HEV are predominantly spread through enteral modes and do not incur chronic disease, and their impact on health appears limited to the acute infection. However, up to 10% of pregnancy-related fatalities in southern Asia are postulated to be attributable to HEV infection.[96]

TABLE 22-4	Major Hepatitis Viruses					
Agent	Family	Genome	Size (nm)	Incubation Periods (d)	Vaccine
Type A	Picornaviridae	ss RNA	27	15–50	Y
Type B	Hepadnaviridae	ds DNA	42	45–160	Y
Type C	Flaviviridae	ss RNA	30–60	15–150	N
Type D	Subviral satellite	ss RNA	35	15–150	Y[a]
Type E	Caliciviridae	ss RNA	27–34	15–60	N

Abbreviations: DNA, deoxyribonucleic acid; ds, double stranded; RNA, ribonucleic acid; ss, single stranded.
[a]Hepatitis B virus vaccination confers protection.
Source: Adapted from Howard.[94]

As a consequence of their parenteral mode of transmission and ability to establish chronic infection, hepatitis types HBV, HDV, and HCV are of particular concern for oral health-care professionals, as chronically infected patients undoubtedly will present for dental care. More importantly, chronic hepatitis is clearly associated with and increased risk of developing cirrhosis and/or hepatocellular carcinoma (HCC). The annual mortality rates for viral-induced cirrhosis and HCC are estimated at 796,000 and 616,000, respectively.[97] Globally, HCC is fifth most common cancer and third most common cause of cancer mortality, and 75% to 80% of cases are attributed to chronic HBV and/or HCV infection.[98,99] This section briefly reviews our current understanding of HBV, HCV, and HDV epidemiology, pathogenesis, and management.

Epidemiology

Over 2 billion people have been infected with HBV, and although effective vaccines against HBV have been available since 1982, an estimated 350 million individuals are chronically infected.[100] The overall risk of developing chronic infection is approximately 5%, but there is significant geographic variability. Chronic infection prevalence rates are highest in sub-Saharan Africa, most of Asia, and the Pacific (8%–20%) and lowest in Western Europe and North America (0.1%–2.0%). In areas of high prevalence, perinatal transmission represents the predominant risk of exposure to HBV. HBV is not directly cytopathogenic,, and the risk of developing chronic infection is inversely correlated with immune competence and correlates well with the patient's age at initial infection.[100] Neonates, whose immune systems are immature, have a 90% chance of developing chronic HBV infection, compared with a 20% to 30% chance during childhood and a <1% chance for adults.[101] HBV transmission in low-prevalence areas is associated with high-risk exposure behaviors such as having multiple sex partners, sex with HBV-infected persons, and intravenous drug use.

For HCV, the worldwide estimates for chronic infection exceed 184 million with the highest prevalence occurring in Central and East Asia, North Africa, and the Middle East.[102] In the United States, an estimated 3.2 million individuals are chronically infected. Although the incidence of new infections has dropped significantly since 1980 (230,000 new infections in 1980 and 16,000 new infections in 2009), the incidence of HCV-related morbidity and mortality has steadily increased.[103] The predominate route of exposure is via injection drug use.[104] Potential, but less likely routes of exposure include receipt of infected blood transfusion, transmission in the health-care setting, sexual transmission, and tattooing or piercing. The risk of transmission via transfusion is estimated to be about 1 per 1 million transfusions. Transmission in the health-care setting most likely occurs as consequence of the reuse of blood-contaminated needles or syringes; the inappropriate use of multidose vials or bags of saline; or inadequate infection control techniques.[105] The risk of sexual transmission is considered small but higher with HIV infection.[104] The risk of HCV transmission associated with tattooing is considered slight when accomplished in a professional parlor, but significant when accomplished by a friend or in a prison settings.[106]

HDV is a defective ribonucleic acid (RNA) virus that requires the hepatitis B surface antigen (HBsAg) coat for virion assembly and subsequent binding to the hepatocyte.[107] Infection almost always occurs as a new infection affecting a patient with chronic HBV (superinfection).[108] Infrequently, infection may occur simultaneously with an HBV infection (coinfection). An estimated 20 million individuals worldwide are chronically infected with HBV/HDV. Prevalence rates are highest in areas with high rates of chronic HBV infection and HDV remains a concern in developed nations, especially among intravenous drug addicts. Coinfected patients tend to progress more rapidly to cirrhosis than patients infected with HBV alone.

HBV, HDV, and HCV all exhibit significant genetic diversity as evidenced by traceable geographic distributions. From a clinical perspective, genotype assessment is useful for monitoring the clinical course, directing therapeutic interventions, and, ultimately, predicting prognosis of infection.[98] For HBV, there are eight genotypes (A–J) and numerous subgenotypes and HbsAg subtypes.[109] Genotypes A and D are predominantly observed in Europe, the United States, and Central Africa, whereas genotypes B and C are more typically observed in Asia.[110] For HCV, there are 11 genotypes (1–11) and numerous subtypes. The predominant

HCV genotype present in the United States is type 1, which accounts for 70% of US cases.[111] Three distinct genotypes of HDV are recognized (I, II, and III), and the predominant HDV genotype observed in the United States is type I.

Diagnosis

For both acute and chronic forms of viral hepatitis, many patients have either no symptoms or symptoms so mild they may be easily overlooked (fatigue, nausea, fever, abdominal pain, loss of appetite). As a consequence, hepatitis is often discovered during routine laboratory screening as part of a physical examination or voluntary blood donation. The likelihood of developing symptomatic illness is inversely related to one's age at the time of infection. The more characteristic signs and symptoms of jaundice, urticaria, dark-colored urine, light-colored stools, and an enlarged/tender liver signal the presence of more extensive liver damage. Other conditions to consider in the differential diagnosis include alcohol abuse, fatty liver, autoimmune hepatitis, primary biliary cirrhosis, hemochromatosis, Wilson's disease, and α_1-antitrypsin deficiency.[112]

Laboratory testing is essential for establishing the diagnosis, monitoring disease progression, and assessing the results of therapeutic interventions. Basic liver function tests include alanine aminotransferase, alkaline phosphatase, aspartate aminotransferase, albumin, and total protein. Although useful, liver function tests must be correlated with specific serologic tests to establish etiology. For HBV, available tests include HBsAg, HBV surface antibody (anti-HBs), and HBV core antibody (anti-HBc and IgM anti-HBc). For HDV, HDV antigen and HDV antibody (anti-HD) may be obtained. For HCV, the only routinely ordered test is for HCV antibody (anti-HCV). (Table 22-5) lists the more common serologic patterns

observed in the course of HBV or HCV infection.[113,114] Viral load testing for all three viruses is available and very useful in assessing disease status, as is liver biopsy.[100,115,116]

Pathogenesis

The pathogenic mechanisms of HBV, HDV, and HCV are only partially understood, and numerous factors such as route of transmission, age of acquisition, viral subtype, and patient's age, immunocompetence, and health influence pathogenesis. Although these viruses are hepatotropic, they do not appear to be directly cytopathic, and the severity of hepatocyte injury reflects the intensity of the host cellular immune response.[97,100] Patients who develop a vigorous cytotoxic T-cell response to infection are more likely to manifest severe, at times fulminant, liver injury, but they are at low risk of developing chronic infection. The mortality rate of fulminant hepatitis is about 70%. In contrast, patients who generate a less vigorous cytotoxic T-cell response to infection manifest little acute liver injury but are at much greater risk for developing chronic infection. Putative mechanisms underlying the ability of these viruses to circumvent the host immune response and establish chronic infection include the suppressive actions of viral antigens on the host immune system, reduced CD4 T-cell help, the suppressive effects of T-regulatory cells, and the high rate of viral mutation.[100,111,117]

Chronic infection is a dynamic process for which the outcome varies from patient to patient. Some patients eventually develop a sufficient immune response to clear the virus; manifest no symptoms throughout their lives; others manifest only occasional flares of clinical illness; and still others experience unrelenting progressive clinical illness.[100,111] Thirty-eight percent to seventy-six percent of chronically infected HCV patients develop at least one extrahepatic

TABLE 22-5 Common Serologic Patterns of Hepatitis B and C Virus Infection[113,114]	
Serologic Result	**Interpretation**
HBV	
HbsAg neg, anti-HBc pos, anti-HBs pos	Immunity from natural infection
HBsAg neg, anti-HBc neg, anti-HBs pos	Immunity from vaccination
HBsAg pos, anti-HBc pos, IgM anti-HBc pos, anti-HBs neg	Acute infection
HBsAg pos, anti-HBc pos, IgM anti-HBc neg, anti-HBs neg	Chronic infection
HBsAg neg, anti-HBc pos, anti-HBs neg	Recovering from acute infection, or False-positive anti-HBc, thus susceptible or "Low level" chronic infection Resolving acute infection
HCV	
Anti-HCV reactive	A repeatedly reactive result is consistent with current HCV infection, or past HCV infection that has resolved, or biologic false positivity for HCV antibody. Test for HCV RNA to identify current infection.
Anti-HCV reactive, HCV RNA detected	Appropriate counseling and referral for medical care and treatment.
Anti-HCV reactive, HCV RNA not detected	No further action required in most cases.

Abbreviations: anti-HBc, hepatitis B core antibody; anti-HBs, hepatitis B surface antibody; HbsAg, hepatitis B surface antigen; HCV, hepatitis C virus; IgM, immunoglobulin M.

autoimmune disorder, typically mixed cryoglobulinemia, Sjögren's syndrome, or autoimmune thyroid disease.[118] It has been postulated that molecular mimicry between viral components and "self" proteins, polyclonal B-cell activation, or genetic predisposition may underlie the autoimmune response. The two main concerns related to chronic viral hepatitis are the increased risks for developing cirrhosis and HCC.

The association between chronic viral hepatitis and HCC, although strong, is complex and poorly understood. A multitude of factors that possibly contribute to the development of HCC include direct virus-induced mutagenesis, the accumulation of genetic and epigenetic lesions associated with continuous hepatocyte necrosis and regeneration, and an increased susceptibility to the carcinogenic actions of aflatoxins, alcohol, and tobacco.[100] Other contributing factors for disease progression include male sex, infection at an early age, heavy alcohol consumption, coinfection with other hepatotropic viruses or HIV, and immunosuppression.

For patients with chronic HBV, the progression to cirrhosis and HCC increases proportionally with increasing viral load, starting at with at least 1×10^4 copies/mL.[100] The annual risk of developing cirrhosis or HCC is 2% to 10% and 1% to 3%, respectively,[119] and integration of HBV DNA into the genome of the host hepatocyte is noted in 85% to 90% of cases.[120] The risk of developing cirrhosis and HCC after 30 years of chronic HCV infection is 15% to 35% and 1% to 3%, respectively.[121] In contrast to HBV, HCV is unable to integrate into the host genome.[122] It is postulated that viral proteins disrupt numerous cellular signal transduction pathways that affect cell survival, proliferation, migration, and transformation.

Medical Management

Preventive measures to reduce viral hepatitis spread include aggressive vaccination protocols (for HBV); adequate screening and handling measures for donated blood and tissues; implementation of proven infection control measures in the health-care setting; and promotional/educational efforts to reduce the practice of unsafe injection drug use and/or high-risk sexual practices. Approximately 90% of healthy adults and 95% of infants, children, and adolescents produce protective antibodies against HBV after vaccination.[123] An adequate response is defined as a serum level of anti-HBs antibody of ≥10 mIU/mL. Although some waning of the anti-HBs response may occur over time, clear guidelines regarding the need for booster immunization have yet to be established. Unfortunately, currently, there exists no vaccine against HCV.

Treatment protocols for acute viral hepatitis are supportive, and there is no consensus on the value or need to provide antiviral therapy during an acute infection. For chronic viral hepatitis, the decision on how and when to institute therapy is complex and must be based on factors such as patient interest, clinical and laboratory findings, risk of disease progression without intervention, odds of therapeutic success, risk of therapeutic adverse effects, and the overall health of the patient.[99,112] The primary goal of therapy is to eliminate or permanently suppress HBV replication to reduce the risk or slow the progression of liver disease and to prevent or reduce the development of hepatic decompensation, cirrhosis, and HCC.[124,125]

Approved drug therapies to treat chronic HBV include IFN-α, pegylated IFN-α$_{2a}$, and the nucles(t)ide analogues (Nucs) adefovir, dipivoxil, lamivudine, entecavir, telbivudine, and tenofovir disoproxil fumarate (TDF).[124] Since these drugs do not typically eradicate HBV, therapeutic protocols tend to be prolonged. IFN-based therapy is modestly efficacious in producing HBeAg loss or seroconversion in patients with HBeAg-positive chronic HBV infection, and in producing sustained HBV DNA suppression (<20,000 copies/mL) in 40% of HBeAg-negative patients.[125] Nucs inhibit HBV DNA synthesis and effectively suppresses HBV replication rapidly in both HBeAg-positive and HBeAg-negative patients. Current guidelines recommend monotherapy with either entecavir or TDF, as they are the most potent available agents and also demonstrate a high barrier to antiviral resistance.[124] Treatment with either drug for up to five years results in a sustained viral response (SVR) in >90% of patients.

The past decade has seen the emergence of new therapies and genomic tests to manage HCV. Therapeutic success is defined by a SVR and is largely predicated on the HCV genotype. The traditional standard regimen of pegylated IFN-α$_{2a}$ and ribavirin has been largely augmented (triple therapy) by the introduction of direct acting antivirals.[126] Currently available drugs are the protease inhibitors (PIs) boceprevir, telaprevir, and simeprevir.[127] All are reversible inhibitors of the HCV nonstructural 3/4A serine protease occurring in genotype 1 HCV. The use of either pegylated IFN-α$_{2a}$ and ribavirin result in an SVR of 70% to 80% in the treatment of naïve patients.[127,128] The most commonly observed adverse events with boceprevir include rash, pruritus, anal-rectal discomfort, anemia, nausea, and diarrhea. The most frequently observed adverse events with telaprevir include anemia and dysgeusia. Commonly observed adverse events with simeprevir include rash, pruritus, nausea, and potentially serious photosensitivity.[127]

Patient response to IFN is largely a genetic trait that is modulated by nucleotide polymorphisms within the *interleukin (IL) 28B* gene.[128] Patients who have cytosine-cytosine (CC) at a specific site within this gene are highly responsive to IFN, whereas patients with thymidine-thymidine (TT) at this specific site within the *IL28B* gene are far less responsive. Nearly 80% of patients with the CC trait can be treated for a shorter duration with boceprevir, telaprevir, or simeprevir-based triple therapy and still develop SVR rates that exceed 90%. In contrast, the SVR for patients with the TT trait is only about 50%.

Emerging direct acting antivirals being investigated to manage chronic HCV infection include second-generation PIs, Nucs, nonnucleoside inhibitors, and NS5A (a membrane-associated phosphoprotein) inhibitors.[129] The goals are to develop drug and regimen protocols that exhibit wide genotypes efficacy, less side effect liability, and less potential for viral resistance. Sofosbuvir is a direct-acting nucleotide polymerase inhibitor approved in December 2013 for use with ribavirin or pegylated IFN-α_{2a} and ribavirin for the treatment of HCV infection.[130] The most commonly observed adverse events with sofosbuvir include headache, fatigue, insomnia, nausea, rash, and anemia.[131]

For patients who develop HCC, treatment options include surgical resection, transcatheter arterial embolization, percutaneous ablation, chemotherapy, and liver transplantation.[132] Cumulative 10-year postintervention survival rates are 22% to 35%. To overcome the lack of cadaveric donors, the living donor transplants of the upper right lobe are becoming more common. Tumor recurrence within five years is clearly influenced by the viral load of the recipient. HCC recurrence is more likely if the HBV DNA levels are ≥10,000 copies/mL.[133] As a consequence, antiviral therapy is recommended.

Oral Health Considerations

Prior to initiating therapy, the clinician should ascertain the patient's overall status with attention focused on the patient's potential for increased hemorrhage and impaired drug metabolism. In general, ambulatory patients who do not manifest signs and symptoms of liver impairment and are not under active medical therapy will tolerate the delivery of routine dental care. However, if there is doubt as to the patient's status, it is prudent to consult the treating physician to develop a treatment plan for the patient that is safe and appropriate. Pertinent laboratory testing includes complete blood count, prothrombin time, partial thromboplastin time, international normalized ratio, bleeding time, and liver function tests.[134] Clinical clues of impaired liver function include jaundice, easy hemorrhage, and the presence of petechiae, hematomas, or ecchymoses. Additional clues to the presence of liver disease include Dupuytren's contracture, palmar erythema, edema, urticaria, gynecomastia, spider nevi, and sialosis.[134,135] Patients with severe liver impairment are best managed in a hospital setting, where close monitoring and indicated supplemental therapies, such as fresh frozen plasma, may be provided. All drugs metabolized by the liver should be avoided when possible or administered cautiously to patients with severely impaired liver function.

An association between the occurrence of oral lichen planus (OLP) and HCV infection, particularly in Japan, Southern European nations, and the United States, has been noted in several studies.[136] Patients with LP have a fivefold higher rate of exposure to HCV infection than controls. Given the association of HCV infection and an increased risk of numerous autoimmune diseases, one might postulate that a similar association may exist for the development of OLP. The strength of association between HCV and OLP has prompted some to recommend patients with OLP be screened for HCV.[137]

As blood-borne agents, HBV, HCV, and HDV pose serious occupational concerns for HCWs, in whom there is a risk of patient to HCW, HCW to patient, and patient to patient transmission.[138–140] The risk of infection is influenced by the route of exposure, the concentration of infectious virions in the source body fluid, and the volume of infected material transferred.[140] For HBV, the risk has been reduced dramatically through HBV vaccination programs. Prior to the availability of HBV vaccination, an estimated 10,000 HCWs became infected annually in the United States. From 2002 to 2009, the estimated number of annual cases affecting HCWs had fallen to 400 and 100, respectively.[141] Another benefit of HBV vaccination is prevention of HDV infection since HDV requires the presence of HBV to establish infection. However, since HBV vaccination is not universally effective and there exists no vaccine for HCV, HCWs must strictly follow established infection control recommendations to minimize the risk of occupational transmission.[138,139,141–143]

For HCWs who either decline HBV vaccination or fail to seroconvert, the risk of HBV infection after a percutaneous exposure is 37% to 62% if the source is HBeAg positive and 23% to 37% if the source is HBeAg negative.[140] For such scenarios, postexposure prophylaxis with hepatitis B immunoglobulin is effective 75% of the time in preventing infection if prescribed within one week of exposure.[144] The risk of occupationally acquiring HCV from an infected patient appears to be much less than HBV, with reported rates of seroconversion ranging from 0.0% to 7.0% after percutaneous exposure. However, no prophylactic postexposure protocols (PEPs) exist.

Patient to patient transmission of viral hepatitis occurs as a consequence of cross-contamination and is unlikely to occur in the dental setting when adequate infection control measures are followed. Reports of HCWs infected with viral hepatitis cross-infecting patients in the occupational setting are fortunately very low, with most cases occurring before the widespread implementation of contemporary infection control measures.[138,139,145] To ensure patient safety, recommendations regarding practice restrictions have been formulated but vary from country to country.[145,146] In general, HBV-infected practitioners who are deemed highly infectious should not perform exposure-prone procedures (EPP).[141,145] The CDC defines EPPs as procedures involving "digital palpation of a needle tip in a body cavity or the simultaneous presence of the HCW's fingers and a needle or other sharp instrument or object in a poorly visualized or highly confined anatomic site."[147] Only extensive oral surgical procedures such as orthognathic surgery fall within the definition of EPP. The two indicators of high HBV infectivity are the presence of HBeAg in the serum or a high viral load of HBV DNA. However, there exists a variant of HBV (precore mutant) that does not express HBeAg but is still capable of producing a high viral load of HBV DNA. As a consequence, most authorities now consider the HBV DNA viral load as the best measure of infectivity. Since the risk of HCV transmission from an infected HCW to a patient is low, most authorities do not recommend preemptive practice limitations.[145,146]

Emerging Putative Viruses

Both hepatitis G virus (GV) and GB virus C (GBV-C) represent two coincidentally discovered isolates of the same virus.[148] A member of the *Flaviviridae* family, it is closely related to HCV, and at least five genotypes have been discovered.[149] Prevalence estimates range from 1% to 3%.[108] However, in contrast to HCV, it appears to not be hepatotrophic but lymphotrophic and does not appear to represent a substantial hepatic risk. Some have postulated that active HGV/GBV-C replication in a patient coinfected with HIV is associated with reduced HIV progression and may represent a protective effect.[148] Others contend such findings simply represent a phase in overall HIV progression and that HGV/GBV-C replication is modulated by overall HIV activity.[150] HGV/GBV-C infection has been reported to be associated with a 10-fold increase in the development of B-cell non-Hodgkin's lymphoma.[151]

The Torque teno virus (TTV) is a circular negative-stranded DNA virus member of *Anelloviridae* family and at least four genotypes are recognized.[108] It has been detected in patients with fulminant non-A-C hepatitis, intravenous drug abusers, HCC patients, cirrhosis patients, and patients receiving blood products or on hemodialysis. TTV has also been isolated in saliva. However, liver enzyme levels of infected patients are similar to those of controls, and there is no conclusive evidence that TTV causes either hepatitis or HCC.

The SEN virus (SEN-V) is a circular single-stranded DNA virus member of *Circoviridae* family.[108] Its rate of mutation is more similar to that of an RNA virus, suggesting it does not possess proofreading capability. Eight genotypes are recognized, and prevalence rates are highest among those exposed to blood or blood products (e.g., intravenous drug abusers, hemophiliacs, HIV patients). SEN-V does not appear to cause either hepatitis or worsen preexisting liver disease.

Recently, a novel single-stranded DNA sequence associated with a newly proposed human hepatitis agent (NV-F) was discovered.[152] The pathogenic potential of NV-F remains to be determined, as it has been found in healthy controls.

Human Immunodeficiency Virus

Over 30 years ago, reports of new outbreaks of the rare opportunistic infection *Pneumocystis carinii* pneumonia and an aggressive form of Kaposi sarcoma (KS) affecting a small number of young homosexual men in California and New York.[153,154] Within the first two years, the CDC formally introduced the term *acquired immune deficiency syndrome* (AIDS) to describe the 593 reports of the disease, which also was detected in hemophiliacs and injection drug users.[155] Independent teams in France and the United States identified isolates of a T-lymphotropic virus they believed to be the primary cause of AIDS and ultimately called it human immunodeficiency virus (HIV).[156,157] In the following decade, diagnostic tests were developed and prevention measures were implemented while the disease continued to spread. In the second decade of the epidemic,

HIV continued to spread rapidly throughout the world, acutely affecting Africa and Asia. During this period, the development of antiretroviral (ARV) drugs and highly active ARV therapy dampened the spread of HIV and led to a reduction in HIV/AIDS-related fatalities. The third decade of the epidemic was marked by an unprecedented global response to the AIDS pandemic by the world's public health officials, community leaders, and politicians. The coordinated and united effort to combat AIDS has resulted in declining rates of new HIV infections in many countries and populations, indicating that the HIV pandemic has passed peak incidence.[158,159] This section briefly reviews our current understanding of the epidemiology (including pathogenesis) and management of HIV.

Epidemiology

There exist two recognized types of HIV: HIV type 1 (HIV-1) and HIV type 2 (HIV-2). Most scientists believe that each type of HIV is a descendant of a specific simian immunodeficiency virus (SIV). SIVs are primate lentiviruses that infect at least 36 nonhuman primate species in sub-Saharan Africa.[160] Contact with nonhuman primates, such as occurs during hunting and butchering, has been shown to allow for species cross-contamination and is believed to have sparked the HIV pandemic.[161] Researchers have established that the immediate precursor to HIV-1 is SIVcpz, whose natural host is the chimpanzee of the subspecies *Pan troglodytes troglodytes*.[162] Similarly, the immediate precursor to HIV-2 is SIVsm, whose natural host is the sooty mangabey.[163]

Both HIV-1 and 2 have the same modes of transmission, and both may cause immunosuppression and AIDS. However, compared with HIV-1, HIV-2 rarely occurs outside Africa and tends to follow a more indolent clinical course. HIV-1 is further classified into four groups: M, N, O, and P. HIV-1 groups M, N, O, and P, as well as chimpanzee and gorilla SIVs, are all part of the (SIV) cpz radiation within the primate lentiviruses. The HIV-1 M group subtypes are phylogenetically associated groups or clades of HIV-1 sequences and are labeled A1, A2, B, C, D, F1, F2, G, H, J, and K. The sequences within any one subtype or sub-subtype are more similar to each other than to sequences from other subtypes throughout their genomes. These subtypes represent different lineages of HIV and have some geographical associations. HIV-1 group M forms collectively account for 95% of human infections.[164–166]

Approximately 35.2 million persons were living with HIV at the end of 2012, with an estimated 0.8% of reproductive age adults globally living with HIV infection.[158] Overall, rates of new HIV infection continues to decline in many countries and populations, and for much of the world, it is now clear that the HIV pandemic has passed peak incidence. The reasons for these declines or stabilization are not always apparent. In its 2012 report, Joint United Nations Programme on HIV/AIDS (UNAIDS) compared incidence rates of 2011 with those of 2001, a period of global expansion and before ARV treatment rollout had begun in most developing countries. Using this approach, UNAIDS reported an overall decline of 20% in new infections globally, with the largest declines in the Caribbean and in sub-Saharan Africa. For much of Africa, the changes have been dramatic, with UNAIDS estimating an overall 25% reduction in HIV incidence from the 2001 peak of 2.4 million new infections across the continent, to 1.8 million new infections.[167]

In the United States, the CDC estimated that there are 1,148,200 persons aged 13 years and older are living with HIV infection, including 207,600 (18.1%) who were unaware of their infection at the end of 2010.[168] The estimated incidence of HIV has remained stable overall in recent years, at about 50,000 new HIV infections per year. In 2011, an estimated 49,273 people were diagnosed with HIV infection in the United States. In that same year, an estimated 32,052 people were diagnosed with AIDS. Since the epidemic began, an estimated 1,155,792 people in the United States have been diagnosed with AIDS. An estimated 15,529 people with an AIDS diagnosis died in 2010, and approximately 636,000 people in the United States with an AIDS diagnosis have died since the epidemic began. The most recent CDC surveillance case

definition criteria for AIDS was published in 2008 (see Table 22-6).[169] The most up-to-date surveillance information on HIV/AIDS in the United States is available at the CDC website: http://www.cdc.gov/hiv/library/reports/surveillance/index.html.

The prime modes of transmission for HIV continue to be (1) unprotected penetrative sex between men, (2) unprotected heterosexual intercourse, (3) injection drug use, (4) unsanitary injections and blood transfusions, and (5) mother to child spread during pregnancy, delivery, or breast feeding. The percentage of adults and adolescents with diagnosed HIV infection attributed to male-to-male sexual contact increased from 55% in 2008 to 62% in 2011.[170] The percentages of diagnosed HIV infections attributed to injection drug use, male-to-male sexual contact and injection drug use, and heterosexual contact remained relatively stable (less than a 5% increase or decrease) from 2008 through 2011. From 2008 through 2011, the largest percentage of diagnoses of HIV infection each year in the United States and six dependent areas was for blacks/African Americans (28%) followed by whites (22%), Hispanics/Latinos (2%), Asians(2%) and persons of multiple races (2%), and less than 1% each for American Indians/Alaska Natives and Native Hawaiians/other Pacific Islanders.

TABLE 22-6 Revised Surveillance Case Definitions for HIV Infection Among Adults, Adolescents, and Children Aged <18 Months and for HIV Infection and AIDS Among Children Aged 18 Months to <13 Years—United States, 2008[169]

Stage	Laboratory Evidence	Clinical Evidence
Stage 1	Laboratory confirmation of HIV infection and CD4+ T lymphocyte count of ≥500/μL or CD4+ T lymphocyte percentage of ≥29	None required (but no AIDS defining condition)
Stage 2	Laboratory confirmation of HIV infection and CD4+ T lymphocyte count of 200–499/μL or CD4+ T lymphocyte percentage of 14–28	None required (but no AIDS-defining condition)
Stage 3	Laboratory confirmation of HIV infection and CD4+ T lymphocyte count of <200/μL or CD4+ T lymphocyte percentage of <14	Documentation of an AIDS-defining condition (with laboratory confirmation of infection)

AIDS-defining conditions

Bacterial infections, multiple or recurrent[a]
Candidiasis of bronchi, trachea, or lungs
Candidiasis of esophagus[b]
Cervical cancer, invasive[c]
Coccidioidomycosis, disseminated or extrapulmonary
Cryptococcosis, extrapulmonary
Cryptosporidiosis, chronic intestinal (>1 month's duration)
Cytomegalovirus disease (other than liver, spleen, or nodes), onset at age >1 mo
Cytomegalovirus retinitis (with loss of vision)[b]
Encephalopathy, HIV related
Herpes simplex: chronic ulcers (>1 month's duration) or bronchitis, pneumonitis, or esophagitis (onset at age >1 mo)
Histoplasmosis, disseminated or extrapulmonary
Isosporiasis, chronic intestinal (>1 month's duration)
Kaposi sarcoma[b]

Lymphoid interstitial pneumonia or pulmonary lymphoid hyperplasia complex[a,b]
Lymphoma, Burkitt (or equivalent term)
Lymphoma, immunoblastic (or equivalent term)
Lymphoma, primary, of brain
Mycobacterium avium complex or *Mycobacterium kansasii*, disseminated or extrapulmonary[b]
Mycobacterium tuberculosis of any site, pulmonary,[b,c] disseminated,[b] or extrapulmonary[b]
Mycobacterium, other species or unidentified species, disseminated[b] or extrapulmonary[b]
Pneumocystis jirovecii pneumonia[b]
Pneumonia, recurrent[b,c]
Progressive multifocal leukoencephalopathy
Salmonella septicemia, recurrent
Toxoplasmosis of brain, onset at age >1mo[b]
Wasting syndrome attributed to HIV

[a]Only among children aged <13 yr.
[b]Condition that might be diagnosed presumptively.
[c]Only among adults and adolescents aged >13 yr.

Pathogenesis

HIV is a RNA retrovirusis. To replicate, the virus must enter a cell, commandeer the cells machinery, and use the cell's reverse transcriptase enzymes to make a DNA copy of its own RNA.[171] The virus itself is spherically shaped with an envelope made up of a lipid bilayer obtained from the cell membrane of the host as newly formed particle buds from the cell. Protruding from the envelope are approximately 72 sets of a complex HIV protein known as Env. Env consists of a stem consisting of three glycoprotein (gp) molecules called gp41 and a cap consisting of three gp molecules called gp120. Both gp120 and gp41 are essential for the recognition and binding of target cells. As HIV enters the host, gp-120 binds to the CD4 molecule on dendritic cells. Cell entry requires the presence of a coreceptor. For macrophage-tropic strains of HIV, the coreceptor is the surface chemokine receptor CCR5 (aka R5), and for T-cell–tropic strains of HIV, the coreceptor is CXCR4 (aka X4). Infected cells then fuse with CD4+ lymphocytes and spread to the deeper tissues.

Within the viral envelope is the bullet-shaped core or capsid, which consists of about 2000 copies of the HIV protein p24.[171] The capsid encircles two single strands of HIV RNA, which codes for the virus's nine genes. Three of which are structural genes (gag, pol, env) needed for the cap and stem on the viral envelope. The remaining seven genes encode proteins necessary to infect a cell, produce copies of the virus and cause disease.

More than 80% of adults infected with HIV are infected through the exposure of mucosal surfaces (linings of the vagina, vulva, rectum, penis, or the oral cavity) to the virus; most of the remaining 20% are infected by percutaneous or intravenous inoculations.[172] The risk of infection varies with different exposure routes. Numerous reports demonstrate that infection can be transmitted across the oral mucosa as a result of genital–oral sex.[173] Breaks in the mucosal barrier and the presence of increased inflammation due to genital ulcer disease, urethritis, or cervicitis increase the risk of acquiring HIV infection. Regardless of the route of viral transmission and the first cells infected, within a few days, viral replication converges on the lymphoreticular system of the GI tract. Rather than being genetically homogeneous, HIV (and other RNA viruses) consists of complex mixtures of mutant and recombinant genomes called quasi-species. In assessing various exposure routes, Lee et al. determined the evidence seems to support that a single virion is responsible for HIV transmission in approximately 80% of heterosexuals but in only about 60% of men who have sex with men and about 40% of injection drug users.[174] In injection drug users, as many as 16 transmitted virions have been found to be responsible for productive infection, which would be consistent with the absence of a mucosal barrier to transmission.

Once the virus breaches the mucosal or cutaneous barrier, the phenotype of the cell most efficiently infected appears to be the resting CD4 T-cell–lacking activation markers and expressing low levels of R5.[172] The preponderance of evidence implicates CD4 T cells and Langerhans's cells as the first targets of the virus, but other dendritic cells may play an important accessory role. Nasopharyngeal tonsil and adenoid tissues are rich in cells of dendritic origin. However, recent observations of mucosally transmitted strains of HIV-1 reveal that monocyte-derived macrophages are generally poor targets for infection as compared with CD4 T cells.

With primary infection, there is a rapid rise in plasma viremia along with the appearance of acute phase reactants in plasma (3–5 days after transmission). The cytokine storm probably contributes to harmful immune activation and the loss of CD4 T cells. Widespread dissemination of the virus is associated with seeding of lymphoid organs and trapping of virus by follicular dendritic cells. Four to eleven days after infection, virus can be detected in the draining internal iliac lymph nodes. Shortly thereafter, systemic dissemination occurs, and HIV-1 can be cultured from plasma five days after infection. High titers of virus are likely to be present in the genital tract during primary infection. After the initial rise in plasma viremia, often to levels in excess of 1 million RNA molecules per milliliter, there is a marked reduction from the peak viremia to a steady-state level of viral replication. The decrease in the viral load during acute HIV-1 infection is probably due to the appearance of HIV-1–specific cytotoxic T lymphocytes. During acute infection, 1 in 17 CD8+ T cells in the peripheral blood may be a cytotoxic T lymphocyte specifically targeted against the virus. This high proportion reflects a vigorous attempt by host cellular immune defenses to contain the massive viral replication. A more broadly directed cytotoxic T-lymphocyte response in the early stages of HIV-1 infection is associated with a subsequently lower viral load and slower progression of disease, suggesting that viremia by this immune response in the early stages of infection may have a clinical benefit. Differences in the virulence of viral strains may modulate a set point. Less virulent strains have attenuated replication, which is associated with lower levels of viremia and slower disease progression. Determining this set point may be related to genetic differences in coreceptors or qualitative differences in the immune response. Studies in animals suggest that lowering the viral load during primary infection results in a lower set point factors.[172]

Neutralizing antibodies are usually detectable weeks to months after the reduction in replicating virus contributing to the second phase, prolonged clinical latency. The initial and ongoing immunologic response to HIV infection is not only unsuccessful in clearing the HIV but is paradoxically paralleled by a progressive reduction in immunocompetence and eventual clinical appearance of the disease. An estimated 10% of patients develop AIDS within 2 to 3 years of exposure to HIV, whereas 10% to 17% of HIV-infected patients may not develop AIDS even 10 years after exposure.[175] Persons with the highest viral loads have the most rapid rates of progression to the acquired immunodeficiency syndrome and death.[172]

Upon initial or acute infection (previously known as "AIDS-related complex" [ARC]), many individuals experience minimal symptoms. An estimated 40% to 90% experience an acute viral syndrome characterized by varying degrees of fever, fatigue, maculopapular rash, headache, lymphadenopathy, pharyngitis, myalgia, arthralgia, GI distress, night sweats, and oral or genital ulcers.[173] However, the symptoms associated with acute HIV-1 infection are often too vague or nonspecific to lead to a diagnosis. Among people enrolled in large epidemiologic studies in Western countries, the median time from infection with HIV to the development of AIDS-related symptoms has been approximately 10 to 12 years in the absence of antiretroviral therapy (ART). This phase is called clinical latency. Researchers have observed a wide variation in disease progression. Approximately 10% of HIV-infected people in these studies have progressed to AIDS within the first 2 to 3 years following infection, while up to 5% of people in the studies have stable CD4+ T cell counts and no symptoms even after 12 or more years. Factors such as age or genetic differences among individuals, the level of virulence of an individual strain of virus, and co-infection with other microbes may influence the rate and severity of disease progression. Drugs that fight the infections associated with AIDS have improved and prolonged the lives of HIV-infected people by preventing or treating conditions such as *Pneumocystis carinii* pneumonia, cytomegalovirus infection, and diseases caused by a number of fungi.[171]

Diagnosis

In April 2013, the US Preventive Services Task Force updated its 2005 guidelines on HIV screening, to recommend that clinicians screen all persons aged 15 to 65 years for HIV infection at least once, regardless of their risk; that younger adolescents and older adults with increased risk also be screened; and that persons with increased risk be screened more frequently (see Table 22-7).[176]

Once screened, it is recognized that the highly infectious phase of acute HIV infection, defined as the interval between the appearance of HIV RNA in plasma and the detection of HIV-1–specific antibodies, contributes disproportionately to HIV transmission.[177] The traditional diagnostic algorithm consists of repeated plasma or serum reactive immunoassay (EIA); followed by a confirmatory Western blot (WB) analysis indirect immunofluorescence assay. This algorithm is highly sensitive and

specific at later stages of infection; however, current laboratory immunoassays (IAs) detect HIV infection earlier than supplemental tests, resulting in reactive IA results and negative supplemental test results very early in the course of HIV infection erroneously interpreted as negative. Furthermore, the algorithm cannot detect acute infections and misclassifies approximately 60% of HIV-2 infections as HIV-1, based on HIV-1 WB results.

To address current testing limitations, the CDC recommends the use of a new diagnostic algorithm (see Figure 22-1).[178] In two screening studies[179,180] for HIV, results yielded 37 and 55 subjects, respectively, who had false-negative results utilizing the traditional algorithm, 32.4% and 55.6% of which were acutely infected. Most laboratories now use either third-generation IAs that detect both immunoglobulin M-class and IgG-class antibodies or fourth-generation combination antigen/antibody IAs that detect both classes of antibody and also p24 antigen (a major core protein of HIV). The p24 antigen can be detected early, before antibody appears, allowing the fourth-generation IAs to identify some HIV infections in the acute phase.

The tests described above require sample transport to centralized laboratory services and a sophisticated referral system. To address this problem, point of care or rapid tests have been developed (see Table 22-8). Results may be obtained in less than an hour, decreasing the numbers of patients lost to follow-up and allowing for a quicker initiation of antiviral therapy. Studies show that those who learn they are HIV positive modify their behavior to reduce the risk of HIV transmission.

The Food and Drug Administration (FDA) has approved a new rapid test for the simultaneous detection of HIV-1 p24 antigen as well as antibodies to both HIV-1 and HIV-2 in human serum, plasma, and venous or fingerstick whole blood specimens. Approved for use as an aid in the diagnosis of HIV-1 and HIV-2 infection, the Alere Determine HIV-1/2 Ag/Ab Combo test is also the first FDA-approved test that independently distinguishes results for HIV-1 p24 antigen and HIV antibodies in a single test. The test is recommended for use by trained professionals in outreach settings to identify HIV-infected individuals who might not be able to be tested in traditional health-care settings.[181]

There are also rapid home-use HIV test kits that do not require sending a sample to a laboratory for analysis currently available. The kits provide test results in 20 to 40 minutes. These in home kits provide opportunities as well as dilemmas including high false-negative rates, results need to be confirmed by a physician, additional costs, and no provisions for psychological support.[182]

Prevention

The first HIV-1 vaccine trial was conducted in 1987, since then, there have since been more than 220 vaccine trials. Recently, only four efficacy studies have been performed. The products have failed to prevent HIV-1 acquisition, delay progression of clinical disease, or reduce HIV viral load among

TABLE 22-7 High-Risk Behaviors for HIV Infection[176]
Injected drugs or steroids or shared equipment (such as needles, syringes, works) with others
Had unprotected vaginal, anal, or oral sex with men who have sex with men, multiple partners, or anonymous partners
Exchanged sex for drugs or money
Been diagnosed with or treated for hepatitis, tuberculosis, or a sexually transmitted disease, like syphilis
Had unprotected sex with anyone who falls into an above category, or with someone whose history is unknown

TABLE 22-8   Currently Available HIV Testing Techniques

Method	Sample	Site	Results
Conventional	Blood	Clinic	<hr-days
Conventional Avioq OraSure	Oral (fluid) swab	Clinic	Days to weeks
Rapid test			
OraQuick Advance HIV 1/2Ab Test	Blood, plasma, oral fluid	Clinic	<20 min
Reveal Rapid HIV ½ Ab Test	Serum, plasma	Clinic	<20 min
Uni-Gold Recombigen HIV Test	Blood, serum, plasma	Clinic	<20 min
Multispot HIV1/HIV2 Rapid Test	Serum, plasma	Clinic	<20 min
INSTI HIV-1 Ab Test	Blood, plasma	Clinic	<20 min
ClearviewHIV1/2 Stat Pak	Blood, serum, plasma	Clinic	<20 min
Clearview Complete HIV 1/2	Blood, serum, plasma	Clinic	<20 min
Calypte	Urine	Clinic	Days to weeks
Home Access HIV1 Test Sys	Blood	Home	3 days
OraQuick In-Home HIV Test	Oral fluid	Home	<20 min

those who seroconverted. Although some of these vaccines were immunogenic, antibodies elicited were not capable of neutralizing genetically diverse circulating HIV strains. One study was halted after the first interim analysis because it failed to achieve its primary end points of preventing HIV-1 infection and/or lowering viral load set point. The evidence from these trials lent support to exploration of a vaccine strategy that may reduce HIV viral load and potentially prolong disease-free survival rather than prevent acquisition. The next generation of vaccines is being screened for their ability to induce IgG antibodies to scaffolded V1V2 of gp120. It is more than likely that an efficacious and durable vaccine will need to elicit a balance of responses and current prime-boost vaccine strategies aim to elicit a combination of B-cell, CD4+, and CD8+ T-cell responses.[183]

Preexposure prophylaxis (PrEP) is a new HIV prevention protocol. PrEP efficacy trials have tested a combination of the ARV drugs TDF and emtricitabine (FTC), taken in a single pill daily for HIV prevention. This combination pill (Truvada®) was approved by the FDA for use as an HIV treatment in 2004 and was approved as PrEP in November 2010 for men who have sex with men. When used consistently, PrEP has been shown to reduce the risk of HIV infection among adults at very high risk for HIV infection through sex, including men who have sex with men and heterosexually active men and women, and most recently, individuals exposed to HIV through injecting drugs. The drug is not intended to be used in isolation, but rather in combination with other HIV prevention methods. If it is used effectively and by persons at very high risk, PrEP may play a role in helping to reduce the number of new HIV infections in the United States.[184–186]

Medical Management

ART for the treatment of HIV infection has improved steadily since the advent of potent combination therapy in 1996. Newer drugs offer new mechanisms of action, improvements in potency and activity even against multidrug-resistant viruses,

dosing convenience, and better tolerability. ART has dramatically reduced HIV-associated morbidity and mortality and has transformed HIV disease into a chronic, manageable condition. In addition, effective treatment of HIV-infected individuals with ART is highly effective at preventing transmission to sexual partners. HIV therapy protocols continue to evolve at a rapid pace. The most current recommendations may be accessed through the AIDS*info* web portal at http://aidsinfo.nih.gov/guidelines.

Current recommendations are that every HIV-infected patient entering into care should have a complete medical history, physical examination, and laboratory evaluation and should be counseled regarding the implications of HIV infection. The goals of the initial evaluation are to confirm the diagnosis of HIV infection, obtain appropriate baseline historical and laboratory data, ensure patient understanding about HIV infection and its transmission, and to initiate care as recommended in HIV primary care guidelines and guidelines for prevention and treatment of HIV-associated opportunistic infections. The initial evaluation also should include introductory discussion on the benefits of ART for the patient's health and to prevent HIV transmission. Baseline information then can be used to define management goals and plans. In the case of previously treated patients who present for an initial evaluation with a new healthcare provider, it is critical to obtain a complete ARV history (including drug-resistance testing results, if available), preferably through the review of past medical records. Newly diagnosed patients should also be asked about any prior use of ARV agents for prevention of HIV infection.[187,188]

The following laboratory tests performed during initial patient visits can be used to stage HIV disease and to assist in the selection of ARV drug regimens: HIV antibody testing, CD4 T-cell count, plasma HIV RNA (viral load), complete blood count, chemistry profile, transaminase levels, blood urea nitrogen, creatinine, urinalysis, serologies for hepatitis A, B, and C viruses; fasting blood glucose and

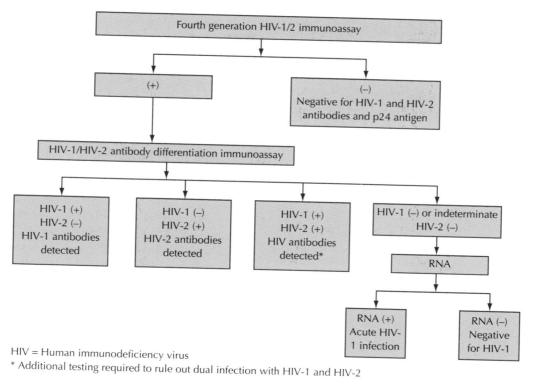

HIV = Human immunodeficiency virus

* Additional testing required to rule out dual infection with HIV-1 and HIV-2

FIGURE 22-1 From Centers for Disease Control. Detection of Acute HIV Infection in Two Evaluations of a New HIV Diagnostic Testing Algorithm — United States, 2011–2013. MMWR Morb Mortal Wkly Rpt 2013;62(24):489-94. Used with permission.

serum lipids; and genotypic resistance testing at entry into care, regardless of whether ART will be initiated immediately. For patients who have HIV RNA levels <500 to 1000 copies/mL, viral amplification for resistance testing may not be always successful.[187]

Genotypic and phenotypic resistance assays are used to assess viral strains and guide treatment strategy selection. Standard assays provide information on resistance to nucleoside reverse transcriptase inhibitors (NRTIs), non-nucleoside reverse transcriptase inhibitors (NNRTIs), and PIs. Testing for integrase and fusion inhibitor (FI) resistance can also be ordered separately from several commercial laboratories. Co-receptor tropism assays should be performed whenever the use of an R5 antagonist is being considered.[187]

Unfortunately, a pool of latently infected CD4 T cells established during the earliest stages of acute HIV infection persist despite prolonged suppression of plasma viremia with ART.[189] Therefore, the primary goals for initiating ART are to reduce HIV-associated morbidity and prolong the duration and quality of survival, restore and preserve immunologic function, maximally and durably suppress plasma HIV viral load, and prevent HIV transmission.

Initiating ART at higher CD4 cell counts may decrease the risk of developing treatment-limiting ARV resistance.[188] ART is now recommended for all HIV-infected individuals to reduce the risk of disease progression, and for the prevention of transmission of HIV, this includes those with early (acute or recent) infection. Early treatment may also decrease

the severity of acute disease and lower the viral set point, which can affect disease progression rates.[190]

More than 20 approved ARV drugs in 6 mechanistic classes are available to design combination regimens. These 6 classes include the NRTIs, NNRTIs, PIs, FIs, R5 antagonists, and integrase strand transfer inhibitors (INSTIs).[191]

NRTIs mimic deoxyribonucleoside triphosphate, the natural substrate for reverse transcriptase. As they become incorporated into the growing DNA chain, they terminate elongation and decrease or prevent HIV replication in infected cells. NRTIs include abacavir (ABC), didanosine (ddI), FTC, lamivudine (3TC), stavudine (d4T), TDF, zalcitabine (ddC), and zidovudine (AZT, ZDV). NNRTIs bind near the catalytic site of reverse transcriptase and inhibit a crucial step in the transcription of the RNA genome into a double-stranded retroviral DNA. NNRTIs include delavirdine (DLV), efavirenz (EFV), etravirine (ETR), nevirapine (NVP), and rilpivirine (RPV). PIs block the cleavage of viral proteins during assembly and maturation, a process essential for the newly formed virus to become infectious. PIs include amprenavir (APV), atazanavir (ATV), darunavir (DRV/r), fosamprenavir (FPV/r), indinavir, lopinavir + ritonavir (LPV/r), nelfinavir (NFV), ritonavir (RTV), saquinavir (SQV, SQV-sge), and tipranavir (TPV). The FI enfuvirtide (T20) is a 36-amino-acid peptide that binds to a region of the envelope gp 41 of HIV-1 that is involved in the fusion of the virus with the membrane of the CD4⁺ host cell to inhibit HIV entry. Maraviroc (MVC) also known as Selzentry acts as an antagonist at the R5 coreceptor to inhibit HIV-1 from entering host cells. It is not effective against a virus that uses the X4 cell coreceptor and has limited effect against HIV that uses both receptors. INSTIs are raltegravir (RAL) and elvitegravir (EVG).[187,191]

An initial ARV regimen generally consists of two NRTIs in combination with an NNRTI, a PI (preferably boosted with RTV), an INSTI, or a CCR5 antagonist (namely MVC). In clinical trials, NNRTI-, PI-, INSTI-, or CCR5 antagonist-based regimens have all resulted in HIV RNA decreases and CD4 cell increases in a large majority of patients. The following are the recommended guidelines for treatment of ARV-naïve patients[187]:

- Efavirenz/tenofovir disoproxil fumarate/emtricitabine (EFV/TDF/FTC)
- Ritonavir-boosted atazanavir + tenofovir disoproxil fumarate/emtricitabine (ATV/r + TDF/FTC)
- Ritonavir-boosted darunavir + tenofovir disoproxil fumarate/emtricitabine (DRV/r + TDF/FTC)
- Raltegravir + tenofovir disoproxil fumarate/emtricitabine (RAL + TDF/FTC)

Alternative and other regimens, to include guidelines for children, older adults, drug abusers and patients with comorbidities, can be found at http://aidsinfo.nih.gov/contentfiles/lvguidelines/adultandadolescentgl.

Oral Health Considerations

Since the initiation of ART, there has been an apparent reduction in the occurrence of some HIV-associated oral lesions among adults and children to include KS, oral hairy leukoplakia (OHL), specific forms of periodontal disease (e.g., linear gingival erythema, necrotizing [ulcerative] gingivitis, necrotizing [ulcerative] periodontitis), and major aphthous ulcers. The occurrence of oropharyngeal candidiasis (OC) has remained stable, whereas the occurrence of oral warts and HIV salivary gland disease appear to have increased.[192–194]

Some patients receiving ART show clinical deterioration despite increased CD4+ T-cell counts[195] and decreased plasma HIV viral loads. This phenomenon has been termed immune restoration disease, immune reconstitution syndrome, or paradoxical reactions, because of clinical deterioration during the apparent recovery of the immune system. Immune reconstitution inflammatory syndrome (IRIS) is another widely used and accepted term because of the role of the host. According to the available literature, about 25% to 35% of HIV-infected patients responding to ART develop IRIS, with the majority of cases occurring within the first 60 days of initiating ART. The increased risk of oral warts that accompanies reductions in viral load may represent a form of IRIS occurring in response to improved cell-mediated immune function.[192,196] The potential increased risk for human papilloma virus–associated oral squamous cell carcinoma in the HIV population should be considered.

For pediatric HIV patients, the most strongly associated oral lesions are candidiasis (e.g., erythematous, pseudomembranous, angular cheilitis), herpes simplex infection, linear gingival erythema, parotid enlargement, and recurrent aphthous stomatitis (e.g., minor, major, herpetiform).[197]

Various topical and systemic antifungal agents exist for the treatment of OC among HIV-infected subjects.[198,199] Fluconazole is the most widely used antifungal agent in the management of OC affecting the HIV patient. Recently, a single-dose regimen of 750 mg fluconazole and in situ fluconazole gel has been shown to be as effective as a standard 14-day regimen in achieving clinical and mycological cure in the treatment for OC in patients with HIV infection.[200,201] Posaconazole is the newest triazole approved for the treatment of acute and/or esophageal candidiasis cases and azole-refractory OC in HIV-infected subjects.[39] Relapse was less common in the posaconazole group. Intravenous anidulafungin, an echinocandin, was shown in a small open-label trial to achieve a high rate of success in the treatment for azole refractory candidiasis; however, this requires intravenous use.[202] The efficacy of treatment with a 14-day course of once daily 50 mg miconazole mucoadhesive buccal tablets was found to be statistically noninferior to 10 mg clotrimazole troches five times a day in a phase-3, multicenter RCT.[199] The safety and efficacy of lemon juice and lemon grass (*Cymbopogon citratus*) was compared with that of 0.5% gentian violet aqueous solution in the treatment for OC in HIV-infected patients in a small study. The lemon juice and lemon grass showed better results than the 0.5% gentian violet aqueous solution in the treatment for OC.[203]

For OHL, topical 25% podophyllin resin, followed by the application of 5% acyclovir cream, showed the same clinical response/recurrence at 12 months posttherapy as podophyllin resin alone[204,205]; however, the addition of acyclovir cream to the regimen resulted in an improved chance of achieving total clinical resolution. Podophyllin-/acyclovir-treated subjects had faster healing and no recurrence compared with 1% penciclovir cream.[194]

Due to the success of ART, most dental consultations for HIV patients are for conventional dental therapy rather than for treatment of oral manifestations HIV.[206] Goals of therapy are to optimize oral hygiene and function, establish a recall schedule, monitor for and manage HIV-associated oral lesions, and monitor for and manage drug-induced oral side effects, such as xerostomia. In a survey of a randomly selected sample of 50 HIV patients at Sandoval STD clinic, 65% admitted to not informing their dentists of their status for fear of rejection or discrimination.[207] Therefore, adherence to standard infection control procedures is warranted on all patients.

Complication rates when performing invasive dental procedures in HIV patients are relatively low (2.2%) and minor in nature. The most common complications observed are infection, prolonged bleeding, and pain.[207] Before initiating therapy, the clinician should ascertain the patient's immune status, presence of comorbidities, current medication profile, and prognosis. In this regard, it may be necessary to obtain permission from the patient to liaise with his or her physician to adequately determine the patient's medical status. The most pertinent criteria related to the provision of oral healthcare are the CD4$^+$ count, HIV viral load, neutrophil count, platelet count, liver function tests (with hepatitis co-infection), and patient's medication profile. The decision to prescribe antimicrobial therapy, either prophylactically or postoperatively, should be based on the patient's overall medical status, such as a risk for subacute bacterial endocarditis or the presence of severe neutropenia.

The most common modes of transmission of HIV infection from patients to health-care worker (HCW) occur after percutaneous (cut injury or needle puncture) as well as mucocutaneous exposure to blood and other body fluids containing blood. A retrospective case-control study found that the risk of infection among HCWs following percutaneous exposure to HIV-infected blood was more likely: (1) in the presence of visible blood on the instrument before injury; (2) if the injury involved a needle, which was placed directly into the patient's vein or artery; (3) if the injury caused by the contaminated instrument or needle was deep; or (4) if the source patient has an increased viral load, that is, was terminally ill.[208] Prospective studies of HCWs estimate that the average risk for HIV infection after percutaneous and mucous membrane (eyes, nose, mouth) exposure to HIV-infected blood is approximately 0.3% and 0.09%, respectively.[209] The transmission of HIV infection after nonintact skin exposure is estimated to be less than the risk following mucous membrane exposure.[210] Similarly, the risk of transmission after exposure to fluids or tissues other than HIV-infected blood is probably considerably lower than the risk following exposure to blood.[209]

HIV PEP call for appropriate initial source patient and exposed provider laboratory testing, procedures for counseling the exposed provider, identifying and having an initial HIV PEP regimen available, and a mechanism for outpatient HCP follow-up. In addition, PEP ARV drugs are now recommended routinely for all occupational exposures to HIV. Examples of recommended PEP regimens include those consisting of a dual NRTI backbone plus an INSTI, a PI (boosted with RTV), or a NNRTI. Other ARV drug combinations may be indicated for specific cases.[211]

As of 2011, in the United States, occupational exposure to HIV was confirmed in 57 HCP and deemed possible in 143 HCP; 6 of whom were dental workers. The last reported documented case of occupational exposure was in 1999, although several cases are in various stages of investigation.[212] Clearly, when adequate infection control precautions are observed, the risk of HIV transmission in the oral health-care setting is extremely low. Data collected on needle stick injuries from the United States may differ from other countries throughout the world. The prevalence of occupationally acquired HIV infection is likely to be underreported in developing countries. This may be due to different infection

control procedures, less common postexposure prophylaxis, and less frequent HIV testing.[213]

Selected Readings

Asselah T, Marcellin P. Long-term results of *treatment with nucleoside and nucleotide analogues (entecavir and tenofovir) for chronic* hepatitis B. Clin Liver Dis. 2013;17(3):445–450.

Baccaglini L, Thongprasom K, Carrozzo M, Bigby M. Urban legends series: lichen planus. Oral Dis. 2013;19(2):128–143.

*Barket S, Coll*ins B, Halusic E, Bilodeau E. A chronic nonhealing gingival mass. Histoplasmosis. J Am Dent Assoc. 2013;144(5):491–494.

Beyrer C, Abdool Karim Q. The changing *epidemiology of HIV in* 2013. Curr Opin HIV AIDS. 2013;8(4):306–310.

Centers for Disease Control and Prevention (CDC). Detection of acute HIV infection in two evaluations of a new H*IV diagnostic testing a*lgorithm—United States, 2011–2013. MMWR Morb Mortal Wkly Rep. 2013;62(24):489–494.

Centers for Disease Control and Prevention (CDC). Testing for HCV *infection: an update of* guidance for clinicians and laboratorians. MMWR Morb Mortal Wkly Rep. 2013;62(18):362–369.

Centers for Disease Control and Prevention (CDC). Trends in tuberculosis—United States, 2012. MMWR Morb Mortal Wkly Rep. 2013;62(11):201–205.

Centers for Disease Control and Prevention (CDC). Update to interim guidance for *preexposure prophylaxis (PrEP) for the preven*tion of HIV infection: PrEP for injecting drug users. MMWR Morb Mortal Wkly Rep. 2013;62(23):463–465.

Centers for Disease Control and Prevention. Aspergillosis. http://www.cdc.gov/fungal/aspergillosis/. Updated May 6, 2013. Accessed December 5, 2013.

Centers for Disease Control and Prevention. Chlamydia Profiles, 2011. *http://www.cdc.gov/std/chlamydia2011/default.ht*m. Updated March 1, 2013. Accessed December 5, 2013.

Centers for Disease Control and Prevention. Crptococcus-neoformans. http://www.cdc.gov/fungal/cryptococcosis-neoformans/. *Updated May 6, 2013. Accessed December* 5, 2013.

Centers for Disease Control and Prevention. Gonorrhea—CDC Fact Sheet. http://www.cdc.gov/std/gonorrhea/STDFact-gonorrhea.htm. Updated February 11, 2013. Accessed December 5, *2013.*

*Centers for Diseas*e Control and Prevention. Gonorrhea. http://www.cdc.gov/std/stats11/gonorrhea.htm. Updated December 13, 2012. Accessed December 5, 2013.

Centers for Disease Control and Prevention. Histoplasmosis. http://www.cdc.gov/fun*gal/histop*lasmosis/. Updated May 6, 2013. Accessed December 5, 2013.

Centers *for Disease Control and Prevention. HIV* in the United States: At a Glance. http://www.cdc.gov/hiv/pdf/statistics_basics_factsheet.pdf. Updated November 2013. Accessed December 4, *2013.*

Centers for Disease Control and Prevention. HIV Surveillance Report. Diagnoses of HIV Infection in the United States and Dependent Areas, 2011 http://www.cdc.gov/hiv/pdf/statistics_*2011_HIV_Su*rveillance_Report_vol_23.pdf#Page=5. Updated July 2013. Accessed November 30, 2013.

Centers for Disease Control and Prevention. Incidence, P*revalence, and* Cost of Sexually Transmitted Infections in the United States. http://www.cdc.gov/std/stats/STI-Estimates-Fact-Sheet-Feb-2013.pdf. Updated February 2013. Accessed December 5, 2013.

Centers for Disease Control and Prevention. Mu*cormycosis. http://www.* cdc.gov/fungal/mucormycosi*s/. Updated May 6, 20*13. Accessed December 5, 2013.

Centers for Disease Control and Prev*ention. Occup*ational HIV Transmission and Prevention Among Health Care Workers. http://www.cdc.gov/hiv/risk/other/occupational.html. Updated August 6, 2013. Accessed November 30, 2013.

Centers for Disease Control and Prevention. Syphilis—CDC Fact Sheet. *http://www.cdc.go*v/std/syphilis/STDFact-Syphilis.htm. Updated February 11, 2013. Accessed December 5, 2013.

Centers for Disease Control a*nd Prevention. T*B Incidence in the United States, 1953–2012. http://www.cdc.gov/tb/stat*istics/tbcase*s.htm. Updated September 16, 2013. Accessed December 5, 2013.

Centers for Disease Control and Prevention. Tuberculosis (TB), Data and Stati*stics. http://www.cdc*.gov/tb/statistics/. Updated September 16, 2013. Accessed December 5, 2013.

Centers for Disease Control and Prevention. Tuberculosis (TB), Testing for TB Infection. http://www.cdc.gov/tb/topic/testing/defau*lt.htm. Updated Septem*ber 6, 2013. Accessed December 5, 2013.

Centers for Disease Control and Prevention. Blastomycosis. http://www.cdc. gov/fungal/blastomycosis/. Updated May 6, 2013. Accessed December 5, 2013.

Centers for Disease Control and Prevention. Chlamydia—CDC Fact Sheet. http://www.cdc.gov/std/chlamydia/STDFact-Chlamydia.htm. Update*d February 11, 2013.* Accessed December 5, 2013.

Department of Health and Human *Services. Pa*nel on Antiretroviral Guidelines for Adults and Adolescents. Guidelines for the Use of Antiretroviral Agents in HIV-1-Infected Adults and Adolescents. http://aidsinfo.nih.gov/contentfiles/lvguidelines/AdultandAdolescentGL.pdf. Updated December 10, 2013. Accessed December 11, 2013.

Food and Drug *Administration.* FDA Approves First Rapid Diagnostic Test to Detect Both HIV-1 Antigen and HIV-1/2 Antibodies. http://www.fda.gov/NewsEvents/Newsroom/PressAnnouncements/ucm364480.htm. Updated August, 2013. *Accessed No*vember 30, 2013.

Food and Drug Administration. FDA approves new treatment for hepatitis C virus. http://www.fda.gov/newsevents/newsroom/pressannouncements/ucm376449.htm. Updated November 26, *2013. Accessed* January 3, 2014.

Food and Drug Administration. FDA Approves Sovaldi for Chronic Hep-at*itis C. http:/*/www.fda.gov/newsevents/newsroom/pressannouncements/ucm377888.htm. Updated December 9, 2013. Accessed January 3, 2014.

Joint United Nati*ons Programme o*n HIV/AIDS (UNAIDS). Global Report—UNAIDS Report on the Global AIDS Epidemic 2013. http://www.unaids.org/en/media/unaids/contentassets/documents/epidemiolog*y/2013/gr2013/UNAIDS_Global_*Report_2013_en.pdf. Accessed December 4, 2013.

Katragkou A, Walsh TJ, Roilides E. Why is mucormycosis more difficult to cure than more common mycoses? Clin Microbiol Infect. 2014;*20*(suppl 6):74–81.

Kew MC. Hepatitis viruses (other than hepatitis B and C viruses) as causes of hepatocellular carcinoma: an update. J Viral Hepat. 2013;20(3):149–157.

Klevens RM, Moorman AC. Hepatitis C virus: an overview for dental health care providers. J Am Dent Assoc. 201*3;144(12):1340–*1347.

Kuhar DT, Henderson DK, Struble KA, et al. Updated US Public Health Service guidelines for the management of occupational exposures to human immuno*deficiency virus and recommenda*tions for postexposure prophylaxis. Infect Control Hosp Ep*idemiol. 2013;34(9):875–892.*

*Liaw YF. Impa*ct of therapy on the long-term outcome of chronic hepatitis B. Clin Liver Dis. 2013;17(3):413–423.

Mohd Hanafiah K, Groeger J, Flaxman AD, Wiersma ST. Global ep*idemi-ology of hepatitis C virus infection: ne*w estimates of age-specific antibody to HCV seroprevalence. Hepatology. 2013;57(4):1333–1342.

Morgan RL, Baack B, Smith BD, et al. Eradication of hepatitis C virus infection and the development of hepatocellular carcinom*a: a meta-analysis of o*bservational studies. Ann Intern Med. 2013;158(5 pt 1):329–337.

Moyer VA; U.S. Preventive Services Task Force. *Screening* for HIV: U.S. Preventive Services Task Force Recommendation Statement. Ann Intern Med. 2013;159(1):51–60.

National Institue of Allergy and Infectious Disease. Tuberculosis (TB). http://www.niaid.nih.gov/topics/*tuberculos*is/Pages/Default.aspx. Updated March 21, 2013. Accessed December 5, 2013.

Pa*tton LL, Ramirez*-Amador V, Anaya-Saavedra G, et al. Urban legends series: oral manifestations of HIV infection. Oral Dis. 2013;19(6):533–550.

Patton LL. Oral lesions associated w*ith human immunod*eficiency virus disease. Dent Clin North Am. 2013;57(4):673–698.

Piot P, Quinn *TC. Response to the AIDS pandemic—a global health model. N* Engl J Med. 2013;368(23):2210–2218.

Radcliffe RA, Bixler D, Moorman A, et al. Hepatitis B virus transmissions associated with a portable dental clinic, West Virginia, 2009. J Am Dent Assoc. 2013;144(10):1110–1118.

Ri*cher SM, Smede*ma ML, Durkin MM, et al. Development of a highly sensitive and specific blastomycosis antibody enzy*me immunoassay using* Blastomyces dermatitidis surface protein BAD-1. Clin Vaccine Immuno*l. 2014;21(2):143–146.*

*Rizzett*o M, Alavian SM. Hepatitis delta: the rediscovery. Clin Liver Dis. 2013;17(3):475–487.

Skiada A, Lanternier F, Groll AH, et al. Diagnosis and treatment of muc*or-mycosis in patients with hematological malignancies: guidelines from the 3rd European Conference* on Infections in Leukemia (ECIL 3). Haematologica. 2013;98(4):492–504.

TB Alliance. MDR-TB/XDR-TB. http://www.tballiance.org/why/mdr-xdr.php. Updated January, 2014. Accessed January 3, 2014.

Tieu HV, Rolland M, Hammer SM, Sobieszczyk ME. Translational res*earch insights f*rom completed HIV vaccine efficacy trials. J Acquir Immune Defic Syndr. 2013;63(suppl 2):S150-S154.

Trembling PM, Tanwar S, Rosenberg WM, Dusheiko GM. Treatment decisions and contemporary *versus pending treatments for* hepatitis C. Nat Rev Gastroenterol Hepatol. 2013;10(12)*:713–728.*

*Ward JW. The epidemiology of chronic hepatitis C and one-time hepatitis C vir*us testing of persons born during 1945 to 1965 in the United States. Clin Liver Dis. 2013;17(1):1–11.

World Health Organization. Global Tuberculosis Report 2013, Executive Summary. http://www.who.int/tb/publications/global_report/gtbr13_executive*_summary.pdf. Updated March* 21, 2013. Accessed December 5, 2013.

Zeng QL, Zhang JY, Zhang Z, et al. Sofosbuvir and ABT-450: terminator of hepatitis C virus? World J Gastroenterol. 2013;19(21):3199–3206.

Zhang X, Gibson B Jr, Daly *TM. Evaluation of commercia*lly available reagents for diagnosis of histoplasmosis infection in immunocompromised patients. J Clin Microbiol. 2013;51(12):4095–*4101.*

Steffen RE, Caetano R, Pinto M, et al. Cost-effectiveness of Quantiferon(R)-TB Gold-in-Tube versus tuberculin skin testing for contact screening and treatment of *latent tuberculosis infection* in Brazil. PLoS One. 2013;8(4):e59546.

World Health Organization. *Multidrug-Resistant Tuberculosis (MDR-TB), October 2013 Update. h*ttp://www.who.int/tb/challenges/mdr/mdr_tb_factsheet.pdf. Updated October, 2013. Accessed January 3, 2014.

For the full reference lists, please go to http://www.pmph-usa.com/Burkets_Oral_Medicine.

CHAPTER 23

Disorders of the Endocrine System and Metabolism

Mark Schifter, BDS, MDSc (Oral Med), M SND, M Oral Med
RCSEd, FFD RCSI (Oral Med), FRACDS (Oral Med)
Mark McLean, BMed, PhD, FRACP
Sunday O. Akintoye, BDS, DDS, MS

INTRODUCTION TO ENDOCRINE DISEASES

Endocrine disorders (endocrinopathies), including obesity and diabetes mellitus (DM), are diseases that affect the endocrine glands and the hormones they produce. The major endocrine glands include the pineal gland, hypothalamus, pituitary gland, thyroid gland, parathyroid gland, gastrointestinal tract, the endocrine pancreas, adrenal glands, and the gonads (ovaries and testes). The term endocrine was coined by Starling, to contrast the actions of hormones secreted internally (hence endocrine) from those that are secreted onto external surfaces (exocrine). Hormones have the ability to induce cellular responses and their regulation of the major physiological processes, of growth, reproduction, metabolism and the maintenance of homeostasis (for example of glucose and calcium). They are among the most abundant and influential chemicals in the human body and in general are secreted by an endocrine gland or group of endocrine cells in one part of the body and then transported by the circulation to their target site of action in another part. Some hormones act only in the region in which they are secreted (termed "paracrine" function).

The release and actions of hormones are controlled by means of feedback processes (Figure 23-1). Therapeutic substitutes for hormones are commonly used as replacements in therapy for endocrine disease.

Hormones

Plasma Transport

Most hormones circulate in association with a serum-binding protein, but only free (unbound) hormones are biologically active. Protein binding buffers against rapid changes in plasma levels of the hormone, and some interactions of binding proteins can regulate hormone action. Many tests of endocrine function measure total, rather than free hormone, making interpretation difficult when the bound proteins are altered by disease or drugs. There are two classes of binding proteins: (1) specific, high-affinity proteins, of limited capacity, which include thyroxine-binding globulin (TBG), cortisol-binding globulin (CBG), sex-hormone-binding globulin (SHBG), and insulin-like growth factor (IGF)-binding proteins (e.g. IGF-BP3); and (2) less specific, low-affinity, transporter proteins, such as prealbumin and albumin.

Mechanisms of Hormone-Receptor Action

The binding of the hormone to its receptor is the first step in a complex cascade of interrelated intracellular events, which eventually lead to the overall effects of that hormone on cell function. The sensitivity and/or the number of hormone receptors can be decreased after prolonged exposure to high or excessive hormone concentrations, with the receptors thus becoming less sensitive (downregulation). The reverse is also true when stimulation is absent or minimal, the receptors increasing in sensitivity and numbers (upregulation).

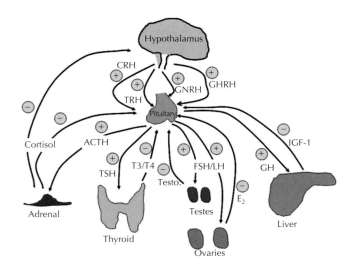

⊕ Stimulatory effect

⊖ Inhibitory effect

FIGURE 23-1   Regulatory loop system. Abbreviations: CRH, corticotropin-releasing hormone; TRH, thyrotropin-releasing hormone; GnRH, gonadotropin-releasing hormone; GHRH, growth-hormone-releasing hormone; ACTH, adrenocorticotropic hormone; TSH, thyroid-stimulating hormone; T3/T4, triiodothyronine/L-thyroxine; FSH, follicle-stimulating hormone; LH, luteinizing hormone; E_2, GH, growth hormone; IGF-1, insulin-like growth factor 1.

Hormone Control and Feedback

Feedback control, either negative or positive, is a fundamental feature of endocrine systems for maintaining hormone levels within a narrow range. This system of one hormone stimulating a second, which, in turn, stimulates a third, and the ability of both the second and the third to feedback on the first, allows for exquisitely sensitive and precise regulation of a hormone within a very narrow physiologic range. It also allows for either positive or negative amplification of any given signal. But, these multilevel positive and negative feedback systems can complicate the understanding of an endocrine pathway and its assessment. Assessing the level of a hormone should be always be done in the larger context of the feedback loop within which it functions. Cortisol (Figure 23-1), for example, which binds to its receptor on cells in the hypothalamus and adenohypophysis, has the effect of inhibiting the secretion of tropic hormones: in this case, CRH (corticotropin releasing hormone) and ACTH (adrenocorticotropic hormone), the hormones responsible for cortisol production and release. Less CRH secretion leads to less ACTH secretion, which leads to less stimulation of cortisol secretion by the adrenal cortex. The value of negative feedback inhibition is that it results in "hormonal homeostasis," with the maintenance of hormone levels within an appropriate physiological range.

Hormonal Rhythms

Circulatory hormonal changes are not only influenced by the feedback mechanisms discussed above but also adapt to environmental changes and fluctuate in response to known but poorly understood biologic rhythms. Seasonal changes, the daily light–dark cycle, sleep, meals, and stress are examples of many environmental events that affect hormonal rhythms. The menstrual cycle is under control of an intrinsic biologic "clock" within the brain that very precisely regulates the timing of pulses of hypothalamic hormones over the 28-day menstrual cycle. In addition, many hormones are under the control of "24-hour clocks." For example, serum cortisol levels peak in the early morning, wane throughout the day, and reach their nadir at night. Recognition and understanding of these rhythms is important for endocrine testing and treatment, so that appropriate hormonal replacement strategies mimic the monthly or diurnal production. For example, replacement cortisol is administered as a larger dose in the morning than in the afternoon. Some endocrine rhythms occur more rapidly, because many peptide hormones are secreted in discrete bursts every few hours. These intermittent pulses of many hormones are required to maintain target organ sensitivity, whereas continuous exposure will cause desensitization.

Furthermore, the levels of one hormone must be interpreted in the context of other hormonal results. For example, the level of PTH, which acts to raise blood calcium levels, must be interpreted in the context of the blood calcium level. A high PTH level may be appropriate in the setting of a low blood calcium level, and, conversely, a low PTH may be appropriate in the setting of a high blood calcium. In conclusion, the interpretation of any given hormone level may be impacted by the developmental stage of the patient, time of day the hormone level is measured, and the point of action of the particular hormone within the feedback loop.

Hormone Measurements and Endocrine Testing

Because the time, day, and condition of measurement will influence hormone levels, so do the method and timing of samples depend on the characteristics of the endocrine system involved, including sex, developmental, and age differences. Hormone levels associated with an endocrine disease or condition may overlap with those in the normal range. Dynamic testing, which includes suppressing or stimulating the level of the hormone, is useful in separating the two groups.

Endocrine Diseases

The most common endocrine disorders after DM and obesity are thyroid disorders (thyrotoxicosis, primary hypothyroidism and goiter), infertility, menstrual disorders such as polycystic ovary disease (PCOS), osteoporosis (especially in post-menopausal women), primary hyperparathyroidism, and disorders in growth and puberty.

Etiology

Syndromes of hormone excess can be caused by neoplastic growth of endocrine cells (e.g., overgrowth of cortisol-producing adrenal cells causing Cushing's syndrome) or autoimmune disorders in which activating antibodies mimic trophic hormones (e.g., Graves' disease of the thyroid gland). Most examples of hormone deficiency can be attributed to glandular destruction caused by infection, inflammation (often immune-mediated), infarction, hemorrhage, tumor infiltration, or replacement and surgery. Autoimmune damage to the thyroid gland (Hashimoto's thyroiditis) and pancreatic islet cells (DM Type 1) are common examples. Common endocrine disorders can be caused by hormone resistance, in which an endocrine gland is resistant to the action of the hormone, usually due to molecular defects in the hormone receptors or molecules in the downstream signaling pathway. These disorders are characterized by defective hormone action, despite the presence of increased hormone levels. The most common acquired form of functional hormone resistance includes insulin resistance seen with Type 2 DM.

Primary and Secondary Endocrine Gland Failure

The pituitary gland orchestrates much of the endocrine system by the release of *trophic hormones*, hormones that promote hypertrophy (and/or hyperplasia) of the tissue being stimulated. Trophic hormones from the anterior pituitary include thyroid-stimulating hormone (TSH or thyrotropin), which stimulates the thyroid gland, and ACTH, which stimulates the adrenal cortex, thus increasing the size and number of cells in each end-organ, respectively. But, excess thyroid-stimulating hormone causes goiter, consisting of hypertrophy with hyperplasia of the cells of the thyroid gland, resulting in palpable or visible enlargement. Importantly, the converse also applies. In pituitary disorders that result in a *lack* of trophic hormone being released, the end-organ atrophies for want of stimulation.

Therefore, in the evaluation and assessment of patients with a suspected endocrinopathy, it is useful to distinguish between "primary" disease of the end-organ gland (e.g., by autoimmune destruction, atrophic change, neoplastic infiltration or replacement, or surgical removal) and "secondary" disorders due to disease of the pituitary gland and the consequent loss of the stimulatory influence of the pituitary-derived trophic hormones downstream. It is useful to consider diseases in the context of the pituitary–end-organ axis. Understanding of the negative feedback system on hormonal control is key to the interpretation of the results of investigations (blood hormone levels) and diagnosing the site of the disease.

Primary hormone deficiency is due to disease in the endocrine end-organ, for example, the thyroid, adrenal glands, or gonads. This will lead to a loss of negative feedback inhibition and consequent elevation in the corresponding anterior pituitary trophic hormone. A patient with atrophic autoimmune thyroiditis (a common cause of hypothyroidism), with consequent immune-mediated destruction of the thyroid glands, will have low levels of circulating T4 and T3, but abnormally high levels of TSH.

Conversely, abnormally high hormone levels due to disease of the primary endocrine gland or excessive exogenous hormone given therapeutically will lead to increased negative feedback and suppression of the corresponding pituitary hormones. The classic example of this is the therapeutic use of exogenous corticosteroids, resulting in decreased ACTH levels. The loss of stimulation by ACTH results in atrophy of the adrenal gland. The atrophied adrenal gland may be able to supply the basal levels of cortisol, but at a time of crisis (e.g., surgical stress) the atrophied adrenal cannot respond and release sufficient cortisol for the body to cope with the crisis. Insufficient cortisol results in inadequate vasoconstriction due to the impaired response by the vasculature to the stimulation by the circulating catecholamines. Cortisol acts to increase vascular sensitivity to epinephrine, resulting in hypotension, potentially leading to circulatory collapse, shock, and even death if not identified and corrected.

Secondary gland failure due to pituitary disease is characterized by low or even "inappropriately" normal levels of the pituitary trophic hormone, despite subnormal end-organ hormone levels. For example, if a patient has low circulating free T3 (fT3) and T4 levels in the context of a low TSH, pituitary disease should be suspected.

Symptoms

As hormones produce widespread and diffuse effects on the body, focal symptoms are uncommon, with many endocrine symptoms diffuse, vague, with a wide range of potential diagnoses (Table 23-1).

Organ specific immune-mediated (autoimmune) disease is common and often associated with stomatognathic manifestations and/or complications. It can affect every major endocrine organ. Characteristic specific antibodies are often present in the patient's serum. Such conditions are more common in women and have a strong genetic component.

Impaired Growth

Multiple hormones and nutritional factors mediate the complex phenomenon of growth. Short stature may be caused by growth hormone (GH) deficiency, hypothyroidism, Cushing's syndrome (excess cortisol), precocious puberty (excess sex steroids), malnutrition or chronic illness, or genetic abnormalities that affect the epiphyseal growth plates. Understanding the interactions of these hormones is essential for proper management of growth abnormalities.

Disturbed Homeostasis

All hormones affect some aspect of homeostasis. For example, thyroid hormone controls approximately 25% of basal metabolism in most tissues; insulin maintains glucose level in the blood; parathyroid hormone (PTH) regulates calcium and phosphorus levels; vasopressin regulates serum osmolality by controlling renal water clearance; and aldosterone controls vascular volume and serum electrolyte (Na+/K+) concentrations.

Infertility and Reproduction

Hormones play a central role in sexual development. Hormones act at different stages throughout life, including gender determination during fetal development, sexual maturation during puberty, conception, contraception, pregnancy,

TABLE 23-1 Diagnosis of Endocrine Disorders		
Gland/Disease	Hormonal Problem	Diagnosis
Adrenal		
Cushing syndrome	Excess cortisol	24 h urinary free cortisol, 1 mg dexamethasone suppression test, midnight serum (or salivary) cortisol
Addison's disease	Low cortisol (and aldosterone)	ACTH stimulation test
Aldosteronism	Excess aldosterone	Plasma renin activity after posture or furosemide test, 24 h urinary aldosterone, saline infusion
Pheochromocytoma	Excess epinephrine and/or norepinephrine	Plasma catecholamines
Thyroid		
Hyperthyroidism	Excess T_4 and/or T_3	Suppressed TSH (most sensitive test)
Hypothyroidism	Low T4 and/or T3	Elevated TSH (most sensitive test)
Gonads		
Male–hypogonadism	Low serum testosterone levels	Low serum free testosterone levels
Male–hypergonadism	Androgen excess	Elevated serum free testosterone (or other androgen) levels
Female–ovarian failure	Loss of ovarian estradiol	Elevated serum gonadotropins (FSH and LH)

lactation, childrearing, and menopause. Many hormones are involved in reproduction, including the pulsatile secretion of estrogen and progesterone from ovaries during the monthly menstrual cycle. During pregnancy, the increased production of prolactin, in combination with placentally derived steroids (estrogen and progesterone), prepares the breast for lactation. The nervous system and oxytocin mediate the suckling response and milk release during breastfeeding.

Hormones as Therapy

Corticosteroid agents are predominantly used in immune-mediated conditions, including those with oral manifestations and complications, such as lichen planus.

Oral Contraceptive Pill

Hormone replacement therapy (HRT), estrogens (as well as progesterone) are used to mitigate post-menopausal signs and symptoms.

Hormonal Therapy in Cancer

Hormonal therapy is one of the major medical modalities used in cancer treatment (others being cytotoxic chemotherapy and biotherapeutics). It entails endocrine manipulation through exogenous administration of specific hormones, particularly steroid hormones, or drugs, that inhibit the production or activity of such hormones (hormone antagonists). Steroid hormones are powerful drivers of gene expression in certain cancer cells, so changing the levels or activity of these hormones can cause related cancers to cease growing, or even undergo cell death.

DIABETES MELLITUS

The term diabetes mellitus (DM) encompasses a group of clinically and genetically heterogeneous metabolic disorders that share a common phenotype, characterized by persistent, abnormally elevated, blood glucose levels (hyperglycemia) with dysregulation of carbohydrate, protein, and lipid metabolism. The primary feature of this disorder is chronic, persistent *hyperglycemia*, resulting from either a defect in the secretion of insulin from the pancreas or resistance to the action of insulin by the body's cells, or both. In essence, DM is disordered glucose homeostasis. Sustained hyperglycemia has been shown to affect almost all tissues in the body and is associated with significant complications of multiple organ systems, including the eyes, nerves, kidneys, and blood vessels. These complications are responsible for the high degree of morbidity and mortality seen in the diabetic population. In the United States (as in other Westernized countries), DM is the leading cause of end-stage renal disease (ESRD); nontraumatic toe, foot, and lower limb amputation; and adult blindness. Clinical presentation of DM covers a wide spectrum from acute onset to asymptomatic cases discovered only during opportunistic screening. The oral healthcare professional is a crucial part of the healthcare team in screening for and monitoring of patients with DM.

Epidemiology

DM, in particular Type 2 DM which accounts for 90-95% of all patients with DM, is now one of the most common noncommunicable diseases worldwide. It is the fourth or fifth leading cause of death in most high-income countries, and substantial evidence exists that it is now becoming epidemic in many low- and middle-income countries. The main risk factor for Type 2 DM is obesity. Obesity is defined as being a condition in which excess body fat has accumulated to the extent that it may have a negative effect on health, leading to reduced life expectancy and/or morbidity. Clinically, it is defined by the body mass index (BMI), a measurement obtained by dividing a person's mass (in kilograms) by the square of the person's height (in meters) that exceeds 30 kg/m^2.[1,2] The usefulness and value of the BMI as a single measure of obesity is contentious, and obesity is usually further evaluated in terms of fat distribution, via the waist–hip ratio.[3]

The global prevalence of DM in 2013 was estimated at 8.3% of adults (382 million people). The prevalence of DM in people between the ages of 60 and 79 is 18.6% representing some 134.6 million people. This accounts for over 35% of all cases of DM in adults, with 6.9% (316 million) having impaired glucose tolerance (prediabetes).[4]

In the United States, for the period 2007–2010, the crude total prevalence of DM was estimated at 11.4%, of the population over 20 years of age. The prevalence is slightly higher for men (13.0%) compared with women (10.1%).[*] It was calculated that 3.3% of the US population had undiagnosed DM, and 12.5% of the total population aged 20 years and above had impaired glycemic control (glycosylated hemoglobin (Hb1Ac) greater than 9%.[5,6] Unfortunately, the incidence of DM rises as the population ages and the prevalence of obesity increases.

Classification

The classification of DM was formerly based on age at onset and type of therapy. The American Diabetes Association has revised the classification, since each type may have an onset at younger or older age and that the classification is now also based on the pathophysiology of DM and not on the basis of the agents used for treatment. Patients with Type 1 DM, previously termed "insulin-dependent DM," and those with Type 2 DM, formerly termed "non–insulin-dependent DM," may take insulin as part of their management. Type 1 DM patients are totally dependent on insulin therapy, whereas Type 2 patients may benefit from insulin therapy, but are not dependent on it for survival.

---

[*] Note: Data obtained by self-report of physician-diagnosed diabetes and excludes women who reported having diabetes during pregnancy.

Other types of DM may occur secondary to genetic disorders, disease, infection and/or injury to the pancreas, and other endocrine diseases. Drug therapy with certain agents, in particular corticosteroids, may also induce DM. Gestational DM occurs during pregnancy and usually resolves after delivery, but it is an established risk factor for the development of DM later in the mother's life.[7]

Hormonal Control of Blood Glucose

In healthy persons, plasma glucose levels are confined to a range of 3.5 – 8.0 mmol/L (63–144 mg/dL), despite physiologic stressors of food, fasting, and exercise. The principal organ of glucose homeostasis is the liver, which absorbs and stores glucose (in the form of glycogen) in the post-absorptive state (after the intake of food) and releases it into the circulation between meals to meet the energy needs (cellular respiration) of the peripheral tissues. The liver is also the site of gluconeogenesis, whereby 3-carbon molecules derived from the breakdown of fat (glycerol), muscle glycogen (lactate), and protein (e.g. alanine) are synthesized into the 6-carbon glucose molecule. About 200 g of glucose is produced and used each day. More than 90% of this is derived from the glycogen stores in the liver and from gluconeogenesis. The remaining 10% is derived from gluconeogenesis undertaken by the kidneys.

The brain is the major consumer of glucose, requiring up to 1 mg/kg bodyweight per min (i.e., 100.8 g daily in a 70-kg man). Glucose uptake by the brain is obligatory and not dependent on insulin, with the glucose used for energy oxidized to form carbon dioxide and water. Other tissues, namely the fat and muscle cells, are facultative consumers of glucose and otherwise rely on fatty acid oxidation for their energy needs. Glucose taken up by muscle cells is stored as glycogen or broken down to lactate, which enters the circulation to become a major substrate for hepatic gluconeogenesis. Glucose is used by fat cells as a source of energy and as a substrate for triglyceride synthesis. Lipolysis is the breakdown of lipids by the hydrolysis of triglycerides into free fatty acids and glycerol. The resulting glycerol also serves as a substrate for hepatic gluconeogenesis.

Insulin

Insulin is the key hormone involved in the storage and controlled release of the energy available from food. Insulin is a peptide hormone, encoded on chromosome 11 and produced by the beta (islet) cells of the endocrine pancreas. After secretion, insulin enters the portal circulation and is transported to the liver. Half of this insulin is degraded by the liver, and the residue is broken down in the kidneys.

Insulin is a major regulator of intermediate metabolism. Although its actions are modified by many other hormones, its importance lies in its differing actions in the fasting and post-prandial states. In the fasting state, insulin functions to regulate the release of glucose by the liver and in the post-prandial state it facilitates the uptake of glucose by fat and muscle. The effect of counter-regulatory hormones (namely glucagon, epinephrine, cortisol, and growth hormone) is to increase release of glucose from the liver and decrease its use by fat and muscle cells. The insulin receptor is a glycoprotein that straddles the cell membrane. When insulin binds with it, the receptor undergoes a conformational change, resulting in the activation of tyrosine kinase and the release of a cascade of intracellular substances. One effect is the migration of the GLUT-4 glucose transporter to the cell surface and the increased intracellular transport of glucose. The insulin-receptor complex is then internalized by the cell, the insulin degraded, and the receptor recycled back into the cell membrane.

Glucagon

Glucagon is a peptide hormone synthesized and secreted from the alpha cells of the islets of Langerhans, which are located in the endocrine portion of the pancreas. Its action is to raise blood glucose levels, so the effect of glucagon is opposite to that of insulin, which lowers blood glucose levels. The pancreas releases glucagon when blood glucose concentrations fall critically low. Glucagon generally elevates blood glucose levels by promoting gluconeogenesis and glycogenolysis in the liver. High blood glucose levels stimulate the release of insulin, which then allows glucose to be taken up and used by insulin-dependent tissues. Thus, glucagon and insulin are part of a feedback system that maintains blood glucose levels at a stable level. Glucagon also regulates the rate of glucose production through lipolysis. Glucagon production appears to be dependent on the central nervous system through pathways yet to be defined.

Pathophysiology of Diabetes Mellitus

The pathophysiology of DM is mediated by alterations of carbohydrate metabolism and insulin action. After a meal, breakdown of carbohydrates leads to hyperglycemia, which stimulates insulin secretion from pancreatic beta cells. Insulin binds to its cellular receptors and facilitates entry of glucose into the cell, resulting in lowered blood glucose and decreased insulin secretion. If insulin production and secretion are altered by disease, glucose entry into cells will be inhibited, resulting in sustained hyperglycemia.

The same effect ensues if insulin is not properly utilized by target cells (insulin resistance). This has potentially serious consequences, as the neurons of the brain rapidly become

---

The pathophysiology of diabetic complications is complex. There is considerable heterogeneity within the diabetic population in regard to the development and progression of diabetic complications. Although poor glycemic control is clearly a major risk factor for complications, not all poorly controlled diabetic patients develop complications. Conversely, some individuals develop complications despite relatively good glycemic control.

starved of the glucose necessary for function. Following meals, the amount of glucose available from carbohydrate breakdown often exceeds cellular demand. The excess glucose is stored in the liver in the form of glycogen. When energy is required, glycogen stores in the liver are converted into glucose via glycogenolysis, elevating blood glucose levels and providing the needed cellular energy source. The liver also produces glucose from fat (fatty acids) and proteins (amino acids) through gluconeogenesis. Glycemia is controlled by a complex interaction between the gastrointestinal tract, the pancreas, and the liver. Multiple hormones also affect glycemia. Insulin is the only hormone that lowers blood glucose levels. Counter-regulatory hormones — glucagon, catecholamines, GH, thyroid hormone, and glucocorticoids — all increase blood glucose levels, in addition to other effects.

Type 1 Diabetes Mellitus

Type 1 DM is characterized by idiopathic autoimmune destruction of pancreatic beta cells, usually leading to absolute insulin deficiency.[5] It comprises 5-10% of DM cases and typically occurs before the age of 25 years in 95% of affected persons, but can occur at any age. It affects both genders equally, and it is more prevalent in Caucasians. The risk of developing Type 1 DM is increased by a family history of Type 1 DM, having gluten enteropathy (celiac disease), or other endocrine diseases.

There are two distinct subclasses of Type 1 DM: (1) the immune-mediated form tends to have a slow onset, with a subclinical prodromal period characterized by cellular-mediated autoimmune destruction of the insulin-producing beta cell in the pancreatic islets. This may be triggered by an environmental event such as a viral infection, but it may be also associated with autoimmune disorders, such as Hashimoto's thyroiditis, Addison's disease, vitiligo, or pernicious anemia. (2) The idiopathic form is acute in onset, not associated with autoantibodies, and the cause of beta cell destruction is unclear. It is prevalent among people of African or Asian origins and has a strong pattern of familial inheritance, but it is not associated with any specific histocompatibility genes.[8]

The risk of Type 1 DM is reflected in the frequency of high-risk human leukocyte antigen (HLA) alleles among certain ethnic groups in different geographic locations. Most Type 1 DM individuals are of normal weight or are thin in build. Since the pancreas no longer produces insulin these individuals are absolutely dependent on exogenously administered insulin for survival. They are highly susceptible to diabetic ketoacidosis, a form of intravascular, extracellular starvation in which glucose is trapped in the circulation and the cells are unable to take it up. To meet cellular energy needs, fat is broken down through lipolysis, releasing glycerol and free fatty acids. Glycerol is converted to glucose for cellular use. Fatty acids are converted to ketones, resulting in increased ketone levels in body fluids and decreased hydrogen ion concentration (pH). Ketones are excreted in the urine, accompanied by large amounts of water. The accumulation of ketones in body fluids, decreased pH, electrolyte loss and dehydration from excessive urination, and alterations in the bicarbonate buffering system result in diabetic ketoacidosis. Untreated diabetic ketoacidosis can result in coma or, eventually, death. Many patients with Type 1 DM are initially diagnosed with the disease following a hospital admission for diabetic ketoacidosis. Periods of stress or infection may precipitate diabetic ketoacidosis. More often, however, diabetic ketoacidosis results from poor daily glycemic control. Patients who remain severely hyperglycemic for several days or longer due to inadequate insulin administration or excessive glucose intake are prone to developing diabetic ketoacidosis.

TYPE 2 Diabetes Mellitus

Type 2 DM is the most common type of DM, comprising 90 to 95% of cases. It is characterized by insulin resistance in the peripheral tissue and/or defective insulin secretion by the pancreatic beta cells.[9] The etiology of Type 2 DM is multifactorial, including genetic predilection, advancing age, obesity, and lack of exercise. About 90% of diabetic Americans have Type 2 DM.[11] It is more prevalent in African Americans, Native Americans, Hispanics, and Pacific Islanders than in Caucasians. Most Type 2 DM patients are overweight, and most are diagnosed as adults. The genetic influence in Type 2 DM is greater than that seen in Type 1 DM. While the concordance rates between monozygous twins for Type 1 DM varies between 30 to 50%, the rate for Type 2 is approximately 90%; however, Type 2 DM has been shown to be associated with a number of genetic defects. The underlying pathophysiologic defect in Type 2 DM does not involve autoimmune beta cell destruction, but rather is characterized by the following three features: (1) peripheral resistance to insulin, especially by the muscle cells; (2) increased production of glucose by the liver; and (3) defective insulin secretion by the beta cells.[6] Increased tissue resistance to insulin generally occurs first, followed by impaired insulin secretion. The pancreas produces insulin, yet insulin resistance prevents its proper use at the cellular level. Glucose cannot enter target cells and accumulates in the bloodstream, resulting in hyperglycemia. The high blood glucose levels often stimulate an increase in insulin production by the pancreas; thus, people with Type 2 DM often have excessive insulin production (hyperinsulinemia). Over several years, pancreatic insulin production usually decreases to below normal levels.

In addition to hyperglycemia, patients with Type 2 DM often have a group of disorders called *metabolic syndrome* that comprises hyperglycemia, hypertension, dyslipidemia, central or abdominal obesity, and atherosclerosis. Despite the strong association of Type 2 DM with genetic factors, the cause of Type 2 DM is considered heterogeneous with environmental and lifestyle factors superimposed on the patients' genetic predilection. Obesity contributes greatly to insulin resistance and may explain its dramatic increase in the incidence of DM in the US and worldwide in the past 10-20 years. The presence of excessive intra-abdominal fat is the factor that conveys the highest risk of Type 2 DM. Other risk factors include advancing age, high caloric intake, sedentary lifestyle, and low birthweight. People with impaired glucose tolerance, impaired fasting glucose, and gestational DM have a high risk of developing Type 2 DM in the future; these conditions are considered its preclinical stages.

Type 2 DM has a slow onset. It may remain undiagnosed for years: some 50% of affected people are unaware of their disease. Unfortunately, the insidious and clinically silent nature of the disease in its early stages results in prolonged periods of hyperglycemia which damage major organ systems. By the time many Type 2 DM patients are diagnosed, complications are already manifest. Although these patients do not require exogenous insulin for survival, insulin injection is often an integral part of medical management. Unlike patients with Type 1 DM, those with Type 2 DM are generally resistant to diabetic ketoacidosis, because their pancreatic insulin production is often sufficient to prevent ketone formation, but severe physiologic stress can still induce diabetic ketoacidosis. Long periods of severe hyperglycemia can result in hyperosmolar nonketotic acidosis. This occurs when hyperglycemia results in the urinary excretion of large amounts of glucose, with attendant water loss. If this fluid is not replaced, dehydration can result in electrolyte imbalance and acidosis.

Other Specific Types of Diabetes Mellitus

Approximately 1 to 2% of DM cases are in this category. It is caused by genetic defects of beta cell function and insulin action; diseases of the exocrine pancreas, endocrinopathies; or pancreatic dysfunction induced by drugs, chemicals, or infections. Other genetic syndromes sometimes associated with DM include Turner's syndrome, Down syndrome, Wolfram syndrome, Klinefelter's syndrome, Friedreich's ataxia, Huntington's chorea, Laurence-Moon-Biedl syndrome, myotonic dystrophy, porphyria, and Prader-Willi syndrome.[10] Thus, the cause of this category of DM is heterogeneous because the abnormal glucose metabolism may be secondary to the precipitating condition, or it may be causal in a manner that remains unclear.

Gestational Diabetes Mellitus

Gestational DM includes the development of Type 1 DM or the discovery of undiagnosed asymptomatic Type 2 DM during pregnancy.[9] It does not include women with DM before pregnancy, which is referred to as pregestational diabetes mellitus. Approximately 2 to 5% of pregnant women in the US develop a mild degree of fasting hyperglycemia or glucose intolerance during the third trimester, which significantly increases perinatal maternal morbidity and mortality. As with Type 2 DM, the pathophysiology of gestational DM is associated with increased insulin resistance. A higher incidence of gestational DM is found in older women, overweight women, and women of specific minority ethnic groups, but older maternal age has the strongest correlation with incidence. Most patients with gestational DM return to a normoglycemic state after parturition; however, some 30 to 50% of women with a history of gestational DM will develop Type 2 DM within 10 years.

Clinical Presentation

Type 1 DM is of sudden onset, whereas Type 2 DM is often present for years without overt signs or symptoms. Patients with undiagnosed DM may present with one or more signs and symptoms of hyperglycemia that include polydipsia, polyphagia, polyuria, and the acute manifestations of hyperglycemia (Table 23-2). Patients may complain of unexplained weight loss, poor wound healing, blurred vision, gingival bleeding, and high susceptibility to infections and may be easily fatigued. When complications of poor glucose control develop, patients complain of visual impairment; neurologic symptoms such as numbness, dizziness, and weakness; chest pain; gastrointestinal symptoms; genitourinary symptoms, especially urinary incontinence; and sexual dysfunction.

Diagnosis and Monitoring of Diabetes Mellitus

The diagnosis of DM is based on specific laboratory findings, as well as the presence of clinical signs and symptoms (Table 23-3). Diagnostic guidelines include testing of the fasting and nonfasting glucose levels, with restricted use of the oral glucose tolerance test (GTT). Diagnosis is not made until the patient has exceeded threshold glucose levels on two separate occasions. Urinary glucose analysis is no longer used for diagnostic purposes.

TABLE 23-2	Signs and Symptoms of Undiagnosed Diabetes Mellitus	
Clinical features	Type 1 diabetes mellitus	Type 2 diabetes mellitus
Polydypsia (excessive thirst)	++	+
Polyuria (excessive urination)	++	+
Polyphagia (excessive hunger)	++	−
Unexplained weight loss	++	+
Weakness, malaise	++	+
Nocturnal enuresis	++	−
Irritability	++	+
Dry mouth	++	+
Chronic skin infections	++	+
Ketoacidosis	++	+
Changes in vision	+	++
Vulvovaginitis or pruritus	+	++
Paresthesia, loss of sensation	+	++
Impotence	+	++
Postural hypotension	+	++
Initially asymptomatic	−	++

++ = more common; + = less common; − = rare

TABLE 23-3 Diagnostic Criteria for Diabetes Mellitus[*][4]

Criterion	Normal	Impaired Fasting Glucose	Diabetes Mellitus
Fasting glucose[**]	< 110 mg/dl	110-126 mg/dl	≥ 126 mg/dl
2-hour post-pandrial plasma glucose	< 140 mg/dl	140-200 mg/dl	≥ 200 mg/dl
OGTT[+] *(not recommended for routine clinical use)*			Plasma glucose at 2 hours ≥ 200 mg/dl

*These criteria should be confirmed by repeat testing on a different day
**Fasting = no caloric intake for at least 8 hours
+OGTT = oral glucose tolerance test performed using an oral load of 75 g anhydrous glucose dissolved in water

Both the fasting and nonfasting plasma glucose tests provide a determination of glucose levels at a single moment in time. It is often useful to assess the long-term control of glycemia, especially in known diabetic patients.

Impaired Glucose Tolerance

Impaired glucose tolerance (IGT) is not a clinical entity or diagnosis, but an accepted, identifiable risk factor for the potential development of DM and cardiovascular disease. It is determined by the GTT, but it is unreliable, as the blood glucose value at the key post two-hour retesting time, is often not reliably reproducible, even in the same test subject. Furthermore, patients determined to have IGT are heterogeneous, some being obese, some have liver impairment or disease, and others taking medication that impairs the performance of the test. Individuals with IGT have the same risk for cardiovascular disease as a patient with frank DM, but they appear to be spared the microvascular complications.

Impaired Fasting Glucose

Impaired fasting glucose (IFG) diagnostic category is not dependent on the glucose tolerance test, but determined by an elevated fasting plasma glucose level of between 5.9 – 6.9 mmol/L, (106 – 124 mg/dL) and yet like the IGT indicates a future risk for the development of DM and/or cardiovascular disease.

Glycosylated Hemoglobin Assay

The glycated or glycosylated hemoglobin assay (Hb1Ac) allows the determination of blood glucose status over the 60 to 90 days before collection of the blood sample. It is now one of the recommended tests for the definitive diagnosis of DM and for screening of individuals suspected to have DM and for population screening. As glucose circulates in the bloodstream, it becomes attached to a portion of the hemoglobin molecule on red blood cells. The higher the plasma glucose levels are over time, the greater is the percentage of hemoglobin that becomes glycated. The American Diabetes

Association recommends that persons with DM attempt to achieve a target Hb1Ac value of less than 7%, whereas an Hb1Ac value of more than 8% suggests that a change in patient management may be needed to improve glycemic control.[5] The Hb1Ac can provide false positive and negative values in rare situations, such as patients with severe iron deficiency and patients with any form of hemoglobinopathy, for example sickle cell disease.

Another assay that can be used to determine long-term glucose control is the fructosamine test. This test is not used as widely as the glycosylated hemoglobin assay but is often helpful in managing women with gestational DM. The fructosamine assay assesses glycemic control over the 2 to 4 weeks preceding the test. The normal range for fructosamine is 200–280 mmol/L (3.6–5 mg/dL). This test may become more widely used in the future since at-home testing is now available.

Patient monitoring, that is, self-testing of blood glucose, has revolutionized the management of DM.[11] The development of small, accurate, handheld glucometers has allowed the diabetic person to take much greater control of the disease. Glucometers use a small drop of capillary blood from a finger-stick sample to assess glucose levels within seconds. Almost all insulin-using patients (and many who are on oral agents) now use glucometers.

Screening

Screening of individuals and populations for Type 2 DM, is recommended, given the large number of persons who are asymptomatic and unaware of their disease, but meet the current criteria for DM. Epidemiologic studies suggest that Type 2 DM may be present for up to a decade before diagnosis. Earlier treatment of Type 2 DM may favorably alter the natural history of DM. The American Diabetes Association recommends screening all individuals >45 years every 3 years and screening individuals at an earlier age if they are overweight (body mass index (BMI) >25 kg/m²) and have one additional risk factor for DM as listed in Table 23-4.

Dental healthcare providers are well placed to undertake screening of their patients for DM. They have the training to recognize systemic diseases like DM from oral manifestations. For many patients who are not on regular medication, the dentist may be the only healthcare professional they see on a regular basis. This strengthens the argument that the dental profession should take on a broader and more active role in screening for DM as well as other common systemic diseases.[12,13,14]

Management of Diabetes Mellitus

Primary treatment goals for DM are to achieve blood glucose levels as close to normal as possible and to prevent diabetic complications.[14] Other goals are to maintain normal growth and development, normal body weight, the avoidance of sustained hyperglycemia or symptomatic hypoglycemia, the prevention of diabetic ketoacidosis and nonketotic acidosis, and the immediate detection and treatment of long-term diabetic complications. Diet, exercise, weight control, and medication are the mainstays of diabetic care. Obesity is very common in Type 2 DM and contributes greatly to insulin resistance. Weight reduction and exercise improve tissue sensitivity to insulin and allow its proper use by target tissues. The principal medication used in Type 1 DM is insulin, on which these patients are dependent for survival.

TABLE 23-4 Risk Factors for Type 2 Diabetes Mellitus

Diabetes-Related Risk Factors

Previously identified with:
- impaired fasting glucose (IFG) or
- impaired glucose tolerance (IGT) or
- an Hb1Ac of 5.7–6.4%

History of gestational diabetes or delivery of a baby >4 kg (9 lb)

Cardiovascular Risk Factors

History of cardiovascular disease
Hypertension (blood pressure ≥140/90 mmHg)
Dyslipidemia
- HDL cholesterol level <35 mg/dL (0.90 mmol/L) and/or a
- triglyceride level >250 mg/dL (2.82 mmol/L)

Conditions/Diseases Associated with the Development of Diabetes

Polycystic ovary syndrome
Acanthosis nigricans

Family History/Lifestyle Risk Factors

Family history of diabetes (i.e., parent or sibling with type 2 diabetes)
Race/ethnicity (e.g., African American, Latino, Native American, Asian American, Pacific Islander)
Obesity (BMI ≥25 kg/m²)
Physical inactivity

Abbreviations: BMI = body mass index; HDL= high-density lipoprotein

Diet

The recommendation of an appropriate, achievable diet, with the involvement of a dietician is essential. The following mix of carbohydrates, fats and protein is recommended: 50–55% carbohydrates; 30% fat and 15% protein as a proportion of the total calories consumed. The diet should favor unrefined carbohydrate rather than simple sugars like sucrose. Foods with a lower glycemic index (GI) are encouraged, as these aid in glycemic control. For patients taking insulin, snacks are required between meals and before retiring to bed at night, to buffer the effect of the injected insulin. The need for patients on insulin to snack needs to be considered in terms of the potential detrimental effects on dental health.

Medications

Drugs used to treat DM lower glucose levels in the blood. With the exceptions of insulin, exenatide, liraglutide, and pramlintide, all are administered orally and are therefore also called *oral hypoglycemic agents* or oral antihyperglycemic agents. There are different classes of anti-diabetic drugs, and their selection depends on the nature of the DM, age, and situation of the person. Type 2 DM persons frequently take oral medications, with metformin considered to be first-line therapy, unless not tolerated or otherwise contraindicated. Many also use insulin to improve glycemic control. Second-line therapy includes the sulfonylureas, thiazolidinediones, dipeptidyl peptidase-IV (DPP-4) inhibitors, glucagon-like polypeptide-1 (GLP-1) agonists, or insulin (Table 23-5a, b).

TABLE 23-5A Drug Therapies Used for Diabetes Mellitus[1,2]

Oral Agents

Insulin Sensitizers

Class	Actions	Generic name	Trade Name(s)[a]	Advantages	Disadvantages/Warnings
Biguanides	↓ hepatic glucose production ↓ intestinal absorption of glucose • improves insulin sensitivity by increasing peripheral glucose uptake and utilization.	metformin	Diabex Fortamet Glucophage Glumetza Riomet	Weight neutral No hypoglycemia	Lactic acidosis with metformin: risk increases with the degree of renal impairment, patient's age, unstable/acute congestive heart failure.
Thiazolidinediones ("glitazones")	↓ tissue sensitivity to insulin ↓ hepatic gluconeogenesis ↓ glucose use ↓ blood glucose levels.	rosiglitazone pioglitazone	Avandia Actos	Lower insulin requirements. No hypoglycemia	May increase risk of congestive heart failure (CHF) and myocardial infarction (MI).

(Continued)

TABLE 23-5A Drug Therapies Used for Diabetes Mellitus[1,2] (*Continued*)

Oral Agents

Insulin Sensitizers

Class	Actions	Generic name	Trade Name(s)[a]	Advantages	Disadvantages/Warnings
Insulin Secretagogues (increase insulin release)					
Sulfonylureas (1st generation)	↓ lowers blood glucose acutely	tolazamide tolbutamide	Tolazamide Orinase	?	Significant adverse side effects (relative to 2nd generation sulfonylureas)
Sulfonylureas (2nd generation)	↑ insulin by stimulating its release from pancreas	gliclazide [b] glimepiride glipizide glyburide	Diamicron [b] Amaryl Glucotrol DiaBeta Glynase	More potent, but less side effects or drug interactions	Hypoglycemia Increased risk of cardiovascular mortality.
Nonsulfonylurea Insulin Secretagogues					
Meglitinides	↓ lowers blood glucose ↑ insulin by stimulating its release from pancreas	nateglinide repaglinide	Starlix Prandin	Acts similar to sulfonylureas but much shorter half-life	Hypoglycemia
Alpha-Glucosidase Inhibitors (have no effect on insulin)					
α-Glucosidase Inhibitors	↓ digestion and ingestion of glucose (in the form of starch) from the GI tract	acarbose miglitol	Precose Glyset	Reduce post-prandial hyperglycemia	Flatulence Inhibits hydrolysis of sucrose to glucose and fructose; use oral glucose (dextrose) instead of sucrose in the treatment of mild-moderate hypoglycemia.
Glycosuric Agents					
Sodium/glucose cotransporter 2 (SGLT2) Inhibitors	↓ reabsorption of renally filtered glucose ↓ lowers the renal threshold for glucose thereby increases urinary glucose excretion ↓ glucose blood levels	canagliflozin dapagliflozin[b]	Invokana Forxiga [b]	Weight reduction Reduced BP	Hypotension Hyperkalemia Genital mycotic infections, urinary tract infections (UTIs), increased urination
Dipeptidyl peptidase-4 inhibitors					
Dipeptidyl peptidase-4 inhibitors	↓ enzymic inactivation of incretin hormones, thereby increasing serum concentrations ↓ fasting and postprandial glucose blood levels	alogliptin linagliptin saxagliptin sitagliptin vildag liptin [b]	Nesina Tradjenta Onglyza Januvia Galvus [b]	No hypoglycemia	angioedema

Notes:

↓ = decreases ; ↑ = increases

[a] Table entry refers to the single agent. Oral anti-diabetic agents are often prescribed and supplied in combination with other anti-diabetic agents.

[b] Not marketed in the United States

XR = extended release; BP = blood pressure; ? = uncertain

TABLE 23-5B Drug Therapies Used for Diabetes Mellitus

Parental Agents

Insulin

Short-acting
Long-acting
Combination (short
  and long acting)
	↑ glucose utilization
	  (and absorption)
	↓ hepatic
	  gluconeogenesis
		Various (see Table 23-6)		Known and
				  predictable safety
				  profile
					Parental: injection
					  needed
					Weight gain (increases
					  hunger)
					Hypoglycemia

Incretin Mimetics

Gastric Inhibitory
Peptide (GLP-1) agonists
	↑ insulin
	↓ glucogon
		Exenatide
		
		Liraglutide
			Bydureon
			(XR)
			Byetta
			
			Victoza
				Slow gastric emptying
				  and so increase
				  satiety leading to
				  weight loss
					Injection
					Hypoglycemia
					Nausea
					Pancreatitis
					? Thyroid carcinoma

Amylin Analogues	• modulation of gastric
	  emptying
	↓ postprandial rise in
	  plasma glucagon
	↑ satiety
		Pramlintide	Symlin	Satiety
				↓ caloric intake
				→ potential weight
				  loss.Regulates food
				  intake
					Parental: injection
					  needed
					Increased risk of
					  insulin-induced
					  severe hypoglycemia
					  (especially in patients
					  with type 1 DM)

Notes:

↓ = decreases; ↑ = increases; →= leads to

a Table entry refers to the single agent.

Oral anti-diabetic agents are often prescribed and supplied in combination with other anti-diabetic agents.

b Not marketed in the United States

XR = extended release

BP = blood pressure

Other Treatments: Interventions for Obesity

Insulin

All patients with Type 1 DM use exogenous insulin, as do many with Type 2 DM. Insulin is taken via subcutaneous injection, most often with a syringe. Insulin infusion pumps deliver insulin through a subcutaneous catheter. Although beef and pork insulin species are still available, most patients currently use recombinant human insulin preparations. Ideally, the use of exogenous insulin provides an insulin profile similar to that seen in a nondiabetic person, with a continuous basal level of insulin augmented by increased availability following each meal. No single insulin preparation can achieve this goal with only one or two injections per day (Table 23-6). Combinations of different insulin preparations taken three or more times daily or the use of a subcutaneous infusion pump more closely approximate the ideal profile, but even with such regimens, blood glucose levels are often unstable.

Human insulin is absorbed slowly, reaching a peak 60–90 min after subcutaneous injection, and its action tends to persist after meals, predisposing patients to hypoglycemia. Absorption is delayed because the soluble insulin is in the form of stable hexamers, with six insulin molecules around a zinc core and it needs to dissociate to monomers, or dimers before it can enter the circulation. Short-acting insulins are used for pre-meal injection in multiple dose

regimens in patients using insulin pumps, in the form of continuous intravenous infusion during childbirth, and for medical emergencies. Short-acting insulin analogues have been engineered to dissociate more rapidly without altering their biological effect. Rapid-acting insulins (insulin lispro, insulin aspart, and insulin glulisine) enter the circulation and also disappear more rapidly than human soluble insulin. Although widely used, the short-acting analogues have little effect on overall glucose control in most patients, because the initially improved postprandial glucose level is balanced by higher levels before the next meal. A Cochrane review has concluded that there is little evidence to support the benefit of rapidly acting insulins in Type 2 DM.

The action of human insulin can be prolonged by the addition of zinc, forming increased numbers of stable hexamers, which then need to dissociate for the insulin to be free and so absorbed, or by the addition of protamine. Protamines are small, arginine-rich, nuclear proteins that replace histones late in the haploid phase of spermatogenesis, and are most readily derived from fish sperm. The most widely used form is NPH (isophane insulin), which is a suspension of crystalline zinc insulin combined with the positively charged polypeptide, protamine. When injected subcutaneously, it has an intermediate duration of action that is longer than that of regular insulin, but shorter than ultralente, glargine or detemir. NPH (isophane insulin) has the advantage that it can be premixed with soluble insulin to form stable mixtures (biphasic insulins), of which the combination of 30% soluble with 70% NPH is most widely used. The intermediate-acting insulins (Lente and Neutral Protamine Hagedorn [NPH]) take several hours after injection to begin having an effect. Peak activity varies among individuals and sites of injection but generally occurs 4 to 10 hours after injection. Thus, a patient who injects intermediate-acting insulin in the early morning will reach peak plasma insulin levels at about lunchtime. Regular insulin is short-acting, with an onset of activity at 30 to 60 minutes after injection and a peak activity at 2 to 3 hours. The rapid-acting insulin (lispro insulin) is rapidly absorbed, becomes active about 15 minutes after injection, and is at peak activity at 30 to 90 minutes. Rapid- and short-acting insulins are usually taken just before or during meals. Thus, regular insulin taken before breakfast will peak at about midmorning; when taken before lunch, it will peak during the midafternoon.

Long-acting analogues have a modified structure in order to delay absorption or to prolong their duration of action. Insulin glargine is soluble in the vial as a slightly acidic (pH 4) solution, but precipitates at subcutaneous pH, to prolong its duration of action. Ultralente insulin is the longest-acting insulin. Commonly called "peakless" insulin, Ultralente has a very slow onset of action, minimal peak activity, and a long duration of action. It is usually taken to mimic the basal metabolic rate of insulin secreted from a normally functioning pancreas. Some examples of common insulin regimens are given in Table 23-7. Insulin detemir has a fatty acid 'tail' which allows it to bind to serum albumin, and its slow dissociation from the bound state prolongs its duration of action. Although widely used, these insulins have little demonstrated advantage over NPH in most clinical situations; however, they are indicated for patients on intensified therapy or with troublesome hypoglycemia.

Insulin - Complications

The most common complication of insulin therapy is hypoglycemia, a potentially life-threatening emergency.[11]

Although, hypoglycemia may occur in patients who are taking oral agents such as sulfonylureas, it is much more common in those who are using insulin. Intensified treatment regimens for DM increase the risk of hypoglycemia. Thus, the long-term benefit of reduced diabetic complications seen with intensive treatment must be weighed against the increased risk of symptomatic low blood glucose. One-third of severe hypoglycemic episodes result in seizure or loss of consciousness and 36% of the episodes occur with no warning symptoms for the diabetic patient. The phenomenon known as "hypoglycemia unawareness" is more common in diabetic patients with good glycemic control than in those with poor control. Hypoglycemia unawareness is characterized by an inability to perceive the warning symptoms of hypoglycemia until the blood glucose drops to very low levels. Signs and symptoms of hypoglycemia are most common when blood glucose levels fall to <60 mg/dL, but they may occur at higher levels in diabetic patients with chronic poor metabolic control.[14] In people with hypoglycemia unawareness, glucose levels can fall to 40 mg/dL or lower before an individual "feels" hypoglycemic.

Emerging Therapies

Pancreas or Beta-Islet Cell Transplantation: an emerging therapeutic option for Type 1 DM is transplantation of the whole pancreas or pancreatic islet cells.[15] Both are still complicated by major side effects and are thereby performed in patients who have already developed significant morbidity from DM.

Complications of Diabetes Mellitus

Life expectancy is considerably reduced in patients with DM. The major causes of death are cardiovascular complications (60–70%), renal failure (10%) and infection(s) (6%). Both the duration and degree of hyperglycemia directly relates to frequency and severity of the complications and morbidity seen in diabetic patients. Better glycemic control reduces the rate and progression of both the nephropathy and retinopathy.

TABLE 23-6 Types of Insulin				
Type	Class	Onset of Activity (h)	Peak Activity (h)	Duration of Activity (h)
Lispro	Rapid acting	0.25	0.5–1.5	<5
Insulin aspart (Novorapid)	Rapid acting	0.25	0.67–1.5	3–5
Insulin glulisine (Apidra)	Rapid Acting	0.2	0.67–1.5	3–5
Regular	Short acting	0.5–1.0	2–3	4–12
Lente	Intermediate acting	3–4	4–12	16–20
NPH	Intermediate acting	2–4	4–10	14–18
Insulin detemir	Long-acting	onset 2 h	no peak	6 to 24
Insulin glargine	Long-acting	onset 2 h	no peak	20 to >24
Ultralente	Long acting	6–10	12–16	20–30

NPH = Neutral Protamine Hagedorn.

TABLE 23-7 Common Insulin Regimens

Insulin(s) Description	Frequency of Injection	Timing of Injection	Characteristics
Intermediate-acting	Single (1x)/daily	Morning - early	• peak insulin activity at midday • can provide enough insulin for mid-day meals only • Hyperglycemia common upon rising, following breakfast and dinner
Mixture of intermediate-acting andregular or rapid-acting	Single (1x)/daily	Morning - early	• peak insulin activity at both midmorning (from regular or lispro insulin) and midday (from intermediate-acting insulin) • can provide enough insulin for breakfast and midday meals • Hyperglycemia common on rising and late afternoon to next morning
Intermediate-acting	Twice (x2)/daily	Prior to breakfast	• peak insulin activity at both midday (from morning injection) and • late evening (from dinner injection)
		Prior to dinner	• can provide enough insulin for lunch and sometimes dinner • prevents early-morning high blood glucose levels • Hyperglycemia common after breakfast and shortly after dinner
Mixture of intermediate-acting andregular or rapid-acting	Twice (x2)/daily	Prior to breakfast	• peak insulin activity after breakfast (from morning regular or lispro insulin), after lunch (from morning intermediate-acting insulin), after dinner (from dinnertime regular or lispro insulin), and late evening or early morning (from dinnertime intermediate-acting insulin)
		Prior to dinner	• can provide enough insulin for all meals • prevents early-morning high blood glucose levels
Regular or rapid-actingand one injection of intermediate-acting	Three (3x)/daily	Prior to each main meal	• peak insulin activity after breakfast, lunch, and dinner (from regular or lispro insulin before each meal) and late evening or early morning (from dinnertime intermediate-acting insulin) • can provide enough insulin for all meal • prevents early-morning high blood glucose levels
	Single (1x/daily)	Bedtime	• provides better glycemic control than once- or twice-daily injection regimens
Ultralente and regular or rapid-acting	Once (morning)	Morning	• peak insulin activity after breakfast, lunch, and dinner (from regular or lispro insulin before each meal) • insulin activity in late evening or early morning (from morning Ultralente insulin)
	Three (3x)/daily	Prior to each main meal	• can provide enough insulin for all meal • prevents early-morning high blood glucose levels • provides better glycemic control than once- or twice-daily injection regimens
Infusion* regular or rapid-acting	Continuous with Bolus (before meals)	See notes	• provides on-demand insulin with meals • Basal metabolic rate most closely mimics normal pancreatic function • often (not always) provides best glycemic control

*Rate set to provide continuous low dose with bolus programmed to be given prior to each meal.

Pathophysiology

Persistent and/or severe hyperglycemia causes a variety of pathologic changes:

- Nonenzymatic glycosylation of proteins: possibly impairing the function of a number of proteins (e.g., hemoglobin, collagen, and tubulin) in peripheral nerves, leading to an accumulation of advanced glycosylated endproducts (AGE's) causing injury and inflammation, via the stimulation of complement and proinflammatory cytokines.
- Polyol pathway: the metabolism of glucose by increased intracellular aldose reductase leads to the accumulation of sorbitol and fructose that causes changes in vascular permeability, cell proliferation, and capillary structure via stimulation of protein kinase C and TGF-β.

It has been hypothesized that all of the above mechanisms stem from a single hyperglycemia-induced process of overproduction of superoxide by the mitochondrial electron chain.

The major cause of the high morbidity and mortality rate associated with DM is a group of microvascular and macrovascular complications affecting multiple organ systems (Table 23-8). People with DM have a greatly increased risk of blindness, kidney failure, myocardial infarction, stroke, the need for limb amputation, and other disorders. These complications are linked to sustained hyperglycemia, which can dramatically alter the function of multiple cell types and their extracellular matrix and thereby cause structural and functional changes in the affected tissues. Other disorders, such as hypertension and dyslipidemia, commonly seen in people with DM increase the risk of microvascular and

TABLE 23-8	Complications of Diabetes Mellitus
System/Organ	**Presentation**
Cardiovascular system	Macrovascular disease (accelerated atherosclerosis) leading to peripheral vascular disease, coronary artery disease and cerebrovascular disease, ischemic ulcers, and gangrenous feet
Nervous system	Sensory: peripheral neuropathy, cranial neuropathy affecting cranial nerves III, IV, VI, VII
	Autonomic: gastroparesis; changes in cardiac rate, rhythm, and dysfunction; postural hypotension; gastrointestinal neuropathy; urinary bladder atony; and impotence
Kidney	Nephropathy, renal failure
Skin and oral mucosa Periodontium	Unusual infections, delayed wound healing Gingivitis and periodontal diseases
Eyes	Retinopathy, cataracts, blindness

macrovascular complications. The vascular complications result from atherosclerosis and microangiopathy. Increased lipid deposition and atheroma formation are seen in the larger blood vessels, along with increased thickness of arterial walls. Proliferation of endothelial cells, alterations in endothelial basement membranes, and changes in the function of endothelial cells induce microvascular damage.

Macrovascular Complications

DM is a risk factor for the development of atherosclerosis. Consequently, occurrence of myocardial infarction is 3–5 times more likely for both diabetic men and women. Also women with DM lose their premenopausal protection from coronary artery disease. Similarly, stroke is two times higher and foot amputation for gangrene is 50 times more likely to occur.

Microvascular Complications

Small blood vessels throughout the body are affected, but the disease process is of particular concern in three sites: retina, renal glomerulus, and nerves (specifically the nerve sheath), the latter resulting in a variety of sensory and autonomic neuropathies.

Infectious Complications

Many common infections in diabetics tend to be more frequent and severe because of DM-associated abnormalities of cell-mediated immunity and impaired polymorphonuclear leucocyte (neutrophil) function. Neutrophil chemotaxis and phagocytosis is diminished, because at high blood glucose concentrations neutrophil superoxide generation is impaired and there is reduced tissue vascularity. Reduced tissue vascularity results in hypoxia and ischemia, which limit neutrophil and antibiotic access. Hyperglycemia also aids in the colonization

and growth of Candida and other fungi and certain bacteria. Conversely, all types of infections may lead to impaired glycemic control and can cause ketoacidosis. Insulin-treated patients need to increase their insulin dose(s) by up to 25% when infection occurs, and non-insulin-dependent diabetics may need insulin during the course of the infection. Distinct rare infections also occur in diabetic populations: malignant, invasive otitis externa, usually secondary to *P. aeruginosa* can lead to osteomyelitis and even meningitis; emphysematous (gas-forming) bacterial infections of the gall bladder and urinary tract; and rhinocerebral mucormyosis.

Stomatognathic Manifestations and Complications of Diabetes Mellitus

The stomatognathic system, comprising the oral cavity, its lining mucosa, the dentition, periodontium and supporting bone, the tempormandibular joints, muscles used in mastication and facial expression, the major and minor salivary glands, and the supporting vasculature, including the lymphatics and nervous system, are all affected in patients with DM. Therefore, oral health professionals have a role in the early recognition of signs and symptoms, diagnosis, and long-term monitoring of DM patients. Dentists also must be prepared to provide surgical treatments for patients with DM that may include the use of general anesthesia (GA). Good oral health, especially the prevention and treatment of infections, such as the various forms of candidiasis, periodontal disease, and odontogenic-related soft tissue infections and cellulitis, is essential for the maintenance of glycemic control and the diabetic patient's overall well-being and health. In the United States, 20% of patients of over 20 years of age in an average dental office have DM, another 20% have undiagnosed DM.[16]

Oral manifestations and complications of DM are related to the impaired immune response. Mycotic (candidiasis) and bacterial infections (periodontal disease) are frequent, severe, and difficult to treat especially in patients with poorly controlled DM. The sensory and autonomic neuropathies characteristic of DM, together with associated impaired renal function, result in dehydration and hyposalivation. The consequences of hyposalivation are increased dental caries, particularly smooth surfaces caries, oral dryness, atrophy of the oral mucosa, and increased frequency and severity in all clinical forms of candida infection. Patients will complain of xerostomia, a subjective feeling of dry mouth (as opposed to hyposalivation). The range of the oral manifestations secondary to DM directly correlates with the degree of glycemic control. Patients who present with any form of candidiasis and/or periodontal disease that is resistant to the usual therapeutic interventions, should be evaluated for DM. Overall glycemic control should be evaluated in patients with established DM. This should include a random (non-fasting) FPG or Hb1Ac. Other oral conditions associated with DM are oral dysesthesia, such as burning mouth syndrome and bilateral sialosis (especially of the parotid glands)

(Figure 23-2), both of which are often related to poor glycemic control.[17,18] Medications taken to control DM and related systemic conditions, such as hypertension, may cause lichenoid drug reactions of the oral mucosa.

According to the World Health Organization (WHO), DM is a stereotypic chronic disease, a permanent disorder that is treatable, but not curable, resulting in residual disability and requiring special training of the patient for rehabilitation. Patients may require a long period of supervision, observation, or care. Chronic diseases have additional characteristics: often preventable, related to life-style factors (diet, exercise, tobacco and alcohol), and inter-related, sharing a common etiology/pathophysiology. Furthermore, DM disproportionally affects the aged and socially/economically disadvantaged and is synergistic with other chronic diseases, including common dental conditions, periodontal disease, and to lesser extent dental caries.

Approach to Dental Care of the Patient with Diabetes

Adults with well-controlled DM have similar risks for oral disease, its progression, and treatment complications as non-diabetic patients. Patients with poor glycemic control are likely to present with more severe, rapidly progressive infections, such as periodontal disease and candidiasis. They also respond poorly to odontogenic-related bacterial infections, involving suppuration, soft tissue collections (of pus), and/or cellulitis spreading to the adjacent soft tissues and tissue spaces (Figures 23-3 and 23-4).

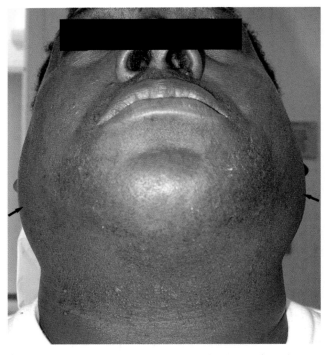

FIGURE 23-2 Bilateral parotid gland enlargement (sialadenitis or sialosis) in a patient with poorly controlled type 2 diabetes mellitus. *Black arrows* point to enlarged parotid glands.

Medical History and Review of Physiological Systems

The focus of a thorough medical history and review of systems is to determine both the severity of the medical condition(s), their stability, and disease control. Stability of DM is the more critical concern. It can be readily assessed by reviewing the patients' ongoing glycemic control, such as their self-assessment of the fasting and nonfasting blood glucose levels using a home glucometer or by arranging Hb1Ac testing. Other important clues to glycemic control are the number and severity of the known complications of DM. For Type 2 diabetic patients, the number of medications they use, recent adjustments in the dose or frequency of their medications, and whether they require insulin as part of their management regimen are also helpful in determining glycemic control. A favourable outcome for dental extractions and surgery within the past 3-6 months indicates the outcome of dental surgery needed in the immediate future.

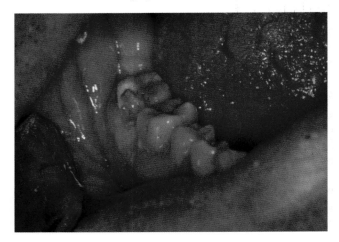

FIGURE 23-3 Advanced periodontal disease and periodontal abscess in the mandibular right first molar that developed in a patient with uncontrolled type 2 diabetes mellitus.

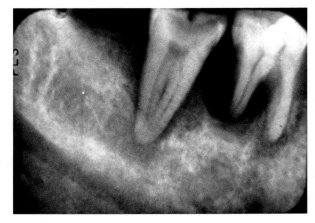

FIGURE 23-4 Periapical radiograph demonstrates extensive bone loss in the mandibular right first molar in the patient with type 2 diabetes illustrated in Figure 23-2. This resulted from a combination of delayed healing, chronic periodontitis, and a protracted periodontal abscess.

The most likely and serious complication is inadvertent hypoglycemia in patients taking their normal medication, especially insulin, but failing to eat, either because of a dental problem associated with discomfort and pain, or the mistaken understanding that they need to fast before a dental procedure. Odontogenic-related infections (periapical periodontitis) that result in either a pus collection in adjacent soft tissue or cellulitis can trigger ketoacidosis. A simple precaution before undertaking invasive dental surgical procedures is to check the patients' blood glucose level. A hypoglycemic patient can be provided with replacement sugar. For a conscious patient, this can be in the form of glucose drink (150 mL carbonated lemonade, two teaspoons of table sugar (sucrose), or preferably glucose (dextrose) in water) followed by a re-checking their blood glucose level.

If a patient exhibits a deteriorating level of consciousness it should be treated as a medical emergency, requiring the prompt institution of first aid including, if necessary, intramuscular administration of glucagon (1 mg/im) (Table 23-9).

Special Considerations and Issues

Burning Mouth

In uncontrolled DM, xerostomia and candidiasis can contribute to the symptoms associated with burning mouth. In addition to treating both conditions, an improvement in glycemic control is essential to alleviate the burning sensations. Treatment guidelines for burning mouth syndrome are well detailed in Chapter 12, Orofacial Pain. Interestingly, amitriptyline, a drug used for burning mouth symptoms, has also been used to treat autonomic neuropathy in DM.[19]

TABLE 23-9	Treatment of Hypoglycemia in the Dental Office
Patient Condition	**Treatment**
Patient is awake and able to take food by mouth	Give 15 g oral carbohydrate 4–6 ounces (125–175 mL) fruit juice or soda (nondiet) 3–4 tsp (equivalent to 15–20 mL) table sugar Hard candy Cake frosting
Patient is unable to take food by mouth and intravenous line is in place	Give 25–30 mL D50 (50% dextrose solution) or 1 mg glucagon
Patient is unable to take food by mouth and intravenous line is not in place	Give 1 mg glucagon subcutaneously or intramuscularly at almost any body site

Infectious Complications

Oral Candidiasis

Candidiasis in in a DM patient is indicative of impaired glycemic control, and the patient's random blood glucose and Hb1Ac should be checked. The treatment of oral fungal infections in DM patients is similar to that for standard patients, except that the topical antifungal medications need to be sugar free. Patients wearing dentures should remove the dentures before going to bed at night. The dentures should be soaked overnight in disinfectants such as dilute sodium hypochlorite solutions, and the tissue-fitting surfaces scrubbed gently to remove any debris. If topical antifungal therapy is not successful within 10 days, systemic antifungal therapy may be required. (See Chapter 5, Red and White Lesions of the Oral Mucosa)

Periodontal Disease

Periodontal disease has been referred to as the sixth sign DM,† and the longer the duration of DM, the greater the likelihood of developing severe periodontal disease.[20,21] Severe periodontitis has also been suggested to be a risk factor for poor glycemic control.[22,23] Since glycemic control is connected to periodontal disease and alveolar bone loss progression,[24] periodontal treatment must be in parallel with DM treatment.[25–26] There is firm evidence of improvement in glycemic control in diabetic patients that receive treatment for their periodontal disease. There is a modest, but significant, improvement in the glycemic control, reflected by 0.4 percentage point reduction of the glycated hemoglobin level. Although this is a modest benefit, it is equal to that of adding one oral hypoglycemic medication.[27] Importantly, this modest benefit in the glycated hemoglobin level, as a result of periodontal therapy, when combined with other interventions, such as diet modification and exercise, may be sufficient to prevent or at least limit the number of medications required for good diabetic control. The evidence in support of improved glycemic control after periodontal treatment is limited, however, because the individual studies lack sufficient statistical power, most of the study participants had poorly controlled Type 2 DM, and there is minimal data from randomized trials on the effects of periodontal treatment in Type 1 DM patients.[28] Primary treatment of periodontal diseases in DM patients is usually nonsurgical, since surgical procedures may require modification of the patient's medications before and after treatment and could result in delayed healing. Periodontal infections may also develop depending on the degree of glycemic control[29]; therefore, antibiotics should be considered.

In controlled clinical trials, a combination of tetracycline or doxycycline with scaling and root planing resulted in

† The classic signs of DM vary in number and order, but are typically described as: (1) polyuria (frequent urination), (2) polydipsia (increased thirst), (3) polyphagia (increased hunger), (4) weight loss, and (5) either disturbed (blurry) vision or peripheral neuropathy.

better periodontal control compared with scaling and root planing alone.[30] Similar results have also been demonstrated in patients who received intrasulcular doxycycline. The mechanism proposed for the additional therapeutic benefit from tetracyclines and doxyclines is that these antibiotics inhibit human matrix metalloproteinases (e.g., collagenase, gelatinase), which are connective tissue–degrading enzymes. For example, a subtherapeutic dose of doxycycline has been shown to inhibit human gingival crevicular fluid collagenase, which significantly eliminated the risk of bacterial resistance.[31] These tetracycline-based drugs can function as inhibitors of bone resorption or bone loss, a property that is independent of their antimicrobial activity.[32]If periodontal surgery is necessary, several factors should be considered depending on the extent of the surgery, anticipated level of postsurgical pain and stress, and level of glycemic control. These include use of antibiotics, nutrition counseling, and changes in DM medications. Supportive periodontal therapy should also be provided at relatively close intervals of 2 to 3 months.

Edentulism

Rate of tooth loss in patients with DM is not only higher compared with nondiabetic patients, but also more rapid, resulting in faster rates of edentulism at a younger age.[33] The main causes of tooth loss are dental caries and periodontal disease, which are exacerbated by the presence of the dental biofilm and dental plaque. It appears that DM per se does not directly contribute to tooth loss, but the combined effects of hyposalivation and peripheral neuropathy that affect manual dexterity are significant contributing factors, because they promote the formation, persistence, and growth of dental plaque. It is also important to note that the same causal lifestyle factors for Type 2 DM—poor levels of health education, personal neglect, and poor lifestyle choices reflected in poor dietary choices—are also contributing factors to dental disease, with poorer levels of oral hygiene seen in this same group of patients.

Dental Implants

DM is not a contraindication for dental implants. Although there is concern that implant survival may be reduced, a long-term cohort study demonstrated that smoking was independently a more significant and adverse factor on implant survival than DM. The study also showed that excellent frequent and regular implant maintenance was a significant factor to ensure and improve long-term implant survival.[34] As in all patients irrespective of DM status, appropriate patient selection and eradication of co-morbidities such as poor oral hygiene, cigarette smoking, and periodontitis are critical to implant success. As dental implant placement is an elective procedure, the best preparation is proper planning by the dentist and the physician responsible for management of the patients' DM.[35] Evidence showing benefits of the use of antibiotics at the time of implant placement for patients with DM is limited.

Dental Treatment Planning Considerations

Well-controlled, stable diabetic patients can undergo all routine dental procedures without modifications to the treatment planning. For protracted dental procedures that involve intravenous sedation or general anaesthesia, adequate planning to address the patients' fasted state and impact of surgical stress on the patients' insulin levels are vital.

Appointment Scheduling

Generally, the best time for dental treatment is either before or after periods of peak insulin activity. This reduces the risk of perioperative hypoglycemic reactions, which occur most often during peak insulin activity. For those who take insulin, the greatest risk of hypoglycemia will therefore occur about 30 to 90 minutes after injecting lispro insulin, 2 to 3 hours after regular insulin, and 4 to 10 hours after NPH or Lente insulin. For those who are taking oral sulfonylureas, peak insulin activity depends on the individual drug taken. Metformin and the thiazolidinediones rarely cause hypoglycemia. The main factors to consider in determining appointment times are the peak action of insulin and the amount of glucose being absorbed from the gut following the last food intake. The greatest risk would occur in a patient who has taken the usual amount of insulin or oral hypoglycemic agent but has reduced or eliminated a meal prior to dental treatment. Patients with poor long-term glycemic control and patients with a history of severe hypoglycemic episodes are at greater risk of future hypoglycemia. Often it may not be possible to plan dental treatment in a way that will avoid peak insulin activity, particularly for patients who take frequent insulin injections because they have greater risks of developing perioperative hypoglycemia. Pretreatment blood glucose level should be measured with a glucometer, and a source of carbohydrates should be available in the dental office. Finally, the dentist must help in modifying a patient's destructive habits, namely, cigarette smoking, poor diet, improper use of DM medications, infrequent glucose monitoring, inadequate visits to physicians, and insufficient oral hygiene and exercise.

Treatment Aims

For patients with suboptimally controlled DM, treatment should be focussed on addressing active infection and likely sources or sites of infection in the immediate future, such as periodontally compromised teeth with questionable prognosis. Odontogenic-related pain should also be aggressively addressed by extraction or root canal therapy (if appropriate) with emphasis on excellent post-operative analgesia through long-acting local anesthetics and opiate-containing analgesics. Elective dental treatment should be delayed until the patient's DM is better controlled. This may require referral of the patient back to the patient's treating physician.

For poorly controlled diabetic patients, only essential treatment should be offered, for example, teeth that are immediate and active sources of infection. This may require aggressive surgical management with drainage of collections in the adjacent soft tissues, and antibiotic coverage. Hospital admission to stabilize the patients' blood glucose levels and manage infection surgically and with intravenous antibiotics may be recommended.

Patients with diabetes must be able to eat and/or drink to replenish their glucose levels. Hypoglycemia occurs more easily and rapidly than hyperglycemia, so is a more critical concern and must be factored into treatment planning. This can be addressed by checking postoperative glucose, providing supplementary glucose in the form of a drink (lemonade, orange juice), ensuring the patient travels home by supervised transport, and that someone can provide home care after discharge.

Because patients with long-standing DM may have developed some degree of autonomic neuropathy with associated orthostatic hypotension, it is vital to raise the patient from the supine to the upright or standing position slowly and carefully.

Drugs Use and Adverse Drug Interactions

Few serious drug interactions exist between agents used for DM control and the drugs commonly used in dentistry and oral medicine. One exception is the interaction between metformin and radiographic iodine contrast, in which case, temporary cessation of the metformin to allow time for the contrast to be administered and the imaging completed is recommended. This may be left to the radiologist to address. Among the anti-infective agents, the azole class of antifungal agents and the NSAIDs can cause hypoglycemia in patients taking sulfonylureas with case reports indicating that topical miconazole can cause serious hypoglycemia. The risk appears hypothetical, with only limited anecdotal information regarding this interaction. The meglitinides (e.g., nateglinide [Starlix] and epaglinide [Prandin]) are cleared by a number of cytochrome enzymes in the liver, so a number of drugs, including the azole antifungals, erythromycin and carbamazepine have the potential to induce hypoglycemia, but again there is limited evidence to support this concern. If these drugs are needed for patients on meglitinides, the prudent course would be to instruct the patient to check blood glucose levels more frequently during treatment (Table 23-10).

Epinephrine (Local Anesthetics)

Under stress, endogenous production of epinephrine and cortisol increases. These hormones can elevate blood glucose levels and interfere with glycemic control. Therefore, during dental treatment, adequate pain control and stress reduction are paramount. Epinephrine is not contraindicated in these patients because it helps promote better dental anesthesia and significantly lowers the amounts of endogenous epinephrine released in response to pain and stress.[42] In a patient with concomitant cardiovascular or renal disease, however, the levels of epinephrine may need to be reduced to two or fewer carpules of local anesthetic containing 1:100,000 epinephrine. Two small-scale studies compared DM patients to controls and found no significant alteration in blood glucose levels after dental treatment that required administration of local anesthetic with epinephrine.[36,37]

Corticosteroids

Topical and systemic corticosteroids have established value in a range of oral dermatoses (see Chapter 3, Pharmacology) because of their physiological actions. Their drug interactions can cause dysregulation of glycemic control. Corticosteroids profoundly affect carbohydrate and lipid metabolism, being designed to protect the glucose-dependant tissues (and their cells), such as the heart (cardiac myocytes) and brain (neurons) from starvation. Corticosteroids increase blood glucose levels by stimulating the liver to form glucose from amino acids and glycerol and to store glucose as glycogen. In the periphery, corticosteroids increase protein breakdown and activate lipolysis. All these contribute to increased blood glucose levels that worsen glycemic control in patients with overt DM and precipitate the onset of hyperglycemias in susceptible patients, potentially leading to frank DM. Corticosteroids should be used with caution in collaboration with the patient's physician. If systemic corticosteroids are required, an adjustment of DM drugs may be necessary. Regular monitoring of glucose levels will be paramount to ensure good glycemic control.

Major Surgery, General Anesthesia, and Hospital Admission

Good glycemic control minimizes the risk of infection and balances the catabolic response to anesthesia and surgery in patients with diabetes.

Type 1 Diabetes Mellitus

Patients with Type 1 DM who are undergoing general anaesthesia (GA) and surgery should receive continuous insulin via intravenous infusion or by subcutaneous administration of a reduced dose of long-acting insulin. Short-acting insulin alone is inappropriate and insufficient. Delay caused by a prolonged surgical procedure or slow postoperative recovery is not uncommon. These may result in periods of insulin deficiency, potentially leading to diabetic ketoacidosis that can be prevented by close monitoring of the patients' blood glucose and maintaining the blood glucose above 4 mmol/l (72 mg/dL). For brief surgical procedures performed under local or regional anesthesia, a reduced dose of subcutaneous long-acting insulin may suffice (30–50% reduction, with short-acting insulin withheld or reduced). This approach facilitates the transition back to long-acting insulin after the procedure. Glucose may be infused to prevent hypoglycemia. The blood glucose should be monitored frequently during the pre-, peri-, and postoperative periods. If the patient is

TABLE 23-10 Diabetic Drug Interactions with Drugs Relevant to Dentistry/Oral Medicine

Insulin Sensitizers

Class	Generic name	Trade Name(s) [a]	Drug Interaction*		Comment
Biguanides	metformin	Diabex Fortamet Glucophage Glumetza Riomet	Iodinated radiographic contrast	S	Recommendation is for temporary discontinuation of metformin

Insulin Secretagogues (increase insulin release)

Class	Generic name	Trade Name(s) [a]	Drug Interaction*		Comment
Sulfonylureas (1st generation)	tolazamide	Tolazamide	Hypoglycemic effects potentiated NSAIDs and miconazole	?	
	tolbutamide	Orinase			See Notes**
	gliclazide [b]	Diamicron [b]			
Sulfonylureas (2nd generation)	glimepiride	Amaryl	Hypoglycemic effects potentiated by NSAIDs, some azoles (miconazole, fluconazole)	?	See Notes**
	glipizide	Glucotrol			
	glyburide	DiaBeta Glynase			

Nonsulfonylurea Insulin Secretagogues

Class	Generic name	Trade Name(s) [a]	Drug Interaction*		Comment
Meglitinides	nateglinide	Starlix	NSAIDs, and CYP2C9 inhibitors: fluconazole, miconazole, may potentiate hypoglycemia	?	
	repaglinide	Prandin	CYP3A4 and/or CYP2C8 inducers: carbamazepine, CYP3A4 inhibitors: erythromycin and OATP1B1 inhibitors: itraconazole, ketoconazole, clarithromycin	?	

Insulin

Class	Generic name	Trade Name(s) [a]	Drug Interaction*		Comment
Short-acting	Various (see Table 23-7)		Epinephrine Corticosteroids	? S	
Long-acting					
Combination (short and long acting)					

Incretin Mimetics

Class	Generic name	Trade Name(s) [a]	Drug Interaction*		Comment
Amylin Analogues	pramlintide	Symlin	Do not administer with agents that alter GI motility (e.g, anticholinergic agents i.e. atropine) and pilocarpine (cholinergic agonists)	S	

* **Corticosteroids all cause loss of glycemic control, but generally not mediated by adverse interaction with drugs used for the management of DM, except for insulin**
S = serious
? = theoretical risk with no or limited case reports documenting an adverse interaction
** Only isolated case reports of severe hypoglycemia with co-administration of miconazole
NSAID's = non-steroid anti-inflammatory drugs; CYP = cytochrome (superfamily of proteins found in hepatocytes and responsible for the metabolism of organic substances); OATP = (organic anion-transporting polypeptide) are membrane transport proteins that mediates the transport of mainly organic anions across cell membranes
[a] Table entry refers to the single agent. Oral anti-diabetic agents are often supplied combined with other agents.
[b] Not marketed in the United States

likely to find alimentation difficult postoperatively, conservative use of insulin, with use of glucose supplied parenterally or in liquid needs to be considered.

Recommendations for Type 1 DM patients undergoing GA and surgery are:

- Long-acting and/or intermediate insulin should be stopped the day before surgery, with soluble insulin substituted.
- Diabetic patients should be first on the morning appointment list.

- Infuse glucose, insulin, and potassium during surgery. The insulin can be mixed into the glucose solution or administered separately by syringe pump. (Standard combination is 16 U of soluble insulin with 10 mmol of KCl in 500 mL of 10% glucose, infused at 100 mL/hour.)

Any other intravenous fluids needed must be given through a separate intravenous line and must not interrupt the glucose/insulin/potassium infusion:

- Postoperatively: the infusion is maintained until the patient is able to eat.
- Glucose levels are checked every 2–4 hours. Potassium levels are monitored and if necessary adjusted by provision of replacement insulin, dextrose and/or potassium.

Type 2 Diabetes Mellitus

Patients with mild hyperglycemia (fasting blood glucose below 8 mmol/L (144 mg/dL)) can be treated as nondiabetics. For patients reliant on oral anti-diabetic agents for management of their DM, they should stop medication two days before the operation. Moreover, these oral agents are of concern if the patient is fasting (in particular the risk of hypoglycemia with sulfonylurea agents).

Those Type 2 diabetics with poorly controlled DM can be managed with an insulin infusion or subcutaneous long-acting insulin (25–50% reduction depending on clinical setting) plus preprandial, short-acting insulin. Oral glucose-lowering agents should be stopped and are of no value in this clinical setting.

Managing the Diabetic Emergency in the Dental Office

The most common emergency related to DM in the dental office is hypoglycemia, a potentially life-threatening situation that must be recognized and treated expeditiously.[50,57,58] Signs and symptoms include confusion, sweating, tremors, agitation, anxiety, dizziness, tingling or numbness, and tachycardia. Severe hypoglycemia may result in seizures or loss of consciousness. Prevention starts with the practitioner being familiar with the general medical risks for hypoglycemic events (Table 23-4) and assessing the patient's risk for developing hypoglycemia (Tables 23-11 and 23-12). Every dental office that treats DM patients should have readily available sources of oral carbohydrates (e.g., fruit juice, nondiet soda, hard candy). As soon as a patient experiences signs or symptoms of possible hypoglycemia, the patient or the dentist should check the blood glucose with a glucometer, which has a typical response time of less than 15 seconds. If a glucometer is unavailable, the condition should be treated presumptively as a hypoglycemic episode. Rapidly absorbed oral carbohydrates are preferable, particularly if the dentist is not trained or adequately equipped to administer intravenous, intramuscular, or subcutaneous glucagon or

dextrose. Following treatment, the signs and symptoms of hypoglycemia should resolve in 10 to 15 min, and the patient should be carefully observed for 30 to 60 min after recovery. A second evaluation with a glucometer should be done to ensure that a normal blood glucose level has been achieved before the patient is released. A medical emergency from hyperglycemia is less likely to occur in the dental office since it develops more slowly than hypoglycemia. Care is initiated by activating the emergency medical system, opening the airway, and administering oxygen. Circulation and vital signs should be maintained and monitored, and the patient should be transported to a hospital as soon as possible. However, under some instances, severe hyperglycemia may present with symptoms mimicking hypoglycemia. If a glucometer is not available, these symptoms must be treated as hypoglycemia, as described above. If it is an actual hyperglycemic event, the small amount of extra glucose delivered will not have any deleterious effect. Emergency measures that will elevate serum glucose should not be delayed or withheld from a DM patient even if hyperglycemia is wrongly suspected in a patient who is actually hypoglycemic. This delay may result in severe adverse outcomes. The best strategy for

TABLE 23-11 Factors that Increase Risk of Hypoglycemia
Skipping or delaying food intake
Injection of too much insulin
Injection of insulin into tissue with high blood flow (eg, injection into thigh after exercise such as running)
Increasing exercise level without adjusting insulin or sulfonylurea dose
Alcohol consumption
Inability to recognize symptoms of hypoglycemia
Anxiety, stress
Denial of warning signs or symptoms
Past history of hypoglycemia
Hypoglycemia unawareness

TABLE 23-12 Determining Risk of Hypoglycemia: Questions for the Dental Patient
1. Have you ever had a severe hypoglycemic reaction?
2. How often do you have hypoglycemic reactions?
3. How well controlled is your diabetes?
4. What diabetic medication(s) do you take? Did you take them today? When did you take them? Is that the same time as usual? How much of each medication did you take? Is this the same amount you normally take?
5. What did you eat today before you came to the dental office? What time did you eat? Is that when you normally eat? Did you eat the same amount you normally eat for that meal? Did you skip a meal?

determining the true nature of a glucose-related emergency is to check the blood glucose level with a glucometer.

ENDOCRINE DISEASES OTHER THAN DIABETES MELLITUS

Pituitary Gland and Hypothalamus

The pituitary gland is a pea-sized structure situated at the base of the brain, within the sella tursica. It plays a key role in the control of the endocrine system and hence has been termed the "conductor of the endocrine orchestra."

Understanding the anatomical relations of the hypothalamus and pituitary is useful in appreciating the clinical signs of pituitary disease, particularly tumors. The optic chiasma is just superior to the pituitary fossa, so any expansile lesion arising from the pituitary or hypothalamus can produce visual field defects. Lateral extension of pituitary lesions may involve the vascular and nervous structures in the cavernous sinus. The pituitary is itself encased in a bony box; therefore any lateral, anterior, or posterior expansion must cause bony erosion that can be seen with appropriate imaging.

Hypothalamus

The hypothalamus contains vital sensors to monitor and control key functions such as appetite, thirst, thermal regulation, the sleeping/waking cycle (circadian rhythm), the menstrual cycle, and the response to stress, exercise, and mood. It serves to integrate the many neural and endocrine inputs to control the release of pituitary hormone-releasing factors. The hypothalamic neurons secrete both pituitary hormone-releasing and pituitary-inhibitory factors (and hormones) via the portal (vein) system, which passes down the stalk into the pituitary.

The Pituitary Gland

The pituitary gland is divided into two anatomically, functionally, and developmentally distinct structures. (1) The anterior pituitary (adenohypophysis): the majority of the anterior pituitary hormones are under predominantly positive control by the hypothalamic-releasing hormones, apart from prolactin, which is under tonic inhibition by dopamine. Therefore, pathologic conditions that interrupt the flow of hormones between the hypothalamus and the pituitary gland result in deficiency of most hormones, but oversecretion of prolactin. The anterior pituitary is a mixture of cells that produce the following hormones: GH, ACTH, thyroid-stimulating hormone (TSH), luteinizing hormone (LH), follicle-stimulating hormone (FSH), and prolactin. ACTH, TSH, FSH, and LH are all intermediaries in their respective endocrine axes; each responds to a specific hypothalamic hormone and, in turn, acts upon an end-organ gland to bring about the endocrine response. There are five major anterior pituitary axes: (1) the gonadotrophin axis, (2) the growth axis, (3) prolactin (lactation) axis, (4) the thyroid axis, and (5) the adrenal axis.

The only established role for prolactin is to initiate and maintain lactation. Prolactin levels are increased during pregnancy, breastfeeding, nipple stimulation, stress, and chest wall injury and by medications with anti-dopaminergic properties (e.g. antipsychotics).

(2) The posterior pituitary (neurohypophysis) is a group of neural cells, an extension of the hypothalamus, that have secretory capacity. The posterior pituitary only secretes two hormones, arginine vasopressin (AVP) also known as antidiuretic hormone (ADH) and oxytocin. Both are nonapeptides (oligopeptides formed from nine amino acids).

The primary physiologic functions of the posterior pituitary hormone oxytocin include contraction of the myoepithelial cells of the alveoli of the mammary gland, which is important during lactation as part of the "let-down response," and contraction of the uterus during childbirth and immediately postpartum. AVP is an important hormone involved in the regulation of water balance (hydration). A decrease in total body water causes high serum sodium (hypernatremia); this increases thirst and the release of AVP from the posterior pituitary, which acts to prevent free water loss from kidneys.

Hormonal Excess

Overgrowth of any of the cell types in the pituitary gland can result in adenomas. Pituitary adenomas are classified on the basis of size and the cells of origin. Lesions smaller than 1 cm are termed microadenomas, and those greater than 1 cm, macroadenomas. Pituitary adenomas can result in increased secretion of the hormone(s) produced by the cells represented in these lesions and/or decreased secretion of other hormones due to compression of other cell types. Symptoms related to the physical enlargement of the adenoma are usually visual impairment or headache. Occasionally, these are detected incidentally as a finding on an MRI or CT scan. Visual impairment is caused by extension of the adenoma in the superior direction, so compressing the optic chiasm. It presents as visual field defects, usually with the loss of peripheral vision, and less often as diminished visual acuity. The course of the visual deficit is usually gradual; many patients are undiagnosed for months or years. Pituitary apoplexy (infarction of the pituitary), on the other hand, has a dramatic manifestation. It presents as a sudden and severe headache, often with diplopia. Apoplexy results from sudden hemorrhage within the tumor. Extension of the tumor inferiorly is rare but can result in cerebrospinal fluid leak through the nose (rhinorrhea) and meningitis. Evaluation of masses within the sella turcica includes anatomic description by MRI and evaluation of the hormonal profile for loss of function. Hormonal assessment of the different axes is described in the relevant sections for each hormone.

Hyperprolactinemia

Hyperprolactinemia can be caused by hyperplasia of the so-called lactotroph cells (prolactinomas) or decreased tonic dopaminergic inhibition of prolactin secretion (e.g., compression by a CNS tumor).[38] Prolactinomas can cause hypogonadism by suppressing gonadotropin secretion. In women, hypogonadism results in low serum estrogen levels that can present as oligomenorrhea, amenorrhea, infertility, and osteoporosis. In men, hypogonadism causes low serum testosterone concentrations that result in decreased libido and energy, decreased facial hair growth, loss of muscle mass, and osteoporosis. Hyperprolactinemia in men may also be associated with impotence even when the serum testosterone concentration is normal. It can cause galactorrhea (leakage of milk from the breast other than during lactation) in women, but this occurs very rarely in men.

Prolactinomas are relatively common, accounting for 30 to 40% of all clinically recognized pituitary adenomas. The diagnosis is made more frequently in women than in men, especially between the ages of 20 and 40 years, presumably because the hyperprolactinemia disrupts their menstrual cycle. However, the adenomas that occur in men are usually larger, due in part to the lack of symptoms or delay in seeking medical attention. Serum prolactin levels in patients with prolactinomas can range from minimally elevated to very high.

Prolactinomas can be treated with dopamine agonists, such as cabergoline or bromocriptine. These drugs have the dual effect of decreasing hormone secretion and tumor size. If the adenoma does not respond to increasing doses of these medications or there is imminent visual loss, transsphenoidal surgery for removal of the tumor indicated.

Growth Hormone Excess

Growth Hormone (GH) is the primary trophic factor responsible for postnatal growth and development. Somatotrophs are the pituitary cells that make GH. GH release is under positive regulation by the hypothalamic peptide GH-releasing hormone. The amount and pattern of GH release changes across the life cycle, with maximal release during the intense growth periods of late childhood and adolescence. Although many cells have GH receptors and may respond to GH, the vast majority of the growth-stimulating effects of GH are mediated by IGF-1. GH is released from the pituitary in a pulsatile fashion, with peak secretion at night. Thus, serum GH values vary considerably over the course of a 24-hour period, so a randomly drawn level may not reliably indicate true GH status. In contrast, IGF-1 serum levels are relatively constant over the course of the day, so an IGF-1 sample for measurement can be taken at any time of the day and is more reliably indicative of the GH status. In normal growth, IGF-1 values also vary considerably across the life cycle, with the highest levels in childhood and low levels in advanced age.

GH excess leads to gigantism if it occurs before the completion of linear growth. The rapid linear growth of gigantism can be distinguished from that of precocious puberty by the fact that the growth occurs in the absence of early secondary sexual characteristics. Indeed, pituitary tumors that lead to GH excess result in the loss of production of other pituitary hormones, such as TSH, FSH, and LH, leading to rapid growth, but without any sexual development. Mild to moderate obesity commonly accompanies the tall stature seen in these patients. Progressive macrocephaly is also seen in children with gigantism and may constitute the presenting complaint, particularly during early childhood.

GH excess results in acromegaly if it occurs after the growth plates have fused. The mean age at diagnosis of acromegaly is usually 40 to 45 years, but because the progression of disease is so slow, the interval from the onset of symptoms until diagnosis can be as much as 12 years. Acral overgrowth is manifested with a classic facial appearance (Figure 23-5), of coarse facies, macrognathia, macroglossia, large diastemas (Figure 23-6), and enlargement of the nose and frontal bones (frontal bossing). Soft tissue edema, due to a direct effect of GH on sodium retention, leads to a "doughy" feel to the hands and feet, as well as an increase in shoe, hat, glove, and ring sizes. Acromegaly has many features, including increased sweating, deepening of the voice due to enlargement of the thyroid cartilage and vocal cords, enlargement of the synovium and cartilages with hypertrophic arthropathy (knees, ankles, hips, spine, and other joints), skin tags, nerve compression (causing paresthesia of the hands, as in carpal tunnel syndrome), enlargement of the soft tissues of the pharynx and larynx (which can lead to obstructive sleep apnea), increased risk of uterine leiomyomata, colonic polyps, and organomegaly (including the thyroid, heart, liver, kidneys, and prostate). Some 50% of patients with GH excess develop hypertension; 10% develop cardiomegaly with heart failure, which accounts for much of the increased mortality associated with acromegaly; and 30% develop insulin resistance or Type 2 DM. Surprisingly, patients seldom independently seek care as the changes are so insidious, but it is often initiated when a relative or friend who has not seen the patient for some time notes the typical changes as described above.

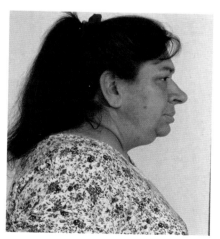

FIGURE 23-5 Characteristic coarse facial features of acromegaly: large, "acral" structures, broad nose, large ears, thickened lips, and slight frontal bossing and large cranium, partially masked by the hair.

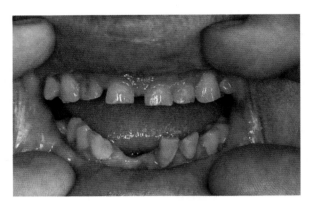

FIGURE 23-6 Dental characteristics of acromegaly (same patient as in Figure 23-5). The maxilla and mandible are enlarged, producing large spaces between the teeth (diastamas). The thrust from the enlarged tongue (macroglossia) caused anterior displacement of incisors.

Diagnosis is confirmed by assessment of serum IGF-1 levels supplemented with dynamic testing by the use of the oral glucose tolerance test. In normal individuals, serum GH concentrations will fall to 1 ng/mL or less within 2 hours after ingestion of 75 g of glucose.

The treatment of choice for patients with a somatotroph adenoma and consequent GH excess is surgical resection via a transsphenoidal approach. Medical therapy consists of somatostatin receptor analogues (octreotide and lantreotide) or use of a GH receptor antagonist, pegvisomant. Somatostatin analogs can inhibit GH secretion and decrease tumor size. External beam irradiation is used in patients whose disease is not controlled by surgery or medical therapy.

Disorders of Antidiuretic Hormone
The Thirst Axis

Thirst and the symptoms of thirst, xerostomia and dehydration, evidenced by hyposalivation and dry oral mucous membranes, are of great relevance to oral healthcare providers. Thirst and water regulation are largely controlled by vasopressin (ADH). ADH is synthesized in the hypothalamus and migrates in neurosecretory granules via axonal pathways to the posterior pituitary. Pituitary diseases that involve the hypothalamus do not lead to ADH deficiency, as the hormone still can "leak," even from the end of a damaged axon.

The kidney, at normal concentrations of ADH, is the predominant site of action of ADH. ADH stimulation of the vasopressin-2 (V2) receptors allows the collecting ducts to become permeable to water, via the migration of aquaporin-2 water channels, resulting in the reabsorption of hypotonic luminal fluid. ADH acts to reduce diuresis (less urine) and results in overall retention of water. At high concentrations ADH can also cause vasoconstriction, via the V1 receptors in the vascular tissue, limiting blood supply to the kidneys and so resulting in a further reduction in diuresis. ADH is regulated by osmoreceptors in the anterior hypothalamus that can sense plasma osmolality. ADH secretion is suppressed at levels below 280 mOsm/kg, thus allowing maximal water diuresis. Above this level, plasma vasopressin increases in direct proportion to plasma osmolality. At the upper limit of normal (295 mOsm/kg) maximum antidiuresis is achieved, with thirst being experienced at about 298 mOsm/kg.

Diabetes Insipidus

Disorders of ADH are in essence disorders of water balance. Too little ADH is termed diabetes insipidus (DI) and is a syndrome characterized by the inability to hold water by the kidneys.[39] It can be caused by inadequate pituitary production of ADH (termed *central DI*), or resistance to the actions of ADH on the kidneys (termed *nephrogenic DI*). DI can also be gestational or present as an iatrogenic artifact of alcohol or some types of drug abuse.

Axis	Replacement Therapy	Comments
Growth	Children: recombinant human GH	• Adults: ? advocated for replacement therapy where rGH has benefits on muscle mass and wellbeing
Thirst	Desmopressin 10–20 µg 1-3x/daily by nasal spray or orally 100–200 µg 3x/daily	• carbamazepine, thiazides and chlorpropamide are very occasionally used in mild DI
Adrenal	Hydrocortisone 15–40 mg daily (Starting dose: 10 mg on rising/5 mg lunchtime/5 mg evening)	• essential • normally no need for mineralocorticoid replacement
Thyroid	Levothyroxine 100–150 µg daily	• essential
Gonadal		
Male	Testosterone imi, orally, transdermally or implant	
Female	estrogen/progestogen (cyclical) orally or as patch	
Fertility	HCG plus FSH (purified or recombinant) orluteinizing hormone (LH) - pulsatile	• to produce testicular development, spermatogenesis or ovulation
Breast (galactorrea → prolactin inhibition)	Dopamine agonist (e.g. cabergoline, 500 µg weekly)	

TABLE 23-13 Replacement Therapies for Hypopituitarism

The primary presenting symptom is polyuria (>3 L/d), and resultant hypernatremia, nocturia, and compensatory polydipsia. Daily urine output may reach as much as 10–15 L, leading to dehydration that may be severe if the thirst mechanism or consciousness are impaired or if the patient is denied fluid. Diagnosis of DI is made by a water deprivation test, which should be done under medical supervision.

Treatment is with synthetic ADH analogue desmopressin, also known as DDAVP (1-desamino-8-*d*-arginine vasopressin, desamino cys-1-*d*-arginine-8 vasopressin), which has the advantages of having a longer duration of action than vasopressin and no vasconstrictive effects. It is most reliably given intranasally as a spray 10–40 μg once or twice daily, but can also be given orally (100–200 μg three times daily or intramuscularly 2–4 μg daily). The response can be variable, and patients must be monitored carefully regarding fluid input/output and with frequent measurement of their plasma osmolality. The main problem is avoiding water overload and consequent hypernatremia. For patients with DI, a reversible underlying cause (e.g. a hypothalamic tumor) should be investigated and, if found, treated.

Of note, DDAVP is also indicated for patients with mild and moderate hemophilia A, von Willebrand's disease, and patients with platelet dysfunction in the setting of uremia or congenital (except in the very rare Glanzmann's thrombasthenia) or drug-induced platelet dysfunction. When given by intravenous infusion DDAVP results in an increase of factor VIII levels, highly suitable for patients undergoing minor surgical procedures, such as dento-alveolar surgery. However it is contraindicated in patients with used in type IIB von Willebrand's disease, since platelet aggregation may be induced.

Other causes of polyuria and polydipsia include DM, hypokalemia, and hypercalcemia and should be excluded. In the case of DM, the cause is an osmotic diuresis secondary to glycosuria, which leads to dehydration and an increased thirst, owing to the hypertonicity of the extracellular fluid.

Syndrome of Inappropriate Antidiuretic Hormone

Excessive ADH (syndrome of inappropriate antidiuretic hormone (SIADH)) is a syndrome of too much total body water, consequent hyponatremia of which the electrolyte disturbance is the main concern and the cause of the presenting clinical features.[40] Major causes of SIADH include central nervous system disturbances such as stroke, infection, trauma, and hemorrhage. Other causes are medications, serious illness (especially in the elderly), and some types of cancer. The clinical presentation tends to be slow, with the patient exhibiting confusion, nausea, irritability, and, later, fits and coma, but with no edema. Mild symptoms usually occur with plasma sodium levels below 125 mmol/L and serious manifestations are likely below 115 mmol/L. The elderly may show symptoms with milder abnormalities. SIADH needs to be differentiated from dilutional hyponatremia due to excess infusion of glucose/water solutions or diuretic administration (thiazides or amiloride). ACTH deficiency can give a biochemical picture very similar to SIADH; therefore, it is necessary to ensure the HPA axis is intact, particularly in neurosurgical patients, in whom ACTH deficiency may be relatively common consequence.

Management entails identifying the underlying cause and correcting this, when possible. Symptomatic relief includes fluid restriction, with an intake of only 500–1000 mL water daily. If complied with, this will usually correct the biochemical abnormalities. Newly available, ADH (V2) antagonists (e.g. tolvaptan) are being used with good effect.

Hypopituitarism

Deficiency of hypothalamic releasing hormones or of the pituitary trophic hormones can be selective or multiple. Selective deficiencies of GH, LH/FSH, ACTH, TSH, and ADH are all seen from a variety of causes. Multiple deficiencies usually result from a tumor. There is generally, a progressive loss of anterior pituitary function, with GH and the gonadotrophins usually being the first trophic hormones affected. Hyperprolactinemia, rather than prolactin deficiency, occurs relatively early, because of loss of tonic inhibitory control by dopamine. TSH and ACTH secretion is usually the last to be affected. Panhypopituitarism refers to deficiency of all anterior pituitary hormones, and it is most commonly caused by pituitary tumors or as a consequence of the surgery or radiotherapy used in the treatment of such tumors. ADH and oxytocin secretion will only be significantly affected if the hypothalamus is involved by a hypothalamic tumor or by suprasellar extension of a pituitary lesion. ADH and oxytocin deficiency is rarely seen with an uncomplicated pituitary adenoma.

In general, the symptoms of deficiency of a pituitary-stimulating hormone are the same as primary deficiency of the peripheral endocrine end-organ.

Treatment entails hormone replacement by synthetic equivalents. Steroid and thyroid hormones are essential for life. Both are given as oral replacement drugs, as in primary thyroid and adrenal deficiency (see Table 23-13).

The Thyroid Axis

Over- or underactivity of the thyroid gland is one of the commonest endocrine disorders. The thyroid gland is found in the neck below the thyroid cartilage, which forms the laryngeal prominence ("Adam's apple"). In a healthy patient the gland is not visible, yet can be palpated as a soft mass. Embryologically, it originates from the base of the tongue and then descends to the middle of the neck. Remnants of functional thyroid tissue can sometimes be found at the base of the tongue (lingual thyroid) and along the line of its embryological descent. The thyroid gland consists of follicles lined by cuboidal epithelioid cells, inside which is the colloid (the iodinated glycoprotein thyroglobulin), synthesized by the follicular cells. Each follicle is surrounded by basement membrane, between the follicles are the parafollicular cells containing the calcitonin-secreting C cells.

The metabolism of virtually all nucleated cells of most tissues is controlled by the thyroid hormones. The thyroid synthesizes two hormones: (1) Triiodothyronine (T3), which is the active hormone that acts at the cellular level and (2) L-thyroxine (T4), which is the prohormone. Iodine is an essential requirement for thyroid hormone synthesis. Inorganic iodide (obtained from dietary sources) is trapped by the gland by an enzyme-dependent system, oxidized, and incorporated into the glycoprotein thyroglobulin to form mono- and diiodotyrosine and then T4 and T3. Globally, dietary iodine deficiency is a major cause of thyroid disease. The recommended daily intake of iodine is at least 140 μg. Dietary supplementation of salt and bread has limited the regions where endemic goiter still occurs, but surprisingly, iodine deficiency is again a concern in Western countries, because adventitious iodine in dairy products is declining, with noniodoform disinfectants used in milk production, and non-iodized rock salt in place of iodized salt in cooking has become popular. In the US, iodine intakes have fallen, and it is uncertain that the iodine status for most pregnant woman is satisfactory, leading to calls for systematic iodine supplementation.[41,42]

Hypothyroidism

Underactivity of the thyroid gland is usually primary, but can be secondary to diseases of the hypothalamic-pituitary axis, resulting in reduced TSH production and/or release. Hypothyroidism is one of the commonest endocrine disorders. Hypothyroidism can be either subclinical, or overt, with one large US population-based survey finding the prevalence of subclinical disease to be 4.3% and that of overt disease 0.3%.[43] The overall UK prevalence for primary hypothyroidism is over 2% in women, but under 0.1% in men. Lifetime prevalence for an individual is higher, perhaps as high as 9% for women and 1% for men, with a mean age at diagnosis around 60 years. The worldwide prevalence of subclinical hypothyroidism varies from 1% to 10%.

TSH levels can usually accurately discriminate between hyperthyroidism, hypothyroidism, and euthyroidism (normal thyroid gland function). Exceptions are hypopituitarism and "sick euthyroid" syndrome when low levels (which normally imply hyperthyroidism) occur in the presence of low or normal T4 and T3 levels. As a single test of thyroid function TSH is sufficiently sensitive in most circumstances, but for an accurate diagnosis of hypothyroidism, TSH plus the serum free T4 levels should be tested. When hyperthyroidism is suspected, the TSH as well as the free T4 and free T3 need to be checked.

Antithyroid antibodies are common and may be destructive or stimulating or both. Destructive antibodies are directed against the microsomes or against the thyroglobulin. The antigen for thyroid microsomal antibodies is the thyroid peroxidase (TPO) enzyme. TPO antibodies are found in up

to 20% of the normal population, especially older women, but only 10–20% of these develop overt hypothyroidism. TSH receptor IgG antibodies (TRAb) typically stimulate, but occasionally block, the receptor.

Primary Hypothyroidism: Etiology

Atrophic (autoimmune) hypothyroidism is the most common cause of hypothyroidism. The pathophysiology involves the development of antithyroid autoantibodies, leading to lymphoid infiltration of the gland and eventual atrophy and fibrosis. It is far more common in women (with a 6:1 female-to-male ratio), and the incidence increases with age. The condition is associated with other autoimmune disease such as pernicious anemia, vitiligo, and other endocrinopathies. Hashimoto's thyroiditis is another form of autoimmune thyroiditis, more common in women and most commonly presenting in late middle age, that produces atrophic changes with regeneration, leading to goiter formation. TPO antibodies are present, often in very high titers (>1000 IU/L), and patients can be hypothyroid or euthyroid, although they may go through an initial toxic phase. Postpartum thyroiditis is usually a transient phenomenon following pregnancy, but such postpartum thyroiditis may be misdiagnosed as postnatal depression, emphasizing the need for thyroid function tests in this context.

Dietary deficiency of iodine is still common and in some areas endemic goiter is still a frequent occurrence. Efforts to prevent deficiency by providing iodine in salt continue worldwide, but often with incomplete success. In India some 500 million have iodine deficiency and about 2 million have cretinism. Cretinism (the preferred term is congenital hypothyroidism) is a condition of severely impaired physical and mental development and growth due to untreated congenital deficiency of the thyroid hormones. The most common cause is maternal hypothyroidism, which occurs as a consequence of dietary deficiency of iodine. It has affected many people worldwide and continues to be a major public health problem in many countries. Iodine deficiency remains the most common preventable cause of intellectual impairment and disability worldwide.[44]

Hypothyroidism may also result from the loss of the TSH-producing cells of the pituitary gland (secondary hypothyroidism). Although less common, it can be caused indirectly by a large, nonfunctioning pituitary adenoma.

Clinical Features

Hypothyroidism produces many symptoms. The alternative term *myxoedema* refers to the accumulation of mucopolysaccharide in the subcutaneous tissues. The hypothyroid patient is the mirror image of the hyperthyroid patient.[73] Patients are chronically fatigued, cold when others are comfortable, gaining weight without eating more, constipated, and bradycardic, with slowed reflexes. A slowed relaxation phase of the Achilles tendon reflex is an accurate physical sign of hypothyroidism. Milder symptoms are, however, more common and difficult to distinguish from other causes of nonspecific tiredness. Many cases are detected through biochemical screening.

Treatment

Treatment is simple: lifetime, replacement therapy with levothyroxine (T4), 100-150 µg given as a single daily dose. The starting dose will depend upon the severity of the deficiency and the age and fitness of the patient, especially cardiac performance. 100 µg/daily is the usual starting dose for the young and fit, 50 µg (increasing to 100 µg after 2–4 weeks) for the small, old, or frail. Patients with ischemic heart disease require even lower initial doses, with only 25 µg/daily given, especially if the hypothyroidism is severe and longstanding. The aim is to restore T4 and TSH to within the normal ranges. Complete suppression of TSH should be avoided because of the risk of atrial fibrillation and osteoporosis. Annual monitoring of thyroid function is mandated.

Myxoedema

Severe hypothyroidism, especially in the elderly, may present with mental confusion or even coma. Myxoedema coma is fortunately very rare. Hypothermia is often present, and the patient may have severe cardiac failure, pericardial effusions, hypoventilation, hypoglycemia, and hyponatremia. The mortality was previously at least 50%, and patients require intensive care. Optimal treatment is controversial, but the current recommendation is for T3 to be given orally or intravenously, initially in doses of 2.5–5 µg every 8 hours, then increased, but titrated to the patients' cardiac status.

Depression is common with hypothyroidism. Rarely, with severe hypothyroidism in the elderly, the patient may become frankly demented or psychotic, so-called "myxoedema madness" with such patients presenting with impressive delusions.

Hyperthyroidism

Hyperthyroidism is common, affecting perhaps 2–5% of women, most frequently between the ages of 20 and 40 years, with a sex ratio of 5 to 1 (women to men). Nearly all cases (>99%) are caused by intrinsic thyroid disease. Pituitary causes of hyperthyroidism are extremely rare.

Graves' disease is the most common cause of hyperthyroidism. Graves' disease is an autoimmune process wherein IgG antibodies to the TSH receptor (TSHR-Ab) bind to the TSH receptors in the thyroid gland, stimulating thyroid hormone production by mimicking the actions of TSH. These TSH receptor antibodies are specific and pathogenic for Graves' disease. Persistent high levels predict relapse if treatment is incomplete. There is an association with HLA-B8, DR3, and DR2 and a 40% concordance rate among monozygotic twins with a 5% concordance rate in dizygotic twins.

Clinical Features

Thyroid Eye Disease (Ophthalmic Graves' Disease). The eye signs, of lid lag and "stare" may occur with all forms of hyperthyroidism. (Figure 23-7). The clinical appearances are characteristic, but thyroid eye disease demonstrates a wide range of severity. A high proportion of people with Graves' disease notice some soreness, painful watering, or prominence of the eyes; and the "stare" of lid retraction is relatively common. Visual impairment due to optic nerve compression is relatively uncommon. The ocular manifestations of Graves' disease are due to specific immune response that causes retro-orbital inflammation. Swelling and edema of the extraocular muscles lead to limitations in eye movement and to proptosis, which is usually bilateral. Ultimately, increased pressure on the optic nerve may cause optic atrophy. Histology of the extraocular muscles shows focal edema and glycosaminoglycan deposition followed by fibrosis. Eye disease is a manifestation of Graves' disease and can occur in hyperthyroid, euthyroid, or hypothyroid patients. Thyroid dysfunction and ocular disease usually occur within two years of each other's presentation. TSH receptor antibodies are almost invariably found in the serum, but their role in the pathogenesis of the eye disease is yet to be fully elucidated. Sight is threatened in only 5–10% of cases, but the discomfort and cosmetic problems can cause great deal of patient anxiety.

Other Clinical Features

Graves' dermopathy is rare, presenting as pretibial myxoedema due to the infiltration of the skin on the shin. Thyroid acropachy is very rare and consists of clubbing, swollen fingers, and new periosteal bone formation. In the elderly, a frequent presentation is with atrial fibrillation, other tachycardias, and/or heart failure, often with few other signs. Thyroid function tests are mandatory in any patient with atrial fibrillation. Children frequently present with excessive stature or excessive growth velocity, or with behavioral problems like hyperactivity.

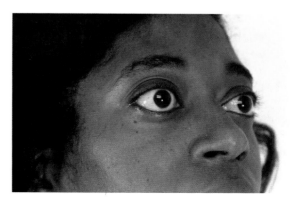

FIGURE 23-7 This patient has the 'stare' and proptosis commonly seen in Graves' disease.

Thyroid Crisis or "Thyroid Storm". This is rare, but can have a mortality rate as high as 10%. The patient presents with rapid deterioration, accompanied by hyperpyrexia, severe tachycardia, extreme restlessness, cardiac failure, and liver dysfunction. It is usually precipitated by stress, infection, following thyroidectomy in an underprepared patient, or after treatment with radioiodine therapy. The control of the cardiac failure and tachycardia is urgent and essential. Propranolol needs to be commenced promptly, together with potassium iodide, antithyroid drugs, corticosteroids (which suppress many of the manifestations of hyperthyroidism), and full supportive measures.

Investigations

Investigations entail measurement of the serum TSH, which is suppressed in hyperthyroidism (< 0.05 mU/L), except for the very rare instances of TSH hypersecretion. A raised free T4 or T3 confirms the diagnosis. TPO and thyroglobulin antibodies are present in most cases of Graves' disease. TSHR-Abs are not routinely measured, but are commonly present. The thyroid-stimulating immunoglobulin (TSI) and TSH-binding inhibitory immunoglobulin (TBII) are also usually positive in Graves' disease.

Treatment

Treatment can be either (1) medical, with the use of antithyroid drugs, (2) by means of radioiodine therapy, or (3) surgical (thyroidectomy). Medical therapy with carbimazole or thiamazole (methimazole), the active metabolite of carbimazole, is more commonly used in the US, and these drugs also have the benefit of modest immunosuppressive activity. Propylthiouracil (PTU) is more commonly used in the UK and Europe. All three agents inhibit the formation of thyroid hormones. The major and concerning adverse effect of drug therapy is agranulocytosis, which occurs in approximately 1 in 1000 patients, usually within 3 months of treatment. In light of this, for patients using these drugs and presenting an unexplained fever or for invasive dental treatment, a full blood count to exclude agranulocytosis is mandated. Radioactive iodine (RAI) can be given to patients of all ages, although it is contraindicated in pregnancy and while breastfeeding. Thyroidectomy is best undertaken only when the patient is rendered euthyroid.

Long-term follow-up studies of hyperthyroidism show a slight increase in overall mortality, which affects all age groups and tends to occur in the first year after diagnosis, regardless of the form of treatment for the hyperthyroidism. People with persistently suppressed TSH levels have an increased likelihood of developing atrial fibrillation and consequently thromboembolic disease; therefore regular cardiac monitoring is recommended, particularly in the first year following a finding of hyperthyroidism. Hyperthyroidism can also lead to a thyrotoxic cardiomyopathy, with measurable ischemic changes on 12-lead ECG, but these can be reversed after the patient is rendered euthyroid.

Stomatognathic Manifestations of Thyroid Gland Disorders
Goiter (Thyroid Enlargement)

Clinical assessment of the thyroid gland, especially of patients with goiter or masses of the thyroid (nodules or tumors) should be a routine part of the comprehensive assessment of oral, facial, and neck structures. Goiter is more common in women than in men and may be either physiological or pathological and present in up to 9% of the population. Most commonly goiter is noticed as a cosmetic defect by the patient or by friends or relatives. The majority are painless, but pain or discomfort can occur in acute varieties. Large goiters can produce dysphagia and difficulty in breathing, from esophageal or tracheal compression. Small goiters are more readily detected visibly (on swallowing) than by palpation.

As part of a routine head and neck examination, the oral health practitioner should palpate the thyroid gland. Clinical examination should entail appreciation of the size, shape, consistency, and mobility of the gland as well as attempting to discern its lower margin (thus implying the absence of retrosternal extension). A bruit may be present. The thyroid gland is best examined with the patient's head extended to one side.[45] The examiner uses the fingers of both hands to palpate the gland. Next, the patient is instructed to swallow, while the examiner evaluates the anatomic extent of the lobules, using the last three fingers of one hand. In healthy patients, the right lobule is usually larger than the left, and the outline of the relaxed gland cannot be easily observed. Associated regional lymph nodes should be palpated, and the tracheal position determined, if possible. The presence of an asymmetric thyroid gland enlargement (Figure 23-8) on routine examination should be referred for follow-up by an internist or endocrinologist. This is particularly true for the patient with a history of hyper- or hypothyroidism. Examination should never omit an assessment of the patient's clinical thyroid status.

There are two major aspects of any goiter: its pathological nature and the patient's thyroid status.

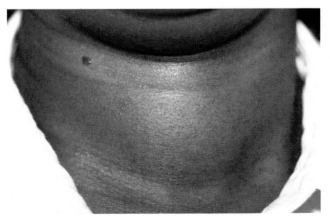

FIGURE 23-8 Asymmetric thyroid gland enlargement was observed in this patient during a routine dental examination. She was referred to her physician for further follow-up.

- Diffuse goiter:

Simple Goiter: no cause is found for the generalised enlargement of the thyroid, which is usually smooth and soft.

Firm diffuse goiter of variable size is usually associated with Hashimoto's thyroiditis and thyrotoxicosis.

Painful, tender goiter with diffuse swelling of the thyroid gland, sometimes with severe pain, is suggestive of an acute viral thyroiditis (*de Quervain's thyroiditis*). It can produce transient clinical features of hyperthyroidism and serological changes, with an increase in the serum T4.

- Nodular goiter:

Multinodular goiter is the commonest goiter found, especially in older patients. The patient is usually euthyroid, but may be hyperthyroid or borderline with suppressed TSH levels but normal free T4 and T3. Multinodular goiter is the commonest cause of tracheal and/or esophageal compression and can cause laryngeal nerve palsy.

Solitary nodular goiter is a difficult clinical problem. Malignancy should be excluded with the presence of any solitary nodule. However, most nodules are cystic or benign and indeed, may simply be the largest nodule of a multinodular goiter. Solitary toxic nodules are quite uncommon and may be associated with T3 toxicosis.

Fibrotic goiter (Riedel's thyroiditis) is rare and associated with a feeling of a 'woody' gland. It can be difficult to distinguish from carcinoma, being irregular and hard. Of interest is that it has been shown to be an IgG4-related disease.

Malignancy presenting as masses is most likely to be a thyroid carcinoma, but the thyroid gland can occasionally be a site for either primary lymphoma or metastases.

Investigations

Blood Tests: thyroid function tests: TSH plus free T4 or T3 and thyroid antibodies to exclude autoimmune causes.

Imaging: Ultrasound can delineate nodules and demonstrate whether they are cystic or solid. Chest and thoracic inlet plain film radiographs or CT scan can detect tracheal compression in patients with large goiters or clinical symptoms indicative of tracheal compression. Thyroid scanning (99mTc, ^{125}I, or ^{131}I) can be useful to distinguish between functioning (hot) and nonfunctioning (cold) nodules, but it has largely been replaced by the use of ultrasound-guided fine needle aspiration (FNA) biopsy.

Thyroid Masses

Thyroid carcinoma, is not common, but these tumors have an annual incidence of 30 000 cases in the USA. Over 75% occur in women. In 90% of cases they present as thyroid nodules (see above), but occasionally with cervical lymphadenopathy (about 5%), or with lung, cerebral, hepatic or bone metastases.

Carcinomas derived from thyroid epithelium may be papillary, follicular (differentiated), or anaplastic (undifferentiated). Medullary carcinomas (about 5% of all thyroid cancers) arise from the calcitonin-producing C cells. The pathogenesis of thyroid epithelial carcinomas is not understood except for occasional familial papillary carcinoma and those cases related to previous head and neck irradiation or exposure to and ingestion of radioactive iodine (e.g. post-Chernobyl). These tumors are minimally active hormonally and so rarely associated with hyperthyroidism, but as over 90% do secrete thyroglobulin, this can be used as a tumor marker after thyroid ablation.

The primary treatment is surgical, normally total or near-total thyroidectomy. Regional or more extensive neck dissection is only needed when there is local nodal spread or involvement of local structures. Most tumors will take up iodine, so current guidelines recommend postoperative use of RAI for ablation of any residual thyroid tissue in patients with well-differentiated thyroid cancer. To further minimize the risk of recurrence, patients are treated with suppressive doses of levothyroxine (sufficient to suppress TSH levels below the normal range). Patient progress is monitored both clinically and biochemically using serum thyroglobulin levels as a tumor marker. Prognosis is extremely good in patients with well-differentiated thyroid cancer confined to the fully excised thyroid gland. Poor prognosis is associated with being 40 years or older, larger primary tumor size (> 4 cm), and macroscopic invasion of the capsule and surrounding tissues.

Medullary carcinoma (MTC) is a neuroendocrine tumor of the calcitonin-producing C cells of the thyroid. This condition is often associated with MEN 2. Patients with MEN2 mutations are advised to have a prophylactic thyroidectomy (as early as 5 years of age) to prevent the development of MTC. Total thyroidectomy and wide regional lymph node dissection is indicated for MTC.

Hypothyroidism

In hypothyroidism, the orofacial findings include myxedema of the skin, an enlarged tongue (macroglossia), compromised periodontal health, delayed tooth eruption, delayed wound healing, and a hoarse voice. Salivary gland enlargement, changes in taste, and burning mouth symptoms have also been reported.[46,47] Hashimoto's thyroiditis has been associated with xerostomia and impaired salivary output.[48,49]

Hyperthyroidism

Hyperthyroidism can exacerbate the patient's response to dental pain and anxiety. Routine examination of the head and neck may disclose signs of thyroid disease, including changes in oculomotor function, protrusion of the eyes, excess sweating, enlargement of the thyroid or the tongue, lingual thyroid tissue, and difficulty in swallowing.

Dental Management of the Patient with Thyroid Gland Disorders

The first concern in treating the patient with thyroid disease is the level of metabolic control and the second concern is the concomitant medications. Well-controlled hyper-/hypo-thyroidism does not present any major risks to the patient undergoing dental care. A complete history and physical examination are necessary to define the particular thyroid disease and assess its level of control. If the thyroid disorder is untreated or unstable the patient's physician should be consulted to determine possible risks associated with the surgical stress due to the use of local anesthetics, infection, bleeding, and wound healing. Inquiry about cardiovascular status, coagulation factors, level of disease control, and a history of other disease complications should be discussed with the patient's physician. Drug interactions may result from the increased metabolic rate associated with hyperthyroidism or the decreased rate in hypothyroidism. Before prescribing any medications for a poorly controlled patient with hyper- or hypothyroidism, the clinician should consult with the patient's physician to determine the appropriate medication regimen.

Patients with a history of thyroid cancer have probably undergone surgery or radioactive iodine therapy that can affect the adjacent regional tissues. Salivary gland dysfunction is one of the most common side effects of high-dose ^{131}I therapy for thyroid cancer.[50,51] [131]I targets the salivary glands, where it is concentrated and secreted into saliva. Dose-related damage to the salivary parenchyma results from the ^{131}I irradiation and causes parotid swelling, pain, and hypofunction.[52,53,54] As with the complications of other head and neck cancer therapies, postsurgical or post-radiation complications may require special oral health care measures. Tooth loss, diminished mandibular bone density, decreased salivary flow, dysgeusia, dysphagia, and skin and mucosal ulceration are potential complications of radiation therapy.[55]

Patients with autoimmune thyroid diseases (Hashimoto's thyroiditis) may also be susceptible to other autoimmune connective tissue disorders, including Sjögren's syndrome. Antinuclear antibodies (ANAs) are found in one-third of patients with autoimmune thyroid disorders, and Sjögren's syndrome is found in nearly one-tenth of ANA-positive patients with autoimmune thyroid disorders.[56] The most common additional autoimmune disease identified in patients with primary Sjögren's syndrome has been identified as hypothyroidism[57]; also, there is a 7-17% prevalence of detectable thyroid antibodies in patients with Sjögren's syndrome and rheumatoid arthritis.[58] Therefore, for the thyroid patient who presents with signs of hyposalivation and xerophthalmia should be evaluated for evidence of Sjögren's syndrome.[59] Similarly, a patient with Sjögren's syndrome should be monitored for developing thyroid disease.[60] Oral health complications resulting from salivary hypofunction are preventable for those patients who have received head and neck radiotherapy or ^{131}I treatment or those with autoimmune thyroid diseases. Patients should be counseled on their increased risk of developing dental caries, gingival and periodontal problems, oral candidiasis, dysgeusia, difficulty wearing dentures, and dysphagia.

Hypothyroidism

Patients with hypothyroidism are susceptible to cardiovascular diseases; therefore, consultation with the patients' medical providers is indicated. Patients who have atrial fibrillation may be taking anticoagulants. Coagulation tests (prothrombin time, partial thromboplastin time, international normalized ratio) are required when the patient is taking an oral anticoagulant and thyroid hormone replacement therapy. The use of epinephrine-containing local anesthetics is not contraindicated if the patient's hypothyroidism is well controlled, but in patients who have cardiovascular disease or who have uncertain control of their thyroid disease, local anesthetic and retraction cord soaked with epinephrine can be used, but cautiously. Hypothyroidism, especially if uncontrolled, can also lead to respiratory depression, so patient positioning should be carefully considered when treating such patients. Consider treating patients in a semi-upright position, with oxygen supplementation via nasal prongs or by means of the nitrous oxide mask.

Hypothyroidism patients are sensitive to CNS depressants and barbiturates, so these medications should be used carefully, with input from the patient's physician. For postoperative pain control, narcotic use should be limited since there is greater susceptibility to these agents in these patients.

Patients with long-standing hypothyroidism may experience increased bleeding after trauma or surgery. The presence of excess subcutaneous mucopolysaccharides (due to its decreased degradation) may impair the ability of small vessels to constrict if severed or traumatized, and this may result in increased postoperative hemorrhage from such infiltrated tissues, including mucosa and skin. The extended application of firm local pressure should control the bleeding from any small vessels affected in such cases.

Patients with hypothyroidism may have delayed wound healing due to decreased metabolic activity of the fibroblasts. However, a study of well-controlled primary hypothyroid patients who had been provided with dental implants demonstrated no significantly increased risk for implant failure when compared with matched normal controls.[61]

Hyperthyroidism

The most important concern in treating the patient with hyperthyroidism is the risk of development of thyrotoxicosis or a "thyroid storm," which includes symptoms of extreme irritability and delirium, hypotension, vomiting, and diarrhea.[62] It can be triggered by surgery, sepsis, and trauma. Emergency medical treatment is required for this condition. Epinephrine is contraindicated, and elective dental care should be deferred for patients who have hyperthyroidism and exhibit signs or symptoms of thyrotoxicosis. In general, stress management and short appointments are recommended for these patients, and treatment should be discontinued if signs or symptoms of a thyrotoxic crisis develop.

Patients who have hyperthyroidism are highly susceptible to cardiovascular diseases, including atrial dysrhythmias, tachycardia, and hypertension. Patients with high arteriolar pressures may require increased attention and a longer duration of local pressure to stop bleeding. Consultation with the patient's physician is required to document these and other organ system problems and to ascertain the level of control of hyperthyroidism.

Chronic medication use for hyperthyroidism brings the risk of developing polypharmacy problems, so the oral health practitioner should be familiar with the patient's current medications. Increased susceptibility to infection may develop as a drug side effect since the antithyroid agents can cause agranulocytosis or leukopenia. Propylthiouracil can also cause sialolith formation and can increase the anticoagulant effects of warfarin. Certain analgesics must be used with caution in these patients. Aspirin and NSAIDs may cause increased levels of circulating T_4, leading to thyrotoxicosis. NSAIDs can also decrease the effect of β-blockers.[52]

The use of epinephrine and other sympathomimetics requires special consideration when treating hyperthyroid patients and those taking nonselective β-blockers. Epinephrine acts on α-adrenergic receptors, causing vasoconstriction, and on β2 receptors, causing vasodilation. Nonselective β-blockers eliminate the vasodilatory effect, potentiating an α-adrenergic increase in blood pressure. This pathophysiology is applicable to any patient taking nonselective β-blockers and those with hyperthyroidism due to concurrent cardiovascular complications.

Disorders of the Adrenal Glands (Cortex)

The normal adrenal glands weigh 6–11 g each and are located above the kidneys; they have their own rich blood supply. Within the glands is the adrenal cortex, which produces three classes of corticosteroid hormones: (1) glucocorticoids (e.g. cortisol), (2) mineralocorticoids (e.g. aldosterone) and (3) adrenal androgen precursor (e.g. dehydroepiandrosterone [DHEA]) prohormones that become the sex steroids. The sex steroids, also known as gonadal steroids, are steroid hormones that interact with androgen receptors that stimulate or control the development and maintenance of male characteristics (testosterone) or with the estrogen receptors (regulating both the menstrual and the reproductive cycles).

Glucocorticoids and mineralocorticoids act through specific nuclear receptors, regulating aspects of the response to physiologic stress, as well as blood pressure, electrolyte, and glucose homeostasis. Adrenal androgen precursors are converted in peripheral target cells, principally found in the gonads, to become the sex steroids that, in turn, act via nuclear androgen and estrogen receptors.

Adrenal steroidogenesis occurs in a zone-specific fashion, with mineralocorticoid synthesis occurring in the outer zona glomerulosa, glucocorticoid synthesis in the zona fasciculata, and adrenal androgen synthesis in the inner zona reticularis. All the steroid hormones are derivatives of cholesterol. The steroidogenic pathway requires the import of cholesterol into the mitochondrion, a process initiated by the action of the steroidogenic acute regulatory (StAR) protein, which shuttles cholesterol from the outer to the inner mitochondrial membrane. The majority of steroidogenic enzymes are cytochrome (cyp) P450 enzymes. Disorders of the adrenal cortex are characterized by deficiency or excess of one or several of the three major corticosteroid classes of hormones. Hormone deficiency can be caused by inherited glandular or enzymatic disorders or by destruction of the pituitary or adrenal gland by autoimmune disorders, infection, infarction, or by iatrogenic causes such as surgery or hormonal suppression. Hormone excess is usually the result of neoplasia, leading to increased production of ACTH by the pituitary or neuroendocrine cells or increased production of glucocorticoids or mineralocorticoids by adrenal nodules. Adrenal nodules are increasingly identified incidentally on abdominal imaging.

Regulation of the production of glucocorticoids and adrenal androgens is under the control of the HPA axis. Mineralocorticoids are regulated by the renin-angiotensin-aldosterone (RAA) system.

Glucocorticoid synthesis is under inhibitory feedback control by the hypothalamus and the pituitary. Hypothalamic release of corticotrophin-releasing hormone (CRH) occurs in response to endogenous or exogenous stress. CRH in turn stimulates the release of ACTH by the cells of the anterior pituitary. ACTH is the pivotal regulator of cortisol synthesis, with additional short-term effects on mineralocorticoid and adrenal androgen synthesis. The release of CRH, and subsequently ACTH, occurs in a pulsatile fashion that follows a circadian rhythm, under the control of the hypothalamus. Reflecting this pattern of ACTH secretion, adrenal cortisol secretion is also circadian, with peak levels in the morning and low levels in the evening.

Diagnostic tests assessing the HPA axis makes use of its regulation by negative feedback. Glucocorticoid excess is diagnosed by the dexamethasone suppression test. Dexamethasone, a potent glucocorticoid, suppresses CRH/ACTH and, therefore, lowers endogenous cortisol levels. If cortisol production is autonomous (e.g. from an adrenal nodule), ACTH is already suppressed, and the dexamethasone has little additional effect. If cortisol production is driven by an ACTH-producing pituitary adenoma, dexamethasone suppression is ineffective at low doses, but usually induces suppression at high doses. If cortisol production is driven by an ectopic source of ACTH, such as an ACTH-producing tumor, these are usually unaffected by dexamethasone suppression. Therefore, the dexamethasone suppression test is useful both in establishing a diagnosis of Cushing's syndrome (corticoid excess) and in differentiating the cause. Conversely, to assess glucocorticoid deficiency, ACTH stimulation of cortisol production is used. The standard ACTH stimulation test involves administration of cosyntropin (Synacthen, a potent ACTH agonist) IM or IV and the collection of blood samples at 0, 30, and 60 min to check the cortisol level. A normal response is defined as a cortisol level >20 μg/dL or an increment of >10 μg/dL over baseline. Alternatively, an insulin tolerance test (ITT) can be used to assess adrenal insufficiency. It involves injection of insulin to induce hypoglycemia, which represents a strong stress signal that triggers hypothalamic CRH release and activation of the entire HPA axis. The ITT involves administration of regular insulin (0.1 U/kg IV—a dose is needed if hypopituitarism is suspected) and collection of blood samples at 0, 30, 60, and 120 min for serum glucose, cortisol, and GH levels. Oral or intravenous glucose is administered once the patient has achieved symptomatic hypoglycemia (usually glucose <40 mg/dL). A normal response is defined as a cortisol >20 μg/dL.

Mineralocorticoid production is controlled by the RAA regulatory cycle, which is initiated by the release of renin from the juxtaglomerular cells in the kidney, resulting in cleavage of angiotensinogen to angiotensin I in the liver. Angiotensin-converting enzyme (ACE) cleaves angiotensin I to angiotensin II, which binds and activates the angiotensin II receptor Type 1 (AT1 receptor), resulting in increased aldosterone production and vasoconstriction. Aldosterone enhances sodium retention and potassium excretion, and increases the renal arterial perfusion pressure, which in turn regulates renin release. As mineralocorticoid synthesis is primarily under the control of the RAA system, disorders of the hypothalamic-pituitary axis generally do not adversely affect adrenal gland synthesis of aldosterone.

Cushing's Syndrome (Glucocorticoid Excess)

Cushing's syndrome reflects a constellation of clinical features that result from the chronic effects of glucocorticoid excess. Cushing's syndrome is rare, with an annual incidence of 1–2 per 100,000 in population. The disorder can be ACTH-dependent (e.g., pituitary corticotrope adenoma) or ACTH-independent (e.g., adrenocortical tumor). Overwhelmingly, the medical use of glucocorticoids is the commonest cause of Cushing's syndrome. Only 10% of patients with Cushing's syndrome have a primary, adrenal cause of their disease. The term Cushing's disease refers specifically to Cushing's syndrome caused by a pituitary adenoma secreting ACTH.

Ectopic ACTH production is predominantly caused by occult carcinoid tumors, most frequently in the lung, but also in thymus or pancreas. Advanced small cell lung cancer can also cause ectopic ACTH production. In rare cases, ectopic ACTH production has been found to originate from medullary thyroid carcinoma or from a pheochromocytoma.

Clinical Manifestations

Glucocorticoids affect almost all cells of the body, so excess cortisol impacts multiple physiologic systems. In addition,

excess glucocorticoid secretion overcomes the ability of a key kidney enzyme system (11β-HSD2) to rapidly inactivate cortisol to cortisone (cortisone has minimal mineralocorticoid activity), thereby exerting mineralocorticoid actions, manifest as diastolic hypertension, hypokalemia, and edema. Excess glucocorticoids also interfere with central regulatory systems, leading to suppression of gonadotropins with subsequent hypogonadism and amenorrhea and suppression of the hypothalamic-pituitary-thyroid axis, resulting in decreased TSH (thyroid-stimulating hormone) secretion.

The diagnosis of Cushing's syndrome (or disease) should be considered when the following key clinical features, are evident in the patient (Figures 23-9 and 23-10): fragility

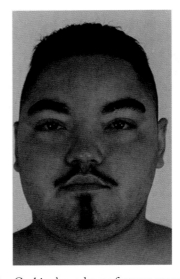

FIGURE 23-9 Cushing's syndrome features appearing as a round (moon) face caused by excessive fat deposition in the temporal fossae. The face is plethoric with fullness in the supraclavicular area.

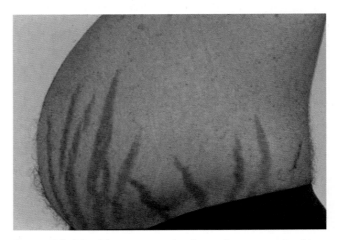

FIGURE 23-10 The presence of wide purple striae on the skin is an additional feature of Cushing's syndrome. The purple hue is due to the proximity of the underlying blood vessels to the surface from thinning of the skin by excess glucocorticoids.

of the skin, with easy bruising and broad (>1 cm), purplish striae, signs of proximal myopathy, with the patient struggling to stand up from a chair (without the use of hands). Patients with Cushing's syndrome may develop marked hypercoagulopathy, so are at acutely increased risk of deep vein thrombosis and subsequent pulmonary embolism. Psychiatric symptoms of marked anxiety and/or depression are also common, but acute paranoia or frank psychosis may also occur.

Overt, untreated Cushing's is associated with a poor prognosis. In ACTH-independent disease, treatment consists of surgical removal of the adrenal tumor. In Cushing's disease, the treatment of choice is selective removal of the pituitary corticotrophic-producing tumor, usually via a transsphenoidal approach.

Mineralocorticoid Excess (Conn's syndrome)

Hyperaldosteronism, the excessive release of the principal mineralocorticoid, aldosterone, typically presents as hypertension, given the adverse effects on the renin-angiotensin system which so powerfully controls renal perfusion and homeostasis and blood pressure. Recent studies have demonstrated that the screening of all patients with hypertension, demonstrates a much higher prevalence aldosterone excess (Conn's syndrome) than was previously thought, ranging from 5 to 12%.

The commonest cause of primary hyperaldosteronism is that of excess production of aldosterone by the adrenal zona glomerulosa, typically occurring with bilateral micronodular adrenal hyperplasia. Infrequently, Conn's syndrome occurs because of an adrenocortical carcinoma. Another rare cause of aldosterone excess is glucocorticoid-remediable aldosteronism (GRA), which is caused by a chimeric gene resulting from the crossover of promoter sequences between the CYP11B1 and CYP11B2, the genes that are involved in glucocorticoid and mineralocorticoid synthesis, respectively. This rearrangement brings CYP11B2 under the control of ACTH receptor signaling so that consequently, aldosterone production is regulated by ACTH rather than by renin.

The clinical hallmark of mineralocorticoid excess is hypokalemic hypertension, but not hypernatremia, with the serum sodium tending to be normal because of concurrent fluid retention, which in some cases can lead to marked peripheral edema. Severe hypokalemia can be associated with muscle weakness, overt proximal myopathy, or in severe cases, hypokalemic paralysis or tetany. Diagnostic screening for mineralocorticoid excess is not currently recommended for all patients with hypertension, but should be considered in hypertensive patients younger than 40 years of age, patients with hypertension resistant to drug therapy, hypokalemia, or the finding of an adrenal mass. The accepted screening test is concurrent measurement of plasma renin and aldosterone with subsequent calculation of the aldosterone-renin ratio, but the serum potassium needs to be normalized prior to testing.

With the diagnosis of hyperaldosteronism, adrenal imaging is needed, best undertaken by fine-cut CT scanning. The treatment provided is dependent on the patients' age and fitness for surgery. Laparoscopic adrenalectomy is the preferred approach. Medical treatment, which can also be considered prior to surgery to avoid postsurgical hypoaldosteronism, is usually with the mineralocorticoid receptor antagonist, i.e. spironolactone.

Adrenal Insufficiency (Addison's Disease)

The US prevalence of adrenal insufficiency is 5 in 10,000 in the general population. Disorders of the hypothalamic-pituitary axis are frequent, with a prevalence of 3 in 10,000 whereas primary adrenal insufficiency has a prevalence of 2 in 10,000, with about half of the cases due to genetic causes (e.g. congenital adrenal hyperplasia). Primary adrenal insufficiency is most commonly caused by autoimmune destruction of the adrenal gland, with some 60–70% developing adrenal insufficiency as part of an autoimmune polyglandular syndrome (APS) APS1, an autosomal recessive disorder also termed APECED (autoimmune polyendocrinopathy-candidiasis-ectodermal dystrophy), is the underlying cause in 10% of patients affected by APS. APS1 patients invariably develop chronic mucocutaneous candidiasis, usually manifest in childhood, which precedes adrenal insufficiency by years or decades. Coincident autoimmune-induced endocrinopathy most frequently includes thyroid autoimmune disease, vitiligo, and premature ovarian failure. Less commonly, Type 1 DM and pernicious anemia (with consequent vitamin B12 deficiency) may occur. Rare causes of adrenal insufficiency involve destruction of the adrenal glands as a consequence of infection; with tuberculous, adrenalitis is still a frequent cause of disease in developing countries; hemorrhage; or more rarely, bilateral bulky metastatic infiltration with replacement of the adrenal glands resulting in hypoadrenalsim.

The commonest cause of adrenal insufficiency is iatrogenic, arising from suppression of the HPA axis as a consequence of exogenous glucocorticoid treatment. This has a reported prevalence of some 0.5–2% of the population in developed countries. Secondary adrenal insufficiency is the consequence of dysfunction of the hypothalamic-pituitary component of the HPA axis. Excluding iatrogenic impairment of the HPA axis (exogenous corticosteroid use) the majority of cases are caused by pituitary or hypothalamic tumors, or their treatment by surgery or radiotherapy.

In principle, the clinical features of primary adrenal insufficiency are characterized by the loss of both glucocorticoid and mineralocorticoid secretion, but in contrast, in secondary adrenal insufficiency, only glucocorticoid deficiency is evident, as the adrenal itself is intact and can still be regulated by the RAA system. Adrenal androgen secretion is disrupted in both primary and secondary adrenal insufficiency.

Hypothalamic-pituitary disease can lead to additional clinical manifestations due to involvement of other endocrine axis or visual impairment with bitemporal hemianopia caused by compression of the optic chiasma. With iatrogenic adrenal insufficiency caused by exogenous glucocorticoid suppression of the HPA axis and their abrupt cessation, this can cause all of the symptoms associated with glucocorticoid deficiency, but the patients will appear Cushingoid from the preceding overexposure to glucocorticoids.

Acute adrenal insufficiency usually occurs after a prolonged period of nonspecific complaints and is more frequently observed in patients with primary adrenal insufficiency, due to the loss of both glucocorticoid and mineralocorticoid secretion. The associated postural hypotension is a red flag, as the patient may then progress to hypovolemic shock. Adrenal insufficiency may also mimic the features of an acute abdomen with abdominal tenderness, nausea, vomiting, and fever. An adrenal crisis can be triggered by an intercurrent illness, surgery, or other stress.

The diagnosis of adrenal insufficiency is established by the short cosyntropin test (Synacthen), a safe and reliable tool with an excellent diagnostic sensitivity. The insulin tolerance test is an alternate test, but can be hazardous to the patient, and should be carried out only under a specialist phyisian's supervision.

Acute adrenal insufficiency requires immediate initiation of rehydration, (1 L/hr saline infusion) with cardiac monitoring and glucocorticoid replacement by bolus injection of 100 mg hydrocortisone, followed by further hydrocortisone supplementation (100–200 mg hydrocortisone over the course of 24 hours). Mineralocorticoid replacement can wait until the daily hydrocortisone dose has been reduced to < 50 mg, because at higher doses the hydrocortisone provides sufficient stimulation of the mineralocorticoid receptors.

Glucocorticoid replacement for the treatment of chronic adrenal insufficiency should be administered at a dose that replaces the physiologic daily cortisol production: typically orally administered hydrocortisone, at a dose of 15–25 mg, in two divided doses: 10–20 mg in the mornings and 5 mg in the evenings, mimicking the natural circadian levels of cortisol. Mineralocorticoid replacement in primary adrenal insufficiency is achieved by the use of 100–150 μg of fludrocortisone, and its efficacy assessed by measuring the blood pressure, sitting and standing, to detect a postural drop indicative of hypovolemia and testing of the serum sodium, potassium, and plasma renin levels. Adrenal androgen replacement is an option for patients with a lack of energy, or with features of androgen deficiency, such as loss of libido.

Pheochromocytoma

Pheochromocytoma consists of tumors that produce epinephrine, norepinephrine, or a combination of both catecholamines. Patients are hypertensive, with headache, sweating, tachycardia, palpitations, and pallor. Occasionally, these can be syndromal, as part of MEN syndrome Type 2B (MEN2B) presenting with a marfanoid habitus, high arched palate, neuromas (of the tongue, buccal mucosa, lips, conjunctivae, and eyelids), and corneal nerve thickening. The diagnosis of pheochromocytoma is confirmed by measuring urinary and plasma catecholamine levels.[63]

Stomatognathic Manifestations and Complications of Disorders of the Adrenal Gland
Hyperadrenocorticism (Glucocorticoid Excess of Cushing's Syndrome)

The primary orofacial feature of Cushing's syndrome is a round, moon face due to muscle wasting and accumulation of fat. Surface capillaries in the face and other skin regions become fragile, rendering them readily susceptible to hematomas after mild trauma. The facial skin has a ruddy color that simulates "glowing health"; acne and excessive facial hair (hirsutism) are also commonly seen. Long-standing Cushing's syndrome produces delayed growth and development, including of the skeletal and dental structures. Many of the systemic findings of Cushing's syndrome are similar to those seen in patients on moderate- to high-dose glucocorticoid therapy, and these patients are considered to be immunosuppressed. Therefore, oral signs and symptoms of immunosuppression can be seen, including oral candidiasis, recurrent herpes labialis and herpes zoster infections, gingival and periodontal diseases, and impaired wound healing.

Hypoadrenocorticism (Glucocorticoid Deficiency or Addison's Disease)

The primary orofacial feature of Addison's disease is unusual skin pigmentation, most intensely of the sun exposed areas. On the face, freckles and moles become darker, as well as the appearance of a tan-like complexion ("bronzing" of the skin and sometimes of the oral mucosa), except that the increased pigmentation does not fade on cessation of sunlight exposure. The mucocutaneous junctions undergo increased pigmentation, including the lips, but hyperpigmentation can also involve the intraoral mucosal surfaces, such as the gingival margins, buccal mucosa, palate, and lingual surface of the tongue. The oral pigmentations appear as irregular spots that range from pale brown to gray or black. The treatment of Addison's disease includes administration of corticosteroids.

Dental Management of Patients with Adrenal Gland Disorders
Hyperadrenocorticism (Cushing's Syndrome)

Dental management of the patient with Cushing's syndrome must take into consideration concomitant medical conditions that include hypertension, heart failure, depression or psychosis, DM, osteoporosis, easy bruising of the skin, impaired wound healing, and immunosuppression. Patients with Cushing's syndrome and those on long-term moderate- to high-dose glucocorticoid therapy are considered to be immunocompromised and are more susceptible to infections.

Antibiotic coverage should be considered for dentoalveolar infections or any scheduled oral surgery, but this decision should be based on the extent and nature of the infection and not solely on dose and duration of the glucocorticoid therapy.

Assessment of the ability to withstand stress is an essential component of dental management of patients with Cushing's syndrome and other patients who have been on long-term moderate- to high-dose glucocorticoid therapy. Stress may be induced by an invasive surgical procedure, the onset of infection, an exacerbation of an underlying disease, or a serious life event, such as the death of a family member.[64] When normal individuals undergo stress, the plasma cortisol levels may double, suggesting an inherent ability of the adrenal glands to increase cortisol production. In a patient with adrenal insufficiency, adrenal function is inadequate to produce sufficient cortisol in response to stress, and so the patient may experience severe hypotension, nausea, cardiovascular events, stroke, coma, and death. Patients with established severe adrenal insufficiency usually require premedication with oral or intramuscular glucocorticoids before an invasive procedure. Dosages must be agreed upon with the patient's physician; a frequent regimen is to double the daily dose of oral glucocorticoids the day before the surgery and on the day of surgery.

Hypoadrenocorticism (Glucocorticoid Deficiency or Addison's Disease)

Dental management is similar to that for the patient who has taken long-term moderate to high doses of glucocorticoids (see above) since Addison's disease is frequently treated with exogenous glucocorticoids. The oral health practitioner must be able to recognize and provide initial management of an acute adrenal crisis (intramuscular or intravenous hydrocortisone) when treating these patients.[65]

Use of Replacement Corticosteroid Therapy ("stress steroids" or "steroid cover")

The "rule of twos" states that adrenal suppression may occur if a patient is taking >20 mg of cortisone (or its equivalent daily) for 2 weeks, for 2 years (or more) requiring invasive dental treatment and that such patients require preprocedural supplemental/replacement corticosteroids. It was thought until recently that failure to provide replacement corticosteroids would lead to acute adrenal insufficiency. Iatrogenic adrenal insufficiency is caused by suppression of the HPA axis due to exogenous glucocorticoid therapy in pharmacological (supra-physiological) doses at >5.7mg/m^2/day (~10mg/day) of cortisol. The resultant atrophied adrenal cortex (caused by the lack of ACTH stimulation) is unable to produce sufficient circulating cortisol, critical at times of stress. Cortisol (hydrocortisone) is essential to maintain vasomotor tone by sensitizing the α-adrenergic receptors (α-1A, -1B, and -1D receptors) of the vasculature to circulating epinephrine (and norepinephrine) and increasing catecholamine release from the adrenal cortex. Therefore, insufficient cortisol is produced

at times of marked physiological stress, and can lead to circulatory vasodilation, reduced cardiac return, and potentially hypotensive cardiac shock, resulting in collapse and death. Significant physiological stressors include severe infection and/or injury, including surgery and intubation associated with GA.[66,67]

The prevalence of therapeutic corticoid use has been assessed over the course of five cycles (1999–2008) of the National Health and Nutrition Examination (NHANE) Survey. Oral glucocorticoids were found to be used by 1.2% of the population, with usage peaking in the 60-69 year age bracket and with a mean duration of oral glucocorticoid use of some 4½ yrs.). Nearly a third (28.8%) had used oral glucocorticoids, in excess of five years.[68] Note that frequent use of highly potent topical and inhaled corticosteroids can also impair the HPA axis, although this is less common than the suppression seen with oral corticosteroid use.[69,70,71]

For patients undergoing invasive dental treatment, the recommendation is for 100-200 mg of hydrocortisone (or its equivalent im or ivi) or to double the patient's current orally administered steroid dose on the morning of the planned surgery. But, there is poor correlation between the degree and level of functional impairment of the HPA axis and the cumulative corticosteroid dose, the highest dose, or even the duration of corticosteroid therapy, with considerable inter-individual variability in the degree and duration of adrenal suppression.

The recommendations for the use of "stress steroids" are largely historical in nature and not well substantiated by laboratory testing or extensive case studies; they appear to have arisen from a single case study published in 1952.[82] The report was of a patient who, following surgery, died from circulatory shock, seemingly as a consequence of secondary adrenal insufficiency. It is worth noting that generally dental procedures are low inducers of surgical stress and stress steroids are detrimental to wound healing, resolution of infections, and glycemic control, especially in diabetic patients. Furthermore, a number of published case studies have failed to demonstrate a clear benefit for the use of steroid supplementation. A number of recent meta-analyses concluded that supplementary steroid use is not indicated for dental procedures done in the chair with local anesthesia for patients using therapeutic corticosteroids, and for invasive dental (surgical) procedures the evidence is considered, at best, equivocal. However for patients with primary hypoadrenalism supplementary corticosteroids are indicated. For patients who have recently (within 2 years) ceased supra-physiological corticosteroid therapy, the evidence is considered to be equivocal. In assessing the need for a patient with hypoadrenalism to receive preprocedure supplemental corticosteroids, the essentials still need to be applied: careful patient assessment and evaluation, including taking a detailed medical history with particular attention on recent surgery and how the patient coped with the procedure.[72,73,74]However, for patients undertaking dental procedures using oral or intravenous sedation with potent-short-acting benzodiazepines (e.g. midazolam) to abrogate the psychological stresses associated with invasive dental treatment, this intended blunting of the emotional stress response may blunt the physiological stress response. For patients considered to be at risk of hypoadrenalism, blunting the emotional stress response may similarly impair stimulation of the limited cortisol release these patients can still marshal. Therefore for those patients with primary hypoadrenalism or on long-term, supra-physiological doses of corticosteroids having dental treatment aided by means of oral or intravenous sedation, supplementary pre- or peri-procedural stress steroids should be considered.

Gonads and Gonadal Dysfunction

The gonads, like most other endocrine organs, are incorporated into an endocrine axis: the hypothalamic-pituitary-gonadal (HPG) axis. The physiologic function and regulation of the HPG axis, especially in women, is complex and changes dramatically over a lifetime. The hypothalamic hormone in the HPG axis is gonadotropin-releasing hormone (GnRH). GnRH is released in a complicated pulsatile fashion that varies widely in a person's lifetime and is significantly different between men and women. The general principles of stimulation and feedback inhibition apply to the HPG axis (see Figure 23-4); however, this axis is complicated by two issues: GnRH is pulsatile, and the pituitary makes two hormones, luteinizing hormone (LH) and follicle-stimulating hormone (FSH). In the male, LH stimulates testosterone production from the Leydig cells of the testicles, and FSH stimulates sperm production by the Sertoli cells. In females, FSH stimulates maturation of the follicle, and LH causes maturation of the follicle into a corpus luteum, as well as the production of ovarian estradiol.

For both males and females, the HPG axis is relatively dormant before the onset of puberty. The onset of puberty in girls occurs approximately 2 years before that of boys. In girls, the average age at which breast development starts is 10.5 years, and menses starts at about 12 years of age. In boys, the peak growth rate and beginning of voice change occur about the age of 14 years, whereas facial hair appears on average at the age of 15 years. In men, from late puberty until about age 60 years, the serum testosterone levels are relatively constant and begin to decline gradually thereafter. In women, serum estradiol levels vary widely over the course of the menstrual cycle, but after the onset of menopause (which occurs on average at the age of 50 years), serum estradiol levels become very low and gonadotropin (LH and FSH) levels are elevated.

Precocious Puberty, Delayed Puberty, Hypogonadism, and Menopause

In both males and females, precocious puberty, delayed puberty, and hypogonadism are clinical diagnoses, made by early or late signs of secondary sexually differentiation or loss of sexual characteristics.[75] Pubertal development is measured clinically by a staging system developed by Tanner.[76] This assesses the development stage of breasts and pubic hair in girls and the pubic hair, testes, and penile length in boys. Puberty is generally considered precocious in boys if it starts before age 10 years and in girls before age 8.5 years or delayed if there are no signs of sexual development by the age of 13 years in girls and 14 years in boys.

Once a clinical diagnosis of gonadal dysfunction is established, the next step is to determine whether the pathophysiologic process is in the gonads (primary), the pituitary (secondary), the hypothalamus (tertiary), or, in the case of precocious puberty, due to an ectopic (or exogenous) source of hormone. Gonadal testing usually involves measuring the appropriate sex steroid (testosterone or estradiol) and the pituitary gonadotropins LH and FSH. The most common cause of precocious puberty in boys and girls is early onset of pituitary hormone production, termed central precocious puberty. If the end-organ hormones are elevated and the gonadotropins are suppressed (gonadotropin-independent precocious puberty), this suggests primary (autonomous) gonadal dysfunction. Finally, the adrenal gland also produces androgens that can lead to early puberty in boys and masculinization in girls.

Premature ovarian failure heralded by the onset of menopause before the age of 40 years, presents as "hot flashes." The commonest associated problem is cessation or marked irregularity of the menstrual cycle. Hypogonadism in men presents with a loss of libido and decreased growth rate of facial hair and can lead to osteoporosis and fractures. Premature ovarian failure is diagnosed by the early loss of menstrual cycles in the setting of an elevated serum FSH. Hypogonadism in men is diagnosed by a low serum testosterone level.

Replacement of the primary gonadal steroid (testosterone or estradiol or one of its analogues) in men and women is straightforward. However, replacement of the missing hormone will not return fertility, which is often the major concern. If the gonad is still functional but disorders or loss of the relevant pituitary hormones leads to a loss of function, the pituitary hormones can be replaced.

Stomatognathic Manifestations of Gonadal Disorders

Hypersecretion of female sex hormones commonly occurs in pregnancy. Several unusual oral manifestations may occur in a pregnant woman, such as bilateral brown facial pigmentation (melasma), which disappears after delivery of the baby. High levels of female sex hormones cause increased capillary permeability, making them susceptible to gingivitis (pregnancy gingivitis), gingival hyperplasia, and pyogenic granuloma (pregnancy tumor). These factors may complicate preexisting periodontal disease. A decrease in gonadal hormones at menopause is associated with a decrease in salivary flow and salivary composition. These may predispose individuals to dental caries, glossodynia, dysgeusia, unpleasant metallic taste, and oral candidiasis. Gingival tissues become atrophic; there is a higher tendency for plaque accumulation and an increased risk of gingivitis and periodontitis. After dental extractions, unrestored edentulous ridges rapidly undergo resorption. Postmenopausal women have increased susceptibility to osteoporosis, so dental radiographs may demonstrate hypocalcified bone. There is also an increase in the incidence of several systemic disorders, including Sjögren's syndrome, pemphigus vulgaris, burning mouth syndrome, and trigeminal neuralgia, but the direct relationship of these conditions with gonadal insufficiency, in particular with estrogen deficiency, has not been established.[77]

Dental Management of Gonadal Disorders

The specific dental management concerns in patients with gonadal disorders are focused on the associated secondary disorders. The pregnant patient is susceptible to gestational diabetes since insulin action is antagonized by estrogens and progesterone. The dental care practitioner should consult with the patient's physician if dental care is required and determine if the patient has been diagnosed with gestational diabetes. Elective and stressful dental procedures should be avoided during the first trimester and the last half of the third trimester. The second trimester is the safest period to provide dental care during pregnancy. During this time, emphasis should be on prevention, maintenance of optimal oral health, and treatment of dental concerns that may lead to complications in late stages of pregnancy.[78] Injudicious use of medications should be avoided in pregnancy; choice of medication should be guided by Food and Drug Administration pregnancy classifications for prescription drugs to avoid those with possible teratogenic effects.[79]

DISORDERS OF BONE AND MINERAL METABOLISM

Bone is a specialized connective tissue serving three major functions: (1) mechanical: attachment for muscles for movement and structure; (2) metabolic: providing the body's primary store of calcium, including a highly active role in calcium homeostasis as well as for phosphate, and as a reservoir for sodium, magnesium, and other critical ions; and (3) protective: of the vital organs as well as enclosing the marrow, containing the essential hematopoietic stem cells which produce red blood cells, leukocytes and platelets.

Bone comprises cells and a matrix of organic protein and inorganic mineral, best characterized as poorly formed hydroxyapatite crystal. Type I collagen is the main protein, forming parallel lamellae of differing density (which impairs spreading of cracks with trauma). Noncollagen proteins that are also found in bone include osteopontin, osteocalcin, and fibronectin. In cortical bone, concentric lamellae form around a central blood supply, and this collectively is termed the Haversian system, with transverse branches (termed Volkmann's canals).

The long bones (e.g., femur, tibia, humerus) and flat bones (e.g. skull, scapula) are variably composed of: (1) compact or cortical bone that forms the shaft of long bones and the outer shell of flat bones. Being formed of concentric rings of bone, it is strong and is particularly resistant to the mechanical strain associated with flexure; (2) trabecular or cancellous bone found at the ends of long bones and inside flat bones and comprising a network of interconnecting rods and plates of bone that provides great strength against compressive forces. It is the main site of bone turnover needed for mineral homeostasis. (3) Woven bone lacks an organized structure. It appears in the first few years of life and at the sites of fracture repair, as well as in bone disorders associated with high turnover, such as Paget's disease. Woven bone is eventually remodeled to be organized and structurally sound bone; and (4) lamellar bone, in which the collagen fibres are arranged in parallel bundles and forms much of the bone found in adults.

The Bone Cells

Osteoblasts are of mesenchymal origin and are initially found on the surface of newly forming bone. The osteoblast secretes an organic matrix, which then is mineralized, encasing the cell, which is then termed an osteocyte; however, the osteocytes remain connected with each other, as well as with the blood supply, through a fine network of canaliculi, distributed throughout the bone. The vast majority of the cells found in bone are osteocytes, which serve to regulate bone formation and resorption and as bone mechanosensors, signaling the surface osteoblasts and their progenitors through the canalicular network. Osteocytes also secrete fibroblast growth factor 23 (FGF23), a major regulator of phosphate metabolism. Mineralization of the matrix, both in trabecular bone and in the osteones (of the Haversian system) of compact cortical bone begins soon after the matrix is secreted and is termed primary mineralization, but only several weeks later or more is it completed by the process of secondary mineralization. Mineralization is a carefully regulated process that is dependent on the activity of osteoblast-derived alkaline phosphatase, and importantly the very high, near saturation concentrations of calcium and phosphate present in the serum. Hormones such as parathyroid hormone (PTH) and 1,25-dihydroxyvitamin D [1,25(OH)2D] activate receptors expressed by osteoblasts so as to regulate mineral homeostasis.

Osteoclasts serve to resorb bone, being multinucleated cells that are formed by fusion of cells derived from the common precursor of macrophages. Multiple factors regulate osteoclast development and function. Macrophage colony-stimulating factor (M-CSF) plays a critical role during several steps in the pathway and ultimately leads to fusion of osteoclast progenitor cells to form multinucleated, active osteoclasts. RANK (receptor activator of nuclear factor kappa-B) ligand, is a member of the tumor necrosis factor (TNF) family, expressed on the surface of osteoblast progenitors and stromal fibroblasts. In a process involving cell-cell interactions, RANK ligand binds to the RANK receptor on the osteoclast progenitors, stimulating osteoclast differentiation and activation. Alternatively, a soluble decoy receptor, referred to as osteoprotegerin (OPG), can bind the RANK ligand and so inhibits osteoclast differentiation. Osteoclastogenesis inhibitory factor, (OCIF) is a cytokine receptor and also a member of the TNF receptor superfamily. Several growth factors and cytokines can also moderate modulate osteoclast differentiation and function (e.g., interleukins 1, 6, and 11, TNF, and interferon γ, which may also have a role in the bone loss seen in periodontal disease). Most hormones that influence osteoclast function do not target these cells directly, but act indirectly, by influencing M-CSF and RANK ligand signaling of the osteoblasts. Both PTH and 1, 25(OH)2D increase osteoclast number and activity, whereas estrogen decreases osteoclast number and activity. Calcitonin, in contrast, binds directly to its receptor on the basal surface of osteoclasts and so inhibits osteoclast function. Osteoclast-mediated resorption of bone takes place in scalloped spaces (Howship's lacunae) where the osteoclasts are attached through a specific αvβ3 integrin to components of the bone matrix, such as osteopontin.

Bone Growth and Remodeling

In the embryo and the growing child, bone develops by remodeling and replacing previously calcified cartilage, termed endochondral bone formation, or bone is formed without a cartilage matrix anlage, by means of intramembranous bone formation. Longitudinal growth occurs at the epiphyseal growth plate, a cartilage structure between the epiphysis and metaphysis. Cartilage production is tightly regulated, with growth arrest and the subsequent mineralization occurring between the ages 18 to 21 years, when the epiphysis and metaphysis fuse.

In adults, bone is constantly being remodeled, to repair microdamage and for the release of calcium and phosphate needed for homeostasis. Signals regulating initiation of remodeling include changes in osteocytes (apoptosis or altered signaling of sclerostin, prostaglandins, and other molecules), resulting in altered balance of RANKL and OPG expression by adjacent osteoblasts. Remodeling is carried out by the basic multicellular unit (BMU). Normal bone remodeling is a coupled process, with bone formation normally following resorption. New bone formation without resorption may occur in the adult skeleton in response to anabolic therapy such as parathyroid hormone peptides. Additional influences include systemic hormones of which estrogen (in both sexes) is particularly involved, by promoting the survival of osteocytes and inhibiting the formation of new osteoclasts.

Calcium Homeostasis

Over 99% of the 1–2 kg of calcium normally present in the adult human body resides in the skeleton, where it provides mechanical stability (in the form of hydroxyapatite) and also serves as a reservoir for maintenance of extracellular fluid (ECF) calcium concentration (Figure 23-11). Only 0.5–1% of the skeletal calcium is freely exchangeable, that is, in chemical equilibrium with the calcium found in the ECF.

The concentration of ionized calcium in the ECF is maintained within a strict narrow range, because of the critical role it plays in a numerous critical cellular functions, particularly neuromuscular activity, secretion, and signal transduction. In the blood, total calcium concentration is normally 2.2–2.6 mM (8.5–10.5 mg/dL), of which some 40% is ionized and physiologically active. The remaining 60% is bound to negatively charged proteins (predominantly albumin and immunoglobulins) or loosely complexed with phosphate, citrate, sulfate, or other anions. Alterations in serum protein concentrations (e.g. hypoalbuminemia) directly affect the total blood calcium concentration, but the ionized calcium concentration tends to remain stable.

Control of the ionized calcium concentration in the ECF is regulated by the effects of PTH and 1,25(OH)2D3 acting on the gastrointestinal tract, kidney, and bone. Ionized calcium in the circulation both directly suppresses PTH secretion by the stimulating the calcium-sensing receptors present in the parathyroid glands, and indirectly suppresses PTH secretion via effects on 1,25(OH)2D production.

Active calcium uptake from the gut by means of highly regulated, energy-dependent, transportation across the gut epithelium that accounts for up to 95% of the daily calcium intake needed. This occurs mainly in the proximal small bowel (duodenum and proximal jejunum). Optimal rates of calcium absorption require gastric acid, particularly for the weakly dissociable calcium salts such as calcium carbonate. Perversely, large boluses of calcium carbonate when taken as supplements are poorly absorbed because of their neutralizing effect on gastric acid. In achlorhydric subjects, usually

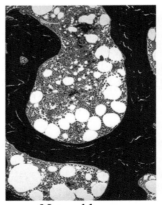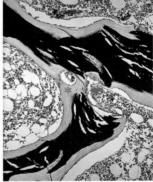

Normal bone   Osteomalacic bone

FIGURE 23-11 Undecalcified, plastic embedded sections of normal and osteomalacic bone stained with Giemsa (*blue*) and Von Kossa (*black*) reveal histological features of osteomalacia. The normal bone (*left panel*) demonstrates complete mineralization of the trabeculae (*black*) whereas osteomalacic bone (*right panel*) is poorly mineralized as demonstrated by a thick layer of un-mineralized osteoid (*stained blue, red star*) around irregular bone trabeculae. There is smooth continuity of normal bone trabeculae compared with irregular discontinuous trabeculae or microfracture in osteomalacic bone (*red arrow*).

those taking drugs that inhibit gastric acid secretion, calcium supplements are best taken with meals to optimize their absorption, or the use of calcium citrate may be preferable. Calcium absorption may also be impaired in diseases such as pancreatic or biliary insufficiency, in which ingested calcium remains bound to unabsorbed fatty acids or food debris, conditions associated with gastrointestinal malabsorption, such as celiac disease, and in patients who have had an extensive bowel resection. At high levels of calcium intake, synthesis of 1,25(OH)2D is reduced, and this then decreases the rate of active intestinal calcium absorption.

The daily net calcium absorption is generally constant at 5–7.5 mmol/daily (equal to 200–400 mg/daily) regardless of variations in the daily dietary calcium intake. This daily load of absorbed calcium is excreted by the kidneys in a tightly regulated manner, with approximately 8–10 g/daily of calcium being filtered by the glomeruli, of which only 2–3% appears in the urine. Most filtered calcium (65%) is reabsorbed in the proximal tubules via a nonregulated, passive, paracellular route that is coupled to concomitant NaCl transporter. The remaining 35% requires active reabsorbtion in the thick loop of Henle and distal tubule.

Calcium and/or vitamin D deficiency contributes to bone fragility in seniors. Intestinal absorption of calcium is reduced by vitamin D deficiency, and in malabsorption states.

Vitamin D Metabolism

The primary source of vitamin D in humans is photoactivation in the skin of 7-dehydrocholesterol to cholecalciferol, which is then converted, first in the liver to 25-hydroxyvitamin D (25(OH)D3) and then subsequently in the kidney to the active form, 1,25(OH)2D3. Regulation of the latter step is by PTH, phosphate and feedback inhibition by 1,25(OH)2D3 itself.

The mounting concern about the relationship between sun exposure and the development of skin cancer has led to increased reliance on dietary sources of Vitamin D. The third NHANE Survey revealed that vitamin D deficiency is widely prevalent in the United States. Vitamin D deficiency can be a result of deficient production of vitamin D in the skin (insufficient UV exposure), lack of dietary intake, accelerated losses of vitamin D, impaired vitamin D activation, or resistance to the biologic effects of 1,25(OH)2D. The elderly and nursing home residents are particularly at risk for vitamin D deficiency, since both the efficiency of vitamin D synthesis in the skin and the absorption of vitamin D from the intestine declines with age.

Regardless of the cause, the clinical manifestations of vitamin D deficiency are predominantly a consequence of the resultant impaired intestinal calcium absorption. Mild to moderate vitamin D deficiency is asymptomatic, whereas long-standing vitamin D deficiency results in hypocalcemia accompanied by secondary hyperparathyroidism, impaired mineralization of the skeleton (osteopenia), with a resultant increased risk for progression to osteoporosis, and proximal myopathy. Vitamin D deficiency has also been shown to be associated with increased mortality rates, including from cardiovascular causes.

Parathyroid Hormone

PTH, an 84 amino-acid hormone, is secreted from the chief cells of the parathyroid glands, which bear calcium-sensing and vitamin D receptors. PTH increases renal phosphate excretion and increases plasma calcium by four principal effects: (1) increasing osteoclastic activity—a rapid response; (2) increasing intestinal absorption of calcium—a slow response; (3) increasing 1α-hydroxylation of vitamin D (the rate-limiting step); and, (4) increasing renal tubular reabsorption of calcium. Hypomagnesemia can suppress the normal PTH response to hypocalcemia.

Calcitonin

Calcitonin is produced by C cells in the thyroid gland. Although, calcitonin inhibits osteoclastic bone resorption and increases the renal excretion of calcium and phosphate, neither excess calcitonin (e.g. from a medullary thyroid carcinoma) nor its deficiency (following thyroidectomy) appear to have any significant effect on the skeleton or bone density. Human calcitonin consists of a peptide chain of 32 amino acids, but there is considerable sequence variability among species, with calcitonin from salmon, which is used therapeutically, being some 10–100 times more potent in lowering serum calcium. Calcitonin is a useful agent for suppressing bone resorption in Paget's disease and osteoporosis and in the treatment of hypercalcemia of malignancy.

Parathyroid Gland and Metabolic Disorders

PTH is secreted by four parathyroid glands found within the thyroid gland in the anterior neck. Secretion of the PTH is in response to the level of serum ionized calcium. Low serum ionized calcium stimulates PTH secretion, whereas high serum ionized calcium suppresses PTH secretion. Another major regulator of PTH is the active form of Vitamin D_3 (1, 25-dihydroxyvitamin D_3 or calcitriol). It suppresses PTH synthesis by its ability to promote intestinal calcium absorption. PTH protects the body from chronic low serum calcium (hypocalcemia); therefore, an individual with chronic hypocalcemia and vitamin D deficiency may develop parathyroid gland hyperplasia.

Hyperparathyroidism

Hyperparathyroidism is chronic excessive secretion of the PTH by the parathyroid glands. It results in uncontrolled chronic hypercalcemia. The condition occurs in 0.1% of adult patients, is more common in the third to fifth decades of life and is three times more prevalent in women than men. The vast majority (90%) of patients with hypercalcemia have either primary hyperparathyroidism or hypercalcemia of malignancy. Modern immunoradiometric and chemiluminometric assays can distinguish between the two, since

PTH is usually elevated or normal in primary hyperparathyroidism, but suppressed when hypercalcemia is caused by a malignancy and its secretion is unrelated to the activity of the parathyroid gland.

Primary hyperparathyroidism refers to excessive PTH secretion. Commonly it is caused by a solitary adenoma (80% of cases), whereas 15% are due to parathyroid hyperplasia and 1% are due to carcinoma of the parathyroid glands. Postmenopausal women are more commonly affected by primary hyperparathyroidism. The amount of PTH secreted usually correlates with the size of glandular enlargement. However, with familial hyperparathyroidism, pathologic parathyroid gland enlargement affects a number of members of the same family. This form of hyperparathyroidism may also be associated with the MEN syndrome types 1, 2A, and 2B or the hyperparathyroid jaw tumor syndrome (HPT-JT). HPT-JT is a rare autosomal dominant disorder consisting of parathyroid cystic adenomas or carcinomas, multiple ossifying fibromas of the mandible and maxilla, and renal disorders that may include cysts, hamartomas, and Wilms' tumors. The risk of developing parathyroid carcinoma is much higher in HPT-JT syndrome.

Secondary hyperparathyroidism occurs with compensatory parathyroid gland enlargement in response to persistent hypocalcemia induced by renal failure (see below), metabolic disorders of deficiency of 1,25-dihydroxyvitamin D, or malabsorption of calcium found in rickets and in some forms of osteomalacia. PTH secretion from enlarged parathyroid glands may become autonomous (secreting without control or response to feedback inhibition), leading to *tertiary hyperparathyroidism.*

The pathophysiology of hyperparathyroidism is related to the tight regualtion of ionized calcium in the extracellular fluid by PTH and vitamin D and the central role of extracellular calcium in both cellular physiology and regulation of metabolism. Specifically, the PTH can be seen as being crucial to the body's defense against hypocalcemia. It binds specific receptors on the surface of PTH-responsive cells such as osteoblasts and renal tubular cells. PTH acts on osteoblastic cells to express RANKL, an inducer of osteoclastic bone resorption. To further maintain normal serum calcium, PTH stimulates renal tubular reabsorption of calcium and magnesium while inhibiting renal tubular reabsorption of phosphate and bicarbonate. This allows elimination of phosphates released from bone during osteoclastic bone resorption so as not to bind to serum ionized calcium. In the kidneys, PTH activates 1-α-hydroxylase, an enzyme that converts inactive vitamin D to the active form. Active vitamin D promotes intestinal absorption of calcium. Therefore, excessive PTH secretion causes diffuse bone resorption, hypercalcemia, and excessive renal excretion of calcium and phosphate. The severity of hypercalcemia is such that it increases calcium in the glomerular filtrate, a process that eventually leads to hypercalciuria and formation of kidney stones. Chronic bone resorption eventually results in patchy cystic bone lesions and pathologic fractures.

Many cases of hyperparathyroidism may be asymptomatic and only detected incidentally by serum analysis during routine serologic evaluation. Clinically, the patients may have manifestations of skeletal and renal disorders and hypercalcemia. The classic quintet of complaints is "bones, stones, abdominal groans, psychic moans, and psychic overtones."

Skeletal presentations include bone demineralization that manifests as reduction in bone mass (osteopenia). Patients complain of bone pains and arthralgia and may develop pathologic fractures. Bone radiographs show well-circumscribed unilocular or multilocular radiolucent lesions known as "brown tumor" of hyperparathyroidism, but brown tumors are now rare occurrences in modern medicine because of early detection. If brown tumors occur, they contain abundant hemorrhagic tissue and hemosiderin, which give them a characteristically dark reddish-brown color. Degeneration of brown tumor leads to patchy osteoclastic bone resorption, cystic lesions, and replacement of bone with abundant vascular cellular fibrous tissue. This transformation is referred to as "osteitis fibrosa cystica." In addition, skull radiographs show patchy regions of demineralization ("salt and pepper" appearance). Due to routine screenings and early detection of hypercalcemia, skeletal presentation is now simply osteopenia, without the classic features of brown tumor. Brown tumors may be seen in developing countries and in patients with parathyroid carcinoma. In patients with HPT-JT syndrome, the multiple fibro-osseous jaw tumors and parathyroid adenomas can occur in isolation. However, unlike the brown tumors of hyperparathyroidism, jaw tumors of HPT-JT are distinct because they do not resolve after parathyroidectomy.

Renal presentations include polyuria and polydipsia as a result of hypercalcemia-induced DI, and 10 to 15% of patients may develop kidney stones consisting of calcium phosphate or calcium oxalate. Nonspecific presentations of hypercalcemia include "abdominal groans" of constipation, indigestion, weight loss, nausea, vomiting, peptic ulceration and pancreatitis, as well as "psychic moans" of lethargy, fatigue, depression, loss of memory, paranoia, neuroses, change in personality, confusion, stupor, and coma. Metastatic calcium precipitation in the cornea may cause keratitis and conjunctivitis, and, if in soft tissues, it may cause calciphylaxis.

The most common laboratory finding in patients with bone lesions is high alkaline phosphatase. Serum calcium is elevated (>10.5 mg/dL), but phosphate may vary from low-normal (<3.5 mg/dL) to low (<2.5 mg/dL). Serum PTH is often elevated, and the level of 1,25-dihydroxyvitamin D may also be high due to the stimulatory effect of PTH on 1-α-hydroxylase. Imaging techniques are required for assessment of a parathyroid adenoma. For symptomatic primary hyperparathyroidism, definitive treatment is surgical parathyroidectomy, which has a 95% success rate. Medical management may involve use of vitamin D when associated with vitamin D deficiency, as well as bisphosphonates and calcimimetics that compete with PTH to decrease its secretion. Medical treatment of hyperparathyroidism also includes the use of the calcium-sensing receptor agonist cinacalcet (Sensipar). As post-menopausal women are commonly affected by hyperparathyroidism, high-dose estrogen replacement therapy is often needed to treat bone lesions and reduce serum calcium, but it does not reduce the PTH level.

Hypoparathyroidism

Hypoparathyroidism is a deficiency in the production, secretion, or action of PTH and is the most frequent cause of hypocalcemia. It usually results when parathyroid glands are surgically removed to correct primary hyperparathyroidism or during thyroidectomy. Hypoparathyroidism can also result from cell-mediated autoimmune glandular destruction associated with mutations of the autoimmune regulator (*AIRE*) gene. It can also occur when there is activating mutations of the calcium-sensing receptor (autosomal dominant hypocalcemia). Radiation to the neck, metastatic cancer, infection, and magnesium deficiency are other unusual causes of hypoparathyroidism. Damage to the parathyroid glands by heavy metals, for example, copper in Wilson's disease or iron in hemochromatosis, and from transfusion hemosiderosis are other unusual causes of hypoparathyroidism. Parathyroid glands may be underdeveloped or completely absent in DiGeorge syndrome, a developmental abnormality of the third and fourth pharyngeal pouches. *Pseudohypoparathyroidism* is a term used to describe a group of disorders that cause hypocalcemia as a result of renal resistance to PTH despite high levels of PTH. Other causes of hypocalcemia in addition to hypoparathyroidism are vitamin D deficiency, hyperphosphatemia, malabsorption of calcium, and chronic renal failure.

Hypocalcemia

Hypocalcemia is often asymptomatic; however, acute hypocalcemia produces symptoms that result from neuromuscular irritability or excitability. This leads to muscular and mental manifestations that include paresthesia of hands, feet, and circumoral muscles; electroencephalographic abnormalities; anxiety; confusion; and depression. A positive Chvostek's sign may be elicited by tapping on the facial nerve in the preauricular region which causes twitching of the facial muscles. Patients may develop tetany characterized by tonic-clonic seizures, carpopedal spasm, and severe laryngospasm. In DiGeorge syndrome, tetany is usually noticed in infancy but may remain undetected until adulthood.

Laboratory findings are of a low PTH and low serum calcium levels, but serum phosphate is elevated and alkaline phosphatase is normal. Most patients with hypocalcemia can be treated with oral calcium and vitamin D supplements, although acute cases may require intravenous calcium infusions.

Chronic Renal Failure

Improved medical management of chronic kidney disease allows many patients to survive for decades and hence potentially have the time to develop renal osteodystrophy and its associated morbidity. Impaired production of 1,25(OH)2D by the diseased kidneys is thought to be the principal factor that causes calcium deficiency, secondary hyperparathyroidism, and bone disease. Hyperphosphatemia typically occurs only in the later stages of chronic kidney disease and lowers blood calcium levels by several mechanisms, including extraosseous deposition of calcium and phosphate, impairment of the bone-resorbing action of PTH, and reduction in 1,25(OH)2D production by remaining renal tissue.

Treatment of the chronic hypocalcemia of renal failure involves the management of patients prior to their commencement of regular dialysis and the adjustment of the treatment regimens once dialysis does become a regular requirement. Treatment entails dietary changes, with the restriction of phosphate in the diet, avoidance of aluminum-containing phosphate-binding antacids to prevent the problem of aluminum intoxication, adequate calcium intake orally, usually 1–2 g/d and supraphysiologic amounts of vitamin D or calcitriol, despite the fact that the uremic state also causes impairment of intestinal absorption of vitamin D. The aim is to restore normal calcium balance to prevent osteomalacia and severe secondary hyperparathyroidism.

Stomatognathic Manifestations of Parathyroid Gland Disorders and Impaired Calcium Homeostasis

Hyperparathyroidism

The primary clinical orofacial signs and symptoms of hyperparathyroidism are reflections of the systemic effects of hypercalcemia. Long-standing hypercalcemia causes generalized osteoporosis, which is visible on dental radiographs. Patients develop cortical resorption and rarefactions, loss of trabeculation presenting as "ground-glass" appearance, partial or total loss of lamina dura, lytic lesions, and metastatic calcifications.[80] The rarefactions occur secondary to generalized osteoporosis when fine trabeculae disappear later in the disease process, leaving a coarse pattern. Alveolar bone is particularly sensitive to increased levels of PTH from either primary or secondary hyperparathyroidism.[81] Thinning and eventual loss of the cortical bone of the maxilla and mandible may occur, especially on the lower border of the mandible. Severe cases may result in spontaneous mandibular fracture.

The lytic jaw lesions or brown tumors[82] can increase in size, causing the bony cortex to expand, ultimately becoming destroyed.[83] These tumors rarely expand into the periosteum but can produce gingival swelling. Biopsy of the lytic lesion is necessary for definitive diagnosis; however, they are histologically similar to central giant cell tumors and giant cell reparative granulomas.[84] Fully developed teeth are not affected except that they appear more radiopaque. Due to bony changes, the teeth become mobile, drift, and cause malocclusion. With gradual loosening of the dentition, periradicular radiolucencies develop, with increased periodontal pocketing, root resorption, and dental pain.

Hypoparathyroidism

In hypoparathyroidism, the resultant hypocalcemia increases muscular and peripheral nerve irritability that may be mistaken for a seizure disorder. Painful muscular spasms affect oral and laryngeal muscles. Despite low serum calcium levels, the maxilla and mandible are abnormally dense, with well-calcified trabeculae. If the hypoparathyroidism is part of an autoimmune polyendocrinopathy syndrome, oral mucocutaneous candidiasis may be readily evident clinically.

If hypoparathyroidism occurs when teeth are still developing, there will be abnormalities in the appearance and eruption pattern. There may be enamel hypoplasia, single or parallel horizontal bands on the enamel, and poorly mineralized dentin. Other dental findings include malformed teeth, anodontia, short blunt root apices, elongated pulp chambers (some occluded by pulp stones, even in the primary dentition), impacted teeth, and mandibular exostoses. If hypoparathyroidism occurs after dental development, there are no abnormalities seen in the erupted teeth.

Dental Management of Patients with Parathyroid Gland Disorders

Hyperparathyroidism

Clinicians must be careful to avoid iatrogenic jaw fractures during oral surgical procedures due to the presence of lytic bone lesions and cortical bone loss. Following successful treatment of hyperparathyroidism, recalcification of the skeleton occurs and serum calcium levels return to normal. Surgical intervention of giant cell tumors is not necessary except to correct large deformities or remove displaced or resorbed teeth.

Hypoparathyroidism

Low serum calcium levels may precipitate cardiac arrhythmias, convulsions, laryngospasm, or bronchospasm. Therefore, consultation with the patient's physicians is required to ascertain the level of metabolic control and update serum calcium and phosphate levels as well as the PTH level. Patients with dental abnormalities require frequent oral examinations due to increased caries risk associated with hypoplastic teeth. Periodic dental radiographs are required to screen for dentigerous cysts that may develop at sites of impacted teeth.

Rickets, Osteomalacia, and Vitamin D Deficiency

The hypocalcemia and hypophosphatemia that accompany vitamin D deficiency result in defective mineralization of newly formed bone matrix or osteoid, a condition known as osteomalacia. Osteomalacia is also a feature of long-standing hypophosphatemia, which may be a consequence of renal phosphate wasting or chronic use of etidronate or phosphate-binding antacids. This hypomineralized matrix is biomechanically inferior to normal bone; as a result, patients are prone to bowing of their weight-bearing extremities and skeletal fractures.

In children, before epiphyseal fusion, vitamin D deficiency results in growth retardation associated with defective mineralization at the epiphyseal growth plate coupled with expansion of the growth plate, known as rickets. Rickets is found in association with osteomalacia in children.

Many factors can result in defective mineralization of the osteoid. For normal mineralization, adequate levels of vitamin D, calcium, and phosphate; adequate activity of alkaline phosphatase; a normal pH at the osteoid surface; and normal osteoid composition are all necessary. The most common cause of osteomalacia is hypophosphataemia due to hyperparathyroidism secondary to vitamin D deficiency. The most common cause of vitamin D deficiency worldwide is dietary deficiency. Ergocalciferol or vitamin D2 derived from plants is insufficient in major food items, so the human daily requirement is supplemented by the formation of cholecalciferol or vitamin D3 in the skin. Dermal synthesis of vitamin D can be impaired by inadequate sunlight in geographic regions of extreme latitude or in cultural regions that wear extensive clothing to cover the whole body. Hepatic and renal disorders can also affect vitamin D metabolism. Bread, milk, and cereals in industrialized countries are now fortified with vitamin D, which has led to a greatly decreased incidence of osteomalacia and rickets.

Osteomalacia may be asymptomatic and identified incidentally. When symptomatic, it characteristically causes muscle weakness and widespread bone pain. The pain is typically a dull ache that is worse on weight-bearing and walking. It can be reproduced by pressure on the sternum or tibia. The muscle weakness is due to a multifactorial proximal myopathy. Patients present with characteristic waddling gait, with difficulty climbing stairs and getting out of a chair and with bone deformities such as bowing of the long bones, scoliosis, bell-shaped thorax, and basilar invagination of the skull. Fractures can also occur. Clinical and radiologic presentations of rickets are skeletal pain and fracture of abnormal bone. Patients with osteomalacia also experience diffuse skeletal pain, especially of the weight-bearing areas. The radiographic presentations are usually nonspecific but may include osteopenia, poorly defined trabecular bone, and masking of the junction between the cortical and trabecular bone. It is common to observe bilateral and symmetric pseudofractures called Looser's zones on several bones (femur, pelvis, ribs, and scapula). Although bone biopsy is usually not necessary for diagnosis, these microfractures are visible in non-decalcified histologic bone sections.

Clinical and radiologic presentations of rickets are usually obvious in children, but diagnosing and identifying the cause of osteomalacia is more challenging. At birth, neonatal rickets may present as craniotabes (thin, deformed skull). In the first few years of life, there may be widened epiphyses at the wrists and beading at the costochondral junctions, producing the "rickety rosary," or a groove in the rib cage (Harrison's sulcus). In older children, lower limb deformities are seen. A myopathy may also occur. Hypocalcaemic tetany may occur in severe cases.

On investigation, the serum alkaline phosphatase is elevated in 90% of cases, with low serum calcium, low phosphate, and elevated PTH, present in approximately half of the cases. The serum 25-(OH)D3 is low, usually less than 25 nmol/L (10 ng/mL), but the serum FGF-23 is elevated in many people with tumor-induced osteomalacia. Plain radiographs demonstrate decreased bone mineralization. The characteristic finding in osteomalacia is Looser's pseudofractures. These are narrow radiolucent lines with sclerotic borders running perpendicular to the cortex. They can be found at any site but are most commonly seen in the femur and pelvis.

Vitamin D replacement is the cornerstone of treatment. Treatment involves two stages: an initial loading stage to replenish body stores of vitamin D and a subsequent maintenance dosing. All patients should also receive supplementary calcium (1000–1200 mg/day). Patients with malabsorption syndrome or those taking barbiturates or phenytoin will require higher doses. Barbiturates and phenytoin cause resistance to 1,25-dihydroxyvitamin D and also accelerate its metabolism.

Stomatognathic Manifestations and Dental Management

Children with rickets/osteomalacia may present with delayed tooth eruption, loss of lamina dura, and enamel and dentine hypoplasia that may progress to periapical infections. Malocclusion and hypoplastic teeth increase the risks of dental caries; therefore, regular oral health evaluation is necessary to monitor dental and periodontal health.

Osteoporosis

Osteoporosis is defined as "a disease characterized by low bone mass and micro-architectural deterioration of bone tissue, leading to enhanced bone fragility and an increase in fracture risk." The WHO defines osteoporosis as a bone density of 2.5 standard deviations (SDs) below the young healthy adult mean value (T-score ≤ –2.5) or lower. Values between –1 and –2.5 SDs below the young adult mean are termed "osteopenia."

Fractures due to osteoporosis are a major cause of morbidity and mortality in elderly populations and a major contributor to rising health costs. Osteoporotic fractures of the spine cause severe, acute pain or deformity and postural back pain. The risk of fracture increases exponentially with age, with one in two women and one in five men aged 50 years, will have an osteoporotic fracture during their remaining lifetime. Caucasian and Asian races are particularly at risk.

Osteoporosis occurs from the increased bone breakdown by osteoclasts and decreased bone formation by osteoblasts, leading to loss of bone mass. Bone mass decreases with age, but will depend on the peak mass attained in adult life (at about the age of 40-45 years) and on the rate of loss in later life. Genetic factors, nutritional status, sex hormone levels, and physical activity all affect peak bone mass.

The main risk factor for osteoporosis is estrogen deficiency. In the elderly, vitamin D insufficiency and consequent hyperparathyroidism are of greater importance. Hyperparathyroidism, hyperthyroidism, and malabsorption each increase the lifetime risk of a person having a low bone mass and low bone mineral density. Additional risk factors are associated with increased bone loss and with increased bone fragility include glucocorticoid therapy and smoking. Falls increase the risk of fracture on top of the risk associated with low bone mass.

Osteoporosis is asymptomatic except after a fracture. Sudden onset of severe pain in the spine radiating anteriorly is indicative of vertebral crush fracture, but in general only about one in three vertebral fractures are symptomatic. Pain also occurs with the mechanical derangement, increasing kyphosis and abdominal protuberances seen with crush fractures of the vertebrae. Colles' fractures typically follow a fall on an outstretched arm. Fractures of the proximal femur usually occur in older persons falling on their side or back. Plain radiographs usually show a fracture and may reveal asymptomatic, but earlier vertebral deformities. Such clinically silent fractures may also be detected during the dual-energy x-ray absorptiometry (DXA) for bone mineral density with additional analysis. Bone density assessment by DXA is the gold standard for the diagnosis of osteoporosis. New vertebral fractures may require bed rest for 1–2 weeks with strong analgesia, muscle relaxants (e.g., diazepam, 2 mg three times daily), and gradual physiotherapy to restore confident mobilization. Intravenous pamidronate can help with severe pain. Nonspinal fractures should be treated by conventional orthopedic means.

Prevention and Treatment of Osteoporosis (and Consequent Fractures)
Lifestyle Modifications

Exercise: lifelong weight-bearing exercise, as little as 30 minutes three times a week, may increase BMD. Gentle exercise in the elderly reduces the risk of falls and improves the protective reflexes needed with falling.

Smoking cessation: should be strongly encouraged as it is associated with lower BMD and increased fracture risk.

Excess alcohol intake (>3 units/day) should be avoided.

Fall reduction: physiotherapy and assessment of home safely, with installation of hand rails and nonslip floor surfaces, especially in wet areas such as the bathroom and toilet.

Vitamin Supplementation

Calcium: research has established that optimal calcium intake reduces bone loss and suppresses bone turnover. For men and women aged 19–50 years, the recommended daily intake is 1000 mg/day and for adults 51 years and older this should be increased to 1200 mg/daily with the best sources being dairy foods, but many patients require calcium supplementation. Optimal calcium supplementation needs to be less than 600 mg at a time, as the calcium absorption decreases at higher doses. Calcium carbonate is best taken with food as it requires acid for solubility, whereas calcium citrate can be taken at any time.

Vitamin D: inadequate vitamin D levels are widely prevalent, hence many adults need supplementation. The Institute of Medicine recommends 200 IU/daily for adults <50 years of age, 400 IU/daily for those 50–70 years, and 600 IU for those >70 years. Multivitamin tablets usually contain 400 IU, and many calcium supplements also contain vitamin D.

Pharmacological Interventions

Estrogen(s): Given the adverse effects of an increased risk for breast cancer and cardiovascular disease risk, hormone replacement therapy (HRT) is a second-line option for osteoporosis except in younger, postmenopausal women at high fracture risk.

Anti-Resorptive Agents

Bisphosphonates are synthetic analogues of bone pyrophosphate that adhere to hydroxyapatite and inhibit osteoclasts. Alendronate, risedronate, and ibandronate are approved for the prevention and treatment of postmenopausal osteoporosis in the US. Aclasta (zoledronic acid) infusion is approved for use in the treatment and prevention of osteoporosis on the UK and Europe. Risedronate and alendronate are approved for the treatment of steroid-induced osteoporosis, with risedronate also approved for the prevention of steroid-induced osteoporosis (in the US).

Bisphosphonates are generally well tolerated, but the orally given agents are associated with upper gastrointestinal side-effects, such as esophagitis, particularly if the dosing instructions are not followed. Bisphosphonates should be used with caution in patients who have severe chronic kidney disease. Bisphosphonate given subcutaneously as an infusion negate the gastrointestinal side effects and ensure patient compliance, thus their increasing popularity for the management of osteoporosis, apart from their established role in malignancy-associated bone diseases (hypercalcemia, bony metastases, and multiple myeloma).

The optimal duration of bisphosphonate therapy is unknown with prolonged suppression of bone turnover having adverse effects, including atypical, low-impact, femoral fractures and osteonecrosis of the jaws (ONJ). Current recommendations are to reassess the need for ongoing bisphosphonate treatment after 3-5 years, although benefits appear to exceed the risk of these complications.

Denosumab (Prolia™, when used for osteoporosis (in contrast to Xgeva when used in the setting of malignancy) is a fully human monoclonal antibody to RANKL. It is given twice yearly by SC administration. Randomized controlled trials in postmenopausal women with osteoporosis has shown to increase BMD in the spine, hip, and forearm and reduce vertebral, hip, and nonvertebral fractures over a 3-year period by 70, 40, and 20%, respectively. Fracture risk reduction is equivalent to bisphosphonates. Interestingly, the risk for osteonecrosis is equivalent to that seen with the more potent bisphosphonates, comparable with the of zolendronic acid in malignancy. In addition to promoting osteoclastogenesis, RANKL has a role in the immune system and denosumab has been associated with exacerbations of eczema and a small increase in severe cases of cellulitis.

Strontium ranelate consists of two strontium atoms linked to ranelic acid. Its mechanism of action remains uncertain, but it has the advantage of being a dual-action agent, with modest antiresorptive activity, coupled with maintenance of bone formation. It increases bone mass throughout the skeleton. Strontium is incorporated into the hydroxyapatite crystal, replacing the calcium atom, a feature that might explain some of its benefits in prevention fracture. In clinical trials, strontium ranelate reduced the risk of vertebral fractures by 37% and that of non-vertebral fractures by 14%. It also reduced the risk of vertebral, hip and other non-vertebral fractures in postmenopausal women with osteoporosis. The dose is 2 g daily, given as granules dissolved in water at night. Nausea, diarrhea and headaches are infrequent side-effects, and the risk of venous thromboembolism is slightly increased. Strontium ranelate is approved in several European countries for the treatment of osteoporosis. To date there has been no ONJ reported with the use of this agent, possibly due to its dual action effects on bone.

Calcitonin preparations are approved by the FDA for Paget's disease, hypercalcemia, and osteoporosis in women >5 years post-menopause. Calcitonin suppresses osteoclast activity by direct action on the osteoclast calcitonin receptor. Osteoclasts exposed to calcitonin cannot maintain their active ruffled border, which is required to maintain close contact with the underlying bone. Calcitonin produces small increments in bone mass of the lumbar spine; however, difficulty of administration, frequent reactions, including nausea and facial flushing, make its general use limited. A nasal spray containing calcitonin (200 IU/d) is available for treatment of osteoporosis in postmenopausal women

Teriparatide (Forteo) is recombinant human parathyroid hormone (rhPTH) peptide 1–34 and is an anabolic agent that stimulates bone formation. Teriparatide reduces vertebral and nonvertebral fractures in postmenopausal women with established osteoporosis, although data on hip fracture is not yet available. It is given by daily subcutaneous injection in a dose of 20 μg for 18–24 months. rhPTH therapy is indicated in severe cases of vertebral osteoporosis or in women who fail to respond to other therapies.

Fluoride has been available for many years and is a potent stimulator of osteoprogenitor cells when studied in vitro. It has been used in multiple osteoporosis studies with conflicting results. Despite increments in bone mass of up to 10%, there are no consistent benefits reported for fluoride on vertebral or nonvertebral fracture rates.

Glucocorticoid-Induced Osteoporosis

Osteoporotic fractures are a well-characterized consequence of the hypercortisolism characteristic for Cushing's syndrome. However, glucocorticoid-induced osteoporosis is a recognized major complication of glucocorticoids used therapeutically and is far more common. The risk of fractures depends on the dose and duration of glucocorticoid therapy, although data now suggests that there may be no completely safe dose.

Patients needing continuous oral glucocorticoid therapy for 3 months or more (at any dose) should be assessed for coexisting risk factors (age, previous fracture, and hormone status). Postmenopausal women and men aged over 50 years, as well as any individuals who have sustained a fracture, should receive treatment for the prevention of osteoporosis and its progression, without awaiting for BMD assessment. To date, only bisphosphonates have been demonstrated to reduce the risk of fractures in patients being treated with glucocorticoids in large clinical trials. Calcium and vitamin D supplementation also needs to be given.

Bisphosphonate-Related Osteonecrosis of the Jaws (BRONJ)[85]

BRONJ is a distinct clinical entity, associated predominantly with the use of the newer, nitrogen-containing (amino-bisphosphonate) agents, wherein patients using these agents developed localized, necrosis of the bones of the jaws (mandible or maxilla), clinically evident in the oral cavity as exposed areas of bone. The condition was described in several case series in 2003 and 2004 and since then has been extensively reported and redefined, to include variants, without frank, clinically exposed bone, but patients have on examination persistent sinus tracts and/or radiographically had patchy radiolucent areas, similar in appearance to that seen with osteomyelitis.

To date, the overwhelming majority of patients with BRONJ have been patients who have received potent amino-bisphosphonate therapy for the treatment and prevention of the lytic bone lesions of multiple myeloma or bony metastases from solid malignancies (generally breast and prostate cancer). However, a small percentage of patients who have received long-term, predominantly oral bisphosphonate therapy for the treatment and prevention of post-menopausal osteoporosis, have also developed BRONJ. Notably, patients are increasingly being given intravenous, potent bisphosphonates, such as zolendronic acid, to improve compliance and avoid gastrointestinal complications seen with the oral bisphosphonates for the treatment and prevention of osteoporosis, but at significantly lower doses than are used in the setting of malignancy.

The incidence of BRONJ in patients taking bisphosphonates for the management of osteoporosis is estimated to be in the range of 0.028 to 4.3%; however, recently published estimates suggests an incidence of only 0.02%, that is

2 in 10,000 patients.[86] This would suggest a very low overall incidence of BRONJ for those patients taking bisphosphonates for osteoporosis, but, from data from case study of patients with BRONJ (admittedly receiving bisphosphonates in the setting of malignancy, advanced age ≥70 years) suggest bisphosphonates increase the risk for the development of BRONJ. Therefore, accepting the risk for BRONJ in patients receiving bisphosphonates the treatment and or prevention of osteoporosis from all causes, postmenopausal, premature menopause, corticosteroid-related osteoporosis and renal osteodystrophy, oral health practitioners need to be mindful of this complication of bisphosphonate and Denosomab use.

Management of Established BRONJ

Initially conservative measures, namely, observation can be used. If signs of infection are evident (active suppuration, the development of facial swelling, in keeping with a collection, or marked regional lymphadenopathy) then provide the patients with antibiotics: amoxicillin in combination with metronidazole or a macrolide (e.g. roxithromycin) with metronidazole or clindamycin. Clindamycin has the advantage of coverage of both gram-positive streptococci and anaerobic bacterial species and good bone penetration. Tetracyclines also have excellent bone penetration, but bacterial resistance is common, limiting these agents' effectiveness. Frequent use of topical antibacterial mouthwashes, such as chlorhexidine-containing mouthwashes should also be instituted (Table 23-14).

Prevention of BRONJ

Poor dental health with active periodontal disease, and/or infectious and inflammatory complications of caries-induced pulpitis is an established risk factor for the development of BRONJ in patients on long-term bisphosphonate therapy. The converse also applies, in that excellent levels of dental health, supported by preventative dental health measures, have been shown to significantly limit the risks of development of BRONJ, even in patients receiving bisphosphonates in the setting of malignancy. This concept needs to be extended, with dental practitioners providing a dentition that patients are best able to maintain and that negates the need for future invasive dental procedures, such as extractions or implant placement,

TABLE 23-14 Interventions to Mitigate the Risk of BRONJ with Invasive Dental Procedures/Treatments of Established BRONJ	
Antibacterial Mouthwashes	– pre- (up to 7 days) and – post-procedural (up to 7 days) frequent (qid) and after meals
Antibiotics	– pre- (up to 7 days) and – post-procedural (up to 7 days)
Antibiotic Regimens	
• amoxicillin (500 mg tds) + metronidazole 400 mg tds • roxithromycin 150 mg bd + metronidazole 400 mg tds • clindamycin 300 mg qid	

given that patients will be in receipt of bisphosphonate therapy for long durations (> 3–5 years) until their BMD score is normalized. For patients needing invasive dental treatment, the risk of such treatment should be carefully balanced against the possible risks of developing BRONJ; however, deferring of extractions of teeth with a poor to dismal prognosis that are otherwise unrestorable, or unmaintable, is also associated with risk since the presence of ongoing infection and associated inflammation in itself increases the risk of BRONJ. So-called "spontaneous" cases of BRONJ have been well documented, occurring in 30% of patients without any invasive dental treatment having been undertaken. Patients will continue to receive further bisphosphonate treatment for their osteoporosis, as the risks of serious bone fracture and their morbid and possible fatal complications outweigh the risks and complications. The risk of BRONJ is now thought to occur in a dose-dependent manner; therefore, it may serve the patient best to undertake the necessary extractions in planned, preemptive fashion, whereby the risk of BRONJ may be mitigated. Mitigation methods include the use of a course of pre-and post-procedural antibiotics with frequent use of antibacterial (chlorhexidine) containing mouthwashes, "gentle" extraction or oral surgical technique, and primary closure. These measures may not prevent BRONJ from developing, but may limit its development to stage 0 or 1, which are highly amenable to conservative and modest surgical interventions.

Table 23-15 with Tables 23-16A and 23-16B assists in estimating and stratifying the risk of BRONJ occurring with invasive dental procedures. For moderate-risk patients,

all the interventions suggested in Table 23-14 should be undertaken after extensive consultation with the patient and the patient's treating physician, including providing detailed and informed consent of the risks for BRONJ occurring. For patients stratified as being at high risk for developing BRONJ, a discussion about the risks versus the benefits of treatment, addressing active pain or infection arising from the involved tooth/teeth, should be undertaken. Referral of such patients to clinicians and or specialized centers experienced in the management of BRONJ should be considered.

There also remains considerable debate regarding the value of "drug holidays" for patients with established BRONJ. Such drug holidays need to be discussed with the patient's treating physician, which should include a an inquiry regarding the use of non-bisphosphonate agents with no known risk for osteonecrosis of the jaws associated with their use (e.g. strontium ranelate, Teriparatide) may prompt consideration of such alternate agents, especially in those patients with BRONJ or with a high risk of developing BRONJ, but requiring invasive dental procedures.

Unfortunately, to date, there appear to be no reliable investigations for determining the optimal time to proceed with invasive dental procedures in patients taking bisphosphonates. Biochemical markers of bone remodeling, such as CTx and NTx, which are present in the blood and can be assessed on serology, are indicative of bone turnover, but this test has not been shown to be reliable in determining the risk for BRONJ occurring; therefore preprocedural serum testing is not presently recommended.[87,88,89,90,91]

TABLE 23-15 Bisphosphonates and Estimated "Window Periods" for Decreased Risk of BRONJ with Invasive Dental Procedures[1]			
Generic Name	Route of Administration	Indication	Window Period: Duration of BP Therap (in months)*
Zoledronic acid	Intravenous	Malignancy-related skeletal events	6
Ibandronate	Intravenous		9
Pamidronate	Intravenous		24
Ibandronate	Oral		24
Etidronate	Oral	Paget's Disease; heterotopic ossification with spinal cord injury; total hip replacement	36
Zoledronic acid	Intravenous	Osteoporosis (non-iatrogenic) treatment/prophylaxis	>36-60?
Pamidronate			
Risedronate	Oral		
Alendronate			

? = uncertain; BP = bisphosphonate
*in which invasive treatment (dental extractions/oral surgery) can be undertaken with a relative <u>lower risk</u> of complications, but not with no risk: risk of BRONJ still is present.

TABLE 23-16A Risk Assessment for BRONJ

Patient Related Factors	Procedural (Surgical) Factors
Amino-Bisphosphonate: • potency • route of administration • duration • clinical indication/usage	• one or more surgical sites • contiguous teeth or multiple separate sites • extent of surgery • mandibular posterior (molar) teeth • proximity of tori

Low Risk Patient
• Amino-Bisphosphonate for Osteoporosis
  - Fosamax (alendronate)
  - any intravenous agent administered only once yearly (or less).
    Eg. Zometa (zoledronic acid)
  - any bisphosphonate agent within designated window period
    (see Table 23-15)
	Low Risk Procedure
	• Routine Office Surgery
	  - routine dental extraction
	  - done under local anaesthetic (LA) in the dental chair
	  - (up to 3 contiguous teeth or 4 separate sites)

High Risk Patient
• Patient on long-term bisphosphonate therapy beyond designated
  window periods (see Table 23-14)
• Bisphosphonate therapy related to malignancy
  - solid cancer metastases; Multiple myeloma
• Aged Patients ≥70 years
• **Immuno-Suppression**
  - recent (within 2 weeks) cytotoxic chemotherapy
  - high-dose corticosteroid administration
  - diabetes mellitus (poorly controlled)
	High Risk Procedure
	• Extensive oral surgery or
	• Extensive number of dental extractions
	  - 5 teeth or more / a dental quadrant
	• Surgical extraction of mandibular molar teeth, impinging on
	  lingual cortical plate &/or mylohyoid ridge
	• Surgery with risk of impinging of tori

TABLE 23-16B Risk Calculator for BRONJ

Risk	Patient-Related Risk Factors	+	Surgical Procedure Risk Factors
Minimal	Low Risk Patient	+	Low Risk Procedure
Medium	Low Risk Patient	+	High Risk Procedure
	High Risk Patient	+	Low Risk Procedure
Significant	High Risk Patient	+	High Risk Procedure

DISORDERS OF INTERMEDIATE METABOLISM

Inheritable Disorders of Connective Tissue: The Skeletal Dysplasias

These include a large group of heterogeneous disorders of collagen adversely affecting the proper development of bone and the connective tissues. All have considerable stomatognathic manifestations and complications.

Marfan's Syndrome (MFS)

This is one of the commonest autosomal dominant inherited disorders of connective tissue, affecting approximately 1 in 5000 of the population worldwide with some 25% of individuals having developed MFS as a consequence of a new mutation. It causes cardiovascular problems, especially of the heart, with sufferers developing aortic aneurysms and dissection, which can be fatal, mitral valve prolapse, and a typical body habitus consisting of a tall, thin body, with long arms, legs and fingers; scoliosis and problems with their the eyes; dislocated lenses; and retinal detachment.

Investigations (are centered on the cardiovascular system and the heart):

- Imaging: image chest x-ray may be normal, but often there are signs of aortic aneurysm, widening of mediastinum, pneumothorax, and scoliosis. CT is useful to detect aortic dilatation and for monitoring its progression.
- Echocardiography demonstrates mitral valve prolapse and mitral regurgitation in the majority of patients.
- ECG: 40% of patients usually have arrhythmia, with premature ventricular tachycardia and atrial arrhythmias.

Management

- Beta-blocker therapy slows the rate of dilatation of the aortic root
- Sedentary activities are encouraged because of the potential adverse effects of exertion on the heart, the pain and potential deformities of the joints, and risk of retinal detachment and lens displacement.
- Annual or more frequent echocardiograms to monitor aortic root dilatation. If the aortic root diameter exceeds 5 cm, this is an indication for aortic root replacement surgery.

Stomatognathic Manifestations and Complications

- Hypermobility with dislocation of the temporomandibular joint.
- High and narrow palatal vault, severe malocclusions with maxillary retrognathy and micrognathia and marked tooth crowding
- Sleep apnea

Ehlers–Danlos Syndrome (EDS)

A highly heterogeneous group of disorders of collagen, with 10 different subtypes recognized; associated with varying degrees of skin fragility, skin hyper-extensibility, and joint hypermobility.

- Types I, II, and III: autosomal dominant inheritance. The biochemical basis for these forms of EDS are yet to be determined.
- Type IV (vascular type): autosomal dominant. It involves the arteries, the bowel, and uterus, as well as the skin. Mutations in COL3A1 gene produce abnormalities in the structure, synthesis, and secretion of Type III collagen.
- Type VI: inheritance is autosomal recessive.
- Type VII: autosomal dominant disorder in which there is a defect in the conversion of procollagen to collagen; *COL1A1* and *COL1A2* mutations delete the N-proteinase cleavage sites.

There are also other rare forms of Ehlers–Danlos syndrome.

Osteogenesis Imperfecta (OI)

A heterogeneous group of mainly autosomally dominant inherited disorders. There are four main types of OI (I-IV), with other clinical subtypes also described (V, VI, and VII). The major clinical feature is bone fragility, but other collagen-containing tissues are also involved, such as tendons, the skin and the eyes and of course the teeth, as dentinogenesis imperfecta.

- Type I: mild bony deformities, blue sclerae, defective dentine, early-onset deafness, hypermobility of joints, and heart valve disorders.

- Type II: perinatal death.
- Type III: severe bone deformity, blue sclerae.
- Type IV: fewer fractures, normal sclerae, normal lifespan.

Treatment involves bisphosphonates (particularly intravenous pamidronate), given from an early age that is stopped at about 18-21 years with growth arrest, and this has considerably improved bone cortical thickness and skeletal development. Overall prognosis is still variable and dependent on the severity of the disease. To date, no cases of ONJ with the use of bisphosphonates in this clinical setting have been reported.

Achondroplasia ("dwarfism")

An autosomal dominant disease, but spontaneous mutations can also occur. The condition is caused by a defect in the fibroblast growth factor receptor-3 gene. The trunk is of normal length, but the limbs are very short and broad due to abnormal endochondrial ossification. The vault of the skull is enlarged, the face is small, and the nose bridge is flat. Intelligence is unaffected. Diagnosis is usually made by fetal ultrasound by progressive discordance between the femur length and the head circumference and diameter. Dental malocclusion is common.

Suggested Readings

Harrison's Principles of Internal Medicine. 18th Edition. Longo, DL, Facui, AS, Kasper DL, Hauser SL, Jameson JL, Loscalzo J. McGraw Hill Medical. 2012. Part 16 Endocrinology and Metabolism. pp 2866-3220.

Kumar and Clark's Clinical Medicine. 8th Edition. Kumar P, Clark M. 2012. Chapters 19 and 20. pp 937-1046.

For the full reference lists, please go to http://www.pmph-usa.com/Burkets_Oral_Medicine.

CHAPTER 24

Neuromuscular Diseases

Eric T. Stoopler, DMD, FDS RCSEd, FDS RCSEng

David A. Sirois, DMD, PhD

Diseases affecting the neuromuscular system have a collective lifetime prevalence rate of 3% to 5%. Thus, every oral health-care provider will encounter a patient who has had, or presently has, a neuromuscular disease diagnosis. The signs and symptoms as well as the complications and implications of these disorders or their treatment can have significant impact on oral health as well as dental management decisions. This chapter focuses on the most common neuromuscular diseases or those with greater impact on the orofacial region and/or dental treatment.

CEREBROVASCULAR DISEASE

Epidemiology and Etiology

Cerebrovascular disease refers to disorders that result in damage to the cerebral blood vessels leading to impaired cerebral circulation. A cerebrovascular accident (CVA), or complete stroke, is a sudden impairment in cerebral circulation resulting in death or a focal neurologic deficit lasting more than 24 hours,[1] neurologic events related to CVA include transient ischemic attack (TIA), defined as a reversible, acute, short-duration, focal neurologic deficit ("mini stroke") resulting from transient (reversible within 24 hours) and localized cerebral ischemia; reversible ischemic neurologic defect (RIND), defined as a reversible, acute, focal neurologic deficit due to transient and localized cerebral ischemia but resulting in neurologic deficits that last more than 24 hours; and stroke in evolution, defined as progressive worsening of stroke symptoms.[1-3]

Despite a 38% decline over the past decade in the relative rate of stroke death and 22.8% decline in actual number of stroke deaths, CVAs remain the fourth leading cause of death and leading neurologic cause of long-term disability in the United States and Europe, with over 795,000

(610,000 first events) strokes and 140,000 stroke-related deaths each year in the United States.[4–6] In 2010, stroke caused approximately 1 of every 19 deaths in the United States. On average, every 40 seconds, someone in the United States has a stroke, and someone dies of a stroke approximately every 4 minutes.[4] Risk for stroke increases with age, with a crude age-adjusted rate per 1000 persons of 0.5 for ages 18 to 44 years, 2.5 for ages 45 to 64 years, 6.9 for ages 65 to 74 years, and 12.4 for ages 75 years and older.[4] As the population ages, it is expected that morbidity and mortality due to stroke will increase, with some estimates of doubling by 2020.[3,5,6] Approximately 15% of all strokes are heralded by a TIA: the short-term risk of stroke after TIA is 3% to 10% at 2 days and 9% to 17% at 90 days. Within 1 year of a TIA, 12% of patients die.[7,8]

Impaired cerebral blood flow leading to ischemia and energy failure is the common pathogenic mechanism for stroke. A 50% decrease in blood flow to the brain for as few as three to four minutes can result in irreversible brain injury. Following infarction, edema and excessive neurotoxic excitation contribute to further regional tissue injury and death. Approximately 15% of strokes result from hemorrhagic events leading to infarction, most often related to hypertension, trauma, substance abuse, or aneurysmal rupture.[1] Eighty-five percent of strokes result from ischemia due to atherosclerotic disease, thromboembolic events, and occlusion of cerebral blood vessels, with neurologic deficits related to the loss of neural function in tissues distal to the event.[1] Three major types of ischemic stroke syndromes have been described: small vessel (lacunar), large vessel (cerebral infarction), and brainstem stroke.

Lacunar strokes result from obstruction of the small (<5 mm diameter) penetrating arterioles supplying the basal ganglia, anterior limb of the internal capsule, and (less commonly) deep cerebral white matter. Age and uncontrolled hypertension are the greatest predisposing factors. Symptoms usually include unilateral motor or sensory deficit without visual field changes or disturbances of consciousness or language. The prognosis for recovery from lacunar infarction is fair to good, with partial or complete resolution usually occurring over four to six weeks.

Cerebral infarction is characterized by extensive downstream ischemia, usually due to a thromboembolic event along the distribution of the internal carotid artery and cerebral arteries. Emboli often originate from the heart after acute myocardial infarction or in hyperdynamic conditions such as chronic atrial fibrillation. Hypertension is an important risk factor in the development of thrombosis, particularly at the carotid bifurcation, and treatment of severe hypertension is essential for the prevention of stroke. High-level brain functions are affected, and the prognosis is poor.

Brainstem infarction results from occlusion of small or large vessels supplying the brainstem, resulting in variable deficits ranging from motor and sensory deficits to death when respiratory centers are affected.

Clinical Manifestations

The clinical manifestations of stroke vary depending on the size and location of the affected brain region. The most common signs and symptoms include sensory and motor deficits, changes (paresis) in extraocular muscles and eye movements, visual defects, sudden headache, altered mental status, dizziness, nausea, seizures, impaired speech or hearing, and neurocognitive deficits such as impaired memory, reasoning, and concentration.[1,9,10]

Diagnosis

Stroke should be considered whenever a patient experiences the clinical manifestations described earlier. Other causes for these signs and symptoms, particularly when focal, may include seizures, hypoglycemia, intracranial tumors, trauma, infection, encephalitis, multiple sclerosis (MS), and prolonged migrainous aura.[9] In addition to a thorough neurologic and cardiovascular examination, anatomic and functional brain imaging is central to the diagnosis of stroke. Time is of the essence for instituting treatment to manage acute stroke. Intracranial hemorrhage must be quickly excluded before life-saving thrombolytic therapy can begin. Although brain magnetic resonance imaging (MRI) provides greater anatomic detail and sensitivity for detection of early infarction, noncontrast computed tomography (CT) scan is the first line of imaging because of its speed, low cost, and availability.[11–13] Laboratory evaluation of the stroke patient includes compete blood count, comprehensive metabolic panel, urinalysis, coagulation profile, and, when indicated, blood culture, echocardiography, and lumbar puncture.[9]

Treatment

The outcome of stroke and related TIAs and RIND is significantly affected by the timeliness of treatment. Early intervention is critical to prevention, treatment, and recovery. TIAs and RIND are treated by reduction in hypertension (lifestyle changes such as diet, exercise, smoking cessation, and stress reduction; medical therapy for hypertension; and anticoagulant or antiplatelet medications).[14] The reader is referred to the chapters in this textbook that describe more thoroughly anticoagulant and antihypertensive therapies.

Management of acute stroke includes medical therapy to reduce bleeding or thromboembolic occlusion, medical therapy to reduce brain edema and neurotoxicity/nerve injury, and surgical interventions (revascularization, hemorrhage control).[9,10,14] Once intracranial hemorrhage has been excluded as the source of acute cerebral ischemia, thrombolysis with intravenous tissue plasminogen activator (t-PA) can improve reperfusion, minimize infarction, and reduce disability.[15] Based on a recent multicenter study demonstrating an expanded window of opportunity for effective t-PA administration following stroke onset,[16] the American Heart Association and the American Stroke Association recently published an advisory statement recommending administration of t-PA from 3 to 4.5 hours after stroke onset.[17] Extensive investigation continues to develop and test new neuroprotective drugs to minimize neurotoxicity, reduce edema, and correct ischemia, mostly among excitatory amino acid antagonists, free radical scavengers, and cytokine inhibitors.[10,14]

Oral Health Considerations

Following stroke, patients may experience several oral problems, including masticatory and facial muscle paralysis, impaired or lost touch and taste sensation, diminished protective gag reflex, and dysphagia. These problems can lead to impairment of food intake, poor nutrition, and weight loss due to diminished taste satisfaction, chewing capacity, and swallowing; choking; and gagging.[18–20] Diminished motor function of masticatory and facial muscles may also reduce food clearance from the mouth and teeth and alone or combined with the presence of diminished dexterity of the arms or hands may adversely affect oral hygiene and increase the risk for caries and periodontal disease.[20,21] Creative and effective use of adjuvant oral hygiene techniques and devices (oral antimicrobial rinse, oral irrigation, floss holders) represent an important approach to oral health promotion and disease prevention, supported by frequent recall examination and prophylaxis. Replacement of missing teeth and adequacy of removable and fixed prostheses are essential to effective chewing and diet.

Dental management of the patient with a history of TIA, RIND, or stroke presents several challenges.[2,18–20] Stroke prevention through routine monitoring of blood pressure is an important step in hypertension risk detection and reduction through referral and effective management. Prior history of TIA or stroke increases the risk of a future or second stroke, with the highest risk during the first 90 days.[5,7,8,22,23] A recent comparative retrospective study[24] examining complications of invasive dental treatment following acute stroke found no evidence to support the historical intuitive guideline[2] to defer elective dental treatment for six months following a stroke or for a patient with active TIAs or RIND. With optimal medical monitoring and poststroke care patients can safely undergo invasive dental treatment, with appropriate consideration for stress reduction, medication interactions and adverse effects, neurologic deficit management, and control of underlying cardiovascular/cerbrovascular risk factors.[24]

Use of antiplatelet and anticoagulant medications is common in patients with a history of stroke, TIA, and RIND. This includes oral aspirin, oral antiplatelet drugs such as ticlopidine and clopidogrel, subcutaneous low-molecular-weight heparin, and, less commonly, warfarin. These medications taken in therapeutic dosages, and for warfarin with an international normalized ratio ≤3.5, rarely require dose modification before routine dental and minor oral surgical treatment.[25–29] For additional information regarding the management of patients taking antiplatelet and anticoagulant medications, the reader is referred to Chapter 19 in this textbook. Concomitant use of nonsteroidal anti-inflammatory drugs (NSAIDs) may increase the risk for bleeding, and their long-term use may reduce the protective effect of aspirin. Potential drug interactions of note include but are not limited to use of metronidazole, erythromycin, and tetracycline, which may alter the bioavailability of warfarin.

Stress reduction and confidence building for the patient during dental visits are important behavioral goals to make the patient comfortable and minimize anxiety-related elevation in blood pressure. Pre- or perioperative inhalation-N_2O-O_2 or oral anxiolytic medication can aid in reducing treatment-related stress and anxiety.

Use of epinephrine-containing local anesthetics is not contraindicated, but they should be used judiciously and follow guidelines recommended for patients with cardiovascular disease; epinephrine-containing impression cord should not be used.[2,24] Blood pressure should be monitored at every visit and within a visit if long and stressful.

MULTIPLE SCLEROSIS
Epidemiology and Etiology

MS is characterized by multiple areas of central nervous system (CNS) white matter inflammation, demyelination, and gliosis (scarring).[30] Myelin is critical for propagation of nerve impulses, and when it is destroyed in MS, slowing and/or complete block of impulse propagation is manifested by abnormal muscular and neurologic signs and symptoms. In Western societies, MS is second only to trauma as a cause of neurologic disability in early to middle adulthood.[31] The clinical course of MS varies from a benign, asymptomatic disease to a rapidly progressive and debilitating disorder.

The age at onset is typically between 20 and 45 years; rarely does MS appear clinically before the age of 10 or after age 60.[30,31] MS is more common among women than men (2:1 ratio); however, in patients with later onset of MS, the sex ratio tends to be more even. The geographic distribution of MS is uneven; in general, the prevalence of MS increases with increasing distance from the equator.[32] When racial differences are correlated with prevalence rated for MS worldwide, white populations are at greatest risk and both black and Asian populations have a low risk of disease.[30]

Although the cause of MS is unknown, genetic susceptibility to MS clearly exists, and it is thought that an initial trigger leads to autoimmune mechanisms causing demyelination. The major histocompatibility complex (MHC) on chromosome 6p21 has been identified as one genetic determinant for MS.[33] The MHC encodes the genes for the human leukocyte antigen (HLA) system, and susceptibility to MS lies with the class II alleles, particularly the class II haplotypes DR15, DQ6, and Dw2.[30] Although other genetic regions have been implicated in MS susceptibility on chromosomal regions 19q35, 17q13, 17q23, and 5q33, recent data suggest that these contribute minimally to the risk of MS compared to the HLA.[33,34]

Substantial evidence suggests that autoimmune mechanisms are involved in the pathogenesis of MS.[34] Myelin basic protein (MBP) is an important T-cell antigen that is critical in the development of experimental allergic encephalomyelitis (EAE) in animals. Certain forms of EAE are pathologically similar to MS, and activated MBP-reactive T cells are often found in the blood or cerebrospinal fluid (CSF) of MS patients, supporting the autoimmune theory of MS pathogenesis.[32] Increased levels of immunoglobulin G (IgG) and cytokines such as tumor necrosis factor are commonly detected in the CSF of patients with MS.[35,36]

Epidemiologic evidence supports the role of an environmental exposure in MS, and two common infectious agents to be implicated in the pathogenesis of this disease are Epstein–Barr virus and human herpesvirus 6.[37] Other viruses that have been implicated in the pathogenesis of MS include measles, mumps, rubella, *Chlaymydia pneumoniae*, parainfluenza, vaccinia, and human T-lymphotropic virus 1.[30,37]

MS lesions or "plaques" vary in size and are characterized by perivenular cuffing with inflammatory mononuclear cells, predominantly macrophages and T cells, that is generally limited to the white matter and periventricular areas of the CNS.[38] Recent studies have established that demyelinated lesions are also commonly found in the cortical gray matter and meningeal inflammation is prominent in early MS.[39] Plaques may be found in both the brain and spinal cord, and within the plaques, there is variable destruction of myelin and neuronal axons with preservation of the ground structure.[30] Uniform areas of incomplete myelination are called shadow plaques and may be evident in chronic lesions of MS.[31]

The major clinical type of MS that affects nearly 85% of those suffering from the disease is termed relapsing/remitting multiple sclerosis (RRMS).[38] This is characterized by discrete attacks that generally evolve over days to weeks and often follows with complete recovery from symptoms. RRMS may evolve into secondary progressive multiple sclerosis (SPMS), which is characterized by a steady deterioration in function unassociated with acute attacks. Approximately 25% to 40% of patients with RRMS will develop SPMS after 20 years.[31,40] Other minor forms of MS include primary progressive multiple sclerosis (PPMS), in which patients display steady functional decline from disease onset without attacks, and progressive/relapsing multiple sclerosis (PRMS) that features clinical characteristics of both PPMS and SPMS.

Clinical Manifestations

The onset of MS may be insidious or abrupt, and symptoms range from trivial to severe. The clinical course of disease generally extends for decades, but a rare few cases are fatal within a few months of onset. The clinical manifestations of MS depend on the areas of the CNS involved, and frequently affected areas include the optic chiasm, brainstem, cerebellum, and spinal cord.[30,38] The sudden onset of optic neuritis (diminished visual acuity, dimness, or decreased color perception), without any other CNS signs or symptoms, is often considered the first symptom of MS. Other common visual signs in patients with MS include diplopia, blurring, nystagmus, gaze disturbances, and visual field defects.[38]

Limb weakness is characteristic of MS and can manifest as loss of strength or dexterity, fatigue, or gait disturbances. Spasticity associated with painful muscle spasms is often observed in the legs of patients with MS and may interfere with a patient's ability to ambulate. Ataxia may affect the head and neck of MS patients and may result in cerebellar dysarthria (scanning speech). Bladder dysfunction and bowel dysfunction frequently coexist and are present in >90% of MS patients. MS patients often demonstrate sensory impairment, including paresthesia and hyperesthesia. Fatigue, sleep disorders, depression, cognitive dysfunction, and chronic pain are often observed in patients with MS.[30,41]

Patients with MS often experience exacerbation of neurologic symptoms in response to an elevation of the body's core temperature. This is referred to as Uhthoff symptom and is often seen in response to increased physical activity.[30] MS patients frequently complain of electric shock–like sensations that are evoked by neck flexion and radiate down the back and into the legs. This is referred to as Lhermitte's symptom and is generally self-limiting but may persist for years.[30]

Diagnosis

There is no definitive diagnostic test for detection of MS. Recent formulations of the diagnostic criteria for MS begin with an initial clinical presentation typical for an MS attack, usually involving the optic nerves, brainstem, or spinal cord.[40] Once MS is suspected, the clinician must evaluate for evidence of dissemination in space (DIS), which requires multiple areas of CNS involvement, and for dissemination in time, which requires ongoing disease activity over time.[40] MRI demonstrates characteristic abnormalities of MS in >95% of patients.[30] MS plaques are visible as hyperintense focal areas on T_2-weighted images that are characteristic of chronic lesions. T_1-weighted images reveal hypointense areas that are usually indicative of active MS lesions.[30] Current DIS MRI criteria requires at minimum only two lesions: at least one T_2 lesion in at least two of four sites typically affected by MS, including periventricular, juxtacortical, infratentorial, and spinal cord.[40,42] Advanced imaging techniques that are currently being evaluated for possible future clinical application include diffusion tensor imaging, magnetization transfer imaging, proton magnetic resonance spectroscopy, and functional MRI.[42] Evoked potentials measure CNS electrical potentials, and abnormalities are detected in up to 90% of patients with MS. CSF is often analyzed in patients suspected of having MS, and positive findings include an increase in total protein and mononuclear white blood cells. In addition, there is often an increase in intrathecally synthesized IgG in patients with MS.[43]

Treatment

Therapy for MS can be divided into three categories: (1) treatment of acute attacks, (2) disease-modifying therapies, and (3) symptomatic therapy.[30,31] Glucocorticoids are used to manage both initial attacks and acute exacerbations of MS. Intravenous methylprednisolone is typically administered at a dose between 500 and 1000 mg/d for three to five days to reduce the severity and length of an attack.[38] Disease-modifying agents include injectable interferon (IFN)-β1a, IFN-β1b, and glatiramer acetate.[44] All four pharmacologic agents slow progression of relapsing disease and reduce the annual relapse rate by 20% to 40%.[44] Natalizumab is a humanized monoclonal antibody that binds α-4 integrin, a cell-surface adhesion molecule on leukocytes, and inhibits early steps of MS pathogenesis.[44,45] It has demonstrated significant efficacy in reducing annualized relapse rates, reduction of disease activity on MRI, and decrease in disability progression.[44,45] Mitoxantrone (Novantrone) is a chemotherapeutic agent administered intravenously that is effective in reducing neurologic disability and frequency of clinical relapses in patients with SPMS, PRMS, and worsening RRMS.[46] Fingolimod, which inhibits T-cell migration, is the first oral drug to receive regulatory approval in North America and Europe to reduce relapses in patients with relapsing MS.[44] Common agents employed for management of specific MS symptoms often include anticonvulsants, benzodiazepines, tricyclic antidepressants, smooth muscle relaxants, anticholinergic agents, and various pain medications.[31,47]

The prognosis for the individual patient with MS is variable. It is difficult to predict the course of MS in an individual patient; however, earlier age of onset, female sex, fewer number of baseline brain MRI lesions at time of clinical diagnosis and less disability five years after onset are generally considered favorable prognostic signs.[30] Most patients with MS experience progressive neurologic disability and gait disturbances and/or difficulty with ambulation are common clinical sequelae for patients with this disease.[48] Mortality as a direct consequence of MS is uncommon, and death usually results from a complication of the disease, such as pneumonia.

Oral Health Considerations

Individuals may present to the oral health-care provider with signs and symptoms of MS. Trigeminal neuralgia (TGN), which is characterized by electric shock–like pain, may be an initial manifestation of MS in up to 5% of cases.[31,49,50] MS-related TGN is similar to idiopathic TGN, and the reader is referred to the chapter in the textbook that describes idiopathic TGN more thoroughly. Features of MS-related TGN include possible absence of trigger zones and continuous pain with lower intensity.[50] Medications often used to manage TGN are similar to those used for treatment of idiopathic TGN, and the reader is referred to the chapter that describes these medications and alternative therapies.

Patients with MS may also demonstrate neuropathy of the maxillary (V2) and mandibular branches (V3) of the trigeminal nerve, which may include burning, tingling, and/or reduced sensation. Neuropathy of the mental nerve can cause numbness of the lower lip and chin.[43] Myokymia may be seen in patients with MS and consists of rapid, flickering contractions of the facial musculature secondary to MS lesions affecting the facial nerve.[51] Facial weakness and paralysis may also be evident in MS patients. Dysarthria that results in a scanning speech pattern is often seen in patients with MS. Other orofacial pain conditions that may be present at higher frequency in patients with MS compared to the general population include temporomandibular disorder and headache.[52,53] If MS is suspected, oral health-care professionals should carefully evaluate cranial nerve function. If cranial nerve abnormalities are detected upon examination, the individual should be referred to a neurologist for further evaluation.

It is recommended to avoid elective dental treatment in MS patients during acute exacerbations of the disease due to limited mobility and possible airway compromise.[54,55] Clinicians must evaluate the level of motor dysfunction of patients with MS as this may affect provision of dental care. Patients with significant dysfunction may require dental treatment in an operating room under general anesthesia due to the inability to tolerate treatment in an outpatient setting. In addition, electric toothbrushes and oral hygiene products with larger handles may be necessary for completing oral hygiene in patients with significant motor impairment. It is critical for oral health-care providers to maintain accurate medication inventories for patients with MS and to be aware of possible interactions of these medications with those commonly used and prescribed in dentistry, as well as oral and systemic side effects of these agents.

ALZHEIMER'S DISEASE

Epidemiology and Etiology

Dementia is defined as an acquired deterioration in cognitive abilities that impairs the successful performance of activities of daily living.[56] Memory is the most common cognitive ability lost with dementia; other mental faculties affected include problem-solving skills, judgment, visuospatial ability, and language. There are an estimated 5.3 million cases of dementia in the United States with an expected increase to 18.5 million cases by 2050.[57] The global prevalence of dementia is estimated at 24 million and has been predicted to quadruple by the year 2050.[58] Alzheimer's disease (AD) is the most common form of dementia in Western countries, accounting for up to 65% of new cases.[56,59,60] The clinical features of AD were first described in 1906 by Alois Alzheimer[61]; more than a century later, the molecular basis of AD has been greatly elucidated, and enhanced diagnostic modalities have enabled clinicians to visualize neurologic changes secondary to AD.

AD is characterized by neuritic plaques and neurofibrillary tangles coupled with a degeneration of neurons and synapses. The most severe pathology associated with AD is usually found in the medial temporal lobe structures and cortical areas of the brain.[59] Neuritic plaques contain a central core of amyloid β (Aβ) peptide derived from amyloid precursor protein (APP), a transmembrane protein that has neurotrophic and neuroprotective effects. An imbalance between the production and clearance of Aβ in the brain, termed the amyloid cascade hypothesis, is thought to be the disease-initiating event that ultimately leads to neuronal degeneration and dementia.[59] Recent studies have suggested a more complex pathophysiology regarding Aβ processing than previously thought.[62,63] Amyloid is deposited around meningeal and cerebral vessels, termed *amyloid angiopathy*, and may lead to cerebral lobar hemorrhages.

Neurofibrillary tangles are twisted neurofilaments in neuronal cytoplasm that represent abnormally phosphorylated tau protein and appear as paired helical filaments by electron microscopy.[56] Tau protein is thought to aid in assembly and stabilization of the microtubules that convey cell organelles and glycoproteins through the neuron. In AD, tau becomes hyperphosphorylated and leads to sequestration of normal tau and other microtubule-associated proteins, thus impairing axonal transport and normal neuronal function. In addition, tau becomes prone to aggregation into insoluble fibrils that develop into tangles, further compromising neuronal function.[59]

The genetic basis of AD has been studied extensively, and specific genetic mutations have been implicated in both the familial and sporadic forms of the disease. Familial AD is an autosomal dominant disorder with onset typically prior to age 65 years. Mutations in the *APP* gene on chromosome 21 were the first to be identified as the cause of familial AD; subsequent investigations have demonstrated mutations in the *presenilin 1 and 2* genes (*PSEN1* and *PSEN2*, respectively) that account for the majority of familial AD cases.[64,65] The most commonly reported gene associated with sporadic AD is apo-lipoprotein E (*APOE*) on chromosome 19, which is involved in cholesterol transport.[56,59,64] The e4 allele accounts for most of the genetic risk in sporadic AD.[59] Mutations of the sortilin-related receptor (*SORL1*) has been associated with both late-onset AD and sporadic AD.[63,66]

Clinical Manifestations

AD is a slowly progressive disorder represented by a continuum of clinical characteristics. Updated clinical criteria recognizes three stages of AD: (1) preclinical AD, (2) mild cognitive impairment due to AD, and (3) dementia due to AD.[67] Preclinical AD occurs before changes in cognition, and everyday activities are observed and primarily used for research purposes.[68] Cognitive impairment (CI) due to AD is characterized by mild changes in memory and other cognitive abilities that are noticeable to patients and families but are not sufficient to interfere with day-to-day activities. Dementia due to AD is characterized by changes in two or more aspects of cognition and behavior that interfere with the ability to function in everyday

life.[67] The initial signs of AD involve retrograde amnesia from progressive declines in episodic memory.[69] This may initially go unrecognized or be viewed as forgetfulness; however, as the disease progresses, memory loss begins to affect performance of daily activities, including following instructions, driving, and normal decision making. As AD progresses, the individual is often unable to work, gets confused and lost easily, and may require daily supervision. Language impairment, loss of abstract reasoning skills, and visuospatial deficits begin to interfere with simple, routine tasks. Advanced AD is characterized by loss of cognitive abilities, agitation, delusions, and psychotic behavior.[56] Patients may develop muscle rigidity associated with gait disturbances and often wander aimlessly. In end-stage AD, patients often become rigid, mute, incontinent, and bedridden.[59] Help is needed for basic functions, such as eating and dressing, and patients may experience generalized seizure activity. Death often results from malnutrition, heart disease, pulmonary emboli, or secondary infections.[56]

Diagnosis

Diagnosis of preclinical AD primarily utilizes biomarker assessment, including markers of Aβ protein deposition in the brain (low CSF Aβ42 and positive positron emission tomography [PET] amyloid imaging), and markers of downstream neurodegeneration (elevated CSF tau [total and phosphorylated], decreased metabolism in temporal and parietal cortex on ^{18}F-fluorodeoxyglucose PET and brain atrophy on MRI.[67] Clinical diagnosis of AD is based on an individual's medical history together with the clinical and neurologic examination findings. Criteria include a history of progressive deterioration in cognitive ability in the absence of other known neurologic or medical problems.[70] Generally, when mental status changes are suspected, a cognitive screening test, such as the Mini-Mental State Examination may be used to assess global cognitive abilities.[69] Definite AD is reserved only for autopsy-confirmed disease. If there is no associated illness, the condition is called probable AD; possible AD refers to those who meet the criteria for dementia but have another illness that may contribute to the neurologic status, such as hypothyroidism or cerebrovascular disease.[64]

Diagnostic analysis of CSF may show a slight increase in tau protein and a lower concentration of Aβ peptide compared with healthy individuals or those with other dementias. Electroencephalographic (EEG) studies typically demonstrate generalized slowing without focal features. Neuroimaging is important in evaluating suspected AD to exclude alternative causes of dementia, such as cerebrovascular disease, subdural hematoma, or brain tumor. MRI and CT typically reveal dilatation of the lateral ventricles and widening of the cortical sulci, particularly in the temporal regions.[64] Volumetric MRI uniformly demonstrates shrinkage in vulnerable brain regions, especially the entorhinal cortex and hippocampus.[64] PET can identify areas of hypometabolism in the temporal, parietal, and posterior cingulated cortices and has a high ability to differentiate AD from other dementias.[59]Slowly progressive decline in memory and orientation, normal results on laboratory tests, and neuroimaging showing only diffuse or posteriorly predominant cortical and hippocampal atrophy are highly suggestive of AD.[56]

Treatment

There is no cure for AD, and therapy is aimed at slowing the progression of the disease. Cholinesterase inhibitors are approved by the US Food and Drug Administration to treat mild to moderate cases of AD and are considered the standard of care.[71,72] The four types of cholinesterase inhibitors currently available are tacrine, donepezil, rivastigmine, and galantamine; tacrine is now rarely used due to its hepatotoxic effects. These medications decrease the hydrolysis of acetylcholine released from the presynaptic neuron into the synaptic cleft by inhibiting acetylcholinesterase, resulting in stimulation of the cholinergic receptor.[64] Common side effects of these medications include nausea, vomiting, diarrhea, weight loss, bradycardia, and syncope.[71]Memantine, a noncompetitive N-methyl-D-aspartate receptor antagonist believed to protect neurons from glutamate-mediated excitotoxicity, is used for treatment of moderate to severe AD.[71] Studies have demonstrated greater cognitive and functional improvement when memantine is used in conjunction with cholinesterase inhibitors compared to monotherapy.[73] Antidepressants, such as selective serotonin reuptake inhibitors, are commonly used to treat depression, which is often seen in the mild to moderate stages of AD.[59,74] Antipsychotic agents are used for those patients who display aggressive behavior and psychosis, especially in the later stages of the disease. Other agents that have been reported to be of clinical value in the treatment of AD include antioxidants, such as selegiline and α-tocopherol (vitamin E), cholesterol-lowering drugs, anti-inflammatories, and herbal remedies, such as Ginkgo biloba.[59,71,73] Currently, disease-modifying agents aimed at reducing Aβ production, preventing Aβ aggregation, promoting Aβ clearance, and targeting tau phosphorylation and assembly are being investigated for future clinical use in the treatment of AD.[73,75] Caregivers of patients with AD must be involved in the overall treatment as they are responsible for maintaining the patient's general health and ensuring a meaningful quality of life; it is often necessary to provide educational, emotional, and psychological support to these individuals as the task for caring for patients with AD can be extremely challenging.

Oral Health Considerations

Oral and dental health is a major issue in patients with AD because significant deterioration in oral health status is commonly observed with advancing disease.[76,77] Patients with AD appear to be at higher risk for developing coronal and root caries, periodontal infections, temporomandibular

joint abnormalities, and orofacial pain compared to healthy subjects.[60,78] Oral health-care providers should be able to recognize symptoms of AD and refer patients for further medical evaluation, if necessary. Patients with AD can become frustrated, irritable, and possibly combative when confronted with unfamiliar circumstances or with questions, instructions, or information that they do not understand.[76] The presence of a caregiver may be beneficial as they can verify patient information, interpret patient behavior, and alleviate anxiety.[78] The oral health-care provider must approach AD patients with empathy and explain all procedures and instructions clearly. Patients with AD should be placed on an aggressive preventive dentistry program, including an oral examination, oral hygiene education, prosthesis adjustment, and a three-month recall.[79] Specially adapted products, such as modified toothbrushes and foam mouth props, may be useful for oral hygiene and provision of dental care in patients with AD.[78] It is recommended to complete restoration of oral health-care function in the earliest stages of AD because the patient's ability to cooperate diminishes as cognitive function declines.[76] Time-consuming and complex dental treatment should be avoided in persons with severe AD.[80]

Medications used to treat AD can cause a variety of orofacial reactions and potentially interact with drugs commonly used in dentistry. Cholinesterase inhibitors may cause sialorrhea, whereas antidepressants and antipsychotics are often associated with xerostomia. In addition, dysgeusia and stomatitis have been reported with use of antipsychotic agents.[76] Antimicrobials, such as clarithromycin, erythromycin, and ketoconazole, may significantly impair the metabolism of galantamine, resulting in central or peripheral cholinergic effects.[76] Anticholinesterases may increase the possibility of gastrointestinal irritation and bleeding when used concomitantly with NSAIDs.[76] Local anesthetics with adrenergic vasoconstrictors should be used with caution in AD patients taking tricyclic antidepressants due to potential risk of cardiovascular effects, such as hypertensive events or dysrhythmias.[73]

SEIZURE DISORDERS
Epidemiology and Etiology

A seizure is a paroxysmal event due to abnormal, excessive, hypersynchronous discharges from neuronal aggregates in the CNS.[81,82] The term *epilepsy* describes a group of neurologic disorders characterized by recurrent seizure activity.[81] The incidence of epilepsy in developed countries is approximately 50 per 100,000 people per year (approximately 1% of the US population) and is higher in infants and elderly people.[81,83]

The International League Against Epilepsy originally developed a classification system of the epilepsies and epileptic syndromes based on the clinical features of seizure activity and associated EEG changes.[84] Subsequent revisions of the classification scheme have taken into consideration several other factors in classifying epileptic syndromes, such as genetics, age at onset, and pathophysiologic mechanisms of disease.[82,85] Focal, generalized and unknown seizures are currently the three major categories of seizure activity used in clinical practice.[82]

The focal seizure category includes partial seizures; this type of seizure activity originates within networks limited to one hemisphere and clinical manifestations of these seizures depend on the site of origin.[82,86] Partial seizures are characterized by two concurrent activities in an aggregate of neurons: high-frequency bursts of action potentials and hypersynchronization.[81] Generalized seizures arise from both cerebral hemispheres simultaneously and have distinctive clinical features that facilitate diagnosis.[81] The underlying pathophysiology of generalized seizures is attributed to abnormal neuronal excitability and is poorly understood. Absence seizures (petit mal) are a type of generalized seizure that is characterized by sudden, brief lapses of consciousness without loss of body tone and may be attributed to abnormal oscillatory rhythms generated during sleep by circuits connecting the thalamus and cortex.[81] Tonic-clonic (grand mal) seizures are generalized seizures that present with dramatic clinical features, most notably, tonic contracture and uncoordinated clonic muscular movements.[83] Other types of generalized seizures include atypical absence, atonic, and myoclonic seizures. Those seizures that cannot be classified as either focal or generalized are termed unknown seizures.[82]

Onset of seizure activity may occur at any point throughout an individual's life, and etiology usually varies according to patient age. The most common seizures arising in late infancy and early childhood are febrile seizures without evidence of associated CNS infection; these usually occur between 3 months and 5 years of age and have a peak incidence between 18 and 24 months.[81,87] Isolated, nonrecurrent, generalized seizures among adults are caused by multiple etiologies, including metabolic disturbances, toxins, drug effects, hypotension, hypoglycemia, hyponatremia, uremia, hepatic encephalopathy, drug overdoses, and drug withdrawal.[83,88] Cerebrovascular disease may account for approximately 50% of new cases of epilepsy in patients older than 65 years.[89] Other etiologies for epilepsy include degenerative CNS disease, developmental disabilities, and familial/genetic factors.[83,89] Epilepsy occurs more frequently in individuals who have neurologic-based disabilities, such as cerebral palsy and autism.[90,91]

Clinical Manifestations
Focal Seizures (Partial Seizures)

Simple partial seizures reflect neuronal discharge from a discrete cortical locus, such as the motor cortex of the frontal lobe, or in subcortical structures, and generally not associated with impaired consciousness.[82] Simple partial seizures consist of clonic activity, which are rapid jerks that also can be accompanied by somato-sensory phenomena, visual changes/distortions, and auditory, olfactory, and gustatory symptoms.[81,86] These seizures can spread over a progressively larger region of the motor cortex, resulting in Jacksonian march, a phenomenon characterized by sequential involvement of the muscles in an extremity.

Complex partial seizures, the most common type of seizure in adults with epilepsy, result in either a loss or a impairment of consciousness.[86] Many of these seizure foci originate within the temporal and inferior frontal lobes, causing patients to appear confused and to experience visual or auditory hallucinations. The seizures frequently begin with an aura (a warning of impending seizure activity) that may consist of a sense of fear, detachment, and/or intense odors/sounds. The patient displays automatisms during the seizure, which are involuntary automatic behaviors that vary from chewing and lip smacking to violent behavior.[92]

Generalized Seizures

Absence seizures are characterized by seconds of unconsciousness with no loss of body tone.[93] In addition, subtle facial twitching and rapid eye blinking are often observed without generalized clinical muscular activity. Patients suffering from absence seizures appear to be "daydreaming," although they often have the ability to continue performing a previously started motor or intellectual activity after cessation of the seizure activity. There is generally no postictal confusion in patients experiencing absence seizures. Absence seizures generally begin in childhood and up to 90% of patients with these seizures have a spontaneous remission before adulthood.[86]

Tonic-clonic seizures characteristically begin abruptly and may or may not be preceded by an aura. The patient loses consciousness, while the entire musculature contracts forcibly, lasting between 20 and 40 seconds.[93] Contraction of the muscles of the larynx and forced expiration can produce a loud moan, often termed "epileptic cry." Patients often become cyanotic during the tonic phase secondary to forceful closing of the mouth accompanied with forced continued expiration. The clonic phase follows with the entire body rhythmically jerking for a period that usually lasts no longer than one minute. In the postictal phase, the patient may be unresponsive for minutes to hours, awakening gradually, often with no memory of the event.[93] Physical injury from falling or muscular convulsions and evidence of bladder emptying, tongue biting, or aspiration pneumonia are often experienced during the postictal phase.[81] Patients gradually regain consciousness and often complain of fatigue and headache after a tonic-clonic seizure. Generalized tonic-clonic seizures may not abate spontaneously or may recur without the patient regaining consciousness. This condition is referred to as generalized convulsive status epilepticus and is considered a medical emergency due to the number of serious sequelae of this condition, including bodily injury, cardiorespiratory dysfunction, metabolic derangements, and irreversible neurologic damage.[94]

Photosensitivity epilepsy is characterized by seizure activity induced by visual stimuli, such as stroboscope illumination, flickering sunlight, and high-contrast black and whitepatterns.[95] Photosensitive epilepsy has been shown to induce generalized tonic-clonic, partial, myoclonic, and atypical absence seizures.[95]

Diagnosis

The primary goals of evaluating a patient with new onset of seizure activity are to establish whether the reported episode was a true seizure, to determine the cause of the seizure by identifying possible risk factors and precipitating events, and to determine the need for antiepileptic drug (AED) therapy in addition to treatment of any underlying illness.[81] An in-depth history and physical examination are critical as the diagnosis of a seizure may be based on clinical findings only. A complete neurologic examination is required for all patients with suspected seizure activity, including testing of cranial nerve function, assessment of mental status, and testing of motor function. Blood studies, such as a complete blood count, electrolytes, glucose, magnesium, and calcium, are performed routinely to identify metabolic causes of seizure activity. Other useful screening tests include toxin screens to identify seizure activity due to drugs and lumbar puncture to rule out any infectious etiologies.

All patients with a possible seizure disorder are referred for brain imaging to determine underlying CNS structural abnormality and/or pathology. MRI is the diagnostic modality of choice for the detection of hippocampal sclerosis, malformations of cortical development, vascular malformations, tumors, and acquired cortical damage, all of which are common etiologies for seizure disorders.[96,97] Functional imaging, including nuclear medicine studies and functional MRI, may help to localize focal structural abnormalities and aid in surgical planning.[97] CT is valuable for investigating intracranial calcification, skull fractures, and suspected CNS infection, which may not be as readily apparent on an MRI.[96]

An EEG is an important diagnostic tool for patients with suspected seizures and is helpful for classifying seizure disorders and to determine the type of AED, if indicated.[86,88] The EEG measures the electrical activity of the brain, and the presence of abnormal, repetitive, rhythmic electrical activity having an abrupt onset and termination during the clinical event ("spike—wave pattern") establishes the diagnosis of seizures.[81]

Treatment

Pharmacologic therapy is considered the mainstay of epilepsy treatment, and the goal is to choose an AED that is most appropriate for the specific type of seizure activity and to administer it in the proper dose to achieve control of seizure activity with minimal side effects.[87,98]

Multiple AEDs are currently available for the treatment of epilepsy, and selection of a particular agent is often influenced by several factors, including medical comorbidities, drug availability, and cost.[86,98] Lamotrigine, carbamazepine, and phenytoin are indicated for the treatment of partial seizures, including those that secondarily generalize.[83] Phenytoin has a long half-life and is dosed less frequently than carbamazepine and lamotrigine, leading to increased patient compliance. Phenytoin is associated with gingival overgrowth, hirsutism, and coarsening of facial features. Carbamazepine can cause hepatotoxicity, leukopenia, and aplastic anemia, whereas lamotrigine has been associated with skin rash. Additional therapies for patients with partial seizures include topiramate, gabapentin, and oxcarbazepine.

Valproic acid is indicated for treatment of generalized tonic-clonic seizures and may cause bone marrow suppression and hepatotoxicity, which requires laboratory monitoring. This AED should be avoided in patients with pre-existing bone marrow or liver disease. Lamotrigine, levetiracetam, carbamazepine, and phenytoin are alternative treatments for generalized tonic-clonic seizures.[98] Ethosuximide has been shown to be particularly effective for the treatment of uncomplicated absence seizures. Recently, perampanel, a novel AED influencing glutamatergic postsynaptic transmission, has been introduced as an adjunctive treatment for refractory partial seizures.[99]

Discontinuation of pharmacologic therapy is considered when seizure control has been achieved. The following patient characteristics yield the greatest chance of remaining seizure free after discontinuation of drug therapy: (1) complete medical control of seizures for one to five years; (2) single seizure type; (3) normal neurologic examination, including intelligence; and (4) a normal EEG.[81] Many patients are often withdrawn successfully from medication after an interval of two to four years without seizures who meet the above criteria and who clearly understand the risks and benefits.[98]

In patients with refractory epilepsy, it often becomes necessary to use a combination of AEDs to attempt seizure control. Patients may use three or more drugs to successfully treat refractory epilepsy; however, up to 30% of patients are resistant to all medical therapies.[99] Surgical procedures may be indicated for these patients, including limited removal of the hippocampus and amygdala, temporal lobectomy, or hemispherectomy.[81] Those patients who are not candidates for resective brain surgery may benefit from vagus nerve stimulation (VNS), which involves placement of an electrode on the left vagus nerve that receives intermittent electrical pulses from an implanted generator. Stimulation of vagal nuclei has been shown to lead to widespread activation of cortical and subcortical pathways and an associated increased seizure threshold.[100] Deep brain stimulation (DBS) and responsive neurostimulation systems are also currently used for treatment of refractory epilepsy.[101] Gene therapy is currently being investigated as an alternative treatment modality for epilepsy refractory to standard therapies.[102]

Oral Health Considerations

Patients with seizure disorders are routinely evaluated and managed in the dental setting. This patient population has a higher rate of physical injuries, including dental and facial trauma, compared to healthy subjects.[103,104] In addition, patients with epilepsy demonstrate poor oral health and dental status compared to age-matched healthy subjects in long-term studies.[105] A complete evaluation of a patient's seizure disorder is necessary prior to initiation of any dental treatment to determine the stability of the condition and an appropriate venue for treatment. Important features for the clinician to assess include the type of seizures, etiology of seizures, frequency of seizures, known triggers of seizure activity, presence of aura prior to seizure activity, and history of injuries related to seizure activity. If a patient demonstrates signs of poorly or uncontrolled seizure disorder, consultation with the patient's physician and/or neurologist is recommended. Patients with poorly or uncontrolled seizure disorder may not be suited for private dental offices and should be referred to a hospital setting for routine dental care. Patients with implanted VNSs do not require antibiotic prophylaxis prior to invasive dental procedures.[106] It is recommended not to use dental devices utilizing diathermy for these patients as it may interfere with VNS function.[107]

While providing dental care, it is prudent to avoid any known triggers of the patient's seizure activity. Patients with poorly controlled seizures often present with signs of intraoral trauma, such as fractured teeth and/or soft tissue lacerations.[106] Patients with poorly controlled disease or stress-induced seizures may require sedative medications prior to treatment; this should be determined in consultation with the patient's physician.[106] To minimize the risk of injury and aspiration during dental treatment, use of dental floss–secured mouth props (which are easily retrievable) and a rubber dam is recommended.[108] Placement of metal fixed prostheses is recommended rather than removable prostheses to decrease the risk of displacement and aspiration risk during seizure activity.[109]

AEDs can induce significant blood dyscrasias that can affect provision of dental care. Several AEDs, including phenytoin, carbamazepine, and valproic acid can cause bone marrow suppression, leukopenia, thrombocytopenia, and secondary platelet dysfunction, possibly resulting in an increased incidence of microbial infection, delayed healing, and both gingival and postoperative bleeding.[98] Patients taking these medications may require laboratory evaluation prior to dental treatment, including a complete blood count with differential to assess white blood cell and platelet counts and coagulation studies to assess clotting ability. Patients on long-term carbamazepine should have serum blood levels evaluated prior to initiating dental treatment as insufficient doses may result in inadequate seizure control and excessive doses have been associated with hepatotoxicity.[98] Aspirin and nonsteroidal anti-inflammatory medications should be avoided for postoperative pain control in patients taking valproic acid as they can enhance the possibility of increased bleeding.[110] There are no contraindications to local anesthetics, when used in proper amounts, in patients with seizure disorders.[54]

Gingival overgrowth is a significant oral complication among seizure disorder patients taking AEDs, most notably phenytoin.[111] The prevalence rate of gingival overgrowth varies and has been reported in up to 50% of individuals taking phenytoin.[111] The anterior labial surfaces of the maxillary and mandibular gingiva are most commonly affected and may be seen within 2 to 18 months after starting the medication. Historically, this condition has been attributed to an increased number of fibroblasts in gingival connective tissue.[111] Studies have shown that phenytoin alters molecular signaling pathways that control collagen degradation by gingival fibroblasts and accumulation of collagen leads to clinically evident gingival overgrowth.[112] Inflammation can exacerbate this condition; therefore, frequent professional cleanings and use of an electric toothbrush are recommended to maintain optimal oral hygiene. Some clinicians advocate the use of chlorhexidine and/or folic acid rinses to minimize gingival inflammation among seizure disorder patients with gingival overgrowth.[113] Surgical reduction of gingival tissue may be necessary if significant overgrowth exists. In addition to gingival overgrowth, other oral side effects of phenytoin include development of intraoral lesions that clinically resemble lupus lesions and lip enlargement.[106,114]

Reduced salivary flow may result from the use of AEDs, and oral health-care providers may observe increased dental caries and oral candidiasis in patients using these agents. Topical fluoride should be considered for patients with seizure disorders who are at increased risk of developing dental caries, and antifungal agents should be prescribed if oral candidiasis develops. Additional oral findings in patients taking AEDs may include stomatitis, glossitis, and ulcerations.[108]

PARKINSON DISEASE

Epidemiology and Etiology

Parkinson disease (PD) is a chronic, progressive, neurodegenerative disorder characterized historically by its cardinal motor symptoms of resting tremor, rigidity, gait disturbance, and bradykinesia. A more contemporary view recognizes PD as a complex neurologic disorder with familiar motor symptoms as well as a broader spectrum of clinical features including cognitive deficits, neuropsychiatric changes, and dysautonomia.[115–119] The American Academy of Neurology has developed diagnostic, assessment, and treatment guidelines to distinguish idiopathic PD from "parkinsonian syndromes" such as corticobasal degeneration, progressive nuclear palsy, dementia with Lewy bodies (LBs) and PD dementia, which share similar symptoms but have different risk factors, pathological processes, and clinical courses.[120,121]

PD is second only to AD as the PD has a prevalence of approximately 1% and an annual incidence of approximately 446 cases per 100,000 population, with 50% fewer cases among African Americans and Asian Americans than among Caucasians.[122,123] Prevalence increases with advancing age to a mean of 1.6% among individuals aged 65 years and older.[122–124] A recent population-based study of US Medicare beneficiaries reported significant differences in regional prevalence with rates as high as 13.8%.[123] Areas with the highest rates included the Northeastern coast and the Midwest/Great Lakes regions where the highest prevalence was attributed to elevated agricultural and industrial exposure. Mortality among elderly PD patients is two to five times that of age-matched controls. The public health and economic burden for PD is significant and growing as the population ages, with annual costs in the US exceeding 14 billion dollars and prevalence projected to more than double by 2040.[125–127]

PD results from degeneration of the dopaminergic cells in the pars compacta of the substantia nigra (SN), leading to depletion of the neurotransmitter dopamine in the basal ganglia (caudate nucleus and putamen). LBs, inclusion structures composed of packed proteins (α-synuclein and ubiquitin) resulting from failed protein degradation, accumulate and displace essential neuronal organelles, and are pathognomonic features of PD.[128,129] A "dual hit" hypothesis has been proposed wherein an unknown (viral) pathogen causing α-synuclein accumulation enters by a nasal route and then along dual pathways to the brain: (1) the olfactory bulb to the temporal lobe and (2) virus in swallowed nasal secretions enter and travel within the vagus nerve and ultimately to the SN.[130] Although provocative, the dual-hit hypothesis is not sufficient alone to explain neuropathological findings in all PD cases.[128,129] Given the growing evidence supporting a heterogenous clinical presentation with complex genetic and environmental interactions, it is unlikely that PD will be understood by a single-disease model. Most agree that the pathogenesis is multifactorial, with environmental factors acting on genetically susceptible individuals.[131–136] Family history is among the strongest disease predictors, clearly suggesting genetic forms of PD, and several genes have been found to be associated with inherited PD: α-*synuclein*, *parkin*, *pink1*, and *UCH-L1*.[137–139] Environmental factors both increase risk for and offer protection from PD.[140] Environmental toxins, particularly pesticides, appear to play an important role in the risk for PD, and the protoxin n-methyl-4-phenyl-1,2,3,6-tetrahydropyridine has been shown to cause parkinsonism in both humans and nonhumans.[132,140,141] Significant protective effects have been demonstrated for tobacco use and caffeine consumption.[140,142]

Clinical Manifestations

PD usually affects people older than 50 years, although it can occur at any age, and earlier cases occur more commonly in the familial forms of PD. Early signs of PD, particularly nonmotor signs, can subtle. The four cardinal motor signs of PD are resting tremor (in hands, arms, legs, jaw, and face); rigidity or stiffness (limbs and trunk), bradykinesia (slowness of movement), and postural instability or impaired balance and coordination. Between 30% and 50% of individuals with PD develop dementia and the majority also exhibit behavioral/psychiatric symptoms including depression, anxiety, apathy, and irritability.[117,122] Autonomic dysfunction is common and can develop early, including orthostatic hypotension, constipation, urinary frequency and urgency, and abnormal sweating.[143] As symptoms become more pronounced, patients become increasingly impaired. Though rate of decline varies widely, PD is inevitably progressive and destructive. Age at onset is the strongest independent predictor of motor decline and is highest with late-onset PD.[120]

Diagnosis

Currently, there are no laboratory tests specific for idiopathic (classic) PD.[115,124] Clinical genetic markers are available for risk assessment where hereditary patterns of PD exist. Therefore, the diagnosis is based on the health history, neurologic examination, and response to levodopa therapy.[120] When symptoms are subtle and the presentation is incomplete, the diagnosis can be difficult. Differentiating classic PD from a variety of parkinsonian syndromes characterized by motor decline and/or dementia can be challenging.[120] Anatomic and functional brain imaging, CSF evaluation, and laboratory testing are often necessary to exclude other diagnoses.

Treatment

Currently, there is no cure for PD, but a variety of medications and procedures provide dramatic relief from the symptoms.[115,120,124,142,144] Dopamine replacement therapy using levodopa (used by neurons to synthesize dopamine) combined with carbidopa (delays the conversion of levodopa into dopamine until it reaches the brain) remains the initial gold standard. Levodopa initially helps about 75% of patients, but not all symptoms respond equally to the drug; bradykinesia and rigidity respond best, whereas tremor may be only marginally reduced and impaired balance and other symptoms may not be alleviated at all. In addition, levodopa often has the unwanted side effect of increasing dyskinesia. Anticholinergics such as scopolamine may help control tremor and rigidity. Dopamine agonists such as bromocriptine, per-golide, pramipexole, and ropinirole, alone or in combination with levodopa, may control PD symptoms and improve daily functioning better than treatment with levodopa alone.[124] Medical management can become challenging as it commonly occurs a medication that improves one symptom may worsen another.

Treatment of dementia, depression, and other psychiatric symptoms in PD can be challenging.[116] Rivastigmine, a cholinesterase inhibitor, is effective in treating PD dementia. Clozapine is effective for treating PD psychosis but worsens motor function. Tricyclic antidepressants are typically avoided for treating depressions due to anticholinergic effects. Similarly, benzodiazepine medications often used to treat anxiety may worsen motor performance and confusion.

Neuroprotective agents such as selegiline and vitamins E and C have not shown any consistent benefit despite early enthusiasm for slowing disease progression.[145,146] Alternative therapy, particularly exercise, has demonstrated significant benefit in physical conditioning, gait, balance, leg strength, and walking speed with fewer falls.[147,148]

Surgical management of PD by DBS has shown excellent efficacy in patients who fail levodopa treatment or have refractory tremor.[149] DBS is more often selected in younger patients with advanced PD or intolerable medication side effects. Additional surgical procedures to reduce symptoms include pallidotomy and thalamotomy. Embryonic stem cell research to provide transplantation, implantation, and gene therapy is an area of active investigation.

Oral Health Considerations

Patients with PD present several challenges to the dental health-care team and to the patient related to both the illness and its treatment.[54] Patients with PD often must be treated in a relatively upright position, making complex dental procedures in the maxillary arch or posterior oral cavity a challenge. Resting tremors and drug-related dyskinesia can complicate procedures, and behavioral techniques to reduce anxiety as well as gentle cradling techniques can help. Dysphagia and impaired gag reflex increase the risk for aspiration of oral and irrigation fluids, and high-speed evacuation of fluids is important in reducing the risk for aspiration pneumonia. Some patients experience sialorrhea, making maintenance of a dry field difficult for some operative and surgical procedures.

Pharmacologic treatment for PD has implications of importance to dentistry. Levodopa and dopamine agonists can lead to both orthostatic hypertension and, rarely, severe hypertension; other side effects of particular importance to the dental team include oromandibular and facial dyskinesia, xerostomia, arrhythmia, and blood dyscrasias. Careful consideration and management include monitoring of blood pressure; correct positioning and repositioning during and after treatment; xerostomia and caries risk reduction through hygiene, sealants, and fluorides when indicated; impact of oromandibular dyskinesia on the design of dental prostheses; and periodic evaluation of the complete blood count to detect drug-related hematologic adverse effects.

MYASTHENIA GRAVIS

Epidemiology and Etiology

Myasthenia gravis (MG) is a chronic neuromuscular disease caused by autoimmune destruction of the skeletal neuromuscular junction resulting in impaired neurotransmission and muscle weakness. Pathogenic antibodies directed against components of the postsynaptic membrane of the neuromuscular junction disrupt neurotransmission. MG is characterized by episodic weakness of the skeletal muscles that increases during periods of activity and improves after periods of rest. Prior to effective therapy death commonly resulted from respiratory failure and pneumonia.[150] Ocular weakness presenting as fluctuating ptosis and/or diplopia is the most common initial presentation of MG, occurring in 85% of patients. Muscles of facial expression, masticatory, and swallowing muscles are also affected early resulting in facial asymmetry, dysarthria, and dysphagia.[150]

Several clinical MG subtypes are defined by clinical presentation, age at onset, autoantibody profile, and presence or absence of thymus pathology.[151] Discrimination among subtypes is important: clinical presentation and disease progression varies significantly and recent evidence suggests differential treatment effectiveness.[151] The most common autoantibody is anti-acetylcholine receptor (AChR) and less commonly a muscle-specific receptor tyrosine kinase (MUSK). A seronegative MG subtype has also been recognized, but recent findings suggest this may represent a distinct subset with low-affinity IgG antibodies to AChR.[152]

The biological and clinical heterogeneity of MG is reflected in a widely accepted classification system: generalized with early (under age 40) and late onset disease or ocular disease only. Generalized early onset tends to be female with anti-AChR antibodies and thymic hyperplasia. Late onset tends to be males with normal thymus glands. Approximately 10% to 15% of MG patients have a thymic tumor (thymoma), and this phenotype occurs equally in men and women, typically older than 50 years, tends to have a more severe clinical presentation and exhibit high anti-AChR titers. As the name implies, ocular MG is limited to the ocular muscles and tends not to generalize if weakness remains limited to ocular muscles for more than 2 years, regardless of anti-AChR titer.[151]

The estimated prevalence rate for MG is 15 to 20 cases per 100,000 population, with an estimated 60,000 affected patients in the United States.[150] However, the rate of MG diagnoses has increased every year for the past 50 years and probably remains underdiagnosed and underreported.[153–156] The most common age at onset is the second and third decades in women and the seventh and eighth decades in men, and as the population ages, males are more often affected than females, and the onset of symptoms is usually after age 50.

Clinical Manifestations

Eighty-five percent of MG patients present with ocular symptoms characterized by diplopia and/or ptosis. Oropharyngeal, facial, and masticatory muscle weakness is common and results in dysphagia, asymmetry, and dysarthria, and are the initial symptoms in one-sixth of patients.[150] Severity of weakness typically fluctuates on a daily and use basis, but tends to worsen as the day progresses. The clinical course of disease is variable but usually progressive.[155] Eighty-eight percent of ocular MG patients go on to generalized weakness one year after onset. Weakness limited to the ocular muscles for more than one year was unlikely to generalize in the future.[150] In general, MG patients experience an initial period of one to two years during which the disease reaches a maximum level of severity, followed by improvement for the majority. Mortality from MG has significantly decreased progressively over the past four decades compared to the preceding two decades. Mortality rates are consistently slightly higher in males (14%) then females (11%).

Diagnosis

The clinical examination and history are highly suggestive of MG. Diagnosis is confirmed by a variety of bedside, electrophysiological and immunological tests. Tensilon (edrophonium) challenge (rapid resulting in immediate elevation of available Ach) administration is highly reliable in patients with ocular weakness. Abnormal (decrease) compound muscle action potential following repetitive nerve stimulation in 75% of generalized and 50% of ocular MG patients.

The most commonly used immunological test to establish a diagnosis of MG quantifies serum anti-AChR, with a reported sensitivity of 85% for generalized MG and 50% for ocular MG.[156,157] The presence of other muscle cytoplasmic antibodies may raise the suspicion for thymoma[158] and CT/MRI imaging of the chest is highly accurate in detecting thymoma.

Treatment

As with many autoimmune illnesses, treatment is directed at several levels: reduction of pathologic antibody production or presence, and/or replacement/preservation of the pathologic antibody target (AChR). Anticholinesterase drugs such as neostigmine and pyridostigmine bromide increase acetylcholine availability and receptor binding and provide symptomatic benefit without influencing the course of the disease. Anti-AChR-positive MG patients with thymus tumors may have dramatic improvement following thymectomy. Plasma exchange and high-dose intravenous immunoglobulin can rapidly and temporarily reduce circulating antibodies and is very effective in crisis management.[159,160]

Patients with more severe symptoms or poor response to treatment have treatment directed at reducing autoantibody production using corticosteroids and nonsteroid immune suppressants to reduce antibody production and/or B-cell/T-cell lymphocyte activation/proliferation. More recently, Rituximab, a monoclonal antibody directed against the B-cell surface marker CD20, like in several other autoimmune disorders has been shown to reduce B-cell counts and disease activity. Several reports have described its benefit for treatment of anti-MUSK MG.[150]

Oral Health Considerations

Orofacial signs and symptoms are prominent presenting features of MG, and the dental provider may be in the position to recognize and refer for diagnosis. Difficulty with prolonged opening and swallowing presents challenges in dental treatment delivery and the ability to tolerate treatment, and difficulty in chewing can affect diet and the design of prostheses. Implant retained removable or fixed prosthesis may be preferable to tissue-supported for improved chewing efficacy.

Aspiration risks can be high and can be reduced by adequate suction, the use of a rubber dam, and avoiding bilateral mandibular anesthetic block. The MG patient may also be at risk for a respiratory crisis from the disease itself or from overmedication; if this is a substantial risk and the dental treatment is necessary, dental treatment in a hospital should be considered where endotracheal intubation can be performed.[161] Avoid prescribing drugs that may affect the neuromuscular junction, such as narcotics, tranquilizers, and barbiturates. Certain antibiotics, including tetracycline, streptomycin, sulfonamides, and clindamycin, can affect neuromuscular activity and should be avoided or used with caution. Esther anesthetics which are metabolized by plasma cholinesterase should be avoided in MG patients on anticholinesterase therapy.

Selected Readings

Asher I. New perspectives in the care of Parkinson disease. *Mo Med.* 2012;109(4):328–332.

Ballard C, Gauthier S, Corbett A, et al. Alzheimer's disease. *Lancet.* 2011;377:1019–1031.

Berg AT, Scheffer IE. New concepts in classification of the epilepsies: entering the 21st century. *Epilepsia.* 2011;52:1058–1062.

Budson AE, Solomon PR. New criteria for Alzheimer disease and mild cognitive impairment. Implications for the practicing clinician. *Neurologist.* 2012;18:356–363.

Carandang R, Seshadri S, Beiser A, et al. Trends in incidence, lifetime risk, severity, and 30-day mortality of stroke over the past 50 years. *JAMA.* 2006;296:2939–2946.

Carr AS, Cardwell CR, McCarron PO, McConville J. A systematic review of population based epidemiological studies in myasthenia gravis. *BMC Neurol.* 2010;10:46–54.

Elad S, Zadik Y, Kaufman E, et al. A new management approach for dental treatment after a cerebrovascular event: a comparative retrospective study. *Oral Surg Oral Med Oral Pathol Oral Radiol Endod.* 2010;110:145–150.

Fatahzadeh M, Glick M. Stroke: epidemiology, classification, risk factors, complications, diagnosis, prevention, and medical and dental management. *Oral Surg Oral Med Oral Pathol Oral Radiol Endod.* 2006;102:180–191.

Fischer DJ, Epstein JB, Klasser G. Multiple sclerosis: an update for oral health care providers. *Oral Surg Oral Med Oral Pathol Oral Radiol Endod.* 2009;108:318–327.

Freedman MS. Present and emerging therapies for multiple sclerosis. *Continuum (Minneap Minn).* 2013;19:968–991.

Grob D, Brunner N, Namba T, Pagala M. Lifetime course of myasthenia gravis. *Muscle Nerve.* 2008;37:141–149.

Henry R, Smith BJ. Managing older patients who have neurologic disease: Alzheimer disease and cerebrovascular accident. *Dent Clin North Am.* 2009;53:269–294.

Katz Sand IB, Lublin FD. Diagnosis and differential diagnosis of multiple sclerosis. *Continuum (Minnep Minn).* 2013;19:922–943.

Levine CB, Fahrbach KR, Siderowf AD, et al. *Diagnosis and Treatment of Parkinson's Disease: A Systematic Review of the Literature.* Evidence Report/Technology Assessment Number 57. (Prepared by

Metaworks, Inc., under Contract No. 290–97–0016.) AHRQ Publication No. 03-E040. Rockville, MD: Agency for Healthcare Research and Quality; 2003.

Meriggioli MN, Sanders DB. Autoimmune myasthenia gravis: emerging clinical and biological heterogeneity. *Lancet Neurol.* 2009;8(5):475–490.

Palace J, Vincent A, Beeson D. Myasthenia gravis: diagnostic and management dilemmas. *Curr Opin Neurol.* 2001;14:583–589.

Phillips LH II. The epidemiology of myasthenia gravis. *Ann NY Acad Sci.* 2003;998:407–412.

Robbins MR. Dental management of special needs patients who have epilepsy. *Dent Clin North Am.* 2009;53:295–309.

Saperstein DS, Barohn RJ. Management of myasthenia gravis. *Semin Neurol.* 2004;24:41–48.

Schachter SC. Seizure disorders. *Med Clin North Am.* 2009;93:343–351.

Straus SE, Majumdar SR, McAlister FA. New evidence for stroke prevention: scientific review. *JAMA.* 2002;288:1388–1395.

Wirdefeldt K, Adami HO, Cole P, et al. Epidemiology and etiology of Parkinson's disease: a review of the evidence. *Eur J Epidemiol.* 2011;26(suppl 1):S1-S58.

For the full reference lists, please go to http://www.pmph-usa.com/Burkets_Oral_Medicine.

CHAPTER 25

Basic Principles of Human Genetics: A Primer for Oral Medicine

Harold C. Slavkin, DDS

Mahvash Navazesh, DMD

Pragna Patel, PhD

Humans have known for several thousand years that heredity affects health. However, it was only 150 years ago when Gregor Mendel first described the mechanism by which genotype results in phenotype. It was less than 100 years ago when Garrod began to apply genetic knowledge to human diseases and disorders. Ironically, for most of the 20th century, clinicians viewed genetics as a somewhat esoteric academic specialty until rather recently with the completion of the Human Genome Project (HGP) in October 2004.[1-3] Meanwhile, rapid advances in high throughput gene sequencing and related bioinformatics have realized that the human genome can be achieved for $1000 per person thereby introducing a tool for diagnostics and prognosis that emphasizes individualized or *personalized* health care.[4-6]

Despite enormous public interest in *genomics* and the thousands of articles published about the completion of the human genome, neither medicine nor dentistry would abruptly change or transform. Medicine and dentistry have not been *gene free* for the last 100 years. Increasingly, a growing and evolving body of knowledge and information has significantly expanded how we think about and how we use human genetics in medicine and dentistry to address epidemiology, public health and risk assessment, single and multiple predictive and prognostic gene-based diagnostics, and pharmacogenomics and pharmacogenetics with customized drug selection specific for individualized metabolism. We are experiencing an expanding knowledge base for Mendelian inheritance, complex human diseases (multifactorial diseases and disorders), and bioinformatics.[7-15] Further, the 21st century has heralded the introduction of inborn errors of development which provides the molecular basis of clinical disorders of human development.[16]

This chapter is a primer for the emerging field of human genetics, and the era of -omics (genomics, transcriptomics, proteomics, metabolomics, diseasomics, phenomics) with oral medicine. The authors and readers acknowledge that the pace of transformation for oral medicine and clinical dentistry and medicine in general is limited not only by the pace of scientific discovery but also by the need to educate practicing dentists, physicians and allied health professions and our patients about the uses and shortcomings of human genetic knowledge and information.[17-22] Human genetic variation is associated with many, if not all, human diseases and disabilities, including the common chronic diseases of major public health impact. Genetic variation interacts with environment and sociocultural influences to modify the risk of disease.

As we look into the future, we must anticipate the logical and rapid advances of human and microbial genomics. This extraordinary progress is already shaping how we consider the etiology and progression of diseases and disorders, how we reach diagnostically useful information, and even how we select therapeutics for particular patients and communities. Today we appreciate the unique interrelationships between the microbiome and the human genome. The average adult consists of 13 trillion cells that coexist with 130 trillion bacterial cells. Our 21,000 human functional genes coexist with 5–8 million bacterial genes in what has recently been termed the *microbiome* or the *second human genome*. In tandem, these advances will also become integrated into the continuum of dental and medical education—predoctoral, doctoral, postdoctoral, residency, and lifelong continuing professional education.

BASIC HUMAN GENETIC PRINCIPLES

The general principles of genetics have been appreciated since the dawn of agriculture some 10,000 years ago when ancient farmers engaged in domestication of plants and animals. The British biologist William Bateson gave the science of inheritance a name—genetics—as recently as 1909. More recently, the use of cytogenetic techniques heralded the technology that enabled cells, intracellular organelles, and chromosomes to be visualized using light microscopy with specific histopathology stains. Karyotyping enabled visualization of the number and fidelity of human chromosomes, and this enabled better diagnostics for chromosomal disorders such as trisomy 21 or Down syndrome.

In the early 1950s, James Watson and Francis Crick discovered the molecular structure of deoxyribonucleic acid (DNA).[7] Thereafter, it became increasingly evident that DNA was arranged in a double-helical structure as an exceedingly long chain of only four units called nucleotides

or bases (adenosine, A; thymidine, T; cytosine, C; and guanosine, G). Three of these nucleotides form codons (e.g., UUA for leucine; U [uracil] substitute for T, thymidine, in ribonucleic acids [RNAs]) and thereby represent the information or code for the ordering of amino acids into forming polypeptides; the so-called *genetic code* was established.

During the last three decades of the 20th century, the fundamental science of DNA accelerated and applications of human genetics rapidly advanced so that a *genetic paradigm* for human diseases and disorders was embraced to a limited extent in many US medical and dental schools.[8-22] Terms such as *susceptibility* versus *resistance* were readily incorporated into the language of health professionals engaged in patient care. Simultaneously, there was also a major acceleration in the study of genes, proteins, and their functions during the human lifespan.[1-15]

The HGP was initiated in 1988 and was completed as of October 2004.[1-6] Exhaustive analyses of the enormous database (the *instruction book* of life) representing the HGP revealed that humans contain 21,000 functional genes and 19,000 nonfunctional pseudogenes within the nucleus of each somatic cell, and another nine genes that are encoded within mitochondria found in all human somatic cells. Genes are discrete units of information encoded within DNA, which, in turn, is localized within chromosomes found in the nucleus of each somatic cell or within mitochondria dispersed through the cytoplasm of all cells. Each cell contains 3.2×10^9 nucleotide pairs per haploid genome in the nucleus and 16,569 nucleotide pairs in each mitochrondrion.[1-15]

Even before a gene's function in disease is fully understood and treatment is available, diagnostic applications can be useful in minimizing or preventing the development of health consequences. The discovery of mutations in the *BRCA1* gene associated with early breast cancer is such an example.[10] The DNA tests used for the presence of disease-linked mutations are proving to be very useful for clinicians. Such tests can assist in the correct diagnosis of a genetic disease, foreshadow the development of disease later in life, or identify healthy heterozygote carriers of recessive diseases. Testing for genetic diseases can be performed at any stage in the human life span.

Importantly, the Mendelian rules that govern the inheritance of many human traits are useful for rare human diseases with highly penetrant changes in a single gene. What is much more difficult is to tease out of the human genome are the multiple genes that are functionally related to complex human diseases such as diabetes, heart disease, oral cancer, periodontal disease, most cleft lip and palate patients, autoimmune disorders (e.g., Sjögren's syndrome), and psychiatric conditions. The challenge is to find multiple, low-penetrance variants, which in the aggregate account for the vast majority of chronic diseases and disorders. This requires new strategies of conceptualizing multifactorial diseases.

There are 46 chromosomes found in every nucleus of every diploid somatic cell in the human body. These chromosomes contain approximately 6 ft in length of the double-stranded DNA and associated proteins (histones and nonhistone chromosomal proteins). These chromosomal proteins insulate and regulate genes and gene expression during the human life span. Specifically, methylation, acetylation, and deacetylation of these proteins are significant posttranslational mechanisms that regulate gene functions and contribute to the relatively new field termed *epigenetics*.

Of the 46 chromosomes that contain DNA, 44 are termed autosomes that exist in homologous pairs (numbered 1–22, with 1 being the largest and the remaining chromosome pairs numbered in descending order of size) and the remaining two chromosomes (designated X and Y) are termed sex chromosomes. In addition, the maternally inherited mitochondria also contain mitochondrial deoxyribonucleic acid (mtDNA), as mentioned.

In either case, whether it is chromosomes in the nucleus of every somatic cell or mtDNA localized within mitochondria, DNA is a polymer macromolecule that is composed of recurring monomeric units called *nucleotides* or *bases*. There are 3.2 billion nucleotides in the haploid genome. Each monomer or base has three components: (1) a phosphate group linked to (2) a five-carbon atom cyclic sugar group, which, in turn, is joined to (3) a *purine* or *pyrimidine* nucleotide or base. The four nucleotides are the purines adenosine (A) and guanosine (G) and the pyrimidines thymidine (T) and cytosine (C). Permutations and combinations of the four nucleotides constitute the DNA sequence within which the genetic code is embedded. Permutations and combinations of A, C, T, and G result in a DNA sequence, and this sequence becomes highly informative within regulatory or structural regions of human genes. Interestingly, only 1%–2% of the entire human genome encodes 21,000 genes, with the vast majority being apparently noninformative or not-as-yet-informative expanses of nucleotides that include repetitive DNA sequences, pseudogenes, and additional DNA whose function is yet unknown.[2,5,6]

The analysis of X-ray diffraction patterns of purified DNA led James Watson and Francis Crick, based on earlier data from Rosalind Franklin on adenoviral DNA, to build three-dimensional models of DNA that represented a right-handed double helix.[7] They showed that the best fit of the data would be two antiparallel chains in a structure that resembles a spiral staircase. Further, they asserted that within these two strands of DNA, A binds to T and C to G—so-called base pairing or hybridization. These rules apply to DNA found within all living organisms, such as microbes (virus, bacteria, and yeast), plants, animals, and people. Watson and Crick conclude the following:

> It has not escaped our notice that the specific pairing we have postulated immediately suggests a possible copying mechanism for the genetic material.[7]

Genes contain the information for proteins. Genes represent hereditary blueprints. All hereditary information is transmitted from parent to offspring through the inheritance of genes, which are identified as the nucleotide sequences within DNA that produce a functional protein product. The largest genetic variance has been determined to be 0.1% between any two people on Earth (or 3 million nucleotides of 3.2 billion found in the haploid human genome), or, from a different perspective, any two humans show 99.9% genetic identity or homology.[1,2]

Genetic variation has phenotypic relevance when considering the impact of this variation on the protein sequence encoded. When comparing protein sequences (of two functionally related proteins or those from two different species), the term *homology* implies that the corresponding amino acid residues in homologous proteins are also homologous. They are derived from the same ancestral residue and, typically, inherit the same function. If the residue in question is the same in a set of homologous sequences, it is assumed that it is evolutionarily conserved. Importantly, protein structure is conserved during evolution much better than protein sequence. For example, lysozyme, the enzyme that hydrolyzes bacterial cell walls, shows little sequence similarity across species but readily adopts similar protein structures, contains identical or related amino acid residues in the bioactive site of the enzyme, and retains a similar catalytic mechanism.[23] Such shared features support the concept that despite low sequence similarities, such proteins are homologous.

Since the completion of the HGP in October 2004,[1,2] numerous other species have also been sequenced with over 300 eukaryotic and nearly 20,000 bacterial genomes in the list (www.genomesonline.org). These genomes include vertebrates such as chimpanzee,[24] rat,[25] mouse,[26] chicken,[27] and dog[28], as well invertebrates such as microbes,[29] malarial parasites,[30] *Anopheles* mosquito,[31] roundworm,[32] fruit fly,[33] and mustard plant.[34] This has been followed by subsequent sequence analysis, comparisons, and interpretations related to structure, function, and evolutionary conservation.[24] Genomic comparisons between human and fruit fly sequences demonstrated that 60% of the human disease genes are conserved between fruit flies and humans.[35] Curiously, two-thirds of the human genes known to be involved in cancers have counterparts in the fruit fly. It would seem counterintuitive that the fruit fly animal organism offers unique opportunities to explore the onset and progression of many human diseases and disorders such as early-onset Parkinson's disease.[36,37] It is now estimated that the number of microbes associated with oral/dental, skin, vaginal, gut, and nasal/lung surfaces is 10-fold greater than the trillions of human somatic cells that comprise an individual adult human being (The International Human Microbiome Consortium, http://www.human-microbiome.org/).[38–47]

It is now accepted that profound similarities or homology exists among genomes of the earth's organisms—microbes (virus, bacteria, yeast), plants, animals, and humans—and that genomes can differ by variations in nucleotide sequences and through duplications or deletions of DNA, through combinations that rearrange the order of genes, and/or by insertions of DNA that may be derived from microbes.[28–37] In humans, the process of sexual reproduction generates new combinations of genes across multiple generations, constituting the fundamental process of evolution.

Surveys of the human genetic code reveal approximately 10 million variations of nucleotides encoded within the DNA found in human chromosomes—about 0.1% variation between two people. Millions of single nucleotide polymorphisms (SNPs) have been well characterized and enable scientific assessment of extremely small variations between people in health and in disease.[48,49] SNPs and haplotype maps enable genetic linkage with specific diseases and disorders using a process referred to as genome-wide association study (GWAS) illustrated in Figure 25-1. These human genetic variants are closely linked with many diseases and disorders, a person's susceptibility or resistance to disease, and individual responses to therapeutics.[48,49] For example, nucleotide variants within genes encoding opioids and opioid receptors can explain why people differ in their responses to pain or pain stimuli.

Briefly, genes function through a complex series of processes. First, encoding sequences of DNA are *transcribed* to messenger ribonucleic acids (mRNAs). These are, in turn, *translated* into proteins. Another class of RNAs termed transfer or tRNAs are guided and instructed by DNA-derived specific mRNAs to assemble amino acids into the correct sequence to produce the functional protein on the ribosomes located in the cytoplasm of cells.

A generic gene (sequence of nucleotides A, C, T, and/or G) begins with a *start sequence* in which the mRNA transcription begins. The region before or *upstream* from this site or location contains the *switches* that turn on the gene and also constitute the gene's promoter *sequence*. Further upstream in a region, typically 2000 nucleotides in length, there are additional control elements that regulate the rates, amplitudes, or quantity of transcription. These elements can be enhancers or repressors that respond to DNA-binding proteins, hormones, certain types of vitamins such as retinoic acid, or growth factors. The body of the gene contains discrete coding sequences that give rise to a protein product; these are called *exons*. These are separated by noncoding sequences termed *introns*. Genes terminate with a *stop sequence*. DNA can be transcribed into RNAs (mRNA) by RNA polymerase II enzyme or can be replicated by DNA polymerase enzyme into copy strands of DNA (as required in mitosis or cell division). These two major processes, *transcription of DNA into mRNA* or *replication of one strand of DNA to a copy strand of DNA*, are enormously important for biologic activities (Figure 25-2).

A process termed *alternative splicing* can modify or alter significantly the gene sequence that is transcribed into mRNAs by producing splices and rearrangements between exons that result in as many as 8–10 different isoforms or variants of the gene. Alternative splicing is a regulatory mechanism by which variations in the incorporation of exons encoded within DNA into mRNAs during transcription can produce different isoforms of the same protein. About 15% of human genetic diseases appear to be caused by point mutations at or near splice junctions located within or between introns and exons that control the fidelity of alternative splicing.

Nucleic acid sequences that encode genes within DNA represent *structural proteins* (e.g., genetically different types of collagens, multiple genes for keratins, globins, amelogenins, enamelins, metalloproteinases, albumins, dentin sialoglycoproteins, dentin phosphoproteins) or *regulatory proteins* (e.g., transcriptional factors, signal transduction–related proteins, growth factors).

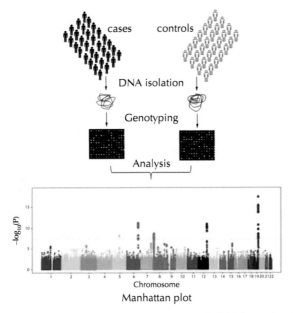

Figure 25-1 Genome-wide association study. DNA is isolated from each individual within an age and gender-matched cohort consisting of cases and controls. Genotypes are determined on a microarray that represents up to 2 million SNPs and subjected to statistical analysis to determine if specific alleles at one or more SNP loci are overrepresented in either cases or controls. A representative resulting "Manhattan" plot is shown at the bottom of the figure. Each dot represents a SNP with the horizontal axis indicating each SNP's chromosomal location, while the vertical axis indicates the statistical significance of disease association; SNPs positioned higher on the plot have stronger association with the disease/trait under study with a SNP yielding a P value $<5 \times 10^{-8}$ (horizontal line) considered as being significant at the genome-wide level.

How Genes Function

How is the information encoded in DNA—sequences of nucleotides—converted into a protein with bioactivity? The process begins with several events: (1) combinations of multiple transcription factors bind to one another (i.e., protein–protein binding) and through binding to DNA (i.e., protein–DNA binding); (2) methylation of cytosine within nucleic acid sequences is highly informative for transcription; and (3) an enzyme, RNA polymerase II, attaches to a specific sequence within DNA and is then followed by the transcription process (DNA to mRNA), followed eventually

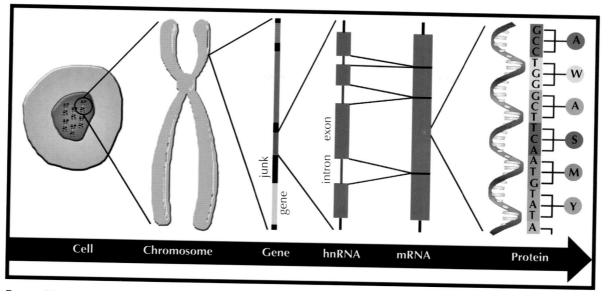

FIGURE 25-2 From gene to protein. Chromosomes are found in the nucleus of the cell. Composed of DNA, these chromosomes contain thousands of genes (colored blocks) which are separated by noncoding, or *junk*, DNA (black blocks). Each gene is composed of both exons (coding DNA; red) and introns (noncoding DNA; blue) which are copied or transcribed (expressed), for the purposes of constructing the protein it codes for, or encodes. There is an intermediary stage between the gene and the protein, where a temporary copy of the gene blueprint is produced as a heterogeneous ribonucleic acid molecule, or hnRNA. The hnRNA consists of both the exons, which are pieced together to form the messenger RNA, or mRNA, and the introns, which are discarded. The mRNA is used as the template for the synthesis of the protein from amino acid building blocks. For this, the DNA is read in three letter blocks, called codons, each of which signifies a single amino acid (colored circles).

by translation (mRNA to protein amino acid sequence) on ribosomes physically located within the cytoplasm of cells.

Transcription defines the process by which genes encoded within the DNA template are copied into mRNAs that, in turn, leave the nucleus and migrate into the cytoplasm. The number and variation of transcripts from a single discrete gene are created by alternative splicing. In addition, genes that encode ribosomal RNA and tRNA are transcribed and also migrate to the cytoplasm, where they participate in the process of protein synthesis.

For example, tooth formation is a complex developmental process that results from a sequence of epithelial–mesenchymal interactions.[50–55] Mutations in one or more transcription factors (e.g., *MSX1, MSX2, DLX5, PAX9*) may inhibit, arrest, or retard tooth development, and these are clinically diagnosed as tooth agenesis (oligodontia or hypodontia).[56–60] Mutations in regulatory genes such as growth factors and their cognate receptors related to signal transduction and/or transcription factors cause a wide variety of abnormalities in tooth number, position, and shape.[50–70]

Translation is the process that defines mRNA being translated into a precise sequence of amino acids termed *polypeptide* or *protein*. Genetic information is stored as the *genetic code*. Each member of the genetic code consists of three bases or nucleotides that represent a *codon* designating a specific amino acid. The three nucleotides within the codon are determined from four possibilities (A, C, T, and

G). Therefore, there are 4^3 or 64 different codons, and all but three specify an amino acid. The functional codons designate 20 different amino acids. Since the alternative splicing of the human 21,000 functional genes is common, the proteome that reflects the human genome is measured in many thousands of distinct proteins well beyond the number of genes in the human genome. For example, the major protein of forming enamel extracellular matrix is amelogenin derived from the AMELX or AMELY gene. In human and other mammals, the number of different amelogenin isoforms is six to eight proteins of varying molecular weights and all cross-reactive with anti-amelogenin rabbit antibodies. Historically, these multiple amelogenins were assumed to be generated by post translational enzymatic steps associated with enamel biomineralization. More recently, it was discovered that AMEL gene produces multiple and different mRNAs through a process termed alternative splicing; one gene produces multiple transcripts which in turn are translated into multiple and different proteins.[14,19,22,71]

Another example is found in dentinogenesis. Dentin formation during tooth development represents secretory odontoblasts engaged in the synthesis, translation, and posttranslation (e.g., glycosylation, phosphorylation) of a number of structural proteins that form the extracellular matrix and control the process of tissue-specific biomineralization. Odontoblasts synthesize and secrete type I collagen and a number of noncollagenous and highly specialized glycoproteins and phosphoproteins. These extracellular matrix structural proteins control the size, shape, and structure of the minerals that engage in biomineralization. The dentin sialophosphoprotein gene (*DSPP*) is located on chromosome 4 (4q21.3) and encodes two different noncollagenous proteins: (1) dentin sialo-protein and (2) dentin phosphoprotein.[61,62] Mutations in type I collagen and/or *DSPP* produce five different patterns of inherited dentin defects termed *dentinogenesis imperfecta* types.[61,62]

Regulation of Gene Expression

The central problem in human genetics is the temporal and spatial expression of the 21,000 functional genes—the organization of the two-dimensional DNA encoded genetic information into the dynamic three-dimensional morpho-genesis and development, cell determination, cell fate, and cytodifferentiation (i.e., growth, development, maturation, senescence). It is now well known that there are *master regulatory genes* (homeotic genes) that control the geometry of body forms.

The most significant level for control is at the level of mRNA production termed *transcriptional control*. Transcriptional control is performed by proteins that bind to DNA, either by modifying cytosine methylation or by *transcription factors* binding to a specific sequence or motif within DNA. A complex of multiple transcription factors often binds to the *TATA box* (a sequence of 8–10 T and A bases) physically located upstream to the formal start sequence of the gene. Other regulatory units encoded within the nucleic acid sequence include the *CAAT box* (a sequence of C, A, and T) and the *GC box* (GGGCGG). Promoters define when and where genes will be expressed, and enhancers define the levels of expression (i.e., copies of mRNA per unit time per cell). In addition to these, molecular tools for regulation, steroids, lipophilic vitamins, and trace elements, also function to control protein–protein and protein–nucleic acid interactions.[1–10]

A number of morphoregulatory or master genes have been identified that are highly conserved from fish to humans. These genes encode highly conserved transcription factors such as *HOX* (homeotic) genes, *PAX* genes, and *T-Box* genes.[50–53] Each of these three types of gene clusters encodes master control genes that regulate the body plan for invertebrates and all vertebrates, including humans.[50–53] Further, each of these three types of transcription factors is transcribed and translated into DNA-binding proteins with high affinities for specific nucleic acid sequence motifs.

For example, two of the morphoregulatory genes are the *FOXC1* and the *PITX2* homeobox genes (Figure 25-3). Mutations in either of these contribute to Axenfeld–Rieger syndrome (ARS), an autosomal dominant developmental disorder that represents a spectrum that involves anomalies of the anterior segment of the eyes, iris hypoplasia, tooth anomalies, craniofacial dysmorphogenesis, cardiac defects,

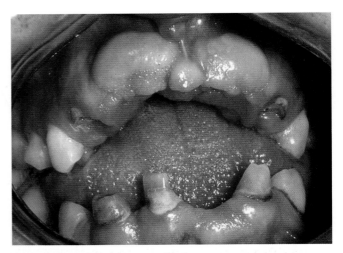

FIGURE 25-3 Mutations in PITX2 (pituitary homeobox transcription factor 2) and/or FOXC1 (forkhead box transcription factor C1) results in Axenfeld-Rieger Syndrome (ARS) which represents a spectrum of diseases and disorders including those of the dentition (i.e., extreme dental hypoplasia as shown in this figure). Courtesy of Dr. Carl Allen.

limb anomalies, pituitary anomalies, mental defects, and neurosensory defects.[63] Mutations in the *PITX2* gene or the *FOXC* gene have been identified in 40% of ARS.[63]

Cell Division

The cell cycle is the process by which the somatic cell divides to form two daughter cells. This process maintains the 46 chromosomes. A complete cell cycle consists of four phases: G_1, S, G_2, and M (mitosis). Progression through these phases is energy dependent and requires phosphorylation and dephosphorylation steps mediated by kinase enzymes. Gene products called cyclins regulate each of these four phases by specific interactions with kinase phosphatases. Loss of cell cycle controls is the signature for carcinogenesis and many birth defects. One of the major conceptual advances in the last decade is the recognition that cancer is largely a genetic disease and that neoplastic cells display a diverse array of genetic rearrangements, point mutations, and gene amplifications.

Epigenetic Controls

Epigenetic controls, molecular controls that are chromosomal protein posttranslational modifications (e.g., methylation, acetylation) and clearly not intrinsic to the nucleic acid sequence within DNA, provide the multiple gene–gene and gene–environment regulatory influences of the human condition. During embryogenesis, fetal development, infancy, childhood, adolescence, and thereafter, multiple combinations of genes are transcribed and translated into protein products that inform, regulate, and build the human organism.[50–53]

Monozygotic twins share an identical genome or genotype. Yet, as monozygotic twin pairs develop and age they present several types of phenotypic discordance, such as differences in susceptibilities to diseases and disorders and even a range of anthropomorphic features. One current explanation for these phenotypic variances is epigenetic control differences. To address this issue, a number of studies examined global and gene or locus-specific differences in DNA methylation and histone acetylation of a large cohort of monozygotic twins. These studies report that monozygotic twins are epigenetically indistinguishable during the early years of life, yet older twins (i.e., fourth decade and beyond) exhibited striking differences in their overall content and genomic distribution of 5-methylcytosine DNA and histone acetylation, affecting their gene expression profile. These findings indicate how an appreciation of epigenetics has been a missing link towards our understanding of how different phenotypes (e.g., arthritis, osteoporosis, periodontal disease, fibromyalgia, Alzheimer's disease and other forms of dementia) can be originated from the identical genotype.

MUTATION AND GENETIC HETEROGENEITY

Mutation is defined broadly as any change in the sequence of nucleic acids within DNA. Mutations or *misspellings* can be silent without clinical symptoms or can be profound, such as a single point mutation in a single nucleotide within one of the codons found in one of the exons for the globin gene that can result in sickle cell anemia. In humans, the mutation rate ranges from 1 to 10 million per gene per cell cycle. Importantly, mutations can be fundamental drivers for evolution as organisms adapt to various environs, or they can become clinically relevant as they delete, inhibit, or truncate specific gene expression during human development from conception through senescence.

Mutations can cause disease by a variety of means. The most common is *loss of function mutations*, resulting in a decrease in the quantity or function of a protein. Other mutations cause disease through *gain of function mutations*, such as the dominantly inherited Huntington's disease.

Single-Gene Mutations

Point mutations affect only one nucleotide with the substitution of one for another (Figure 25-4) (e.g., GAG is codon for glutamic acid in the sixth exon of the β-hemoglobin(HbB) gene; a point mutation or substitution of the A for a T in the codon changes meaning to valine and results in sickle cell anemia). *Missense mutation* describes a point mutation that results in the change of a codon, resulting in a change in the primary structure of the protein product resulting from translation. This is clinically observed in select examples of hemoglobinopathies such as sickle cell anemia (globin), craniosynostosis (e.g., fibroblast growth factor receptor), osteogenesis imperfecta (collagen), and amelogenesis imperfecta (AI; amelogenin). *A silent mutation* is a point mutation that has no effect on transcription or translation.

Mutations that abolish protein expression or function are termed *null alleles*. Mechanisms that produce null alleles include mutations that interfere with transcription in general, termination of transcripts, or mutations within splice sites related to alternative splicing. Human carriers of a null allele are often asymptomatic or can have clinical phenotypes if and when the mutations directly inhibit structural protein structure and function. Hypodontia involving primarily molar teeth is associated with mutations in the *PAX9* gene and a repertoire of mutations ranging from point mutations of the missense type to a small insertion within the exon to deletion of the entire gene result in the same clinical phenotype.[59,60]

Chromosomal Mutations

Mutations that involve large alterations in chromosome structure are readily visible microscopically by karyotypic analysis. These macromolecular mutations include deletions, duplications, inversions, and translocations from one chromosome to another. These chromosomal mutations affect large numbers of genes encoded in specific regions of DNA.

Single Nucleotide Polymorphisms

One of the derivatives from the federally funded HGP (1988–2004) is a comprehensive catalog of common human sequence polymorphisms. Every person, with the exception of monozygotic twins, has a unique genome with the variance between any two people on the planet being 0.1% or we are 99.9% identical. That reality still leaves many millions of differences among the 3.2 billion base pairs. Present evidence has confirmed that within these several million bases resides what explains our differences with respect to risk or susceptibility to a variety of diseases and disorders. Most of these differences are actually in the form of single nucleotide or base and are termed *single nucleotide polymorphisms* (SNPs). Today the international SNP map working groups have identified and mapped several million SNPs and also discovered a mutation rate of 2×10^{-8} per base pair per generation within the total 6 billion bases that are found in an individual human genome. These tools, still in their infancy, will enable critical dissection of human genetic variance in health as well as in disease. The reader is encouraged to follow this area of inquiry and to appreciate that genetics is the study of variation, and the prospect of carrying it on this level of resolution is heady while being remarkable.

GENETIC DISEASES AND DISORDERS

Approximately 2%–3% of all newborns are born with a serious congenital anomaly, and an additional 2%–3% of infants and children are found to have birth defects by the age of 5 years. Genetics plays a role in 40%–50% of childhood

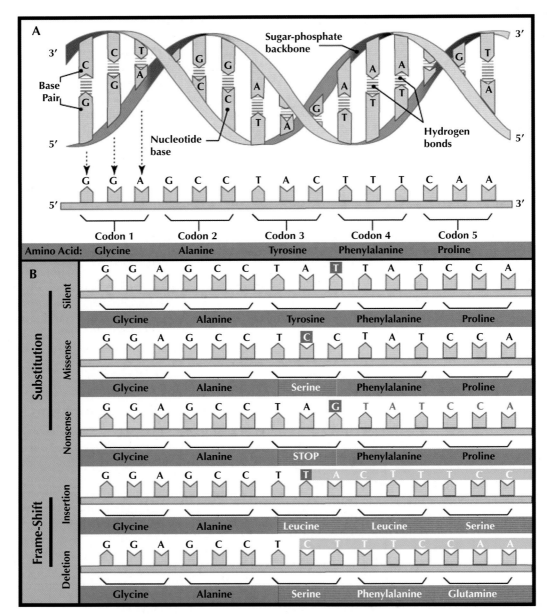

FIGURE 25-4 (A) The structure of DNA, which is composed of just four chemical, or nucleotide, building blocks; A, C, G and T. Adenine always associates with thymine whilst guanine always associates with cytosine. To form individual genes, these nucleotide bases are placed in a unique order, or sequence, upon a poly-sugar backbone that determines their unique characteristics. This is sectioned into triplet nucleotide groups, called codons, which code for the different amino acids. (B) The five major types of mutation. Silent mutations cause no change in the encoded amino acid sequence due to redundancy in the codons. Missense mutations lead to a single change in the encoded amino acid sequence. Nonsense mutations result in the formation of one of the three translation stop codons (TAA, TAG and TGA) that result in truncation of the encoded amino acid sequence. Frame-shift mutations (insertions or deletions) result in a change in the encoded amino acid sequences from the point of the mutation as they shift the nucleotide positions in each triplet codon such that they form different codons. Mutated nucleotides are highlighted in red, affected nucleotides are highlighted in yellow and affected amino acids are highlighted in pink.

deaths, 5%–10% of common cancers, and >50% of the older population's medical problems. About 4% of human genes contribute to disease in a major way. Of the over 5000 genetic syndromes known, over 700 have dental-oral-craniofacial defects and over 250 have associated clefting.[50–55,61–70] Facial

clefting is a clinical phenotype associated with Mendelian gene inheritance (single-gene mutation), and facial clefting is also presented in complex human diseases that are polygenic, involving multiple genes and multiple environmental factors.[72,73] Mutations in many different classes of

TABLE 25-1   Examples of Genetic Disorders in Newborn Screening Programs

Genetic Disorder	Screening Method	Treatment
Phenylketonuria	Guthrie bacterial inhibition assay	Diet restricting phenyl alanine
	Fluorescence assay	
	Amino acid analyzer	
	Tandem mass spectrometry	
Congenital hypothyroidism	Measurement of thyroxine and thyrotropin	Oral levothyroxine
Hemoglobinopathies	Hemoglobin electrophoresis	Prophylactic antibiotics immunization against *Diplococcus pneumonia* and *Haemophilus influenza*
	Isoelectric focusing	
	High-performance liquid chromatography	
	Follow-up DNA analysis	
Galactosemia	Beutler test	Galactose-free diet
	Paigen test	
Maple syrup urine disease	Guthrie bacterial inhibition assay	Diet restricting intake of branched-chain amino acids
Homocystinuria	Guthrie bacterial inhibition assay	Vitamin B12
		Diet restricting methionine and supplementing cystine
Biotinidase deficiency	Colorimetric assay	Oral biotin
Congenital adrenal hyperplasia	Radioimmunoassay	Glucocorticoids
	Enzyme immunoassay	Mineralocorticoids
		Salt
Cystic fibrosis	Immunoreactive trypsinogen assay followed by DNA testing	Improved nutrition
	Sweat chloride test	Management of pulmonary symptoms

All of these genetic screening tests for newborn infants are well established.

Tests are offered throughout the United Sates. The other tests are available in a limited number of states.

genes cause craniofacial-dental-oral defects, and these genes include those encoding transcription factors, hormone receptors, cell adhesion molecules, growth factors and their receptors, G proteins, enzymes, transporters, and collagens.[50–55,59–71]

Genetic disorders are broadly categorized as (1) single-gene or Mendelian disorders that are typically rare and familial (e.g., hemophilia); (2) chromosomal anomalies that are typically sporadic (e.g., Down syndrome); (3) multifactorial disorders or complex human diseases in which multiple genes are involved with a role played by environmental factors (e.g., many congenital craniofacial malformations, arthritis, hypertension, many cancers, diabetes, osteoporosis, temporomandibular disorders); and (4) acquired somatic genetic disease (e.g., many cancers) (Tables 25-1 and 25-2).

Mendelian Diseases and Disorders

The Online Mendelian Inheritance of Man (OMIM) catalogues approximately 11,000 monogenic or Mendelian traits. These inherited human diseases, typically caused by a mutation in a single gene, can be transmitted within families in a dominant or recessive mode. A dominant disease results if one copy of the two copies of a given gene bears a deleterious mutation. Examples of dominant diseases include achondroplasia (or short-limb dwarfism), myotonic dystrophy, and neurofibromatosis. Certain forms of hypodontia involving molar or premolar teeth also display autosomal dominant inheritance.[54–71] Even though one copy of the gene is normal, the abnormal copy of the gene is able to override it, causing disease. Dominant diseases can be traced through family pedigrees and appear to spread vertically because everyone carrying a dominant mutant allele (form of the gene) generally shows the disease symptoms. Individuals with disease are present in successive generations. There are an equal number of males and females with disease, and each affected individual has only one parent with disease. Individuals mating with an unaffected individual rarely have an affected offspring. Over 200 autosomal dominant diseases are known and can manifest in any organ system and occur at different frequencies.

A disease displays a recessive inheritance pattern when two abnormal copies of the gene are present for the individual

TABLE 25-2   Selected Examples of Genetic Tests for Neurological Diseases, Connective Tissue Diseases, Cancer, and Renal Diseases

Condition	Genes	Testing Utility
Neurologic		
Spinocerebellar ataxias	SCAI, SCA2, SCA3, SCA6, SCA7, SCAI0, DRPLA	Diagnostic, predictive
Early-onset familial Alzheimer's disease	PSENI, PSEN2	Diagnostic, predictive
Canavan's disease	ASPA	Diagnostic, prenatal
Nonsyndromic inherited congenital hearing loss (without other medical complications)	GJB2	Diagnostic, prenatal
Fragile X syndrome	FMRI	Diagnostic, prenatal
Huntington's disease	HD	Diagnostic, predictive, prenatal
Neurofibromatosis type 1	NFI	Prenatal
Neurofibromatosis type 2	NF2	Predictive, prenatal
Connective tissue		
Ehlers–Danlos syndrome, vascular type	COL3AI	Diagnostic, prenatal
Marfan's syndrome	FBNI	Diagnostic, prenatal
Osteogenesis imperfect types I–IV	COLIAI, COLIA2	Diagnostic, prenatal
Oncologic		
Familial adenomatous polyposis	APC	Diagnostic, predictive
Hereditary nonpolyposis colorectal cancer	MLHI, MSH2, PMS2, MSH3, MSH6	Diagnostic, predictive
von Hippel–Lindau disease	VHL	Diagnostic, predictive
Li–Fraumeni syndrome	TP53	Diagnostic, predictive
Hematologic		
β-Thalassemia	HbB	Carrier detection, prenatal diagnosis
Hemophilia A	F8C	Prognostic, carrier detection, prenatal
Hemophilia B	F9C	Carrier detection, prenatal
Renal		
Nephrogenic diabetes insipidus	AVPR2, AQP2	Diagnostic, carrier detection, prenatal
Polycystic kidney disease (autosomal dominant and autosomal recessive)	PKDI, PKD2, PKHD I	Predictive, prenatal

This table is intended to be illustrative, not exhaustive. Most entries are based on information from GeneTests-GeneClinics at <http://www .geneclinics.org>. This Web site includes a comprehensive list of available molecular genetic tests and further clinical information about these and other genetic conditions.

to be affected. Over 900 autosomal recessive diseases that manifest in a wide range of organs are known. Examples of recessive diseases include phenylketonuria, cystic fibrosis, Tay–Sachs disease, and Gaucher's disease. Recessive diseases that are rare are seen more often in communities in which consanguineous marriages are quite common since there is a high probability of mating between two carriers of the mutant gene. Parents of the affected individual show no symptoms even though they carry one mutant copy of the gene. If both parents are carriers of the gene, the child has a one in four chance of receiving a recessive allele from each parent and inheriting the disease. The distinctive features of an autosomal recessive disease are unaffected parents having affected offspring, equal numbers of affected males and

females, all offspring being affected when both parents are affected, and, frequently, the presence of consanguinity or origin of the population from a small group of founders.

Common population traits can be recessive, such as the blood group O; it may be brought into a pedigree by two parents independently and may appear dominant, but it is really pseudodominant and is a recessive trait. Therefore, it occurs in successive generations. Many dominant diseases may appear to skip a generation owing to a phenomenon referred to as nonpenetrance. Thus, even though a dominant disease should be apparent in all gene carriers, this is true only when the disease is 100% penetrant. The molecular basis of incomplete penetrance is unclear but is likely due to the effect of modifier genes that have an impact on the disease-causing mutation. Many psychiatric diseases, such as schizophrenia and bipolar mental disease, show incomplete penetrance owing to the effect of environmental factors and modifier genes. Late-onset diseases such as spinocerebellar ataxias demonstrate an age-related penetrance, with gene carriers being symptom free until midlife. This is the result of slow cell death—the inability to restore the normal cellular state on environmental damage or accumulation of a toxic product over time. In contrast to penetrance, which refers to the all-or-one state with respect to disease phenotype, variable expressivity is the variable expression of the disease phenotype within the same family. Many dominant diseases (e.g., Charcot–Marie–Tooth disease, neurofibromatosis) display variable expressivity, and the phenomenon is attributed to the effect of modifier genes since each member of the family who carries the same disease mutation can have a unique complement of genes other than those related to the disease that do interact with the disease gene.

Clinicians know that a major feature of gingivitis and periodontitis is the destruction of the collagenous matrix of the connective tissues by microbe-derived and/or host enzymes. Proteolytic cathepsins B, D, and L are biomarkers for the progression of disease.[63] What was quite surprising to many clinicians was the discovery that cathepsin C mutations appear to cause Papillon–Lefèvre syndrome.[74,75]

Sex-linked or X-linked diseases arise when there is a mutation in 1 of more than 285 genes that are located on the X chromosome. In X-linked dominant disease, both males and females are affected, although the females are usually less severely affected. This is because females have two X chromosomes, and during development, one of the two X chromosomes is selected at random and inactivated to allow X-chromosome gene dosage between males and females to be balanced. Thus, in some cells of the body, the X chromosome carrying the disease allele is inactivated, and in others, the *normal* X chromosome is inactivated. An example of an X-linked dominant disease is anhidrotic ectodermal dysplasia characterized by the absence of sweat glands, abnormal teeth, and sparse hair.[50] X-linked dominant inheritance can manifest in either sex, with more affected females than males. Females are more mildly affected than males. All female children of an affected male are affected, and all children of an affected female have a 50% chance of being affected. Most importantly, there is no male-to-male transmission of the disease since males receive their only X chromosome from their mother.

In X-linked recessive inheritance, only males are affected. Females are typically carriers with no symptoms or very mild symptoms. Affected males are usually born to unaffected parents, and the mother is normally an asymptomatic carrier. There is no male-to-male transmission of the disease. Occasionally, females may be affected if by misfortune most cells in a critical tissue have inactivated the normal X (referred to as nonrandom X-inactivation). Examples of such diseases are Duchenne muscular dystrophy and fragile X syndrome.

One example of a clinical phenotype that appears to be caused by either X-linked or autosomal inherited mutations is AI. There are three types of this genetic disorder: (1) type 1, hypoplastic AI; (2) type 2, hypocalcified AI; and (3) type 3, hypomaturation AI.[64–70] AI also shows three types of inheritance patterns: X-linked, autosomal dominant and autosomal recessive with mutations in any of nine genes to date, attributed to the disorder. X-linked AI is associated with mutations in the *AMELX* gene (amelogenin), the most prevalent protein in forming enamel extracellular matrix with genes located on both the X and Y chromosomes.[71] In most cases, males with X-linked AI are more severely affected than affected females. Autosomal dominant AI is associated with mutations in either the *ENAM* gene (enamelin) encoding the second most prevalent protein in the forming enamel matrix, or in the FAM83H gene whose function is unknown. Autosomal recessive AI is associated with mutations in both copies of the genes encoding *ENAM, MMP20, KLK4, FAM20A, C4orf26 or SLC24A4* in each ameloblast cell. Of these, *MMP20* and *KLK4* encode proteases that allow time- and position-specific protein degradation related to calcium hydroxyapatite crystal formations[68–71] while *SLC24A4* encodes a calcium transporter that mediates calcium transport to developing enamel during tooth development. The function of the remaining genes is presently unknown. Additional genes yet unidentified are expected to bear mutations leading to AI.

Y-linked inheritance implies that only males are affected. An affected male transmits his Y-linked trait to all of his sons but none of his daughters. Deletions of genes on the Y chromosome have been linked to infertility owing to azoospermia (or absence of sperm in semen) in males.

Chromosomal Diseases and Disorders

Chromosomal disorders are categorized into three general areas. The first is incorrect chromosomal number such as trisomy 21 (Down syndrome) of chromosome 21; this type is termed *aneuploidy*. Trisomies of chromosomes 13 and 18 are additional examples. Turner's syndrome occurs in women who acquire only one X chromosome. Klinefelter's syndrome occurs in men who receive two X chromosomes in addition to one Y chromosome. The second type is large chromosomal structural defects including microdeletions. DiGeorge syndrome is characterized by T-cell immunodeficiency and cardiac anomalies and is caused by a microdeletion of chromosome 22. The third type of anomaly is uniparental disomy, which refers to the presence of two copies of a chromosome (or part of a chromosome) from one parent and none from the other parent. One example of an adverse outcome of a uniparental disomy is the consequence of genetic imprinting. This term is used to describe when a genetic trait is inherited only when transmitted by the mother in some diseases, such as Beckwith–Wiedmann syndrome, or the father in others, such as glomus tumors. Genetic imprinting can be described as *parent of origin differences* in the expression of inherited genetic traits. Other examples of such genetic imprinting are presented with Prader–Willi and Angelman's syndromes, caused by a deficiency of paternal and maternal contributions, respectively, to a segment of the long arm of chromosome 15.

Mitochondrial Diseases and Disorders

Mitochondria are exclusively inherited from the mother since only maternal mitochondria are transmitted to the forming zygote in early embryogenesis. mtDNA is a small circular piece of DNA consisting of 16,569 nucleotides that encodes nine genes. Each mitochondrion normally contains multiple copies of mtDNA, whose total amount per cell is typically in the range of 40–2,000 copies. Most of these genes encode information for oxidative phosphorylation and energy production for the individual somatic cell type. Mitochondria contain a small fraction of the genes required for mitochondrial functions. Therefore, the remainder of genes is those found within the nucleus. Curiously, several codons are used for mtDNA differently from codons used for nuclear DNA.

Mitochondrial diseases frequently affect organs that are dependent on relatively high levels of energy, such as the nervous system, muscle, and beta cells in the pancreas. Each somatic cell contains different mixtures of mutant or partially deleted mitochondria that exist along with normal mitochondria. This interesting condition is known as heteroplasmy. The hallmark of mitochondrial inheritance, aside from maternal origin, is a broad spectrum of symptoms within a family segregating the same mitochondrial mutation, extreme variability in severity, and delayed onset with age. Examples of mitochondrial genetic diseases include mitochondrial encephalomyopathy or myoclonic epilepsy with ragged red muscle fibers, Leber's hereditary optic neuropathy with bilateral loss of central vision, and Kearns–Sayre syndrome, which presents retinal disease and cardiac disease (Tables 25-3 and 25-4).

Complex Human Diseases and Disorders

Complex human diseases or *multifactorial genetic disorders* are the most common forms of human genetic disease; they do not present a well-delineated Mendelian pattern of inheritance but *tend to run in families.* These disorders include many types of craniofacial malformations, tooth decay, periodontal disease, atherosclerosis, cardiovascular disease, osteoporosis,

TABLE 25-3 Craniofacial Dysmorphology Associated With Chromosomal Abnormalities

Syndrome	Chromosomal Defects	Craniofacial Features
Disorders affecting the autosomes		
Down syndrome	Trisomy 21	Mongolism, brachycephaly, mental retardation, upslanting palpebral fissures, epicanthus, iris brushfield spots, small mouth, protruding tongue, small ears, folded helix, short nose, flat nasal bridge, short neck
Edwards' syndrome	Trisomy 18	Prominent occiput, small chin, narrow palpebral fissures, occasional cleft lip, mental defect
Patau's syndrome	Trisomy 13	Cleft lip and palate, broad nasal bridge, sloping forehead, mental retardation, microcephaly, occasional holoprosencephaly, microphthalmia, forehead hemangiomas
Partial trisomy 22	Trisomy 22, partial	Microcephaly, hypertelorism, epicanthus, coloboma, preauricular pits and tags, mental retardation
9p Trisomy	Trisomy 9p	Microcephaly, small deep-set eyes, thin protruding upper lip, bulbous nose, mental retardation
Killian–Pallister mosaic syndrome	Mosaic tetrasomy of short arm of chromosome 12	Coarse facial features, broad forehead, hypertelorism, saggy cheeks, droopy mouth, prominent upper lip, sparse hair, mental retardation
Wolf–Hirschhorn syndrome	Deletion of short arm of chromosome 4	Frontal bossing, high hairline, prominent glabella, short prominent philtrum, occasional cleft lip, mental retardation
13q Syndrome	Deletion of long arm of chromosome 13	Minor dysmorphic face, trigonocephaly, microcephaly, broad nasal root, mental retardation, retinoblastoma
18q Syndrome	Deletion of long arm of chromosome 18	Midface hypoplasia, deep-set eyes, preauricular pits, short philtrum, carp-shaped mouth, narrow or atretic external auditory canal
Disorders affecting the sex chromosomes		
Turner's syndrome	45(XO)	Minor dysmorphic face, narrow maxilla, small chin, curved upper lip, straight lower lip, prominent ears, neck webbing
Females with multiple X chromosomes	47 (XXX) 48(XXXX)	Resemble Down syndrome features, broad flat nose, hypertelorism, epicanthus, prominent jaw, mental retardation

TABLE 25-4 Selected Examples of Craniofacial-Oral-Dental Mendelian Genetic Diseases and Disorders

Type	Gene Name	Gene Symbol	Chromosomal Location	Omim Number for Gene	Syndrome	OMIM Number for Syndrome	Inheritance	Description of Craniofacial-Oral-Dental Features*
ECM	Collagen, type I, alpha-1 chain	COL1A1	17q21.31-q22.05	120150	Osteogenesis imperfecta, type I	166200	AD	Hypoplasia of dentin and pulp, translucent teeth with yellow or blue–gray coloration, delayed tooth eruption, irregular placement of teeth, susceptibility to caries, wormian bones, occasional deafness, otosclerosis, blue sclerae
					Osteogenesis imperfecta, type III	259420	AR	Dentinogenesis imperfecta, macrocephaly, trianglar facial appearance, wormian bones, occasional deafness
					Osteogenesis imperfecta, type IV	166220	AD	Dentinogenesis imperfecta, multiple caries, wormian bones, occasional hearing loss, otosclerosis
					Ehlers-Danlos syndrome, type VII	130060	AD	Narrow maxilla, small mandible, occasional hypodontia and microdontia, wide nasal bridge, epicanthus
ECM	Collagen, type I, alpha-2 chain	COL1A2	7q22.1	120160	Osteogenesis imperfecta, type I	166200	AD	Hypoplasia of dentin and pulp, translucent teeth with yellow or blue–gray coloration, delayed teeth eruption, irregular placement of teeth, susceptibility to caries, wormian bones, occasional deafness, otosclerosis, blue sclerae
					Osteogenesis imperfecta, type III	259420	AR	Dentinogenesis imperfecta, macrocephaly, triangular facial appearance, wormian bones, occasional deafness
					Osteogenesis imperfecta, type IV	166220	AD	Dentinogenesis imperfecta, multiple caries, wormian bones, occasional hearing loss, otosclerosis
ECM	Collagen, type III, alpha-1 chain	COL3A 1	2q31	120180	Ehlers-Danlos syndrome, type IV	130050	AD	Narrow maxilla, small mandible, occasional hypodontia and microdontia, wide nasal bridge, epicanthus, large eyes, pinched nose, thin lips
ECM	Collagen, type VII, alpha-1 chain	COL7A 1	3p21.3	120120	Epidermolysis bullosa dystrophica	226600	AR	Defective tooth enamel, lingual adhesions, microstomia, bullae of conjunctiva and cornea

(Continued)

TABLE 25-4 Selected Examples of Craniofacial-Oral-Dental Mendelian Genetic Diseases and Disorders (Continued)

Type	Gene Name	Gene Symbol	Omim Number for Gene	Chromosomal Location	Syndrome	OMIM Number for Syndrome	Inheritance	Description of Craniofacial-Oral-Dental Features*
ECM	Collagen, type XI, alpha-2 chain	COL11A2	120290	6p21.3	Stickler syndrome, type II	184840	AD	Cleft palate, micrognathia, glossoptosis, severe myopia, flat facies, dental anomalies, deafness
ECM	Keratin 16	KRT16	148067	17q12-q21	Pachyonychia congenita, Jadassohn–Lewandowsky type	167200	AD	Oral leukoplakia, neonatal teeth, early loss of secondary teeth
ECM	Keratin 17	KRT17	148069	17q12-q21	Pachyonychia congenita, Jackson-Lawler type	167210	AD	No oral leukoplakia, neonatal teeth, early loss of secondary teeth
ECM	Amelogenin	AMELX	301200	Xp22.3-p22.1	Amelogenesis imperfecta 1, hypoplastic type	301200	XD	Hypoplastic-type amelogenesis imperfecta, very hard enamel, thin enamel, small teeth, rough tooth surface
ECM	Dentinogenesis imperfecta 1 gene	DGI1	125490	4q13-q21	Dentinogenesis imperfecta 1	125490	AD	Dentinogenesis imperfecta, blue-gray or amber brown opalescent teeth, enamel splitting, teeth have bulbous crowns, narrow roots with small or obliterated pulp chambers and root canal
ECM		Fibrillin 1		FBN1	15q21.1	134797 syndrome	Marfan's	154700	AD Dolichocephaly, high arched palate, narrow palate, crowded teeth, micrognathia
ECM					Shprintzen-Goldberg syndrome	182212	AD	Craniosynostosis, microcephaly, maxillary and mandibular hypoplasia, palatal shelf soft tissue hypertrophy, cleft palate, prominent nose, narrow palpebral fissures
ENZ	Alkaline phosphatase, liver/bone/kidney type	ALPL	171760	1p36.1-p34	Hypophosphatasia, infantile	241500	AR	Generalized lack of ossification, craniostenosis, microcephaly, leptomeningeal hemorrhage, absent bony cranial vault, poorly formed teeth
ENZ	Iduronate 2-sulfatase	IDS	309900	Xq28	Mucopolysaccharidosis, type II (Hunter's syndrome)	309900	X	Scaphocephaly, macrocephaly, frontal bossing, coarse facies, enlarged tongue, deafness
ENZ	Galactosamine (N-acetyl)-6-sulfate sulfatase	GALNS	253000	16q24.3	Mucopolysaccharidosis, type IVA (Morquio's syndrome)	253000	AR	Dense calvarium, broad mouth, wide-spaced teeth, thin enamel

	Gene	Symbol	Location	OMIM	Syndrome	Inheritance	OMIM	Clinical features
IS	Guanine nucleotide-binding protein, alpha-stimulating activity polypeptide 1	GNAS1	20q13.2	139320	Pseudohypoparathyroidism, type Ia	AD	103580	Round face, low nasal bridge, short neck, cataracts, delayed tooth eruption, enamel hypoplasia
					McCune-Albright syndrome	AD	174800	Cranial foramen impingement, craniofacial hyperostosis, facial asymmetry, prognathism
IS	Retinoblastoma 1	RB1	13q14.1-q14.2	180200	Retinoblastoma	AD	180200	Cleft palate, high forehead, prominent eyebrows, broad nasal bridge, bulbous tip of the nose, large mouth with thin upper lip, long philtrum, prominent earlobes
IS	Cyclin-dependent kinase inhibitor 1C	CDKN1C	11p15.5	600856	Beckwith-Wiedemann syndrome	AD	130650	Coarse facial features, linear earlobe creases, posterior helical indentations, macroglossia, midface hypoplasia
NP	Small nuclear ribonucleoprotein polypeptide N	SNRPN	15q12	182279	Prader-Willi syndrome	AD	176270	Narrow bitemporal head dimension, thin upper lip, down-turned corners of mouth, viscous saliva
NP	Werner's syndrome gene	WRN	8p12-p11.2	277700	Werner's syndrome	AR	277700	Wide face, prematurely aged face, beaked nose
NP	CREB binding protein	CREBBP	16p13.3	600140	Rubinstein-Taybi syndrome	AD	180849	Microcephaly, hypoplastic maxilla, beaked nose, slanted palpebral fissures, hypertelorism, short upper lip, pouting lower lip
SEC	Sonic hedgehog	SHH	7q36	600725	Holoprosencephaly, type 3	AD	142945	Cyclopia, ocular hypotelorism, proboscis, midface hypolasia, single nostril, midline cleft upper lip, premaxillary agenesis
NP	Eyes absent 1 gene	EYA1	8q13.3	601653	Branchio-otorenal Syndrome	AD	113650	Branchial cleft fistulae; external, middle, and inner ear malformations; hearing loss
TM	Fibroblast growth factor receptor 1	FGFR1	8p11.2-p11.1	136350	Pfeiffer's syndrome	AD	101600	Mild craniosynostosis, flat facies, acrocephaly
TM	Fibroblast growth factor receptor 2	FGFR2	10q26	176943	Crouzon's craniofacial dysostosis	AD	123500	Craniosynostosis, parrot-beaked nose, short upper lip, hypoplastic maxilla, relative mandibular prognathism, shallow orbit
					Jackson-Weiss syndrome	AD	123150	Craniosynostosis, midfacial hypoplasia Craniosynostosis, brachysphenocephalic acrocephaly, flat facies, high narrow palate

(Continued)

TABLE 25-4 Selected Examples of Craniofacial-Oral-Dental Mendelian Genetic Diseases and Disorders (Continued)

Type	Gene Name	Gene Symbol	Chromosomal Location	Omim Number for Gene	Syndrome	OMIM Number for Syndrome	Inheritance	Description of Craniofacial-Oral-Dental Features*
					Apert's syndrome	101200	AD	Mild craniosynostosis, flat facies, acrocephaly
					Pfeiffer's syndrome	101600	AD	Craniosynostosis, cloverleaf skull, cleft palate or uvula, craniofacial anomalies
					Beare-Stevenson cutis gyrata syndrome	123790	AD	
TM	Fibroblast growth factor receptor 3	FGFR3	4p16.3	134934	Achondroplasia	100800	AD	Frontal bossing, megalencephaly, midfacial hypoplasia, low nasal bridge
					Hypochondroplasia	146000	AD	Normocephaly or occasional brachycephaly, mild frontal bossing
					Thanatophoric dysplasia	187600	AD	Megalencephaly, small foramen magnum, cloverleaf skull, depressed nasal bridge
					Crouzon's disease with acanthosis nigricans	134934	AD	Craniosynostosis
					Craniosynostosis,nonsyndromic	134934	AD	Craniosynostosis
TM	Insulin receptor	IR	19p13.2	147670	Leprechaunism, insulin-resistant diabetes mellitus with acanthosis nigricans	147670	AD	Bitemporal skull narrowing, supernumerary teeth, severe premature caries, prominent lower canines and upper incisors, thickened lips, prominent ears
TM	Parathyroid hormone receptor	PTHR	3p22-p21.1	168468	Metaphyseal chondrodysplasia,Murk Jansen type	156400	AD	Sclerosis of cranial base, wide cranial sutures, supraorbital hyperplasia, prominent supraorbital ridges, frontonasal hyperplasia, micrognathia, high arched palate, deafness
TM	RET oncogene	RET	10q11.2	164761	Neuromata, mucosal, with endocrine tumors	162300	AD	Neuromata of lips and tongue, conjunctival and nasal mucosa neuromas, diffuse lip hypertrophy, high arched palate, coarse facies
TM	Ectodermal dysplasia gene, anhidrotic	EDA	Xq12.2-q13.1	305100	Ectodermal dysplasia, anhidrotic	305100	X	Absent teeth, small pointed incisors, saddle nose, sparse hair, prominent forehead, prominent lips

TM	Patched	PTC	9q22.3	601309	Basal cell nevus syndrome (Gorlin's syndrome)	109400	AD	Macrocephaly, broad facies, frontal and biparietal bossing, mild mandibular prognathism, odontogenic keratocysts of jaws, misshapened and/or carious teeth, cleft lip and palate, ectopic calcification of falx cerebri
TF	Msh homeobox homolog 1	MSX1	4p16.1	142983	Tooth agenesis, familial	142983	AD	Hypodontia
TF	Msh homeobox homolog 2	MSX2	5q34-q35	123101	Craniosynostosis, type 2	123101	AD	Craniosynostosis, forehead retrusion, frontal bossing, turribrachycephaly, Kleeblattschaedel deformity (cloverleaf skull, trilobular skull anomaly)
TF	Microphthalmia-associated transcription factor	MITF	3p14.1-p12.3	156845	Waardenburg's syndrome, type IIA	193510	AD	Wide nasal bridge, short philtrum, cleft lip or palate, deafness
TF	GLI-Kruppel family member 3 oncogene	GLI3	7p13	165240	Greig's cephalopoly-syndactyly syndrome	175700	AD	Peculiar skull shape, expanded cranial vault, high forehead and bregma, frontal bossing, macrocephaly, hypertelorism
					Pallister-Hall syndrome	146510	AD	Short nose, flat nasal bridge, multiple buccal frenula, microglossia, micrognathia, cleft palate, malformed ears
TF	Paired box homeotic gene 3	PAX3	2q35	193500	Waardenburg's syndrome, type I	193500	AD	Wide nasal bridge, short philtrum, cleft lip or palate, occasional deafness, dystopia canthorum
					Waardenburg's syndrome, type III	148820	AD	Microcephaly, wide nasal bridge
					Craniofacial-deafness-hand syndrome	122880	AD	Flat facial profile, hypertelorism, hypoplastic nose and maxilla, slitlike nares, hearing loss
TF	Solurshin	RIEG	4q25-q26	601542	Rieger's syndrome, type I	180500	AD	Maxillary hypoplasia, mild prognathism, protruding lower lip, short philtrum, microdontia, hypodontia, cone-shaped teeth
TF	Core-binding factor, runt domain, alpha subunit 1	CBFA1	6p21	600211	Cleidocranial dysplasia	119600	AD	Brachycephaly, frontal and parietal bossing, wormian bones, persistent open anterior fontanel, midfacial hypoplasia, delayed eruption of deciduous and permanent teeth, supernumerary teeth

(Continued)

TABLE 25-4 Selected Examples of Craniofacial-Oral-Dental Mendelian Genetic Diseases and Disorders (Continued)

Type	Gene Name	Gene Symbol	Chromosomal Location	Omim Number for Gene	Syndrome	OMIM Number for Syndrome	Inheritance	Description of Craniofacial-Oral-Dental Features*
TF	Twist	TWIST	7p21	601622	Saethre-Chotzen syndrome	101400	AD	Craniosynostosis, acrocephaly, brachycephaly, flat facies, thin long pointed nose, cleft palate, cranial asymmetry, ptosis, malformed ears
UNK	DiGeorge's syndrome chromosome region	CATCH22	22q11	188400	DiGeorge's syndrome	188400	AD	Low-set ears, short ears, small mouth, submucous or overt palatal cleft, cleft lip, bulbous nose, square nasal tip, short philtrum, micrognathia
					Velocardiofacial syndrome	192430	AD	Pierre Robin syndrome, cleft palate, small open mouth, myopathic facies, retrognathia, prominent nose with squared-off nasal tip
UNK	Treacle	TCOF1	5q32-q33.1	154500	Treacher Collins mandibulofacial dysostosis	154500	AD	Malar hypoplasia, cleft palate, mandibular hypoplasia, macrostomia, malformed ears, sensorineural deafness, coloboma of lower eyelid

AD, autosomal dominant; AR, autosomal recessive; ECM, extracellular matrix protein; ENZ, enzyme; IS, intracellular signaling protein; NP, nuclear protein; TF, transcription factor; TM, transmembrane protein; UNK, unknown; X, X-linked; XD, X-linked dominant.

aThe following description is a summary of the craniofacial-oral-dental features of the diseases and disorders. For detailed information regarding defects in other affected tissues and organs, refer to Online Mendelian Inheritance in Man (OMIM) at <http://www.ncbi.nlm.gove/omim/>.

autoimmune disorders, hypertension, emphysema, diabetes, peptic ulcers, numerous mental diseases, and numerous birth defects, such as clefting, spina bifida, limb deformities, and congenital heart disease (Figure 25-5).[10,15] These conditions are caused by multiple genes with environmental factors and appear to cluster in families over multiple generations. Further, these examples are more prevalent in females versus males or males versus females, depending on the specific disease or disorder. For example, autoimmune diseases (e.g., Sjögren's syndrome, lupus) are more prevalent in females. These and other areas of interest have led to the emerging field of *gender biology* and *gender medicine.*

This section focuses on selected examples of complex human diseases and disorders that demonstrate multigene and multigene–environment interactions and that are of importance to oral health care providers in the everyday practice of dentistry.

The etiology, pathogenesis, manifestations, management, and treatment outcomes of *complex human diseases* or *multifactorial genetic disorders* represent a dynamic interplay between regulatory and structural genes and environmental and behavioral factors. The results from international, multicenter studies of cleft lip and/or palate suggest that many genes (e.g., *MSX1*, interferon regulatory factor 6 [*IRE6*]) and their expression are coupled with several environmental factors.[73] Protein–calorie malnutrition, vitamin deficiencies such as those related to folic acid and retinoic acid, and alcohol and tobacco consumption are a few of the environmental factors that relate to specific sets of genes essential for morphogenesis.[10,15,50–53]

The sex chromosomes were previously assumed to be the determinants of the sex of a child. Currently, it is believed that gender identity vis-à-vis sex chromosomes not only influences gender sexuality but also has profound influences on multigene and complex human disorders. Individual gene expression, multiple gene–gene interactions, and multigene–environment interactions are fundamentally different between men and women.

Gene networks that regulate metabolism, drug absorption, and drug use differ between genders. Gene circuits in the immune and endocrine systems show gender variance. These emerging observations may also reflect physiologic effects influenced by genes encoded within the two X chromosomes of the female, albeit with only one of the two active in any given cell, versus the one X and one Y chromosome of the male. Multiple gene–gene and gene–environment interactions demonstrate significant differences in many aspects of growth, development, maturation, and senescence between genders. As increasing numbers of men and women live longer within industrial nations, data are emerging that demonstrate gender differences in the prevalence and incidence of many complex conditions, such as cardiovascular diseases, diabetes, periodontal diseases, osteoporosis, and pulmonary diseases. Risk factors such as diet, lack of exercise, and stress seem to have different influences on the incidence, onset, and progression of cardiovascular diseases between men and women. Examples involve relationships such as low birth weight premature infants and periodontal diseases,[76,77] osteoporosis, and cardiovascular diseases.[78–80] Women's diseases are no longer viewed as those limited to diseases of the reproductive system and related hormones (e.g., estrogen and progesterone).

The function of multiple genes encoded within both sex chromosomes and autosomes, the specific gender of the individual (i.e., XX versus XY), and multiple environmental influences serve as the foundation for increased susceptibility to different manifestations of diseases. Further, gender-based genetic differences are also implicated in pharmacogenomics and individual responses to the absorption, diffusion, use, and metabolism of many therapeutics, including analgesics for pain management.[81,82] Gender differences in analgesic absorption, diffusion, and binding to specific sets of receptors suggest strong gender-specific differences, and these are important in oral medicine and other disciplines. Collectively, these and many other scientific discoveries herald the new fields of *gender biology* and *gender medicine.* A primer in modern human genetics for health professionals must include *gender oral medicine.*

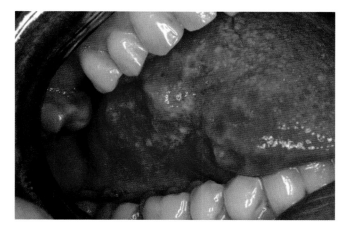

FIGURE 25-5 Multiple mutations in multiple genes, genes often associated with cell cycle regulation during mitosis and/or tumor suppressor genes, are implicated in squamous cell carcinoma as presented in numerous head and neck cancers (i.e., advanced oral cancer as shown in this figure). (Courtesy Dr. Parish Sedghizadeh.)

Respiratory Diseases

Asthma is an inflammatory disease of the small airways of the lung. Adult-onset asthma is more commonly seen in women than in men. In the United States, since 1990, mortality from chronic lower respiratory diseases remained relatively stable for men, whereas it increased for women. Genetic susceptibility and environmental factors weigh equally in contributing to this finding. Asthma affects one child in seven in some societies and approximately 15 million individuals worldwide. Although identification of all asthma genes is incomplete, five asthma susceptibility genes have been identified by positional cloning: *ADAM33*, *PHF11*, *DPP10*, *GRPA*, and *SPINK5*. Approximately a third of the genetic predisposition to asthma has been uncovered. Genetic findings will lead to the development of new therapy and new treatments for individuals with severe asthma who do not respond to commonly available steroid inhalers.[83–86]

Cardiovascular Disease

Cardiovascular disease is one of the leading causes of death in the world. The 2002 World Health Report demonstrated a higher prevalence and incidence of cardiovascular diseases (rheumatic heart disease, hypertension, cerebrovascular disease, and inflammatory heart disease) in women than in men.[87] The risk for cardiovascular diseases also increases with age at a faster rate in women than in men. Genetic and environmental factors and biologic and anatomic differences have been considered as possible contributory factors to these differences. A genetic predisposition to cardiovascular disease results from gene mutations that alter the biologic function expressed by the original gene(s) and increase an individual's risk for cardiovascular diseases. A region on chromosome 13 in Caucasians and on chromosome 19 in African–Americans has been linked to hypertension and stroke.[88–90]

In addition to gene mutations that directly increase susceptibility, there are multiple genes that indirectly increase the risk of cardiovascular diseases. These indirect predispositions are in the form of genes that are related to unhealthy behaviors, such as metabolic pathways related to tobacco use and alcohol consumption. For example, the complications associated with the angiotensin-converting enzyme (*ACE*) gene in ischemic cerebrovascular disease were investigated in smoking and nonsmoking patients. The *ACE* gene mutation was a risk factor only in individuals who smoked but did not appear to behave as a risk factor in those individuals who did not smoke.[91,92]

Endocrine Disease

Oral diseases and disorders are associated with systemic diseases.[93–95] Oral infections are closely linked with diabetes, and management of diabetes is related to the management of oral infections.[78–80,93–95] At present, there is evidence that more than 20 regions of the genome may be involved in susceptibility to type 1 diabetes.[96] The genes in the human leukocyte antigen region of chromosome 6 are currently considered to have the highest influence on susceptibility to type 1 diabetes. To date, more than 50 genes have been studied for their possible association with type 2 diabetes in different populations worldwide. The most noteworthy genes are *PPAR8*, *ABCC8*, *KCNJ11*, and *CALPN10*.[96–98] For more information on diabetes, see Chapter 21, "Diabetes Mellitus and Endocrine Diseases."

The prevalence of type II diabetes is significantly higher in populations within Mexico and Latin America. A newly discovered gene sequence mutation or variant in *SLC16A11* revealed disease risk alleles in Mexican and other Latin American populations using a panel of SNPs (analysis of 9.2 million SNPs) and no risk alleles in other populations.[99] Currently, the variant gene for *SLC16A11* produces a mRNA that is localized to hepatocytes and the protein product functions in lipid metabolism causing an increase of intracellular triacylglycerol levels leading to the type II diabetic phenotype.[99]

Autoimmune Diseases

Women are 2.7 times more likely than men to acquire an autoimmune disease. Women have enhanced immune systems compared with men, which increases women's resistance to many types of infection but also makes them more susceptible to autoimmune diseases.[100–102] Men appear to have higher levels of natural killer cell activity than women. This difference in bioactivity may be associated with reduced levels of autoimmune disease in men. The plasma activity level of phospholipase A_2, a key enzyme in causing chronic inflammatory diseases, is significantly higher in Caucasian and Asian Indian women than in their male counterparts.[103–105] A molecule involved in reducing the inflammatory response, interleukin (IL) 1 receptor II, is present in higher concentrations in blood fractions from men than from women.[100–105]

The most striking sex differences for complex human diseases are observed in Sjögren's syndrome, lupus, autoimmune thyroid disease (Hashimoto's thyroiditis, Graves' disease), and scleroderma; these represent a spectrum of diseases in which the patient population is greater than 80% female. In rheumatoid arthritis, multiple sclerosis, and myasthenia gravis, the sex distribution is 60%–75% female.[100–102,106]

In addition to increased susceptibility to autoimmune disorders, women experience certain viral infectious conditions that affect their immune system disproportionately when compared with men.[106,107] For example, human immunodeficiency virus (HIV) infection that was more prevalent in men in the early 1980s is currently affecting women at an alarming rate.[106] Women account for almost 50% of the 40 million people living with HIV-1 worldwide, with an even higher percentage in developing countries. In the United States, the estimated number of acquired immune deficiency syndrome (AIDS) cases increased 15% among women and only 1% among men from 1999 to 2003.[106] The major burden of the disease was in young women, particularly African–American and Hispanic women.[106]

Heterosexual transmission is now the most commonly reported mode of HIV transmission in women. Women's increased susceptibility has been linked to physiologic factors such as hormonal changes, vaginal microbial ecology, and a higher prevalence of sexually transmitted diseases. These factors, in combination with other factors, such as gender disparities, poverty, cultural and sexual norms, lack of education, and sexual and domestic violence, make women vulnerable to this and other viral infections.[107,108]

Women develop signs and symptoms of AIDS, including oral manifestations, at a lower HIV viral load than men.[109] They also seem to benefit from the initiation of antiretroviral therapy at a lower HIV viral load than men.

Cancer

The role of genetics in cancer is widely recognized. The prevalence of cancer is projected to increase 50% worldwide within the next 20 years. According to the World Cancer Report, 10 million new cancer cases are diagnosed annually. Cancer contributes to 12.6% of the global mortality rate.[110] All cancers have genetic determinants. Cancers are usually caused by a sequence of multiple genetic mutations, and this is highlighted by neoplastic diseases of the head and neck.[111-116] There are three categories of cancer: inherited, familial, or sporadic. *Inherited* cases of a dominant type are often caused by direct mutations of genes that are passed successively from parents to offspring throughout generations. These are often regulatory genes required for the control of the cell cycle and cell division, as well as genes that regulate tumor suppression. *Familial* cases involve mutations of multiple susceptibility genes that increase an individual's risk for cancer (so-called multigene–gene and gene–environment interactions). *Sporadic* cancer cases are those in which an individual randomly develops cancer in the absence of any familial pattern, such as chronic exposure to carcinogenic substances.

Three of the most studied cancers with susceptibility genes are breast, colorectal, and prostate cancers. *BRCA1, BRCA2, TP53* (breast cancer), *hMLH1, hMLH2, IGF2* (colorectal), *BRCA1, BRCA2, hMLH1, hMLH2* (ovarian), *CYP1A1* (lung), and *HPC2* (prostate) are among the genes of interest.[117-119] Further, molecular studies of development has revealed that gene products associated with embryonic pattern formation and morphogenesis in most organs can also be causative to the process of neoplasia. One example is found associated with Wnt signaling that may lead to cancer. Severe permanent tooth agenesis (oligodontia) and colorectal neoplasia are found to segregate with dominant inheritance. Both oligodontia and predisposition to cancer are caused by a nonsense mutation, Arg656Stop, in the Wnt-signaling regulator $AXIN_2$.[120]

Tumor suppressor genes are involved in regulating the cell cycle and activate cell apoptosis or cell death.[111,112] The gene mutation results in the production of altered protein that is no longer capable of initiating apoptosis. Although great progress is being made in the discovery of genetic susceptibility to cancer, little attention had been paid to gender and sex disparities in cancer. For most common cancers, men seem to have a higher incidence than women. Men and women are predisposed to different anatomic, biochemical, and genetic features, and these factors may play a role in the susceptibility to and onset of cancer. Men and women respond differently to stress-inducing environments, which may make them more susceptible to certain behaviors (e.g., tobacco use and alcohol consumption) that might enhance their susceptibility to neoplastic diseases, such as oral and pharyngeal cancers (see Figure 25-5).[112-116]

Neurodegenerative Diseases and Mental Diseases

Research in neurodegenerative and mental diseases and disorders is focusing on tracing positions of gene mutations coupled with environmental factors that lead to the causes of these profound chronic disease conditions. Alzheimer's disease constitutes about two-thirds of all cases of dementia. Alzheimer's disease is a progressive neurologic disease that results in irreversible loss of neurons, particularly in the cortex and hippocampus.[121,122] There are missense mutations in three genes in families with early-onset autosomal dominant Alzheimer's disease: beta-amyloid on chromosome 21, presenelin 1 on chromosome 14, and presenilin 2 located on chromosome 1. The *APOE* gene on chromosome 19 has been linked to late-onset Alzheimer's disease, which is the most common form of the disease. This gene has three different forms: *APOE2, APOE3,* and *APOE4. APOE3* is the most common form in the general population. *APOE4* occurs in 40% of all late-onset Alzheimer's disease patients but is not limited to those whose families have a history of Alzheimer's disease. Patients with no known family history (sporadic Alzheimer's disease) are also more likely to have an *APOE4* gene.

Parkinson's disease is the second most common neurodegenerative disorder after Alzheimer's disease. The exact cause of Parkinson's disease remains unknown, but genetic factors have been identified as potential contributing factors in the onset and severity of the disease.[123] Studies with monozygotic twins show a very high level of concordance in the early-onset (before age 50 years) type of Parkinson's disease. The early onset version appears to be autosomal dominant in families of the Mediterranean and German regions and has several missense mutations in the gene coding for α-synuclein located on chromosome 4q21.

Genetics studies are also contributing toward enhanced understanding of mental diseases and disorders. For example, men are more likely to express depression or severe unhappiness through an *externalizing pathway* of physical behaviors, including drinking, drug abuse, and violence, whereas women are more likely to *internalize*, leading to depression and anorexia. This sex difference is more prominent during puberty. Epidemiologic studies have shown that in families of women with bulimia, the men often have alcoholism and other addictions. Men may cope with disasters by drinking. In some cultures, it is not acceptable for women to drink, and they may cope with disasters by developing anxiety disorder and depression. More than half of all female suicides worldwide take place in China.[117-119,124]

It has been have proposed that sex hormones are responsible for a higher incidence of mental disorders in women.[125] A comprehensive evaluation of women's mental health is currently ongoing in 28 countries as part of an epidemiologic study sponsored by the World Health Organization.[87] New emerging information by genetic epidemiologists reveals a number of structural and functional differences between men's and women's brains. Men's brains are more lateralized, whereas women's brains are not. This makes it more likely for women than for men to overcome language deficits resulting from strokes in the left hemisphere, where language is centered. This structural difference has also been linked to the lower likelihood of childhood developmental and mental disorders in girls than in boys. Sex differences are also present in substance abuse. Female substance abusers are more likely to report psychiatric symptoms before the onset of substance abuse, whereas male substance abusers are more likely to report depression and other psychiatric symptoms after chronic substance abuse. Recently, bioimaging studies have provided information about the neural processes underlying differences in the manifestations of substance abuse.[118,119,124]

GENETICS, GENDER, AND TREATMENT RESPONSES (PHARMACOGENOMICS)

Human genetic variance, the 200–300 million base differences (SNPs) between human genomes, can explain why all patient responses to therapy are not always the same.[12,81,82] For example, despite appropriate management of hypertension and accomplishment of target blood pressure, some hypertensive patients still develop myocardial infarction or stroke, and, despite appropriate management of these conditions, some patients survive and some do not. Similarly, not all patients respond to behavioral modifications in the same way. It is known that regular exercise alleviates hypertension in some patients but not all. In summary, human genetic variations contribute to these differences. Recent investigations have identified five sources of genetic variation between multiple families receiving medications for the management of cardiovascular diseases.[126]

The birth and evolution of pharmacogenetics and pharmacogenomics have contributed significantly to a better understanding of individual variations in therapeutics. The genetics of pharmacokinetics and pharmacodynamics and physiologic regulation that is influenced by ethnicity, age, and gender all affect an individual's discrete response to a drug therapy. Men and women may respond to the same drug differently. For example, intake of certain antibiotics, antihistamines, antiarrhythmics, and antipsychotics places women at a higher risk than men for drug-induced arrhythmias.[127,128]

The differences in responses to drugs have been missed in the past because women were not always included in clinical trials; if they were, the data were not broken down by sex.[129,130] Recently, based on a long-term clinical trial, it was shown that aspirin, which protects men against heart attack but not stroke, has exactly the opposite effect in women. Evidence shows that men and women differ in the activity of liver enzymes that metabolize drugs. Women are, on average, smaller in size and have a higher percentage of body fat. Therefore, women may absorb and/or excrete drugs more slowly or may retain fat-soluble drugs longer than men. Furthermore, women were reported to have a significantly higher likelihood than men of being admitted to a hospital as a direct consequence of adverse drug reactions.[131]

Traditionally, health care providers have used a combination of history, clinical evaluation, and diagnostic tests as a basis for their diagnoses and patient management. Often multiple patients who presented with similar histories and had similar clinical and laboratory findings received the same treatment. Today, with the availability of different genetic tests, the level of risk for or susceptibility to different diseases can be identified. This will change the practice of medicine and dentistry in the future because risk factors will be the driving force for treatment selection, not merely the clinical signs and symptoms. Patients with clinical risk factors will be treated differently even though the presenting signs and symptoms are the same.

Advances in genomics and molecular tests for assessments and diagnoses, as well as pharmacogenomics and pharmacogenetics, will change the future of the practice of medicine and dentistry.[8,10,14,15,51–55,61–73,76–81,94,132–134] Efforts should be made to incorporate *genomic* information in continuing education programs for current practitioners and in medical and dental school curriculums for future health care providers.[111,135,136] The interpretation of genetic test results, the provision of appropriate counseling, and the solutions to potential ethical and confidentiality-related issues need adequate training and expertise involving all health care providers.

PHENOTYPIC (PHENOMICS) AND GENETIC HETEROGENEITY (GENOMICS) IN DISEASES AND DISORDERS

Human disorders are heterogeneous as the result of complex interactions between multiple genetic loci and environmental factors during the life span resulting in phenotype. This interpretation is true for human diseases that segregate as simple Mendelian traits as well as for non-Mendelian multifactorial conditions. There are many examples of single gene disorders in which identical mutations result in widely different clinical phenotypes, referred to as variable expressivity. For example, monozygotic twins, two siblings with identical genetic inheritance, show phenotypic heterogeneity with age and varying environments.[137,138] This nonintuitive realization has become the rapidly advancing field of *epigenetics*, which refers to the posttranslational alteration of gene function through methylation, acetylation, sulfation, or phosphorylation of histone and non-histone chromosomal proteins without altering the nucleic acid sequence of DNA.

Single-gene mutations can have pleiotropic or multiple effects. For example, patients who present with xeroderma pigmentosum are unusually sensitive to sunlight, and patients with α_1-antitrypsin deficiency often have a predisposition to developing emphysema and are more sensitive to tobacco smoke.[139] Single-gene mutations may also be associated with serious and inappropriate responses to certain therapeutics. Mendelian and non-Mendelian multifactorial diseases may also present clinical complexities with drug use, absorption, and metabolism.[12,15,48,49,81,82] For example, glucose-6-phosphate dehydrogenase deficiency is inherited as an X-linked recessive disorder and can induce hemolytic anemia in response to various drug therapies.[139] Mendelian and non-Mendelian multifactorial diseases and pharmacogenomics are remarkably linked to genetic variations in drug metabolism in a growing array of patients. Distinct alleles of the cytochrome P-450 network of genes that function in drug metabolism have an impact on drug efficacy and toxicity.[81,82,140]

In addition to genetic heterogeneity resulting from gene–gene and gene–environment interactions, other factors serve to enhance or increase the phenotypic heterogeneity of human disorders, such as *penetrance*. The varying degree of severity and incomplete penetrance of gene expression need to be appreciated by all clinicians. Many autosomal dominant diseases often display varying severity owing to variable expressivity and incomplete penetrance. Examples of disorders with reduced penetrance are tuberous sclerosis and Marfan's syndrome.

It is important to recognize the phenomenon of locus heterogeneity wherein mutations in different genes can cause remarkably similar clinical phenotypes. One classic example is that forms of hemophilia can be caused by genetic mutations in either the gene for factor VIII (so-called classic hemophilia) or the gene for factor IX (Christmas disease). Both of these two genes are located on the X chromosome, and both of these diseases or conditions are inherited as X-linked recessive disorders. Similarly, the enamel disorder AI can be caused by mutations in *AMELX*, *ENAM*, or *MMP20*.[63–71] In addition, different point mutations in the same gene can result in very different clinical phenotypes. One example is the gene fibroblast growth factor receptor 2 (*FGFR2*). Different point mutations in *FGFR2* result in very different craniofacial dysmorphogenesis syndromes with craniosynostosis.[51–53,135,138] Similarly, severe mutations within the dystrophin gene, such as deletion of large portions of the gene, result in Duchenne muscular dystrophy, whereas milder mutations, such as certain point mutations, result in the milder Becker dystrophy.

THE "OMICS" REVOLUTION AND A SYSTEMS BIOLOGY APPROACH TO DISEASE

Within the fields of molecular biology and genetics, the *genome* is the entirety of an organism's hereditary information. It is encoded either in DNA or, for some viruses, in RNA. The genome includes both genes, pseudogenes, and the noncoding nucleic acid sequences of DNA and RNA. The literature describes the human genome as inclusive or highlights the mitochondrial genome (mitDNA) in juxtaposition to the nuclear genome (nuclear DNA + mitochondrial DNA = human genome). More recently, the human genome term also implies the inclusion of the total bacterial genomes that coexist with the human condition (*microbiome*).

The advent of genomics and other -*omics* technologies have begun to revolutionize biomedical research and clinical practice. The term *genomic medicine* or *personalized medicine* that refers to a clinical decision guided by knowledge of an individual's DNA sequence is ever expanding in scope and now includes information from derivatives of genomes that include RNAs (*transcriptome*), proteins (*proteome*), and metabolites (*metabolome*). The progress in part has been the result of inexpensive high-throughput sequencing and array-based solutions that address genomic complexity. From a clinical perspective, a patient's nuclear and mitochondrial genome can be completed within 24 hours at a cost less than $5000 using leading-edge technology.[4–6,9] The curious reader is encouraged to study Kevin Davies provocative book *The $1,000 Genome: The Revolution in DNA Sequencing and the New Era of Personalized Medicine*. Soon to be added to this compendium will be a detailed profile of an individual's *epigenome*, that reflects modifications that occur in the genome that do not change the sequence of the bases in the DNA an individual is born with but that can change the DNA conformation and as a consequence, change the expression of genes. Exact descriptions of a person's every physical and behavioral characteristic constitutes his *phenome*. Compilation of phenome data on humans is underway but is much more challenging than it is for model organisms such as the mice, rats or yeast as the same symptoms may have different descriptors such as *caries* or *tooth decay* or *cavity* which could make construction of databases akin to those with other -omic data more difficult. Astute clinical observations and annotations coupled with standardized electronic patient records that fully integrate a patient's total health information are imperative to advance phenomics.

The advent of next-generation (or third-generation) sequencing (NGS) has greatly enhanced the ability to examine the genomes and transcriptomes of humans and other species at a pace and cost that was not possible with earlier sequencing technologies. These rapid advances were made possible through federal funding from the HGP (1988–present) as well as industry and venture capital investments that has resulted in the development, manufacture and marketing of life science tools and integrated systems for large-scale analysis of human, viral, bacterial and yeast genomes.[4–6,9] DNA sequencing using the NGS approach has focused on either only exons of genes (*exome*) representing 1%–2% of the genome or the entire genome (*whole genome*).[6] The choices are largely driven by cost and the extent of data storage required with costs for the latter often surpassing the cost of the actual sequencing! Exome sequencing has had a great impact on rare Mendelian diseases, particularly autosomal recessive ones, by enabling the identification of a gene underlying a disease by identification of candidate mutations by the analysis of a single affected individual. For instance, at least four novel genes associated with recessive amelogenesis imperfecta have been identified using exome sequencing of single patients within unrelated families.

The 1000 Genomes Project was launched in 2008, to establish a detailed catalog of human genetic variation by sequencing the whole genomes of at least 1000 anonymous participants from a number of different ethnic groups. Although Mendelian diseases are considered rare, genetic mutations are estimated to occur at a rate of 40–82 per 1000 live births. This catalog has been an invaluable resource for GWA studies (Figure 25-1) on common diseases as knowledge about the frequency and types of sequence variants and their order on chromosomes in different populations is necessary for the success of these studies. The data have also been instructive on tracing the history of world populations by examination of the nature and pattern of variants amongst different world populations.

Knowledge of DNA variants however, is not sufficient to understand disease mechanism ultimately needed for design of both prevention as well as treatment regimens. The approach for achieving these goals is a systems-based approach which is a type of analysis that examines changes across the expanse of the entire genome at the DNA, RNA, and protein level and the interactions between these elements that result in changes in biochemical molecules (e.g., Cytokines) and clinical outcomes (e.g., Hypertension). Systems Biology encompasses studies that aim to define the interactions between molecules within a cell on a large-scale (*interactome*) as well as those that relate genomic, transcriptomic, and metabolomic data to each other and to phenome data at the level of the whole organism such as yeast or a whole organ level such as liver (Figure 25-6).

SALIVARY DIAGNOSTICS

Saliva as a screening and/or diagnostic tool has received significant visibility in recent years due to the advancements in biomedical, translational, and clinical sciences. Salivary biomarkers have a promising future and may eventually be used routinely for risk assessment, disease prevention, and identification of systemic and oral diseases in clinical settings.[145–148] Several laboratory-based tests are currently

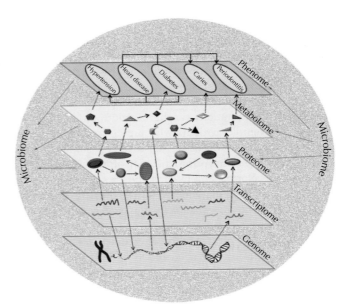

FIGURE 25-6 Systems biology.

available to assess the presence of microbial components, viruses, drugs and hormones in saliva.[149] In addition, scientists are utilizing salivary biomarkers to assess genetic risk factors for the development of common oral diseases such as dental caries, periodontal disease, and oral cancer.[150,151]

The term salivaomics was introduced to the literature in 2008 as a result of the rapid knowledge that was emerging based on the study of salivary biologic molecules.[152] Since then terms such as salivary proteome, transcriptome, microRNA (mi RNA), metabolome, and microbiome have been added to the nomenclature associated with salivary-related research. The metabolome is the complete set of small molecules found in a biologic sample. Salivary transcriptome consists of 180 mRNAs. The core salivary proteome contains 1,166 proteins, as determined by the collective efforts of three scientific groups with support from the National Institute of Dental and Craniofacial Research.[145,152–154] Scientists are utilizing salivary metabolome for early detection of oral and systemic diseases. Potential variation in the salivary microbiome has recently been used as a vehicle for detection of early resectable pancreatic cancer. Two microbial markers (*Neisseria elongate* and *Streptococcus mitis*) have been successfully used in one study to identify those individuals with early-stage resectable pancreatic cancer from study participants without cancer.[155] Scientists are developing informatics and statistical models to determine the most discriminatory combination of salivary biomarkers for specific diseases.

Abundant salivaomics data has been generated utilizing evolving high-throughput technologies in recent years.[156–159] In order to facilitate access to information, compare data sets from different studies, and support salivary diagnostic research, the Salivaomics Knowledge Base (SKB) data management (*UCLA WEB SITE ACCESSED 2013*) system and

Web resource was developed by a group of scientists at the University of California at Los Angeles (UCLA).[160] Ontologies are controlled structured vocabularies designed to provide consensus-based means to ensure consistent descriptions of data by scientists working in different domains. The Saliva Ontology (SALO) is used in an attempt to facilitate salivaomics data retrieval and integration across multiple fields of research together with data analysis and data mining. The SKB and the SALO initiatives are devoted to the translation of saliva data into saliva knowledge, and to the task of enabling saliva data and knowledge sharing in the broadest possible communities of researchers. The SALO is being created through cross-disciplinary interaction among saliva experts, protein experts, diagnosticians, and ontologists.[161]

In 2004, the US Food and Drug Administration (FDA) approved an over-the-counter saliva-based test for HIV antibody screening that can be used in the comfort of one's home.[162] There is growing interest in the development of saliva-based rapid tests for screening and/or diagnosis of hepatitis C virus (HCV) and human papilloma virus (HPV) infection. However, no test as yet has received FDA approval.[163]

Several other saliva-based laboratory tests are commercially available for the detection of periodontal pathogens and genetic risks of developing periodontal diseases. Infection, inflammation and tissue destruction are cause and consequences of periodontal diseases. Biological phenotypes could be of value to determine disease progression and response to therapy at the individual patient level. Emerging data support the predictive value of genetic microbial and protein saliva-based byproducts in gingival inflammation and periodontal bone destruction. Salivary biomarkers of periodontal diseases in the presence of comorbidities such as rheumatoid arthritis,[164,165] as well as patients' responses to therapies such as periodontal surgery combined with matrix metalloproteinase (MMP) inhibition or to oral tissue engineering, have also been topics of investigations by scientists in recent years.[166–168]

Furthermore, wound repair biomarkers have been utilized to determine the tissue-healing response of patients undergoing intraoral soft tissue transplant procedures.[169] Matrix metalloproteinase-8 (MMP-8) is an enzyme for tissue destruction. In 2010, a commercial test with reasonable sensitivity and specificity became available for the identification of active or stable periodontal lesions in smokers and nonsmokers.[170] More recent scientific approaches have focused on the utilization of multiple salivary biomarkers including MMP-8, microbial factors, viruses, and pro-inflammatory cytokines such as IL-1B[171] or IL-17 from a single saliva sample to predict diseases.[172–174] It is estimated that variations in more than 70 genes are associated with periodontitis.[175] In assessing risks for the development and progression of periodontal disease, a patient's DNA can be captured through a saliva-based oral rinse sample and analyzed for the genotypic status of IL-1. This test can be further complemented by other laboratory tests that focus on the

microbial biofilm in the patient's dental plaque. Collectively these sources of information can enhance the prediction of risk assessment based on the patient's genetic make-up modulated by the microbial infection.

A new saliva test for caries risk assessment was introduced by scientists in recent years.[176] The test integrates a variety of host factors to predict individual risk levels that are tooth-group specific. These various host factors correlate with caries history, decayed and filled teeth (DFT), or decayed and filled surfaces (DFS) in young adults. The test is based on the pattern of genetically determined oligosaccharides present on salivary glycoproteins. The mechanism behind the test is believed to be centered on the specific oligosaccharides that either facilitate bacterial attachment and colonization at the surface of teeth or protect against colonization by promoting agglutination and removal of free bacteria. It is the ratio of the two classes of oligosaccharides that is very strongly correlated with the numerical range of DFS or DFT observed in a young adult population. Sensitive DNA-based methods such as DNA–DNA hybridization, genomic finger printing, 16S rRNA gene cloning and sequencing, or Terminal Restriction Fragment Length Polymorphism are also being investigated in identification and classification of dental caries microbiota.[177] The real-time quantitative polymerase chain reaction technique is believed to be more sensitive for enumeration of cariogenic salivary pathogens as compared to the traditional culture-based methods.[178]

Salivary biomarker panel inclusive of thioredoxin, IL-8, SAT, ODZ, and IL-1b has been used successfully in the detection of oral cancer. Breast cancer, Alzheimer disease, myocardial necrosis, and stomach cancer are other areas of interest and investigation.[179,180]

PROSPECTUS: HUMAN GENETICS, PHENOMICS, GENOMICS, MICROBIOME, AND ORAL MEDICINE

It was 61 years ago (1953) when Watson and Crick published a one-page presentation of the structure of DNA with biological implications. It was 39 years ago when the international recombinant DNA conference was held at Asilomar, California, that established regulations for biotechnology using viral, bacterial, plant, animal, and human DNA. It was 26 years ago when the US Congress authorized and funded the National Institutes of Health to initiate the ambitious HGP. It was 14 years ago when a 95% draft of the complete human genome was published (under budget and under time) and 10 years ago the HGP was completed revealing the functional and pseudogenes as well as noncoding regions of the human genome. Last year the FDA authorized the first high throughput DNA and RNA sequencer that can complete a patient's genome within 24 hours at a cost less than $5000.

It is readily apparent that genetics will continue to dominate dental and medical education, health care, industry. and continuing health professional education in the 21st century. Human and microbial genomics, proteomics, and metabolomics, coupled with pharmacogenomics, will continue to shape the future in the health professions.[4–6,10–22,132–137,148,151,152] Mendelian and non-Mendelian patterns of inheritance are clinically important. Genetic screening assays for individual and multiple genes as found in multifactorial conditions will become more specific, more sensitive, faster, and cheaper.

High-throughput phenotype testing on single cells is increasingly important for assessment of viruses, bacteria, yeast, and animal as well as human cells. Phenotype microarrays now make it possible to quantitatively identify and measure many thousands of cellular phenotypes all at the same time. Phenotype microarrays enable simultaneous assays of the phenotype of living cells in response to environmental challenges. This and many other revolutionary advances in molecular assays further enhance the astute clinician with clinical diagnostics and prognostics to improve clinical outcomes.

Our future is even brighter when we consider the emerging opportunities to be found within phenomics, which expands the role of astute clinical observations and evaluations coordinated with genomics. A number of currently employed innovations in imaging and bioassays have already advanced the precision of comprehensive health care. Genotype to phenotype correlations are advancing. In order to realize *personalized health care* that includes mental, vision, and oral health care, significant progress will be made from analysis of large data bases that align and further coordinate genotype with phenotype. In this sense, clinicians are crucial to increase the study power while decreasing observational or measurement errors. Phenomics is the systematic measurement and analysis of qualitative and quantitative traits, including physical observations, vital signs, blood, urine and saliva chemistries, and biochemical real-time metabolic data that collectively define phenotype.[181–183]

Diagnosis will encompass the cardinal features of the all-inclusive clinical phenotype, differential diagnosis, and sensitive and specific tests for the detection of one or more biomarkers (e.g., genes and/or gene products). Risk assessment will increasingly be used, coupled with patient, family and community patterns of disease, environmental insults, and carrier detection within individuals and populations. Molecular epidemiology will emerge as increasingly useful for individuals, families, and populations to define people at risk for disease as well as for the precise diagnosis of diseases and disorders. Moreover, increasing evidence indicates that the human microbiome plays a major role in health ranging from obesity, infectious oral diseases to a patient's susceptibility to cancer or diabetes. Genetic counseling will encompass the human genome, human microbiome as well as the psychosocial management issues. Legal, regulatory, and ethical issues will continue to surface related to genetic screening, privacy and confidentiality, disclosure of unexpected and unwanted findings, and obligations to identify and communicate difficult issues.

The field of genetics should no longer be limited to syndromes of the head and neck as a chapter in a textbook. It should be considered as the essential primer for all aspects of health care and should become encoded within medicine, dentistry, pharmacy, nursing, and the allied health professions and beyond. Oral medicine specialists are instrumental in closing the gap between medicine and dentistry. These specialists serve as a resource to the medical and dental communities in the detection, prevention, and management of conditions that affect systemic and oral health. Greater interaction is necessary among all health professionals in planning systemic and oral care for patients.

Molecular microbial studies led to the emergence of the concept of biofilm formation on tooth surfaces, mucosal surfaces, stents, catheters, medical and dental implants, and even water lines.[141] Biofilms contain microbial species within a three-dimensional structure. Immunology and targeted pharmaceutical developments must address antimicrobial resistance within biofilms, coupled with an aging population in the industrial nations of the world.[140] DNA microarray technology is useful for the purposes of disease diagnosis and drug development.[142] The emerging information on molecular epidemiology will facilitate the assessment of an individual's risk profile based on the host's susceptibility genotype and risk behaviors (smoking, drinking, diet), as well as exposure to common pathogens (bacterial, viral, fungal) and other environmental factors (heavy metals, allergens).

An individual's response to foreign chemicals (xenobiotics) is genetically controlled. This explains why some individuals are at risk for oral conditions such as oral cancer, dental caries, periodontal disease, and soft tissue disorders. Understanding the molecular pathogenesis of squamous cell carcinoma will provide the basis for improved risk assessment, as well as diagnostic and therapeutic approaches.[142,143] Infectious pathogens and dietary factors influence dental caries and periodontal diseases, but genetic variance also contributes to host susceptibility in different populations. Tooth morphology, tooth structure, salivary composition, response to microbial pathogens, and response to fluoride and other anti-caries (tooth decay) products, as well as susceptibility to head and neck cancers and cardiovascular, respiratory, and autoimmune disorders, are all genetic in nature. Recent studies analyzing the genetic and epigenetic changes in preneoplastic head and neck squamous cell carcinoma (HNSCC) indicated that 46% of HNSCC tumors demonstrate mutations in mtDNA.[144]

Except for monozygotic twins, each person's genome is unique. All dentists and physicians need to understand the concept of genetic variability, its interactions with the environment, and its implications for patient and population health care. In the near future, genomics will become a fundamental tool for health professionals to enhance prevention, diagnostics and therapeutics. As nucleic acid sequencing technology becomes *faster, smarter, cheaper* and becomes fully integrated into health care, can we ensure the availability of genetic counseling to guide patients through complex decision making? What role will oral health professionals play in genomics and counseling? How can we be educated and trained to address the potential reality that whole genome sequencing may produce unexpected findings with as yet unknown clinical significance?

Suggested Readings

Amur S, Parekh A, Mummaneni P. Sex differences and genomics in autoimmune diseases. *J Autoimmun*. 2012;38(2–3):J254–J265.

Brady KT, Randall CL. Gender differences in substance use disorders. *Psychiatr Clin North Am*. 1999;22:241–52.

Chambers DA. editor. *DNA: The Double Helix: Perspective and Prospective at Forty Years.* New York: New York Academy of Sciences; 1995.

Collins FS. *The Language of Life: DNA and the Revolution in Personalized Medicine*. New York, NY: HarpersCollins Publisher; 2010.

Collins FS, Hamburg MA. First FDA authorization for next-generation sequencer. *N Engl J Med*. 2013;369:2369–2371.

Collins FS, McKusick VA. Implications of the Human Genome Project for medical science. *JAMA*. 2001;285:540–544.

Collins FS, Patrinos A, Jordan E, et al. New goals for the U.S. Human Genome Project: 1998–2003. *Science*. 1998;282:682–9.

Conrado DJ, Rogers HL, Zineh I, Pacanowski MA. Consistency of drug-drug and gene-drug interaction information in US FDA-approved drug labels. *Pharmacogenomics*. 2013;14(2):215–223.

Davey ME, O'Toole GA. Microbial biofilms: From ecology to molecular genetics. *Microbiol Mol Biol Rev*. 2000;64:847–67.

Davies K. *The $1,000 Genome: The Revolution in DNA Sequencing and the New Era of Personalized Medicine*. New York, NY: Free Press; 2010.

DeAngelis CD, Glass RM, eds. Women's health. [Theme Issue]. *JAMA*. 2006;295:1339–1474.

Epstein CJ, Erickson RP, Wynshaw-Boris A, eds. *Inborn Errors of Development*. 2nd ed. London, UK: Oxford University Press; 2008.

Feero WG, Guttmacher AE, Collins FS. Genomic medicine—an updated primer. *New Engl J Med*. 2010;362(21):2001–2011.

Guttmacher AE, Collins FS, Drazen JM, eds. *Genomic Medicine: Articles from the New England Journal of Medicine*. Baltimore, MD: The Johns Hopkins University Press; 2004.

Hart TC, Marazita ML, Wright JT. The impact of molecular genetics on oral health paradigms. *Crit Rev Oral Biol Med*. 2000;1:26–56.

Ilana R, Yurkiewicz BS, Korf BR, Lehman LS. Prenatal whole-genome sequencing—is the quest to know a fetus's future ethical? *New Engl J Med*. 2014;370:195–197.

International Human Genome Sequencing Consortium. Finishing the euchromatic sequence of the human genome. *Nature*. 2004;431:931–945.

Kuo WP, Whipple ME, Sonis ST, et al. Gene expression profiling by DNA microarrays and its application to dental research. *Oral Oncol*. 2002;38:650–656.

Lander ES, Linton LM, Birren B, et al. Initial sequencing and analysis of the human genome. *Nature*. 2001;409:860–921.

Mark S. Sex- and gender-based medicine: Venus, Mars, and beyond. *Gend Med*. 2005;2:131–136.

McDermott U, Downing JR, Stratton MR. Genomics and the continuum of cancer care, 2011. *New Engl J Med*. 364(12):340–350.

Mendelsohn ME, Karas RH. Molecular and cellular basis of cardiovascular gender differences. *Science*. 2005;308:1583–1587.

Pemberton TJ, Gee J, Patel PI. Gene discovery for dental anomalies: a primer for the dental professional. *J Am Dent Assoc*. 2006;137:743–752.

Quinn TC, Overbaugh J. HIV/AIDS in women: an expanding epidemic. *Science*. 2005;308:1582–1583.

Ross MT, Grafham DV, Coffey AJ, et al. The DNA sequence of the human X chromosome. *Nature*. 2005;434:325–337.

Schmutz J, Wheeler J, Grimwood J, et al. Quality assessment of the human genome sequence. *Nature*. 2004;429:365–368.

Shum L, Takahashi K, Takahashi I, et al. Embryogenesis and the classification of craniofacial dysmorphogenesis. In: Fonseca R, ed. *Oral and Maxillofacial Surgery*. Vol 6. Philadelphia, PA: WB Saunders; 2000:149–194.

Slavkin HC. *Birth of a Discipline: Craniofacial Biology*. Newtown, PA: Aegis Communications; 2012.

Slavkin HC. The evolution of the scientific basis for dentistry 1936 to now and its impact on dental education. *J Dent Educ*. 2012;76(1):28–35.

Slavkin HC. The human genome, implications for oral health and diseases, and dental education. *J Dent Educ*. 2001;65:463–479.

Slavkin HC. Recombinant DNA technology in oral medicine. *Ann NY Acad Sci*. 1995;758:314–328.

Venter JC. *A Life Decoded: My Genome: My Life*. New York, NY: Penguin Group; 2007.

Venter JC, Adams MD, Myers EW, et al. The sequence of the human genome. *Science* 2001;291:1304–1351.

Wang L, McLeod HL, Weinshilboum RM. *Genomics and drug response. New Engl J Med*. 2011;364(12):1144–1153.

Watson JD, Crick FH. Molecular structure of nucleic acids. A structure for deoxyribose nucleic acid. *Nature*. 1953;171:737–738.

Web-based Resources

The reader is encouraged to access the expanding human, animal, plant, and microbial genomic databases using the Internet: National Center for Biotechnology Information (NCBI) http://www.ncbi.nlm.nih.gov

Arachaea and *Eubacteria* microbial genome projects sorted by taxonomic groups, present in GenBank, annotation in progress and "in progress" http://www.ncbi.nlm.nih.gov/Taxonomy/

Ethical, legal, and social implications of genome research on privacy/confidentiality http://www.ornl.gov/hgmis/elsi/elsi.html

GenBank, current status of human, animal, plant, and microbial genomics http://www.ncbi.nlm.nih.gov/Genbank/index.html

Gene expression in teeth http://bite-it.helsinki.fi/

Human Genome Map compiled by the National Center for Biotechnology Information http://www.ncbi.nlm.nih.gov/gen-emap/

Human Microbiome Project http://commonfund.nih.gov/hmp/

Genome Programs of the US Department of Energy Office of Science http://www.doegenomes.org/

National Coalition of Health Professional Education in Genetics http://www.nchpeg.org

OMIM, Online Mendelian Inheritance in Man http://www.ncbi.nlm.nih.gov/entrez/query.fcgi?db=OMIM

Agency for Healthcare Research and Quality http://www.ahrq.gov

Centers for Disease Control and Prevention http://www.cdc.gov

GeneTests-GeneClinics http://www.genetests.org/

National Human Genome Research Institute http://www.nhgri.nih.gov

National Institute of Dental and Craniofacial Research http://www.nidr.nih.gov

National Institutes of Health http://health.nih.gov

National Center for Biotechnology Information projects with Cancer Genome Anatomy Project data http://www.ncbi.nlm.nih.gov/ncicgap/

The International Human Microbiome Consortium http://www.human-microbiome.org/

For the full reference lists, please go to http://www.pmph-usa.com/Burkets_Oral_Medicine

CHAPTER 26

Geriatric Oral Medicine

Katharine Ciarrocca, DMD, MSEd

Nidhi Gulati, MD

People older than 65 years are the fastest growing segment of the population, a fact that will have a dramatic impact on general and oral health in the future. In 1900, less than 5% of the US population was older than 65 years.[1] As recently as 2010, however, 13% of Americans were older than 65 years—a percentage that is estimated to increase to over 20% by 2030.[2] This demographic trend is even more significant for the "oldest old" population (individuals older than 85 years) who are projected to undergo a nearly fourfold increase in numbers from 2006 to 2050.[3] The growth in the number of older Americans is unmatched in US history and can be attributed to a variety of reasons. First, advances in medicine have led to a significant increase in life expectancy, as Americans are living longer than in previous generations.

The average life expectancy in 1900 was only 58 years, but in 2013, was nearly 80 years.[3] Another reason for the "graying" of our population is the aging of the baby boomer generation. The first baby boomer turned 65 in 2011, beginning an exponential increase that will continue for nearly 20 years: Each day approximately 10,000 Americans will turn 65.[4] The last baby boomer will turn 65 in 2030, creating a demographic where one in every five Americans will be older than 65 years.[4] With this dramatic change in the landscape of our nation and the improved medical management of disease, oral health-care professionals must possess the tools and knowledge to manage older adults, their oral manifestations of systemic disease, and their age-related specific oral changes (see Table 26-1).[3]

TABLE 26-1 Population Growth Projections[3]
Population aged 65 and older and aged 85 and older, selected years 1900–2010 and projected 2020–2050

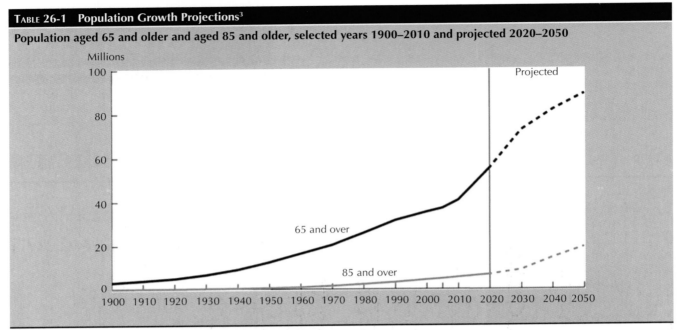

Reference population: These data refer to the resident population
Source: US Census Bureau, 1900 to 1940 ,1970, and 1980, US Census Bureau, 1983, Table 42; 1950, US Census Bureau, 1953, Table 38; 1960, US Census Bureau, 1964, Table 155; 1990, US Census Bureau, 1991, 1990 Summary Table File; 2000, US Census Bureau, 2001, Census 2000 Summary File 1; US Census Bureau, Table 1: Intercensal Estimates of the Resident Population by Sex and Age for the US: April 1, 2000 to July 1, 2010 (US-ESTIINT-01); US Census Bureau, 2011. 2010 Census Summary File 1; US Census Bureau, Table 2: Projections of the population by selected age groups and sex for the United States: 2010–2050 (NP2008–002).

CONCEPTS OF AGING

The age 65 was selected as the dividing line between middle aged and elderly individuals in the late 1880s in Germany as a criterion for Social Security and was adopted by the United States in the early 1900s due to state pension systems in place.[5] It is now the accepted chronological age for the elderly; this number is arbitrary as aging is both chronologic and functional. The chronologic definition of age is simply a number. However, the functional definition is based on the ability of the individual to travel to seek services, making this definition of age much more appropriate than a chronological one.[6–8] The aging population can be categorized into three broad functional groups: (1) functionally independent older adults or those who are physically well despite advanced age, (2) frail older adults or those at high risk for major adverse outcomes, and (3) functionally dependent older adults or those who have experienced deterioration of physical capacities and must rely on assistance from others.[9] The majority of older adults (95%) live in the community, approximately 5% of these people are homebound and another 17% have a major limitation in mobility due to a chronic condition.[10] This leaves about 70% of the elderly population living in the community and capable of traveling to seek services independently, including the dental office for oral healthcare.

Today's older adult is more likely to have natural teeth compared with previous age cohorts. It is estimated that less than 27% of people older than 65 are edentulous,[11] whereas 60 years ago, over 50% were edentulous. Therefore, older adults are at a higher risk of developing serious systemic complications of dental origin, but at the same time, older adults are more likely to utilize dental health-care services and perform regular oral hygiene compared with previous older generations.[12] Aging and medical illness as well as their management directly influence oral health, function, and the provision of dental care.[12] It is vital that oral health professionals are able to recognize, diagnose, and manage oral conditions in the aging patient. This chapter will provide background on the etiology, clinical manifestations, and treatment of common oral conditions that affect older individuals. In addition, a comprehensive review of age-related oral changes and the impact they have on oral health and the provision of dental care will be reviewed.

GERIATRIC PATIENT ASSESSMENT

The medical assessment of an older adult can be quite different and significantly more complicated than the medical workup of a younger patient. First, older persons commonly present with both atypical symptoms and responses to illness. For example, a patient presenting with confusion may not actually have a neurologic problem, but instead have an infection.[13] In addition, social and psychological factors can disguise classic disease presentations. Patients are able to mask a disease process, such as dementia, which can lead to physicians missing the diagnosis. A structured assessment, which incorporates a multidimensional, multidisciplinary approach that includes the patient's functional ability, physical health, cognition, and mental health, as well as socioenvironmental circumstances, is required for these patients. This assessment should also include a thorough review of prescription and over-the-counter medications and supplements, and also a review of immunization status. The medical assessment of a geriatric patient differs from a typical medical assessment because it includes nonmedical domains, such as the patient's functional ability and quality of life. A multidisciplinary team including a physician, nutritionist, social worker, physical and occupational therapists, and oral health-care professional yields a more complete and relevant list of medical problems, functional problems, and psychosocial issues.[14]

Treatment planning and managing the oral healthcare for elderly patients can also be complicated, as a multitude of factors can affect decision making and provision of care. Limitations due to social, economic, financial, family, medical, physical, and transportation constraints must all be considered when formulating a comprehensive oral health-care plan for an older patient.[15] In addition, the sequencing of a dental treatment plan can be difficult and ultimately explain to a patient, as there are a variety of issues that complicate the progression of care, making the final outcome difficult to predict. Treatment plans must always be dynamic, but especially so for older adults. The older patient's health may change as treatment proceeds, thus resulting in new treatment modifications that necessitate reassessment as well as communication based on these needs.[14] Patients, their family, and their caregivers must continually be informed about their oral condition and the fact that treatment needs may change as treatment progresses. Individualized and personalized care for the geriatric patient should occur only after evaluating all the modifying factors, making this approach more complicated but much more appropriate than planning for idealized care.[15]

A systematic approach to managing an older patient is imperative to provide the most comprehensive treatment.[16] This approach starts with an assessment that answers several basic questions specific to older adults: (1) how does the patient function in their environment, (2) what role does pharmacotherapy play in the patients' medical and oral health, (3) what social support systems for the patient exist, (4) what diverse sociologic variables exist, and (5) how does oral healthcare fit into the patient's environment? Dental management of the geriatric patient is consistent with any medically complex patient and involves the evaluation of four risks and the modification to the provision of dental care. Risk of infection, risk of bleeding, risk of drug actions, and interactions and risk of medical emergency in the dental chair all need to be evaluated before routine dental treatment begins.[17] The elderly can be immunosuppressed or nonadherent with medications and instructions and these actions therefore place them at an increased risk of infection. In addition, they may be taking anticoagulation medications or have a systemic disease that alters hemostasis. Depending on the invasiveness of the procedure, these patients can be at an increased risk of bleeding. The elderly are often on more medications, are more sensitive to medications, may need renal dosing, and have difficulty with drug adherence and accuracy.[18] The oral health professional plays a role in improving drug adherence with these patients.[19] Finally, it is imperative to evaluate their ability to withstand treatment based on their systemic disease, their compliance in control of their disease, and also ensure that the office is prepared for a potential emergency.

OSCAR is a multidimensional assessment tool for planning oral healthcare for the older patient, which has been developed by the American Academy of Oral Medicine.[20] This tool is called OSCAR, a five-item pneumonic for oral, systemic, capability, autonomy, and reality. OSCAR serves to guide dentists in identifying the dental, medical, pharmacologic, functional, ethical, and fiscal factors that need to be considered before dental treatment of older patients. This approach enables the clinician to evaluate each older patient in a comprehensive manner, incorporating all factors that may affect care. The OSCAR approach starts with the patient's oral needs and can include issues such as oral mucosal disease, periodontal issues, and dental problems. Assessment of systemic factors is next and incorporates medical problems, medications, and even communication with other healthcare providers into the treatment plan. Evaluating a patient's capability is very important and involves the assessment of a patient's functional capacity, their ability to transport, and even their skill in performing oral hygiene. Next is evaluation of the patient's autonomy, which is vital as it assesses the patient's decision-making ability, their ability to communicate and understand, and even their ability to consent to care. Finally, the assessment of reality will demonstrate the patient's medical stability, prognosis, life expectancy, financial limitations, and ability to maintain oral hygiene. Taking each of these facets into consideration enables the clinician to provide patient-centered care that is specific for each older patient (see Table 26-2).[20]

TABLE 26-2	"OSCAR" Approach to Evaluation and Treatment of the Older Dental Patient[20]
	Areas of Concern
Oral	Dentition, restorations, fixed and/or removable prostheses, periodontium, oral mucosa, salivary glands
Systemic	Medical problem list, medications, age-related changes, interprofessional communication
Capability	Ability to perform IADLs, ADLs, caregivers, oral hygiene, transportation, mobility
Autonomy	Decision-making ability, consent to care, dependence on others for decisions
Reality	Financial limitation, life expectancy, prognosis, ability to maintain dental treatment, medical stability

Abbreviations: ADL, Activity of daily living; IADL, instrumental activity of daily living.
Source: Adapted from Laudenbach and Ship.[20]

PHARMACOTHERAPEUTICS IN OLDER ADULTS

Older adults make up approximately 14% of the US population but consume one-third of all prescribed medications.[21] Due to increased exposure to medication, older adults are at an increased risk for drug-related complications. Problems such as drug–drug interactions, adverse drug reactions (ADRs), undermedication, polypharmacy (use of multiple medications or use of more medications than appropriate), and nonadherence are common among this population.[22,23] In addition, numerous changes occur as a result of physiologic aging that alter the way medications are absorbed, distributed, metabolized, and eliminated.[24] Therefore, medications often need to be prescribed differently in this population by carefully choosing medications to avoid adverse effects or drug interactions and adjusting doses to allow for changes to organ function such as the liver and kidneys. Finally, certain medications may not be safe to use at all in older adults, which are delineated in the Beers List of Medications to Avoid in Older Adults.[25] (A more in-depth explanation of the Beers List is addressed later in this chapter.)

Pharmacokinetics

The pharmacokinetics of medications—the absorption, distribution, metabolism, and elimination—can be altered in an older patient due to the aging process. The absorption of medications is least affected by the aging process. Most drugs are absorbed passively, simply by being in the stomach or intestine. If absorption is affected in older adults, it is usually decreased either due to increased amount of acid in the stomach or due to decreased movement of the muscles of the digestive system or even decreased surface area for absorption.[24,26,27] Many medications are not significantly affected by these changes; but the co-administration of medications can further decrease absorption (e.g., antacids). Distribution and metabolism of medications can be greatly affected by the aging process. Many medications are metabolized in the liver, and older adults generally have a decline in liver function. As the body ages, the overall size of the liver decreases and there is less blood flow to the liver; therefore, there is a decrease in the break down and distribution of medications by the liver.[24] Ultimately, the dosing interval of medications may need to be increased since the body will take longer to break down the medication in patients with decreased liver function.[24] Finally, elimination is affected due to deteriorating function of the kidneys—the major route of elimination for medications from the body. As the body ages, kidney function declines due to (1) decreased kidney size, (2) decreased blood flow to the kidneys, or (3) long-standing diseases such as diabetes or hypertension.[23,24] The medication dose or dosing frequency may need to be altered; usually, less frequent administration is needed, as it will take longer by the body to eliminate the medication.[24]

Pharmacodynamics

The pharmacodynamics of medications—the drug's action on the body—can also be affected by the aging process. As we age, multiple changes occur, such as changes in body composition (increased body fat, decreased lean muscle mass, and decreased body water), which can change the effective dose of pharmaceuticals. Medications that are lipophilic may have prolonged effects due to increased amount of body fat. Drugs that are hydrophilic may have a more rapid increase in concentrations in the blood because of less water. These changes often necessitate the lower dosing of medication.[23,24] Drugs that are highly protein bound, however, have less protein upon which to bind; therefore, more of that medication may be required for it to be effective. Finally, older adults may experience decreased or enhanced effects of drugs compared to younger populations. Changes occur at the medication's receptor site of action and can ultimately affect the way the body responds to the medication. For example, some older patients are susceptible to medications that cause sedation as a side effect. Sedation can have multiple comorbidities: risk of falls, confusion, and the inability to perform daily tasks.[23,24] In these patients, medications that cause sedation could be inappropriate and in the end, influence the care for multiple providers including medicine, nursing, physical or occupational therapy, speech therapy, and nutrition.

Drug-related Complications

Polypharmacy is the use of multiple medications and/or the administration of more medications than are clinically indicated, representing unnecessary drug useage.[27,28] Polypharmacy may also be described as the use of one medication to treat the side effects of another medication, rather than changing to another medication that may be better tolerated.[27] Polypharmacy is common among geriatric patients, as these patients are taking 34% of all prescribed medications and 30% of all over-the-counter drugs.[27,28] The likelihood of receiving a prescription increases with age.[22] In one study of older nursing home patients, around 40% of patients had at least one inappropriate medication.[26] Polypharmacy may increase the incidence of ADRs, as well as drug–drug interactions. The incidence of adverse drug events is 13% for a patient taking two medications, 58% for five medications, and 82% for seven medications.[24]

Medication adherence is the extent to which a patient's use of medications coincides with medical or health advice[29] and is a significant problem among the geriatric population. Ninety percent of Medicare beneficiaries take prescription medications, but as many as 55% are nonadherent.[30] Complex medication regimens, confusion over directions, not understanding medication importance, and cost may contribute to decreased adherence.[22] In addition, older patients tend to have more than one prescribing physician and use more than one pharmacy, making it more difficult to track their medications and identify potential problems (e.g., drug interactions, harmful doses, unnecessary medications with no health benefits).[31]

Finally, undertreatment—when a necessary medication is omitted—can occur in the medical management of older patients. Some medications may be underutilized for conditions such as pain because of concerns about adverse effects or polypharmacy in the aging population.[32] One study of ambulatory older patients indicated that 50% had more than one necessary medication missing from their regimens.[32]

The Beers Criteria

The Beers Criteria for Potentially Inappropriate Medication Use in Older Adults was originally developed in 1991 by the late geriatrician, Mark Beers, MD, as a catalogue of medications that cause adverse drug events in older adults due to their pharmacologic properties and physiologic changes of aging.[25] Beers formulated an explicit list of medications, doses, and durations that should be avoided in patients older than age 65 (in nursing homes), which was developed from expert consensus through extensive literature review. Beers revised the list in 1997 and again in 2003, to be applicable to all adults aged 65 years and older regardless of where they lived, and also included criteria specific to diagnosis and condition. In 2011, the American Geriatrics Society (AGS) undertook an update of the criteria and developed the AGS 2012 Beers Criteria, using an enhanced, evidence-based methodology.[25] The AGS Updated Beers Criteria for Potentially Inappropriate Medication Use in Older Adults was published in 2012 to assist health-care providers in improving medication safety in older adults. Each criterion on the list of medications is rated by quality of evidence and strength of evidence using the American College of Physicians' Guideline Grading System.[25] This updated list contains 53 medications divided into 3 categories: (1) medications to avoid in *any* patient older than 65, (2) medications to avoid in patients older than 65 with certain diseases, and (3) medications to use with caution in patients older than 65. In addition, this update eliminated 19 medications from list that were no longer deemed as a threat. Printable Beers Pocket Cards are available for download.[33]

Tools for Medication Assessment

Medication use in older adults can be complicated. Each person is different, and all geriatric patients may not have the same degree of impairment, so an individualized approach is of utmost importance. Evaluation of medications in the geriatric population is vital to ensure that medications are used appropriately and safely. Studies have shown that as many as 40% of nursing home residents in the United States were prescribed inappropriate medications.[31] In addition, a meta-analysis in 2002 showed older people are four times as likely as younger people to be hospitalized due to problems related to ADRs, with up to 88% of those ADRs being preventable.[34] There are a variety of different screening tools used to assess medication appropriateness, both implicit tools and explicit tools. Implicit tools utilize patient-specific information and the users' clinical judgment and experience

to address questions, statements, and algorithms, with the goal of optimizing medication regimens.[22] Implicit tools enable health-care providers to identify both the medications that should be avoided, as well as the incorrect doses, drug interactions, and patient preference. Examples of implicit tools—the Medication Appropriateness Index (MAI) and the ARMOR tool—are discussed below.[35–37] Explicit tools, on the other hand, do not consider patient-specific factors in determining medication appropriateness and are composed of lists of medications developed by consensus panels after extensive literature and database searches. An example of an explicit tool is the Beer's Criteria for Potentially Inappropriate Medication Use in Older Adults, which was discussed earlier.[25] Explicit tools can be used by anyone regardless of discipline to determine the appropriateness of prescribing but are limited to the medications recognized by the tools' developers.[31] In contrast, implicit tools can be applied to any medication but require clinical judgment and an understanding of physiology and pharmacology.

The MAI is a tool that uses implicit criteria to rate medications to reduce polypharmacy and inappropriate prescribing.[35,36] The MAI is very reliable and is structured in a way to evaluate medication use in geriatrics. Even when different clinicians evaluate the regimen, the results will generally be similar.[32] The MAI covers 10 elements of appropriate prescribing and is useful in a variety of situations, including patients in the community and hospital settings.[35,36]

The ARMOR tool is used to Assess, Review, Minimize, Optimize, and Reassess medication regimens[37] (see Table 26-3). The goal of ARMOR is to improve functional status and mobility of a patient. The tool was designed for use in nursing home residents and can be used in patients receiving greater than nine medications, seen for initial assessment, with falls or behavioral disturbance, or who are admitted for rehabilitation.[37] This tool was tested in a long-term care facility and evaluated by a team that included health-care team members from the areas of medicine, nursing, physical/occupational therapy, recreational therapy, and social work. The use of ARMOR led to a reduction in polypharmacy, reduced cost of care, and decreased hospitalization.[37,38]

Many geriatric patients are likely to be on numerous medications, many of which can complicate the provision of oral care. Therefore, it is imperative for oral health-care professionals to evaluate the patient's medications, their pharmacokinetics and pharmacodynamics, their adverse reactions, and their complications as a part of the comprehensive oral/medical evaluation of the geriatric patient. In addition, the dental office can serve as location for medication adherence and reconciliation.[39]

HEALTH LITERACY

Health literacy—a significant problem for health-care professionals—is defined as "the degree to which individuals have the capacity to obtain, process, and understand basic health information and services needed to make appropriate health decisions."[40]

TABLE 26-3 ARMOR Tool of Medication Assessment[37]
Assess the patient for the total number of medications with a potential for adverse effects (beta blockers, antidepressants, antipsychotics, pain medications, medications on the Beers Criteria).
Review medications for possible drug–drug interactions, drug–disease interactions, pharmacodynamic (how drugs act in the body) interactions, impact on function, and adverse effects.
Minimize the number of nonessential medications, particularly medications with a clear lack of evidence or if the risk outweighs the benefits of using the medication.
Optimize therapy. Evaluate duplicative treatments, adjust doses for kidney or liver function, and adjust doses to achieve treatment goals.
Reassess the patient and medications using information such as heart rate, blood pressure, oxygen saturation, functional status, cognitive status, and medication compliance.

Source: Adapted from Haque.[37]

Health literacy is not only the ability to read, as it involves a variety of skills—reading, listening, analyzing, and decision making—and using them together in health-care situations. It is important to distinguish health literacy from literacy because patients may be well educated and knowledgeable in any number of areas while having limited knowledge about their health and healthcare. Findings of the National Assessment of Adult Literacy (NAAL), conducted in 2003, revealed that although the majority of adults in the United States had intermediate or proficient health literacy, 36% had only basic or below basic health literacy.[41] Results of this survey also revealed that compared to adults in younger age groups, adults aged 65 years and older had lower average health literacy. Among adults aged 60 years and older, 71% have difficulty using print materials, 80% have difficulty using documents such as forms or charts, and 68% have difficulty interpreting numbers and performing calculations.[42] In addition, estimates suggest that two-thirds of older adults are not able to understand information received about their prescription medications.[19,42] Activities requiring health literacy include communicating with clinicians about health and illness, reading and understanding health information, taking medications, making appointments, and filling out medical forms.[42,43]

Health literacy is especially important among the geriatric population because it affects a patient's ability to navigate the health-care system, share personal and health information with providers, engage in self-care in chronic disease management, and even adopt health-promoting behaviors. Low health literacy is associated with increased use of inpatient and emergency care, decreased use of some preventive and primary care, and deficits in self-care, including medication management.[43] Limited health literacy also leads to underutilization of services, poor understanding of health, poor health outcomes, and increased health-care costs.

There are a variety of important strategies for healthcare providers, including dentists, and their staff to ensure that patients have a baseline understanding of their health.[44] The entire oral health-care team must be aware and sensitive to the effect health literacy has on provision of care. It is important to explain things clearly to the patient using plain language, starting with the most important information first and limiting new information.[45,46]

TABLE 26-4 TEACH-BACK Method: Confirmation of Understanding[48]
Do not ask a patient, "Do you understand?"
Ask patients to explain or demonstrate.
Ask questions that begin with "how" and "what," rather than closed-ended yes/no questions.
Organize information so that the most important points stand out and repeat this information. Ensure agreement and understanding about the care plan. This is essential to achieving adherence.

Source: Adapted from Stein et al.[48]

- Emphasize one to three points and encourage patients to ask questions.
- Have written instructions for important information and provide useful educational materials.
- Use the teach-back method to confirm the patient's understanding (see Table 26-4). With the teach-back method, the provider asks the patient to explain or demonstrate what they were just taught by asking questions that begin with how and why rather than close-ended yes or no questions. (Do not ask the patient, "Do you understand?")[47,48]
- Organize the information so that the most important points stand out and repeat this information.
- Ensure agreement and understanding from the patient about the care plan; this is essential to the achieving adherence.[48]

CHRONIC CONDITIONS AND LEADING CAUSES OF DEATH

Advances in medical treatment and effective public health strategies have contributed to a striking increase in average life expectancy in the United States.[49,50] Within the span of a century, a 30-year increase in life expectancy was realized, something that has never been achieved before.[49,50] Diseases that were fatal 100 years ago are no longer the leading killers of American adults. However, other diseases such as heart disease, stroke, and cancer have continued to be the leading causes of death every year for over a century. Since 1910, heart

TABLE 26-5 Chronic Conditions That Were the Leading Causes of Death Among US. Adults Aged 65 or Older in 2007–2009[4]

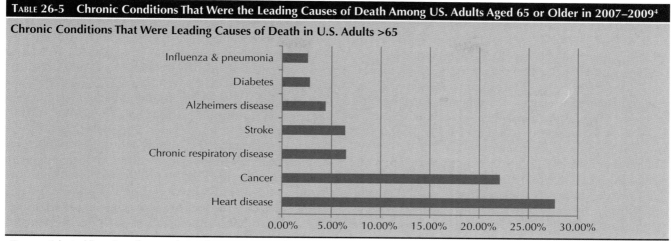

Source: Adapted from http://www.cdc.gov/features/agingandhealth/. Accessed March 21, 2014.

TABLE 26-6 Instrumental Activities of Daily Living Versus Activities of Daily Living[52]

IADLs	ADLs
Handling transportation (driving or navigating public transit)	Toileting
Shopping	Selecting proper attire
Preparing meals	Grooming
Using the telephone and other communication devices	Maintaining continence
Managing medications	Putting on clothes
Housework and basic home maintenance	Bathing
Managing finances	Feeding
	Walking and transferring (such as moving from bed to wheelchair)

Abbreviations: IADLs, instrumental activities of daily living; ADLs, activities of daily living.
Source: Adapted from Pol et al.[51]

disease has been the leading cause of death every year except 1918 to 1920, when there was an influenza epidemic.[49] Since 1938, cancer has been the second leading cause of death every year. Chronic diseases such as heart disease, cancer stroke, chronic respiratory diseases, Alzheimer's disease, and diabetes pose their greatest risk as people age.[50] Influenza and pneumonia also continue to contribute to death among older adults despite the availability of effective vaccines (see Table 26-5).[49]

The burden of chronic disease is much more than death alone. People suffering from even one chronic disease can experience a poorer quality of life, and this quality only diminishes as other diseases develop. Ultimately, there is a long period of disability and decline due to the disease which affects all aspects of life. Even essential activities, both inside and outside home, can be affected. At first, a person may have trouble with the instrumental activities of daily living, such as money management, grocery shopping, preparing meals, and taking medications properly.[51] As physical and/or mental ability declines, the capability to perform the most basic activities called activities of daily living (ADLs) is affected and can include tasks such as personal hygiene, self-feeding, getting dressed, and toileting.[52] The inability to perform ADLs can alter social engagement with family and friends. Restriction of mobility in the home and engagement in the community can greatly narrow an older person's world and ability to do the things that bring pleasure and satisfaction. The inability to care for oneself in a safe and appropriate manner leads to further dependence on others and very often leads to the need for care in an institutional setting (see Table 26-6).[52]

AGE-RELATED SYSTEMIC CHANGES

Changing demographics and improved medical management of disease are placing increased demands on oral health professionals for improved knowledge of oral manifestations of systemic disease and the provision of dental care including those for older patients. Many of these patients have age-related specific oral changes that are the responsibility of the oral health professional to diagnose and treat.[53] In addition to age-related oral changes, the aging patient has systemic changes with which the oral health-care provider should be familiar, as well. In the cardiovascular system, there is stiffening of the aorta, decreased baroreceptor sensitivity, changes in electrical conduction, reduction in maximal cardiac output, coronary artery disease, and valvular fibrosis and calcification.[54] The respiratory system declines with stiffer lungs with numerous calcifications, decreased diaphragmatic muscle efficiency, structural changes in the alveoli with increased dead space, and decreased central nervous system control of ventilation.[55] With aging, 30% of neurons are lost and 20% or more of brain parenchyma are being reduced between the ages of 18 to 80. Furthermore, decreased cerebral blood perfusion and decreased nerve transmitter function lead to loss of sensory function, delirium, and confusion.[56] Renal function declines approximately 1% per year after the age of 30, and there is a decrease in renal mass of approximately 30% with concurrent diminished glomerular filtration rate.[57] The endocrine system is affected by thyroid changes, alterations in glycemic control, and adrenal function. Vitamin D production from the skin is decreased, and a significant loss of skeletal mass happens after the fourth decade.[58] Gastrointestinal and hepatic systems experience reduced gastric emptying and splanchnic blood flow with decreased motility and absorption. Hepatic blood flow as well as hepatic mass decrease, thus affecting drug metabolism.[59] As more people live longer and as their organ systems gradually decline, there will be an increase in chronic conditions and illnesses that influence the provision of oral care.

All of these acute and chronic conditions have potential oral sequelae, particularly in an older and more medically complex adult. Moreover, the treatment of these diseases with pharmacotherapy, chemotherapy, and radiotherapy has implications for the maintenance of oral health. In addition, chronic impairments are common among the geriatric population, with frequently encountered hearing, visual, orthopedic impairments, and speech disorders.[60] These chronic impairments can directly affect oral health and impair dental treatment, and simple steps can be taken by oral health professionals that will help improve communication with these patients.

MOST COMMON SYSTEMIC DISEASES IN OLDER ADULTS

The 10 most common systemic diseases among functionally independent older adults include arthritis, head and neck cancer, chronic obstructive pulmonary disease, diabetes mellitus, mental health, cardiovascular diseases, hypertension, osteoporosis, Parkinson disease, and cerebrovascular accidents.[61] These medical conditions are discussed in detail in various chapters throughout this book. However, three of these chronic diseases deserve particular mention within the geriatric context: mental health (dementia, Alzheimer's disease), Parkinson disease, and arthritis, as they most often affect the elderly.

Dementia

Dementias are a considerable problem among the elderly population. There are estimates that the prevalence is about 1% at the age of 60 years and doubles every 5 years

to reach more than 50% by the age of 85 years.[62] Dementias are characterized by both mental and physical decline. With increased severity of dementia, there is progressive cognitive and memory loss, development of social and behavioral problems, and inability to perform daily activities.[63] Dementias comprise more than 55 different illnesses with the most common being Alzheimer's disease and Parkinson disease.[64] Progression of dementia is accompanied by a gradual inability to perform self-care, including adequate oral hygiene due to self-neglect and loss of cognitive and motor skills. Persons with dementia, and even those living in the community and experiencing few medical problems, have impaired oral health as a result of poor oral hygiene. For example, patients with Alzheimer's disease have more gingival plaque, bleeding and calculus compared to age- and gender-matched adults, and submandibular saliva output is impaired in nonmedicated persons with Alzheimer's disease.[64] Poor gingival health and oral hygiene have been found to increase with the severity of dementia.[65]

Oral care, treatment planning, and behavioral management for persons with dementia must be designed with consideration of the severity of disease and may involve family members or caregivers.[65,66] The definition of competency and who can consent for care usually depends on the state of residence. Early in the disease process, aggressive preventive and interceptive steps need to be formulated to preserve existing oral health. As dementia progresses, treatment becomes problem based. Frequent recalls and preventive measures must be instituted. The role of the caregiver becomes more critical in providing symptomatic and objective information, as well as in help to performing daily oral hygiene.[64-66] Complex and time-consuming dental treatment should be avoided in persons with severe dementia. The emphasis should be on keeping the patient free of pain and able to maintain adequate nutritional intake, particularly if the patient is no longer able or willing to wear removable prosthesis.

A comprehensive preventive dental plan is crucial for individuals with dementia. Involving the caregiver as a co-therapist is also important. Patients with dementia may forget to perform routine oral hygiene procedures, dental appointments, and oral hygiene or postoperative instructions unless the caregiver is involved.[66-68] Dental treatment should preferably be provided in the morning, when cooperation tends to be best, with the usual caretakers present. Treating the patient in an upright or semi-upright position aid in the prevention of aspiration and postural hypotension.[69]

Arthritis

It is estimated that about 49% of people older than 65 years in the United States have arthritis, and this condition may limit the activity of nearly 12% of this segment of the population.[70] Patients with arthritis often have diminished manual dexterity, which can then affect their ability to maintain adequate oral hygiene. These individuals may need to perform oral hygiene activities with modified hygiene tools.[71,72] Toothbrushes with specially adapted handles, such as a bicycle handle grip or the addition of a tennis ball, enables the patient to hold and maneuver the brush more easily. In addition, these patients may benefit from electric or sonic toothbrushes to make the burden of oral hygiene less.[73]

Short appointments in the late morning or in the early afternoon are recommended for patients with arthritis, as joint stiffness and pain tends to improve during the day. Supine positioning may be uncomfortable for them, and they may need neck and leg support. Finally, these patients may need assistance ambulating as well as transporting into and out of the dental chair. Caution must be taken to minimize adverse outcomes, such as falls, as well as maximize patient comfort.

Parkinson Disease

Parkinson disease is a progressive degenerative disorder of the central nervous system and is usually seen in people older than 55 years.[64] Some of the typical signs and symptoms of Parkinson—tremors, muscle rigidity, spasmodic head and neck movements, and drooling—can make the provision of all phases of dentistry quite difficult for the practitioner. Involuntary movements, especially in the head and neck region, can make the use of sharp and rotating instruments hazardous. The neuronal degeneration that accompanies Parkinson disease also impacts negatively on oral health, mainly due to inadequate oral hygiene and the medical management of the disease with medications that cause salivary dysfunction.[74] For maximal patient comfort, dental treatment should be performed during the time of day at which their medication has maximum effect, usually two to three hours after administration, as it helps to minimize tremors and improve patient safety. In addition, short appointments and use of mouth props with a floss ligature can aid in providing high-quality dental treatment. Patients with Parkinson disease are at a greater risk for falls due to muscle rigidity and bradykinesia, thus assistance may be needed ambulating and transporting in and out of the dental chair.[75] Finally, of utmost importance is utilizing the patient's caregiver as a co-therapist, giving oral hygiene and postoperative instructions to both patient and caregiver.[48] More frequent hygiene recall and fluoride supplementation can help prevent further disease.

AGE-RELATED ORAL CHANGES

Oral health is particularly important among the geriatric population. Older adults are more susceptible to medical conditions that predispose them to oral and maxillofacial diseases that can directly or indirectly lead to malnutrition, altered communication, increased susceptibility to infection, and diminished quality of life. Age alone, however, does not play a major role in impaired oral health. Instead, oral diseases such as decay, gingivitis and periodontitis, oral mucosal diseases, salivary dysfunction, and resorptive bone disease couple with systemic conditions and the use of medications, placing older adults at risk of developing

TABLE 26-7 Common Oral Disorders in Older Adults[53]

Oral Structure	Common Disorder Associated With Aging
Oral mucosa	Cancers Vesiculobullous diseases Ulcerative diseases Inflammatory diseases
Dentition	Root caries Coronal caries Attrition Fracture/chipping
Periodontium	Gingivitis Periodontitis Abscesses Tooth loss
Salivary glands	Hypofunction Cancers
Sensory function	Olfactory dysfunction Disgeusia
Motor dysfunction	Dysphagia Aspiration Masticatory muscle weakness
Pain sensation	Atypical facial pain "Burning mouth" syndrome Trigeminal neuralgia Temporomandibular disorders
Prosthesis	Atrophic mandible Ill-fitting dentures Inflammatory lesions secondary to ill-fitting dentures Poor denture hygiene

Source: Adapted from De Rossi and Slaughter.[53]

a variety of oral disorders. Therefore, this complex interplay makes the dental management of the geriatric patient challenging. Some oral diseases can become significant in terms of morbidity and mortality, bringing about severe and even life-threatening consequences. The effects of these oral diseases are not limited to the oral cavity and its functions. Oral diseases give rise to pathogens which can become aspirated into the lungs, causing severe even life-threatening consequences. Systemic, mucocutaneous, dermatologic, and neurologic diseases can manifest initially in the oral cavity which can predispose older individuals to additional oral problems. Therefore, oral health-care providers must be able to recognize, diagnose, and treat oral conditions in elderly patients that are caused by age-related changes and systemic influences (see Table 26-7).[53]

Oral Motor and Sensory Function

As we age, olfactory function declines. Not only does our sense of smell diminish but also the ability to discriminate between smells decreases. Greater than 75% of people older than 80 years have evidence of major olfactory deterioration, with that decline being most significant after the age of 70.[76] However, taste disorders are far less prevalent than olfactory losses with age. Gustatory dysfunction may be attributed to the normal aging process, but many times, a perceived defect in taste is actually a primary defect in olfaction. Other frequent causes of taste dysfunction are upper respiratory infection, head injury, drug use, and idiopathic causes.[76] Mastication problems associated with tooth loss and ill-fitting dentures or reduction in saliva production can also inhibit proper taste sensation. Patients who have diminished food recognition and enjoyment as well as altered smell and taste function can therefore have significant quality of life issues and malnutrition.[77] The dentist can play an important role in nutritional counseling to prevent malnutrition, dehydration, and diminished quality of life.[77]

Alterations in mastication, swallowing, and oral muscular posture also occur with aging. The most commonly reported oral motor dysfunction is altered mastication.[78] Even fully dentate elderly patients are less able to prepare food for swallowing due to decreased muscular strength. This muscle weakness can be exacerbated by various systemic diseases such as Parkinson disease, a history of head and neck cancer and its treatment, multiple sclerosis, and cerebrovascular accidents. Subsequent effects on swallowing and deglutition may lead to choking and aspiration. The dentist must be aware of these changes, especially when approaching restorative care. The motor issues, themselves, may cause challenges to actual restorative treatment; therefore, extra time should be allowed and extra patience should be exercised. In addition, the dentist should eliminate dental factors that might further inhibit the patient's ability to eat properly. Finally, patients may need counselling or care that would go beyond the scope of a dental office; therefore, referral to appropriate health-care providers is imperative. Practitioners such as speech and swallow experts, otolaryngologists, and nutritionists can provide treatment and information of great benefit to elderly patients suffering from oral and maxillofacial motor and sensory dysfunction.

Orofacial Pain

An accurate diagnosis of a painful condition is more difficult in the elderly due to a greater frequency of multiple chronic diseases and an altered pain response in this population.[79] Epidemiologic studies suggest that both acute and chronic orofacial pain are significant problems in the aging population. Understanding the nature and prevalence of pain in this group is paramount to a correct diagnosis, being cautious to avoid the oversimplification that "pain decreases with age."[80] The most prevalent types of pain in the orofacial complex include pain associated with the dentition, periodontium, oral mucosa, and bone. In addition, peripheral neuropathies such as burning mouth syndrome and atypical odontalgia are common. Extraoral pain disorders may include temporomandibular disorders, neuralgias, and persistent dentoalveolar pain from a neuropathic process (such as atypical facial pain or persistent idiopathic facial pain).[20] Many elderly patients have diminished pulpal sensitivity making an accurate diagnosis difficult.[81] A prompt and

correct diagnosis is key, however, as it is important to minimize treatment and avoid unnecessary therapy in patients with persistent dentoalveolar pain that is neuropathic in origin. Pain assessment can be made by means of pain scales and specific open- and closed-ended questions. In patients who suffer from temporomandibular pain, the dentist should schedule short appointments with frequent resting of the jaw. In patient with neuralgias, keen avoidance of the trigger areas is imperative. Some practitioners may underestimate the severity of pain in older adults and subsequently do not prescribe appropriate analgesics when indicated.[80] When analgesics are prescribed, though, a detailed analysis of the patients' current medications and medical conditions should lead to an accurate medication and dosage. In general, the management of geriatric patients with acute or chronic orofacial pain is not significantly different than their younger counterparts; however, it requires thorough examination and management, often involving multiple healthcare providers.

For more information about temporomandibular disorders and orofacial pain, please see Chapters 11 and 12.

Dentition

Elderly people in the past century have composed a relatively small proportion of the total population, but the majority was edentulous and received dental care infrequently or only when their dental needs could no longer be ignored. The rate of edentulism in the United States, however, has declined from over 40% in the early 1990s, to approximately 23% in 2010.[82] Geriatric dental care is no longer simply denture care, but must also include complex restorative procedures, as well as aesthetic dentistry and implants. Because older adults are retaining their teeth into much advanced ages, a multitude of age-related changes to the dentition can be observed. Occlusion attrition, pulpal recession, fibrosis, and decreased cellularity are some of the more common changes seen— all of which may lead to diminished tooth sensitivity and reduced perception of painful stimuli.[83] In addition, staining, chipping and cracking, and increased susceptibility to tooth fracture are common in older patients.

Most commonly, however, is recurrent coronal and root surface caries.[84,85] The United States has become an aging industrialized society, with decreased caries rate in children and increased coronal and root caries rate in the aging population.[86] The percentage of teeth with decayed or restored root surfaces increases with each decade of adulthood, affecting more than one-half of all remaining teeth by age 75 years.[87] As people live longer and retain more natural teeth, the complexity of their treatment increases. Over time, dentin undergoes a reduction in thermal, osmotic and electrical sensitivity, and pain perception and its susceptibility to caries decreases.[83] Cementum thickness and pulp dimensions are also reduced with age.

Root caries lesions initiate at the cemento–enamel junction and create darker than normal dentin tissues. Any exposed root surface is at risk; enamel becomes secondarily involved. Root caries occur as a result of increased gingival recession, salivary gland dysfunction, less effective oral hygiene, and diminished oral motor function. These lesions are especially common in institutionalized patients. Risk factors for root caries include root exposure, decreased salivary flow, a history of other caries, oral hygiene status, bacterial virulence, and fluoride exposure. Mandibular molars, premolars, and maxillary canines are most commonly affected, with the surfaces affected most often being facial and proximal.

Strategies to prevent root caries include gingival recession prevention, plaque control, use of multiple fluoride sources (including rinses, sprays, mouthwashes, and varnishes), dietary and nutritional counseling, and improvement of salivary flow. A literature review and clinical case study by Lazarchik and Haywood, published in *The Journal of the American Dental Association* in 2010, noted that 10% carbamide peroxide gel delivered in custom-fitted trays can be an effective treatment for caries prevention in patients with compromised oral hygiene.[88] Plaque is suppressed, and therefore, caries is controlled due to a carbamide peroxide–induced increase in salivary and plaque pH. This increase in salivary pH results from a urea component and from possible antimicrobial activity via physical debridement and a direct chemical effect of hydrogen peroxide.[88] In addition, frequent use of fluoride is essential for root caries prevention. Fluoride provides important antimicrobial and remineralization actions, and it also alters tooth surface energy.[89] Fluoride has the ability to concentrate in carious lesions as well as increase salivary pH.[89,90]

Restorative management of root caries lesions involves multifaceted considerations: isolation, gingival morphology, lesion location, preparation design, and choice of restorative material. Rubber dam is an ideal form of isolation; however, due to the often subgingival extension of root caries, cotton roll isolation or a VAC-ejector system may be indicated. Removing gingival obstructions with a gingivectomy or retraction cord or even a full-thickness flap may also be indicated. Restorative material options include (1) amalgam, which is effective when isolation is poor but requires gross mechanical retention and has minimal plaque resistance, (2) glass ionomer, which sets up fast, needs moderate isolation, has sufficient chemical bonding, and has good plaque resistance, and (3) composite, which has strict isolation requirements for bonding, has poor plaque resistance, and requires a rubber dam.[90] Restorative maintenance for these patients includes a low carbohydrate diet, patient education with intense hygiene instruction, and frequent recall. Addressing the cause of decay (through a caries risk assessment) as well as remineralizing therapies with both office- and home-based fluoride therapy is important. The dentist should consider fluoride-releasing restorative materials when evaluating treatment options.[91] Finally, conservative treatment plans in high caries risk patients, especially among those who are unable to maintain their restorations, is vital.

Periodontal Tissues

Aging is accompanied by a variety of periodontal changes: the periodontal tissues themselves show signs of aging, the composition of plaque changes, and the reaction of the periodontium to the presence of plaque changes as well. The degree of periodontal breakdown increases with increasing age, most likely due to the interplay of the factors.[92] Change in the periodontium, however, is not solely due to the aging process. A combination of gingival recession with loss of periodontal attachment and poor oral hygiene predispose the aging patient to tooth loss and thus masticatory insufficiency.[8,92] Problems with deglutition soon follow, as does malnutrition. In geriatric patients with a compromised periodontium, more conservative treatment plans should be formulated. In addition, these patients need more frequent recall and oral health maintenance. Improved oral hygiene can result from the use of a variety of oral hygiene aids for those with motor difficulties. A variety of different tooth brushes are available: toothbrushes with modified handles, electric toothbrushes, three-sided brushes, finger toothbrushes, and suction brushes may be indicated. Of utmost importance, however, is patient and caregiver education by the oral health-care team.

Oral Mucosa

The clinical appearance of oral mucosa in healthy older adults is indistinguishable from that in younger patients. Changes over time, however, including mucosal trauma, mucosal diseases, oral habits, and salivary gland hypofunction can alter the clinical appearance and character of the oral tissues in older adults. Declining immunologic responsiveness further increases their susceptibility to oral mucosal infection and trauma.[10,54] The increased incidence of oral and systemic disorders in older patients along with the increased use of medications can also lead to oral mucosal disorders. Both normal aging changes and pathologic factors can contribute to oral pathology. Oral epithelium becomes thinner, loses elasticity, and atrophies with age.[10] The oral mucosa is a common site for various desquamative, ulcerative, and malignant lesions. The most common oral lesions among the elderly include trauma, lichen planus and lichenoid reactions, inflammatory processes such as papillary hyperplasia, epulis fissurata, candidiasis, vesiculobullous conditions such as pemphigoid, pemphigus, herpes, and finally premalignant and malignant lesions.[20]

Traumatic Ulcers

Traumatic ulcerations of the oral mucosa are commonly seen in the geriatric population. These ulcerations most frequently affect the labial and buccal mucosa and are associated with lip and cheek biting, facticial habits, motor dysfunction, pressure necrosis, improper hygiene, broken teeth, irritation by faulty restorations, and ill-fitting removable prostheses. Traumatic ulcerations appear as shallow ulcerations with a necrotic center and varying degrees of erythema at the periphery. Treatment of these lesions involves identifying the etiology and removing it. If no resolution occurs within a two-week time period, an incisional biopsy for histologic diagnosis is prudent. Palliation with topical emollients and anesthetics may be helpful.

Lichen Planus

One of the more common ulcerative disorders of the oral mucosa is lichen planus, which also includes lichenoid reactions caused by medications. Although the etiology may be idiopathic or virally induced, most lichenoid lesions are likely due to some precipitating event that leads to a T-cell–mediated chronic inflammatory response in the oral tissues, resulting in a reticular striated, plaque-like, or ulcerative mucosal condition.[93] These lesions need to be diagnosed with the help of an histopathologic assessment. There have been reports in the literature of associated malignant transformation in patients with chronic oral lichen planus.[94] The possibility of experiencing a lichenoid reactions to dental materials exists, and more frequent recalls in patients with desquamative gingivitis is important as painful, sore and tender gingiva often affect oral hygiene, exacerbate intraoral inflammation, and create a cycle of inflammation and poor oral hygiene.

Inflammatory Lesions

Inflammatory lesions in older adults occur often as a result of poorly fitting dentures. Papillary hyperplasia is a common finding in patients with loose maxillary dentures. Clinically, these lesions represent multiple, polypoid, and papillary nodules, found typically on the hard palate, giving a cobblestone appearance. There also may be comorbid candidiasis. Treatment includes decreased or discontinued use of the denture. Tissue conditioners may reduce papillary hyperplasia along with concomitant treatment with an antifungal agent. Occasionally, surgical removal of the hyperplastic tissue is needed or the construction of new prostheses may be indicated.

Another denture-related inflammatory lesion is epulis fissurata, which are lesions that appear as hyperplastic, redundant tissue in the vestibule. This hyperplastic granulation tissue surrounds the denture flange and can be associated with pain, bleeding, and ulceration, oftentimes appearing quite ominous. The etiology is overextended denture flanges either due to the resorption of the alveolar bone that makes the denture borders overextended or in patients who have lost weight and whose dentures no longer fit. Treatment of these lesions depends on their size. Small lesions may resolve if denture flanges are reduced. However, surgical excision is necessary for larger fissurata prior to rebasing or relining a denture.

Candidiasis

Older patients are at an increased risk of developing intraoral yeast infections. This opportunistic infection is seen commonly due to systemic disease, poor immune function, dry mouth secondary to disease or because of multiple medications, and patients with removable prostheses.[95] Pseudomembranous candidiasis is the most common clinical presentation and appears as a white cottage cheese-like plaque on any intraoral mucosal surface that can be often wiped away leaving an erythematous base. Less commonly, candida infections appear as generalized, diffuse erythema throughout the oral tissues. Patients may complain of pain or burning in the oral cavity as well as a change in taste sensation. However, many cases of intraoral candidiasis are asymptomatic. The diagnosis of intraoral candidiasis includes a thorough review of systems along with disease history and can be made clinically in many instances. Direct cytologic smear for periodic acid–Schiff staining is helpful to confirm a diagnosis. In severely debilitated patients, extension of the yeast to the esophagus and trachea may lead to significant morbidity and mortality. Use of both topical and systemic antifungals is indicated in the geriatric patients as well as direct topical treatment of any prostheses.

Angular Cheilitis

Angular cheilitis is a common variant of a candida infection that is seen very commonly in the older patient. Angular cheilitis can occur not only due to candidiasis but also due to diminished occlusal vertical dimension or nutritional deficiencies, such as vitamin B or iron deficiencies. Commonly, patients have wrinkled and sagging skin at the lip commissures with desiccation and mucosal cracking along the corner of the vermillion border. The most effective treatment includes a combination antifungal and steroid cream applied to the affected areas several times daily. The clinician needs to rule out vitamin deficiencies and address any vertical dimension of occlusion issues. For further information on oral candidiasis, please see Chapter 5.

Vesiculobullous Disease

Oral vesiculobullous diseases in older adults include pemphigus vulgaris, mucous membrane pemphigoid, and lesions related to the human herpes virus. Pemphigus vulgaris is a potentially serious life-threatening autoimmune vesicular bullous disorder that usually affects individuals after their fifth and sixth decade of life (see Chapter 4). Cicatricial or mucous membrane pemphigoid is another immunologically mediated disorder that primary effects older women (see Chapter 4).[96] Prolonged use of removable prostheses in any of these conditions can cause exacerbation of oral mucosal lesions. More frequent hygiene recall and early and accurate diagnosis of these lesions with biopsy for both routine and direct immunofluorescence study is vital. Geriatric patients diagnosed with these two vesiculobullous diseases require the same topical and/or systemic treatments as their younger counterparts; however, drug–drug interactions and comorbid systemic disease must be considered when choosing treatment.[97] Recurrent herpes labialis, recurrent intraoral herpes, and herpes zoster reactivation along any of the three distributions of the trigeminal nerve can cause vesiculobullous ulcerations and significant oral pain in the older patient.[98] It is important for the dentist to avoid elective dental care during these acute flares and to consider prophylactic antiviral medications in patients with a history of reactivation of the virus and oral lesions secondary to dental treatment. Treatment of recurrent herpetic lesions is more effective when started in the prodromal stage before lesions ulcerate and crust. Topical ointments and creams as well as systemic antiviral therapies are often indicated in these patients. Occasionally, prophylactic systemic antiviral therapy may be appropriate. Herpes zoster, or shingles, most commonly occurs in people older than 50 years and those who are immunosuppressed. The shingles vaccine is recommended by the Advisory Committee on Immunization Practices to reduce the risk of shingles and its associated pain in people aged 60 years or older.[98]

Oral Cancer

Oral cancer is the most significant oral mucosal disease in older adults (see Chapter 8). Incidence rates of oral cancer increase with age. Over 90% of all oral cancers in the United States occur in individuals older than 50 years.[99] Five-year survival rates for oral cancer decrease with age and are low compared with those of other cancers. Oral cancer has an overall five-year survival rates of approximately 62%, a rate that increases significantly with both advanced staging and delay in diagnosis.[99] Typical sites of oral malignancy in the elderly include the tongue, lips, buccal mucosa, floor of mouth, and posterior oropharynx. The most common risk factors other than increased age are the use of tobacco and alcohol. Approximately 90% of all oral cancers are squamous cell carcinomas.[100] These lesions can appear as exophytic, poorly demarcated and ulcerated, erythroplakic, or leukoplakic masses that can metastasize to regional lymph nodes before involving distant organs. It is imperative that the dentist perform an oral cancer screening examination each time the patient is seen and also reinforce prevention by means of limiting risk factors such as sun exposure, alcohol intake, and tobacco use.

Salivary Glands

Salivary glands are known to undergo histologic changes with age. Secretory components of the glands are replaced by fibrous and adipose tissue making them less effective at producing saliva.[8,101] Actually, clinically significant decreases in major salivary gland flow do not occur in healthy older people, although age-related changes in salivary quality and electrolytes have been demonstrated.[101] Changes in salivary quantity and quality cannot be attributed only to aging, as it is more likely that changes in saliva occur due to the effects of medications and systemic disease. Saliva serves a vital role in the maintenance of oral health, with diminished output causing dental decay, oral mucosal infections, sensory disturbances, speech dysfunction, decreased nutritional intake, and difficulty in chewing, swallowing, and denture retention.[101] Hyposalivation is defined as a measurable decrease in the function of one or more salivary glands as measured by flow rate. Hyposalivation has validated clinical measures for diagnosis including dry lips, dry buccal mucosa, absence of saliva produced by parotid gland palpation, and high decayed/missing/restored dental score.[102] Xerostomia, on the other hand, represents a patient's subjective feeling of oral dryness and may or may not be a result of decreased saliva. Older adults can experience a dry mouth for a variety of reasons. Systemic diseases, medications, and therapeutic head and neck radiation are common causes of salivary gland dysfunction.

Clinicians should not attribute an older patient's symptoms of a dry mouth and signs of salivary hypofunction to age; an appropriate diagnosis is required. A plethora of both salivary and nonsalivary causes for symptoms of oral dryness exist, thus making it imperative for oral health-care professionals to determine the cause of the symptoms.[101] In addition, the management of salivary gland hypofunction and dry mouth is multidisciplinary and multimodal requiring communication and collaboration among multiple practitioners as well as the patient and the patient's caregiver. A comprehensive discussion of salivary gland diseases and decreased salivary flow and their management is found in Chapter 10.

INSTITUTIONALIZED OLDER ADULTS

Although most of the world's population lives independently, a significant number of older adults are completely dependent for all aspects of life. For example, in 2005, over 7% of the Medicare-covered adults in the United States, aged 65 and older, were living in long-term care facilities and community housing with services, such as retirement communities or assisted living environments.[103] Approximately 1.5 million elderly reside in 16,000 nursing homes in the United States.[103] These individuals are likely to have many vulnerabilities including diminished physical capabilities as well as cognitive impairment, which together can compromise general and oral health status. Multiple studies have reported that large proportions of nursing home residents have a host of dental diseases and rarely seek dental care services.[16,18] Currently, on admission to a nursing home, residents are to receive a comprehensive health assessment that includes an oral evaluation. This evaluation is federally mandated for all facilities that receive either Medicaid or Medicare reimbursement, which is about 98% of all US long-term care facilities.[66] These oral evaluations are typically performed by dietitians, clinical nurse assistants, or other health-care professionals who are not necessarily able to accurately identify oral problems and cannot always recommend appropriate follow-up care.[65,66] Among nursing homes in the United States, over 80% have a formal contract for pharmacy services as well as a medical director; however, dental and other oral services are contracted at a far lower rate.[103] In addition, oral healthcare is not adequately considered in most protocols on personal hygiene for the elderly in hospitals or long-term care units.

Oral health is rarely life threatening; however, it plays an essential role in the management of medical problems, nutrition, social interaction, and ultimately the quality of life of older adults. It was not until the year 2000, that this link between oral health and general health was brought to the forefront, when the US Surgeon General released the report on "Oral Health in America."[104] This report highlighted the "silent epidemic" of oral disease that affects our nation's most vulnerable citizens, among whom are the elderly. One example of this relationship seen especially in older, institutionalized adults is the fact that oral hygiene itself appears to be related to subsequent lung infection.[105] Multiple studies support the notion that institutionalized subjects are at greater risk not only of developing pneumonia but of also having dental plaque colonization by respiratory pathogens.[106] Although federal legislation that funds payments to nursing homes for the care and housing of their residents requires that there should be no oral neglect, the absence of a consensus definition of oral neglect means that there can be no systematic enforcement of this legislative mandate.[107] An ideal definition of oral neglect would provide minimum standards for the oral health status of nursing home residents, provide operational oral health standards for nursing home administrators, provide enforceable guidelines for agencies responsible for quality, and provide the general public with a clear statement of dentistry's ethical and professional stance on this topic.[107]

Special Considerations for Dental Care and Strategies for Education of Institutionalized Older Adults

Older adults have various functional and behavioral changes that require special consideration during dental treatment and oral hygiene education. Communication between dentist and patient very often needs to be enhanced so that the patient gleans the most out of both the treatment and the instruction.[48] Oftentimes, there is a slowing of voluntary responses in the elderly, thus necessitating the dentist to make suggestions gradually, even over a series of appointments.

TABLE 26-8	Strategies for the Aging Patient[72]
Bridging	Involves engaging the individual's senses, especially sight and touch, to help understand the task you are trying to do for them
Chaining	The caregiver begins the oral hygiene task and the individual then helps to finish it
Hand-over-hand	Technique that helps to improve sensory awareness of takes and gives individuals' the sensation that they are performing the task with you
Rescuing	Used to help with completing hygiene task for individuals with dementia
Distraction	Involves placing a familiar item in his/her hands during oral hygiene care

Source: Adapted from Weening-Verbree et al.[72]

There can be slowing of the speed of thought or associations in older adults, and to combat this problem, it is best for the dentist not to demand the patient learn a new procedure, but instead adapt the patient's current approach to make it more effective. Many times older adults have difficulty in timing sequential events; therefore, their skills become separate movements. In this situation, it is best to guide the patient's demonstration of their oral hygiene to avoid embarrassment. As we age, our rate of learning changes, even though our ability to learn does not change. In addition, there are changes in vocalization speed. Therefore, it is important not to expect perfection from the patient, but to go slowly and anticipate difficulties while giving clues and cues to the patient. Simply because a patient is slow to learn does not mean he or she cannot learn.

There are specific strategies that are useful in teaching oral hygiene for the aging patient. Bridging involves engaging the patient's senses, especially sight and touch, to help them understand the task that is being taught.[48] There is chaining, which is when the caregiver begins the oral hygiene task and the oral health-care professional then helps to finish. Hand-over-hand technique helps to improve sensory awareness of the task and gives the patient the sensation that they are doing the task with you. Rescuing is used to help with completing hygiene tasks for patients with dementia. Finally, distraction involves placing a familiar item in the patient's hands during hygiene care[48] (Table 26-8).[72]

SUMMARY

Older adults are the most rapidly growing segment of the population. In the absence of major medical problems and interventions, aging is associated with few dramatic and deleterious consequences to the health and function of the oral cavity. However, oral and systemic diseases concurrently interact to produce a myriad of oropharyngeal disorders. Thus, many older persons will experience oral mucosal, dental, periodontal, and alveolar diseases and chemosensory, masticatory, salivary, and swallowing disorders. Most of these problems can be treated to diminish morbidity and mortality in this population. Therefore, health-care practitioners must be able to identify, manage, and prevent these problems to enhance the quality of life of older adults.

ACKNOWLEDGMENT

I would like to acknowledge the late Jonathan Ship for his inspiration and contribution to geriatrics.

Selected Readings

Abdulla A, Adams N, Bone M, et al. Guidance on the management of pain in older people. *Age Ageing*. 2013;42 (suppl 1):i1-i57.

American Cancer Society. *Cancer Facts and Figures 2013*. Atlanta, GA: American Cancer Society; 2013. http://www.cancer.org/acs/groups/content/@epidemiologysurveilance/documents/document/acspc-036845.pdf. Accessed March 29, 2014.

American Geriatric Society. *AGS Beers Criteria for Potentially Inappropriate Medication Use in Older Adults*. http://www.americangeriatrics.org/files/documents/beers/PrintableBeersPocketCard.pdf. Accessed March 29, 2014.

Anand S, Johansen KL, Kurella Tamura M. Aging and chronic kidney disease: the impact on physical function and cognition. *J Gerontol A Biol Sci Med Sci*. 2014;69(3):315–322.

Bultink IE, Lems WF. Osteoarthritis and osteoporosis: what is the overlap? *Curr Rheumatol Rep*. 2013;15(5):328.

Burnett A, Abdo AS, Geraci SA. Geriatrics: (women's health series). *South Med J*. 2013;106(11):631–636.

Centers for Disease Control and Prevention. *The State of Aging and Health in America 2013*. Atlanta, GA: Centers for Disease Control and Prevention, US Department of Health and Human Services; 2013. http://www.cdc.gov/features/agingandhealth/. Accessed March 21, 2014.

Drenth-van Maanen AC, Wilting I, Jansen PA, et al. Effect of a discharge medication intervention on the incidence and nature of medication discrepancies in older adults. *J Am Geriatr Soc*. 2013;61(3):456–458.

Gallagher JC. Vitamin D and aging. *Endocrinol Metab Clin North Am*. 2013; 42(2):319–332.

Gluzman R, Katz RV, Frey BJ, McGowan R. Prevention of root caries: a literature review of primary and secondary preventive agents. *Spec Care Dentist*. 2013;33(3):133–140.

Hurria A. Management of elderly patients with cancer. *J Natl Compr Canc Netw*. 2013;11(5 suppl):698–701.

Hwang U, Platts-Mills TF. Acute pain management in older adults in the emergency department. *Clin Geriatr Med*. 2013;29(1):151–164.

Lalley PM. The aging respiratory system—pulmonary structure, function and neural control. *Respir Physiol Neurobiol*. 2013;187(3):199–210.

Lee JK, Slack MK, Martin J, et al. Geriatric patient care by U.S. pharmacists in healthcare teams: systematic review and meta-analyses. *J Am Geriatr Soc*. 2013;61(7):1119–1127.

Lee W, Kim SJ, Albert JM, Nelson S. Community factors predicting dental care utilization among older adults. *J Am Dent Assoc*. 2014; 145(2):150–158.

López-Otín C, Blasco MA, Partridge L, et al. The hallmarks of aging. *Cell*. 2013;153(6):1194–1217.

Musiek ES, Schindler SE. Alzheimer disease: current concepts & future directions. *Mo Med*. 2013;110(5):395–400.

National Institute of Dental and Craniofacial Research. *Tooth Loss in Seniors (Age 65 and Over)*. http://nidcr.nih.gov/DataStatistics/FidDataByTopic/ToothLoss/ToothLossSeniors65andOlder. Accessed March 29, 2014.

National Network of Libraries of Medicine (NNLM). *Health Literacy*. http://nnlm.gov/outreach/consumer/hlthlit.html. Accessed Match 29, 2014.

Noble JM, Scarmeas N, Papapanou PN. Poor oral health as a chronic, potentially modifiable dementia risk factor: review of the literature. *Curr Neurol Neurosci Rep*. 2013;13(10):384.

Pasina L, Brucato AL, Falcone C, et al. Medication non-adherence among elderly patients newly discharged and recurring polypharmacy. *Drugs Aging*. 2014;31(4):283–289.

Pol MC, Poerbodipoero S, Robben S, et al. Sensor monitoring to measure and support daily functioning for independently living older people: a systematic review and roadmap for further development. *J Am Geriatr Soc*. 2013;61(12):2219–2227.

Roett MA, Coleman MT. Practice improvement, part II: health literacy. *FP Essent*. 2013;414:19–24.

Social Security. *Frequently Asked Questions*. http://www.ssa.gov/history/age65.html. Accessed March 29, 2014.

Stein PS, Aalboe JA, Savage MW, Scott AM. Strategies for communicating with older dental patients. *J Am Dent Assoc*. 2014;145(2):159–164.

Stine JG, Sateesh P, Lewis JH. Drug-induced liver injury in the elderly. *Curr Gastroenterol Rep*. 2013;15(1):299.

van der Maarel-Wierink CD, Vanobbergen JN, Bronkhorst EM, et al. Oral health care and aspiration pneumonia in frail older people: a systematic literature review. *Gerodontology*. 2013;30(1):3–9.

Weening-Verbree L, Huisman-de Waal G, van Dusseldorp L, et al. Oral health care in older people in long term care facilities: a systematic review of implementation strategies. *Int J Nurs Stud*. 2013;50(4):569–582.

Willis AW. Parkinson disease in the elderly adult. *Mo Med*. 2013;110(5):406–410.

For the full reference lists, please go to http://www.pmph-usa.com/Burkets_Oral_Medicine

CHAPTER 27

Pediatric Oral Medicine

Juan F. Yepes, DDS, MD, MPH, MS, DrPH, FDS RCSEd

<table>
<tr><td>

❑ EVALUATION OF THE PEDIATRIC PATIENT
General Evaluation
Clinical Examination
Laboratory Tests in Children
Informed Consent

❑ MEDICAL AND DENTAL ISSUES ASSOCIATED WITH CRANIOFACIAL ABNORMALITIES
Hemifacial Microsomia
Treacher Collins Syndrome
Robin Sequence
Ectodermal Dysplasia
Cleidocranial Dysplasia
Dentinogenesis Imperfecta and Dentin Dysplasia
Amelogenesis Imperfecta
Cherubism

❑ PEDIATRIC ORAL PATHOLOGY

❑ DEVELOPMENTAL VARIATIONS OF NORMAL STRUCTURES
Cyst of the Newborn
Natal and Neonatal Teeth
Congenital Epulis of the Newborn
Lymphangioma
Melanotic Neuroectodermal Tumor of Infancy
Congenital Ranula

</td><td>

❑ DISEASES OF THE TONGUE
Macroglossia
Ankyloglossia
Lingual Tonsil
Benign Migratory Glossitis
Strawberry Tongue

❑ DISEASE OF THE GINGIVA AND PERIODONTUM
Pyogenic Granuloma
Peripheral Giant Cell Granuloma
Peripheral Ossifying Fibroma
Localized Juvenile Spongiotic Gingival Hyperplasia
Giant Cell Fibroma

❑ SALIVARY GLAND PATHOLOGY
Mucoceles

❑ DISEASES WITH ALTERED IMMUNE SYSTEM
Erythema Multiforme
Recurrent Aphthous Stomatitis

❑ INFECTIONS
Fungal
Bacterial
Viral
Cytomegalovirus
Epstein-Barr Virus
Human Papilloma Virus
Coxsackie Virus Infections

</td></tr>
</table>

EVALUATION OF THE PEDIATRIC PATIENT

In infants, the age of the eruption of the first primary teeth (mandibular incisors) is typically around six months.[1] The American Academy of Pediatric Dentistry and the American Academy of Pediatrics recommend that a child's first visit to the dentist occur around the age of 12 months. The oral evaluation of a child should consist of infant risk assessment and anticipatory guidance—guidance that helps parents to understand expected evolving physical and intellectual development of the child. A key component of the first encounter with a child, in a pediatrician or dentist office, is the establishment of the child's dental home (equivalent to the medical home). The purpose of the dental home is to provide an opportunity for the child, the parents, and the dentist to start anticipatory guidance as soon as possible and to begin necessary preventive programs.

General Evaluation

The initial exam of the newborn starts with the past medical history, including prenatal, birth, and maternal information, as well as developmental screening information. The birth history provides important information about a child's current health. Babies who are born significantly before term are at risk for multiple medical issues. The parents should be queried about the estimated gestational age at birth and the birth weight. Maternal history, including illness (e.g., gestational diabetes, hypertension), medications, or drug or alcohol abuse must be recorded. Children with prenatal infections (e.g., syphilis, rubella) are usually small in size, have a low birth weight, and are at risk for developmental or congenital abnormalities. Developmental milestones are also evaluated, including speech acquisition.

Clinical Examination

The clinical examination is a key component of comprehensive oral assessment of the young patient. The dentist must perform an intraoral and an extraoral examination. The extraoral examination should include the skin of the head and neck, the presence of palpable lymph nodes, the palpation of the thyroid gland, the palpation of the salivary glands, and an assessment of the temporomandibular joint.[2] Furthermore, the dentist should record the patient's stature, weight, and gait. The intraoral examination should be all-inclusive.[3] The intraoral examination includes the presence of abnormalities in the soft tissues, the floor of the mouth, the soft palate and hard palate, the teeth and surrounding gingiva, and the occlusion. Periodontal screening must be included in the intraoral examination of the pediatric patient after the eruption of the first permanent teeth.[4] The tongue and the oropharynx should be closely evaluated. Enlarged tonsils accompanied by purulent exudate may be an initial sign of streptococcal infection, which can lead to rheumatic fever. The teeth should be inspected after the evaluation of the soft tissues. Presence of caries lesions or evidence of acquired or hereditary anomalies should be recorded. The teeth should be counted and identified individually to ensure recognition of supernumerary or missing teeth.[3] Finally, after examination of the oral soft tissue and teeth, the dentist should inspect the occlusion and note any dental or skeletal irregularities.

Oral Examination of the Newborn and Infant

It is not always necessary to conduct an infant's oral examination in the dental chair, but it should take place where there is adequate light for a visual examination.[3] Before the examination is performed, like with any other dental procedure, the dentist must obtain consent from the parents or guardian. The examination is called a "lap to lap" exam. The infant or newborn is held on the lap of the parent. The involvement of the parents provides emotional support to the child and allows the parent to help restrain the child. The dentist's behavior should reassure the child and alleviate the parent's anxiety concerning this first dental procedure. Parents should be informed of the behavior expected by the newborn or infant during the examination.

The examination of the oral cavity of the newborn or infant can be performed by direct observation and digital palpation. The dentist will need good lighting for visibility and gauze for drying or debriding tissues. Sometimes a tongue depressor or a small toothbrush can be helpful. The mouth of the normal newborn is lined with an intact, smooth, and moist mucosa. The alveolar ridges are continuous and relatively smooth.

Laboratory Tests in Children

Laboratory tests are usually not indicated for healthy children undergoing routine dental treatment including simple oral surgical procedures. If indicated, the laboratory exams prescribed for a child must have a reason based on the medical history and the clinical examination. For example, an infant (2 years old) with persistent oral infections, including yeast, may need a full laboratory panel to evaluate the immune status. Any test ordered in children must be individualized based on a child's history, physical examination, and the proposed treatment plan. A hematocrit and hemoglobin concentration is obtained, in consultation with the pediatrician, if there is clinical evidence of anemia, or if the child is scheduled for a surgical procedure that is likely to result in significant blood loss (bone graft, major reconstructive orthognathic surgery, and multiple extractions). A white blood cell count with differential is indicated for the pediatric patient with an orofacial infection with systemic signs and symptoms. Studies to assess hemostatic impairment, such as platelet count, prothrombin time, and partial thromboplastin time, are not routinely indicated for healthy children. During the initial evaluation, a bleeding history must be obtained. This should include episodes of spontaneous nosebleeds, prolonged bleeding after minor surgical procedures (simple extractions), unusual bruising history, and hemarthrosis. A family history of specific bleeding disorders should also be obtained. Positive findings should encourage the dentist to refer the child to a pediatrician for evaluation and appropriate management. Normal common laboratory values in children are presented in Table 27-1.

Informed Consent

The process of informed consent is different in children than with adults. A competent adult patient is capable, after consultation with the dentist, to decide the best treatment alternative. Furthermore, an adult patient has the full cognitive capacity to balance the benefits and risk of the different treatment proposed by the dentist. Obviously, a child does not have the capacity of *self-determination* and the opportunity to use the principle of *autonomy*. The dentist must include the parents and/or legal guardian in the decision process of the best treatment for the child (including no treatment). Depending on the cognitive age, the child must be included in the discussion, a process known as *assent*. Using different words and analogies, an explanation of the treatment to the child is mandatory. Two interesting issues are associated with the informed consent in children, the first is related to the legal age that a child can use the principle of self-determination. This varies state to state, and it is beyond the focus of this chapter to discuss the complex factors associated with the right of the patient

TABLE 27-1 COMMON LABORATORY VALUES

Complete Blood Count

Test	Normal Value	Function	Significance
Hemoglobin	12–18 g/100 mL	Measure oxygen carrying capacity of the blood	Low: hemorrhage, anemia High: polycythemia
Hematocrit	35%–50%	Measure relative volume of cells and plasma in blood	Low: hemorrhage, anemia High: polycythemia, dehydration
Red blood cell	4–6 million/mm³	Measures oxygen-carrying capacity of blood	Low: hemorrhage, anemia High: polycythemia, heart disease, pulmonary disease
White blood cell		Measures host defense against inflammatory agents	Low: aplastic anemia, drug toxicity, specific infections High: inflammation, trauma, toxicity, leukemia
Infant	8,000–15,000/mm³		
4–7 y	6,000–15,000/mm³		
8–18 y	4,500–13,500/mm³		

Differential Count

Test	Normal Value	Differential Count
Neutrophils	54%–62%	Increased in bacterial infections, hemorrhage, diabetic acidosis
Lymphocytes	25%–30%	Viral and bacterial infections, acute and chronic lymphocytic leukemia, antigen reactions
Eosinophils	1%–3%	Increased in parasitic and allergic conditions, blood dyscrasias
Basophils	1%	Increased in types of blood dyscrasias
Monocytes	0%–9%	Hodgkin's disease, lipid storage disease, recovery from severe infections, monocytic leukemia

Bleeding Screen

Test	Normal Value	Function	Significance
Prothrombin time	1–18 s	Measures extrinsic pathway	Prolonged in liver disease, impaired vitamin K production, surgical trauma with blood loss
Partial thromboplastin time	By laboratory control	Measures intrinsic pathway	Prolonged in hemophilia A, B and C, Von Willebrand's disease
Platelets	140,000–340,000/mL	Measures clotting potential	Increased in polycythemia, leukemia, severe hemorrhage; decreased in thrombocytopenic purpura
Bleeding time	1–6 min	Measure quality of the platelets	Prolonged in thrombocytopenia
International Normalized Ratio	Without anticoagulant therapy: 1; Anticoagulant therapy target range: 2–3	Measure extrinsic pathway function	Increased with anticoagulant therapy

Reproduced with permission from the American Academy of Pediatric Dentistry Reference Manual.[138]

to decide the best treatment alternative. The second issue is related with the potential conflict between the parent's desire and the options proposed by the dentist. Both the parents and the dentist have the obligation to act in the best interest of the child, even if this places the dentist in a conflict with the parent. If the consent from the parents is refused, the dentist has the legal and ethical obligation to act in the best interest of the child, and legal advice must be obtained if the time permits.

MEDICAL AND DENTAL ISSUES ASSOCIATED WITH CRANIOFACIAL ABNORMALITIES

There is a long list of craniofacial abnormalities that include head and neck (including the oral cavity) features. These are some of the most common conditions present in children with oral/dental manifestations or implications:

Hemifacial Microsomia

Hemifacial microsomia is the second most common congenital condition after cleft lips and palates. It is estimated to occur in 1:3000 to 1:5000 live births.[5] The typical features are unilateral hypoplasia of the mandible (including lack of development of the normal structures of the ear), deformed ears, facial nerve paralysis, macrostomia, and malformations of the temporal bone, zygoma, and facial musculature.[6] The aplasia or hypoplasia of the mandibular condyle is associated with severe malocclusions.[7] The mandibular deformities tend to increase with age. Complex craniofacial surgical procedures are indicated to minimize the deformities.

Treacher Collins Syndrome

Treacher Collins syndrome is an autosomal dominant disorder of craniofacial development that has an incidence of approximately 1 in 50,000 newborns.[8] The main features of this condition are hypoplasia of the facial bones, including the mandible and the zygomatic complex, cleft palate, abnormalities of the external auditory canal, and an inclination of the palpebral fissures with structural defects of the lower eyelids. The palatal vault may be either high or cleft. The teeth may be widely separated, hypoplastic, displaced, or have an open bite. Orthodontic treatment is usually indicated.

Robin Sequence

Robin sequence (RS) is a congenital condition characterized by a small mandible, macroglossia and airway obstruction. Approximately 90% of the children with RS have cleft palates.[9] The incidence of RS ranges from one in 8500 to one in 20,000 newborns.[10] The etiology of RS is unknown. It has been suggested that the small mandible causes posterior displacement of the tongue, and prevents closure of the palatine processes as approximately 10 weeks of age.[11] The most common syndrome associate with RS is Stickler syndrome (a connective tissue disorder with characteristic ocular, orofacial, auditory, and articular anomalies).[12] In some patients with RS, the only alternative to maintain an open airway is the tracheostomy. However, for some patients, the risk for airway obstruction can be treated with an adequate position of the child (prone position).[13]

Ectodermal Dysplasia

Ectodermal dysplasia (ED) is a spectrum of a large group of inherited developmental syndromes. An estimated seven of 10,000 newborns meet the criteria for ED.[14] ED is defined as a disorder involving structures developing from the ectoderm (skin, hair, nails, teeth, sweat glands) as well as structures that interact with the ectoderm. The oral manifestations in ED range from minimal to complex involvement. The teeth range from normal on one side of the spectrum to absent on the other side of the spectrum. If teeth are not present, the normal development of the alveolar bone is limited and can be partially or totally absent.[15] Facial development in ED is not altered. Teeth, when present, can range from normal to small and conical. Dryness and irritation of the oral mucosa can be present if the salivary glands are affected. Children with ED, depending on the severity of the condition, may need partial or complete dentures (Figure 27-1).

Cleidocranial Dysplasia

Cleidocranial dysplasia (CCD) is an autosomal dominant skeletal dysplasia characterized by skeletal changes, abnormal clavicles, supernumerary teeth, and short stature.[16] The nature of bone changes in CCD that include alterations in the shape and number of bones suggest that the gene involved is active during fetal and postnatal growth. The most important oral features of CCD are mandibular prognathism, broad nasal base, and frontal bossing. The normal eruption process of the teeth is delayed in the majority of patients with CCD. Interestingly, primary teeth are usually over-retained.[17] Restorations of the erupted primary and permanent teeth should be performed when carious lesions are present.

Dentinogenesis Imperfecta and Dentin Dysplasia

Dentinogenesis imperfecta (DGI) and dentin dysplasia (DD) are two autosomal dominant genetic conditions characterized by abnormal dentin structure affecting either the primary or both the primary and the permanent dentition. Non-syndromic DGI is reported to have an incidence of one in 6000 newborns, whereas the incidence of DD is one in 100,000 newborns.[18] Some of the common dental features of these conditions include changes in the normal color of the teeth (amber to brown/blue), large crowns, and radiographically, the pulp chambers are small or obliterated. The root canals are difficult to identify and the roots are short (Figure 27-2).[19] The underline defect in mineralization often results in shearing of the overlying enamel, leaving exposed weakened dentine that is prone to wear. Currently, three subtypes of DGI and two subtypes of DD are recognized. DGI type I is inherited with osteogenesis imperfecta. All other forms of DGI and DD appear to result from mutations in the gene encoding the formation of the dentin. Treatment of DGI and DD includes removal of sources of infection,

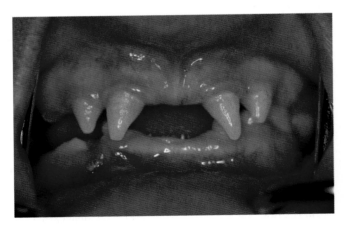

FIGURE 27-1 Ectodermal dysplasia.

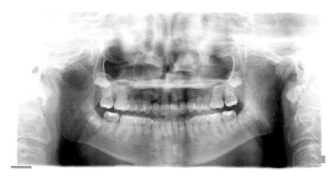

FIGURE 27-2 Dentinogenesis imperfecta.

improvement of the esthetics, and protection of the posterior teeth from wear using stainless steel crowns.

Amelogenesis Imperfecta

Amelogenesis imperfecta (AI) is a condition that affects the dental enamel as well some extraoral and oral tissues.[20] The enamel may be hypoplastic, hypomineralized or both, and teeth affected may be discolored, sensitive, or too fragile to support the normal masticatory function.[20] The prevalence varies from one in 700 to one in 14,000 newborns, according to the geographical area.[21] AI may be inherited in an X-linked manner or as an autosomal dominant or recessive trait. Many different classifications have been proposed for AI. The classification that primary accounts for the mode of inheritance should be the mode of classification, with the phenotype as the secondary parameter.[22] The treatment of AI requires a multidisciplinary team and involves prevention and restorative dentistry.

Cherubism

Cherubism is a rare inherited disease affecting the jaws. The main feature is the replacement of normal bone by fibrovascular tissue.[23] Cherubism presents in childhood and tends to regress spontaneously after puberty. Patients with cherubism typically report a history of progressive swelling of the lower face during early childhood, which eventually tilts the eyes upward, giving the "cherubic" appearance. Cherubism is more common in males than females. Usually, there is no needed of active treatment for cherubism. Since the lesions may undergo spontaneous regression, if surgical intervention is indicated, it is delayed until after puberty.

PEDIATRIC ORAL PATHOLOGY

Oral medicine includes several areas of knowledge, from the dental treatment of medically complex patients, to the correct use of laboratory examinations and the diagnosis of soft tissue lesions. Several articles and book chapters are available that review the most common oral lesions in adults. However, few studies are available on the most common oral lesions in children, including newborn and infants.

Shulman, in the United States, performed 10,030 oral examinations in children between 2 and 17 years old. Nine percent (914 out of 10,030) presented with oral lesions. The most common anatomical site for lesions was the lips (30%). The dorsum of the tongue (14%) and the buccal mucosa (13%) were the second and the third most common locations. Males are more often affected than females. Lip/cheek bite (1.9%), recurrent aphthous stomatitis (RAS) (1.6%), recurrent herpes labialis (1.4%), and benign migratory glossitis (BMG) (1%) were the most common lesions.[24] Bessa, in Brazil, examined 1112 pediatric patients from birth to 12 years of age. He diagnosed oral lesions in 25% of the children under the age of 4 years, and in 30% of children between 5 and 12 years old. In contrast to Shulman's study, the most prevalent lesion was BMG (9%) followed by cheek bite (6%) and melanotic macules (2.6%).[25] Gultelkin et al.[26] in Turkey, reviewed 472 oral biopsies from children below 15 years of age. They found that reactive and inflammatory lesions were the most common diagnoses (49%).

A detailed examination of the oral mucosa of newborns, children, and youths is an essential part of a visit to the dentist. Often, the examination of the oral cavity is brief, especially in the context of an uncooperative child. Dentist must know that the oral lesions in children can be different from lesions in adults. A number of oral lesions seen in infants and children are benign and of no medical significance. In these instances, the ability of the dentist to confidently ascertain a diagnosis and reassure parents that a lesion is not worrisome carries significant value. Likewise, the ability to recognize an underlying systemic illness or genetic disease based on an oral examination can also be an important value, particularly when oral involvement is the presenting feature.

DEVELOPMENTAL VARIATIONS OF NORMAL STRUCTURES

Cyst of the Newborn

Inclusion cysts of transient nature during the neonatal period are developmental lesions, which are seen in the oral cavity of the newborn infant. These developmental variations of the oral mucosa are subdivided in three subtypes depending on the location: Epstein's pearls, dental lamina cyst (gingival cyst of the newborn), and Bohn's nodules. When notice by the parents on the gingival surfaces, they are often mistaken for natal teeth. Developmental cysts are observed in 50%–85% of newborns.[27–29]

Epstein's Pearls and Bohn's Nodules

Epstein's pearls are developmental cysts that are located at the junction of the hard and soft palate. It is likely that this developmental cyst represents epithelial tissues entrapped during palatal fusion. *Bohn's nodules* develop from salivary gland located in abnormal places such as the lingual surfaces of the alveolar ridges and on the palate away from the midline.[30] The cysts are small (1–3 mm), white or yellow papules, and a cluster of two to six cyst are frequently observed. No treatment is required for these developmental cysts. They are self-healing and usually disappear several weeks after birth.

Dental Lamina Cyst (Gingival Cyst of the Newborn)

Lesions on the crest of the alveolar ridge are known as dental lamina cysts. They are derived from dental lamina, the ectodermal aspect of the tooth bud. Clinically, they are small and translucent (similar to Epstein's pearls and Bohn's nodules), and include one or multiple lesions. Dental lamina cysts usually resolve spontaneously and no treatment is indicated.[31]

Natal and Neonatal Teeth

Natal and neonatal teeth are very similar. The difference is the time of eruption. Natal teeth are present at birth and neonatal teeth (less common) erupt during the first month of life. A positive family history is noted in 8%–46% of patients with natal and neonatal teeth.[32] The teeth are mobile with poorly calcified enamel secondary to the premature eruption. The radiographic examination is critical to differentiate the premature eruption of a primary tooth from a supernumerary tooth. The majority of natal and neonatal teeth are prematurely erupted primary teeth (90%). Only 1%–10% of natal and neonatal teeth are supernumerary.[33] The most common place for natal and neonatal teeth is in the incisors region of the mandible followed by the maxillary incisors, and less commonly, the mandibular molars. There is a slight predilection for females.[34] The exact etiology for the premature eruption is unknown. It has been suggested that they occur due to inheritance as dominant autosomal traits or endocrine disturbances resulting from the thyroid gland.[33] Ulceration of the sublingual aspect of the tongue, also known as *Riga-Fede disease*, can result from trauma from these teeth.[35] Other complications are injury to mother's breast and difficulty during breastfeeding. Because most of these teeth are part of the normal complement of the primary dentition, it is helpful for normal dental development to maintain them if possible. If the tooth is extremely mobile and there is an aspiration risk, or if the crown is poorly developed, extraction is indicated.[32] It is important to assess with the pediatrician the risk of bleeding before the extraction because of the risk of hemorrhage in the newborns due to hypoprothrombinemia (Figure 27-3).

Several syndromes are reported to be associated with natal and neonatal teeth.[36] Some of these syndromes include Ellis-Van Creveld, Pachyonychia Congenital, Rubinstein-Taybi, and Cleft Lip and Palate.

Congenital Epulis of the Newborn

Congenital epulis (CE) of the newborn is also known as a congenital gingival granular cell tumor.[37]. It is an uncommon tumor present only in the newborn. CE presents in the mucosa of the maxillary alveolus. The typical presentation is a smooth,

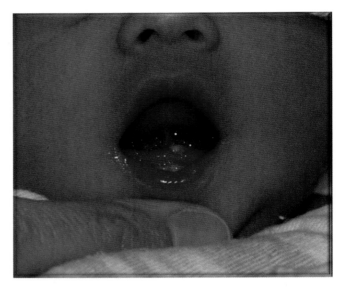

FIGURE 27-3 Natal tooth in a 3-month-old baby.

pedunculated, protuberant, pink surface mass, usually not associated with any other abnormality of the teeth or other congenital abnormalities.[38] CE is more common in females (8:1) and the most common place is the maxillary alveolar mucosa.[39,40] The size of the CE varies from a few millimeters to 8–9 cm. In cases of large lesions, mechanical oral and nasal obstruction can impair fetal swallowing and neonatal respiratory efforts.[41] It is hypothesized that intrauterine hormonal stimulus is the etiological factor of CE.[42] The differential diagnosis includes: lymphangioma, fibroma, heterotopic gastrointestinal cyst, hemangioma, and rhabdomyoma.[43] The lesion does not increase in size after birth and spontaneous regression is unlikely.[44] Surgical excision of the lesion is the treatment of choice. Damage to the future dentition and recurrence have not been reported (Figure 27-4).[42,45–47]

Lymphangioma

Orofacial lymphangioma, or lymphatic malformation, is a benign, unusual, congenital malformation of the lymphatic system.[48] The incidence is estimated in 1.2–2.8 cases per 1000 newborns.[49] It has a predilection for females and the most frequent location is the dorsum of the tongue, but it may also arise on the lips, buccal mucosa, soft palate, and floor of the mouth.[50–52] Superficial lesions have a papillated surface that can appear vesicular in nature.[27] Deeper lesions in the tongue can result in macroglossia. Although often asymptomatic, lymphangiomas may enlarge, leading to increased difficulty and pain with speech and feeding. They can become secondarily infected. Surgical excision is the treatment of choice.[31] However, because of the possible surgical complications, such as nerve damage or facial deformity, other treatment options, such as cryotherapy, electrocauterization, drainage aspiration, radiofrequency ablation, and laser therapy have been proposed.[53] After excision of the lesion, recurrences have been reported in 20% of the cases.[49]

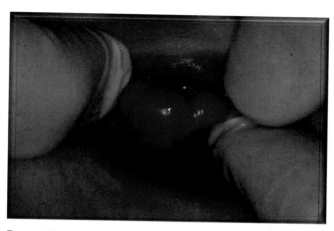

FIGURE 27-4 Congenital epulis of the newborn.

Melanotic Neuroectodermal Tumor of Infancy

Melanotic neuroectodermal tumor of infancy (MNTI) is an uncommon condition that occurs in infants within the first six months of life.[54] MNTI is a benign neoplasia of neural crest origin composed by primitive pigment producing cells. Several hypotheses have been suggested as the etiology of this tumor. Some authors speculate that this tumor derives from epithelial islands trapped during embryonic fusion of the facial buds.[54] The tumor has a smooth surface, and a color that varies from blue to black. The most common location is the maxillary alveolar ridge.[27] Differential diagnosis includes Ewing's sarcoma, rhabdomyosarcoma, peripheral neuroepithelioma, lymphoma, and neuroblastoma.[55] Surgical excision is the treatment of choice.

Congenital Ranula

Congenital ranula is a cyst caused by saliva and fluid collection either due to disruption of minor salivary glands ducts or by obstruction of the duct producing expansion.[56] The clinical presentation is a soft tissue swelling in the anterior floor of the mouth lateral to the lingual frenulum. The overlying mucosa may have a blue discoloration or be normal in appearance.[27] Treatment is controversial. Early surgical marsupialization to prevent potential complications such as sialadenitis is advocated by some authors.[57] Others suggest periodic examination with surgical intervention only if airway obstruction or feeding difficulties are present.[56]

DISEASES OF THE TONGUE

Macroglossia

Macroglossia is an uncommon condition that occurs in children for a variety of causes and is associated with several functional problems.[58] In infants and small children, macroglossia decreases tongue mobility and at the same time increases aspiration risk. In older children, macroglossia can cause problems with mastication and also can cause speech dysfunction. Multiple etiologies cause macroglossia. The most common reason is probably tissue overgrowth and tongue muscle hypertrophy (like in patients with Beckwith-Wiedemann syndrome).[59] Infiltration of the tongue by ectopic tissue, such as venous or lymphatic malformations, can also be the reason for macroglossia.[60] Local tumors, such as lingual thyroid gland, can enlarge the tongue base and cause dysfunction. Amyloidosis and mucopolysaccharidoses are also associated with tongue enlargement due to deposition of abnormal substances within the tongue tissue.[61] The tongue can be relatively enlarged if the mandible or maxilla is small or if there is muscular hypotonia, like in patients with Down syndrome.[62] Less common in children, macroglossia related with infection can occur acutely from bleeding or odontogenic infections spreading into the floor of the mouth.

Macroglossia can lead to psychological distress, other maxillofacial abnormalities, impaired swallowing and speech, and even airway obstruction.[27] Evaluation of macroglossia is complex and includes an evaluation of all structures and functions affected by the tongue.[58] Medical management may be beneficial if the macroglossia is caused by an underlying systemic disease such as hypothyroidism. Surgical removal of a causative tumor or reduction glossectomy is another therapeutic option.[63]

Ankyloglossia

Ankyloglossia, also known as tongue-tie, results from an abnormally short lingual frenulum. This congenital anomaly is relatively common affecting up to 5% of newborns.[64] Although many believe ankyloglossia is rarely of medical significance, other report breastfeeding difficulties and advocate neonatal frenulectomy.[65]

Lingual Tonsil

The lingual tonsil is a developmental anomaly found in the posterior third of the tongue between the epiglottis and the circumvallate papillae. Although often small and asymptomatic, lingual tonsils can become enlarged creating dyspnea, dysphonia, and the sensation of a lump in the throat. The treatment of symptomatic lingual tonsils is tonsillectomy.[66]

Benign Migratory Glossitis

BMG is a chronic condition characterized by loss of epithelium, particularly of the filiform papillae on the dorsum of the tongue. In children, it is one of the most common conditions clinically observed in the oral mucosa.[24] The etiology of BMG is not clear. Several etiological factors have been proposed. However, none of the suggested causes is solid enough to probe a causal relationship. Some of the conditions associated with BMG include psoriasis, allergy, hormonal disturbances, type I diabetes, Reiter syndrome, Down syndrome, nutritional deficiencies, psychological upsets, fissure tongue, and lichen planus.[67] Although the majority of patients are asymptomatic, during active episodes, the lesions may be accompanied by burning, foreign body sensations or discomfort.[68] Clinically, the lesions are characterized for multifocal, well-defined or irregular erythematous patches that represent loss of the papillae. As the name suggests, the lesions tend to migrate to different places within the tongue. Any location on the dorsum or the lateral borders of the tongue may be affected. This clinical appearance can lead to a geographic configuration or map-like appearance, hence the name geographic tongue.

The diagnosis of BMG is based on the clinical examination and history consistent with migratory lesions in the dorsum of the tongue that change in size, color, and position.[69] Routine laboratory tests, including complete blood count, sedimentation rate, and levels of C-reactive protein and glucose, are usually normal. Biopsy and histologic examination of the lesions may assist in reassuring patients of the benign nature of the condition.[67] The differential diagnosis of BMG is complex and includes psoriasis, Reiter syndrome, lichen planus, systemic lupus erythematosus, candidiasis, herpes simplex virus (HSV), neutropenia, erythema multiforme (EM), and local trauma. Reassurance is usually the only treatment needed. Symptomatic treatments, all of which are unproven, include, fluids, pain medications, mouth rinsing with topical anesthetic agents such as lidocaine, antihistamines, and in severe cases, corticosteroids.[68]

Strawberry Tongue

Both scarlet fever and Kawasaki's disease have been associated with strawberry tongue. The strawberry tongue is a red-inflamed tongue with a white exudate and covers the entire dorsum of the tongue with the exception of prominent fungiform papillae. In scarlet fever, this white coating quickly resolves, leaving a smooth, deep-red tongue. Dramatic hyperemia of other oral mucosa surfaces and the oropharynx is also observed in both diseases.[70]

DISEASE OF THE GINGIVA AND PERIODONTUM

Pyogenic Granuloma

Pyogenic granuloma (PG) is a frequent vascular tumor of the skin and mucous membranes. The clinical presentation of oral PG is soft mass, lobulated or smooth, sessile or pedunculated. The color of the lesions varies from pink to red to purple and hemorrhage may occur either spontaneously or after minor trauma.[30] The majority of PGs (65%–70%) occur in the gingiva, most commonly the maxillary anterior labial gingiva, followed by the lips, tongue, buccal mucosa, palate, mucolabial or mucobuccal fold, and alveolar mucosa of edentulous areas.[71] The term "pyogenic granuloma" was incorrectly applied by Hartzell,[72] in opposite to what the name implies, the lesion does not contain pus. PG is a reactive inflammatory tumor in which an exuberant fibrovascular proliferation of the connective tissue occurs secondary to some low-grade, chronic irritation.[3] The differential diagnosis of PG includes

peripheral giant cell granuloma (PGCG), peripheral ossifying fibroma (POF), hemangioma, and inflammatory gingival hyperplasia. The recommended treatment is surgical excision with a recurrence rate around 10% (Figure 27-5).[73]

Peripheral Giant Cell Granuloma

PGCG is a lesion unique to the oral cavity, occurring only in the gingiva. Like the PG and the POF, this lesion may represent an unusual response to tissue injury. It normally presents as a soft tissue purple-red nodule. Clinically it appears very similar to the PG and the POF. The biopsy is essential for the differentiation. The PGCG occurs mainly during the mix dentition years.[74] It has a slightly predilection for females.[75] The mandible is affected more often than the maxilla.[75] Multinucleated giant cells in combination with mesenchymal and red blood cells are the typical histological presentation. The recommended treatment is surgical excision. The recurrence is rare.

Peripheral Ossifying Fibroma

POF is a reactive lesion believed to be of periodontal ligament origin that occurs exclusively in the gingival.[3] Excessive proliferation of fibrous tissue can occur in response to gingival irritation, subgingival calculus, gingival injury or the presence of a foreign body in the gingival sulcus. Half of the cases occur in individuals between 5 and 25 years of age. The most common age is at 13 years.[76] POF is composed of a cellular fibroblastic connective tissue stroma, which is associated with the formation of randomly dispersed foci or mineralized products, which consists of bone, cementum-like tissue, or dystrophic calcification.[77] POF accounts for approximately 10% of all gingival lesions.[78] It has a predilection for females and Caucasians. In most cases, the lesion affects the maxilla (60%), more often in the anterior region.[79] A POF may closely resemble a pregnancy tumor, epulis, inflammatory hyperplasia, a PGCG or a central giant cell granuloma.[80] The recommended treatment is surgical excision. A recurrence rate of 20% has been reported, mainly due to incomplete removal of the lesion and persistence of the etiology factor.[81]

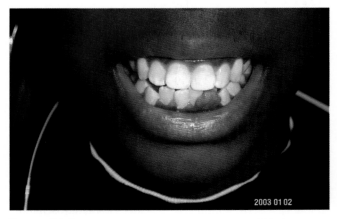

FIGURE 27-5   Pyogenic granuloma in a 12-year-old boy.

Localized Juvenile Spongiotic Gingival Hyperplasia

Localized juvenile spongiotic gingival hyperplasia (LJSGH) is a subtype of inflammatory hyperplasia that affects the anterior gingiva mainly in children.[82] The condition occurs more often in females who are approximately 12 years old.[83] Clinically LJSGH may present as either as multifocal plaques or solitary, multiple, or slightly raised popular lesions with a pebbly, mottled, granular, or velvety surface texture.[84] The lesion is painless and may bleed easily during oral hygiene procedures. The cause is not clear. However, some authors hypothesize that the ectopic tissue interrupts the layer of normal keratinized tissue and its protection from mechanical damage, resulting in the clinical features of LJSGH.[85] The natural history is unknown, however, the majority of the cases are self-limited. An incisional biopsy is adequate to rule out other periodontal pathologies and to establish a diagnosis. Recurrence after excisional biopsy has been reported in approximately 25% of cases (Figure 27-6 and Figure 27-7).[84]

Giant Cell Fibroma

Giant cell fibroma is a benign tumor of connective tissue. It represents 2%–5% of all oral fibrous lesions.[86] The condition

occurs slightly more frequent in females, and it is most commonly found in Caucasians in the first two decades of life.[87] Giant cell granuloma was named for it characteristically large mononuclear and multinucleated giant cells.[87] The clinical presentation is usually an asymptomatic sessile or pedunculated papillary fibrous lesion, often less than 1 cm in size. The most common presentation is in the gingiva, particularly in the mandible. The clinical differentiation with irritation fibroma is not straightforward. Irritation fibroma is usually found in older adults and located commonly on the buccal or labial mucosa along with the line of occlusion.[88] PG is also included in the differential diagnosis. However, PG appears red and lobulated and bleeds easily if manipulated.[89] An excisional biopsy is the treatment of choice with a low probability of recurrence.[90]

SALIVARY GLAND PATHOLOGY

Mucoceles

Mucoceles are one of the most common soft tissue lesions found in the oral cavity of children. Mucoceles account for 12%–26% of all pediatric oral biopsies.[91] Mucoceles commonly affect children but are rarely found in neonates and infants.[92] The clinical presentation of mucoceles is an intramucosal lesion, which is "dome-shaped" and often located on the lower lip.[93] Other places include the palate, upper lip, buccal mucosa, and retromolar region.[94] Mucoceles occur because of a break of a minor salivary gland duct and leakage of mucin into the surrounding tissue that then becomes encapsulated by granulation tissue. The cause of mucocele is often attributed to trauma. Spontaneous resolution of a mucocele is possible, especially when small or superficially located. The treatment for the majority of mucoceles is surgical excision. In some cases, and depending on the size and location, other treatment options are marsupialization and decompression (Figure 27-8 and Figure 27-9).[95]

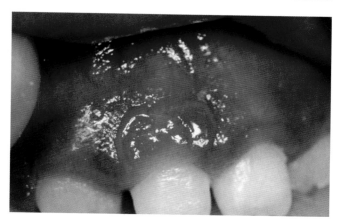

FIGURE 27-6 Localized juvenile spongiotic gingival hyperplasia in an 8-year-old boy.

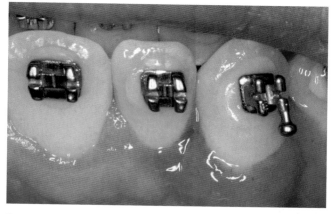

FIGURE 27-7 Localized juvenile spongiotic gingival hyperplasia in a 13-year-old girl.

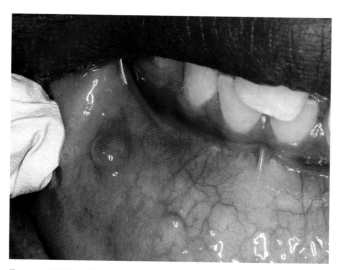

FIGURE 27-8 Mucocele in an 8-year-old boy.

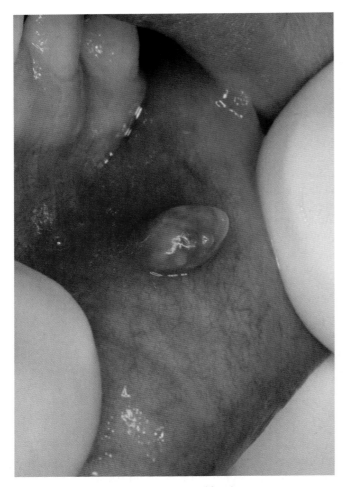

FIGURE 27-9   Mucocele in a 9-year-old girl.

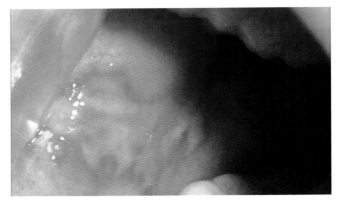

FIGURE 27-10   Erythema multiforme: Buccal mucosa in a 12-year-old girl.

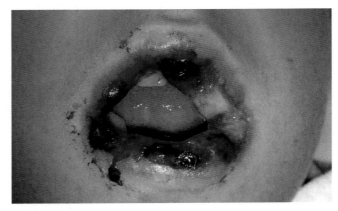

FIGURE 27-11   Erythema multiforme: Lips of a 7-year-old boy.

DISEASES WITH ALTERED IMMUNE SYSTEM

Erythema Multiforme

EM is a reactive mucocutaneous condition that affects the skin, mucous membranes, or both.[96] EM includes a spectrum of reactions that are acute and self-limiting. Approximately 20% of EM cases are found in adolescents and children.[62–64] EM can exhibit varying signs and symptoms, making the diagnosis difficult. EM's typical clinical presentation consists of acrally distributed target lesions, which are considered the landmark feature.[96] As skin lesions are a major component in diagnosing the disease, cases where the skin lesions are absent makes diagnosis more difficult.[97] The severe forms of EM are characterized by a prodrome of nonspecific symptoms such as malaise, headache, and sometimes fever as much as one week before the ulcers appear. A key clinical feature of EM is the acute onset, often within one or two days. This is a critical feature in the differential diagnosis from other clinical conditions that mimic EM such as aphthous ulcers, pemphigus vulgaris, primary herpes, Behcet's disease, systemic lupus erythematosus, acute necrotizing gingivitis, cyclic neutropenia, and allergies.[98–100] The oral severity is variable, and the condition tends to be generalized and in some way symmetrical in its distribution. Lesions range from erythema to full thickness ulceration.[96] The lesions tend to affect non-keratinized mucosa (Figure 27-10), but occasionally the gingiva and hard palate are affected. The ulceration and crusting of the lips is one of the most characteristic features of EM (Figure 27-11).

EM generally results from an immune-mediated reaction to different antigenic factors and has a tendency to recur.[101,101] Several factors have been proposed as possible causes of EM, including viral and bacterial infections, drugs, and several associated neoplastic conditions.[103] The more severe and widespread the reaction, the more likely it is to be drug induced.[104] HSVs are considered the primary trigger for EM in children.[103] A possible genetic predisposition has also been implicated, together with other viral and bacterial possibilities.[105] Drugs have been also reported as potential trigger factors. The most commonly reported associated with EM are amoxicillin, sulfamethoxazole, cephalosporins, and tetracyclines. Nonsteroidal anti-inflammatory drugs and anticonvulsants have been implicated as well.[106]

If untreated, EM is self-limited within two to eight weeks. The target of the treatment is to improve the symptoms. An attempt should be made to explore the underlying cause, especially if the episode is related to a drug, which should be discontinued and not prescribed again. Several treatment options have been discussed in the literature for the symptomatic treatment of EM in children. Liquid antacids, antihistamines, topical corticosteroid suspensions, and anesthetics may reduce symptoms; however, they have limited impact on its course.[107] Systemic use of corticosteroids has been controversial. For many years, several authors considered the use of steroids the standard of care.[103,108] However, on the other hand, some evidence showed that the use of corticosteroids did shorten the disease course.[109] In a prospective study by Kakourou et al.[110] it was concluded that an early and short course of corticosteroids in children is favorable.[110] There is some agreement among authors that corticosteroid therapy might be most appropriate in early stages of the disease, and in patients with complicated and potentially serious cases of EM.[111] The use of antivirals has been also included in the treatment options for EM. It has been shown that oral acyclovir may prevent EM and the continuous prophylaxis with acyclovir for a 6–12 month period is highly effective at limiting episodes of EM.[112,103] Finally, up to 37% of patients with EM experience recurrence episodes.[114]

Recurrent Aphthous Stomatitis

RAS is the most common inflammatory ulcerative condition of the oral mucosa in the U.S. patients. It is frequently seen in the pediatric population. It is estimated that 20% of the general population has RAS during childhood or early adult life.[115] This topic is discussed in detail in Chapter 4 (Ulcerative, vesicular, and bullous lesions). RAS can be classified according to the morphology of the lesions into types: (1) minor, (2) major, and (3) herpetiform. Seventy-five percent to 85% of patients who suffer from RAS have minor ulcers. This form is characterized by the infrequent development of one or more small (<1 cm) oval or round shallow ulcers with a gray to tan fibromembranous slough surrounded by a peripheral area of erythema. They are moderate to severely painful and usually heal without scarring in one to two weeks. Most patients suffer two to four episodes per year. Another helpful classification of RAS is based on the clinical course and includes simple aphthosis and complex aphthosis.[115] Most pediatric patients with RAS suffer from simple aphthosis. This term refers to the common presentation of a few lesions that heal in one to two weeks and usually do not recur. Several conditions can mimic RAS. These conditions include cyclic neutropenia, aplastic anemia, hematologic disorders, severe combined immunodeficiency disease, chronic granulomatous disease, inflammatory bowel disease, and nutritional deficiencies. In those patients where an underlying nutritional deficiency or gluten sensitivity is found, treatment of the underlying associated disease can sometimes lead to remission (Figure 27-12 and Figure 27-13).

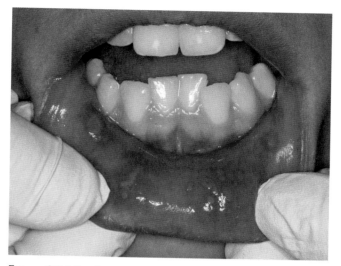

FIGURE 27-12   Recurrent aphthous stomatitis. Minor. 13-year-old boy.

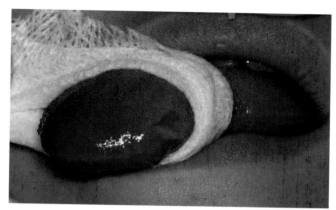

FIGURE 27-13   Recurrent aphthous stomatitis. Major. 9-year-old girl.

INFECTIONS

Fungal

Fungal infections are frequent in infants and children and can be precipitated by broad-spectrum antibiotic therapy, oral corticosteroids, or compromised immune system. Candidiasis (or thrush) is an opportunistic fungal infection of the oral mucosa caused by *Candida albicans*. The condition presents with superficial white curd-like plaques on the mucous membranes, which can be wiped off. For infants, nystatin suspension applied to a gauze and held on the affected areas can be an effective treatment. A child may be able to swish and expectorate a nystatin solution or use a clotrimazole lozenge (Figure 27-14).[116]

Bacterial

Acute necrotizing ulcerative gingivitis / periodontitis mainly affects adolescents and young adults but can rarely also be seen in children. Necrotizing periodontal disease (NPD) occur with low frequency (less than 1% in North American and European children).[117] The typical features of NPD are

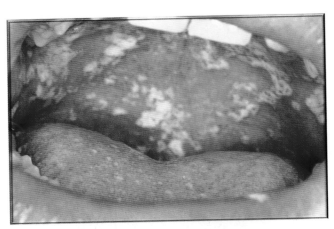

FIGURE 27-14 Candidiasis in a 7-year-old girl.

the presence of interproximal gingival ulceration followed by necrosis. NPD is extremely painful and associated with halitosis due to a lack of an adequate oral hygiene, which is limited by the pain. Children and adolescents with NPD can often present with fever. The bacteria associated with NPD are spirochetes and *Prevotella intermedia*.[118] Several factors have been proposed to increase the risk of NPD development in children. These factors include malnutrition, emotional stress, viral infection (including HIV), lack of sleep, and a diversity of systemic conditions.[119] The treatment of NPD involves mechanical debridement, oral hygiene instructions, and follow-up. If the patient is febrile, not eating and drinking well, antibiotics may be an important adjunct therapy. Metronidazole and penicillin have been suggested as the antibiotics of choice.[120]

Viral

Herpes Simplex Virus

HSV-1 and HSV-2 are the main types of HSV and are responsible of the most common intraoral herpes virus infections.

Primary Herpes Simplex Infections

Herpes simplex is a neurotropic virus that infects the skin and neurons of the dorsal root ganglia. Several factors are associated with reactivation of the virus including stress, hormonal changes, sun, and so forth. Primary HSV-1 infection presents when a susceptible person, usually a child, comes into close contact with a person previously infected by the virus. Primary infection in children is often asymptomatic. However, in some cases the infection can cause severe herpetic gingivostomatitis that often requires hospitalization for fluid management due to dehydration.[121] Symptomatic primary HSV disease is preceded by generalized symptoms that may include fever, headache, malaise, nausea, and vomiting. In the oral cavity, vesicles and ulcers appear on the oral mucosa, and generalized acute marginal gingivitis occurs one or two days after the prodromal symptoms appear. The generalized gingivitis is an important clinical feature in the differential diagnosis of other conditions that present with oral ulcers such as aphthous stomatitis. Primary HSV in healthy

children is usually a self-limiting disease with fever for three to four days and oral lesions healing in 7–10 days.

The treatment of primary HSV infection is symptomatic. The treatment includes supportive care, including fluids, acetaminophen to reduce the fever, and topical anesthetics such as viscous lidocaine to decrease oral pain. Use of aspirin and nonsteroidal medications is not recommended for patients with acute, systemic viral infections, especially in children, because of the risk of development of Reye's syndrome.[122] If the patients presents to the clinic within 72 hours of the beginning of the vesicles, antiviral medications may be helpful in decreasing healing time of the lesions by inhibiting DNA replication in HSV-infected cells.[123] Acyclovir has been shown to decrease symptoms of primary HSV infection in children, including days of fever and viral shedding.[124,125] Newer antiherpes drugs are available, including valacyclovir and famciclovir; both drugs have a better bioavailability allowing fewer daily doses. The majority of HSV infections are diagnosed clinically. However, there are several conditions that mimic the lesions produced by HSV. RAS is commonly misdiagnosed as an HSV infection; however, there are clinical characteristics that are unique to each disease. HSV typically has a prodrome of fever and malaise before vesicles and ulcer eruption. RAS generally does not have the same prodromal symptoms before ulcer formation. HSV infection usually presents with gingival erythema, which is not common in RAS. HSV lesions can also be similar to coxsackie viral infection, the most common being herpangina and hand-foot-and-mouth disease (HFMD). Herpangina lesions are typically located in the posterior aspect of the oral cavity, including the soft palate, uvula, tonsils, and pharyngeal wall. Additionally, herpangina infections are typically milder than HSV infections, generally occur in epidemics and do not cause acute gingivitis. Laboratory tests may be necessary to diagnose atypical presentation of HSV infections. The diagnosis of herpes virus infections can be made quickly and accurately by using immunomorphologic techniques.[126]

Cytomegalovirus

Human cytomegalovirus (CMV) belong to the herpes virus family and produces infections early in life. Usually the infections are asymptomatic.[127] However, CMV may cause significant clinical disease in immunosuppressed patients. CMV is transmitted by contaminated blood and bodily secretions, including breast milk, saliva, and genital fluids.[128] Approximately 20% of children in the United States will have contact CMV before puberty. Infection is also common during adolescence and is associated with the beginning of sexual activity.[129] Primary infection is often asymptomatic. As other herpes viruses, CMV stays latent within the host, reactivating and shedding when the host's immune system is altered.

CMV is acquired from close personal and body fluids (saliva, urine, blood, breast milk, semen, and even transplanted organ tissue) contact. Initial infection in newborns and reactivation of the virus in immunocompromised persons can result in severe pathology. CMV produces a mononucleosis syndrome, which is very difficult to distinguish from Epstein–Barr-induced mononucleosis. The syndrome consists in an acute febrile illness with an increase of 50% or more in the number of lymphocytes. Patients may also present with nonspecific skin rashes, lymphadenopathy, splenomegaly, and pharyngeal erythema. However, these features are less common than in primary Epstein–Barr virus (EBV) infection.[123] The differential diagnosis of the infection caused by CMV is difficult and many of the clinical features overlap with other conditions, such as mononucleosis by EBV, toxoplasmosis, acute viral hepatitis, human herpes virus 6, and rug reaction.

Epstein-Barr Virus

EBV typically infects and replicates in B lymphocytes. After primary infection, EBV-specific T lymphocytes are usually acquired. EBV infection is usually asymptomatic or occasionally symptomatic in infectious mononucleosis (IM). The virus is acquired by contact with oral secretions. The virus replicates in cells of the oropharynx, and almost all seropositive persons actively shed virus in the saliva.[130] EBV is associated as etiological factor with IM, different malignancies including nasopharyngeal carcinoma and Burkitt's lymphoma, and oral hairy leukoplakia.

Infectious Mononucleosis

IM is particularly common in children and adolescents. The clinical presentation includes pharyngitis, malaise, adenopathy, fever, and an atypical increase in the number of lymphocytes. Splenomegaly, hepatomegaly, jaundice, and splenic rupture can occur in patients with IM, but these conditions are rare.[131] The infection is spread primarily by saliva, and the incubation period is four to eight weeks. The majority of children with IM present with painful lymph nodes, fever, and tonsillar enlargement. Other common physical signs include transient palatal petechiae and pharyngeal inflammation.[131]

Human Papilloma Virus

Human papillomaviruses (HPV) are small DNA viruses. Approximately 90 types of HPV have been recognized and related with particular lesions. The "low risk types" of HPV are found in mucosal and cutaneous places and can cause benign lesions as verrucae vulgaris or "warts" (HPV-2, HPV-4, and HPV-7), papillomas and condylomata (HPV-6 and HPV-11), and the lesions of focal epithelial hyperplasia (FEH) (HPV-13 and HPV-32).[132]

Squamous Cell Papilloma

The squamous cell papilloma is a benign, common intraoral neoplasm that presents as a pink to white verrucous papule. The most common location is the junction of the hard and soft palate, although lesions may occur anywhere. Treatment options include cryotherapy, electrodessication, and surgical excision. (Figure 27-15)

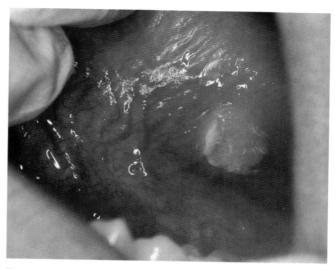

FIGURE 27-15 Squamous papilloma in a 9-year-old girl.

Verruca Vulgaris

Verruca vulgaris is the most common HPV lesion of the skin. The lesion is also found in the mouth (oral papilloma) but the most common place is the skin. The term "verrucae vulgaris" is usually applied when a crop of lesions develops, sometimes in association with similar skin lesions. In the oral cavity, the lesions are located in areas of heavy keratinization such as the lips, hard palate, and less common, in the gingiva.[133]

Focal Epithelial Hyperplasia

FEH or Heck's disease, is a rare, benign epithelial hyperplasia that appears clinically as multiple, soft nodular elevations, most commonly affecting buccal mucosa, tongue, and lips. Children are most commonly affected and present with multiple, soft, smooth-surfaced, well-demarcated, irregular papules on the mucosa of the lips, the buccal mucosa, the tongue, and the hard palate.[27] They can be white, gray, or the color of normal surrounding mucosa. Greater than 90% of all FEH lesions have been found to harbor either HPV-13 or HPV-32.[134] Although spontaneous remissions have been reported, CO_2 laser and cryotherapy have also been used to treat this condition (Figure 27-16).[134]

Coxsackie Virus Infections

Coxsackieviruses are RNA enteroviruses and are named for the city in upper New York State where they were first discovered. Coxsackieviruses have been separated into two groups, A and B. There are 24 known types of coxsackie group A and six types of coxsackie group B. These viruses cause hepatitis, meningitis, myocarditis, pericarditis, and acute respiratory disease. Three clinical types of infection of the oral region that have been described in children and are usually caused by group A Coxsackieviruses: *herpangina, HFMD, and acute lymphonodular pharyngitis.*

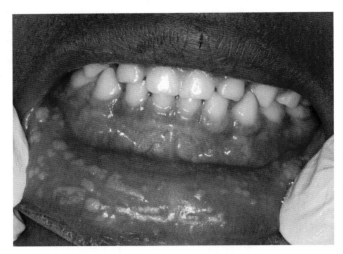

FIGURE 27-16 Focal epithelial hyperplasia in a 6-year-old child.

Herpangina

Herpangina is a common condition in the childhood. It is characterized by sore throat and fever, followed by multiple, small round ulcers located mainly in the soft palate and tonsil pillars. The gingiva is usually not affected (differential diagnosis with herpetic gingivostomatitis). Herpangina frequently occurs in epidemics that have their highest incidence from June–October. The oral ulcerations will last for three or four days and, unlike herpes infections, there will be no recurrences of that particular type of virus. Coxsackievirus A4 has been shown to cause the majority of cases of herpangina, but types A1 to A10 as well as types A16 to A22 have been also been implicated.

After a 2–10 days incubation period, the infection begins with generalized symptoms of chills, fever, and anorexia. The fever and other symptoms are generally milder than those experienced with primary HSV infection. The patient will typically complain of sore throat, dysphagia, and occasionally sore mouth. Lesions starts as punctuate macules, which in hours progress into papules and vesicles involving the posterior pharynx, tonsils, pillars, and soft palate. Within 24–48 hours, the vesicles rupture, forming small 1–2 mm ulcers. The disease is usually mild and heals without treatment in one week. Herpangina could be difficult to distinguish from herpes simplex infection. However, there are some important differences that help the clinician to establish the correct diagnosis: herpangina occurs in epidemics, herpangina is milder than the infection for HSV, herpangina usually is not associated with gingival lesions, and finally the lesions in herpangina tend to be smaller than those of HSV.[135] The diagnosis of herpangina is based on the clinical presentation; however, a smear taken from the base of a fresh vesicle will not show ballooning degeneration or multinucleated giant cells. The treatment of herpangina is supportive, including hydration and topical anesthesia. Specific antiviral treatment is not available.

Hand-foot-and-mouth Disease

HFMD affects children under the age of 10 years old. The disease is highly contagious and is spread by oral-oral and fecal-oral routes. In geographical areas with seasons, as in the United States, the infection is more common during late summer and early fall.[136] The initial viral invasion is in the oral mucosa and ileal mucosa and is followed by a spread to regional lymph nodes within 24 hours. The incubation period is three to six days, followed by a short 12–36 hour prodrome of malaise, cough, abdominal pain, low-grade fever, difficulty to eat, and sore mouth. The ulcers in the oral cavity are found more often on the buccal mucosa, tongue, and hard palate. Oral lesions resolve without treatment in one week. The exanthema in the hands and feet usually follow the oral ulcers. Lesions are elliptical, with the long axis running parallel to skin lines, and may be asymptomatic or painful. They slowly disappear over 5–10 days without scarring. Treatment of HFMD is palliative and includes acetaminophen, viscous lidocaine, diphenhydramine, magnesium hydroxide, and sucralfate.[137]

Acute Lymphonodular Pharyngitis

Acute lymphonodular pharyngitis is a variant of herpangina caused by Coxsackievirus A10. The distribution pattern is similar to herpangina. However, the yellow-white nodules do not progress to vesicles or ulcers. The disease is self-limiting, and only supportive care is necessary.

Selected Readings

Akkara F, Chalakkal P, Boyapati CM, Pavaskar R. Peripheral ossifying fibroma secondary to pulpo-periodontal irritation. *J Clin Diagn Res*. 2013;7(9):2076–2077.

American Academy of Pediatric Dentistry. Clinical Affairs Committee S, General Anesthesia S. Guideline on use of anesthesia personnel in the administration of office-based deep sedation/general anesthesia to the pediatric dental patient. *Pediatr Dent*. 2012;34(5):170–172.

Birgfeld CB, Heike C. Craniofacial microsomia. *Semin Plast Surg*. 2012;26(2):91–104.

Kempton J, Wright JM, Kerins C, Hale D. Misdiagnosis of erythema multiforme: a literature review and case report. *Pediatr Dent*. 2012;34(4):337–342.

Knaudt B, Volz T, Krug M, et al. Skin symptoms in four ectodermal dysplasia syndromes including two case reports of Rapp-Hodgkin-Syndrome. *Eur J Dermatol*. 2012;22(5):605–613.

Laudenbach JM. Oral medicine update: infectious oral lesions. *J Calif Dent Assoc*. 2013;41(4):257–258.

Linder M, Fittschen M, Seidmann L, Bahlmann F. Intrauterine death of a child with Goldenhar syndrome: a case presentation and review of the literature. *Arch Gynecol Obstet*. 2012;286(3):809–810.

Mhaske S, Yuwanati MB, Mhaske A, et al. Natal and neonatal teeth: an overview of the literature. *ISRN Pediatr*. 2013;2013:956269.

Prajapati VK. Non-familial Cherubism. *Contemp Clin Dent*. 2013; 4(1):88–89.

Reddy ER, Kumar MS, Aduri R, Sreelakshmi N. Melanotic neuroectodermal tumor of infancy: a rare case report. *Contemp Clin Dent*. 2013;4(4):559–562.

Shapira M, Akrish S. Mucoceles of the oral cavity in neonates and infants-report of a case and literature review. *Pediatr Dermatol*. 2014;31:e55–e58.

Solomon LW, Trahan WR, Snow JE. Localized juvenile spongiotic gingival hyperplasia: a report of 3 cases. *Pediatr Dent*. 2013;35(4):360–363.

Soni A, Suyal P, Suyal A. Congenital ranula in a newborn: a rare presentation. *Indian J Otolaryngol Head Neck Surg*. 2012;64(3):295–297.

Uloopi KS, Vinay C, Deepika A, et al. Pediatric giant cell fibroma: an unusual case report. *Pediatr Dent*. 2012;34(7):503–505.

Yepes JF, White D. A young patient with persistent gingival bleeding. *JAMA*. 2012;307(22):2430–2431.

For the full reference lists, please go to http://www.pmph-usa.com/Burkets_Oral_Medicine.

CHAPTER 28

Panoramic Image Interpretation

Ernest W.N. Lam, DMD, MSc, PhD, FRCD(C)

❏ REVIEW OF THE PANORAMIC IMAGE   ❏ IMAGE INTERPRETATION

Panoramic radiography or orthopantomography is a tomographic imaging modality that relies on the complex simultaneous movement of an X-ray source and receptor around the jaws. The tomographic slice that is created mirrors the curvature of the jaws and produces an image that is a section or slice through the jaws that displays the anatomy of the bones, the teeth and their supporting structures is called the focal trough. Given the movement pattern of the X-ray source and receptor during image acquisition, the panoramic image can be fraught with artifacts that can make interpretation both challenging and at times, confusing. Having an elementary understanding of panoramic image production is, therefore, a useful first step in the interpretation of these images.

The panoramic X-ray beam is collimated (or limited) to a thin, tall slit that is directed upward at a positive angle toward the patient from the X-ray tube housing of the machine. Collimation of the X-ray beam occurs at two locations, first where the X-ray beam exits the X-ray tube housing (the incident beam), before it interacts with the patient. And second, after the X-ray beam has been attenuated by the patient, but before the X-ray beam strikes the image receptor (the attenuated beam). Image acquisition begins with the receptor positioned adjacent to one of the mastoid processes of the temporal bones and with the incident X-ray beam adjacent to the facial surface of the contralateral maxilla. At the start of this process, the incident X-ray beam is directed with a small anterior angulation. As acquisition begins, the X-ray source and receptor move through a series of short, but discrete arcing movements around centers of rotation located lingual/palatal to jaws. These arcs, when taken together, scribe, albeit roughly, the "average" patient curvature of the jaws. Because of this, the incident beam may not meet the buccal surface

of the mandible or maxillae, or the buccal or labial surfaces of the teeth at a 90 degree angle. The obliquity of the beam may result in distortion of some structures, in particular the mandibular condylar heads, and overlap tooth contacts.

Contemporary panoramic systems use an infinite number of continually moving rotational centers and short arcing movements rather than the limited number of fixed rotational centers and arcs that earlier systems used, thus optimizing both the shape and the location of the focal trough through the jaws. To further optimize the image, some newer systems may incorporate changes to the speed of movement of the X-ray source and receptor, and voltage output (kVp). These changes to the incident X-ray beam may improve visualization of the area near the anatomical midline, minimizing the image of the cervical spine on the resulting image. Newer systems also allow the operator to further refine the shape and location of the focal trough by defining multiple trajectories based on the clinician's perceived curvature of the patient's jaws; this can vary the curvature from one that is more "V" shaped to one that is more "U" shaped.

Patients should be carefully positioned in the panoramic system so that the resulting image is optimized as much as possible and to avoid unnecessary image artifacts. For patients with an intact anterior dentition, the patient's maxillary central incisor teeth should contact the shallow groove located within the upper surface of the most panoramic bite registration devices, and their mandibular central incisors should contact, as symmetrically as possible, the groove on the underside of the bite registration. When the positioning lights are activated, the vertical positioning light should pass through the embrasure space and contact between the maxillary central incisors (Figure 28-1A). If the patient's mandible has closed symmetrically, the vertical positioning light should

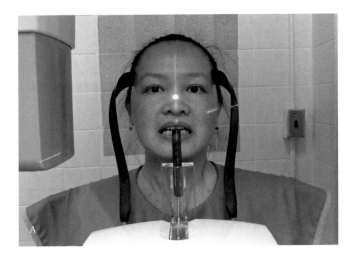

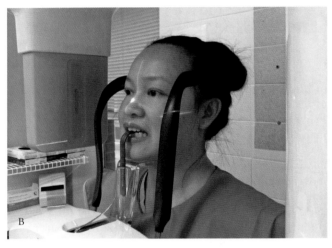

FIGURE 28-1 Both the vertical (A) and horizontal (B) positioning lights should be used to optimize patient positioning.

also pass through the embrasure space and contact between the mandibular central incisors, although this may be difficult to verify. For patients without anterior teeth, the tip of the nose can be used as a midline reference point. The horizontal component of the positioning light is oriented such that the tragus of the ear and either the ipsilateral inferior orbital rim or ala of the nose (Figure 28-1B) are aligned. The choice of using orbital rim or ala depends mostly on personal preference; the former produces a curvature to the occlusal plane on the image that some may find excessive. Finally, some sort of spring-loaded device closes bilaterally and symmetrically on the head, applying equal pressure to the temporal regions of the skull to ensure that the head is not tipped to one side or the other. Unfortunately, such devices do little to correct head rotation; this is still best assessed by the operator. The small additional amount of time it takes to ensure that the patient is correctly positioned in the panoramic system will ultimately pay off, given the additional amount of time the procedure may require should it have to be repeated if the

initial image is not of high enough diagnostic quality. Finally, before the exposure button is depressed, the patient should be instructed to lay the dorsum of their tongue against the hard palate, breathing gently through their nose during the approximately 15-second acquisition.

The most common problems associated with suboptimal patient positioning result in the appearances of the teeth and jaws (in particular, the mandibular rami) appearing relatively larger or smaller than their true anatomical dimensions. For example, if the patient's maxillary anterior teeth have not engaged the groove in the bite registration device, the incisor teeth may fall outside the focal trough and appear distorted mesial-distally, or simply blurred. If the patient's head is rotated to the right or the left, even by as little as 5 degrees, the teeth and mandibular ramus on one side may appear magnified relative to the other.[1] If the patient's head is positioned too far forward or back in the machine, the mesial-distal dimensions of the anterior teeth may appear very narrow or very wide. Both errors result from the abnormal positions of the jaws within the focal trough and the relative changes to the X-ray source-to-object and object-to-receptor distances. And finally, should the patient's chin be tipped too far down or too high up, the curvature of the dental arches may appear less or more pronounced.

During image acquisition, the slit-shaped incident X-ray beam sweeps around the patient. Although the X-ray beam passes through both the right and left sides of the jaws, only one side is captured and recognizable on the image. Because the rotation centers of the panoramic system are located closer to the structures nearer the receptor than the X-ray source, the images of the anatomical structures on this side appear "in focus" rather than the structures closest to the incidental X-ray beam. The images of structures located closest to the incident X-ray beam (and farthest from the receptor) are magnified (due to the relatively short X-ray source-to-object and long object-to-receptor distances), and blurred because they lie outside the focal trough.

Most humans receive an approximately 3 milli-Sievert dose of radiation per year from naturally occurring cosmic and terrestrial sources. Whether the receptor is film or a digital sensor, the reported doses from panoramic imaging vary up to approximately 24 micro-Sieverts.[2] As with all imaging techniques that involves the use of ionizing radiation, patients are subject to a dose, and with it, the potential risk of radiation injury. And while the dose from panoramic imaging is a relatively small one, the dose is not zero, so some form of radiation protection should be used. Many jurisdictions mandate the use of a lead apron that covers at the least, the upper chest and upper back of the patient. The use of a thyroid collar may, however, be difficult, as the top edge of the collar may be captured on the receptor and obscure a portion of the anterior mandibular image. Although lead aprons may incorporate different thicknesses of lead, a thickness of 0.25 mm has been shown to be effective for intraoral imaging.[3]

Structures that are strongly attenuate radiation (e.g., metal and cortical bone) but are outside of the focal trough may still appear on the panoramic image, but they are blurred and are projected a short distance more superiorly on the contra-lateral side of the image as a "ghost image." Such is the case of right mandibular ramus when the receptor is located adjacent to the left mandibular ramus, and the right and left greater arms of the hyoid bone in a similar fashion. Another structure whose image may also appear on the final panoramic image is the cervical spine, blurred because of its position well-outside of the focal trough. An elementary step in the interpretation of the panoramic image must then exclude ghost images and similar acquisition artifacts as being potential pathoses.

After a panoramic image is acquired, the image should be viewed under dimly lit conditions without interference from extraneous or ambient light, even when viewing on a computer monitor. To ensure that the panoramic image is completely reviewed in its entirety, a systematic approach should be used. This is particularly important for novice clinicians. Although experienced clinicians have likely developed their own approaches to viewing panoramic images, all approaches are equally valid as long as the entire image is reviewed in its entirety in the same way each time so that nothing is missed.

Panoramic images, like any other radiologic image, should be ordered only when there is a historical or clinical sign, or a symptom that requires further investigation; panoramic imaging should not be used as a "screening tool" for asymptomatic patients.[4] To this end, when an abnormality is identified on a panoramic image, it is important to undertake a systematic approach to the interpretation of the image and the abnormality being investigated. Only in this way, one can be assured that the image and features of any abnormality contained in the image are comprehensively and fully characterized.

REVIEW OF THE PANORAMIC IMAGE

Although panoramic images may appear to be rather simple depictions of the jaws, the complexity of the image requires that clinicians have a firm grasp of the range of appearances of normal panoramic anatomy, the so-called range of normal. Indeed, recognizing the range of normal anatomical appearances contained on these images is the most elementary step in image interpretation. Therefore, at a minimum, clinicians must have a firm understanding of the fundamental principles that underlie image production and normal radiologic appearances of anatomical structures portrayed on the image. And certainly, the experience of having viewed many images is also very useful. Because of the complexity of such images, it is important that the clinician develop a systematic approach to image review and interpretation so that nothing is overlooked.

1. The dentition (Figure 28-2).
   a. Count the teeth depicted on the image, and account for those that have erupted, are developing, or are

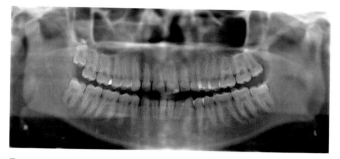

FIGURE 28-2 The dentition. Count the teeth, and account for their sizes and shapes, their positions and alignment, the relative radiopacity and radiolucency of the tissues, and their associated pericoronal and periradicular structures.

unerupted or impacted in the jaws. As supernumerary teeth commonly develop in the maxillary midline where the image of the cervical spine is superimposed, follow-up intraoral images may be necessary to confirm their presence.
   b. Account for the sizes and shapes of the teeth. Teeth on one side of the dental arch should be compared with teeth on the contralateral side, and in the opposing arch. Should the image of a tooth be unclear or if there is a seemingly unexplainable disparity between the positions of teeth on the right and left sides, these areas should be assessed clinically or with further imaging. If abnormalities are identified, the clinician should determine if an anomaly is isolated or generalized, as the latter may reflect a genetically acquired condition of the dentition.
   c. Assess the positions and alignments of the erupted, developing, unerupted or impacted teeth. If a tooth is developing in an unusual position or location in the jaws, a portion of the root and/or crown may fall outside of the focal trough causing it to appear distorted or magnified. Commonly, the anterior teeth in both the mandible and maxillae may appear foreshortened or display what appear to be blunted root apices. These appearances may reflect excessive tooth torque or an obtuse interincisal angle. If there is uncertainly, a follow-up intraoral image may be useful.
   d. Assess the relative thicknesses, radiopacities and radiolucencies of the enamel and dentin, and the calibers of the pulp chambers, keeping in mind that both genetic and developmental anomalies of the dental hard tissues may be localized or generalized.
   e. Assess the appearances of the periodontal ligament spaces and lamina dura. Both should be uniform in thickness and completely encircle the tooth root. Should the image of these structures

not be clear, the area may be assessed with intraoral imaging.

   f. Assess the size(s) of the follicle spaces surrounding the crowns of any unerupted and developing teeth, and the root apices of developing roots. Enlarged follicles, whether symmetrical or asymmetrical, could represent hyperplastic follicles, or odontogenic cysts or tumors, making definitive interpretation difficult. Follow-up images may be needed, and these may include intraoral or advanced imaging, such as cone beam computed tomography (CBCT) or medical multidetector computed tomography (MDCT).

2. The mandible (Figure 28-3).

   a. Choose a convenient anatomical landmark as a starting point, such as the superior surface of the right mandibular condylar head (white asterisk). From this point, trace (black arrows) the ipsilateral sigmoid notch, coronoid process, and the crest of the alveolar process of the mandible to the contralateral condylar head. From here, continue along the posterior border of the mandibular ramus, the inferior border of the mandible, returning to the starting point along the superior surface of the right condylar head. The traced border should be smooth and free from surface irregularities.

   b. Compare the appearances of the different processes of the mandible (i.e., the condylar, coronoid, alveolar, body, and ramus) from the right side to the left, and assess the mandible for symmetry. It should be noted that the appearances of the mandibular condylar heads are invariably distorted on panoramic images given the disparities between the incident X-ray beam and the condylar angles. Consequently, panoramic imaging is not a reliable tool for assessing subtle morphological changes or asymmetries to the mandibular condylar heads. The evaluation of these structures is most reliably accomplished with advanced imaging.

   c. Evaluate the inferior cortex of the mandible (+). This structure should be depicted as a thick, robust, and homogeneously radiopaque line in adults, feathering more thinly toward the gonial notches. For children and older adults, one may see an alternating pattern of linear radiolucent and radiopaque lines. This is a normal feature in growing children but a potential early sign of osteopenia in older adults.

   d. Investigate the internal trabecular pattern of the mandible, noting that there should be more trabeculae around the roots of the anterior teeth than the posterior teeth (white arrowheads). This often gives the anterior mandible, the superimposition of the cervical spine notwithstanding, a more radiopaque appearance than the posterior mandible with its larger marrow spaces. Also note that there should be more trabeculae located around the tooth roots than more apical to them, giving the areas of the mandible near the inferior border a more radiolucent appearance.

   e. Follow the course of the inferior alveolar canals (black asterisks). The canals should have symmetrical pathways on both sides, and typically the inferior cortices are more easily visualized than the superior cortices due to fenestrations within this surface.

3. The maxillae (Figure 28-4).

   a. Like the mandible, choose a convenient starting point like the posterosuperior border of the right maxillary sinus near the apex of the pterygomaxillary fissure (white asterisk). From here, trace (black arrows) the posterior border of the right maxilla, which in most cases is coincident with the posterior border of the maxillary sinus, the maxillary tuberosity, the alveolar crest to the contralateral tuberosity, and the posterior border of the left maxillary sinus, ending at the apex of the left pterygomaxillary fissure. Identify the right and left (black asterisk)

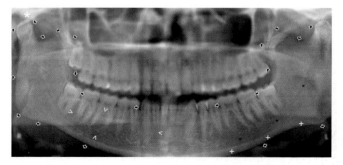

FIGURE 28-3 The mandible. Beginning at the superior border of the right mandibular condylar head (white asterisk), trace the external borders of the mandible (black arrows), and evaluate the inferior cortex (+), the cancellous bone pattern (arrowheads) and the inferior alveolar canals (black asterisks).

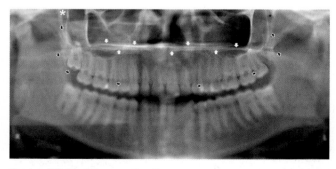

FIGURE 28-4 The maxillae. Beginning near the superior border of the right pterygomaxillary fissure (white asterisk), trace the external borders of the maxillae (black arrows), and locate the floors of the nasal fossae and the hard palate (white arrows). The left pterygomaxillary fissure is also shown (*).

pterygomaxillary fissures, inverted tear drop-shaped radiolucent entities near the top border of the image. The trabecular bone pattern of the maxillae should be uniform, with marrow spaces approximately 2–3 mm in size. Finally, the radiopaque image of the hard palate/floors of the nasal fossae should be seen extending horizontally over the root apices of the maxillary teeth (white arrows).

4. The maxillary sinuses (Figure 28-5) and nasal fossae (Figure 28-6).

The maxillofacial air spaces, the maxillary sinuses, and nasal fossae should be the most radiolucent areas on a panoramic image. Because of the way in which the maxillary sinuses are imaged, only the posterior, inferior, medial, and superior borders may be seen. Begin by examining the posterior border of the right maxillary sinus beginning at the apex of the pterygomaxillary fissure (Figure 28-5, white asterisk). Trace (black arrows) the posterior border of the maxillary sinus inferiorly toward the tuberosity, the inferior (alveolar recess) and medial borders of the sinus, and if visible, the superior borders. Repeat this process with the left maxillary sinus beginning at the apex of the left pterygomaxillary fissure. The borders should be continuous and intact, and flow over or between the roots of the maxillary premolar and molar tooth roots; this is referred to "draping" of the sinus floor.

The nasal fossae are located superior to the root apices of the maxillary incisor teeth in the anatomical midline. Begin by the lateral border of the right nasal fossa at its most superior point (Figure 28-6, white asterisk). Trace (black arrows) the lateral, inferior, and then left lateral border of the nasal fossa. The radiopaque cartilaginous portion of the nasal septum is visible in the anatomical midline, superior to the roots of the maxillary central incisor teeth (white arrows).

5. The soft tissues (Figure 28-7).

Some soft tissue structures in the oral and maxillofacial region can have very prominent appearances on panoramic images; some structures are thick and others simply dense. The conchae (also known as the turbinates) may appear as prominent "sausage-shape" structures (white arrows) extending from anterior-posteriorly along the lateral wall of the nasal fossa. In some instances, the posterior border of the inferior conchae may be seen in the nasopharynx. Encircling the inferior conchae are air spaces (white asterisks), the middle meatus, and the inferior meatus, respectively. Identify the nasopharyngeal (and oropharyngeal, if possible) surfaces of the soft palate immediately posterior to the hard palate (white arrowheads) and the dorsum of the tongue on both the right and left sides of the image (black arrowheads).

6. Miscellaneous structures (Figure 28-8 and Figure 28-9). Depending on the size of the patient, one may be able to identify structures within the middle cranial fossa such as the greater wing of the sphenoid bone (Figure 28-8, black arrows), the mastoid process of the temporal bone (Figure 28-9, white arrows), components of the cervical spine (Figure 28-9, black arrowheads) and the external auditory meatus (Figure 28-9, black arrow). Because of their positions within the focal trough and receptor, these structures may appear blurred or only portions of them may be seen;

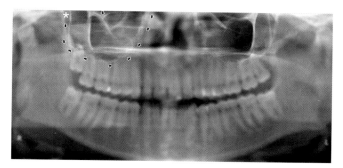

FIGURE 28-5 The maxillary sinuses. Beginning near the superior border of the right pterygomaxillary fissure (white asterisk), trace the borders of the maxillary sinuses (black arrows), and appreciate their relationship to the teeth.

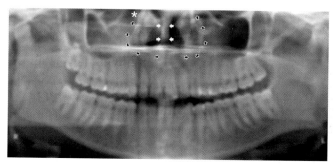

FIGURE 28-6 The nasal fossae. Beginning at the white asterisk, trace the borders of the nasal fossae (black arrows), and identify the nasal septum (white arrows).

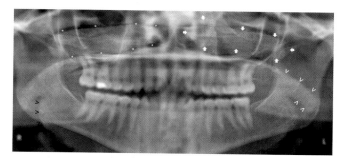

FIGURE 28-7 The soft tissues. Trace the borders of the inferior conchae (white arrows), the soft palate (white arrowheads) and the dorsum of the tongue (black arrowheads). The middle and inferior meatus are indicated by white asterisks.

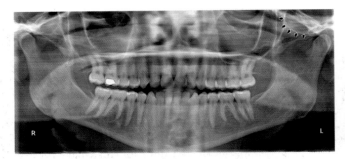

FIGURE 28-8 The panoramic image shows the greater wing of the left sphenoid bone (black arrows).

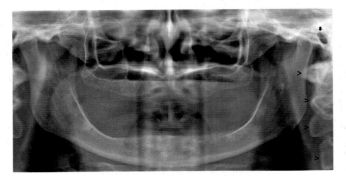

FIGURE 28-9 The panoramic image shows the right mastoid process of the temporal bone (white arrows), the left external auditory meatus (black arrow), and some cervical vertebrae (black arrowheads).

these structures should, however, be assessed for gross asymmetry.

Should a review of these normal anatomical structures appears outside the range of normal, the areas of perceived abnormality should be further investigated, clinically and/or radiologically. Additional radiologic investigations may range from periapical and occlusal images if the area in question is one that is located within the tooth-bearing areas of the jaws and if a high degree of image detail is sought. For more extensive abnormalities, skull images or advanced imaging such as CBCT, MDCT, or magnetic resonance imaging (MRI) may be useful depending on the perceived nature and scope of an abnormality.

IMAGE INTERPRETATION

If an entity has been identified as falling outside of the range of normal, a systematic evaluation of its radiologic features or characteristics should be performed to arrive at an interpretation or diagnosis that supports the patient's signs or symptoms, and/or the dentist's clinical findings. As with the systematic evaluation of the panoramic image described above, experienced clinicians will have likely developed their own approaches to image interpretation, all of which are equally valid as long as the features of an entity are described comprehensively in their entirety in the same way each time so that no feature is missed.

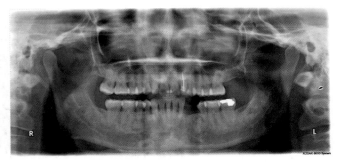

FIGURE 28-10 Florid osseous dysplasia, a bone dysplasia, is characterized by multiple mixed radiolucent and radiopaque entities located at or superimposed over the roots of the teeth. As well, these entities may occur in edentulous areas. The entities have well-defined, corticated peripheries. The cortices are relatively thick and exhibit a sclerotic type of character, blending into the normal adjacent bone. Internally, the entities have a mixed radiolucent and radiopaque appearance with the globular radiopaque component located centrally, and the radiolucent component rimming the periphery. An important imaging feature is the presence of this radiolucent rim surrounding the more centrally placed radiopaque component of the entities.

The clinician's ability to comment confidently on radiologic features may, however, be dependent on the type and quality of the image being viewed.

1. Number of entities.
   Account for the number of similarly appearing entities on the image. There are relatively few abnormalities that may arise in the jaws that are multifocal. Appearances of multiple, similarly appearing entities may commonly reflect a bone dysplasia, or less commonly, a genetic or underlying systemic disease that may require further radiologic investigation. The panoramic image shown in Figure 28-10 shows multiple similarly appearing entities in both the maxillae and mandible. These are seen at or superimposed over the roots of the maxillary right second molar and the maxillary left first molar teeth, the mandibular premolar and molar teeth, and the edentulous mandibular left first premolar and third molar areas. The imaging appearance of these entities is consistent with florid osseous dysplasia, a bone dysplasia.

2. Location(s) of the entity(ies).
   The geographic center, sometimes referred to as the "epicenter," may provide valuable information about the biological nature of an entity. For example, an entity that arises in a location coronal or pericoronal to the crown of an unerupted tooth generally has its origins from odontogenic ectoderm or ectomesenchyme, as does an abnormality that arises along a tooth root surface. Figure 28-11A is a panoramic image that shows an area of increased soft tissue radiopacity overlying the occlusal surface of an unerupted and potentially impacted mandibular right second molar. An intraoral

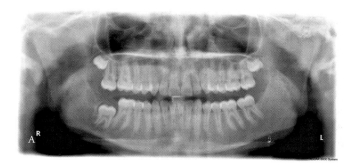

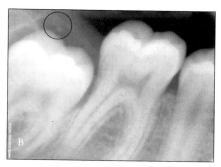

FIGURE 28-11 Panoramic (A) and periapical (B) images of a mixed radiolucent and radiopaque mass with bone soft and hard tissue elements overlying the occlusal surface of the impacted mandibular right second molar. Periapical imaging may be useful in identifying small calcifications (black circle) associated with odontogenic lesions like this ameloblastic fibro-odontome because of the high resolution of these receptors. (Courtesy Dr. H. Grubisa.)

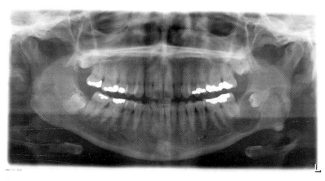

FIGURE 28-12 This dentigerous cyst is located in a pericoronal location around the crown of the mandibular left third molar. This entity has a well-defined, corticated periphery and is radiolucent. It is associated with the crown of an impacted and posterosuperiorly displaced mandibular left third molar. The entity has a round or "hydraulic" appearance, which is suggestive of a cyst or cyst-like entity. Unfortunately, the image detail is such that one cannot determine if the entity has resulted in a loss of periodontal ligament space or lamina dura around the roots of the adjacent second molar. Of note is the association of the entity with the cemento-enamel junction areas of the impacted third molar, and that the anterior border of the mandibular ramus is intact. This suggests that the entity is slow growing and rather more indolent than aggressive. The round or "hydraulic" character is a feature of cysts or cyst-like entities. The association of the entity with the cemento-enamel junction of the tooth is an important feature of this cyst.

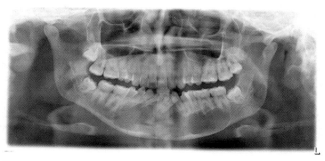

FIGURE 28-13 This entity has a periapical location to many of the teeth in the mandible. The entity has a well-defined, corticated periphery. Internally, the entity is radiolucent. Its growth is "hydraulic" and minimally expansile, extending from the root apices of the mandibular left second molar to the mesial root apex of the mandibular right first molar. Note how the entity has displaced teeth away from the midline and the scalloped appearance of the inferior cortex. In the mandibular left molar area, the inferior border of the mandible may have also been displaced. Although the entity extends to the contralateral mandible yet is confined to the mandibular body without any concomitant increase in the height of the mandible. The ability of the entity to tunnel through the mandibular bone, scalloping the inferior cortex is a characteristic feature of the keratocystic odontogenic tumor. (Courtesy Dr. R. Witzke.)

image of the same area (Figure 28-11B) shows two small radiopaque entities overlying the distal cusps of this tooth within its follicular space. Of note is the discontinuity of the superior border of the follicle. This is an abnormality of odontogenic origin; an ameloblastic fibro-odontome. The panoramic image in Figure 28-12 shows an entity that is located pericoronal to the crown of the impacted mandibular left third molar. This appearance is an example of another entity of odontogenic origin, a dentigerous cyst.

An abnormality with an epicenter located just apical to a tooth root apex may be either odontogenic or nonodontogenic in origin. The panoramic image in Figure 28-13 shows an entity with an epicenter that is located midway between the root apices of the involved mandibular teeth and the inferior cortex of the mandible. This entity is well defined and corticated with a round or "hydraulic" shape to its borders. The entity scallops the inferior cortex of the mandible, but given its mesial-distal extensions, it has caused only a minimal amount of superior-inferior expansion of the bone. As well, the entity has produced both movement and external resorption of the adjacent teeth. These shapes and effects on the adjacent teeth are consistent with the features of a keratocystic odontogenic tumor, an entity of odontogenic origin. In contrast, the entity shown in Figures 28-14A and 14B have had no effect whatsoever on the inferior cortex or the teeth. Figure 28-14B shows the lamina dura and periodontal ligament spaces are intact. This appearance is consistent with an extremely indolent

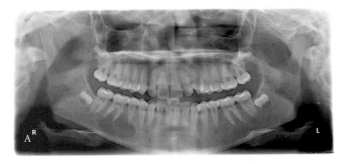

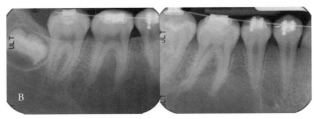

FIGURE 28-14 Panoramic (A) and periapical (B) images of a simple bone cyst in the right posterior mandible. This entity has well-defined, but delicately corticated borders and is radiolucent. The intraoral images (B) are useful because they demonstrate that the superior cortex of the entity scallops around the roots of the mandibular premolar and molar teeth in such a way that the lamina dura and periodontal ligament spaces around these tooth roots are intact and, in fact, undisturbed. That the lamina dura around the roots of the adjacent teeth are undisturbed, and the scalloping effects of the superior border of this entity around the roots of the teeth are characteristic features of a simple bone cyst. (Courtesy Dr. E. Selnes.)

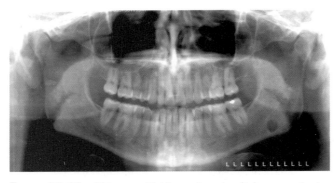

FIGURE 28-15 This very thickly corticated radiolucent entity is located inferior to the inferior alveolar canal in the mandible. This feature is characteristic for a Stafne mandibular lingual cortical defect. (Courtesy Dr. J. Lovas.)

entity. The round or "hydraulic" shape of this entity and its propensity to scallop around the adjacent premolar and molar teeth are features consistent with a simple bone cyst, an entity of odontogenic. This appearance is consistent with a simple bone cyst.

Should an abnormality have an epicenter well apical to the tooth roots, for example overlying the inferior alveolar canal or near the inferior cortex of the mandible, these entities are generally nonodontogenic in

origin. The panoramic image in Figure 28-15 shows an entity located inferior to the mandibular canal, near the inferior border of the mandible. This is a well-defined, but thickly corticated, round, radiolucent entity whose inferior border is continuous with the thick inferior cortex of the mandible. This is a Stafne lingual mandibular cortical defect.

3. Border characteristics.

The definition of an entity's border reflects its growth behavior, slow or fast growing, indolent or aggressive. The terms well-defined, moderately well-defined, poorly or ill-defined are among those generally used to describe this feature. Entities that have well-defined or moderately well-defined peripheries show a slower, more indolent, or controlled pattern of growth. As such, osteoblasts in the surrounding bone may be better able to isolate the abnormality from the surrounding normal structures as it grows. Abnormalities with poorly defined peripheries grow faster with have a more aggressive pattern of growth, easily infiltrating the adjacent normal tissue.

Scribe the periphery of an abnormality with an imaginary pencil or pen. If the majority of the abnormality's periphery can be traced, the abnormality likely has a well-defined periphery. For example, many of the entities already discussed have well-defined peripheries (e.g., the dentigerous cyst, the keratocystic odontogenic tumor, the simple bone cyst, and the Stafne mandibular lingual cortical defect). Another term used to describe the peripheries of entities is "punched-out." This term has been used to describe the peripheries of entities with very discrete border transitions from lesion to adjacent normal bone.

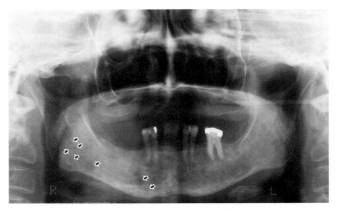

FIGURE 28-16 Multiple myeloma is characterized by multiple "punched out," discrete radiolucent regions throughout the jaws (black arrows). These entities are well-defined, noncorticated and radiolucent, and located throughout the mandible. The borders of these entities are very discrete. Where these lesions engage the inferior cortex of the mandible, the uniform density of the cortex is disturbed by small focal scallops to the endosteal surface. (Courtesy Dr. L. Lee.)

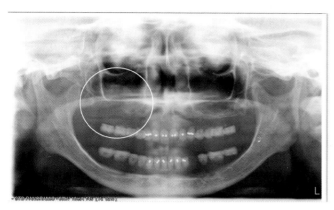

FIGURE 28-17 The loss of the cortex overlying the maxillary right tuberosity and alveolar crest, and the floor of the adjacent maxillary sinus (white circle) is an ominous sign of an aggressive entity, a malignancy. (Courtesy Dr. I. Hernández.)

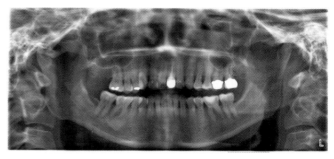

FIGURE 28-18 There is an area of sclerosing osteitis located at the root apices of the mandibular right first molar tooth. The periphery of the sclerotic bone reaction blends into the adjacent trabecular pattern.

Moreover, the term further implies that there has been a concomitant reaction (i.e., sclerosis) of the adjacent normal bone. The term "punched out" has been ascribed to the blood borne disease multiple myeloma. Figure 28-16 shows multiple entities (black arrows) within the mandible where there are no intervening radiologic features between the entity and the adjacent normal bone; the transition is sudden and without any bone reaction at the entity's periphery.

For an entity where much but perhaps not all of its peripheries are easily identifiable and therefore traceable by an imaginary pen or pencil, this periphery may be moderately well defined. For entities where the location of the abnormality's edge is difficult to determine, the abnormality's periphery is likely poorly defined. Figure 28-17 is a panoramic image of an entity centered in the maxillary right alveolar process. The entity has a poorly defined, noncorticated periphery. Indeed, the cortices of the alveolar crest, the maxillary tuberosity and the floor of the adjacent maxillary sinus have been lost. This appearance is one that reflects an aggressive, infiltrating mass lesion, a malignancy. This image is of a maxillary squamous cell carcinoma that has extended from the gingiva of the alveolar process into the underlying bone.

A cortex is a discrete radiopaque line that scribes the outer border of an entity. The presence of a cortex infers that such an entity is growing slowly, indolently, and at a controlled rate. It should be noted that a well-defined periphery does not infer that the entity has a corticated border; an entity with a well-defined border may or may not have a visible cortex. In the past, some clinicians have used the word "sclerotic" as a synonym for "corticated"; this is incorrect. Sclerosis, from which the term sclerotic is derived, refers to a diffuse peripheral area of radiopacity in bone, commonly, but not always associated with inflammation. In contrast to a corticated border, a sclerotic

border transitions to the adjacent normal cancellous bone in a more gradual way, with the periphery of the sclerotic reaction blending into the surrounding cancellous bone. Figure 28-18 shows an area of sclerosis (sclerosing osteitis) located at the apices of the mandibular right first molar tooth.

The periphery of an abnormality can also take on other features, depending on the local effects an abnormality has had on adjacent tissues such as the periosteum. Should an abnormality have the capacity to stimulate adjacent periosteum overlying a nearby bone cortex, that periosteum may lift away from the surface of the bone, resulting in additional peripheral features. For example, when the products and mediators of an inflammatory response developing within the bone are conducted to the bone's surface through the Haversian system and Volkmann canals, the overlying surface periosteum may be mechanically stripped and lifted away from the bone surface and elevated. Osteoprogenitor cells located within the endosteal surface of the periosteum are stimulated to differentiate and deposit new bone on the deep surface of the displaced periosteum. The result is the development of a single layer of new bone superficial to the cortex. Multiple cycles of activation and quiescence result in the production of additional layers of new bone being laid down. Such a response is often referred to as a lamellar or "onion skin" type of periosteal response and is a characteristic radiologic feature of osteomyelitis. Figure 28-19 shows coronal cross-sectional cone beam CT renderings through a mandibular ramus that demonstrates the radiologic correlate of the biologic process described above. More intense stimulation of the periosteum may occur with other disease processes such as vascular tumors, blood dyscrasias, or intraosseous osteoblastic metastases. In these instances, the development of a "hair-on-end" or sunray type of periosteal new bone formation may be seen at the bone surface (Figure 28-20).

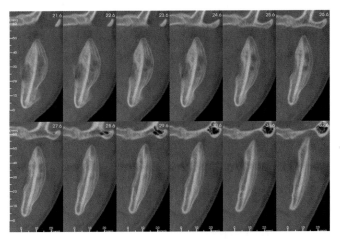

FIGURE 28-19 Coronal cone beam CT reconstructed images through the left mandibular ramus show the lamellar, alternating high-attenuation (radiopaque) and low-attenuation (radiolucent) pattern that is characteristic of osteomyelitis.

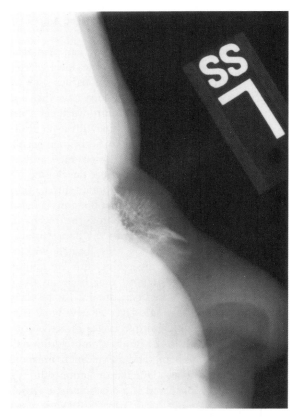

FIGURE 28-20 A "sun-ray" type of periosteal reaction is seen in this collimated lateral image of a vascular lesion of the nasal bones. The image has been purposely underexposed to demonstrate the fine detail of the bone emanating from the surface of the nasal bones.

4. Internal structure.

Radiolucent and radiopaque are relative terms that describe the attenuation or absorption of radiation by a tissue; entities that are radiolucent have not attenuated radiation to any significant degree, whereas

radiopaque entities do. Because these terms are "relative," the identification of an entity as being radiolucent or radiopaque is ultimately dependent on what other tissues are located adjacent to the object or area of interest.

Among the tissues or materials that may appear on panoramic images, metal, whether in the form of a dental material or a foreign body, is always the most radiopaque entity on any image. This is followed by radiopaque composite restorative materials and cements, and then enamel and dentin (and cementum, if visible due to hyperplasia or neoplasm). Cortical and cancellous bone trabeculae are next in this sequence of relative radiopacities and radiolucencies, followed by calculus. Nearest the bottom of the list are the soft tissues, including mucosa and cartilage, body fluids, and radiolucent composite restorative materials and cements. At the very bottom of this hierarchy of material radiopacities and radiolucencies are fat and air; both are radiolucent relative to all other materials and tissues found on panoramic images.

Cells within some abnormalities have developed some specialized capability to produce a mineralized substances including bone (Figure 28-10) or tooth (Figure 28-11B). The deposition of such materials onto a background soft tissue matrix may give an abnormality a mixed radiolucent and radiopaque appearance on a panoramic image. Where the X-ray beam interacts with these mineralized deposits, a focal area of radiopacity may be visualized. Initially, the deposition of bone or dental hard tissue can be a diffuse process over a relatively small area or volume. With time, separate smaller areas may coalesce forming larger aggregate regions of radiopacity. For other abnormalities, the mineralization may appear more discrete and appear to have a high degree of organization. To the extent that enough of the normal bone pattern is removed or replaced, and the nature of the tissue deposited, the bone may take on an appearance that is more radiolucent than cortical bone, but more radiopaque than cancellous bone.

Internal structure may also occur in the form of septation, regions of entrapped remnant bone between different growth centers within the same abnormality. Figure 28-21A shows an entity with numerous curvilinear radiopaque structures that subdivide the larger radiolucent entity into smaller compartments. As some entities may not have the capacity to lay down a mineralized matrix, the presence of septae should not be misinterpreted as conveying that ability; the cells within such entities do not have the capacity to lay down a mineralized matrix. Many of the abnormalities that have the appearance of internal septation are soft tissue tumors growing in bone. Figure 28-21B shows that the entity imaged in Figure 28-21C has broached the buccal cortex of the mandible as

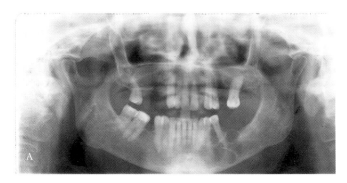

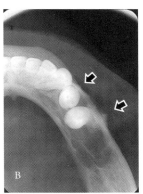

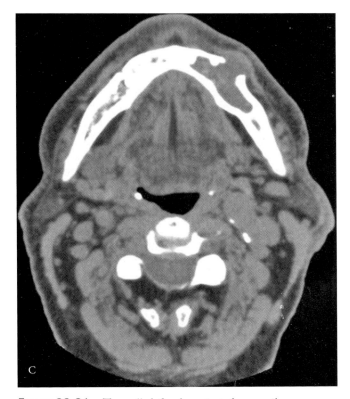

evidenced by the two small extensions of bone (black arrows) that emanate from the buccal cortex. Medical multidetector spiral computed tomography (MSCT) (Figure 28-21C) or MRI is useful to demonstrate the extension of the soft tissue mass into the adjacent tissue planes; this is a feature that panoramic imaging is not capable of demonstrating.

5. Effects on adjacent and/or surrounding structures, and the teeth.

Some abnormalities may grow to a size where their peripheries begin to impinge on adjacent normal anatomic structures like the teeth and their supporting structures, or bone boundaries. Where an intraosseous abnormality increases in size to an extent where it begins to impact on a nearby bone boundary, the bone may begin to expand to accommodate the growing entity, the borders of the bone may become displaced, the overlying cortex may become thinned or even lost (Figure 28-16B) as a result. In the case of the floors of the maxillary sinus or nasal fossa, displacement of these cortices is visible on a panoramic image, and this may result in a loss of air volume within these cavities. Figure 28-22 is a panoramic image that shows an area of abnormal bone in the right maxilla. This region of expansile bone has a "ground glass" type of internal pattern. The floor of the right maxillary sinus has been displaced superiorly, although the general shape of the air sinus appears intact but just smaller. A similar process can also be observed at the inferior border of the mandible when an entity enlarges inferiorly. In order to observe buccal-lingual expansion of the mandible or buccal-palatal expansion of the maxillae, other imaging modalities may be required. Entities that have a faster, more aggressive growth pattern may introduce discontinuities or fenestrations in a bone cortex boundary should the growth of the abnormality outstrip the ability of osteoblasts to maintain the integrity of that bone boundary (Figure 28-21B).

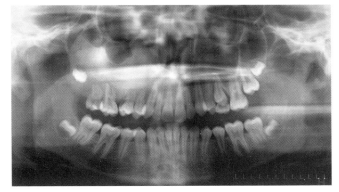

FIGURE 28-21 The well-defined, corticated, expansile entity located in the mandibular left premolar and molar areas demonstrates the thick, curvilinear septations that are characteristics of ameloblastoma (A). The cross-sectional occlusal image (B) shows "flow-around" sign (arrows) as the entity has extended through the buccal cortex of the mandible and into the adjacent soft tissues (C).

FIGURE 28-22 Elevation of the floor of the right maxillary sinus while maintaining the general shape of the sinus in a patient with fibrous dysplasia. Note the ground glass bone pattern that is characteristic of this bone dysplasia.

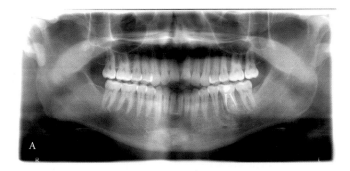

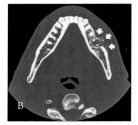

FIGURE 28-23 Focal widening of the periodontal ligament spaces without an epicenter around the roots of the mandibular left second premolar, and first and second molars, is a characteristic sign (Garrington's sign) of a sarcoma (in this case, an osteosarcoma) developing in the bone (A). The axial CT image shows enlargement of the tumor mass through the buccal cortex and the dystrophic deposition of mineralized tissue beyond the buccal surface of the mandible (B).

Benign space-occupying abnormalities also have a tendency to displace the teeth. Where the peripheries of such entities contact the teeth directly, there can also be both displacement (Figure 28-13) and directional external resorption of the teeth. This process, which is a very slow one, involves the localization of osteoclast-like cells at the expanding front of the entity, contacting and then slowly resorbing tooth materials. Although patients may develop gross asymmetries due to the enlarging abnormality, changes may also occur to the dental occlusion, and there may be a loss of normal interproximal tooth contacts.

The appearance of an abnormality having an association with the apex of a tooth and/or its supporting structures may indicate derivation of the abnormality from an odontogenic source. Unfortunately, such an association may be difficult to ascertain on the basis of a panoramic image alone. Additional images (intraoral, occlusal, or a limited field-of-view cone beam CT volume) may be required to demonstrate an association. An abnormality that arises within the periodontal ligament space in close association with a tooth root is more likely to be of odontogenic origin. The same can also be said for an entity that arises with an attachment to a tooth root.

Some entities can grow into the periodontal ligament space, resulting in an increase in the ligament space along the length of a tooth surface. Such an appearance known as Garrington's sign is associated primarily with sarcomas that invade or metastasize to the adjacent bone. Figure 28-23A is a panoramic image that demonstrates focal periodontal ligament space enlargement around the roots of the mandibular left second premolar, and first and second molars. As well, there is a disruption in the normal cancellous bone pattern in the furcation of the first molar. An axial MSCT shows the expansile and poorly mineralized growth extending from the buccal cortex of the mandible (Figure 28-23B). This appearance is consistent with a primary malignancy of bone, an osteosarcoma. When enough of the supporting bone around a tooth has been lost due to malignant cell proliferation, the teeth may appear as if to be "standing in space." Although not a common feature, some sarcomas have the capacity to externally resorb tooth roots.

Panoramic image interpretation is a multistep process that begins with a fundamental understanding of image formation. Developing an appreciation for normal anatomical appearances on panoramic images is a necessary second step in the process. The development of a systematic search strategy for abnormalities on the panoramic image and finally feature identification complete the set of necessary skills required to competently interpret panoramic images.

References

1. McKee IW, Glover KE, Williamson PC, et al. The effect of vertical and horizontal head positioning in panoramic radiography on mesiodistal tooth angulations. *Angle Orthod.* 2001;71(6):442–451.
2. Ludlow JB, Davies-Ludlow LE, White SC. Patient risk related to common dental radiographic examinations: the impact of the 2007 International Commission on Radiological Protection recommendations regarding dose calculations. *JADA.* 2008;139:1237–1243.
3. Wood RE, Harris AMP, van der Merwe EJ, Nortjé CJ. The lead apron revisited: does it reduce gonadal radiation dose in dental radiology? *Oral Surg Oral Med Oral Pathol.* 1991;171:642–646.
4. The American Dental Association and the U.S. Department of Health and Human Services. *The Selection of Patients for Dental Radiographic Examinations.* http://www.fda.gov/Radiation-EmittingProducts/RadiationEmittingProductsandProcedures/MedicalImaging/MedicalX-Rays/ucm116504.htm. Updated November 28, 2012. Accessed December 10, 2013.

Note: Page numbers followed by f or t refers to figures or tables respectively.